Thieme

Head and Neck Cancer Recurrence

Evidence-based, Multidisciplinary Management

Hisham M. Mehanna, PhD, BMedSc (Hons), MBChB (Hons), FRCS, FRCS (ORL-HNS)
Director, Institute of Head and Neck Studies and Education
Consultant Head–Neck and Thyroid Surgeon
Chair, Head and Neck Surgery at the School of Cancer Sciences
The University of Birmingham
Birmingham
UK

K. Kian Ang, MD, PhD, FACR, FASTRO
Professor
and holder of the Gilbert H. Fletcher Memorial Distinguished Chair
Department of Radiation Oncology
The University of Texas MD Anderson Cancer Center
Houston, Texas
USA

With contributions by
Oludolapo O. Adesanya, K. Kian Ang, R.J. Baatenburg de Jong, Alfonsus J.M. Balm, Beth M. Beadle, Jan Paul de Boer, Maarten F. de Boer, Lenine Garcia Brandão, Augusto Caraceni, Claudio R. Cernea, Kevin S. Choe, Ezra E.W. Cohen, Marc A. Cohen, Ralph Gilbert, David P. Goldstein, Patrick Gullane, Kevin J. Harrington, Jarrod Homer, Julie Howle, N. Gopalakrishna Iyer, Charles G. Kelly, Lai Wan Dora Kwong, Lisa Licitra, Julia Maclean, Hisham M. Mehanna, Gary Morgan, Dan Munday, Ramez Nassif, Christopher M. Nutting, Marinella P.J. Offerman, Vinidh Paleri, Alison Perry, Jean F.A. Pruyn, Alexander D. Rapidis, Coen R.N. Rasch, Joseph Kamel Salama, M.P. van der Schroeff, Cherith J. Semple, Ashok R. Shaha, Priyamal Silva, Nick Slevin, Pol Specenier, Miroslav Tedla, R. Michael Tuttle, Michael Veness, Jan B. Vermorken, Randal S. Weber, Eduardo Weltman, William I. Wei, Mark E. Zafereo

358 illustrations

Thieme
Stuttgart • New York

Library of Congress Cataloging-in-Publication Data is available from the publisher.

Illustrator: Dr. Katja Dalkowski, Buckenhof, Germany

Important note: Medicine is an ever-changing science undergoing continual development. Research and clinical experience are continually expanding our knowledge, in particular our knowledge of proper treatment and drug therapy. Insofar as this book mentions any dosage or application, readers may rest assured that the authors, editors, and publishers have made every effort to ensure that such references are in accordance with **the state of knowledge at the time of production of the book**.
Nevertheless, this does not involve, imply, or express any guarantee or responsibility on the part of the publishers in respect to any dosage instructions and forms of applications stated in the book. **Every user is requested to examine carefully** the manufacturers' leaflets accompanying each drug and to check, if necessary in consultation with a physician or specialist, whether the dosage schedules mentioned therein or the contraindications stated by the manufacturers differ from the statements made in the present book. Such examination is particularly important with drugs that are either rarely used or have been newly released on the market. Every dosage schedule or every form of application used is entirely at the user's own risk and responsibility. The authors and publishers request every user to report to the publishers any discrepancies or inaccuracies noticed. If errors in this work are found after publication, errata will be posted at www.thieme.com on the product description page.

Rüdigerstrasse 14, 70469 Stuttgart, Germany
http://www.thieme.de
Thieme Medical Publishers, Inc., 333 Seventh Avenue,
New York, NY 10001, USA
http://www.thieme.com

Cover design: Thieme Publishing Group
Typesetting by le-tex publishing services GmbH, Leipzig, Germany
Printed in China by Asia Pacific Offset, Hong Kong

ISBN 978-3-13-147391-2
eISBN 978-3-13-164571-5

Contributors

Oludolapo O. Adesanya, PG Dip (Nucl Med), MRCP, FRCR
Consultant Radiologist
Department of Radiology
University Hospital Coventry and Warwickshire (UHCW)
Coventry
UK

K. Kian Ang, MD, PhD, FACR, FASTRO
Professor
and holder of the Gilbert H. Fletcher
Memorial Distinguished Chair
Department of Radiation Oncology
The University of Texas MD Anderson Cancer Center
Houston, Texas
USA

R. J. Baatenburg de Jong, MD
KNO-Heelkunde
Erasmus MC
Rotterdam
Netherlands

Alfonsus J. M. Balm, MD
Professor
The Netherlands Cancer Institute
Antoni van Leeuwenhoek Hospital
Amsterdam
Netherlands

Beth M. Beadle, MD
Assistant Professor
University of Texas
M. D. Anderson Cancer Center
Houston, Texas
USA

Jan Paul de Boer, MD
Department of Medical Oncology
The Netherlands Cancer Institute
Antoni van Leeuwenhoek Hospital
Amsterdam
Netherlands

Maarten F. de Boer, MD
KNO-Heelkunde
Erasmus MC
Rotterdam
Netherlands

Lenine Garcia Brandão, MD, PhD
Professor
Head and Neck Surgeon
Brazilian Institute for Cancer Control (IBCC)
Sao Paulo
Brazil

Augusto Caraceni, MD
Palliative Care, Pain Therapy and Rehabilitation Unit
Fondazione IRCCS Istituto Nazionale Tumori
Milan
Italy

Claudio R. Cernea, MD
Professor of Surgery
Department of Head and Neck Surgery
University of Sao Paulo Medical School
Sao Paulo
Brazil

Kevin S. Choe, MD
Assistant Professor
Department of Radiation Oncology
University of Texas
Southwestern Dallas, Texas
USA

Ezra E.W. Cohen, MD
University of Chicago Medical Center
Chicago, Illinois
USA

Marc A. Cohen, MD
Department of Otolaryngology
Princess Margaret Hospital
Toronto, Ontario
Canada

Ralph Gilbert, MD
Professor of Otolaryngology—Head and Neck Surgery
Princess Margaret Hospital
University of Toronto
Toronto, Ontario
Canada

David P. Goldstein, MD, MSC, FRCSC
Assistant Professor
Department of Otolaryngology—Head and Neck Surgery
Princess Margaret Hospital
University of Toronto
Toronto, Ontario
Canada

Patrick Gullane, CM, MB, FRCSC, FACS, Hon FRACS, Hon FRCS
Professor and Chair
Department of Otolaryngology—Head and Neck Surgery
University Health Network
Toronto General Hospital
University of Toronto
Toronto, Ontario
Canada

Kevin J. Harrington, MD
Institute of Cancer Research
Chester Beatty Laboratories
London
UK

Jarrod Homer, MD, FRCS
ENT / Head and Neck Surgeon
Manchester Royal Infirmary
Manchester
UK

Julie Howle, MB, BS, FRACS
Staff Specialist
Surgical Oncology Unit
Westmead Cancer Care Centre
Wentworthville, New South Wales
Australia

N. Gopalakrishna Iyer, MD
Department of Surgical Oncology
National Cancer Centre
Singapore

Charles G. Kelly, MD
Consultant Clinical Oncologist
Degree Program Director and Honorary Clinical Senior Lecturer
Newcastle University
Northern Centre for Cancer Care
Freeman Hospital
Newcastle-upon-Tyne
UK

Lai Wan Dora Kwong
Professor
Department of Clinical Oncology
Queen Mary Hospital
University of Hong Kong
Hong Kong
China

Lisa Licitra, MD
Department of Otolaryngology
National Cancer Institute
Milan
Italy

Julia Maclean
Cancer Care Centre
St. George Hospital
Kogarah, New South Wales
Australia

Hisham M. Mehanna, PhD, BMedSc (Hons), MBChB (Hons), FRCS, FRCS (ORL-HNS)
Director, Institute of Head and Neck Studies and Education
Consultant Head–Neck and Thyroid Surgeon
Chair, Head and Neck Surgery at the School of Cancer Sciences
The University of Birmingham
Birmingham
UK

Gary Morgan
Head and Neck Cancer Service
Westmead Hospital
Westmead
Sydney
Australia

Dan Munday, MD
Associate Clinical Professor
Honorary Consultant in Palliative Medicine
Health Sciences Research Institute
University of Warwick/Myton Hospice
Coventry
UK

Ramez Nassif, MD
ENT Department
Norfolk and Norwich University Hospital
Norwich
UK

Christopher M. Nutting, MD
Director Head and Neck Unit
Royal Marsden Hospital
London
UK

Marinella P. J. Offerman, MSc
KNO-Heelkunde
Erasmus MC
Rotterdam
Netherlands

Vinidh Paleri
Consultant Head Neck Surgeons
ENT Department
Freeman Hospital
Newcastle-upon-Tyne
UK

Alison Perry
Professor
Head of Department of Clinical Therapies
Faculty of Education and Health Sciences
University of Limerick
Limerick
Ireland

Jean F. A. Pruyn, PhD
Professor
Department of Pulmonary Medicine and Tuberculosis
Erasmus MC
Rotterdam
Netherlands

Alexander D. Rapidis
Professor and Chairman
Department of Head and Neck / Maxillofacial Surgery
Greek Anticancer Institute
St. Savvas Hospital
Athens
Greece

Coen R. N. Rasch, MD, PhD
Department of Radiation Oncology
The Netherlands Cancer Institute
Antoni van Leeuwenhoek Hospital
Amsterdam
Netherlands

Joseph Kamel Salama, MD
Department of Radiation and Cellular Oncology
University of Chicago Hospitals
Chicago, Illinois
USA

M. P. van der Schroeff
KNO-Heelkunde
Erasmus MC
Rotterdam
Netherlands

Cherith J. Semple, MD
Cancer Services
Ulster Hospital
Belfast, Northern Ireland
UK

Ashok R. Shaha
Professor of Surgery
Chair of Head and Neck Surgery Department
Memorial Sloan-Kettering Cancer Center
New York
USA

Priyamal Silva, MD
Department of Head and Neck Surgery
John Radcliffe Infirmary Oxford
Wallingford, Oxfordshire
UK

Nick Slevin, MD
Director of Clinical Oncology
The Christie NHS Foundation Trust
Withington, Manchester
UK

Pol Specenier
Department of Oncology
Antwerp University Hospital
Edegem
Belgium

Miroslav Tedla, MD
Post CCT Fellow in Head and Neck Surgery
Coventry
UK

R. Michael Tuttle
Professor of Medicine
Endocrinology Service
Memorial Sloan-Kettering Cancer Center
New York
USA

Michael Veness, MD (UNSW), MB, BS, MMed FRANZCR
Clinical Associate Professor
Senior Staff Specialist
Department of Radiation Oncology
Westmead Hospital
University of Sydney
Wentworthville, New South Wales
Sydney
Australia

Jan B. Vermorken, MD
Department of Medical Oncology
Antwerp University Hospital
Edegem
Belgium

Randal S. Weber, MD
University of Texas
M. D. Anderson Cancer Center
Houston, Texas
USA

Eduardo Weltman, PhD
Department of Radiation Oncology
Hospital Israelita Albert Einstein
Morumbi, Sao Paolo
Brazil

William I. Wei
Professor
Queen Mary Hospital
Hong Kong
China

Mark E. Zafereo, MD
T. Boone Pickens Academy
Houston, Texas
USA

Preface

The head and neck region contains numerous delicate, intricately organized organs essential for basic physiological functions and critical for appearance, expression, and social interactions. Although representing less than 5% of cancers, a variety of neoplasms with diverging natural histories arise in this relatively small region of the body. Many advances have been made during the past few decades in the understanding of the biology, natural history, and treatment of head and neck cancer through thorough basic, translational, and clinical investigations. Although improvement in overall survival has been modest, substantial progress has been made in terms of organ preservation and toxicity reduction by incorporating new treatment technologies, such as intensity-modulated radiotherapy (IMRT) and transoral laser and robotic surgery, and establishing new multimodality therapy regimens.

Early-stage head and neck cancer can now be successfully cured with modern therapy modalities. Unfortunately, a substantial proportion of patients with locally advanced head and neck cancer still develop local recurrence despite aggressive multimodality therapy. These patients die of the distressing consequences of uncontrolled local tumor growth. An increasing body of data reveals that some of the patients with local relapse can be successfully salvaged with surgery or combined therapy including re-irradiation, when selected and managed properly, albeit at the cost of some severe morbidity. In addition, well-organized supportive and symptomatic care can reduce suffering of those with progressive disease.

Many textbooks focus on the biology, diagnosis and work-up, and frontline management of various head and neck cancers. So far, little published work has specifically addressed assessment and management of patients with recurrent disease. That need prompted us to edit this textbook, which is intended to serve as an evidence-based reference book for oncologists in day-to-day practice and also for trainees interested in the field.

The first few chapters of the book discuss the general principles and techniques underpinning the investigation and management of recurrence in head and neck cancer. These cover the molecular biology, radiological investigations, re-irradiation, chemotherapy, surgical reconstruction, and patient selection in the setting of head and neck recurrence. The rest of the chapters provide detailed evidence-based, multidisciplinary guides to the management of recurrence at each site within the head and neck. Each chapter is written by at least one surgeon and one clinical oncologist. Emphasis has been given to providing the evidence in a structured and systematic manner. Each chapter outlines the epidemiology of the disease, the risk factors, and the outcomes of treatment. It then discusses the recommended investigations followed by the principles of the management of recurrence following previous treatment with surgery and/or chemoradiotherapy. The authors then discuss any specific practical techniques, pitfalls, and potential complications relevant to management of recurrence in that particular area. Real case histories illustrate important and/or practical aspects of management. Each chapter has a summary of the important points, as well as recommendations for further reading, further research, and indications of the most important reference articles on the topic. The final chapters give detailed practical reviews of rehabilitation and palliative care for head and neck recurrence.

We have selected the contributors for their world-renowned expertise and extensive experience in their fields. We are indebted to all of them for their efforts in putting together a comprehensive review and providing practical guidelines in these rather difficult and challenging topics.

We sincerely hope that you will find this book of practical use in your day-to-day clinical practice.

Hisham M. Mehanna
K. Kian Ang

Acknowledgments

We thank all the contributors who have very generously given their time and effort to put this book together. Their contributions have been invaluable and are much appreciated. We would also like to thank all the staff at Thieme Publishers who have worked on the book, especially Stephan Konnry, editor, and Dr. Sibylle Toenjes, freelance editor, who have been very helpful and patient throughout. We would also like to thank our PAs, Gemma Jones and Cathy Ramirez for their help with the manuscripts. Finally, last but not least, we would like to thank our families who have had to endure the time we spent away from them while putting the book together.

Contents

1 Introduction

K. Kian Ang, Hisham M. Mehanna

Recurrence is unfortunately still a common occurrence, experienced by up to 50% of patients treated for locally advanced head and neck cancer. The management of recurrent head and neck cancer is without doubt challenging. Indeed, recurrence in the head and neck is often regarded as untreatable and, accordingly, is managed with palliative intent. However, as you will read in later chapters, a substantial proportion of patients with head and neck cancer recurrence are responsive to salvage treatment that prolongs survival or may even achieve cure.

We feel that one of the reasons there is a large variation in the management of recurrence of head and neck cancers is that there is relatively little research in the field. In addition, and possibly as a consequence, there are also very few publications that address the topic of recurrence in a holistic and comprehensive way. Indeed, the issue is often addressed as a single chapter in a book on the management of a particular tumor or of a particular site.

Our aim for this book was that it would bring together all the current evidence and expertise on the epidemiology, risk factors, clinical and imaging evaluation, and management of recurrent head and neck cancer tumors. We have tried to take a holistic, multidisciplinary approach to the management of recurrence of head and neck cancers. We have endeavored to include both curative and palliative approaches, and include surgical, radiotherapeutic, and chemotherapeutic options where they exist. Each site-specific chapter has at least one surgical and one oncological contributor. Specialists in speech and language therapy, palliative care, psychology, epidemiology, and clinical cancer nursing have also contributed substantially.

Clinical Assessment and Imaging Evaluation of Recurrence

Accurate diagnosis and staging is the essential first step in the management of recurrent head and neck cancer. Not only does it determine the presence of tumor, but it should also determine the extent and the likelihood of successful salvage, the best modality or modalities of treatment, and the potential impact on function.

Patients treated for head and neck cancer will usually undergo surveillance in the form of clinical examinations and in some centers routine investigation such as ultrasound or computed tomography (CT) scans.[1,2] The aim of these surveillance visits is in part to attempt to identify recurrence, or a second primary tumor, at an early stage, and therefore to institute salvage treatment where possible.[2] There is no clear evidence of what the optimum surveillance regimen or frequency is, or whether self-surveillance is as effective as clinician-led, regular surveillance.[3]

It is important to note that a report of a change in symptoms, whether initiated by the patient or reported at a routine follow-up consultation, should be treated with a high index of suspicion and considered a sign of recurrence until proven otherwise.[3] Pain, hoarseness, dysphagia or odynophagia, otalgia, weight loss, and node enlargement should all be regarded as symptoms suspicious for recurrence.[4]

Principles of the Assessment of Potential Recurrence

Careful assessment of patients who present with potential recurrence is mandatory. As part of a comprehensive assessment, it is important to ascertain the following aspects:

- What was the previous treatment?
- Is there any evidence of distant metastases?
- Is there recurrence at the primary site and in the neck?
- What is the extent of the primary recurrence and the distribution of the nodal recurrence?
- Is there evidence of soft tissue extension or nodal extracapsular extension by physical examination and on imaging?
- Is there evidence of, and what is the extent of, involvement of the carotid arteries, brachial plexus, and prevertebral muscles?
- Can the recurrence be excised surgically with no gross tumor left behind?
- What are the potential functional deficits of excision of the recurrence?

The above questions must be addressed and answered as comprehensively as possible, through a combination of investigations, to allow the formulation of a treatment plan.

History and Examination

The history should elicit the duration of any symptoms suggestive of recurrence. It should also elicit previous treatments in as much detail as possible, including the length of time between last treatment and recurrence. The patient's current medical history and performance status should be assessed, as that is often one of the main determinants of eligibility for surgical and nonsurgical treatments. Risk factors, such as continuing smoking, should also be ascertained.

The extent of the tumor should be assessed on examination, as well as the number, distribution, and fixity of any nodal recurrence. A full clinical examination of the primary site and the rest of the upper aerodigestive tract should also be undertaken to exclude second primaries.

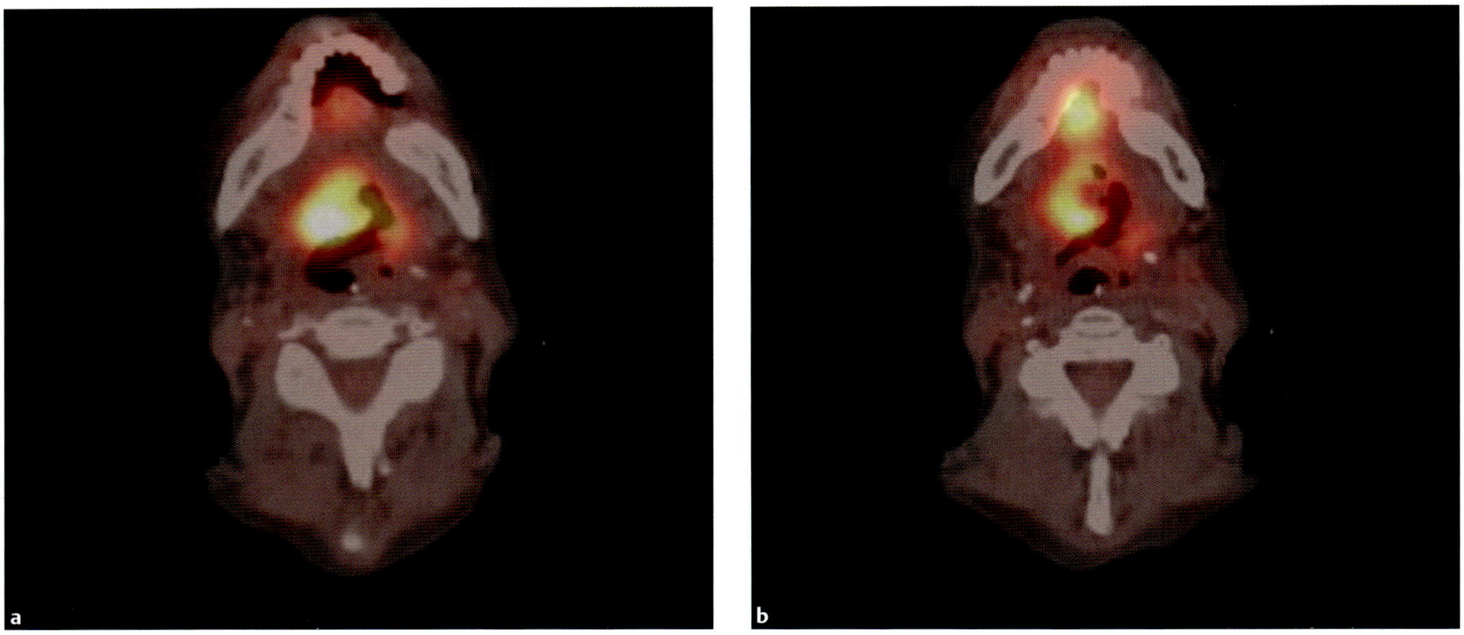

Fig. 1.1a, b Axial PET-CT scans of a recurrent tongue base tumor (with kind permission of Dr. Olu Adesanya, Coventry, UK).

Previous Treatment Records

It is important to attempt to obtain the patient's previous treatment records, including details of their operations, radiotherapy plans including isodose distributions, all chemotherapy given, and any documentation of toxicity, complications, and compliance with the treatments. Relapse within high radiation dose regions, for example, indicates that the tumor may be relatively radioresistant, which decreases the expectation for successful outcome with re-irradiation. A short duration between the end of treatment and recurrence is indicative of an aggressive tumor that is relatively resistant to treatment. It is also important to obtain the original diagnostic and resection histopathology specimens, and to submit them for review by a pathologist specializing in head and neck cancer to confirm the initial histological diagnosis and identify any poor prognostic factors the patient may have had that predisposed them to developing recurrence, for example, poor tumor differentiation, vascular and perineural invasion, extranodal extension, and involved resection margins.

Imaging

Computed tomography (CT) or magnetic resonance imaging (MRI) with contrast is an appropriate first-line investigation. These allow assessment of the recurrence both at the primary site and in the neck, as well as the relationship to the vital structures, especially the carotid artery. It can also allow assessment of the likelihood of soft tissue or extranodal extension. In patients who have had previous surgery, the extent of the previous operations, as well as sacrificed and preserved structures, should be carefully ascertained. For example, it should be ascertained whether both internal jugular veins are present and patent.

However, both of these imaging modalities may be unable to accurately assess recurrence at the primary site in some cases. Therefore, we recommend that additional assessments of the primary site should be undertaken. If available, PET-CT scanning would be the preferred diagnostic modality, as it has been shown to be the most accurate method for assessment of nodal recurrence, exceeding the accuracy of CT or MRI. A systematic review and meta-analysis by our group examined 1871 papers and found 27, mainly reporting retrospective cohorts, that were eligible for inclusion.[5] Most studies reported on a combination of patients with persistent nodal disease and patients with recurrent disease. The mean sensitivity of detection of nodal recurrence by PET was 74% (95% CI, 50%–89%), and the mean specificity was 88% (95% CI, 74%–95%). The pooled mean positive and negative predictive values for the detection of recurrent disease in the neck were 49% (95% CI, 29%–70%), and 96% (95% CI, 84%–99%) respectively. Importantly, the sensitivity of the PET-CT scan was significantly higher for scans performed more than 10 weeks after treatment ($P = 0.002$). **Figure 1.1a, b** shows axial PET-CT scans of a recurrent tongue base tumor.

A further important advantage of PET-CT is that it may detect distant metastases that are not detected by other modalities, as its sensitivity and specificity for this are very high (92% and 82% respectively). **Figure 1.2a, b** shows distant metastasis in an unusual site—the liver—from a recurrent nasopharyngeal carcinoma. **Figure 1.3a–d** shows PET-CT scans of a markedly avid focus in the right inferior articular process of the L4 vertebra corresponding to the focal lucency on CT (**Fig. 1.3d**) in keeping with bone metastasis following multiple thyroid cancer recurrences. Importantly, the negative predictive value of PET-CT has been reported to be up to 98% in a follow-up cohort of 80 patients with head and neck cancer.[6] Accordingly, a PET-CT scan that is positive only in the head and neck region is generally considered a strong indication for the absence of distant metastases, which increases the enthusiasm to embark on potentially morbid treatments.

If PET-CT is not readily available, then in addition to an examination under anesthetic, the assessment may include serial CT or MR, comparing the posttreatment scan with the pretreatment scan and/or a baseline posttreatment scan of the primary site.[7,8] **Figure 1.4a, b** shows tumor recurrence in a parotid bed on MRI.

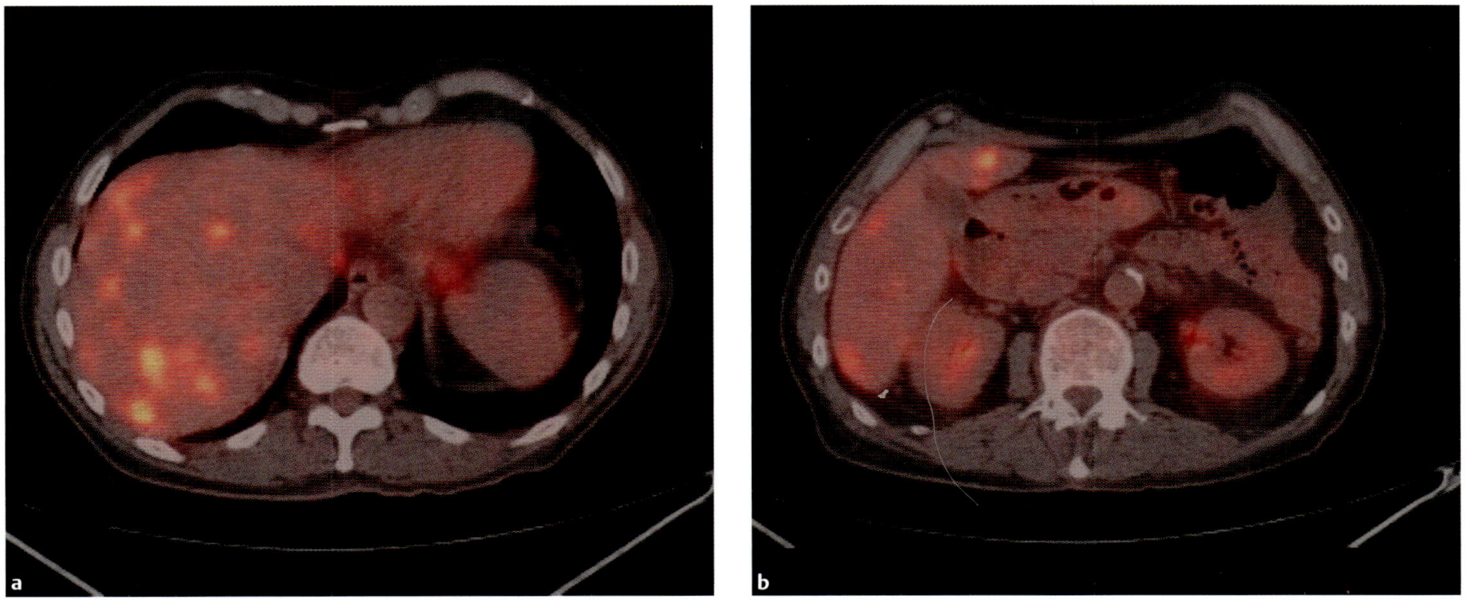

Fig. 1.2a, b Distant metastasis in the liver from a recurrent nasopharyngeal carcinoma (with kind permission of Dr. Olu Adesanya, Coventry, UK).

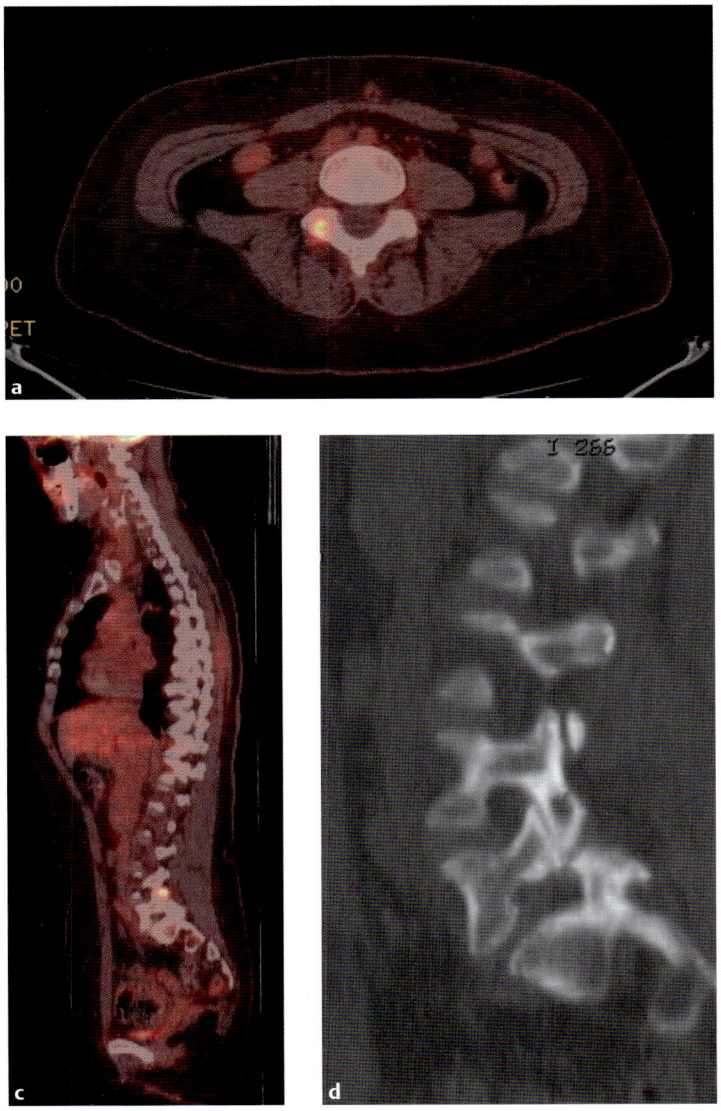

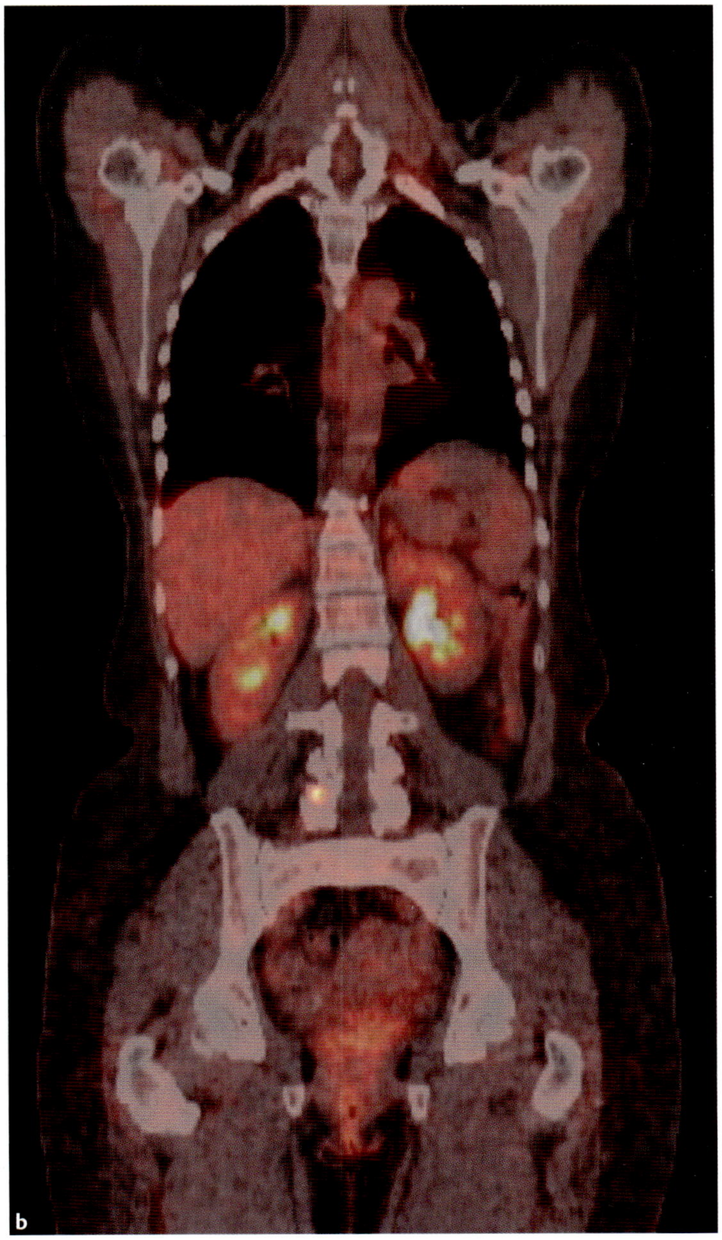

Fig. 1.3a–d PET-CT scans of a markedly avid focus in the right inferior articular process of the L4 vertebra corresponding to the focal lucency on CT (**d**) in keeping with bone metastasis following multiple thyroid cancer recurrences (with kind permission of Dr. Olu Adesanya, Coventry, UK).

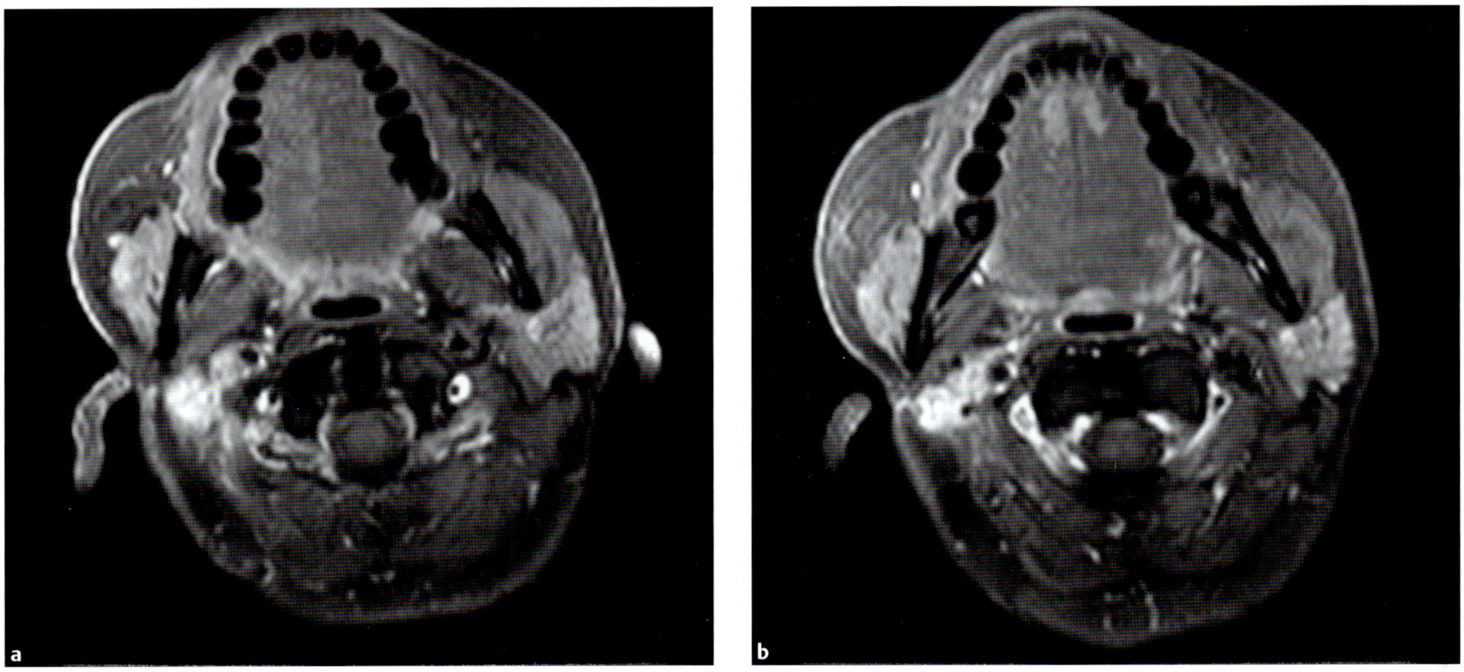

Fig. 1.4a, b Tumor recurrence in a parotid bed on MRI (with kind permission of Dr. Olu Adesanya, Coventry, UK).

MRI scanning has been shown to improve the accuracy of the detection of primary site recurrences. Hermans et al. demonstrated that a follow-up CT scan, following a baseline CT scan taken after primary treatment had ended, helped identify 40% of recurrences earlier than clinical examination.[8] Van den Broek et al. found in a series of 82 patients that serial MRI scanning was effective in avoiding unnecessary examination under anesthetic, with a positive predictive value for recurrence of 55% and a negative predictive value of 82%.[7]

Examination under Anesthetic

Occasionally, examination under anesthetic (EUA) is not necessary if the patient has isolated nodal metastases that have been confirmed on needle biopsy, and where the primary site can be assessed carefully by clinical examination and the quality of detailed imaging, as described above, is excellent. However, an EUA is recommended in the majority of cases where only limited assessment of the primary site has been possible (e.g., due to the presence of fibrosis or flap) and because it generally allows accurate assessment of the extent and potential resectibility. It is also frequently necessary to obtain samples for histological confirmation of the diagnosis.

It is of note that EUA with biopsy can miss detection of recurrence. In a series of 131 patients undergoing 207 of such investigations, the EUA and biopsy was falsely negative in 31% of patients in whom the recurrence was detected within 6 months at the site of the initial biopsy.[9]

Needle or Open Biopsy

It is important to obtain a cytological or histological diagnosis of recurrence, as diagnostic imaging investigations often have a low specificity. If a primary site recurrence is present, then histological confirmation can be obtained by biopsy during the EUA. Diagnosis in the case of isolated nodal metastases can be obtained by fine-needle aspiration or core biopsy of the neck nodes, often guided by ultrasound or CT.[10] **Figure 1.5a, b** shows ultrasound, and **Fig. 1.5c, d** shows cytological features consistent with recurrent squamous carcinoma on cytology of lymph nodes in the neck. It is important that the cytological specimen is examined by head and neck pathologists to decrease the risk of false-positives and false-negatives. If a result cannot be confirmed on needle biopsy, then a diagnosis can often be obtained by open biopsy or frozen section. Care should be taken when undertaking open biopsy to plan incisions with potential further surgical treatments in mind.

Recommended Reading[1]

- Joshi A, Calman F, O'Connell M, Jeannon JP, Pracy P, Simo R. Current trends in the follow-up of head and neck cancer patients in the UK. Clin Oncol (R Coll Radiol) 2010;22(2):114–118*
- Kothari P, Trinidade A, Hewitt RJ, Singh A, O'Flynn P. The follow-up of patients with head and neck cancer: an analysis of 1,039 patients. Eur Arch Otorhinolaryngol 2011;268(8):1191–1200
- Paniello RC, Virgo KS, Johnson MH, Clemente MF, Johnson FE. Practice patterns and clinical guidelines for posttreatment follow-up of head and neck cancers: a comparison of 2 professional societies. Arch Otolaryngol Head Neck Surg 1999;125(3):309–313
- Isles MG, McConkey C, Mehanna HM. A systematic review and meta-analysis of the role of positron emission tomography in

1 References with asterisks indicate the most important reference articles on the topic.

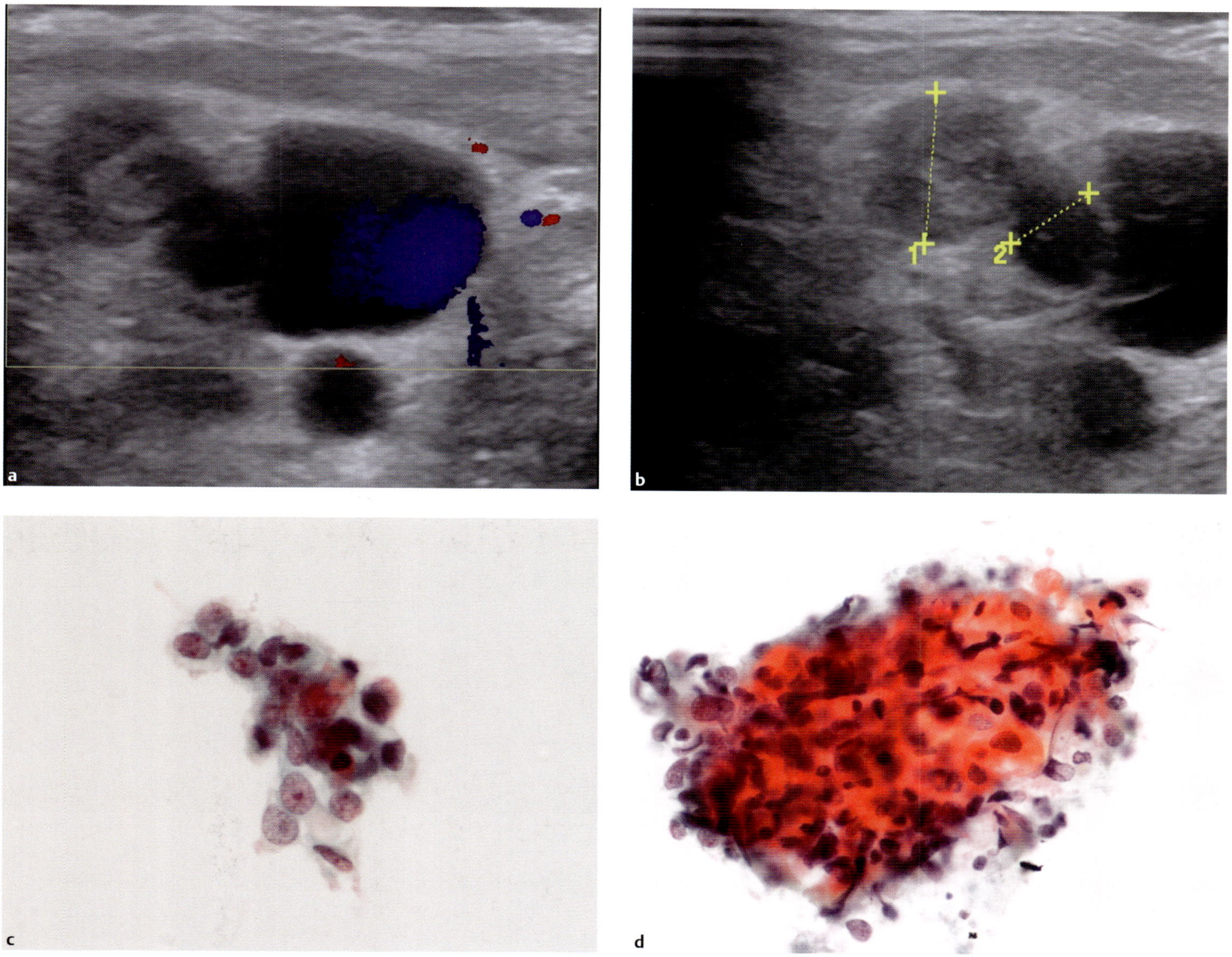

Fig. 1.5a–d Recurrent squamous carcinoma of lymph node in the neck.
a, b Ultrasound (images courtesy of Dr. Olu Adesanya, Coventry, UK).
c, d Cytological features (images courtesy of Dr. Yen Ching Yeo, Coventry, UK).

the follow up of head and neck squamous cell carcinoma following radiotherapy or chemoradiotherapy. Clin Otolaryngol 2008;33(3):210–222 (A systematic review and meta-analysis of the role of positron emission tomography in the follow up of head and neck squamous cell carcinoma following radiotherapy or chemoradiotherapy.)

References[1]

1. Joshi A, Calman F, O'Connell M, Jeannon JP, Pracy P, Simo R. Current trends in the follow-up of head and neck cancer patients in the UK. Clin Oncol (R Coll Radiol) 2010;22(2):114–118
2. National Comprehensive Cancer Network. Guidelines for the treatment of head and neck cancer 2010. www.nccn.org/clinical.asp.* Accessed 1 Dec, 2010
3. Kothari P, Trinidade A, Hewitt RJ, Singh A, O'Flynn P. The follow-up of patients with head and neck cancer: an analysis of 1,039 patients. Eur Arch Otorhinolaryngol 2011;268(8):1191–1200
4. Paniello RC, Virgo KS, Johnson MH, Clemente MF, Johnson FE. Practice patterns and clinical guidelines for posttreatment follow-up of head and neck cancers: a comparison of 2 professional societies. Arch Otolaryngol Head Neck Surg 1999;125(3):309–313
5. Isles MG, McConkey C, Mehanna HM. A systematic review and meta-analysis of the role of positron emission tomography in the follow up of head and neck squamous cell carcinoma following radiotherapy or chemoradiotherapy. Clin Otolaryngol 2008;33(3):210–222
6. Kao J, Vu HL, Genden EM, et al. The diagnostic and prognostic utility of positron emission tomography/computed tomography-based follow-up after radiotherapy for head and neck cancer. Cancer 2009;115(19):4586–4594
7. van den Broek GB, Rasch CR, Pameijer FA, Peter E, van den Brekel MW, Balm AJ. Response measurement after intraarterial chemoradiation in advanced head and neck carcinoma: magnetic resonance imaging and evaluation under general anesthesia? Cancer 2006;106(8):1722–1729

1 References with asterisks indicate the most important reference articles on the topic.

8. Hermans R, Pameijer FA, Mancuso AA, Parsons JT, Mendenhall WM. Laryngeal or hypopharyngeal squamous cell carcinoma: can follow-up CT after definitive radiation therapy be used to detect local failure earlier than clinical examination alone? Radiology 2000;214(3):683–687
9. Brouwer J, Bodar EJ, De Bree R, et al. Detecting recurrent laryngeal carcinoma after radiotherapy: room for improvement. Eur Arch Otorhinolaryngol 2004;261(8):417–422
10. Som PM, Silvers AR, Urken ML. Surveillance CT and the prompt use of CT-guided fine-needle aspiration in patients with head and neck cancer who have undergone surgery. AJR Am J Roentgenol 1999;173(6):1505–1508

2 Molecular Biology of Recurrence

Kevin J. Harrington

Summary

- Disease recurrence following nonsurgical treatment of head and neck cancer occurs as a result of the tumor having intrinsic or acquired insensitivity to radiotherapy/chemotherapy or because the disease has metastasized to distant sites.
- Cancer stem cells reside in a "hypoxic niche" in tumors and display intrinsic resistance to both irradiation and chemotherapy.
- Resistance to cisplatin chemotherapy in head and neck cancer can be multifactorial—involving decreased drug uptake/retention, increased DNA repair, and reduced drug-induced apoptosis.
- Resistance to agents that target the epidermal growth factor receptor (EGFR) can occur through mutation of the receptor or through changes in patterns of activity in other signal transduction pathways.
- Hematogenous metastasis is a complex process that may involve secretion of tumor factors that precondition a metastatic niche in advance of tumor cell colonization.
- Lymphatic metastasis of head and neck cancers is promoted by expression of chemokine receptors on tumor cells that allow them to migrate along chemokine gradients to locoregional lymph nodes.

Introduction

Securing locoregional disease control is of central importance when managing patients with squamous cell carcinoma of the head and neck (SCCHN). Failure to achieve this goal leads to persistent or recurrent disease at the primary tumor site or in the regional lymph nodes. In addition, patients can develop metastatic disease, either as a consequence of spread from the primary tumor before the initial diagnosis or from treatment-resistant persistent or recurrent locoregional disease. Both of these clinical scenarios (persistent/recurrent locoregional or metastatic disease) represent extremely difficult management problems. Salvage treatment of the former situation is possible, but in practice this is frequently unsuccessful—especially in patients in whom macroscopic disease is evident at or within 6 months of the end of initial chemoradiotherapy—and usually entails very significant acute and long-term morbidity. Systemic metastatic disease may be palliated by cytotoxic chemotherapy, biological agents, or low-dose radiotherapy, but it remains incurable with a median survival of ca. 6–9 months.

Until recently, clinicians and researchers had a very limited picture of the factors that contribute to disease persistence, recurrence, and metastasis; as a consequence, they had few clues about the best approaches to targeting these events to improve therapeutic outcomes. The molecular biology revolution has furnished us with a growing understanding of the mechanistic bases of recurrent/metastatic SCCHN and we now have the prospect of predicting such adverse biological behavior and designing specific therapeutic strategies to counter it. Elucidation of the factors that mediate resistance to standard cancer therapies (radiotherapy and chemotherapy) may allow clinicians to design specific therapies capable of sensitizing tumors to these modalities or, alternatively, accurately to select patients for more appropriate surgical management, even if this involves loss of organ function. Furthermore, early identification of tumor characteristics that are involved in the process of systemic metastasis may enable us to design treatment strategies that reduce its incidence. Of course, this approach will only be successful in preventing metastasis occurring between diagnosis and the end of the therapy period. More importantly, early identification of the likelihood or the presence of systemic metastasis will allow clinicians to evaluate targeted therapies that are capable of arresting (cytostatic agents) or killing (cytocidal agents) micrometastatic disease to improve progression-free and overall survival rates. Key to this approach will be an improved understanding of the factors involved in allowing tumor cells to establish, maintain, and expand metastatic colonies.

This chapter will focus on the biological bases of disease recurrence with specific emphasis on factors that mediate resistance to standard anticancer therapies and lead to metastatic disease. In doing this, potential avenues for future therapeutic advances will be highlighted and discussed.

The Biology of Treatment Resistance

The term *treatment resistance* pertains to a situation in which malignant cells within a tumor are able to survive exposure to therapy. This ability can be an intrinsic property of the tumor cells or may be acquired after exposure to a specific therapeutic modality. In either case, the cells that remain following treatment will be resistant to re-challenge with the initial therapeutic modality, but may also be resistant to other, unrelated treatments. It is this multiresistant phenotype (best exemplified in terms of drug resistance) that underlies the clinical observation that recurrent cancer is more aggressive and refractory to treatment than the primary lesion at initial diagnosis.

The concept of "resistance" to surgical intervention is not helpful, given the fact that the only reasons for surgery to fail are either inadequate margins of excision of the primary or nodal disease (due either to poor surgical planning/conduct or widely infiltrative locoregional disease) or prior metastatic spread of the tumor to sites beyond the surgeon's reach. When disease is found to be close to (1–5 mm) or at (<1 mm) the surgical margin, there is still the option of using postoperative radiotherapy or chemoradiotherapy successfully to reduce the risk of locoregional recurrence.[1,2] Disease that persists after such adjuvant treatment behaves in a similar fashion to disease that shows persistence/recurrence after primary nonsurgical management and carries a very poor prognosis. In the rest of this chapter, the discussion will be confined to considering mechanisms of resistance to the main nonsurgical treatments for head and neck cancer and their role in causing disease recurrence or spread.

■ Radiation Resistance

The early practitioners of radiation therapy rapidly came to understand that some tumor histotypes are intrinsically more radioresponsive and radiocurable than others. Thus, most radiation oncologists will recognize that lymphomas and seminomas are very radiocurable, while glioblastomas and melanomas are not. Within the epithelial malignancies, squamous cell carcinoma of the head and neck is regarded as sensitive to radiation therapy, especially when it presents as early-stage disease (American Joint Committee on Cancer [AJCC] Stage I and II). Later-stage SCCHN (AJCC Stage III and IV) is recognized as likely to show initial sensitivity, but with a relatively high risk of recurrence following either radiation or chemoradiation therapy. The whole issue is made significantly more complicated by the fact that individual head and neck cancers may appear to be identical at diagnosis, but following treatment may exhibit very different responses. This difference in the intrinsic biological behavior of tumors in response to radiotherapy was recognized by the incorporation of "radiosensitivity" into the Five Rs of radiobiology.[3] At that time, the term radiosensitivity denoted little more than a phenotype with no underlying biological basis. Over the last two decades, many of the processes that govern the response of tumor cells to radiation therapy have been elucidated and they now provide us with a framework for understanding how we might be able to improve therapeutic outcomes in SCCHN.

The other determinants of the radiation response (repopulation, repair, redistribution, and reoxygenation) can also explain, at least in part, why tumors respond differently to radiotherapy. Each of these factors can be viewed as a double-edged sword such that changes can occur in either direction to increase or decrease the net therapeutic effect.[4] For example, if a tumor cell has acquired a defect in its DNA repair pathways, it is more likely than an adjacent normal cell to be killed by a dose of radiation. However, the abnormal DNA repair pathway may already have enabled the tumor cell to accumulate nonlethal mutations in other important genes that allow it to tolerate unrepaired DNA damage (or to repair it in an inaccurate fashion that only serves to enhance genetic instability). Similarly, the enhanced tumor cell division that occurs during a course of radiotherapy is generally viewed negatively as the driving force behind accelerated repopulation, but it may also make a tumor cell more susceptible to radiation-induced death by causing it to enter mitosis with unrepaired DNA damage (so-called mitotic catastrophe).

■ Role of Clonogenic Cells and Cancer Stem Cells

Classical radiobiological teaching holds that a tumor is made up of several different cellular compartments and that the most important of these comprises the so-called clonogenic cells (defined in in-vitro studies as cells with the capacity to undergo repeated division to generate a colony of 50 or more cells). There was no clear understanding of the phenotype of these clonogenic cells and no appreciation that they might be preferentially located in specific compartments within the tumor. Because of this, all of the cells within a tumor were judged to pose a threat to the patient through their potential ability to mediate tumor regrowth after radiotherapy. The success or failure of radiotherapy was thought to rest with the ability of the treatment to eradicate all tumor cells by the end of treatment.

More recently, this concept has been refined and has crystallized around the notion that tumors contain cancer stem cells (CSCs) that are capable of limitless replication and have the capacity to self-renew. They can therefore give rise to all of the heterogeneous lineages of cancer cells that comprise a tumor. Importantly, these cells comprise a very small minority of the total cell burden within a cancer. The remaining cells in the so-called transit-amplifying and postmitotic differentiated compartments may have only limited replicative capacity and are incapable of mediating the regrowth of an entire tumor. The CSC concept has resulted in a paradigm shift so that these cells are now seen as the primary target of therapeutic irradiation.[5,6] It is hypothetically possible for a single surviving CSC to serve as the seed for the regrowth of a tumor—even after a clinically complete response (**Fig. 2.1**).

Initially, CSCs were described in non–head and neck cancers, but there have also been several publications that have reported the existence of such cells in SCCHN. In-vitro and in-vivo studies in animals have reported that CSCs show a specific pattern of surface markers and gene expression profiles. The surface mark-

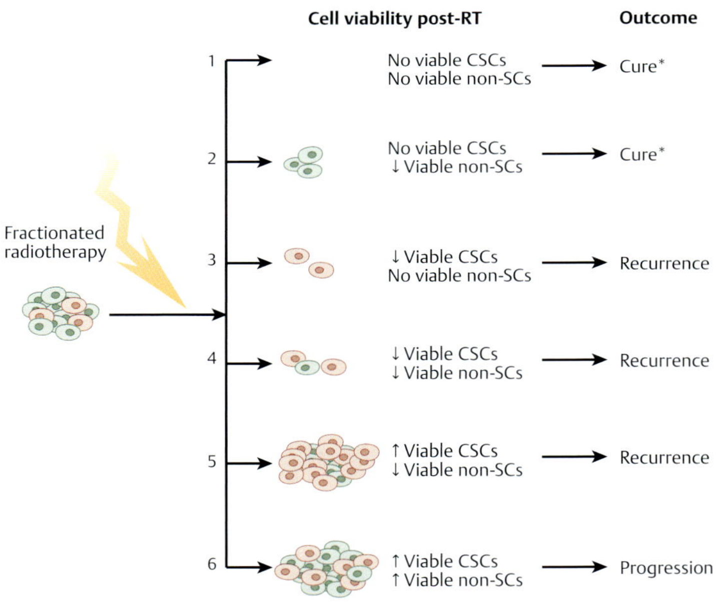

Fig. 2.1 The effect of cancer stem cells (CSCs) on therapeutic outcomes of fractionated radiotherapy. Note that for illustrative purposes the number of CSCs relative to non-SCs has been exaggerated. Most estimates suggest that fewer than 1 cancer cell in 1000 is a CSC. Six potential outcomes are depicted based on the potential ability of radiotherapy to kill CSCs (orange) or non-SCs (green). In scenarios 1 and 2, complete elimination of all CSCs results in cure (*unless metastasis has occurred before radiotherapy). In scenarios 3–6, the persistence of CSCs after completion of the course of fractionated radiotherapy means that the disease will recur at the locoregional site. In scenario 6, the expansion of both CSC and non-SC compartments during radiotherapy is likely to be manifest as disease progression on treatment.

ers expressed by CSCs from different tissues vary, but for SCCHN many sources agree that expression of CD44, Oct-4, aldehyde dehydrogenase, and Bmi-1 are features of CSCs.[7,8] In addition, the ability of CSCs to extrude certain dyes (e.g., Hoechst 33342) has facilitated their identification as a so-called "side population" by fluorescence activated cell sorting. These various markers identify a population of cells that are capable of repeated division without replicative senescence and that form tumors after injection into mice.

The ability to isolate CSCs has allowed researchers to define some of their biological properties. There are suggestions that CSCs may be preferentially localized to hypoxic niches within tumors. It has been known for more than 50 years that cells are less sensitive to the effects of ionizing radiation at low levels of oxygen tension. Simply residing in sites where the ambient oxygen level is low may assist CSCs in surviving radiation therapy. Therefore, radiation techniques, such as dose-painting intensity-modulated radiotherapy, which aim to increase radiation dose delivery to hypoxic areas may provide better targeting of hypoxic CSCs and, hence, improved cancer control rates.

In addition, however, CSCs have also been shown to be resistant to radiation therapy irrespective of the oxygen effect. One of the principal mechanisms by which CSCs are radioresistant is through upregulation of the DNA damage response (DDR). The DDR is a series of interlinked cell signaling pathways that are activated in normal (and cancer) cells following genotoxic stresses (such as damage from radiation and chemotherapy). Early studies in cell lines derived from glioblastoma multiforme revealed that CSCs upregulate expression of the key DNA damage sensor ataxia telangiectasia mutated (ATM) and, as a result, have very robust signaling through the DDR.[9] These findings suggest that targeted agents that are able to inhibit DNA repair may be particularly effective against CSCs and this is certainly an area that deserves further research.

Resistance to Cytotoxic Chemotherapy

Platinum Resistance

The most important cytotoxic agent in the treatment of SCCHN is cisplatin. It has a well-established role as part of concomitant chemoradiotherapy regimens and in palliative chemotherapy schedules, and an emerging role in induction chemotherapy.[10–12]

Mechanism of Action

Cisplatin (*cis*-dichlorodiammine platinum (II)) exerts its antitumor effects through binding to DNA, where it forms adducts. Specifically, cisplatin has a propensity to react with the N7 position of the imidazole ring of guanine and adenine to form mono- or bifunctional adducts that may involve one DNA strand (intrastrand) or both (interstrand). The relative importance of the different types of DNA adducts in mediating cellular toxicity has not yet been fully resolved, but the so-called 1,2-intrastrand and interstrand crosslinks are thought to be particularly important. The effect of these adducts is to block replication and/or prevent transcription and, as a result, to induce cell death.

Mechanisms of Resistance

Several mechanisms of resistance to platinum-based chemotherapy agents have been described in in-vitro experiments (see the box). In general, resistance mechanisms are subdivided into two types:

- **Failure of the platin agent to reach the DNA target:** The resistant cells appear to be able to reduce platinum uptake (either through decreased cellular entry or increased efflux) and to increase detoxification of the drug before it reaches the DNA.
- **Increased ability of the target cell to survive the damage induced by platinum:** Likely mediated by intracellular sulfydryl-containing agents such as glutathione or metallothioneins.

However, even if platins are able to gain access to the DNA and cause chemical alterations, there are several processes that are associated with an enhanced ability of tumor cells to survive the genotoxic insult. These include mechanisms involved in repairing or ignoring the DNA–platinum adducts and those that allow tumor cells to resist the pro-apoptotic effects of DNA damage.

! Mechanisms of Resistance to Platinum-based Cytotoxic Agents

- Reduced cellular uptake of platins
- Increased cellular efflux of platins
- Increased cytoplasmic detoxification of platins before they reach DNA targets
- Enhanced nucleotide excision repair
- Replicative bypass
- Decreased platin-induced apoptosis
- Promoter hypermethylation in genes required for drug sensitivity

DNA Repair

Platin-resistant cancer cells have been shown to exhibit increased DNA repair through the nucleotide excision pathway, which is able to remove platinum adducts from the DNA sequence. There are some suggestions that this process is preferentially active in regions of the genome that are actively transcribed (so-called transcription-coupled DNA repair). In addition, a separate mechanism seems to shield platin adducts from attempted cellular repair and this may be coupled to enhanced replicative bypass (the ability of the replication machinery to synthesize DNA past a platin adduct). This phenomenon may also involve abnormalities in mismatch repair genes.

Nucleotide Excision Repair Pathway

The clinical relevance of components of the nucleotide excision repair pathway has been reported in a study involving tumor specimens from patients who received cisplatin-based induction chemotherapy.[13] Pretreatment tumor samples were available from a cohort of 96 patients in whom the response to induction chemotherapy had been documented. Immunohistochemical staining for excision repair cross complementation group 1 (ERCC1) and *p53* was performed and correlated with response. Patients whose tumors expressed low levels of ERCC1 were four times more likely to achieve a clinical response to cisplatin-based chemotherapy than those whose tumors expressed high levels of the protein. When the data were analyzed using a Cox proportional hazard model that was adjusted for patient age, TNM stage, tumor differentiation, and tumor site, low levels of ERCC1 expression were associated with a significantly lower risk of death from cancer (hazard ratio = 0.42).

Cell Signaling Pathways

In addition, resistance to cisplatin may involve changes in cell signaling pathways that mediate cytotoxic drug-induced cell death. For example, tumor cell lines with mutations in the *p53* gene are more resistant to cisplatin than those with wild-type *p53*, presumably due to an inability to activate intrinsic apoptotic signaling pathways. *p53* is very frequently mutated in head and neck cancers and may play an important role in clinical platin responsiveness. Similarly, downstream effectors of apoptosis, such as bcl2 family members, frequently show aberrant patterns of expression in cancers and this can be associated with resistance to cisplatin-based chemotherapy by breaking the link between drug-induced DNA damage and cell death.

DNA Hypermethylation

Recently, attention has focused on the hypothesis that treatment-related DNA hypermethylation may be involved in the acquisition of cisplatin resistance through inactivation of genes that are required for drug-induced cytotoxicity. Chang et al. used a pharmacological approach in an attempt to detect hypermethylated genes whose inactivation may contribute to cisplatin resistance in three pairs of isogeneic, cisplatin-sensitive, or cisplatin-resistant cell lines derived from two parental squamous cell cancers (KB-3–1 and SCC25).[14] Several hundred genes were downregulated in each resistant cell line and reactivated by the DNA methyltransferase inhibitor 5-aza-2′-deoxycytidine. Thirty of these genes were common to two or more of the cell lines or had been reported to be downregulated in other studies. This was narrowed down further to 14 genes that were confirmed as hypermethylated by bisulfite sequencing in resistant but not in sensitive parental cell lines. Finally, 6 of the 14 genes (SAT, C8orf4, LAMB3, TUBB, G0S2, and MCAM) were induced by cisplatin in sensitive but not in resistant cell lines. Subsequent studies using small interfering RNA (siRNA) knockdown of SAT and S100P resulted in increased cell viability with cisplatin treatment in sensitive parental cell lines.

These findings support the hypothesis that treatment-induced epigenetic silencing of key genes may play a role in the development of resistance to cytotoxic chemotherapeutic agents. The availability of targeted drugs that are capable of modulating DNA methylation status offers new therapeutic options for maintaining or even restoring platinum sensitivity in patients with head and neck cancers.

Taxane Resistance

Docetaxel has an emerging role in the management of head and neck cancers, with data from at least two large clinical trials supporting its use as part of induction treatment protocols.[15,16] As a class of drugs, the taxanes act by stabilizing microtubules (both through promoting tubulin polymerization and through inhibiting its depolymerization) and, as a result, interfere with cell cycle progression and successful cell division.

Many factors may contribute to resistance to taxane chemotherapy. Taxanes as a class of drugs have been shown to be substrates for the multidrug resistant (MDR) efflux pump, at least in in-vitro studies. The significance of this in mediating taxane resistance in vivo in all tumor types remains uncertain. There are suggestions that variations in the isotypes of tubulin that are expressed by tumors appears to be a better indicator of taxane sensitivity/resistance than total tubulin expression. This is exemplified by observations in vitro that taxane-resistant cell lines tend to express β-tubulin-II or III isotypes. Recently, the importance of this mechanism was validated in patients enrolled in the phase III TAX 324 study, which randomized between two arms of induction chemotherapy comprising either docetaxel, cisplatin, and 5-fluorouracil (TPF) or cisplatin and 5-fluorouracil (PF).[16,17] By evaluating tumor markers in pretreatment biopsies from 265 of the 501 participants, the authors demonstrated that low β-tubulin-II expression was associated with an improved outcome. Thus, the median overall survivals for the low and high β-tubulin-II-expressing groups were highly statistically significantly different at 58.6 versus 18.2 months, respectively. Similar data were obtained after analysis of median progression-free survivals (43.2 vs. 9.8 months) in low and high-expressing tumors, respectively. These data potentially provide a rational basis on which to select patients for taxane-based induction chemotherapy in future clinical protocols.

Resistance to Epidermal Growth Factor Receptor Inhibitors

The emergence of epidermal growth factor receptor (EGFR) inhibitors as potentially valuable new therapeutics in the setting of SCCHN has been a significant development in recent years. In combination with radiotherapy, these agents have been shown to yield significant improvements in locoregional control and progression-free survival.[18] In the context of metastatic disease, EGFR blockade has been shown to be capable of enhancing the therapeutic activity of standard palliative chemotherapy, resulting in a 2.7-month increase in median overall survival.[19] However, as stand-alone therapies these agents have limited efficacy, with several tumors demonstrating primary resistance or developing it rapidly during treatment. By understanding the mechanisms underlying this resistance to therapy, we may be able to improve therapeutic options in this group of patients.[20]

Mechanism of Action

Epidermal growth factor receptor is a member of the ErbB/HER family of receptor tyrosine kinases that plays a major role in the biology of SCCHN. The family comprises four members: EGFR or c-erbB-1, c-erbB-2/neu/HER-2, c-erbB-3/HER-3, and c-erbB-4/HER-4. The receptors consist of a glycosylated extracellular ligand-binding domain, a hydrophobic transmembrane component, and an intracellular domain with tyrosine kinase activity. SCCHN very frequently (>90%) usurps normal EGFR-mediated cell signaling pathways and, in doing so, obtains a growth and survival advantage over neighboring normal tissues. Three main mechanisms are at the heart of the ability of SCCHN to deregulate normal EGFR signaling (**Fig. 2.2**):

- Tumors manufacture and release growth factor ligands that stimulate their own receptors (autocrine signaling) and those of their immediate neighbors (paracrine signaling).
- Tumors alter the number, structure, or function of the recep-

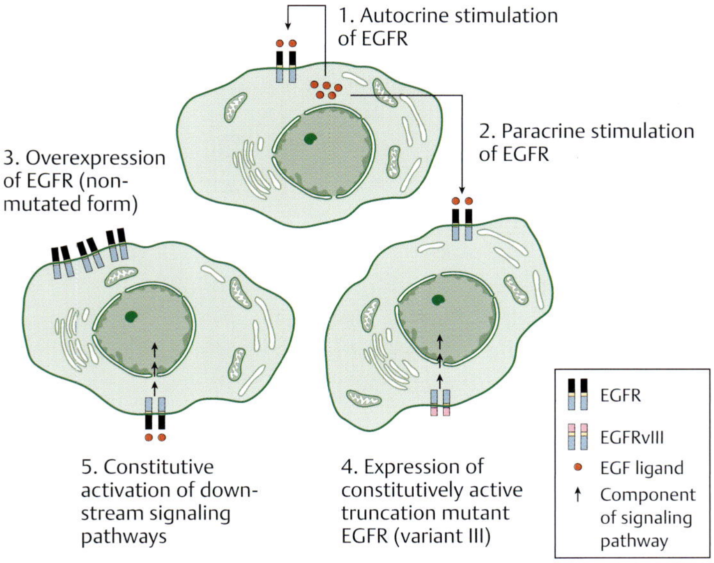

Fig. 2.2 Mechanisms of EGFR-driven head and neck cancer. Several processes have been shown to enable EGFR to mediate cancer growth, invasion, metastasis, and treatment-resistance. Cancer cells can secrete EGFR ligands to activate receptors on their own (autocrine signaling) or neighboring cells' (paracrine signaling) surfaces. SCCHN frequently overexpresses nonmutated forms of EGFR, but is also uses a truncation mutation (EGFRvIII) that is constitutively active. Even in the absence of aberrant signaling at the level of the ligand–receptor interaction, SCCHN can exploit constitutive activation of downstream elements of the signaling pathway.

tors on their surface such that they are more likely to transmit growth signals (even in the absence of the cognate ligand).

- Tumors deregulate the signaling pathways downstream of the receptor so that it is permanently switched on (constitutively active).

EGFR-driven Oncogenesis

SCCHN is an excellent example of EGFR-driven oncogenesis, since this signaling pathway can account for all of the malignant features of the disease. Overexpression of EGFR correlates with treatment resistance, tumor spread, and poor survival. The consequences of ligand binding, receptor dimerization and activation, and subsequent intracellular signaling provide mechanistic explanations for many of the features that characterize SCCHN. In contrast to certain tumor types in which amplification or mutation of the EGFR gene is implicated, overexpression of the protein without gene amplification is the dominant process in SCCHN. Several studies have shown links between EGFR overexpression and head and neck cancer oncogenesis and progression.

Expression of Receptors

The c-erbB-2 receptor is a 185 kDa receptor-like phosphoglycoprotein with no known exogenous ligand. When highly overexpressed it may spontaneously dimerize and autoactivate, but it is more frequently activated by heterodimerization with other erbB receptors. The contribution of c-erbB-2 expression to the pathogenesis of SCCHN is less well defined than in other solid cancers, such as breast and ovarian cancer.

However, c-erbB-2:c-erbB-3 heterodimers are potent inducers of the PI3-kinase antiapoptotic pathway as c-erbB-3 can bind directly to the PI3-kinase p85 subunit. Increasing expression of c-erbB-2 has been shown in parallel with acquisition of a more malignant phenotype in a series of oral carcinomas, which may imply a role in disease progression. The distribution of c-erbB-3 protein in tissues is different from that of EGFR and c-erbB-2. It does not have intrinsic tyrosine kinase activity but it can be trans-phosphorylated by both EGFR and c-erbB2. Its overexpression (but not amplification) has been reported in head and neck cancer cell lines and in some cases it has been related to malignant potential.

There has been comparatively little investigation of erbB-3 and erbB-4 in clinical samples from head and neck cancers, probably due to the low detection (~10%) in immunohistochemical surveys of clinical specimens. It has been suggested that expression of all four receptors is associated with shortened survival in patients with oral cancers, with the combination of EGFR, erbB-2, and erbB-3 (but not erbB-4) giving the greatest prognostic information.

Mechanisms of Resistance

A striking feature of the biology of EGFR in SCCHN is the fact that even in tumors that express high levels of the target protein, targeted drugs with the capacity to block receptor signaling appear to exhibit only very modest activities. Thus, single-agent response rates to gefitinib, erlotinib, or cetuximab have all been disappointingly low in the setting of relapsed/metastatic disease. Tumors manifest either primary (intrinsic) or acquired drug resistance. Primary resistance can usefully be defined as failure to achieve stable disease or progression within a short period of achieving an initial response, whereas acquired resistance occurs after a prolonged period of medication. Several mechanisms of resistance to EGFR inhibitors have been described and will be discussed below.

EGFR Mutations

The mutated version of EGFR (EGFRvIII or EGFR variant III) is the most common of seven known variants of EGFR. In this version of the protein, deletion of exons 2–7 of the EGFR gene results in a truncated extracellular domain that is associated with ligand-independent constitutive activation of the intracellular tyrosine kinase and, consequently, multiple downstream phosphorylation cascades. It has been hypothesized that the change in the extracellular domain of the receptor affects the conformation of the intracellular domain and, in particular, the ATP binding pocket. EGFRvIII can associate with and activate wild-type EGFR in the absence of ligand. This particular mutation is common in tumor types such as glioblastoma multiforme and non–small cell lung cancer, and has been reported to be present in 42% of head and neck cancers.[21] The alteration in the conformation of the receptor renders it resistant to targeted therapy with monoclonal antibodies (presumably because of loss or deformation of their specific binding epitopes), but some of the irreversible EGFR inhibitors (such as BIBW2992) have shown activity against EGFRvIII in preclinical studies.

In direct contrast to non–small cell lung cancer, EGFR tyrosine kinase domain mutations have not been shown to be correlated with response to EGFR inhibitors in SCCHN and seem to be very rare events. Similarly in non–small cell lung cancer, amplification of EGFR, which results in high gene copy number, has been associated with response to EGFR inhibition. Such findings were not replicated for SCCHN in a randomized phase III trial of two doses of gefitinib (250 and 500 mg/day) versus methotrexate 40 mg/m² per week in which EGFR gene copy number was measured by fluorescence in-situ hybridization (FISH) in 212 patients.[22] The incidence of EGFR FISH-positivity was similar between the study arms and median survivals for EGFR FISH-positive patients receiving gefitinib 250 mg, gefitinib 500 mg, and methotrexate were 6.1, 5.9, and 7.6 months, respectively. These data were essentially identical to the EGFR FISH-negative patients in whom median survivals were 6.0, 6.0, and 6.8 months, respectively.

Activation of Alternative Signaling Pathways

Blockade of EGFR signaling can lead to unanticipated changes in the activity in other downstream cytoplasmic signaling pathways. Several in-vitro and in-vivo studies have drawn attention to a diverse array of potential determinants of treatment sensitivity or resistance but, as yet, no clear consensus has emerged regarding which pathways play a dominant role.

The observation that patients with colon cancers that harbor activating mutations of KRAS/HRAS are less likely to respond to EGFR targeted small molecule or monoclonal antibody therapies is clinically important. However, KRAS/HRAS is very seldom mutated in SCCHN and is not a clinically relevant mechanism of treatment resistance. As such, in contrast to colon cancers, screening for KRAS/HRAS mutation will not be the basis for a test for suitability for EGFR targeted treatment in SCCHN. Mutations in KRAS/HRAS may be more common in SCCHN, but this issue has not yet been sufficiently assessed to evaluate its role in determining resistance to anti-EGFR therapies.

It has become increasingly clear that signaling through other receptor and non–receptor kinase pathways, such as insulin-like growth factor 1 receptor, c-Met, Src family kinases and G-protein-coupled receptors, can antagonize the antiproliferative and pro-apoptotic effects of EGFR blockade. In addition, increased activity on the PI3K/AKT pathway—through activating mutations of PI3KCA, Akt amplification, or loss of PTEN—has come into focus as a means by which cancer cells can circumvent the therapeutic effects of EGFR blockade.

Biological Processes Involved in Metastasis

The initial description of metastasis as the "transfer of disease from one organ or part to another not directly connected to it" was made nearly 200 years ago. The "seed and soil" hypothesis to explain clinical patterns of metastatic disease was first proposed by Paget in 1889 on the basis of postmortem observations in more than 700 women with breast cancer.[23] However, it is only since the 1980s that the mechanistic basis of tumor metastasis has been understood. We now have a relatively clear, but still evolving, view of the main steps in the metastatic process and some important leads in how we may be able to interrupt it. For SCCHN, there is a great difference in the relative significance of lymphatic and hematogenous metastasis: the former is prognostically important but can be curable, the latter is universally fatal. In light of this fact, the different biological processes underlying these events in SCCHN will be discussed separately.

Hematogenous Metastasis

The individual components of the metastatic process involve the following events:

- Detachment of malignant cells from neighboring cells and the local stroma
- Digestion of the extracellular matrix
- Migration/motility through the digested stroma
- Intravasation into the blood or lymphatic vessels
- Survival in the circulation
- Attachment to the endothelium/basement membrane in blood vessels at the site of metastasis
- Extravasation from the blood vessels in to the metastatic site
- Establishment of a secondary tumor deposit in the metastatic niche

The general scheme of these events has been known for some years, but recently several observations have shed new light on the metastatic process.

By using an in-vitro culture system that partially reproduces the physiological situation (surface exposed to a gaseous interface; base in contact with a matrix of fibrillar collagen I, laminin, and collagen IV), Gaggioli et al. reported that the movement of malignant head and neck cancer cells through the extracellular matrix was a collective process that required the involvement of cancer-associated fibroblasts. Using elegant imaging and molecular biology techniques, they were able to show that fibroblasts generate tunnels in the extracellular matrix, by enzymatic (protease) digestion and force-mediated matrix remodeling, through which carcinoma cells follow.[24] The carcinoma cells use Cdc42 and MRCK (myotonic dystrophy kinase-related CDC42-binding protein kinases) to regulate intracellular myosin light chain as a means of controlling their directional motility behind invading fibroblasts. Several of these signaling events are controlled by proteins that may be druggable targets and this offers some real hope of developing agents that may be able specifically to inhibit the ability of malignant cells to invade normal tissues.

The details of the processes by which tumor cells are able to escape from the primary tumor and establish metastatic colonies elsewhere in biologically favorable secondary tissues have also received significant attention. Indeed, much of this work has completely rewritten the way in which we think about the biology of tumor metastasis. One such example has been provided by studies that show that far from being a passive game of chance whereby a metastatic "seed" trusts to fortune to wash it ashore on what Paget called "congenial soil," metastasis involves a degree of forward planning on the part of the tumor. In breast cancer models, it has been shown that metastasis is facilitated by the formation of "premetastatic niches" in target organs by bone marrow–derived cells that serve as an advanced party to condition the environment in the metastatic site to make it favorable to tumor cells that subsequently arrive there and establish a secondary colony. This process is triggered by a secreted enzyme called lysyl oxidase (LOX) that is released in to the circulation by hypoxic tumor cells and subsequently accumulates at premetastatic sites where it regulates the crosslinking of structural proteins in the extracellular matrix.[25] Specifically, LOX catalyzes oxidative deamination of the primary amines of lysine and hydroxylysine in proteins such as collagen and tropoelastin to generate peptidyl-α-aminoadipic-δ-semialdehyde, an aldehyde that spontaneously condenses to form both interchain and intrachain crosslinks. As a result, LOX regulates maturation of proteins in the extracellular matrix, thereby contributing to its tensile strength and function and playing an important part in connective tissue remodeling. LOX-mediated tissue remodeling appears to be an essential prerequisite for subsequent recruitment of CD11b+ myeloid cells, which adhere to crosslinked collagen IV and produce matrix metalloproteinase-2, which cleaves collagen and enhances the invasion and recruitment of bone marrow–derived cells and metastasizing tumor cells. Therefore, LOX is a critical mediator of invasion and metastatic tumor spread and its expression is increased in breast cancer, non–small cell lung cancer, and pancreatic cancer. Elevated LOX expression is associated with the formation of metastases but it also appears to be required for their continued survival and growth. Importantly, it has been demonstrated that inhibition of LOX can prevent CD11b+ cell recruitment and, thus, prevent metastatic growth. Le et al. have recently validated LOX as a bone fide marker of metastasis in head and neck cancer patients using standard immunohistochemical staining and automated quantitative analysis.[26] They studied 66 head and neck cancer patients from a single institution and 306 of 1113 patients treated in the RTOG 90–03 phase III trial of four different radiation fractionation schedules in locally advanced disease. LOX expression was predictive for time to metastasis in the initial 66 patients. In addition, multivariate analysis, controlling for significant parameters such as nodal stage and performance status, revealed that LOX expression was a statistically significant independent predictor for time to metastasis, time to progression, and overall survival in the patients treated in RTOG 90–03. Their data translated into a 259% increase in metastatic risk for a patient at the 75th percentile of LOX expression compared with one at the 25th percentile.

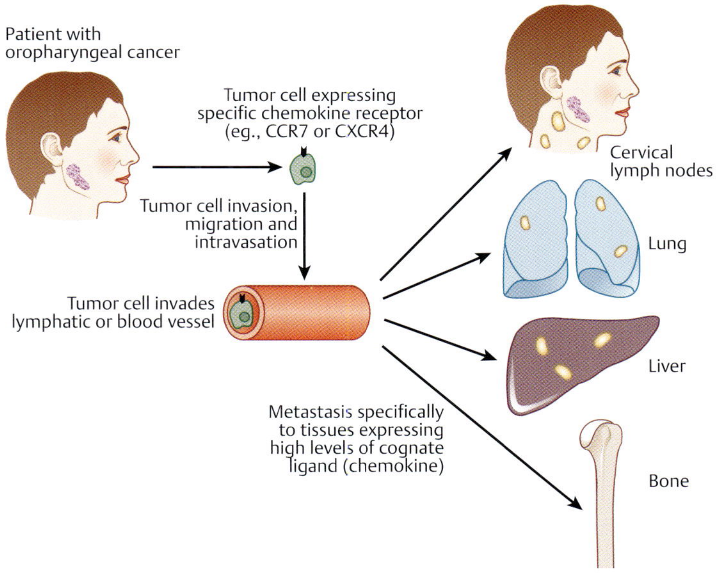

Fig. 2.3 Chemokine-mediated metastasis of SCCHN. Invasion and metastasis of tumor cells results from upregulated expression of molecules that mediate digestion of the extracellular matrix and subsequent migration and intravasation into blood vessels. Spread to locoregional (or distant) lymph nodes via the lymphatic system or to systemic sites via the bloodstream may be governed by the expression of specific chemokine receptors by cancer cells. These receptors allow the cancer cells to migrate along gradients of the secreted cognate ligand to find suitable sites in which to establish secondary deposits.

■ Lymphatic Metastasis

Head and neck cancer shows a specific predilection for nodal metastasis and this event in itself reduces the chance of cure by approximately 50% (at least for non–human papilloma virus–related SCCHN). The presence or absence of lymphatic metastasis is the single most important prognostic factor for patients with SCCHN. In an analogous fashion to the findings for blood-borne tumor spread, it has recently become clear that the ability of tumors to metastasize to locoregional lymph nodes is governed by specific biological processes.

Chemokines are small, secreted proteins with characteristic cysteine motifs in their amino-acid sequences. Most chemokine superfamily members have four cysteines and accordingly they have been classified into four groups (CXC or α, CC or β, C or γ, and CXC3 or δ) depending on the motif displayed by the first two cysteines. Chemokines are ligands for cognate G-protein-coupled, seven-transmembrane receptors and were initially shown to be involved in controlling targeted migration of hematopoietic cells.[27] More recently they have been reported to be involved in a diverse range of physiological and pathological functions including wound healing, the control of angiogenesis, and the development of tumor metastases. The initial study that demonstrated a role for chemokines and chemokine receptors in metastasis was in the setting of experimental breast cancer, where it was shown that tumor cells expressing the chemokine receptors CXCR4 and CCR7 were capable of preferentially homing to particular tissues.[28] Subsequently, CCR7 was shown to play an important role in nodal metastasis in 84 patients with squamous cell cancers of the tonsil in whom a significant association between CCR7 immunopositivity and synchronous cervical nodal metastasis was seen.[29] Relapse-free, overall, and disease-specific survival rates were significantly lower in patients whose tumors expressed high levels of CCR7. On multivariate analysis, high-level CCR7 staining predicted relapse-free and disease-specific survival. Interestingly, 15% of patients with the highest level of tumor CCR7 immunopositivity relapsed with systemic disease, suggesting that this chemokine receptor was also involved in mediating more widespread dissemination of head and neck cancer through the bloodstream (**Fig. 2.3**).

As with many aspects of tumor biology, further analysis reveals added layers of complexity. Thus, chemokines and their receptors have been shown to play a role not only in cell migration, invasion, and homing, but also in tumor cell survival and in angiogenesis.[30] As such, attempts to inhibit chemokine function in head and neck cancers represent a promising potential therapeutic avenue in this disease. Attempts to block ligand–receptor interactions are an obvious first choice, but clearly there will be concerns about the risks of interfering with normal immune cell trafficking. An alternative strategy might be to target the signal transduction pathways that mediate expression of chemokines and their receptors. For example, NFκB controls the expression of many chemokines and is constitutively active in many tumor types. As such, it has been viewed as a legitimate druggable target and the effects of anti-NFκB agents might include downregulation of chemokine signaling. However, remembering some of the lessons from targeting EGFR signaling (reviewed above), it will be important to define specific indications for use of anti-chemokine therapies and to ensure that activity in parallel pathways does not abrogate their activity.

Conclusions

Recurrent and/or metastatic head and neck cancer represents a life-threatening condition for patients and poses extremely difficult management problems to clinicians. Through detailed analysis of some of the biological processes involved in treatment resistance, we are gaining new insights into ways in which we may be better able to target SCCHN to secure disease control at the locoregional site. However, the issue of systemic relapse—either from disease dissemination from the initial primary tumor or from sites of persistent/recurrent disease—remains an apparently insoluble problem. Currently available systemic therapies are purely palliative, although recent data from the addition of an EGFR-targeted monoclonal antibody to standard chemotherapy yielded the first evidence of an improvement in overall survival in decades. More importantly, we are now beginning to understand the mechanisms behind hematogenous and lymphatic metastasis and this information may enable us to develop specific therapies that can prevent the establishment, maintenance, and growth of metastatic foci. Although a great deal of work remains to be done, there is cause for cautious optimism that we may have new therapeutic modalities available to us in the foreseeable future.

Future Research

- Molecularly targeted therapies are in development with the aim of increasing the efficacy of standard radiotherapy and chemotherapy approaches.
- Combining different molecularly targeted agents may prevent the emergence of treatment resistance (e.g., resistance to an EGFR inhibitor may be prevented by combining it with an insulin-like growth factor-1 receptor antagonist).
- Better understanding of the processes involved in hematogenous and lymphatic metastasis will drive the development of novel classes of antimetastatic drugs (e.g., lysyl oxidase inhibitors).

Recommended Reading[1]

- Weinberg RA. The Biology of Cancer. Garland Science, Taylor & Francis Group, New York, USA; 2007
- Koch U, Krause M, Baumann M. Cancer stem cells at the crossroads of current cancer therapy failures—radiation oncology perspective. Semin Cancer Biol 2010;20(2):116–124
- Harrington K, Jankowska P, Hingorani M. Molecular biology for the radiation oncologist: the 5Rs of radiobiology meet the hallmarks of cancer. Clin Oncol (R Coll Radiol) 2007;19(8):561–571
- Chen LF, Cohen EE, Grandis JR. New strategies in head and neck cancer: understanding resistance to epidermal growth factor receptor inhibitors. Clin Cancer Res 2010;16(9):2489–2495
- Talmadge JE, Fidler IJ. AACR centennial series: the biology of cancer metastasis: historical perspective. Cancer Res 2010;70(14):5649–5669
- Handra-Luca A, Hernandez J, Mountzios G, et al. Excision repair cross complementation group 1 immunohistochemical expression predicts objective response and cancer-specific survival in patients treated by Cisplatin-based induction chemotherapy for locally advanced head and neck squamous cell carcinoma. Clin Cancer Res 2007;13(13):3855–3859 ** (Key study describing mechanistic basis of platinum-resistance in patients with head and neck cancer.)
- Cullen KJ, Schumaker L, Nikitakis N, et al. beta-Tubulin-II expression strongly predicts outcome in patients receiving induction chemotherapy for locally advanced squamous carcinoma of the head and neck: a companion analysis of the TAX 324 trial. J Clin Oncol 2009;27(36):6222–6228 * (Study describing predictive biomarker of taxane response in patients treated with induction chemotherapy.)
- Sok JC, Coppelli FM, Thomas SM, et al. Mutant epidermal growth factor receptor (EGFRvIII) contributes to head and neck cancer growth and resistance to EGFR targeting. Clin Cancer Res 2006;12(17):5064–5073 ** (Description of a mutant form of EGFR as a driver of resistance to EGFR inhibition in head and neck cancer.)
- Erler JT, Bennewith KL, Nicolau M, et al. Lysyl oxidase is essential for hypoxia-induced metastasis. Nature 2006;440(7088):1222–1226 ** (Landmark description of a novel process of metastasis from the hypoxic niche.)
- Le QT, Harris J, Magliocco AM, et al. Validation of lysyl oxidase as a prognostic marker for metastasis and survival in head and neck squamous cell carcinoma: Radiation Therapy Oncology Group trial 90–03. J Clin Oncol 2009;27(26):4281–4286* (Proof-of-concept study of lysyl oxidase as a prognostic biomarker of metastasis in head and neck cancer.)

References[1]

1. Bernier J, Domenge C, Ozsahin M, et al. European Organization for Research and Treatment of Cancer Trial 22931. Postoperative irradiation with or without concomitant chemotherapy for locally advanced head and neck cancer. N Engl J Med 2004;350(19):1945–1952
2. Cooper JS, Pajak TF, Forastiere AA, et al. Radiation Therapy Oncology Group 9501/Intergroup. Postoperative concurrent radiotherapy and chemotherapy for high-risk squamous-cell carcinoma of the head and neck. N Engl J Med 2004;350(19):1937–1944
3. Steel GG, McMillan TJ, Peacock JH. The 5Rs of radiobiology. Int J Radiat Biol 1989;56(6):1045–1048
4. Harrington K, Jankowska P, Hingorani M. Molecular biology for the radiation oncologist: the 5Rs of radiobiology meet the hallmarks of cancer. Clin Oncol (R Coll Radiol) 2007;19(8):561–571
5. Baumann M, Krause M, Hill R. Exploring the role of cancer stem cells in radioresistance. Nat Rev Cancer 2008;8(7):545–554
6. Koch U, Krause M, Baumann M. Cancer stem cells at the crossroads of current cancer therapy failures—radiation oncology perspective. Semin Cancer Biol 2010;20(2):116–124
7. Clay MR, Tabor M, Owen JH, et al. Single-marker identification of head and neck squamous cell carcinoma cancer stem cells with aldehyde dehydrogenase. Head Neck 2010;32(9):1195–1201
8. Zhang P, Zhang Y, Mao L, Zhang Z, Chen W. Side population in oral squamous cell carcinoma possesses tumor stem cell phenotypes. Cancer Lett 2009;277(2):227–234

1 References with asterisks indicate the most important reference articles on the topic.

9. Bao S, Wu Q, McLendon RE, et al. Glioma stem cells promote radioresistance by preferential activation of the DNA damage response. Nature 2006;444(7120):756–760
10. Pignon JP, Bourhis J, Domenge C, Designé L. Chemotherapy added to locoregional treatment for head and neck squamous-cell carcinoma: three meta-analyses of updated individual data. MACH-NC Collaborative Group. Meta-Analysis of Chemotherapy on Head and Neck Cancer. Lancet 2000;355(9208):949–955
11. Monnerat C, Faivre S, Temam S, Bourhis J, Raymond E. End points for new agents in induction chemotherapy for locally advanced head and neck cancers. Ann Oncol 2002;13(7):995–1006
12. Vermorken JB, Mesia R, Rivera F, et al. Platinum-based chemotherapy plus cetuximab in head and neck cancer. N Engl J Med 2008;359(11):1116–1127
13. Handra-Luca A, Hernandez J, Mountzios G, et al. Excision repair cross complementation group 1 immunohistochemical expression predicts objective response and cancer-specific survival in patients treated by Cisplatin-based induction chemotherapy for locally advanced head and neck squamous cell carcinoma. Clin Cancer Res 2007;13(13):3855–3859
14. Chang X, Monitto CL, Demokan S, et al. Identification of hypermethylated genes associated with cisplatin resistance in human cancers. Cancer Res 2010;70(7):2870–2879
15. Vermorken JB, Remenar E, van Herpen C, et al. EORTC 24971/TAX 323 Study Group. Cisplatin, fluorouracil, and docetaxel in unresectable head and neck cancer. N Engl J Med 2007;357(17):1695–1704
16. Posner MR, Hershock DM, Blajman CR, et al. TAX 324 Study Group. Cisplatin and fluorouracil alone or with docetaxel in head and neck cancer. N Engl J Med 2007;357(17):1705–1715
17. Cullen KJ, Schumaker L, Nikitakis N, et al. beta-Tubulin-II expression strongly predicts outcome in patients receiving induction chemotherapy for locally advanced squamous carcinoma of the head and neck: a companion analysis of the TAX 324 trial. J Clin Oncol 2009;27(36):6222–6228
18. Bonner JA, Harari PM, Giralt J, et al. Radiotherapy plus cetuximab for locoregionally advanced head and neck cancer: 5-year survival data from a phase 3 randomised trial, and relation between cetuximab-induced rash and survival. Lancet Oncol 2010;11(1):21–28
19. Vermorken JB, Mesia R, Rivera F, et al. Platinum-based chemotherapy plus cetuximab in head and neck cancer. N Engl J Med 2008;359(11):1116–1127
20. Chen LF, Cohen EE, Grandis JR. New strategies in head and neck cancer: understanding resistance to epidermal growth factor receptor inhibitors. Clin Cancer Res 2010;16(9):2489–2495
21. Sok JC, Coppelli FM, Thomas SM, et al. Mutant epidermal growth factor receptor (EGFRvIII) contributes to head and neck cancer growth and resistance to EGFR targeting. Clin Cancer Res 2006;12(17):5064–5073
22. Stewart JS, Cohen EE, Licitra L, et al. Phase III study of gefitinib compared with intravenous methotrexate for recurrent squamous cell carcinoma of the head and neck [corrected]. J Clin Oncol 2009;27(11):1864–1871
23. Talmadge JE, Fidler IJ. AACR centennial series: the biology of cancer metastasis: historical perspective. Cancer Res 2010;70(14):5649–5669
24. Gaggioli C, Hooper S, Hidalgo-Carcedo C, et al. Fibroblast-led collective invasion of carcinoma cells with differing roles for RhoGTPases in leading and following cells. Nat Cell Biol 2007;9(12):1392–1400
25. Erler JT, Bennewith KL, Nicolau M, et al. Lysyl oxidase is essential for hypoxia-induced metastasis. Nature 2006;440(7088):1222–1226
26. Le QT, Harris J, Magliocco AM, et al. Validation of lysyl oxidase as a prognostic marker for metastasis and survival in head and neck squamous cell carcinoma: Radiation Therapy Oncology Group trial 90-03. J Clin Oncol 2009;27(26):4281–4286
27. Gerard C, Rollins BJ. Chemokines and disease. Nat Immunol 2001;2(2):108–115
28. Müller A, Homey B, Soto H, et al. Involvement of chemokine receptors in breast cancer metastasis. Nature 2001;410(6824):50–56
29. Pitkin L, Luangdilok S, Corbishley C, et al. Expression of CC chemokine receptor 7 in tonsillar cancer predicts cervical nodal metastasis, systemic relapse and survival. Br J Cancer 2007;97(5):670–677
30. Yeudall WA, Miyazaki H. Chemokines and squamous cancer of the head and neck: targets for therapeutic intervention? Expert Rev Anticancer Ther 2007;7(3):351–360

3 Imaging Modalities for Head and Neck Cancer Recurrence

Oludolapo O. Adesanya

Summary

- Major risk factors for recurrence on imaging include tumor histology, grade, N stage, extracapsular spread, and perineural spread.
- Imaging of tumor recurrence in head and neck cancer requires a multidisciplinary approach and the choice of imaging modality as well as interpretation are influenced by previous disease and the type of treatment.
- A combination of different imaging modalities may be required to adequately image the recurrent tumor and demonstrate various aspects such as skull base invasion and perineural spread.
- Skull base and cranial nerve anatomy are valuable in the interpretation of perineural involvement.

Most head and neck cancer recurrences occur within 2 years of therapy.[1] Recurrence rates vary and depend on several factors including tumor histology, grade, and stage. For the most part, the nodal stage determines prognosis and disease outcome.[2] Other risk factors for recurrence include extracapsular spread and perineural spread, both of which may be detected on staging scans.[3]

Tumor recurrence in the head and neck region can be illustrated optimally by a combination of different imaging methods. Both the primary and nodal masses may recur. Furthermore, some of the main modes of spread may be demonstrated on imaging, including local invasion by perineural spread, direct skull base invasion, extracapsular spread, lymphatic spread, and hematogenous as well as in-transit metastasis.[4] As a result, recurrence may be demonstrated on imaging locally at the primary site, in transit, or in local draining or distant nodes, as well as in the form of distant metastases.

Therapy-related Changes in the Head and Neck Region

Imaging modalities commonly used to detect recurrence in the head and neck include plain radiography, ultrasound, magnetic resonance imaging (MRI), computed tomography (CT), fluoroscopy, and functional imaging. Determination of the best modality for detection of a particular suspected recurrence and the successful imaging interpretation of the posttherapy neck is by and large reliant on constructive exchange of information between clinicians and radiologists.[5] Information such as dates of surgery, chemoradiotherapy, and biopsies should be considered. Attention should also be paid to surgical techniques such as the type of flap as well as its expected appearance.[6] The radiologist should be able

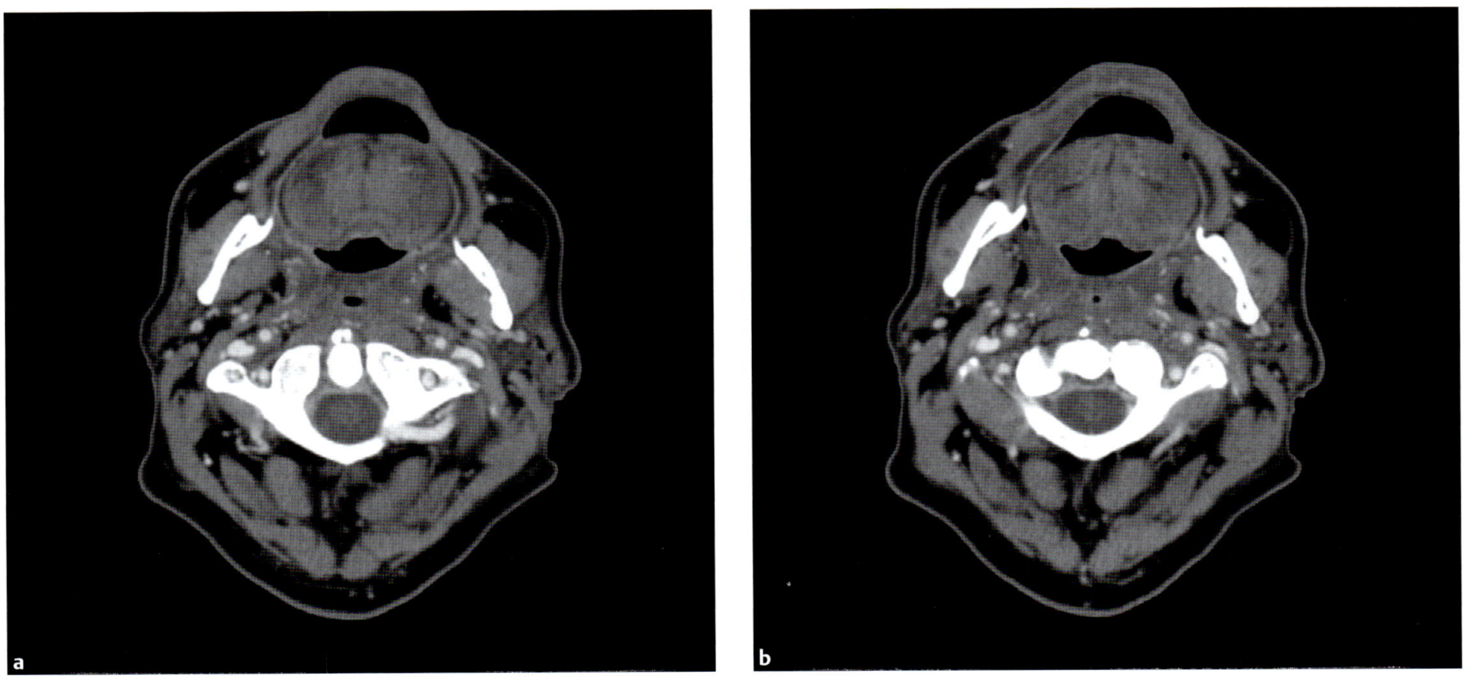

Fig. 3.1a, b Axial CT demonstrates left-sided facial swelling due to the presence of air in the left parotid duct (pneumoparotitis), following chemoradiotherapy for squamous cell carcinoma of the tongue base.

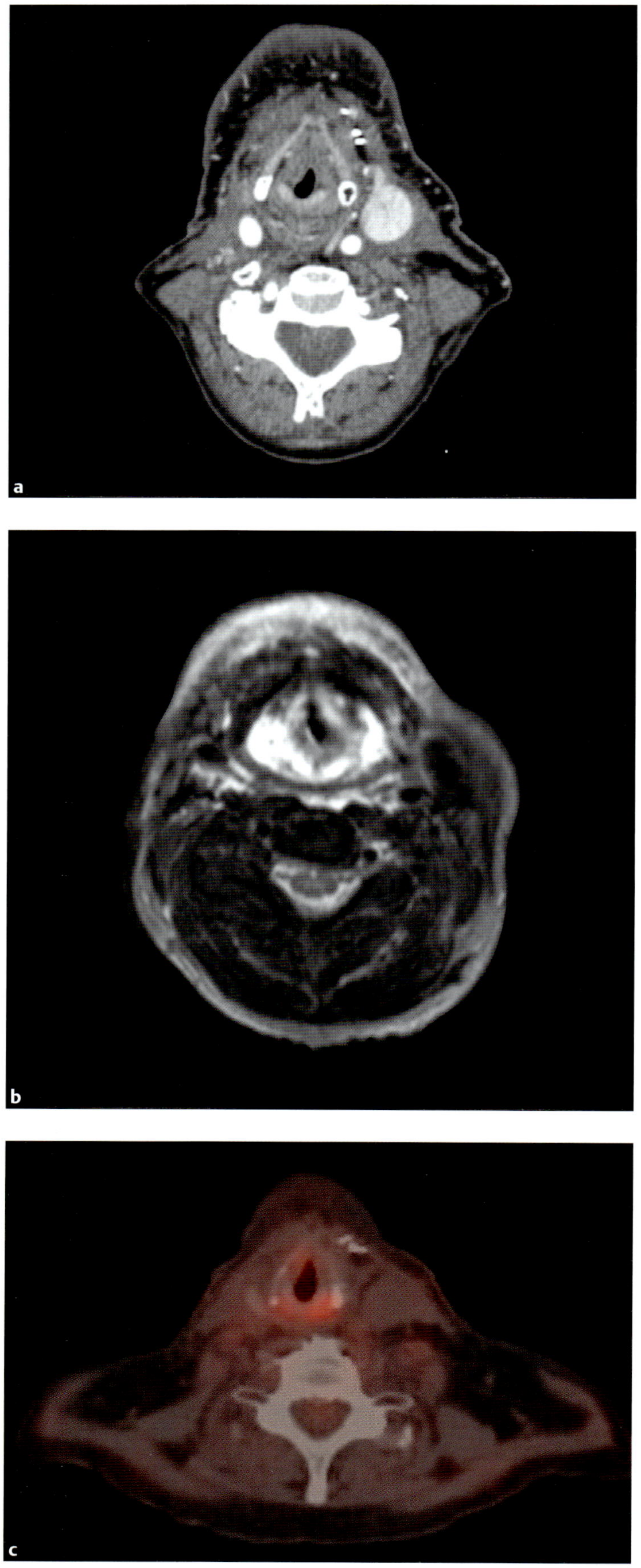

Fig. 3.2a–c A 69-year-old woman with acute swelling of the face and neck during postsurgical radiotherapy for squamous cell carcinoma of the anterior floor of the mouth. The images demonstrate postradiotherapy edematous mucosal swelling with increased enhancement and associated low-level increased metabolic activity due to postradiotherapy soft tissue inflammation/mucositis.
a Axial CT.
b Axial T2-weighted MRI.
c Axial FDG PET-CT.

to decide which imaging modality to utilize after consideration of these facts.

Imaging characteristics of treatment-related features result from surgery, radiotherapy, or chemoradiotherapy and include soft tissue–related and bony manifestations. These can mimic malignant recurrence. Distinguishing tumor recurrence from treatment-related features requires knowledge of the treatment type and time span as well as an understanding of the possible appearances of treatment-related changes.

■ Radiation-induced Changes in the Neck

The damage induced by radiation is related to radiation dose, fraction size, volume of irradiated tissue, fractionation scheme, and the type of ionizing irradiation.[7]

Soft tissue swelling develops as a result of acute inflammation within a fortnight of radiotherapy and later gives way to fibrosis. All fascial compartments may be affected, resulting in thickening of the dermis and platysma, reticulation of subcutaneous and deep compartments of fat due to generalized edema, and increased enhancement of mucosal regions and the salivary glands (**Figs. 3.1 and 3.2**). These changes are clearly demonstrated on both CT and MRI, and can persist for up to 12–18 months after treatment.[8,9]

In comparison to soft tissue change, bony change is a much slower process. These changes include marrow fatty change, paranasal sinus inflammation, and osteoradionecrosis (**Fig. 3.3**).[9] Radiation injury induces vascular injury. It also affects osteocytes, osteoblasts, and osteoclasts; osteoblasts are more radiosensitive, leading to imbalance in bone turnover and increased bone lysis.[7] Thus, an initial state of hyperemia is followed by endarteritis, thrombosis, and vascular occlusion. Resultant reduction in cellularity and vascularity leads to fibrosis and fatty degeneration.[7] Endosteal and periosteal atrophy ensues with loss of osteoblasts and osteoclasts.[7]

Osteoradionecrosis (ORN) (**Fig. 3.4**) is defined as bone death secondary to radiotherapy.[7] It affects the mandible more often than any other bone in the head and neck region, with a peak incidence at 6–12 months following irradiation.[8,10] Its incidence in other bones, such as the cervical spine and skull, is much lower.[11] ORN incidence is lowest in the maxilla and hyoid.[7,12] The most common risk factors for ORN comprise inclusion of the mandible in the radiation field, use of over 60 Gy of radiation, dental extractions after radiotherapy, and alcohol and tobacco abuse.[13] The addition of chemotherapy to treatment regimens does not necessarily increase the incidence of osteoradionecrosis. On the other hand, steroids may be protective in the initial inflammatory phase. Other preventive measures include prophylactic dental extraction of carious or periodontal compromised dentition prior to radiotherapy.[13] Bisphosphonates are a recognized cause of jaw osteonecrosis that can mimic ORN.[14] Imaging features of ORN include bony fragmentation and focal lysis on CT, as well as abnormal marrow signal and cortical destruction on MRI. Other features on CT include bony fragmentation, cortical disruption, and intraosseous air adjacent to soft tissue ulceration.[7,9,12] ORN can often mimic tumor recurrence. However, the absence of soft tissue enhancement on CT and MRI, as well as the absence of avid soft tissue on FDG PET-CT suggest that ORN is more likely than tumor recurrence.[12] Radiation induces generalized increased uptake on FDG PET-CT. These changes persist for up to 3 months and

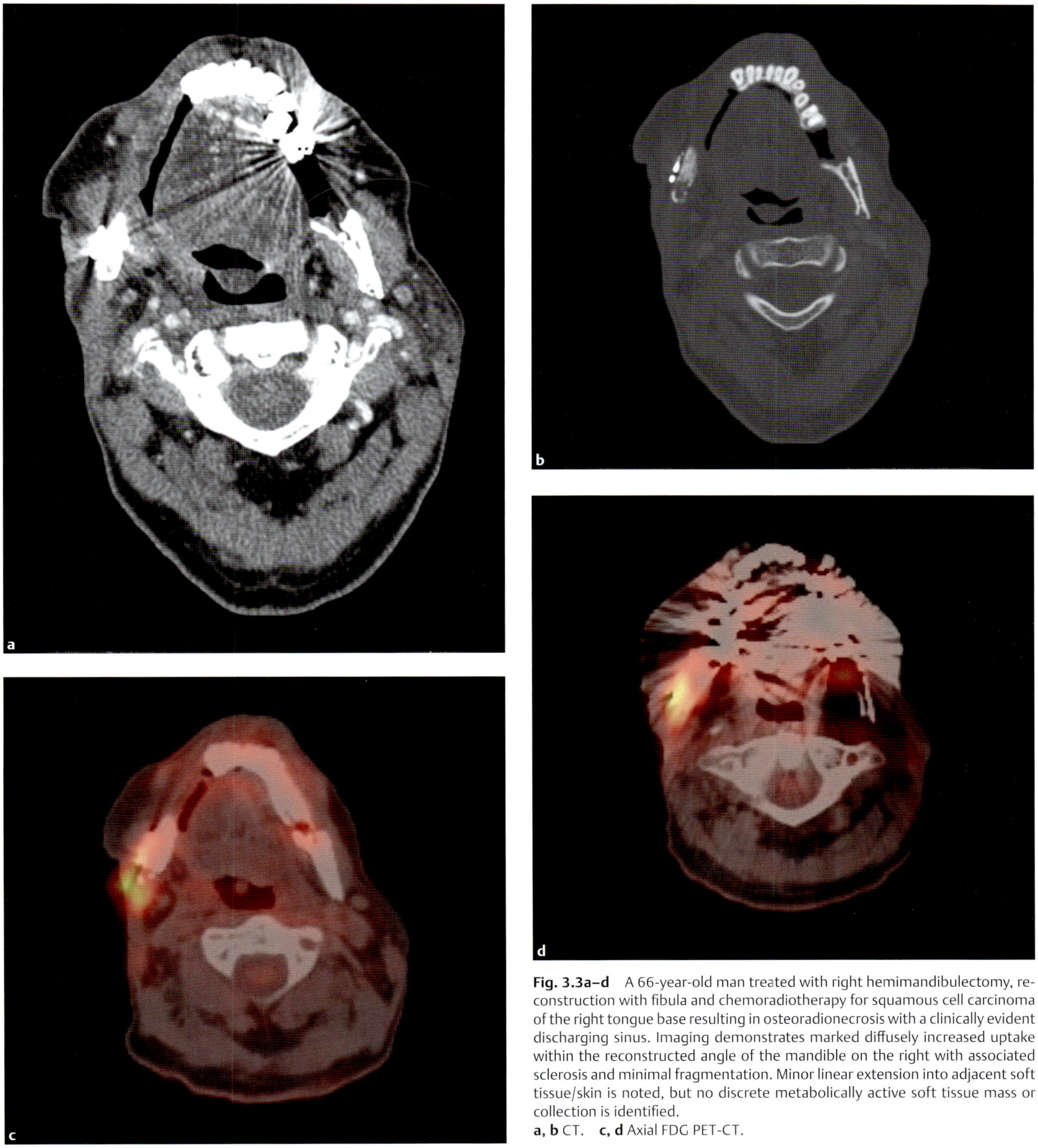

Fig. 3.3a–d A 66-year-old man treated with right hemimandibulectomy, reconstruction with fibula and chemoradiotherapy for squamous cell carcinoma of the right tongue base resulting in osteoradionecrosis with a clinically evident discharging sinus. Imaging demonstrates marked diffusely increased uptake within the reconstructed angle of the mandible on the right with associated sclerosis and minimal fragmentation. Minor linear extension into adjacent soft tissue/skin is noted, but no discrete metabolically active soft tissue mass or collection is identified.
a, b CT. **c, d** Axial FDG PET-CT.

therefore the optimal time to image is about the 3rd or 4th month after radiotherapy.[15] FDG PET-CT features are also nonspecific and may also mimic recurrent malignancy due to increased metabolic activity in the affected areas.

Cartilage lacks blood vessels, which makes it less vulnerable to the effects of radiotherapy. However, tumor or trauma may damage the perichondrium, resulting in exposure to laryngeal bacteria, with resultant perichondritis[16] and chondroradionecrosis. Chondroradionecrosis (**Fig. 3.5**) affects the larynx and peaks around 12 months after radiotherapy.[8,16] Radiological features are nonspecific and include the presence of gas bubbles, cartilage fragmentation, and sclerosis.

Radiotherapy fields commonly include the salivary glands, resulting in a reduction in salivary flow, xerostomia, fall in pH, and increased occurrences of parotitis.[17,18] This can often be seen on imaging (**Figs. 3.6 and 3.7**).

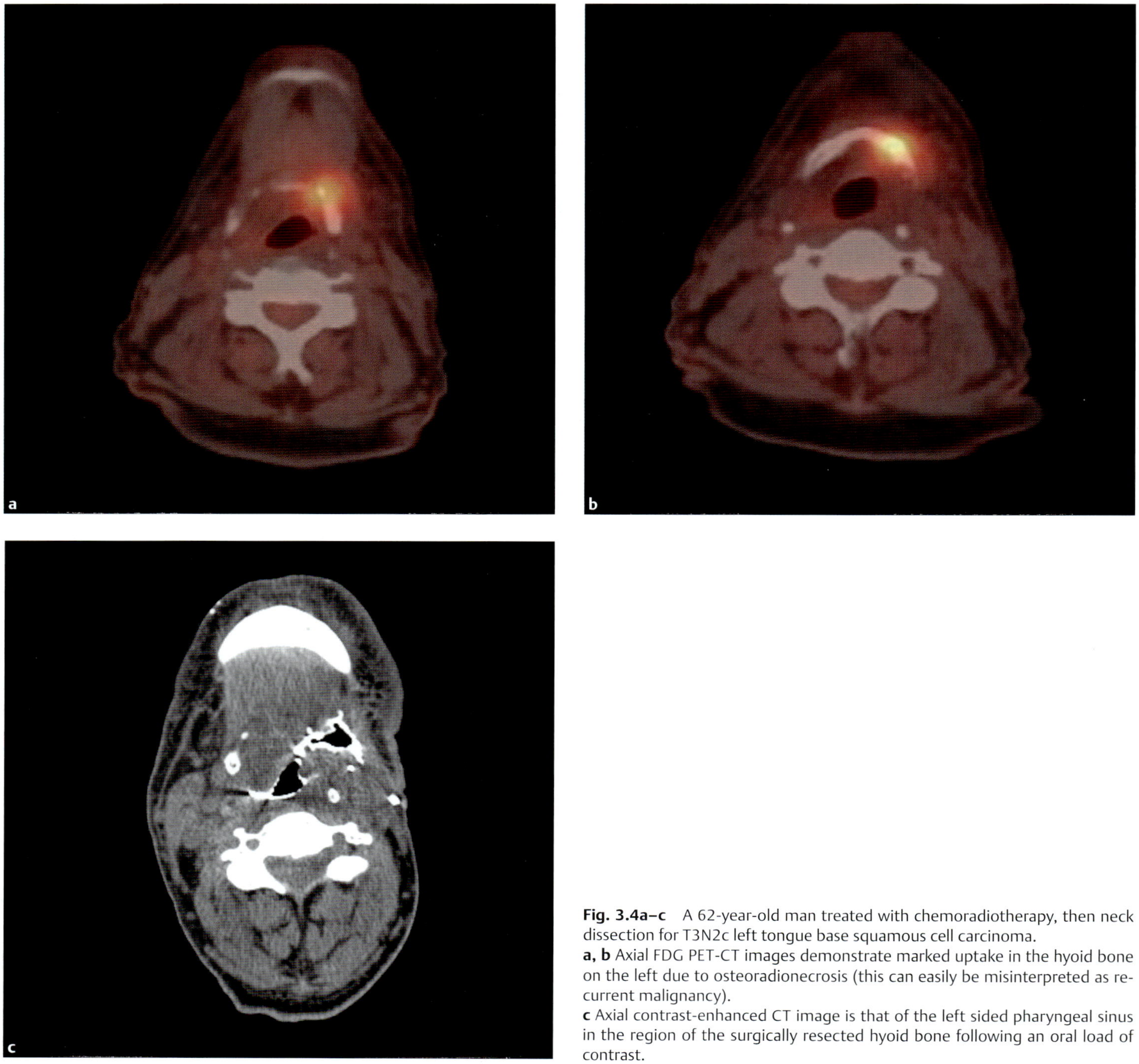

Fig. 3.4a–c A 62-year-old man treated with chemoradiotherapy, then neck dissection for T3N2c left tongue base squamous cell carcinoma.
a, b Axial FDG PET-CT images demonstrate marked uptake in the hyoid bone on the left due to osteoradionecrosis (this can easily be misinterpreted as recurrent malignancy).
c Axial contrast-enhanced CT image is that of the left sided pharyngeal sinus in the region of the surgically resected hyoid bone following an oral load of contrast.

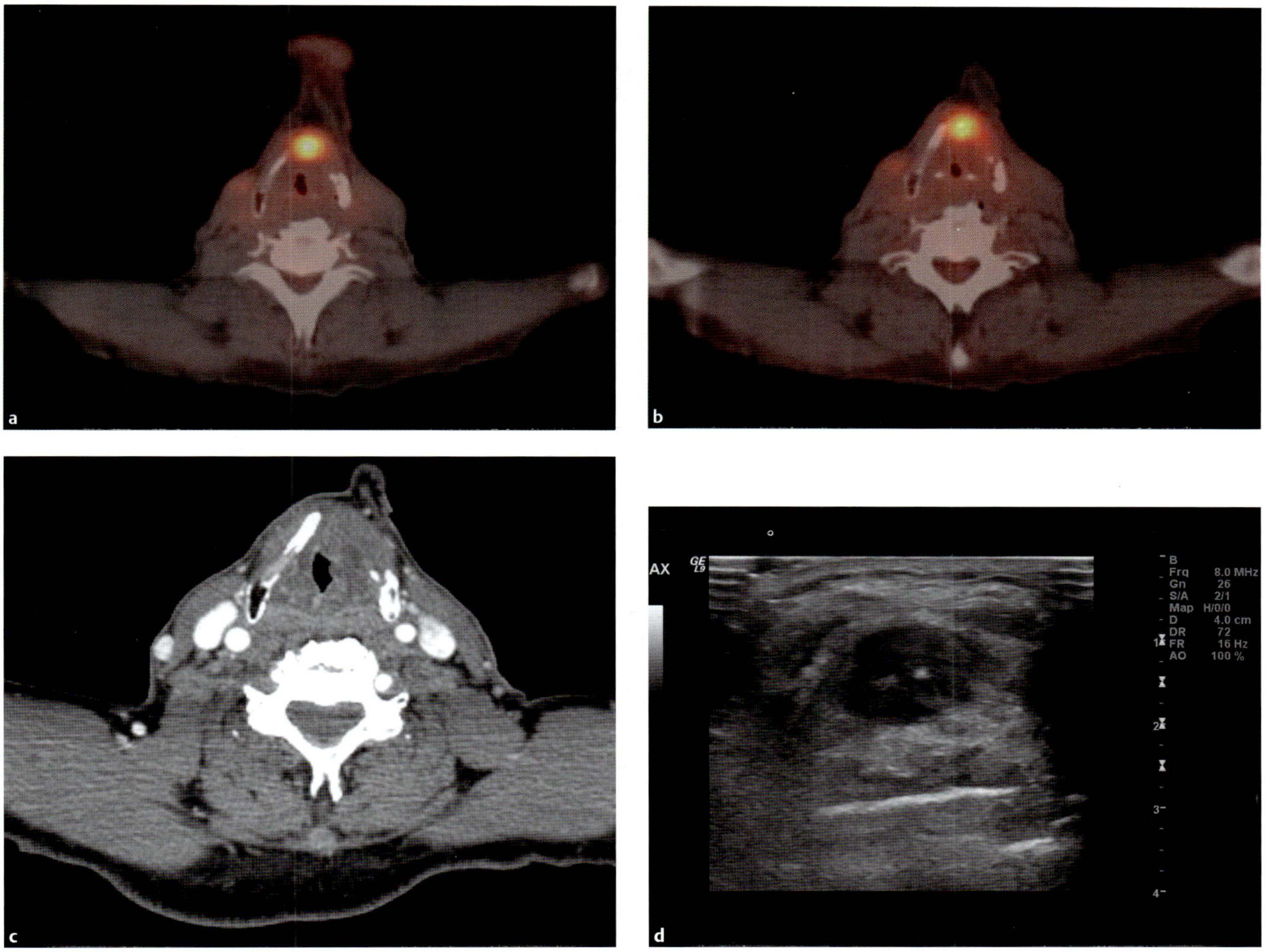

Fig. 3.5a–d A patient with chondroradionecrosis of the larynx. The patient was treated 3 years previously for carcinoma of the larynx with radiotherapy only. Subsequently, an ultrasound-guided aspiration yielded pus and neither cytology nor histology showed any evidence of malignancy. He subsequently improved with conservative treatment.

a, b Axial FDG PET-CT demonstrates marked focal uptake in the thyroid cartilage.

c Axial CT demonstrates corresponding ring enhancement and thickening in the anterior larynx anteriorly.

d Parasagittal ultrasound shows a thick-walled collection in the anterior larynx.

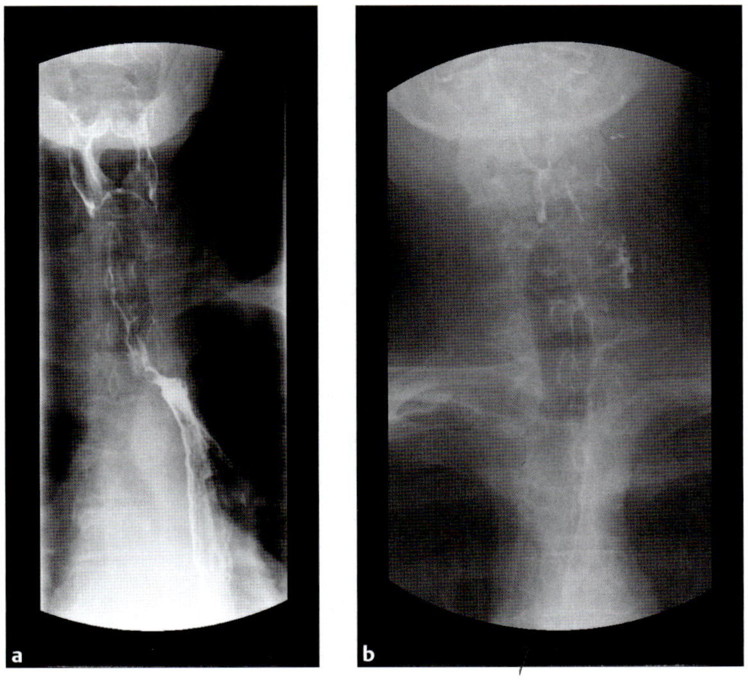

Fig. 3.6a, b Esophageal strictures.

a AP contrast swallow image of an irregular malignant proximal esophageal stricture.

b AP water soluble contrast swallow image of a postradiotherapy proximal esophageal smooth benign stricture (subtle) as well as left sided pharyngeal contrast leakage.

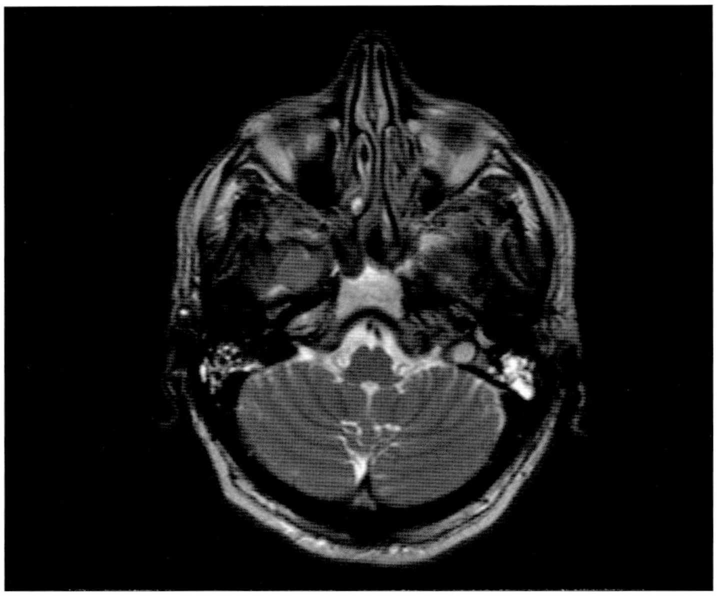

Fig. 3.7 A 60-year-old man treated with chemoradiotherapy for tongue base carcinoma, presenting soon afterward with left hearing loss. Clinically, the postnasal space was very inflamed. Axial T2-weighted MR image through the mastoid region shows bilateral secretory otitis media (slightly worse on the left), secondary to recent radiotherapy.

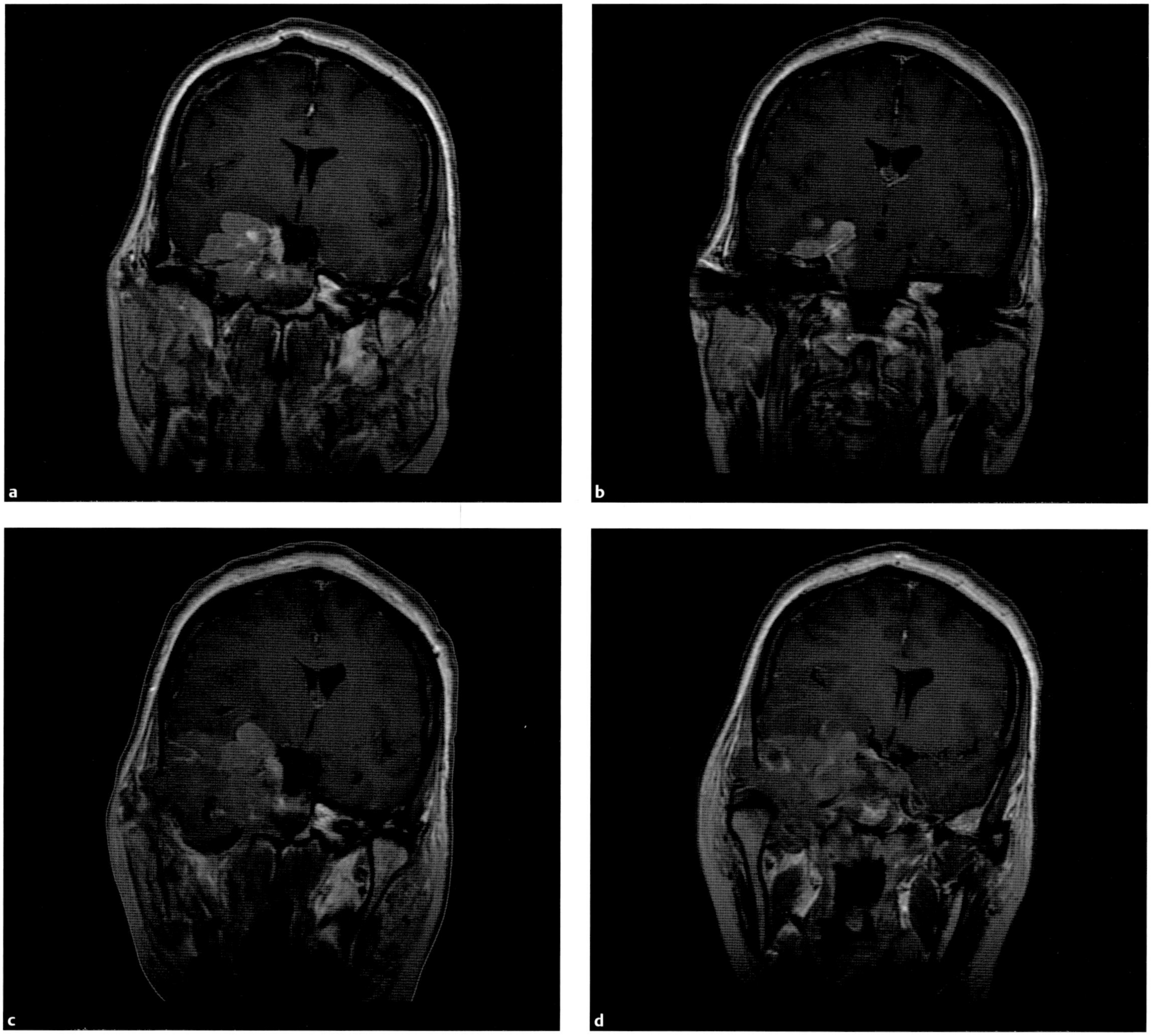

Fig. 3.8a–d A woman with right temporal and sphenoid meningioma. **a, b** Coronal T1-weighted MRI, postcontrast images. **c, d** Coronal T1-weighted MRI, postcontrast images 6 months later after transformation into malignant meningioma following radiotherapy.

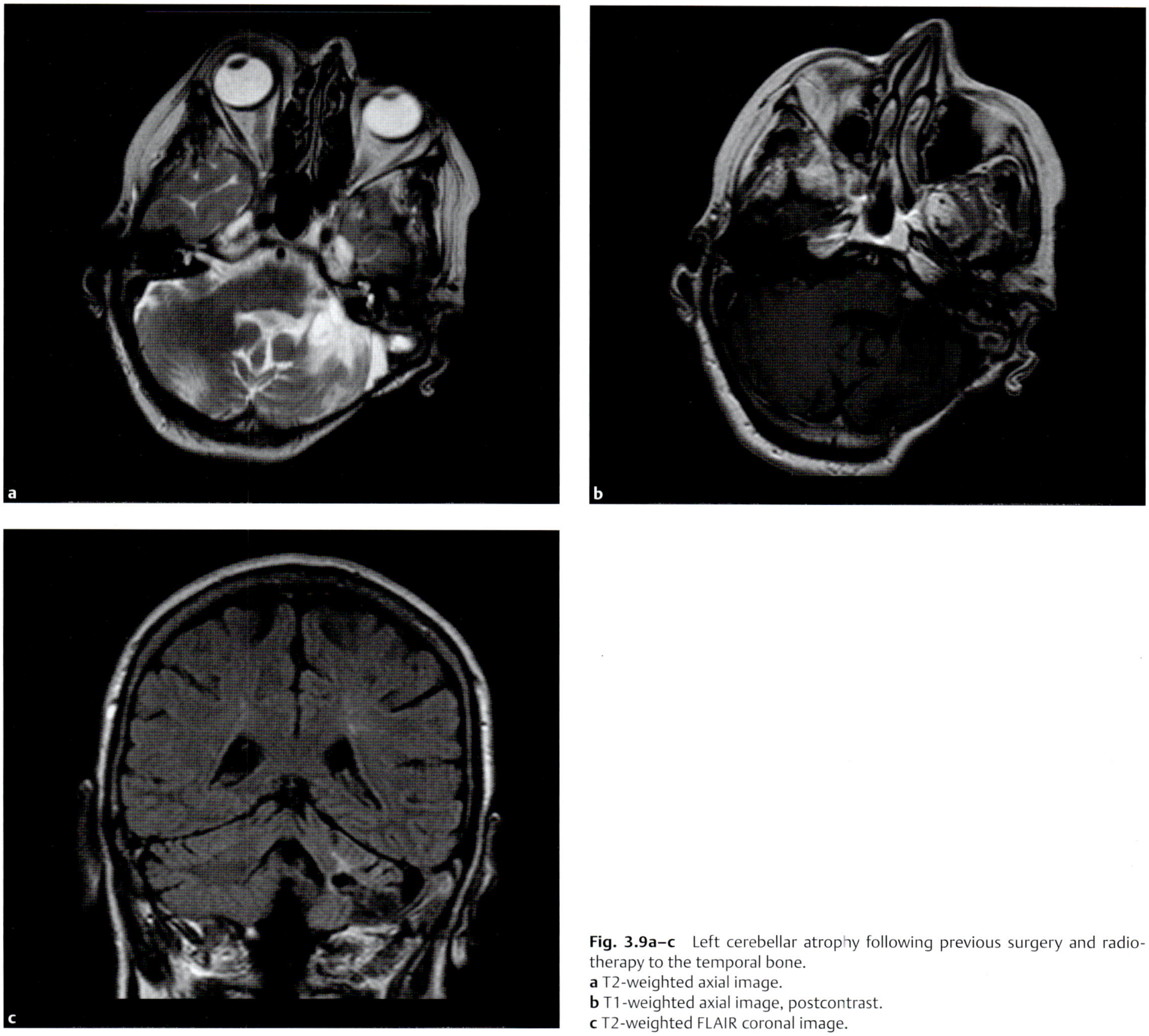

Fig. 3.9a–c Left cerebellar atrophy following previous surgery and radiotherapy to the temporal bone.
a T2-weighted axial image.
b T1-weighted axial image, postcontrast.
c T2-weighted FLAIR coronal image.

Radiation may also induce tumors. In the skull base region, meningioma is the most common radiation-induced central nervous system tumor (**Figs. 3.8 and 3.9**).[9]

Postchemotherapy Change

Cancer chemotherapy agents continue to evolve and increase in number. Mucositis is a cytotoxic side effect of chemotherapy and/or radiotherapy that may affect any part of the gut.[19] Oral mucositis results in erythema, edema, atrophy, and ulceration of the oral mucosa, which can be disabling and which may result in reduced oral intake and even cessation of therapy (**Figs. 3.10 and 3.11**). Several techniques for reducing ORN have been tried, with varying success.[20] Marked thickening and increased enhancement in affected mucosal areas can be seen on postcontrast MRI in mucositis. Other changes include mucosal atrophy and ulceration.[21] FDG PET-CT changes include false-positive uptake of low to moderate levels, of uptake as well as mucosal thickening.[22]

There is a well-established direct relationship between chemotherapy and downregulation of hexokinase II mRNA and hexokinase protein receptor as an immediate consequence.[23] Theoretically these result in false-negative results on PET-CT, due to reduced accumulation of FDG in tumors, known as PET-CT stunning. It is therefore common practice to allow an interval of a few weeks following chemotherapy before arranging a PET-CT scan.[24]

Postsurgical Change

Excision biopsies, resections, neck dissection, and flap reconstruction result in neck asymmetry and complicated imaging features. Changes associated with neck dissection depend on the extent of neck dissection performed (radical neck dissection, modified radical neck dissection, selective neck dissection, extended neck dissection) as well as the side and level involved. In the immediate postsurgical period, edema, fluid collections, and hematoma can mimic residual tumor.

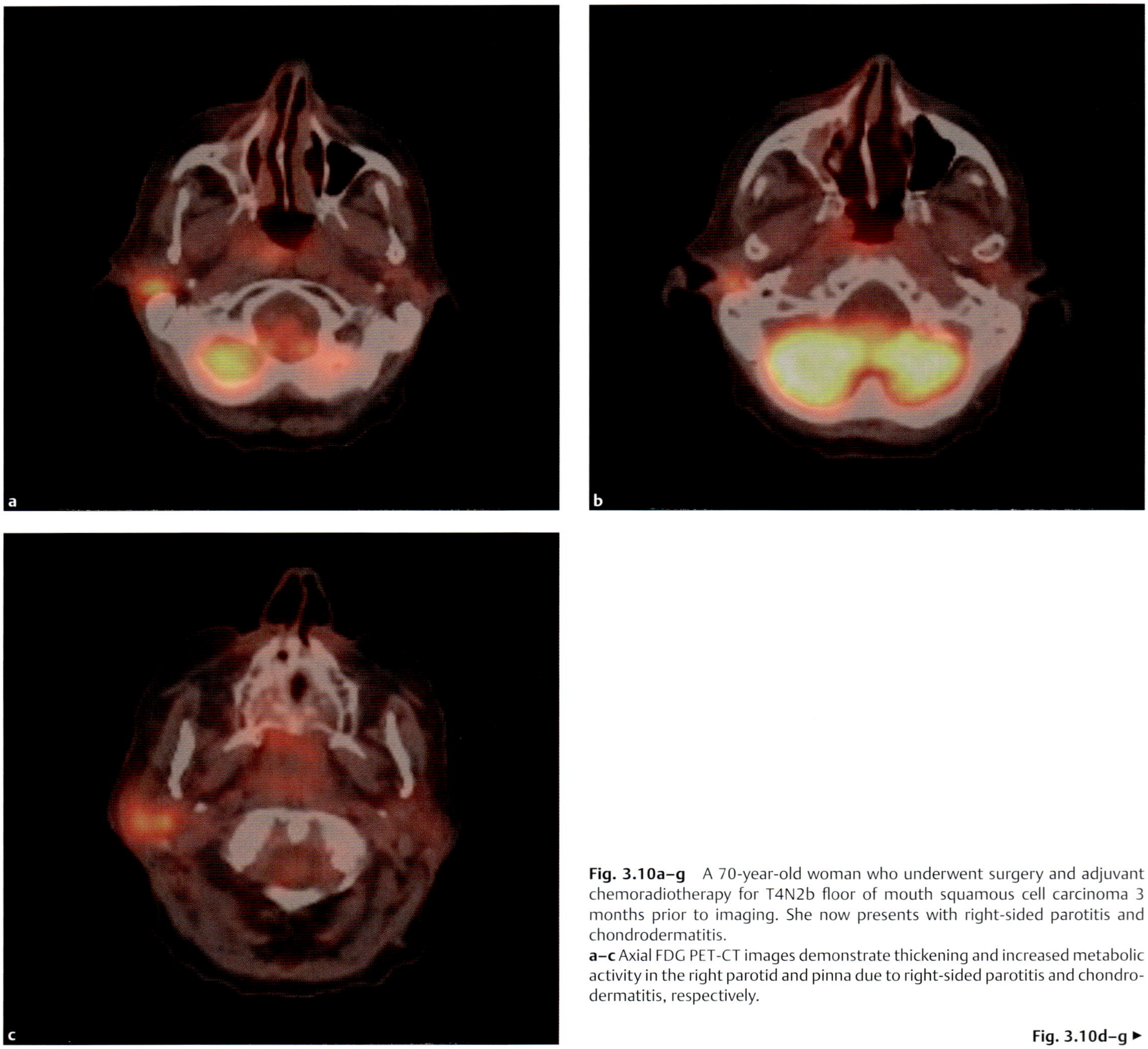

Fig. 3.10a–g A 70-year-old woman who underwent surgery and adjuvant chemoradiotherapy for T4N2b floor of mouth squamous cell carcinoma 3 months prior to imaging. She now presents with right-sided parotitis and chondrodermatitis.
a–c Axial FDG PET-CT images demonstrate thickening and increased metabolic activity in the right parotid and pinna due to right-sided parotitis and chondrodermatitis, respectively.

Fig. 3.10d–g ▸

The process of harvesting and transferring fasciocutaneous flaps results in disruption of muscle nerve supply, which leads to muscle atrophy and fatty change evident on both CT and MRI scans. Flaps demonstrate a variety of differing T2-weighted signal characteristics and contrast enhancement. This considerably limits their use in the detection of tumor recurrence or nonviable free flaps. The use of fat-saturation MRI sequences and attention to CT density may be useful in this situation.[8,25] Local recurrence at the vascular pedicle is a recognized feature that may occur along lymphatic and hematogenous channels of transposed myocutaneous flaps (**Fig. 3.12**).[26]

Late changes after exposure to heat from laser therapy may result in sclerosis of arytenoid and cricoid cartilages in a similar manner to sclerosis secondary to malignancy and must not be confused with malignancy (**Fig. 3.13**).[8] Other late changes after surgery include atrophy secondary to nerve sacrifice, such as of the spinal accessory nerve, which may result in atrophy of the ipsilateral trapezius and compensatory hypertrophy of ipsilateral levator scapulae muscle (**Figs. 3.13–3.21**).[8]

Iatrogenic injury induced by endotracheal tubes and by tracheostomy affects the stomal, subglottic, and glottic regions resulting in fibrotic scar tissue and stenosis (**Fig. 3.22**).[27] Vocal cord paralysis is a known complication of neck and cardiac surgery.[28] However, other mediastinal causes must be excluded with cross-sectional imaging (**Figs. 3.23 and 3.24**).

Finally, clinical monitoring plays a key role in the assessment of flap viability.[8] However, osseous flap viability can be monitored in the first week after surgery with radionuclide bone scans with a high degree of accuracy that outperforms clinical methods of monitoring, particularly when SPECT is employed (**Fig. 3.25**).[29,30]

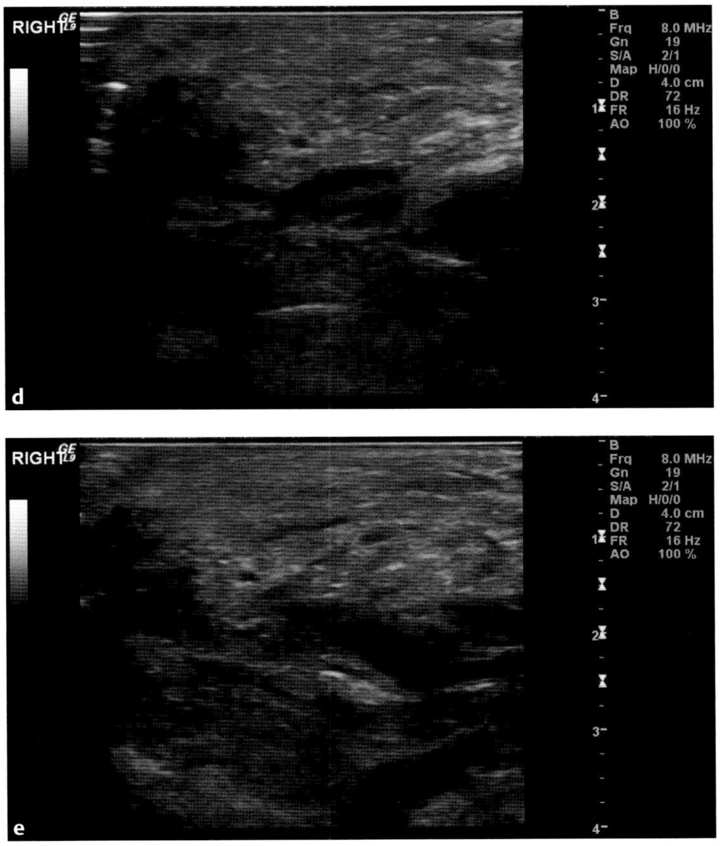

Fig. 3.10d–g
d, e Ultrasound images show corresponding subcutaneous thickening in the right pinna.
f, g T1-weighted, postcontrast MRI: thickening and increased enhancement and thickening in the right parotid and pinna due to right-sided parotitis and chondrodermatitis, respectively.

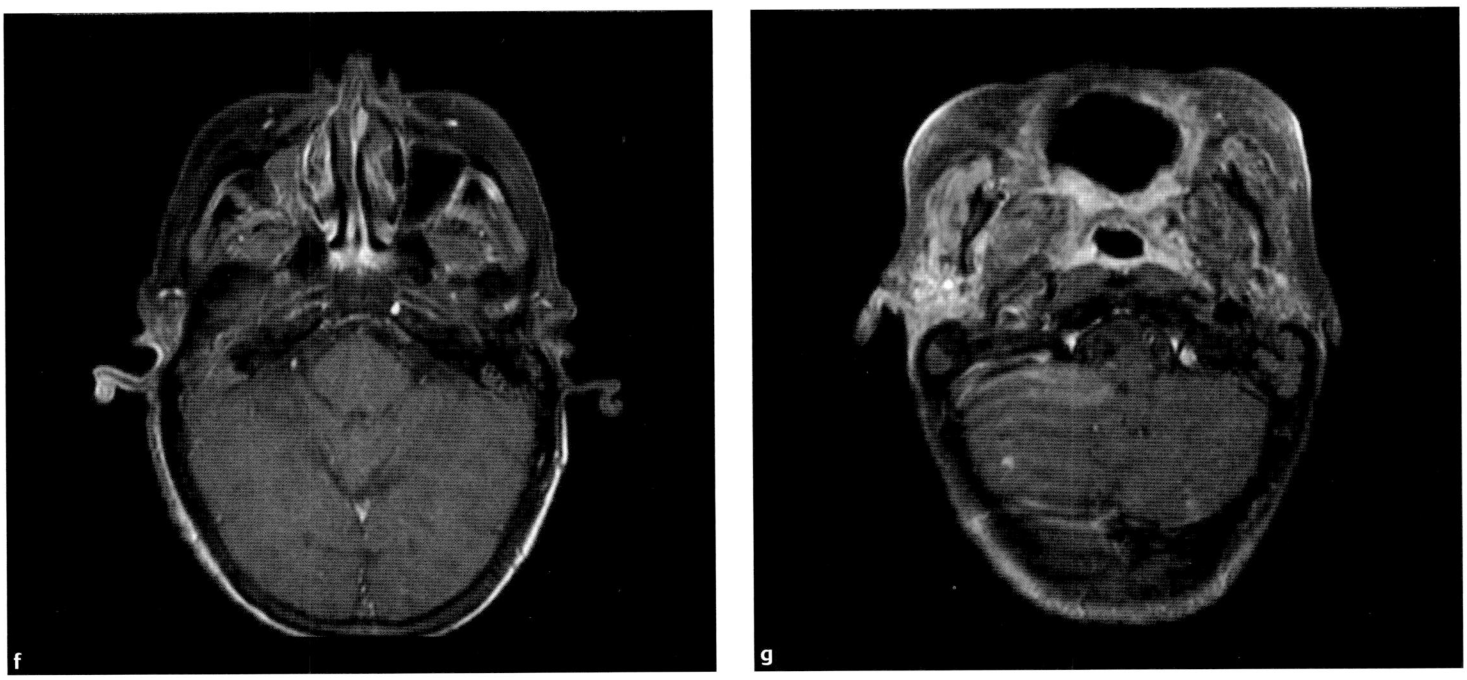

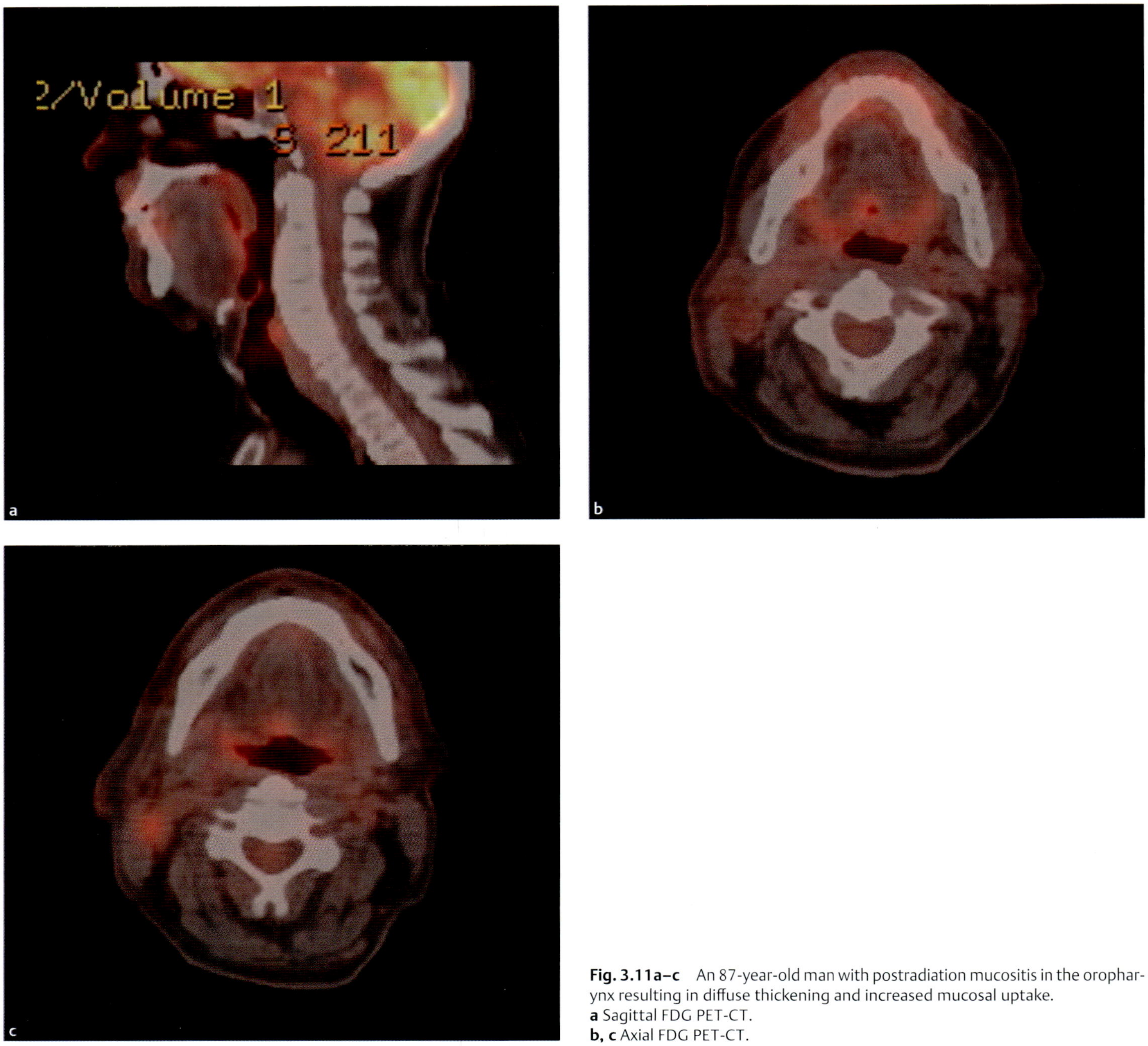

Fig. 3.11a–c An 87-year-old man with postradiation mucositis in the oropharynx resulting in diffuse thickening and increased mucosal uptake.
a Sagittal FDG PET-CT.
b, c Axial FDG PET-CT.

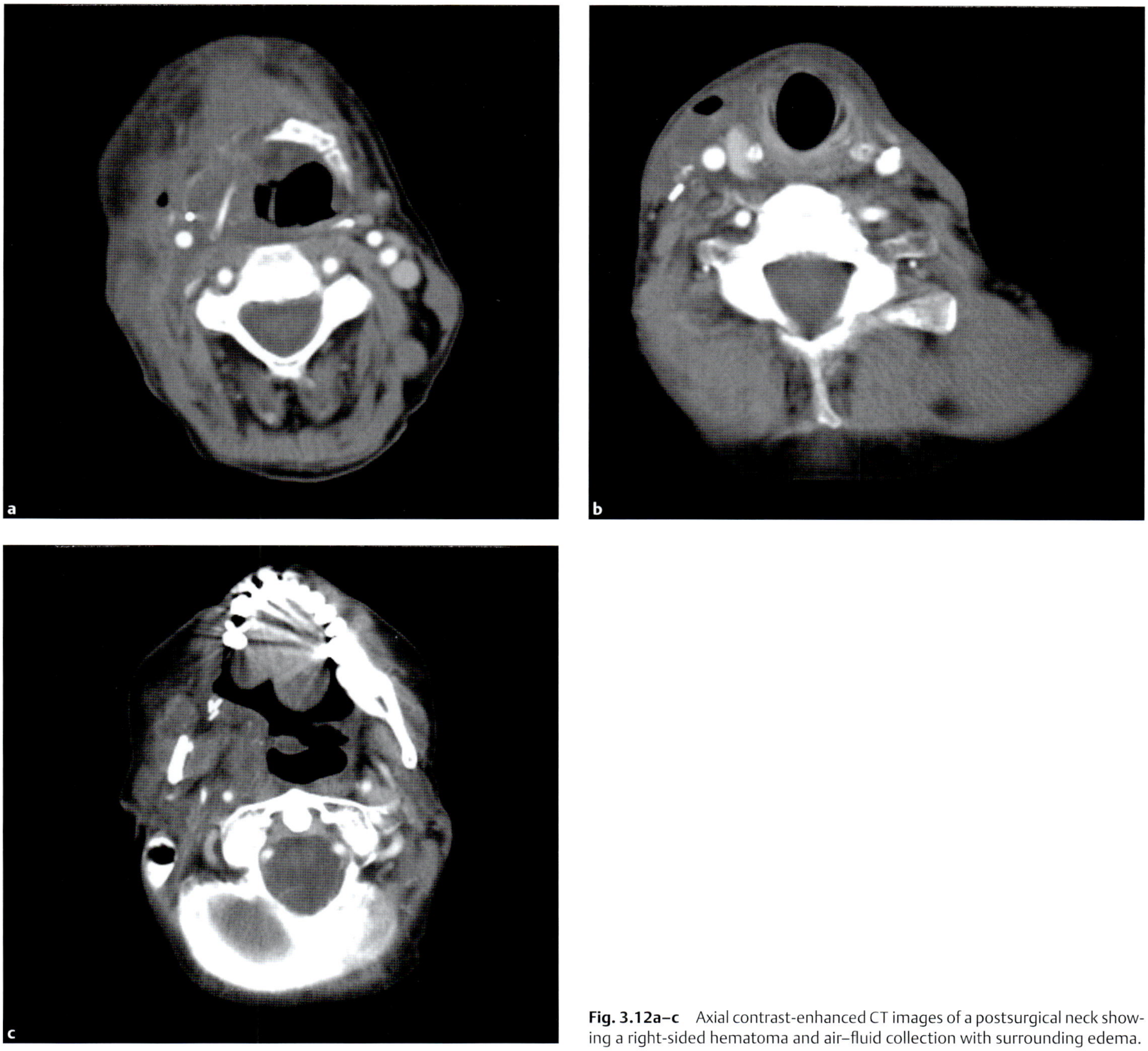

Fig. 3.12a–c Axial contrast-enhanced CT images of a postsurgical neck showing a right-sided hematoma and air–fluid collection with surrounding edema.

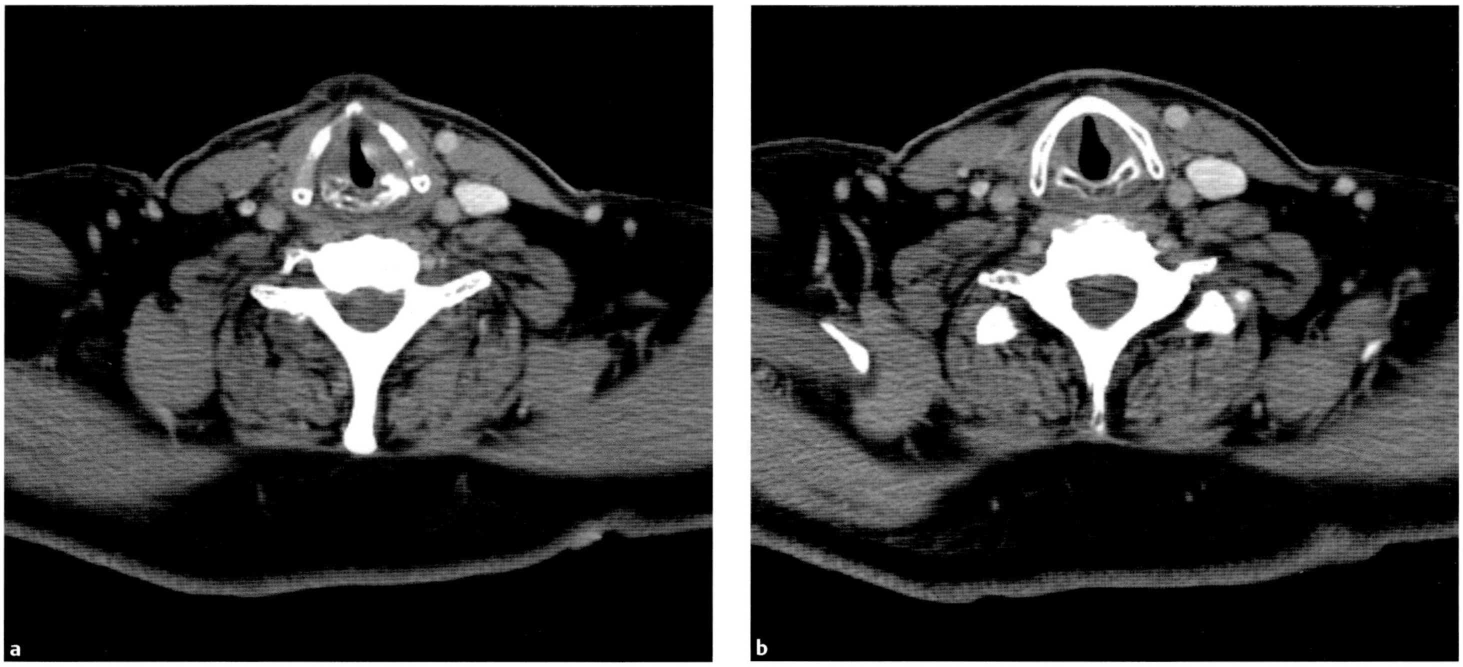

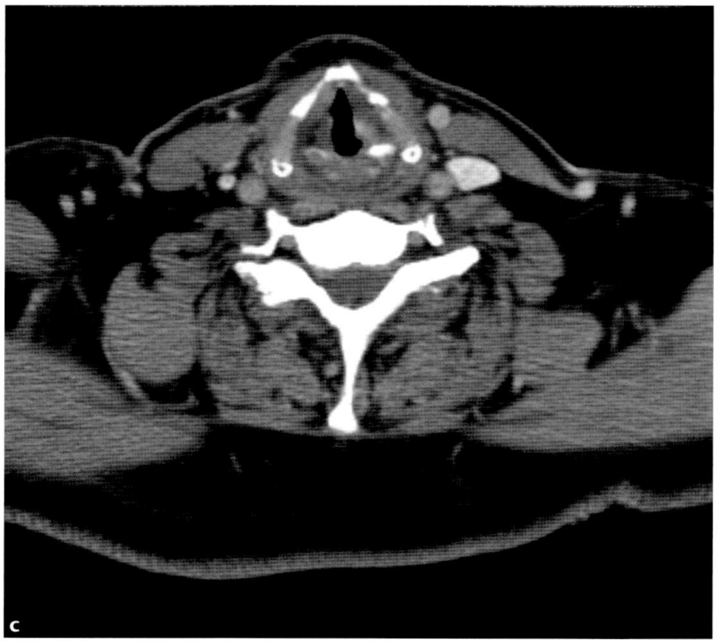

Fig. 3.13a–c Axial contrast-enhanced CT images of a 62-year-old man 2 weeks after laser polypectomy on the left vocal cord. Note the asymmetry and thickening of the true cord as well as sclerosis of the left arytenoid cartilage.

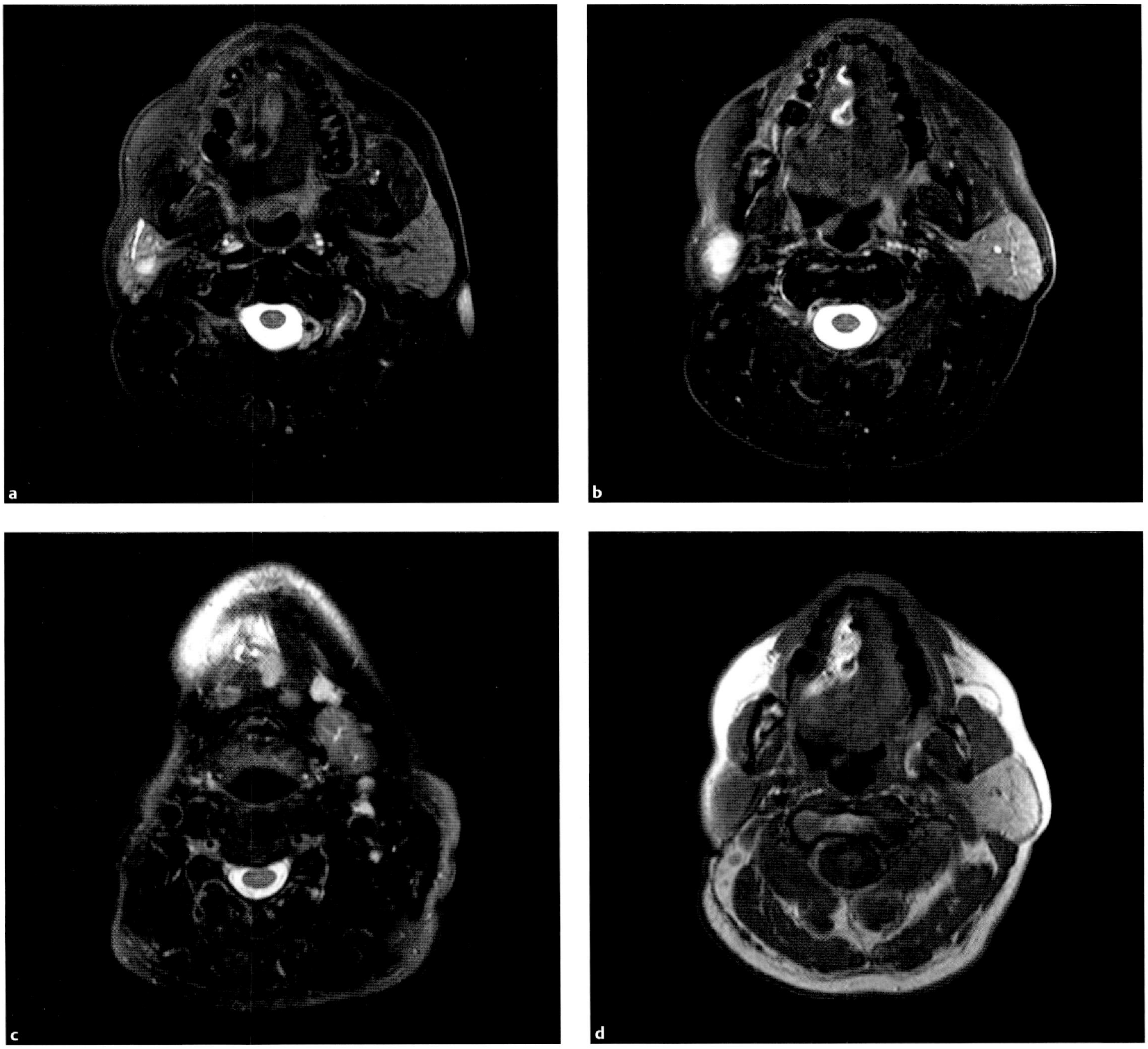

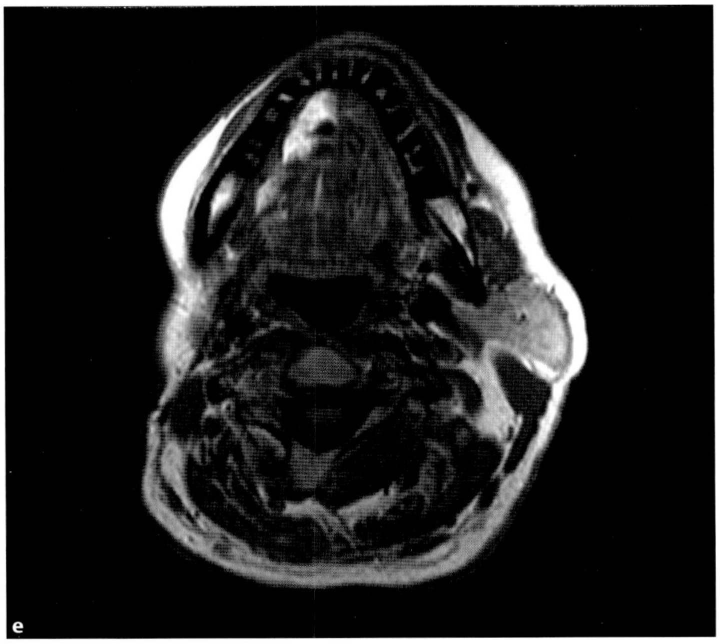

Fig. 3.14a–e Axial MR images in a 49-year-old man with previous squamous cell carcinoma of the right tongue, treated with flap, neck dissection, and post-operative radiotherapy about 20 years previously. Images demonstrate right tongue resection, right-sided flap with fatty signal, and right neck dissection. Small to slightly enlarged level I nodes can be seen. Note right parotid atrophy.
a–c Axial T2-weighted, fat-suppressed images.
d, e Axial T1-weighted images.

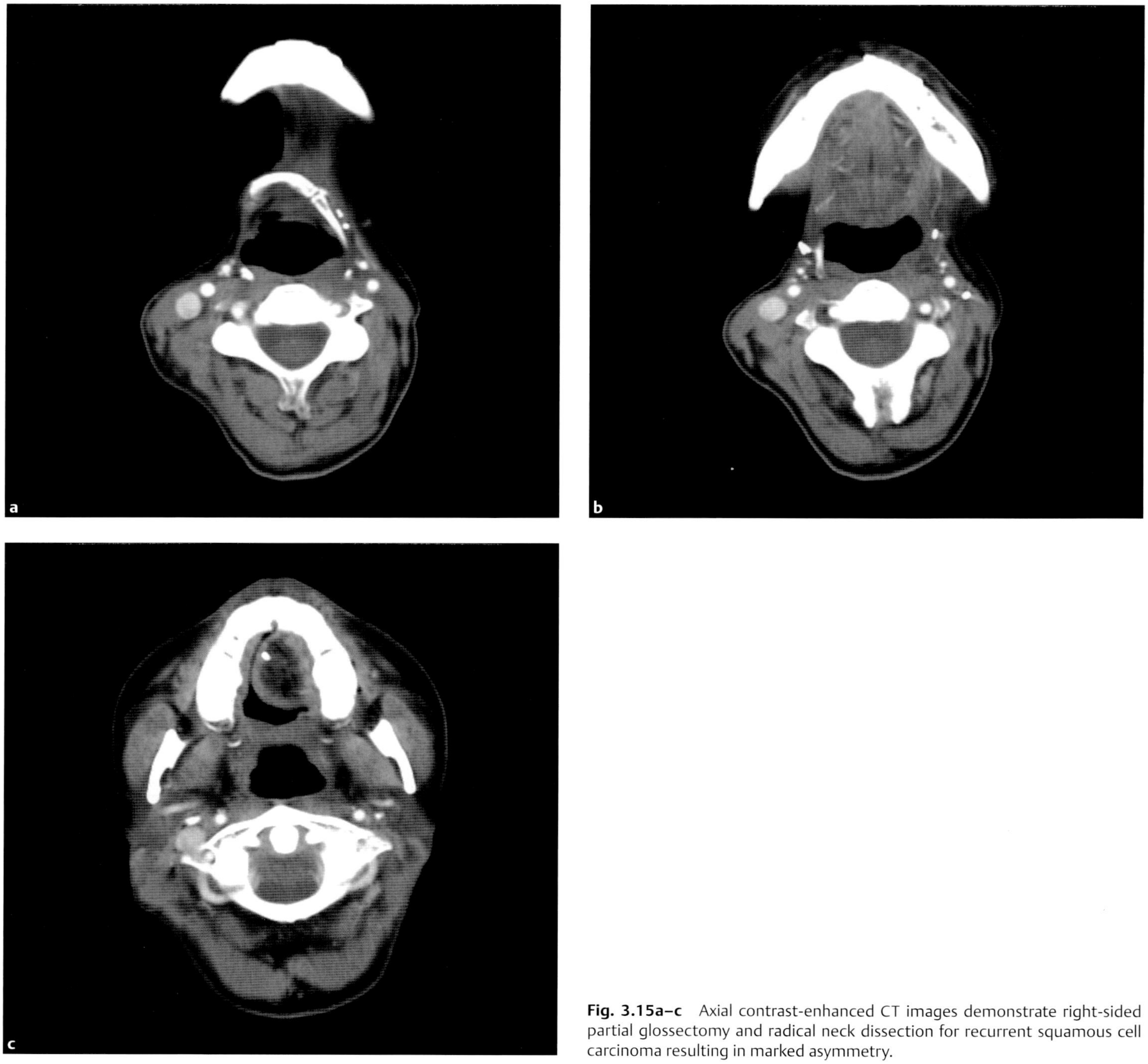

Fig. 3.15a–c Axial contrast-enhanced CT images demonstrate right-sided partial glossectomy and radical neck dissection for recurrent squamous cell carcinoma resulting in marked asymmetry.

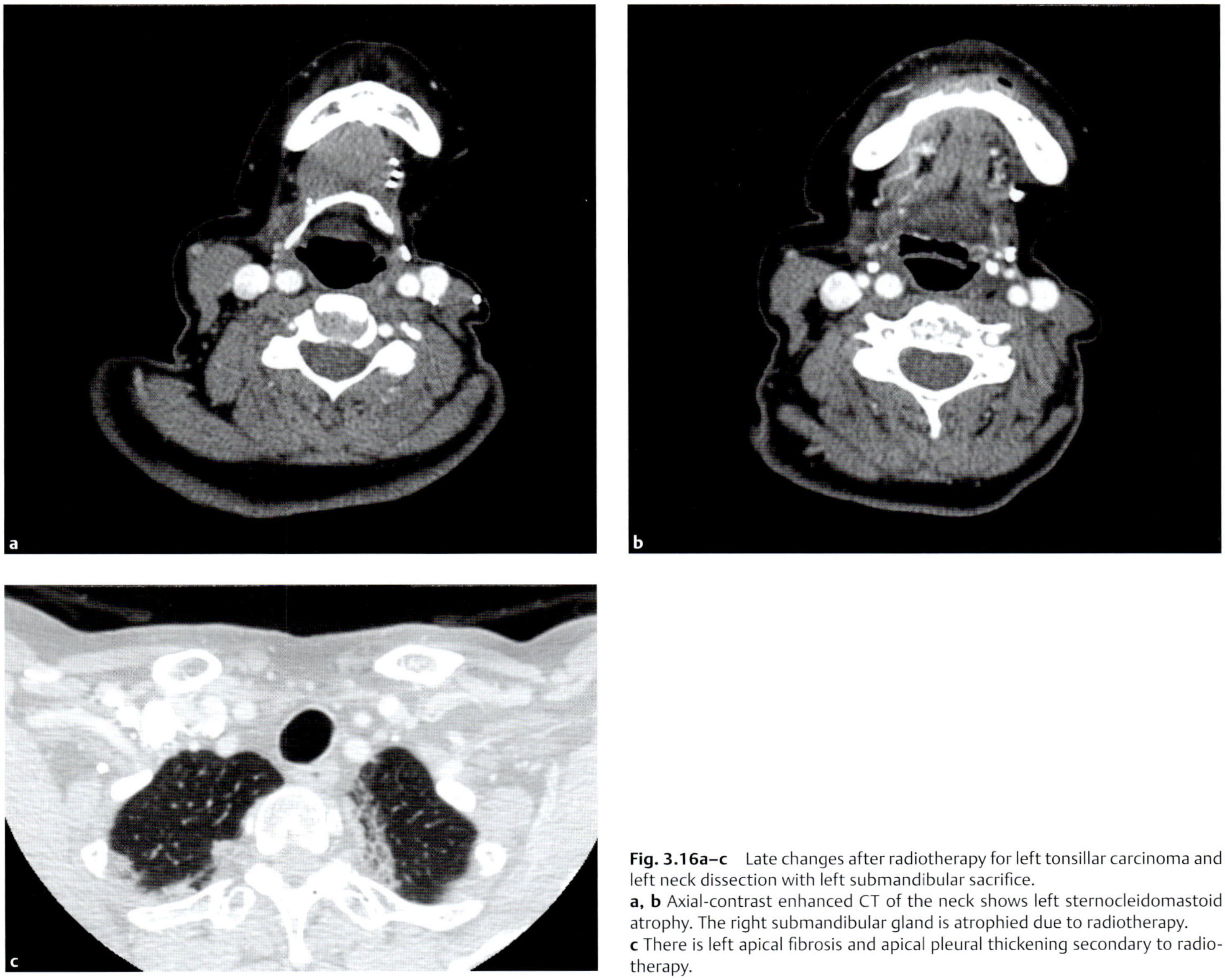

Fig. 3.16a–c Late changes after radiotherapy for left tonsillar carcinoma and left neck dissection with left submandibular sacrifice.
a, b Axial-contrast enhanced CT of the neck shows left sternocleidomastoid atrophy. The right submandibular gland is atrophied due to radiotherapy.
c There is left apical fibrosis and apical pleural thickening secondary to radiotherapy.

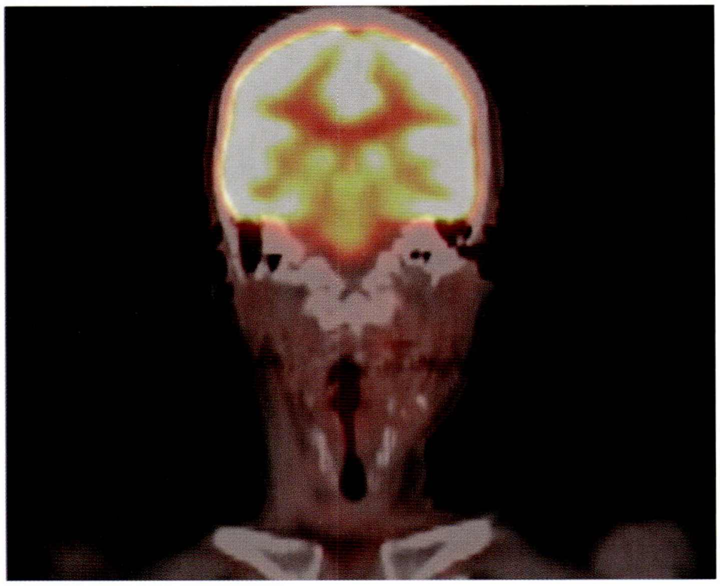

Fig. 3.17 Previous left radical neck dissection for thyroid carcinoma demonstrated on coronal FDG PET-CT. Note surgical clips, asymmetry, and the sacrificed left sternocleidomastoid muscle.

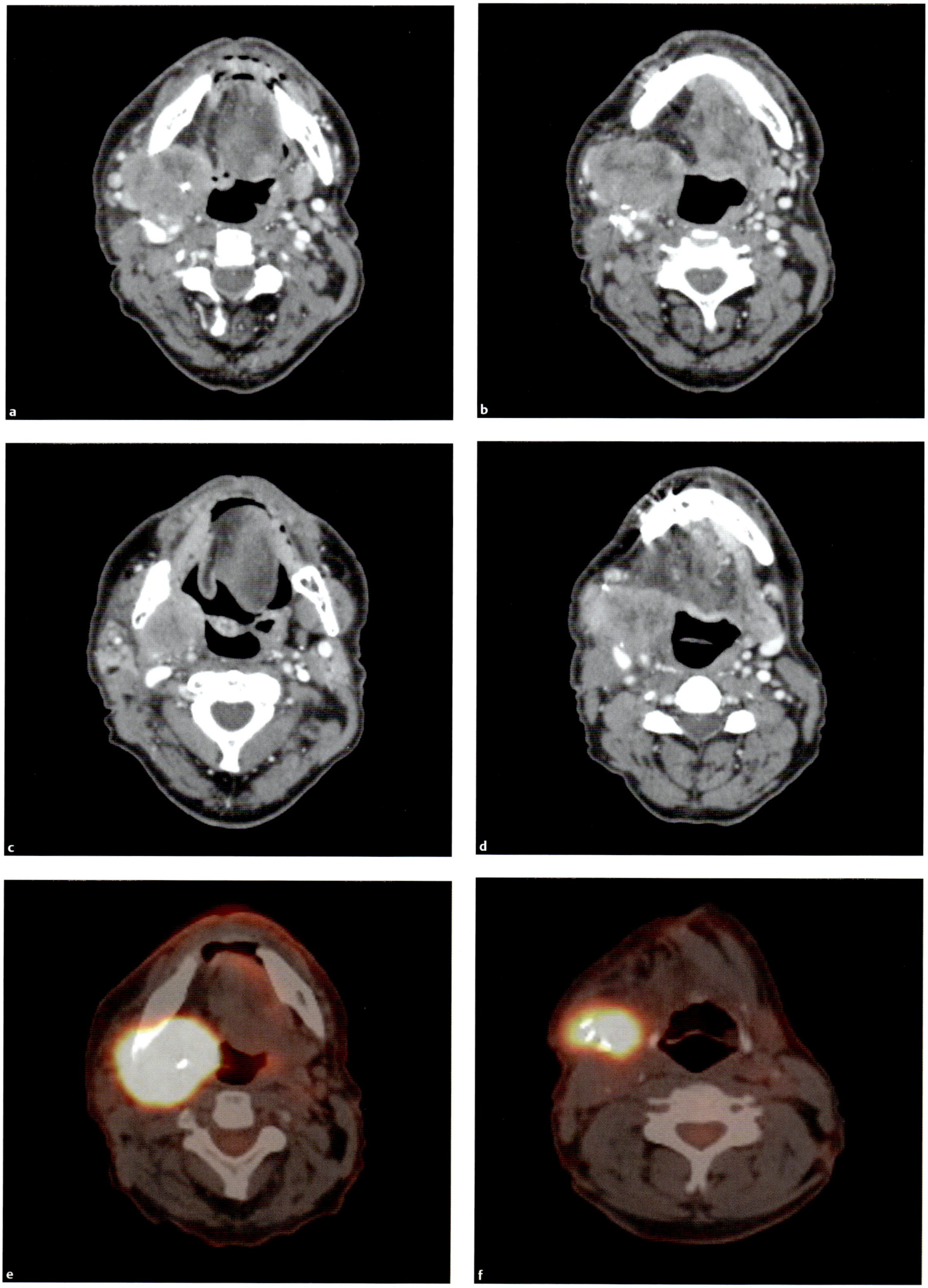
a
b
c
d
e
f

◀ **Fig. 3.18a–f** A 59-year-old man with local recurrence following previous neck dissection and free flap for T2N1 moderately differentiated squamous cell carcinoma of the tongue. **a–d** Axial contrast-enhanced CT images show nodal recurrence in the surgical bed infiltrating the right medial pterygoid muscle. **e–f** Axial FDG PET-CT shows marked increased metabolic activity in the recurrent mass.

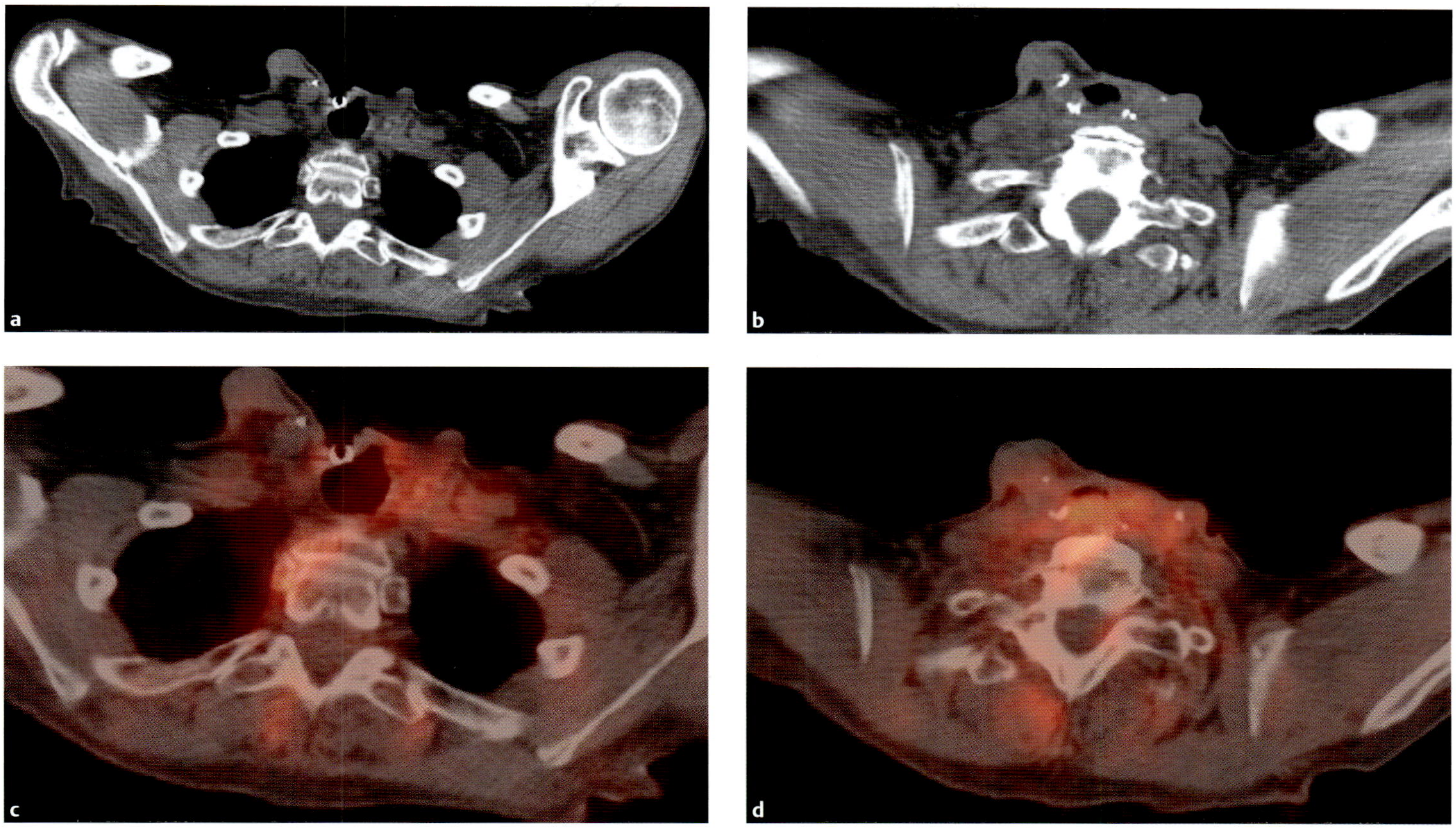

Fig. 3.19a–d Changes after previous laryngectomy, neck dissection, and tracheostomy for laryngeal carcinoma in a 68-year-old man.
a, b Axial contrast-enhanced CT shows no evidence of local recurrence clinically or on follow-up.
c, d Axial FDG PET-CT shows no marked uptake and low-level physiological activity in the proximal esophagus.

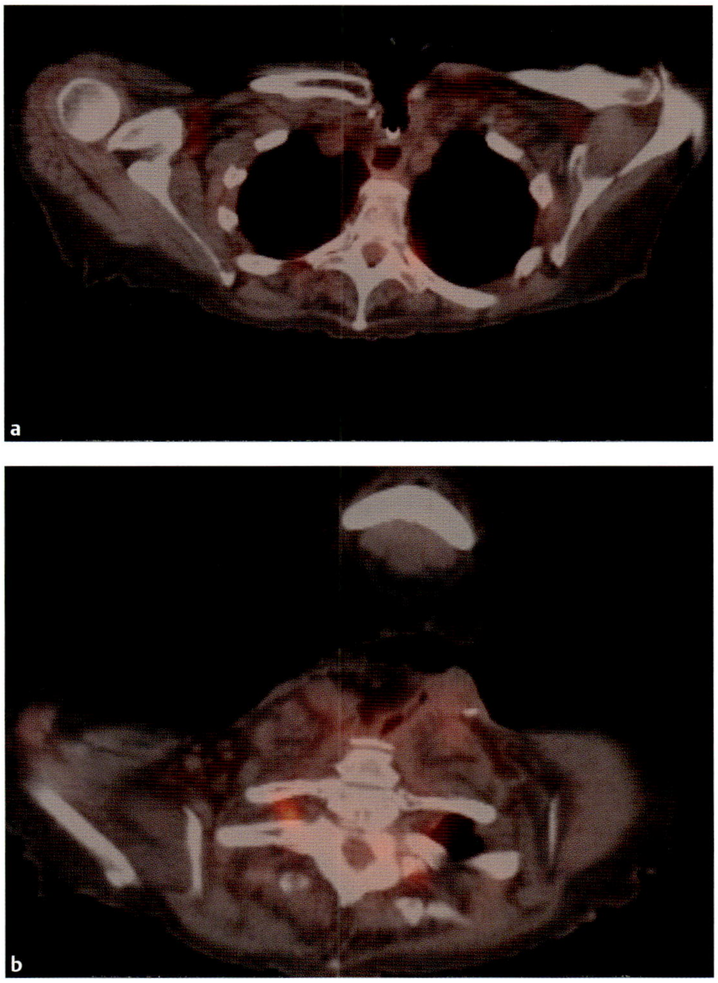

Fig. 3.20a–c Axial FDG PET-CT in a 77-year-old woman with prior laryngopharyngectomy, resected trachea, tracheostomy, free flap, and speech valve in situ for recurrent poorly differentiated thyroid carcinoma. Note the absence of marked uptake, there was no recurrence.

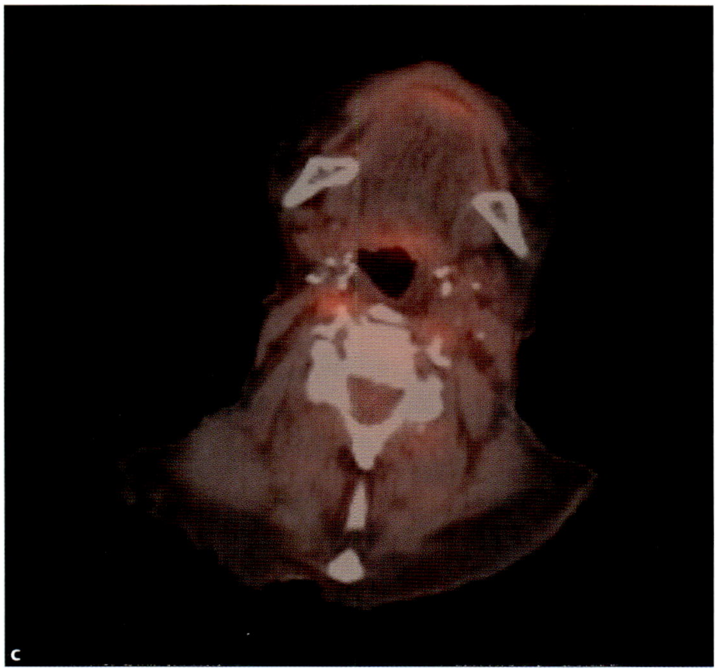

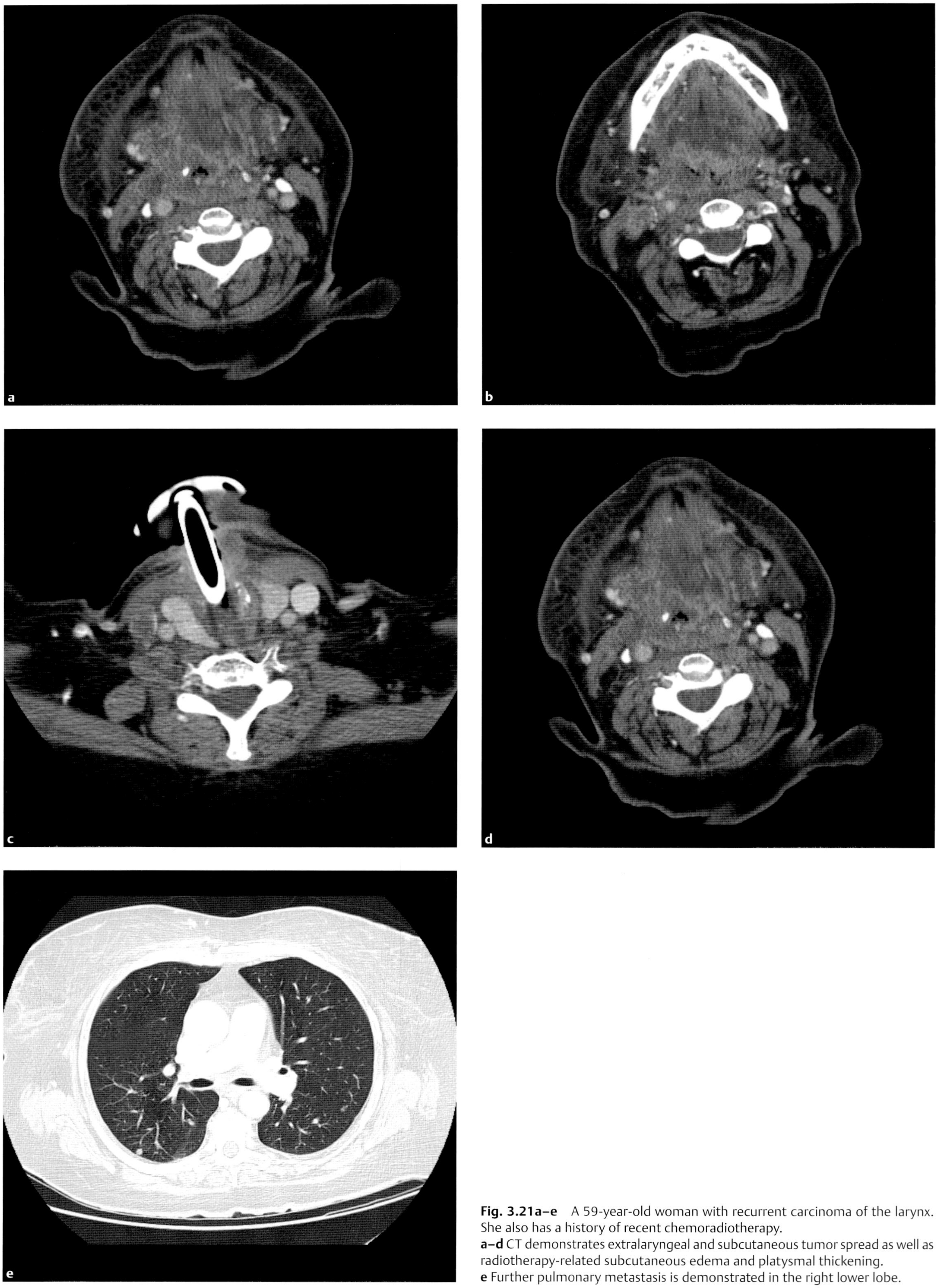

Fig. 3.21a–e A 59-year-old woman with recurrent carcinoma of the larynx. She also has a history of recent chemoradiotherapy.
a–d CT demonstrates extralaryngeal and subcutaneous tumor spread as well as radiotherapy-related subcutaneous edema and platysmal thickening.
e Further pulmonary metastasis is demonstrated in the right lower lobe.

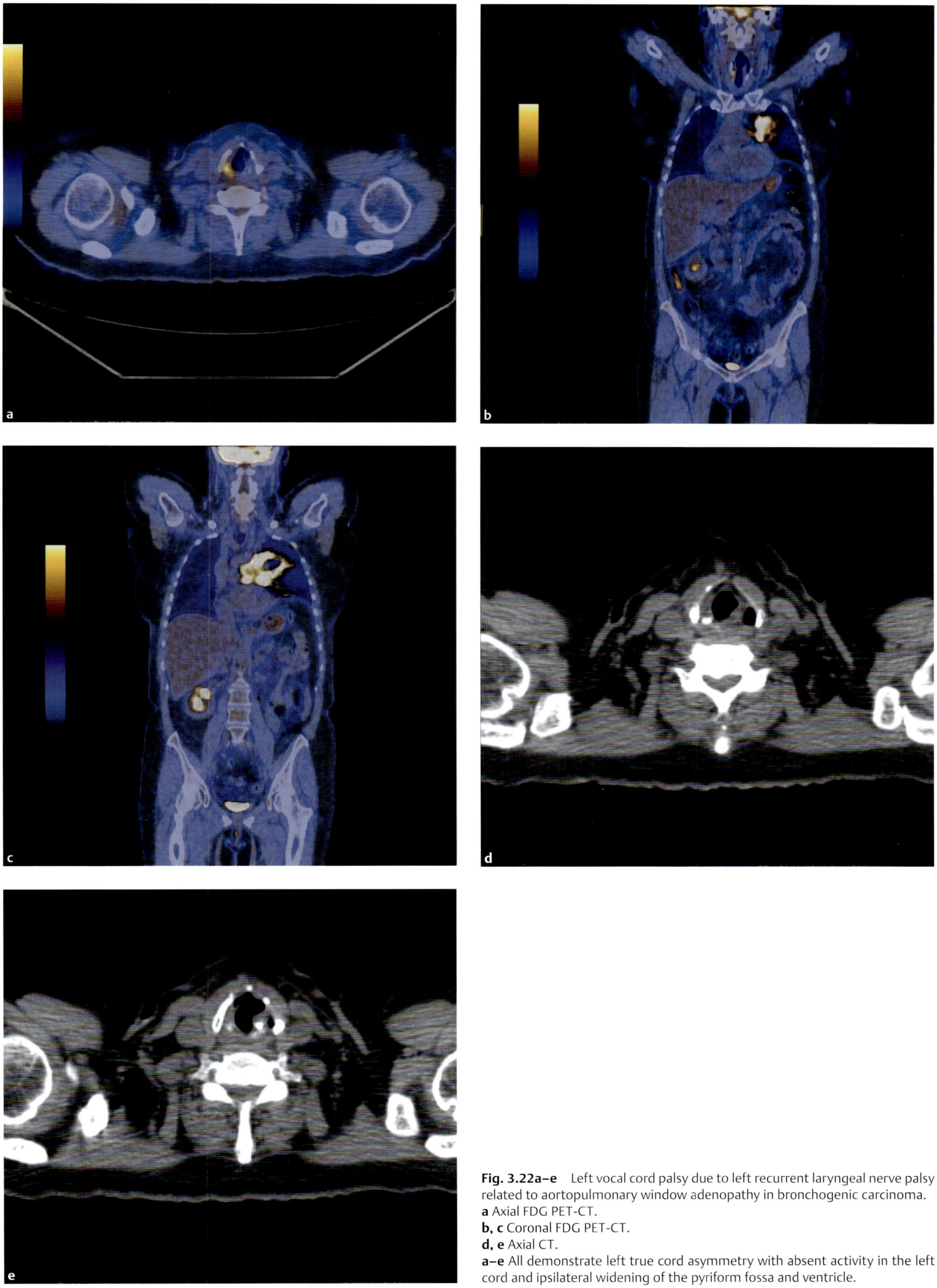

Fig. 3.22a–e Left vocal cord palsy due to left recurrent laryngeal nerve palsy related to aortopulmonary window adenopathy in bronchogenic carcinoma.
a Axial FDG PET-CT.
b, c Coronal FDG PET-CT.
d, e Axial CT.
a–e All demonstrate left true cord asymmetry with absent activity in the left cord and ipsilateral widening of the pyriform fossa and ventricle.

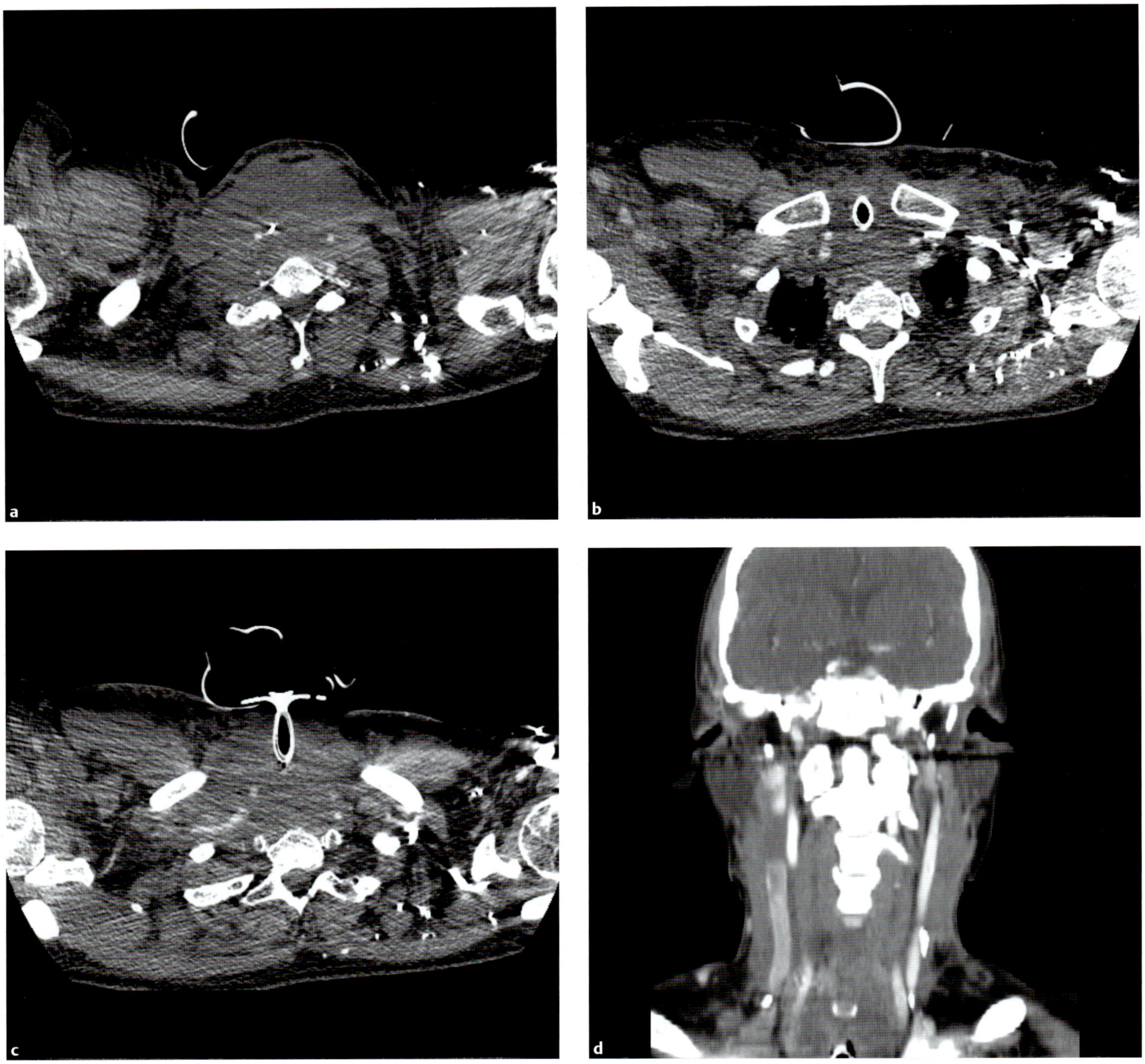

Fig. 3.23a–d Prior laryngectomy and tracheostomy, with recurrent locally advanced carcinoma resulting in right subclavian and right internal jugular venous occlusion.

a–c Axial contrast-enhanced CT images.
d Coronal reformatted image.

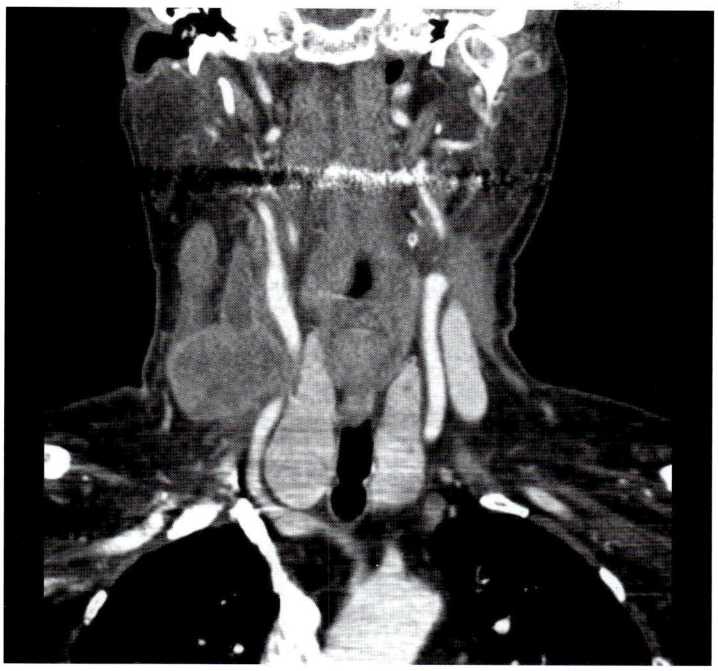

Fig. 3.24 Previous SCC left tongue border. Coronal reformatted CT image with a right level III large necrotic lymph node mass with extracapsular spread and right internal jugular vein invasion.

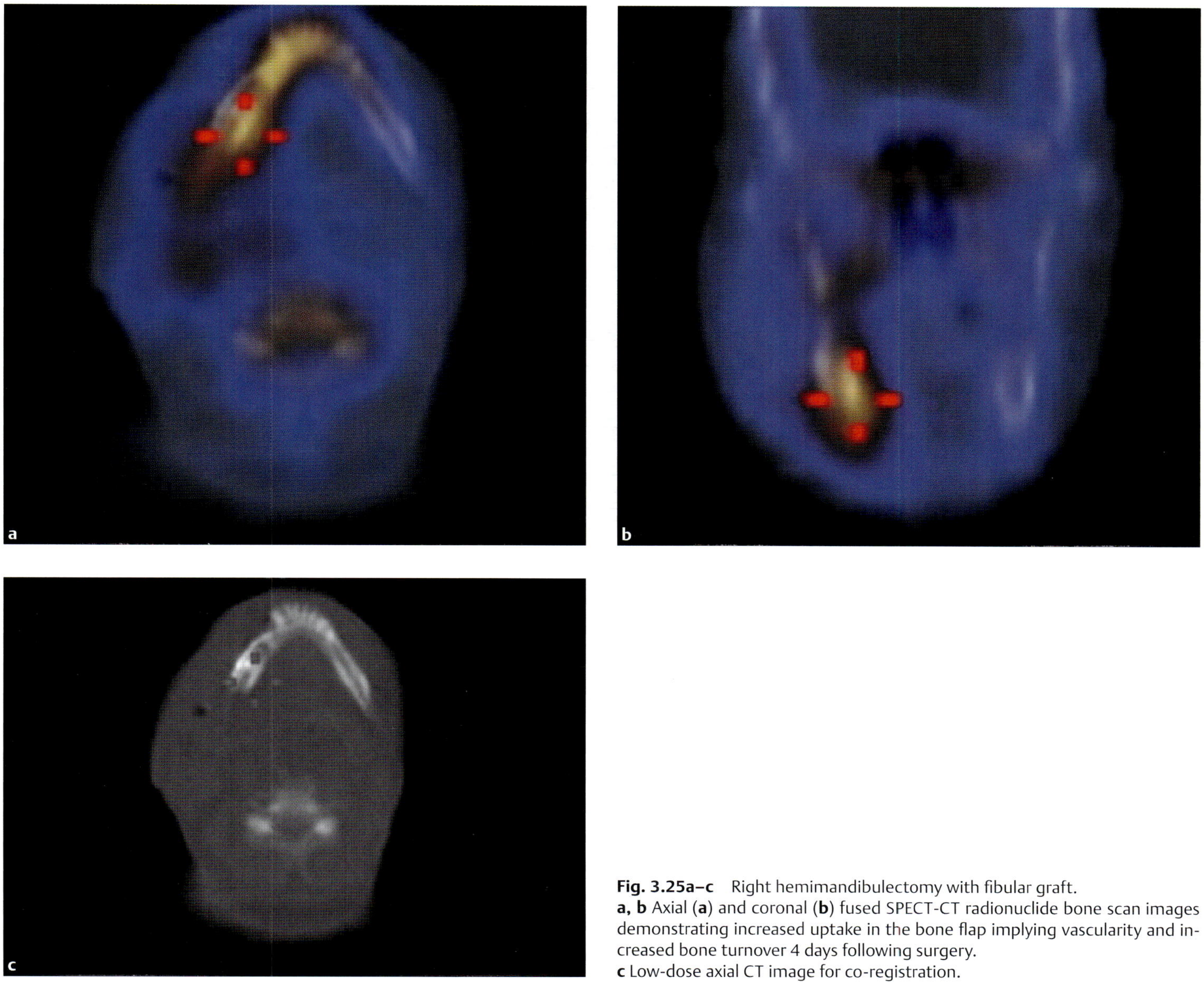

Fig. 3.25a–c Right hemimandibulectomy with fibular graft.
a, b Axial (**a**) and coronal (**b**) fused SPECT-CT radionuclide bone scan images demonstrating increased uptake in the bone flap implying vascularity and increased bone turnover 4 days following surgery.
c Low-dose axial CT image for co-registration.

Imaging Modalities for Detection of Recurrence

Plain Radiography and Fluoroscopy

Although plain radiographs have a limited role in the imaging of patients with head and neck cancer, they still have specific roles such as the chest radiograph (**Fig. 3.26**) and mandibular orthopantomogram (**Fig. 3.27**). They are relatively cheap and widely available, and require less skill for interpretation. Fluoroscopy is particularly useful in diagnosing anastomotic leakage and other postsurgical defects, especially in the oral cavity, oropharynx, and hypopharynx (**Fig. 3.28**).

Ultrasound

High-frequency ultrasound is extremely useful in the detection of superficial recurrences such as skin, parotid, and thyroid local recurrence as well as the detection of nodal recurrence. Some of its drawbacks include its operator-dependent features.[31]

Ultrasonography is usually able to distinguish between reactive and malignant nodes. Ultrasound assessment of nodal disease is based on nodal size, shape, and echogenicity as well as the absence of hilar vascularity, absence of hilar fat, and central nodal necrosis. Other features that may aid sonographic diagnosis include calcification and elastography.[32] When combined with fine-needle aspiration for cytology (FNAC), ultrasonography has a high accuracy rate, leading to a higher detection rate for nodal recurrence than with CT (**Fig. 3.29**). However, cytology can be difficult to interpret

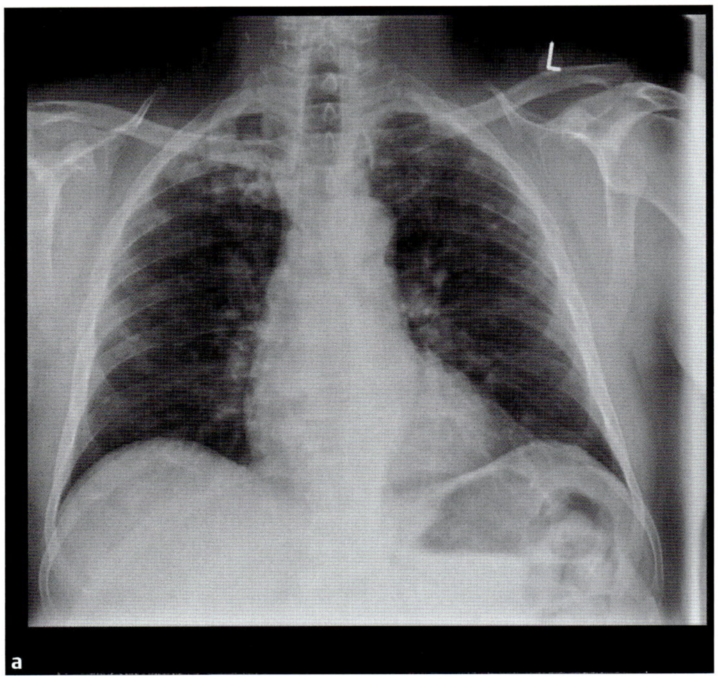

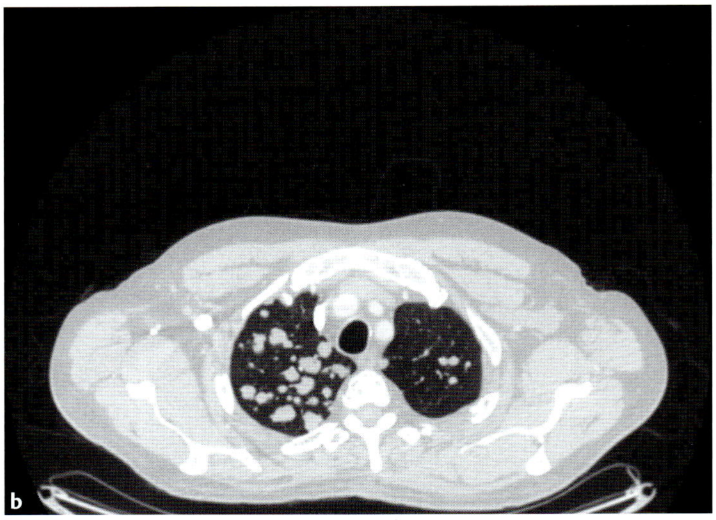

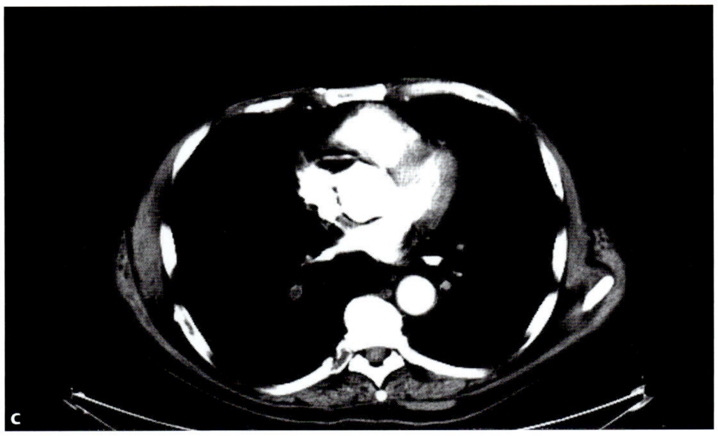

Fig. 3.26a–c Pulmonary metastases in a 57-year-old man with parotid gland acinic cell carcinoma resulting in lung metastases and bone metastases (not shown). Status: post surgery and chemotherapy.
a Frontal chest x-ray (CXR).
b, c Axial CT images.

after recent chemoradiotherapy.[33] Although ultrasound examination alone is more accurate than clinical palpation, follow-up with ultrasound alone risks missing up to 18% of cases of occult recurrences.[34] Palpable head and neck masses less than 3 cm in size are more successfully sampled with FNAC when performed under ultrasound guidance as opposed to palpation-guided fine-needle aspiration, with a tissue adequacy rate of 84% for ultrasound guidance versus 58% for standard palpation technique (**Figs. 3.30 and 3.31**). This is more relevant for the thyroid gland than for lymphatic and salivary tissue.[35]

■ Computed Tomography

Computed tomography (CT) is the workhorse of cross-sectional imaging and is readily available in most departments. Dental amalgam may result in streak artifacts, but this can be reduced by angling the CT gantry.[36,37] The relatively low scan time lends itself to less susceptibility to movement-related artifacts compared with MRI. Modern CT scanners produce better spatial resolution than MRI and are also able to match multiplanar images.[38] However, following radiotherapy of the neck, MRI and CT have similar rates of accuracy.[39] Posttherapy edema and postsurgical change can be difficult to distinguish from recurrence but comparison with baseline posttherapy CT scans is very useful. CT is therefore able to detect local and nodal recurrence, as well as detect lung metastases.[40] CT is also particularly useful for skull base erosion (**Fig. 3.32**).

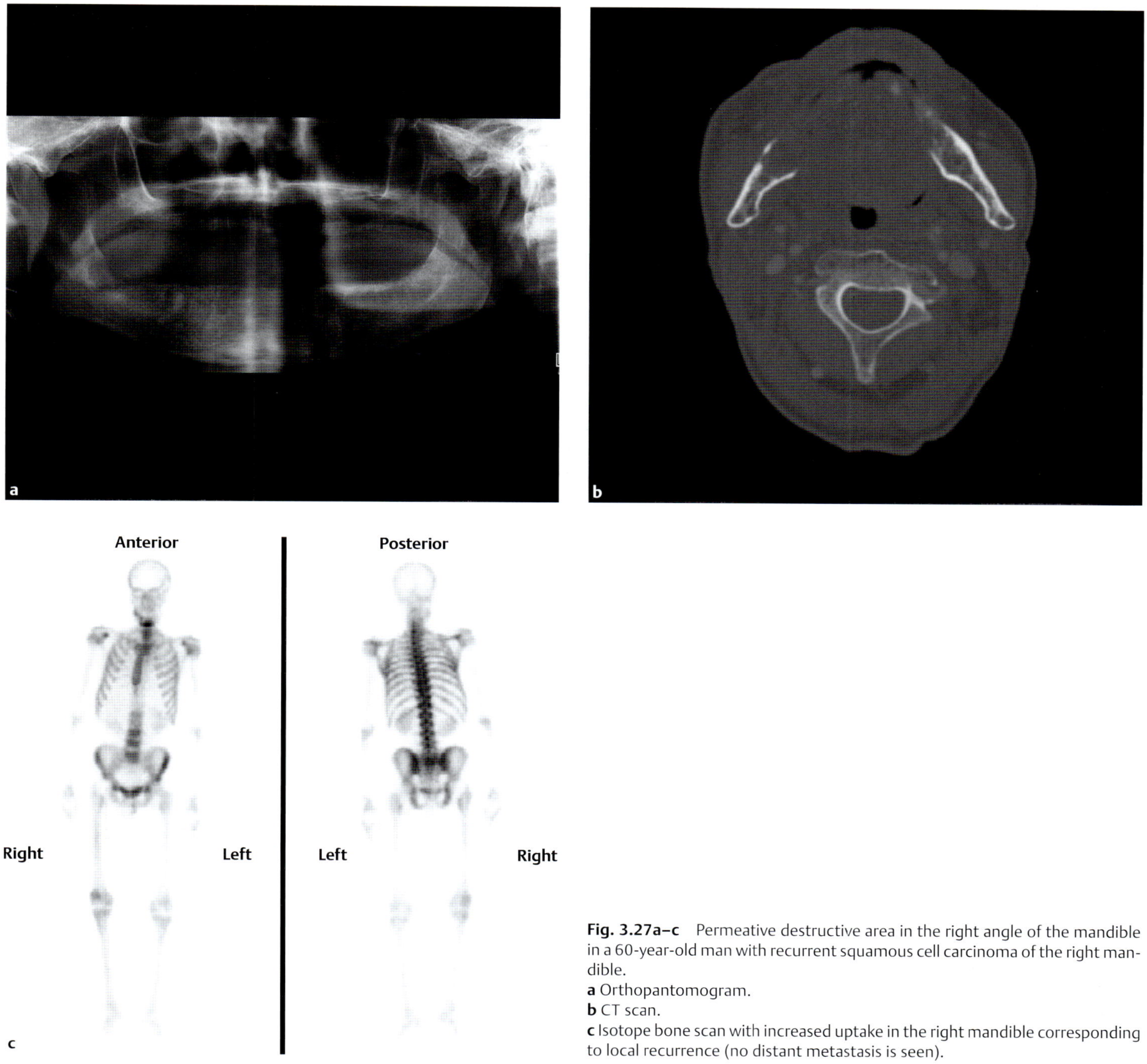

Fig. 3.27a–c Permeative destructive area in the right angle of the mandible in a 60-year-old man with recurrent squamous cell carcinoma of the right mandible.
a Orthopantomogram.
b CT scan.
c Isotope bone scan with increased uptake in the right mandible corresponding to local recurrence (no distant metastasis is seen).

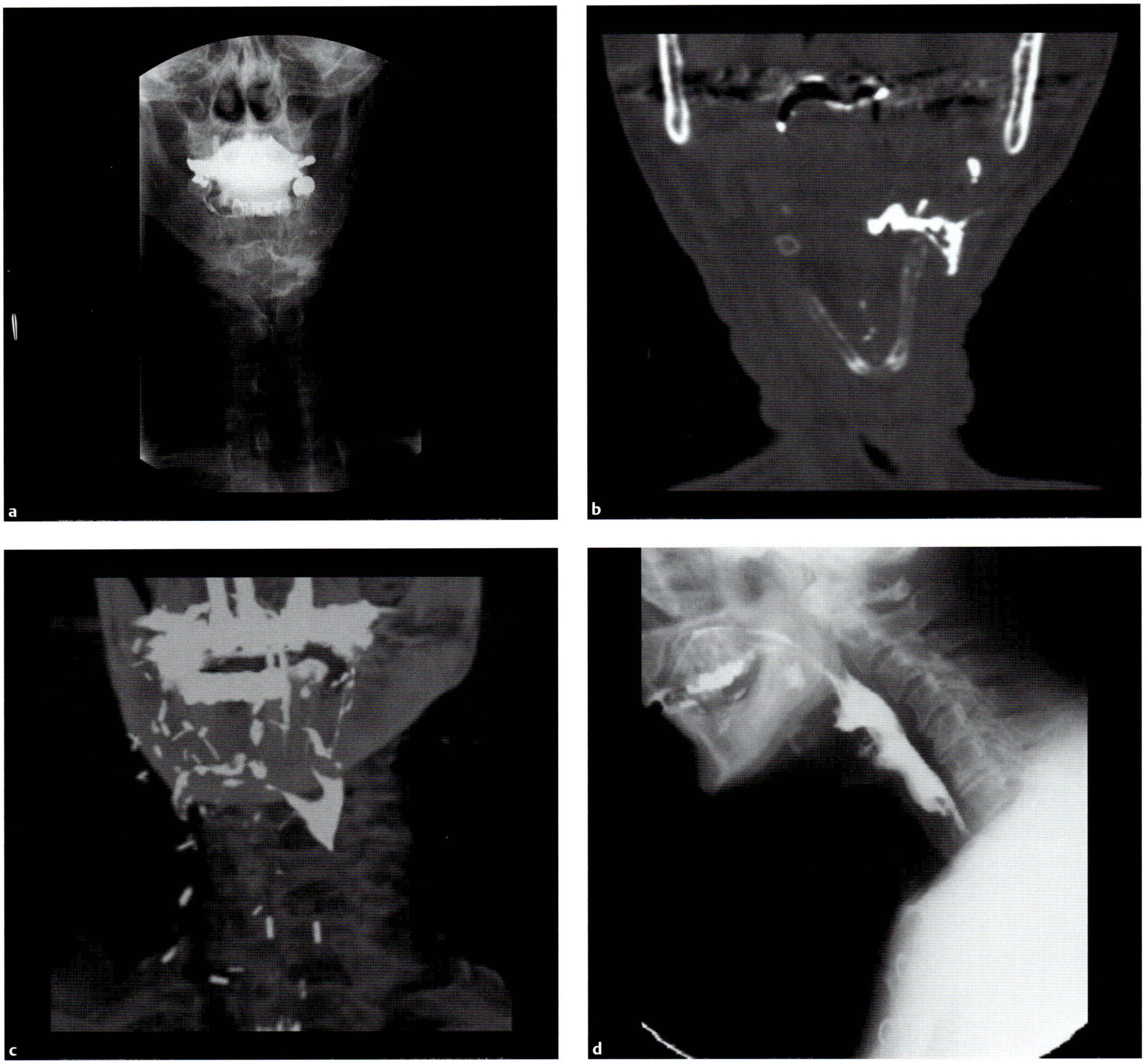

Fig. 3.28a–d Findings on contrast swallow.
a–c A 62-year-old man treated for T3N2c left tongue base squamous cell carcimona (SCC) with chemoradiotherapy then neck dissection demonstrating left-sided leakage and sinus crater.
a Frontal water soluble contrast swallow.
b Coronal reformatted CT with oral contrast.
c Volume rendered reformatted CT with oral contrast.
d Lateral barium swallow in a different 83-year-old man demonstrating a malignant postcricoid and proximal esophageal mass.

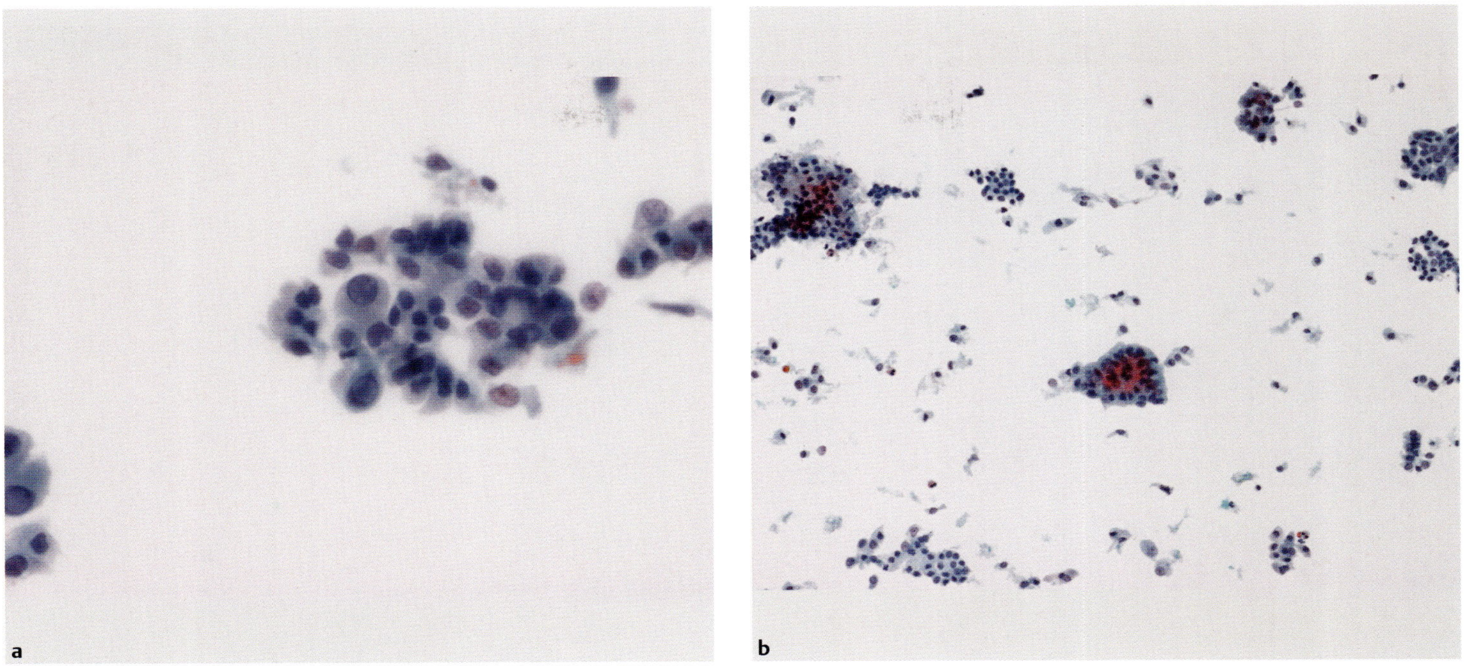

Fig. 3.29a, b Fine-needle aspiration (FNA) of locally recurrent thyroid carcinoma comprising colloid mixed with abundant cohesive papillary groups and clusters of follicular epithelial cells showing nuclear overlapping, nuclear clearing, conspicuous nucleoli, occasional pseudo-intranuclear inclusion, and grooving. Multinucleate giant cells are present. (Image courtesy of Dr. Yen Ching Yeo, Coventry, UK.)

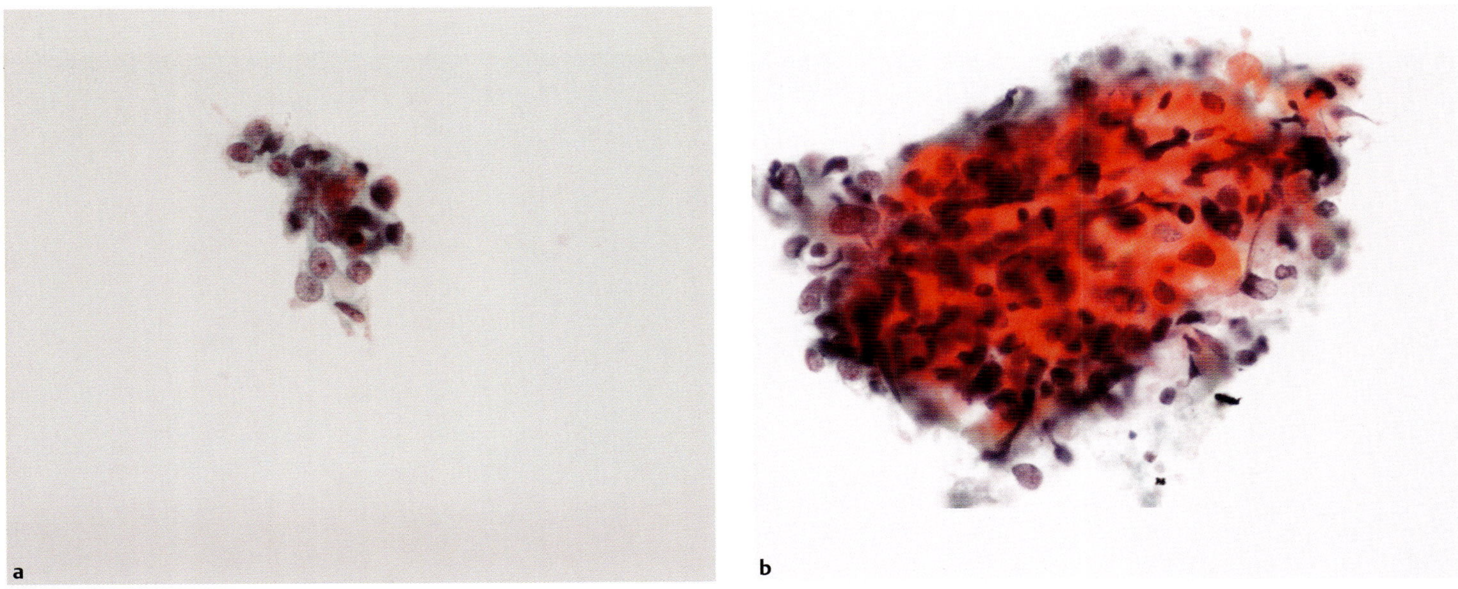

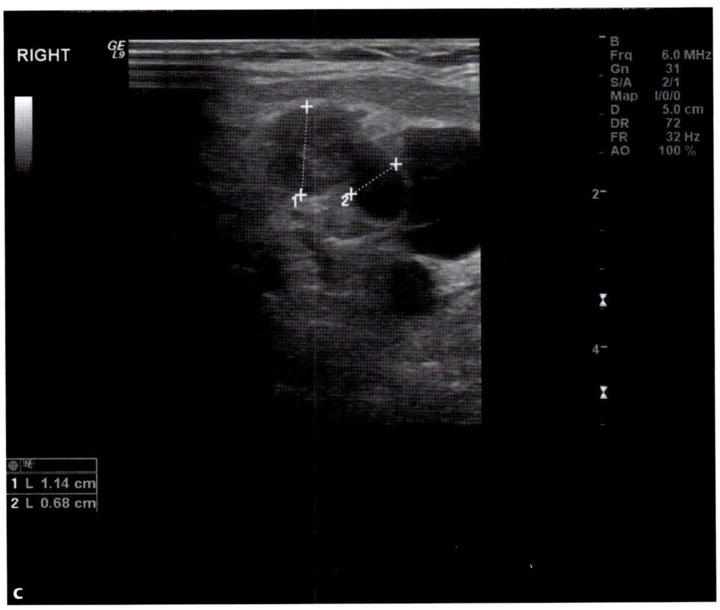

Fig. 3.30a–c A 68-year-old woman post chemoradiotherapy for supraglottic squamous cell carcinoma, presenting with palpable right level III enlarged node.
a A group of malignant cells with enlarged nuclei, coarsely granular chromatin and conspicuous nucleoli. (Image courtesy of Dr. Yen Ching Yeo, Coventry, UK.)
b A group of malignant cells showing squamoid differentiation with dense orangeophilic cytoplasm and large irregular nuclei. Occasional hyperchromatic and pyknotic nuclei are present. (Image courtesy of Dr. Yen Ching Yeo, Coventry, UK.)
c High-resolution ultrasound of the neck showing a cluster of morphologically abnormal and enlarged right-sided cervical lymph nodes.

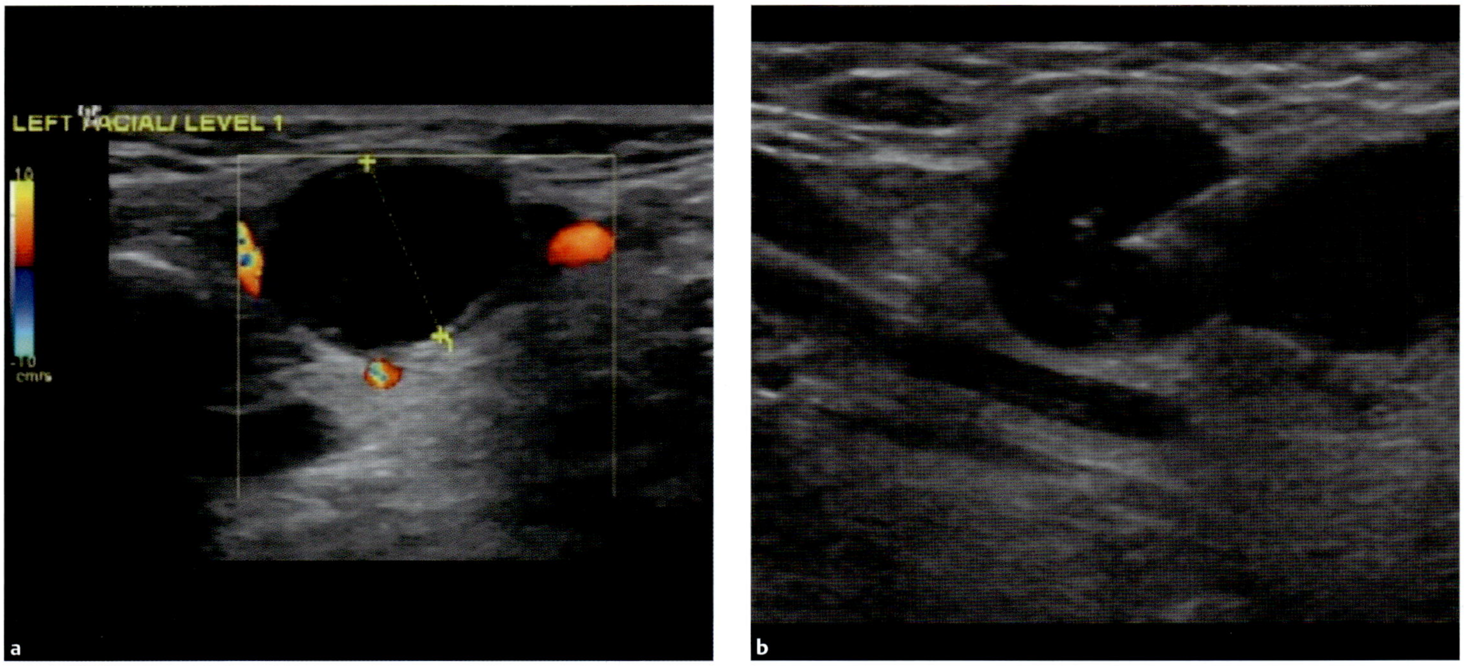

Fig. 3.31a, b Recurrent lymphadenopathy in a patient with previously resected nasal angiosarcoma.

a Ultrasound-detected recurrence of pathologically enlarged cervical nodes with abnormal morphology.
b FNA of pathologically enlarged cervical nodes.

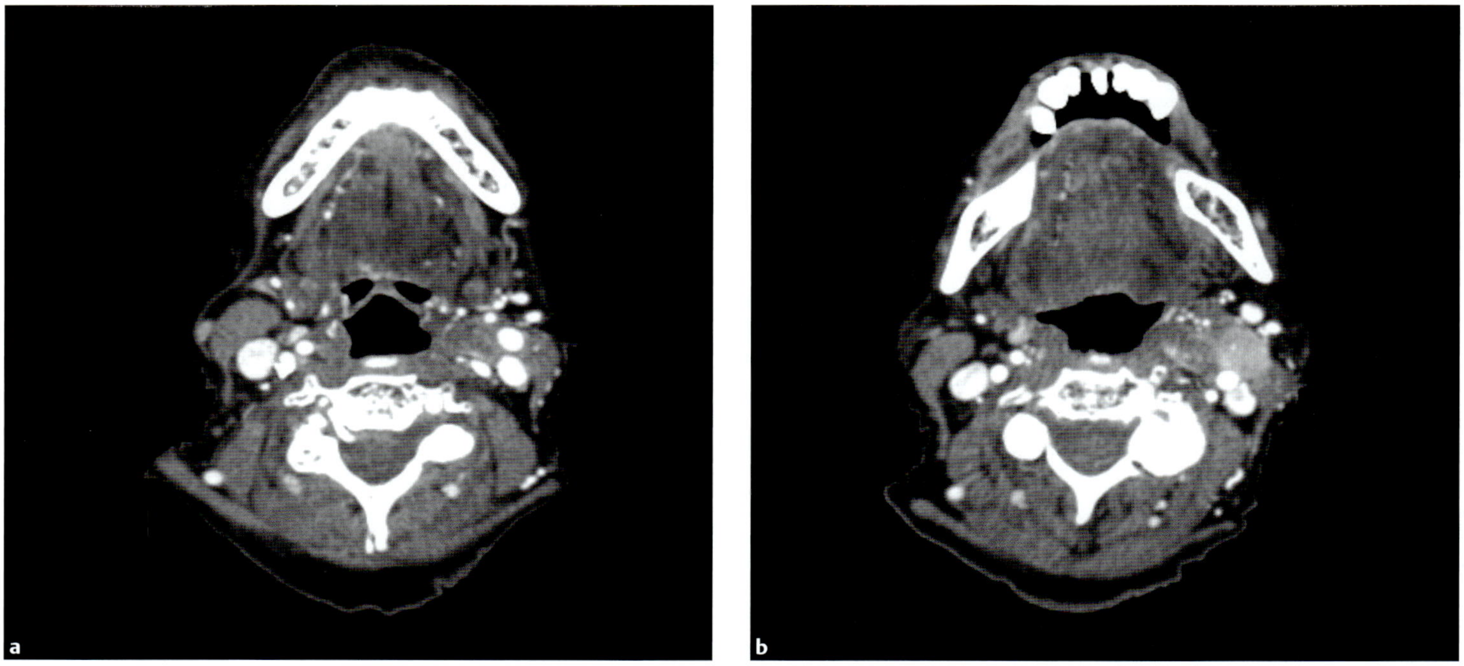

Fig. 3.32a–g An 84-year-old woman with recurrent left carotid body tumor. She had been treated with radiotherapy 2 years previously; current symptoms included ataxia, hoarse voice, and mass in the upper neck. Axial contrast-enhanced CT demonstrates a large avidly enhancing infiltrative left carotid space mass with skull base and jugular foraminal invasion as well as mass effect on the left middle cerebellar peduncle and brainstem.

Fig. 3.32c–g ▸

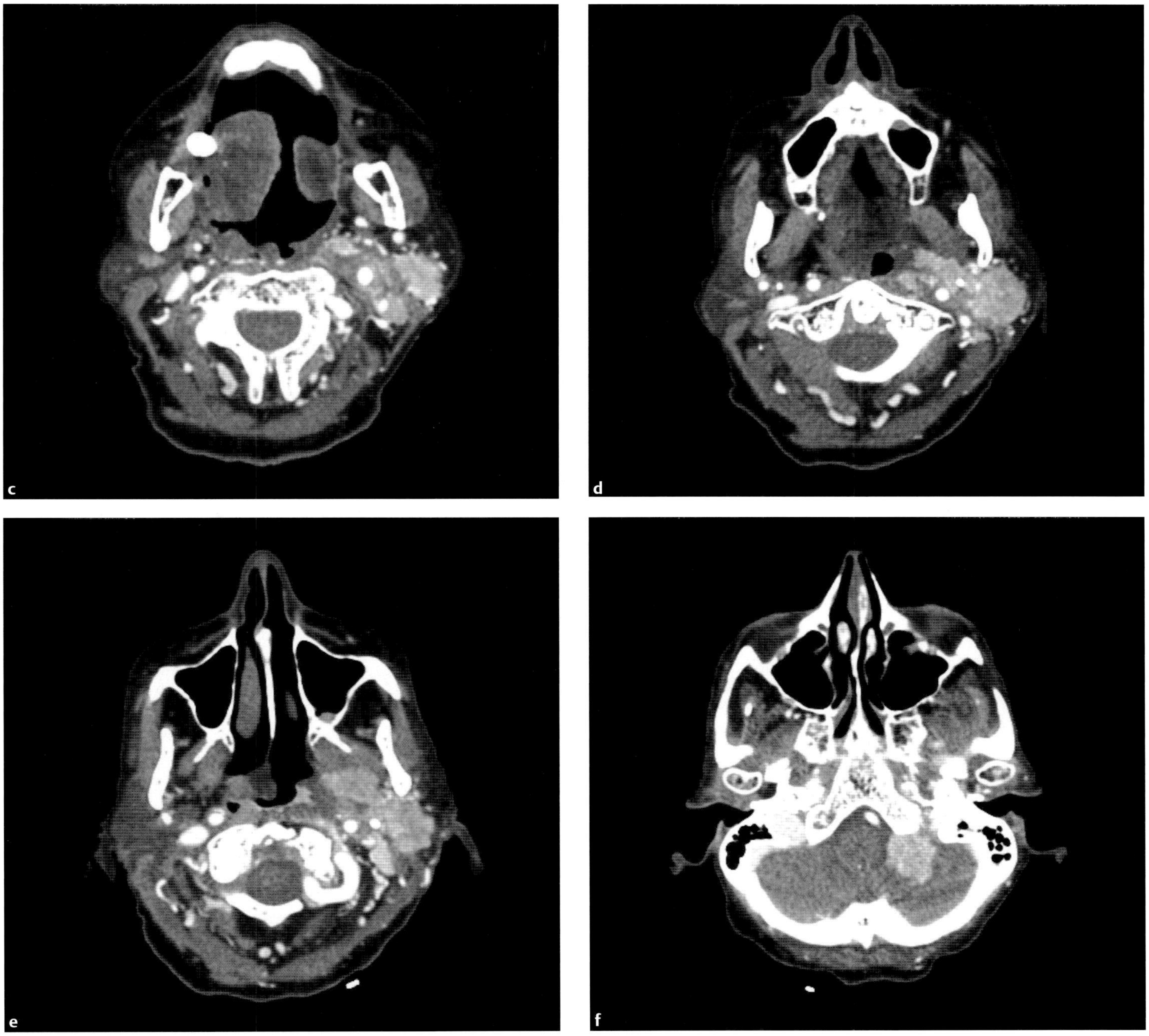

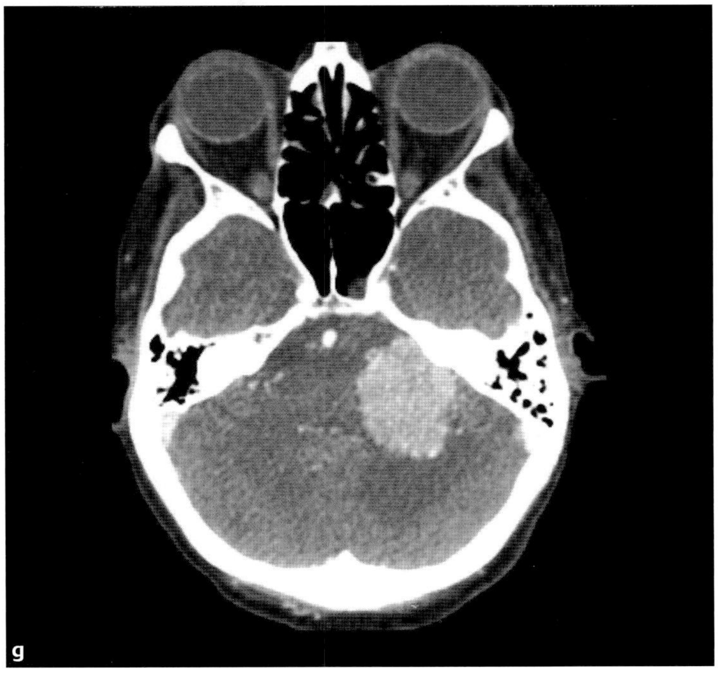

◄ ▲ **Fig. 3.32c–g**

■ Magnetic Resonance Imaging

Magnetic resonance imaging (MRI) has good soft tissue contrast resolution. However, it has its limitations due to swallowing and movement-related artifacts as well as dental amalgam–related artifact. There is also the well-recognized complication of nephrogenic systemic fibrosis as a result of the use of gadolinium-based contrast agents in patients with impaired renal function.[41] MRI is also contraindicated in patients with permanent pacemaker devices, cardioverter-defibrillator devices, or ferromagnetic vascular clips.

MRI is the modality of choice for demonstrating perineural spread. MRI is therefore recommended for the follow-up of tumors with a high risk for perineural spread such as adenoid cystic carcinoma and desmoplastic type melanoma as well as sinonasal, nasopharyngeal, and skull base tumors (**Figs. 3.33 and 3.34**).[1,40] Some authors report that the addition of dynamic contrast-enhanced and diffusion-weighted imaging sequences improves MRI accuracy.[39,42] A study based on a cohort of 33 patients revealed that diffusion-weighted imaging (DWI) may be better than turbo spin-echo MR imaging in staging of lymph node spread in head and neck squamous cell carcinoma when performed using apparent diffusion coefficient (ADC) with wide-ranging b values between 0 and 1000 s/mm^2.[43] Furthermore, it added value in lymph nodes less than 10 mm in shot-axis diameter.[43]

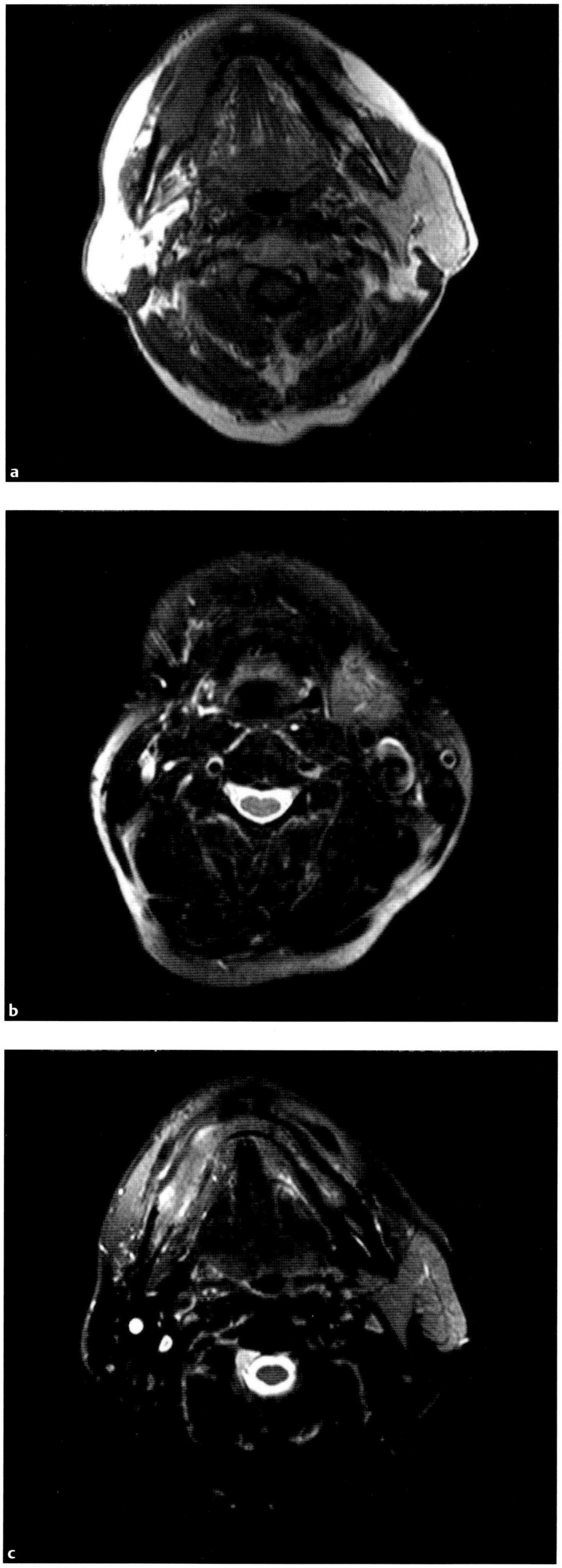

Fig. 3.33a–c A 63-year-old man with recurrent squamous cell carcinoma in the right mandible. History of previous squamous cell carcinoma of the right maxilla treated with resection, soft tissue reconstruction, and radiotherapy.
a Axial T1-weighted MR image.
b, c Axial T2-weighted MR images with fat suppression. Note the infiltration of the right mandible and right parotid atrophy secondary to prior radiotherapy.

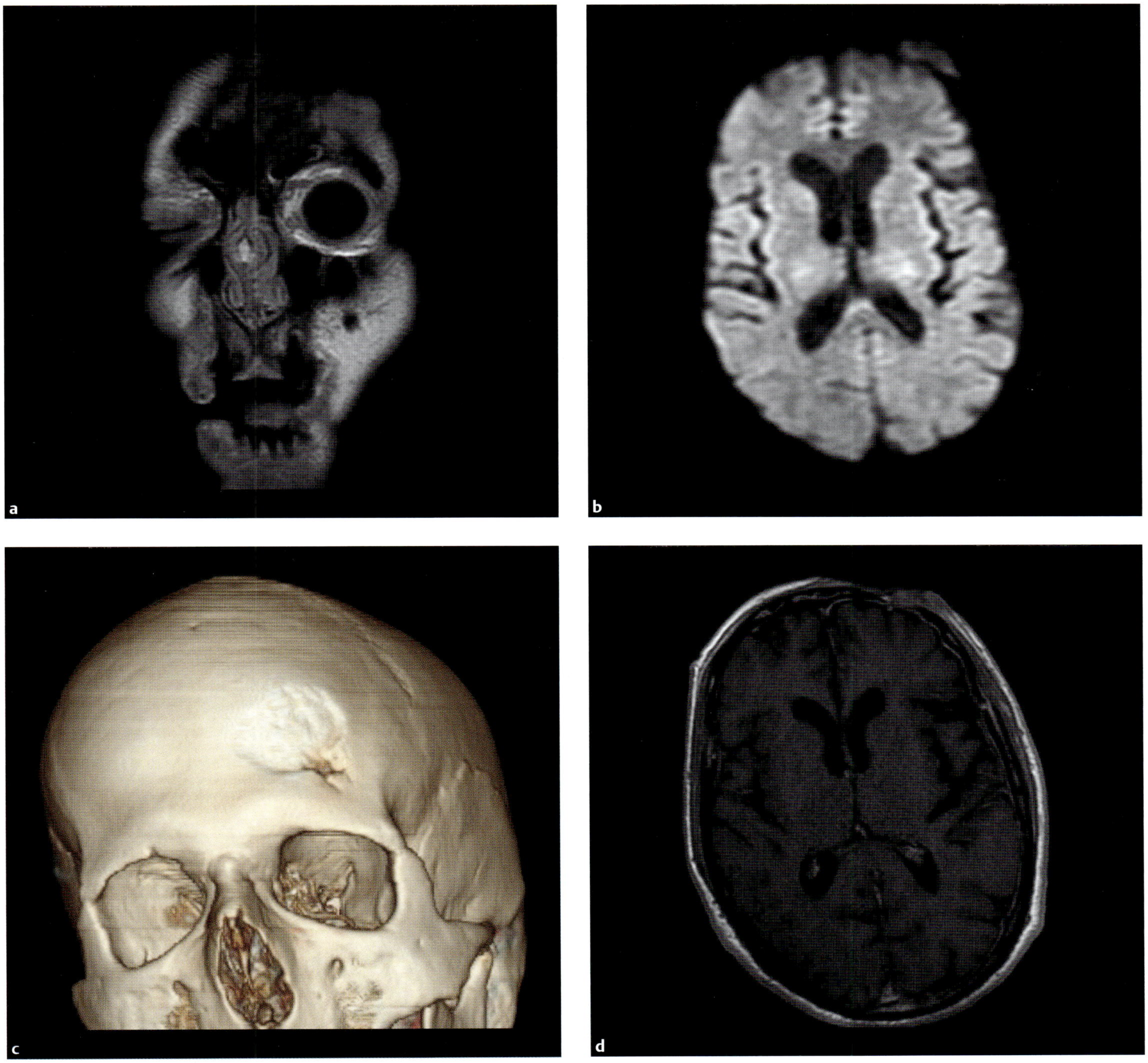

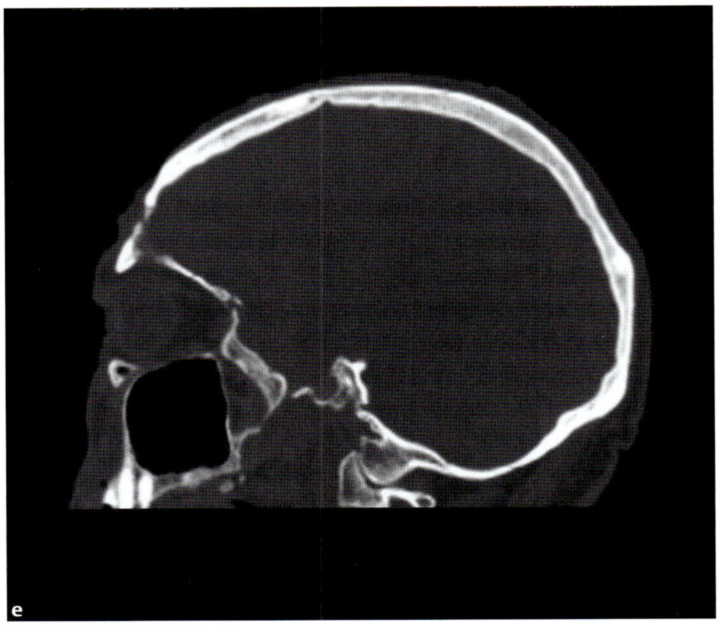

Fig. 3.34a–e Recurrent aggressive squamous cell carcinoma of the left forehead despite previous burring of frontal bone and postoperative radiotherapy.
a Coronal T1-weighted MR image, post contrast.
b Axial diffusion-weighted image.
c Reformatted maximum-intensity projection CT image.
d Axial T1-weighted MR image, post contrast.
e Sagittal reformatted CT image demonstrates an infiltrating left forehead skin lesion with intracranial extension and erosion of the left orbital roof. (There is restricted diffusion of protons in the solid tumor.)

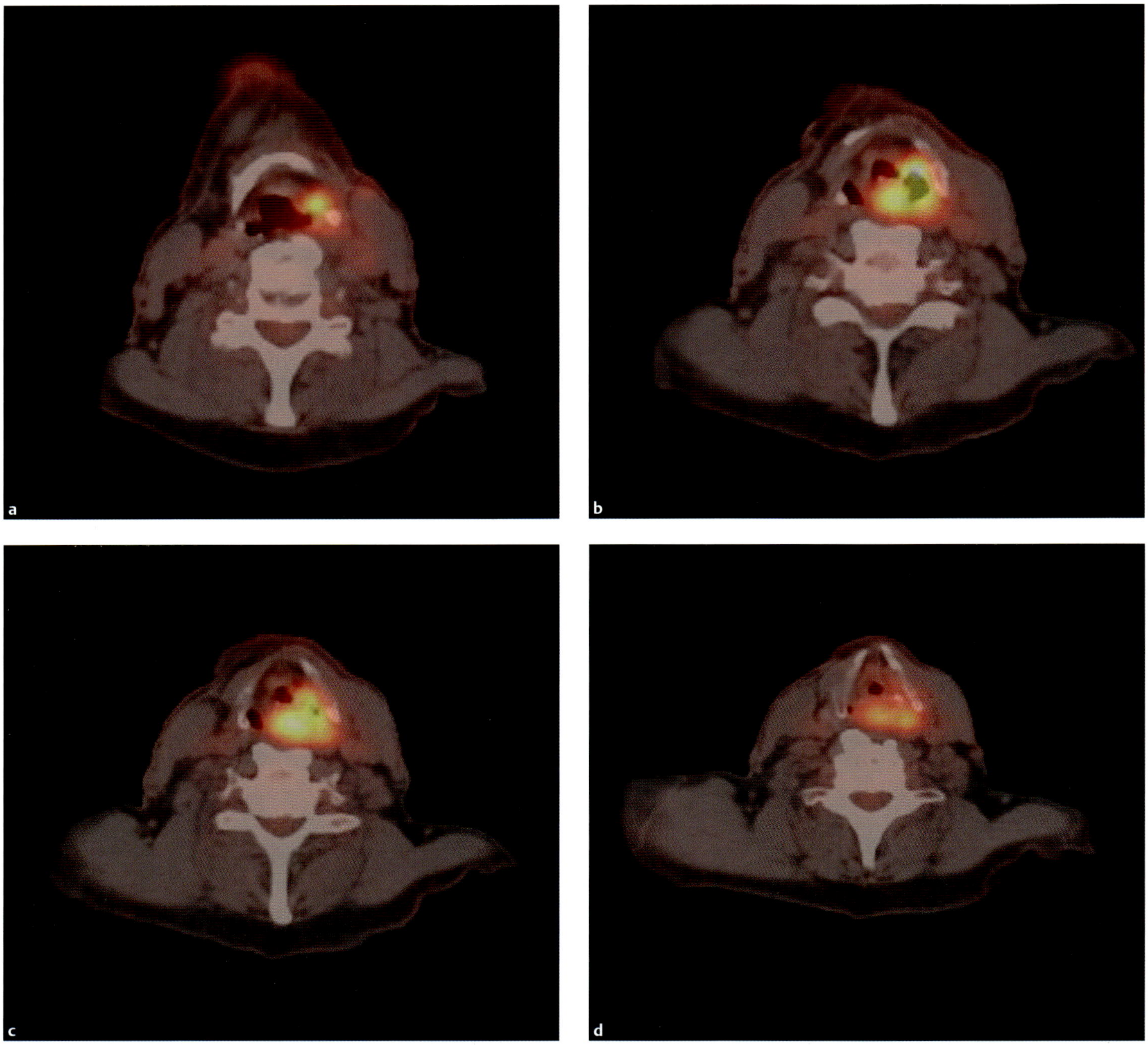

Fig. 3.35a–g Axial FDG PET-CT images in a 70-year-old male with previous oropharyngeal cancer. He now has a new diagnosis of a second tumor, a left-sided hypopharyngeal carcinoma recurrence with extralaryngeal spread. Note the incidental focal thyroid gland uptake on the left, which is unrelated to the tumor.

Fig. 3.35e–g ▸

Positron Emission Tomography and Computed Tomography (PET-CT)

The fusion of positron emission tomography (PET) and computed tomography (CT) was successfully pioneered in 2001. It combines the detailed high spatial resolution anatomical data from CT with the low-resolution but highly informative functional data from PET.

Advantages of PET-CT over PET and CT individually come from the added information provided by the fusion of functional and morphological information and from better localization,[1] which lessens the impact of PET-related artifacts such as physiological muscular, tonsillar, and salivary gland uptake which can easily be excluded on fusion.[44] FDG PET-CT is more accurate (100% sensitivity and 66% specificity) than CT or MRI in detecting suspected recurrent head and neck cancer (**Fig. 3.35**) due to its high negative predictive value.[45] Hence, a negative PET-CT scan is a strong indication of the absence of recurrence/residual disease. However, false-positive uptake in inflamed and infected tissues results in reduced FDG PET-CT specificity. It is therefore common practice to allow 12–16 weeks after completion of radiotherapy before performing a FDG PET-CT scan.[46,47]

Some of the drawbacks include the fact that mis-registration may occur in patients who are unable to lie still, and in lesions smaller than 10 mm, and in necrotic lesions and may produce false negative results. False positive uptake may also occur in aneurysms, in infection, and post treatment.[1]

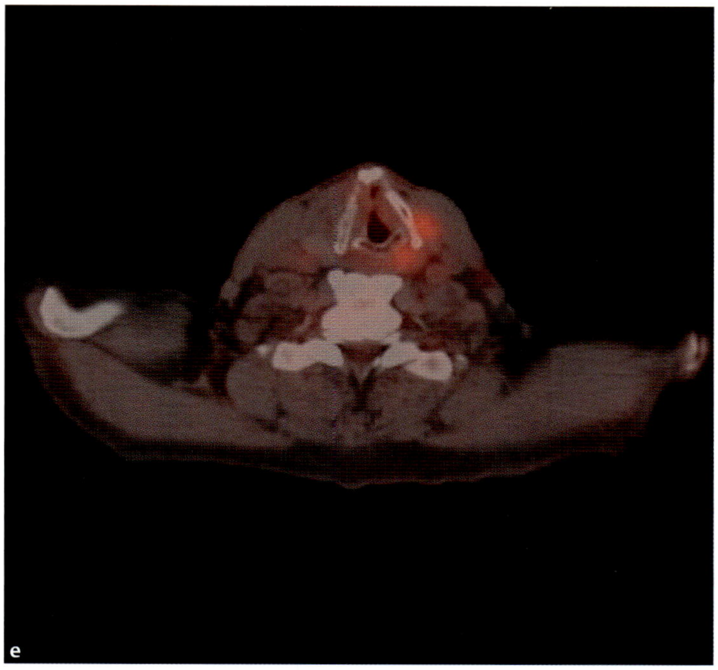

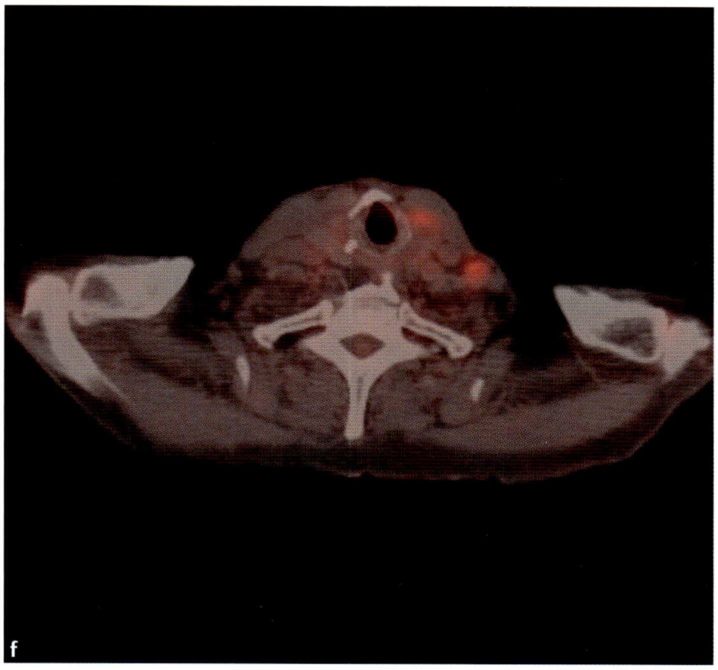

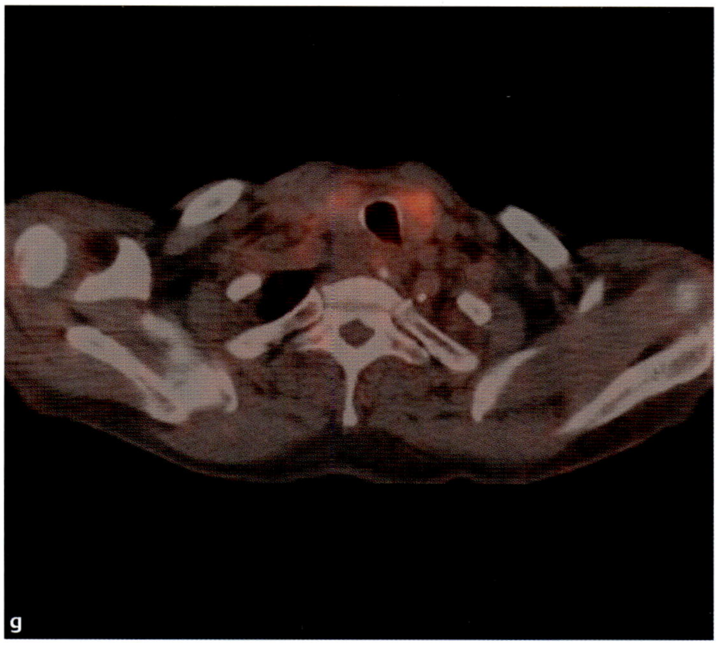

Fig. 3.35e–g

Imaging for Recurrence at Specific Sites

Differentiated Thyroid Cancer Recurrence (Figs. 3.36–3.40)

After total thyroidectomy, the accuracy of radioiodine I-131 scans is increased by postoperative adjuvant radioiodine ablation, which also enhances the value of serum thyroglobulin as a marker of carcinoma recurrence.[48] It should be noted that sensitivity of the radioiodine scan is reduced within 1–3 months of intravenous iodinated contrast.[48] Furthermore, endogenous or exogenous TSH

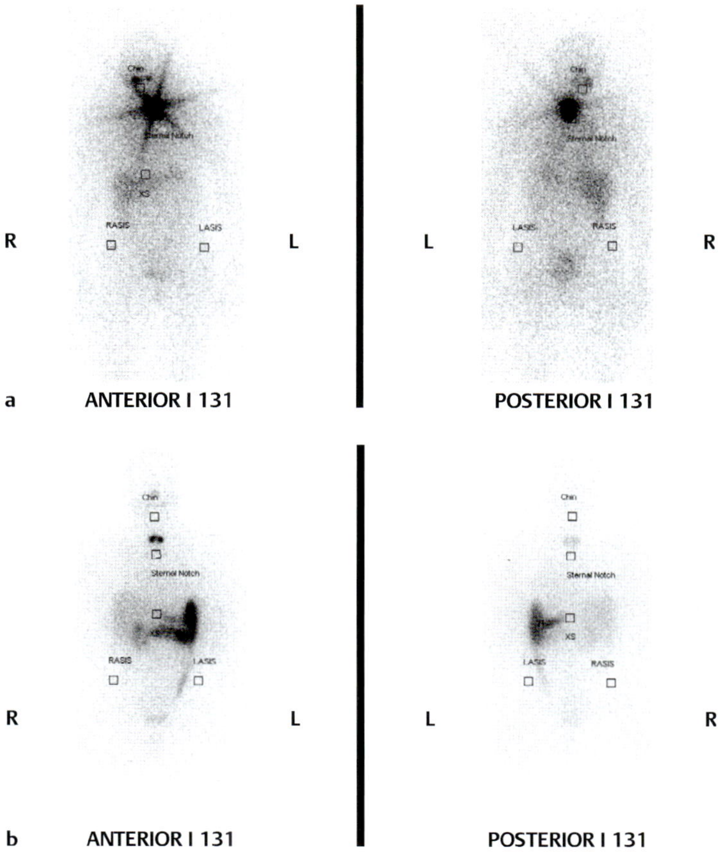

Fig. 3.36a, b Thyroid I-131 scan.
a Planar anterior and posterior images with metastatic recurrent thyroid cancer showing septal penetration star artifact.
b Planar anterior and posterior images of a normal thyroid I-131 scan with normal physiological uptake only.

levels should be high and iodine-rich food or medication should be avoided.[48] Posttreatment I-131 scans have a higher sensitivity for the detection of metastasis than preablation diagnostic scans, partly because of the direct relationship between sensitivity and the radioiodine dose given.[48,49] Evidence of metastatic disease on posttreatment I-131 scans can help clinicians decide on the need for future diagnostic procedures and treatment requirements.[50,51]

Differentiated thyroid carcinoma (DTC) may be followed with serial serum thyroglobulin measurements following total thyroidectomy and radioiodine ablation. Iodine-131 whole-body scintigraphy may be employed when the serum thyroglobulin levels become raised during follow-up. Focal uptake away from the usual physiological sites is an indicator of metastatic disease.[52]

A comparison of I-123 diagnostic study and I-131postablation scans revealed high concordance for detection of recurrence in the thyroid bed and for detection of bone metastasis, but discrepancy and lower sensitivity in cervical nodes and lung secondaries on I-123 images.[49] I-131 is much cheaper and has a longer half-life enabling prolonged imaging periods. However, I-123 produces higher image quality and the whole-body dose is lower.[53] CT has a role to play in the detection of thyroid cancer recurrence in the lungs and bone and local recurrence of thyroid cancer, while MRI is able to detect local and bony recurrence.

FDG PET-CT is useful for localizing recurrent thyroid cancer in patients with rising thyroglobulin who have had negative I-131 scans, particularly when the thyroglobulin levels are above 10 ng/mL.[54] This is known as the flip-flop phenomenon and is usually an indication of de-differentiation.[55,56]

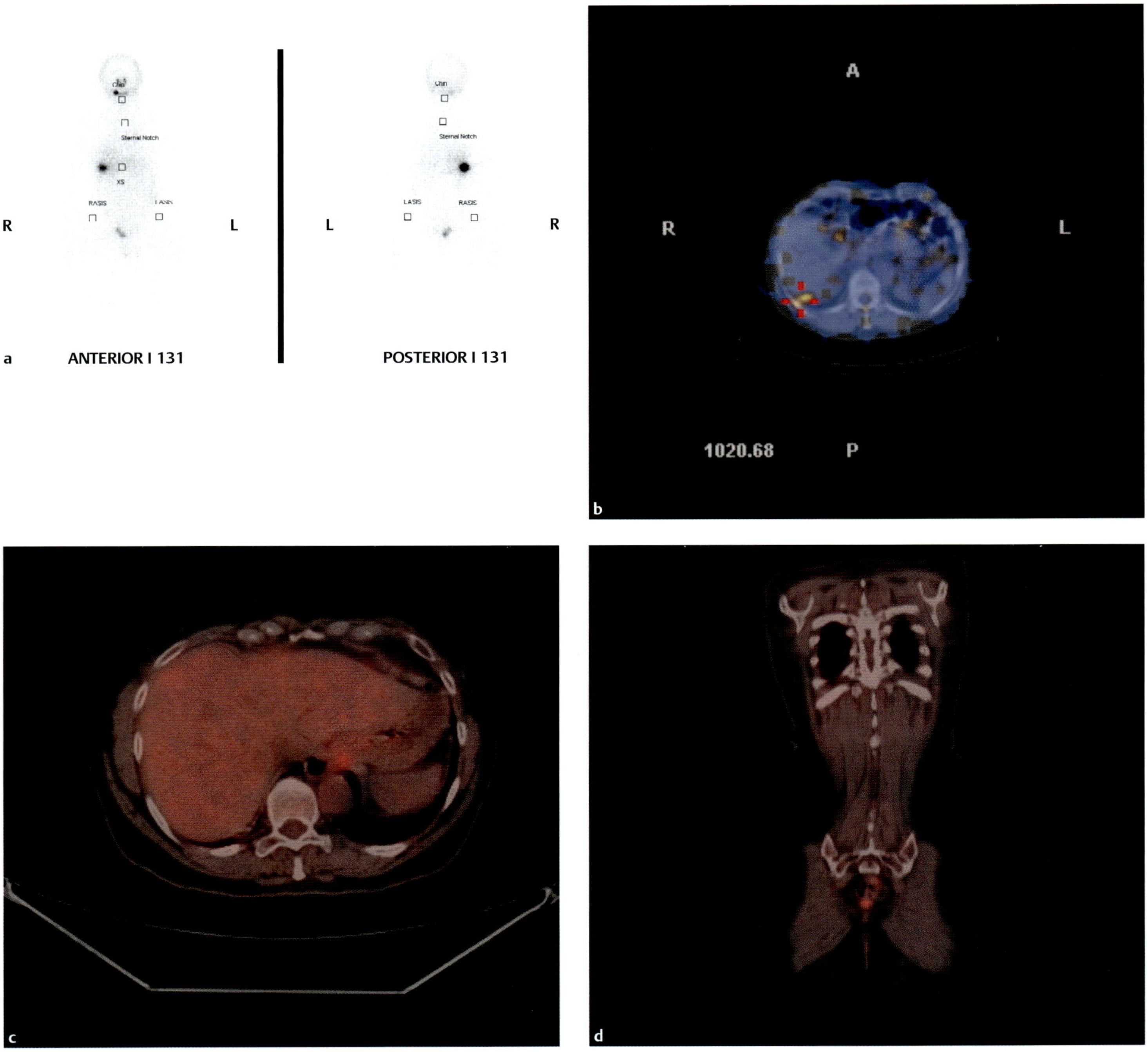

Fig. 3.37a–d Well-differentiated thyroid cancer with flip-flop phenomenon: right posterior rib recurrence.

a I-131 planar scan image is positive.
b Fused SPECT-CT is positive.
c Axial FDG PET-CT image is negative.
d Coronal FDG PET-CT image is negative.

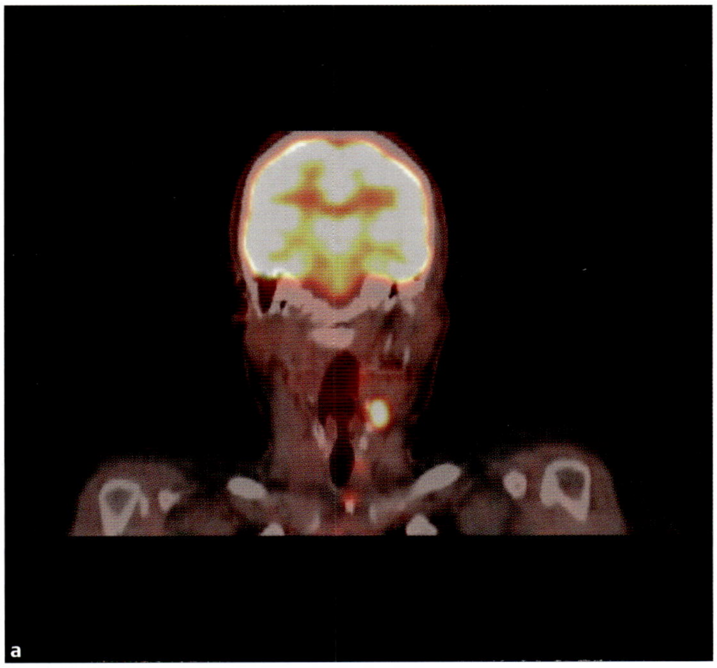

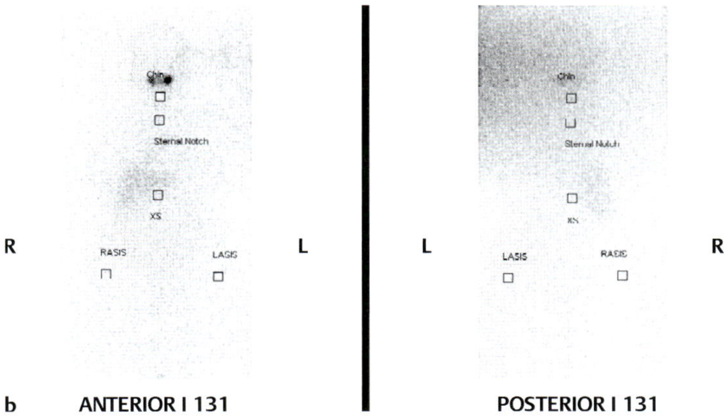

Fig. 3.38a, b Thyroid with flip-flop phenomenon: right neck recurrence in the lower left neck.
a Coronal FDG PET-CT images are positive.
b I-131 anterior and posterior planar images are negative.

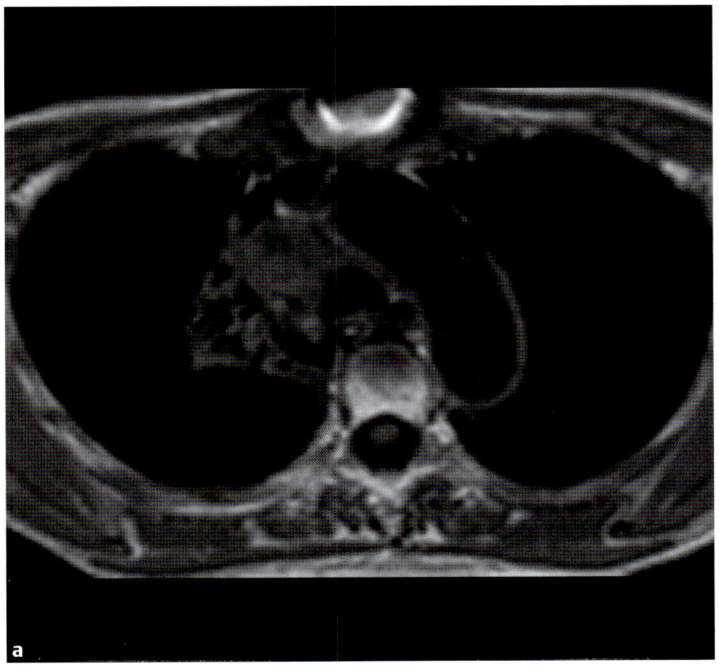

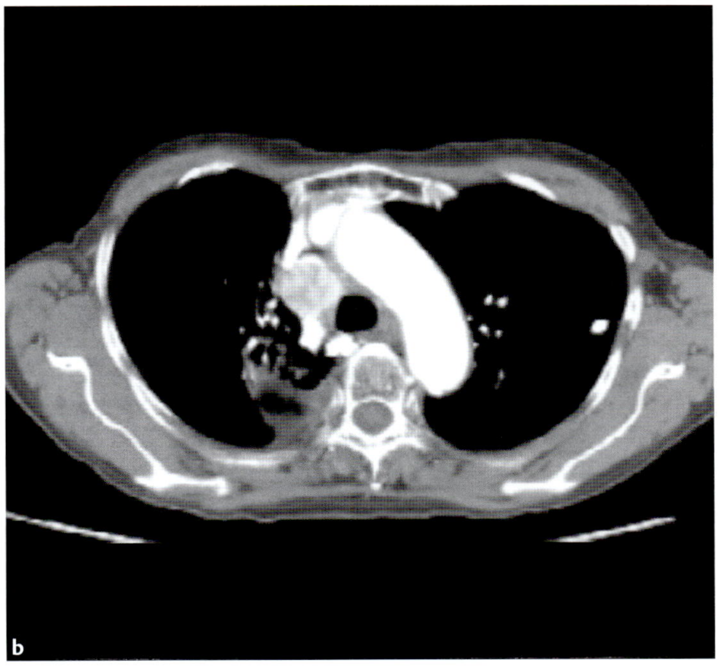

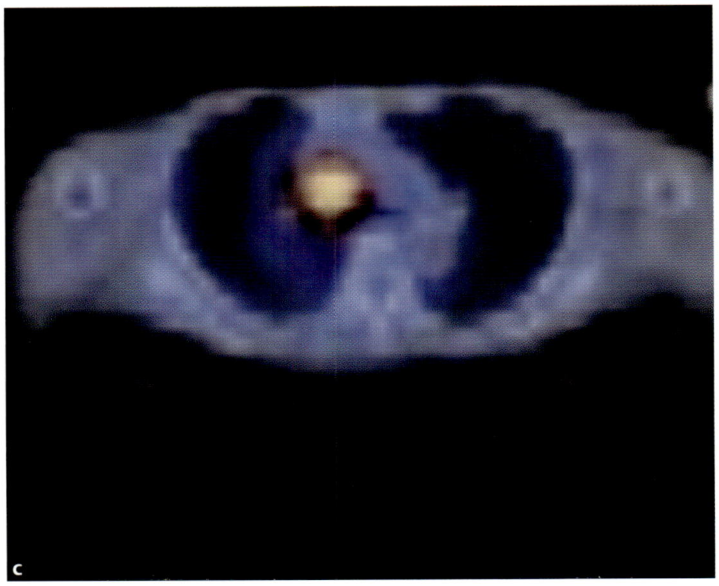

Fig. 3.39a–c Mediastinal recurrence in a 74-year-old woman with a family history of hyperparathyroidism and four previous operations for hyperparathyroidsm. Patient has suspected multiple endocrine neoplasia I (MENI).
a Axial T1-weighted MRI, with fat-suppression and contrast.
b Axial contrast-enhanced CT.
c In-111-labeled octreotide fused axial SPECT-CT.

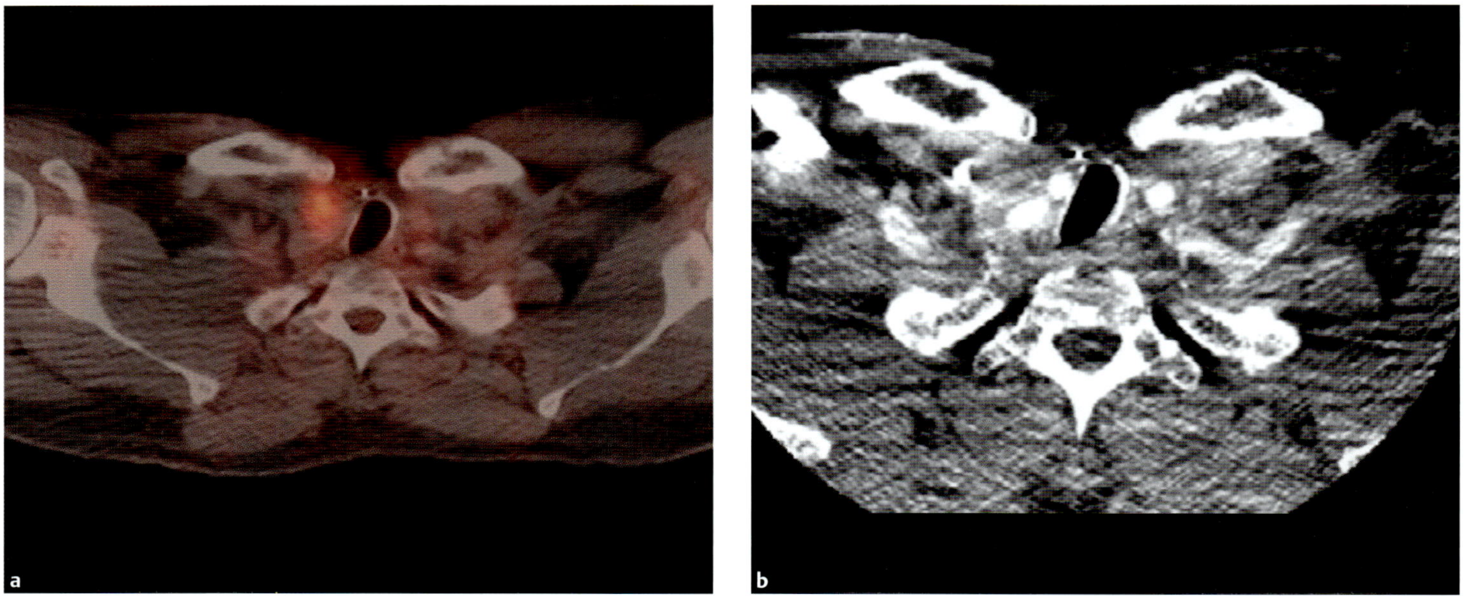

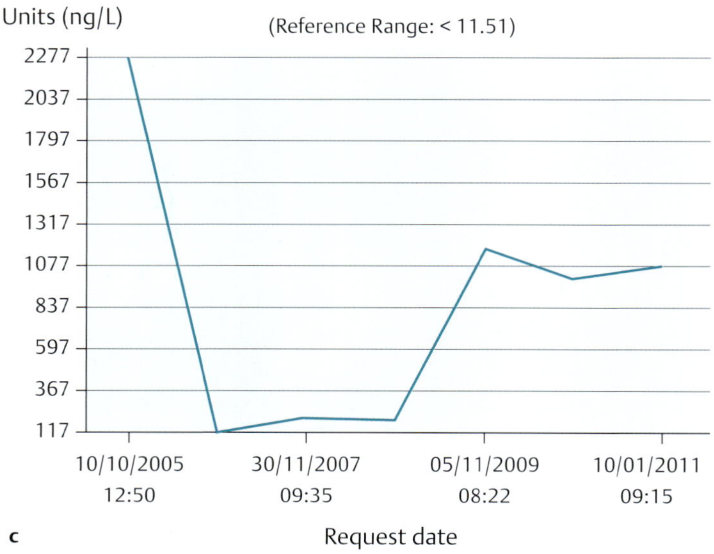

Fig. 3.40a–c Right thyroid bed recurrence in a 39-year-old man with known medullary thyroid carcinoma. He has a history of multiple operations and chemoradiotherapy 2 years before the scans. He re-presents with persistently rising serum calcitonin levels. Although the scar tissue seen in the right thyroid bed demonstrated no interval increase on serial MRI and CT, the focal increased metabolic uptake on FDG is in keeping with recurrence.
a Axial CT.
b Axial FDG PET-CT.
c Graphical representation of rising serum calcitonin.

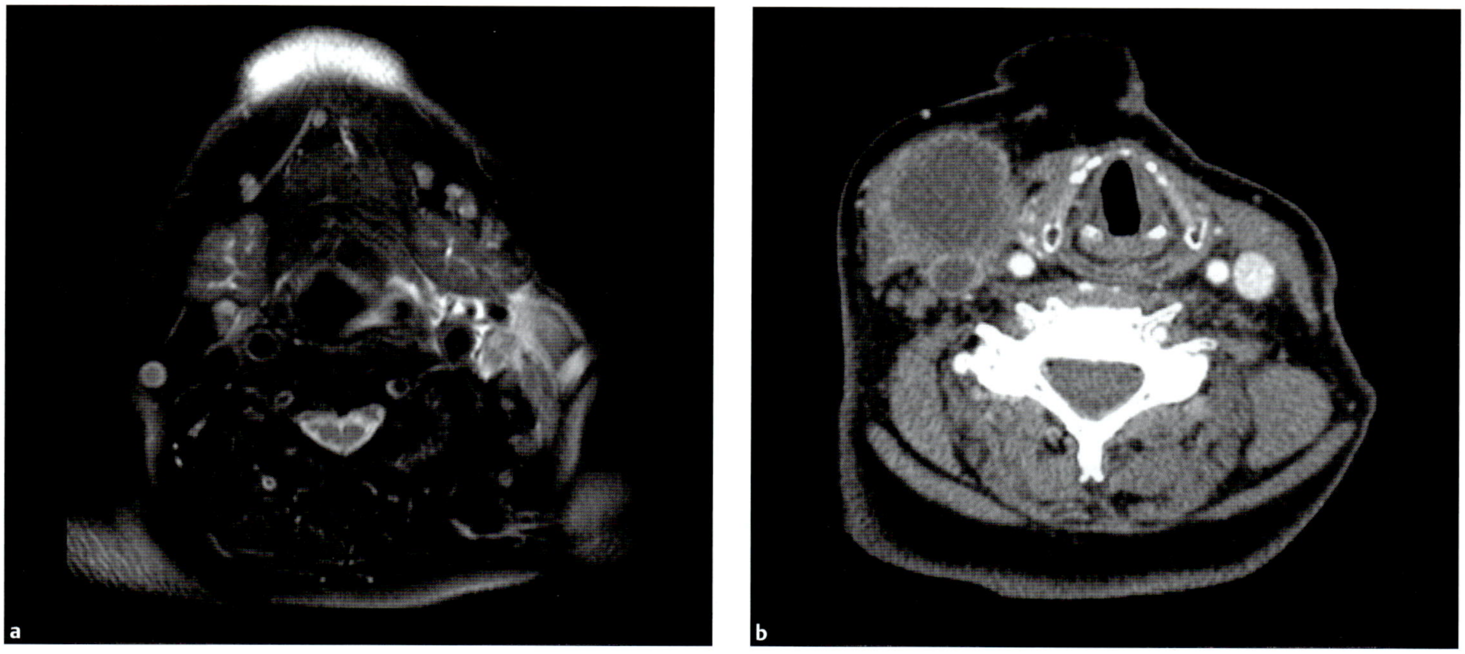

Fig. 3.41a, b Recurrent carcinoma with cervical adenopathy.
a Axial T2-weighted MR images of recurrent carcinoma with left cervical adenopathy and gross extracapsular extension of tumor.
b Axial CT scan with right level III cervical nodal recurrence. Note the indistinct margins and extranodal haziness which are indicative of extracapsular spread.

■ Medullary Thyroid Carcinoma

Medullary thyroid carcinoma (MTC) makes up 3%–12% of all thyroid malignancies. MTC originates from the parafollicular cells (or C cells), which are of neural crest origin and thus act as neuroendocrine tumors.[57] These highly functional tumors secrete carcinoembryogenic antigen (CEA) as well as calcitonin and express serotonin receptors. Most MTC recurrences present as occult tumors. Consequently, ultrasound is useful in detecting local and neck recurrence. CT is also helpful in detecting recurrences in the neck, chest, abdomen, and pelvis but has reduced sensitivity in scar tissue. MRI is useful in detecting recurrences in the neck, liver, and spine.

The fusion of single-photon emission computed tomography (SPECT) with CT allows improved localization of neuroendocrine tumors in general,[58] resulting in a change in diagnostic interpretation in a third of cases and altered patient management in 14% of cases. This same technique is applied to radionuclide sestamibi scanning for improved localization of parathyroid lesions.[59] Selective venous catheterization for serum calcitonin estimation has a sensitivity reaching 89% and may help detect occult recurrences.[60]

■ Lymph Node Extracapsular Spread

The lymph node status is an important prognostic factor in squamous tumors of the head and neck.[61] Additionally, the presence of extracapsular spread on imaging has both therapeutic and prognostic implications and should be conveyed to clinicians.[61,62] The detection of macroscopic extracapsular spread is based on the presence of spiky contours or irregular lymph node margins, the loss of fat planes around the lymph nodes, and the blurring and thickening of nearby fascial planes. Other features include a suggestion of infiltration of nearby structures such as the sternocleidomastoid muscle and the internal jugular vein. These features may be demonstrated on CT and MRI (**Fig. 3.41**), ultrasonography, and FDG PET-CT.[63] Lymph nodes with extracapsular spread generally demonstrate higher levels of metabolic activity as depicted by demonstrably higher mean standardized uptake values (SUV_{max}).[64] This is clearly illustrated by the fact that, in patients with oral cavity squamous cell carcinoma and pathologically positive lymph nodes, an SUV_{max} of 5.7 within lymph nodes, either alone or in combination with extracapsular spread, is an important independent prognostic factor for the 5-year disease-free survival, disease-specific survival, and overall survival.[65] In borderline-sized nodes, it can be hard to tell malignant nodes from reactive nodes, but the presence of extracapsular spread or necrosis is a helpful distinguishing factor indicating the presence of malignancy.[66]

Retropharyngeal lymphadenopathy is clinically silent and only detectable on cross-sectional imaging. These patients are particularly at risk for regional recurrence, resulting in worse disease-free survival, and therefore these nodes must be accounted for in treatment plans.[67] MRI is more accurate than CT for retropharyngeal adenopathy and PET-CT may not detect necrotic nodes and those of less than 5 mm (**Fig. 3.42**).[68,69] A short-axis diameter above 6 mm and abnormal enhancement patterns and central necrosis on either CT or MRI, as well as marked uptake on PET-CT, are usually indicators of retropharyngeal adenopathy.[70]

Four percent of head and neck malignancies present as metastatic lymph nodes where the primary remains unknown, with squamous cell carcinoma accounting for 80% of these lesions.[71] PET-CT is able to detect just under a quarter of primary tumor sites after negative endoscopy and anatomical imaging techniques, remaining negative in just over 75% of cases.[72] The occult primary site may eventually reveal itself years later after treatment (**Fig. 3.43**).[73]

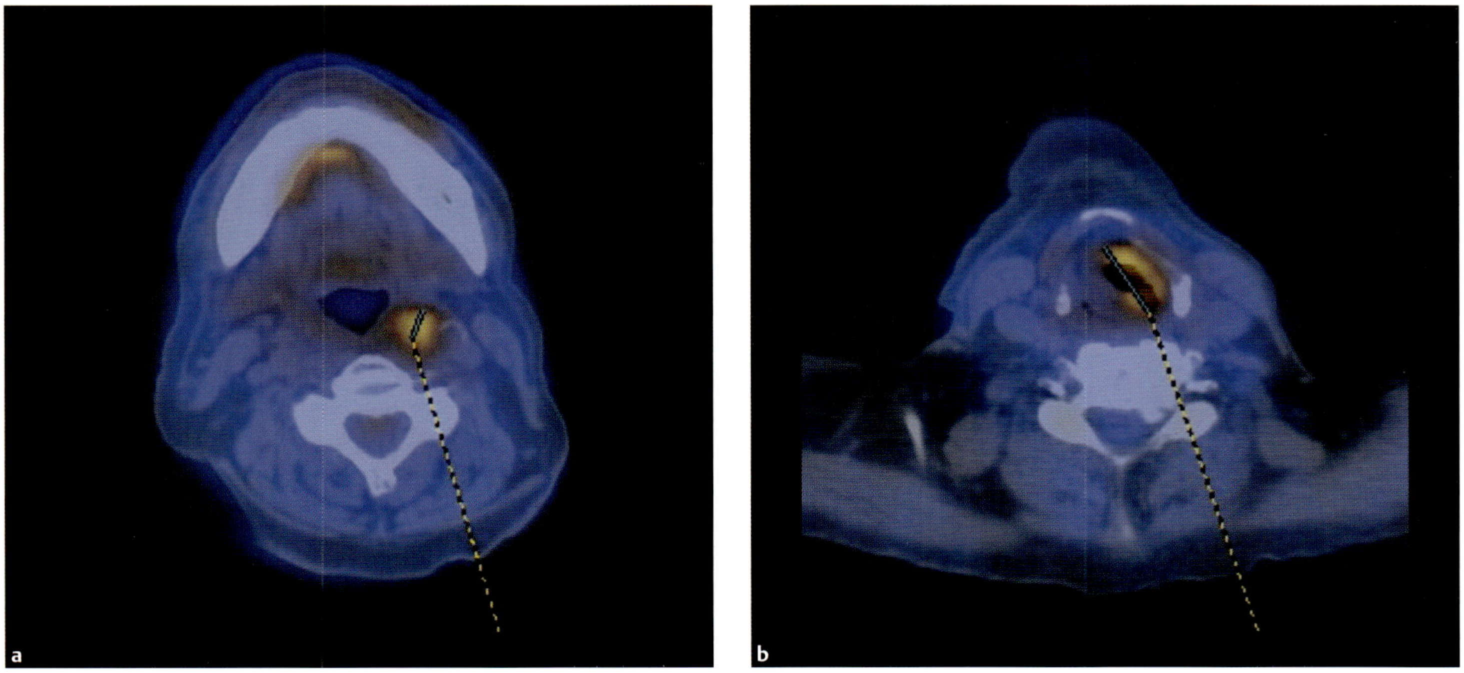

Fig. 3.42a, b Axial FDG PET-CT images of a markedly avid supraglottic tumor and left retropharyngeal lymph node with residual malignancy following chemoradiotherapy.

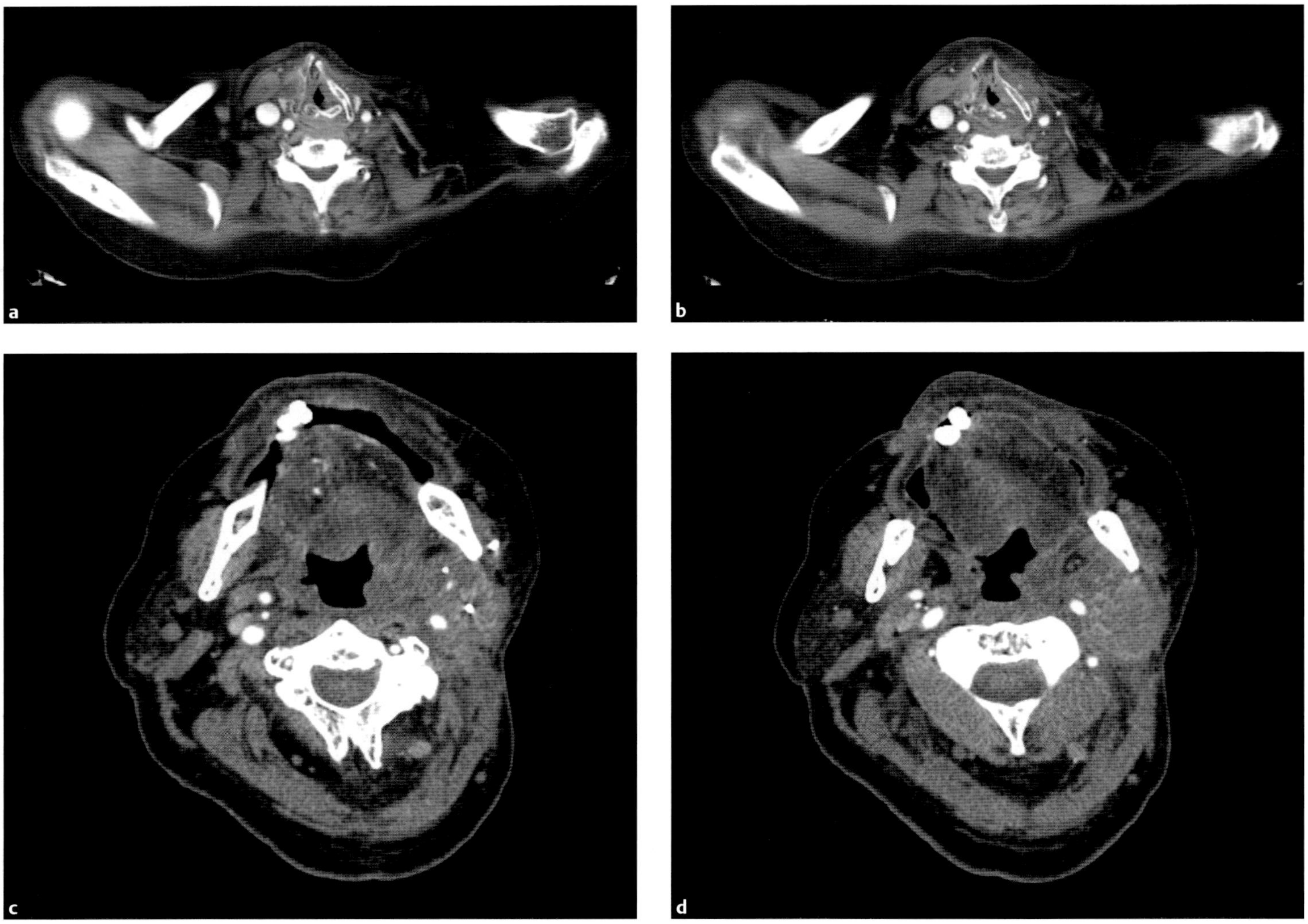

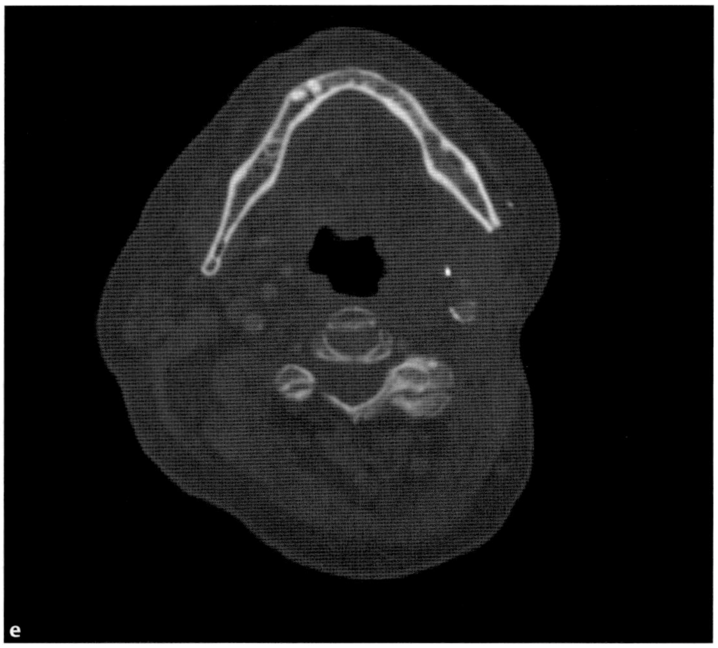

Fig. 3.43a–h A 67-year-old man with recurrent carcinoma of the larynx with extensive metastatic disease in the left parotid and neck resulting in left internal jugular vein invasion. There has been prior radical neck dissection, superficial parotidectomy, resection of mandible and flap pectoralis major myocutaneous. Note the left-sided trapezius muscle atrophy due to previous left level V block dissection and spinal accessory nerve sacrifice.
a–e Axial contrast-enhanced CT images.

Fig. 3.43f–h ►

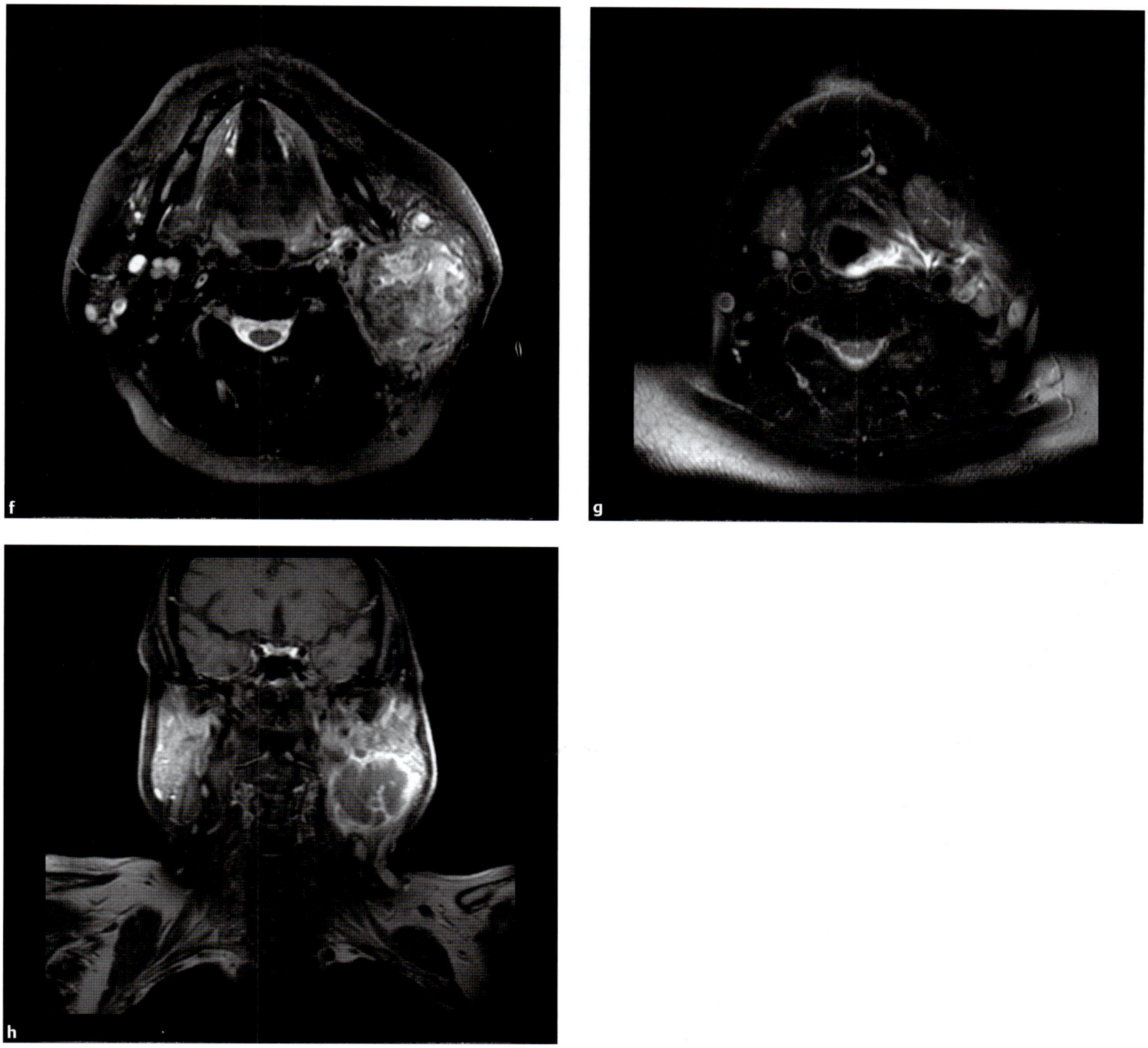

Fig. 3.43f–h
f, g Axial T2-weighted MR images.
h Coronal T1-weighted, postcontrast image.

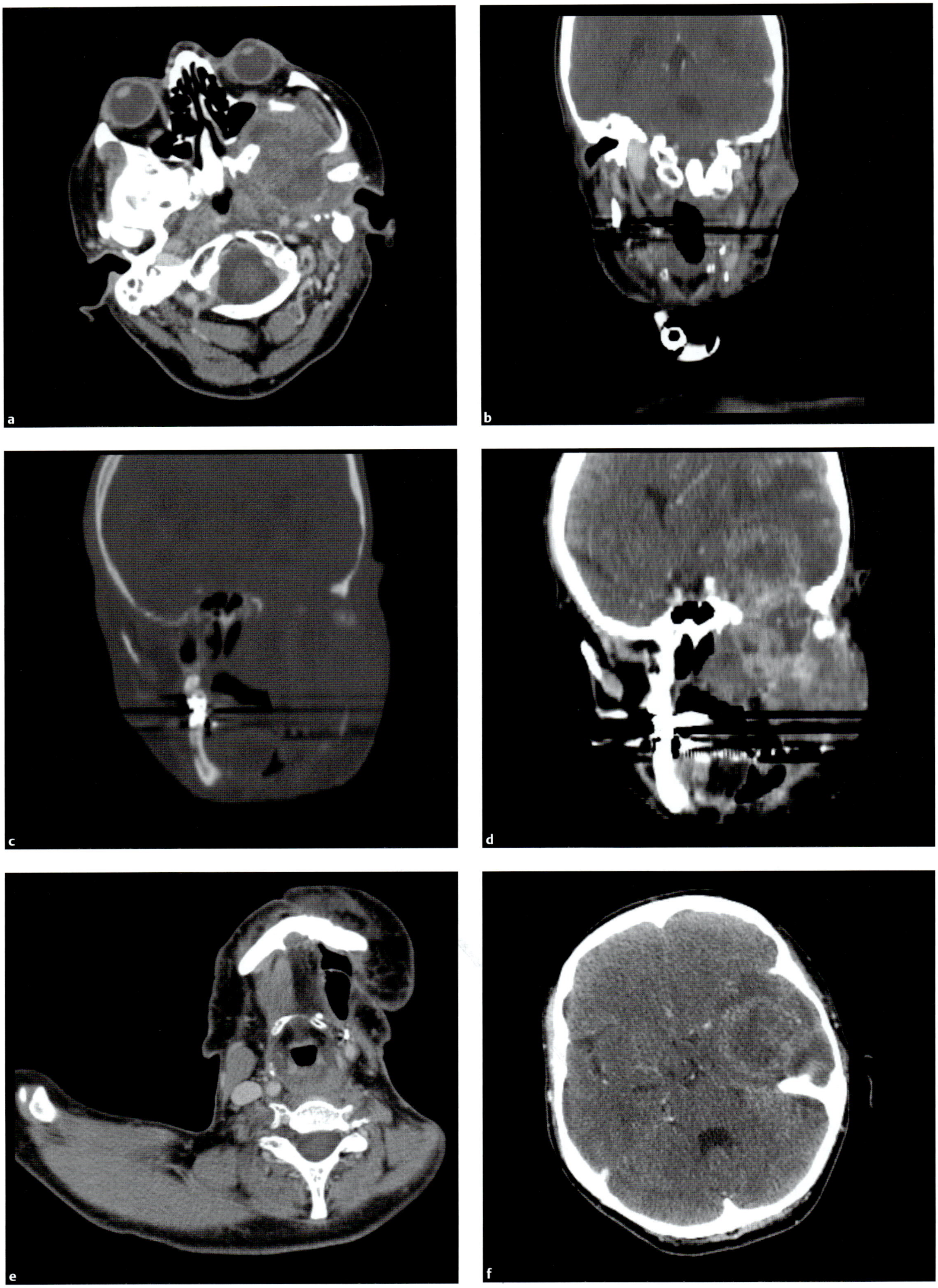
a
b
c
d
e
f

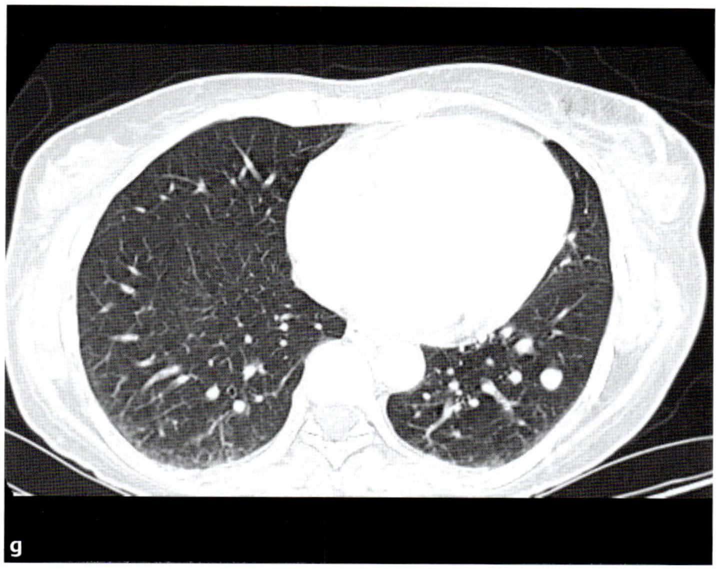

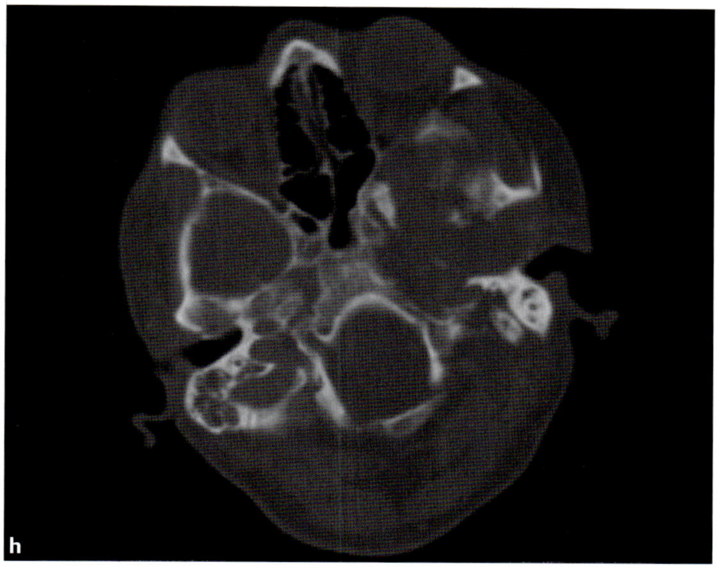

◄ ▲ **Fig. 3.44a–h** A 49-year-old woman with previous resection, flap, and adjuvant radiotherapy. The axial and coronal CT images demonstrate left infratemporal recurrence and posterior auricular lymph nodal recurrence. There is skull base erosion and intracranial invasion of this malignantly transformed neurofibroma as well as pulmonary metastasis. Histology (not shown) demonstrates malignant peripheral nerve sheath sarcoma on a background of neurofibroma.

Skull Base Invasion

Skull base infiltration may occur from below or from above. There are different degrees of skull base invasion, i.e., minor erosion, minor involvement of anterior and posterior cranial nerves, involvement of both anterior and posterior cranial nerves, and intracranial invasion. This occurs because neck tumors that infiltrate the skull base can result in dural infiltration and ultimately parenchymal involvement.[74] Foraminal invasion occurs more easily compared with direct erosion. CT and MRI play complementary roles in skull base invasion (**Fig. 3.44**) and their combination may be required to define the full extent of disease.[75]

Perineural Spread in Head and Neck Malignancy

Perineural spread refers to the gross macroscopic retrograde or antegrade extension of tumor cells along nerve sheaths. This spread occurs through the endoneurium, perineurium, or perineural lymphatics.[76,77] In contrast, perineural invasion refers to the microscopic finding of tumor cells encasing tiny nerve branches and cannot be demonstrated radiologically (**Fig. 3.45**). Although both may result in similar symptoms, perineural spread is a macroscopic feature which may be diagnosed radiologically and perineural invasion is a histopathological diagnosis.[76,77] Clinically, approximately slightly less than half of patients with perineural spread may be symptom free or present with nonspecific symptoms.[76] Alternatively, they may demonstrate clinical features related to the specific cranial nerve branch involved. Pain is a frequent feature with involvement of the trigeminal nerve; this may spread sequentially from the more peripheral branches to central branches.[78] Paresthesia, anesthesia, dysesthesia, and formication may also manifest in the various nerve distributions. Motor weakness may be encountered as lower motor facial weakness when cranial nerve VII is involved or as masticator muscle weakness when V3 is implicated.[76] Total ophthalmoplegia is a crucial pointer to the possible presence of perineural spread in the cavernous sinus.

Perineural tumor spread in the head and neck region occurs most commonly in the trunk and various terminal branches of divisions of the trigeminal nerve, particularly V2 and V3, as well as the facial nerve (VII). Tumor may also involve the pterygopalatine ganglion as well as spread between the facial (**Fig. 3.46**) and trigeminal divisions via the auriculotemporal nerve, vidian nerve (nerve of the pterygoid canal), and the greater (superficial) petrosal nerve.[79] Spread between cranial nerves may present as multiple cranial neuropathy. Other head and neck tumor–related causes of multiple cranial neuropathies include leptomeningeal spread and cavernous sinus involvement.[76,79] The head and neck malignancies that are most likely to demonstrate perineural spread are squamous cell carcinoma, adenoid cystic carcinoma (**Fig. 3.47**), and melanoma (usually of the desmoplastic type).[80]

It is generally accepted that contrast-enhanced MRI is considered more sensitive than other cross-sectional imaging modalities for demonstrating perineural tumor spread.[77,81] However, FDG PET-CT underestimates perineural tumor spread.[82,83] PET-CT may demonstrate perineural spread when MRI is contraindicated, such as in patients with cardiac pacemakers and implanted cardioverter-defibrillators.

A good understanding of cranial nerve anatomy is important to facilitate the detection of perineural tumor spread while it may still be potentially curable. The detection of perineural spread on imaging may result in a change of outcome and allows alteration of treatment planning.[84] Regardless of the type of cross-sectional modality employed, particular attention should be paid to the anatomy of the facial nerve as well as the three divisions of the Trigeminal nerve (V1, V2, V3) as well as interconnecting nerves that pass between the facial, mandibular and maxillary nerves, i.e., the auriculotemporal, greater superficial petrosal, and vidian nerves (**Figs. 3.48–3.52**).

Plain radiographs such as the orthopantomogram can demonstrate perineural spread in the inferior alveolar nerve.[85] On MRI, perineural spread appears as nerve thickening and abnormal nerve enhancement on fat-suppressed T1-weighted MRI sequences as well as obliteration of perineural fat on T1-weighted sequences and foraminal widening.[79,81,86] Foraminal widening and cortical destruction are features of perineural spread that are elegantly demonstrated on CT and hence comparison with the contralateral side is important.[81,86] Ipsilateral muscle atrophy such as in masticator muscles, cavernous sinus enlargement, and replacement of the trigeminal subarachnoid cistern with soft tissue are other features demonstrated on MRI and CT.

FDG PET-CT combines anatomical CT and functional PET data subsets. Imaging features of perineural spread on PET-CT therefore include CT characteristics of perineural spread as well as PET features that include abnormal linear increased metabolic activity corresponding with the known nerve anatomy or foramina.[87,88] Perineural spread may also be inferred from the mode of spread or linear increased metabolic activity along the path of the evaluated nerve[89] or the associated CT findings of obliteration of perineural fat or all of the methods.[79] Imaging findings should be correlated with clinical features such as facial weakness and numbness. High

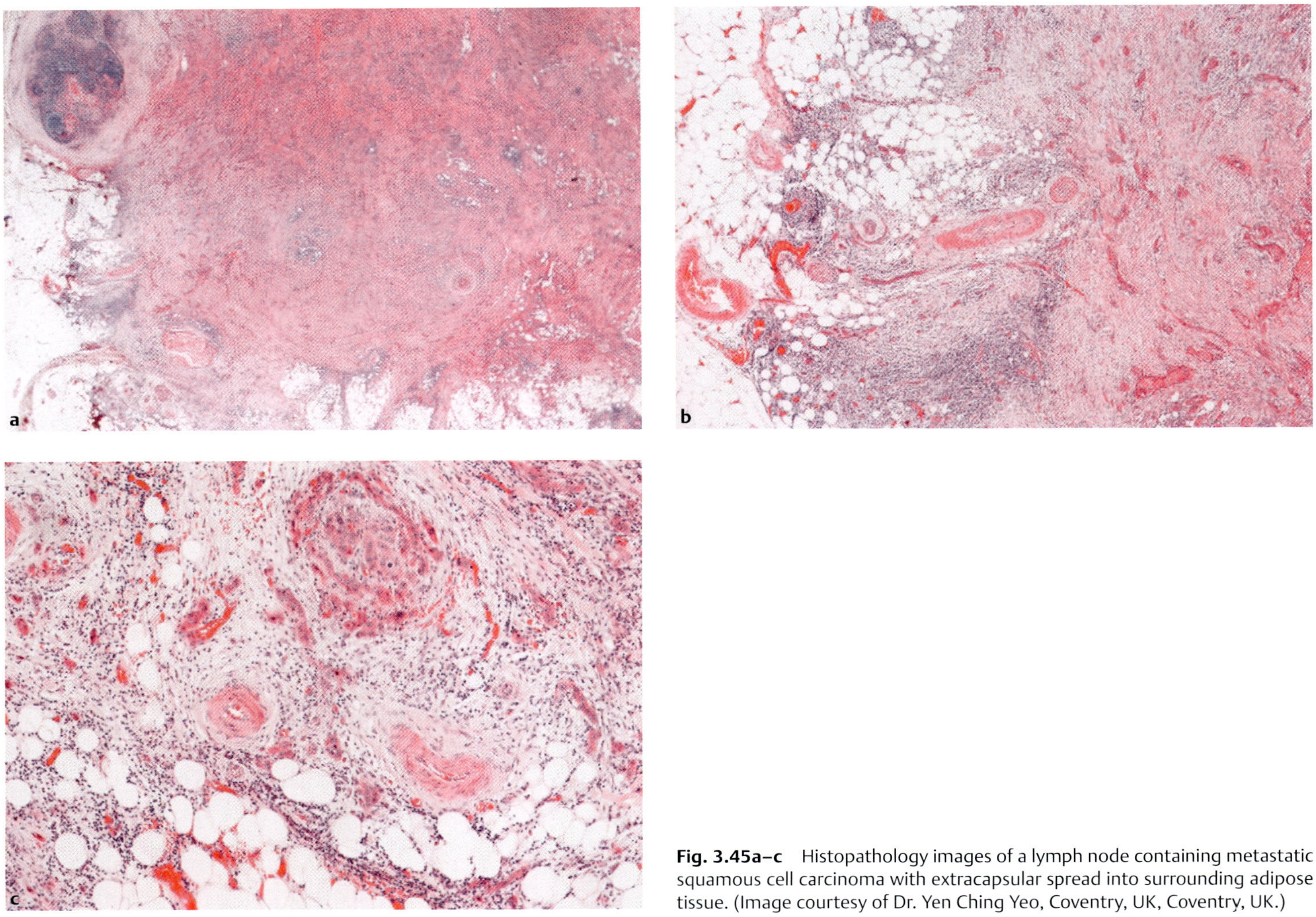

Fig. 3.45a–c Histopathology images of a lymph node containing metastatic squamous cell carcinoma with extracapsular spread into surrounding adipose tissue. (Image courtesy of Dr. Yen Ching Yeo, Coventry, UK, Coventry, UK.)

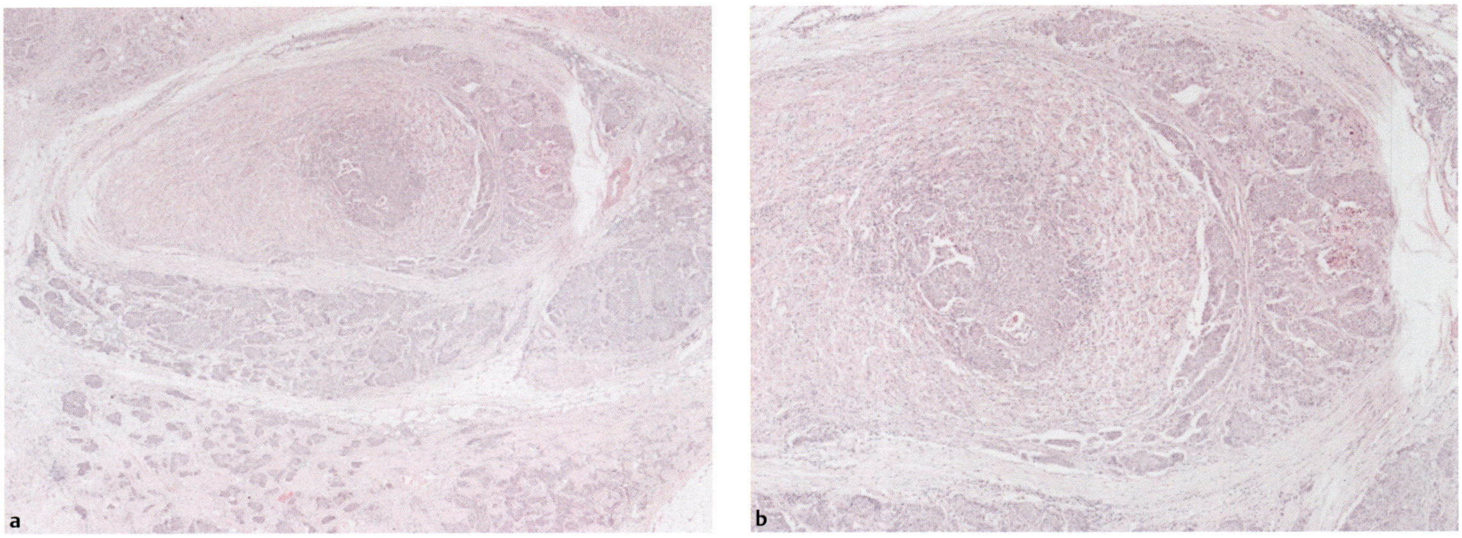

Fig. 3.46a, b Histopathology images of invasive squamous cell carcinoma involving facial nerve with invasion into the perineurium and endoneurium. (Image courtesy of Dr. Yen Ching Yeo, Coventry, UK.)

tumor volume, density, vascularity, and favorable histology such as adenoid cystic carcinoma, squamous cell carcinoma, and melanoma[80,83] lead to higher sensitivity, but sensitivity is lower in the region of the skull base due to relatively marked background uptake in the brain.[83]

Anatomy of Cranial Nerves V and VII

The trigeminal ganglion is located in the so-called Meckel cave, a dural enclosure between the anterior pons and the cavernous sinus. Two of its three divisions, V1 (ophthalmic) and V2 (maxillary), carry on forward into the cavernous sinus, while the third division, the V3 (mandibular) nerve, exits the skull base inferiorly through foramen ovale.

V1 courses through the cavernous sinus and via the superior ophthalmic fissure into the orbit. The three branches of V1 (sensory) are the frontal, lacrimal, and nasociliary nerves, of which the lacrimal is smallest and the frontal is the largest. The lacrimal gland receives its sensory innervation from the lacrimal nerve.[89] The lacrimal nerve receives parasympathetic twigs from the facial nerve, via the greater superficial petrosal nerve; these nerve fibers hitchhike via V2, but documented spread along this path is rare.[76,90]

The maxillary nerve V2 is a sensory nerve to the sinuses, palate, and mid-facial region. V2 courses through the cavernous sinus and leaves the skull base via foramen rotundum into the pterygopalatine fossa in the infratemporal region.[76,90]

The mandibular nerve V3 is a mixed nerve (sensory and motor); the only trigeminal division that does not course through the cavernous sinus but exits the skull via the foramen ovale. Extracranially, it divides into anterior and posterior trunks, which are respectively mainly motor and mainly sensory. V3 sensory roots supply the lower third of the face, the preauricular skin, the mandibular teeth; the inferior alveolus, the floor of mouth, the oral tongue, and the buccal mucosa[76,90] via the auriculotemporal, inferior alveolar, and lingual nerves among others. The motor roots of V3 innervate the masticator muscles, the mylohyoid muscle, the anterior belly of the digastric muscle, and the tensor veli palatini muscle.[76,90]

The facial nerve is a motor nerve to the muscles of facial expression as well as a sensory nerve to the external auditory canal and concha of the pinna, taste from the anterior two-thirds of the tongue, parasympathetic to the lacrimal, submandibular salivary and sublingual salivary glands, and sympathetic vasomotor to the tongue and salivary glands.[89,90] Briefly, the cisternal segment facial nerve runs from the cerebellopontine angle to the porus acousticus of the internal auditory meatus (IAM). The labyrinthine segment runs laterally through the IAM in the superior and anterior portion and exits the IAM as the relatively short labyrinthine segment. After a 70° turn, it continues as the tympanic segment in the middle ear. The geniculate ganglion is located at the genu. The mastoid portion runs inferiorly in the facial recess and exits the skull base through the stylomastoid foramen and onwards into the parotid gland.[89,90]

There are several cross-connections between various cranial nerves. Distal branches of divisions of the trigeminal nerve act as pathways for branches of other cranial nerves, especially the facial (seventh cranial) nerve.[76,90] The greater superficial petrosal nerve (GSPN) is a branch of the facial nerve that arises at the geniculate ganglion[76,91] and runs anteriorly into the middle cranial fossa. It merges with the deep petrosal nerve to form the vidian (pterygoid) nerve which runs through the vidian canal located in the sphenoidal sinus wall. The vidian nerve carries on forward and inferiorly to the pterygopalatine ganglion and hence postganglionic fibers merge with V2 and ultimately supply the palate, nasopharynx, and lacrimal gland.[76] The path of the GSPN runs close to the Meckel cave and hence tumor could extend from the gasserian ganglion to the GSPN.[76] Other interconnections include the chorda tympani branch of the mastoid segment of the facial nerve, which sends fibers to the lingual nerve, a sensory branch of V3.[90]

The auriculotemporal nerve, a branch of the posterior division of the mandibular nerve also provides small branches to the facial nerve.[79]

■ In-transit Metastasis

In-transit metastasis is a unique manifestation of intralymphatic tumor dissemination characterized by satellite deposits in cutaneous or subcutaneous tissue located between the primary tumor and the primary lymph node basin.[92,93] In-transit metastasis occurs in skin tumors such as melanoma, probably when cancer

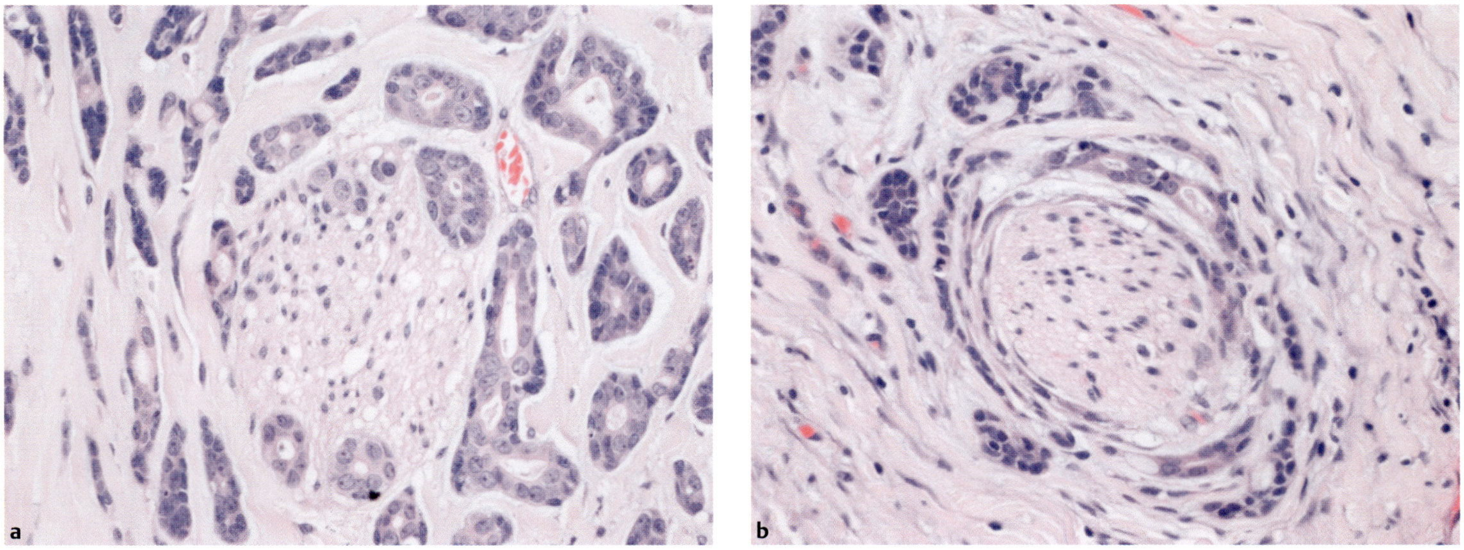

Fig. 3.47a, b Histopathology images of perineural spread in adenoid cystic carcinoma; ×40 magnification. (Image courtesy of Dr. Yen Ching Yeo, Coventry, UK.)

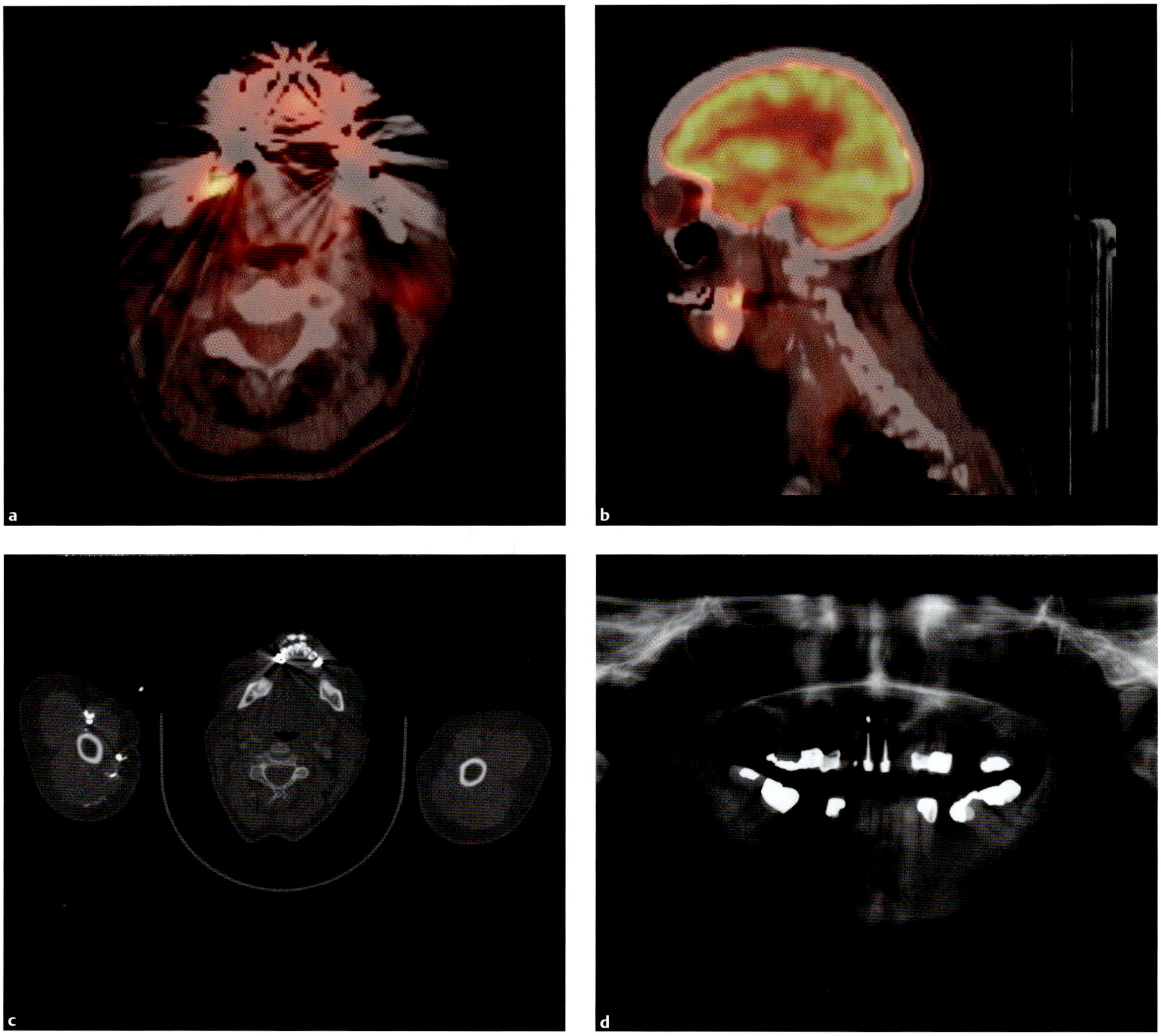

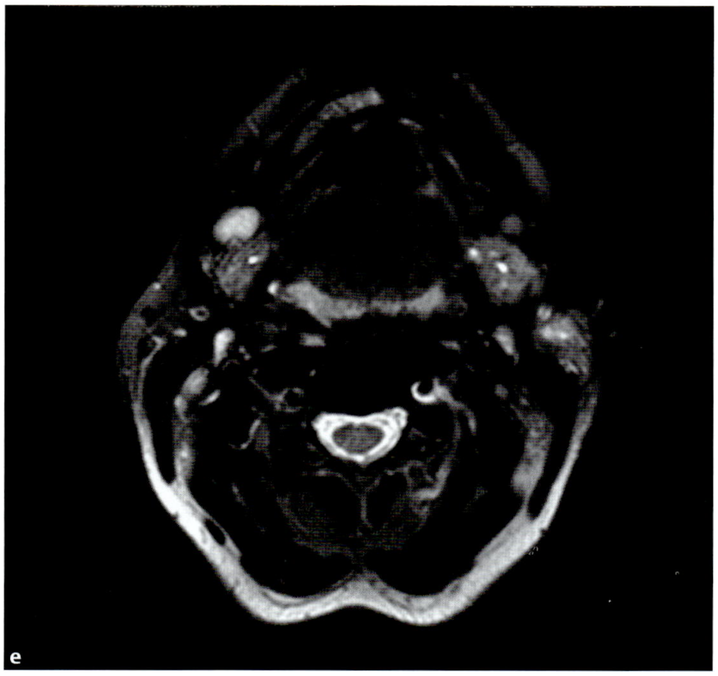

Fig. 3.48a–e Patient with grade 3 follicular lymphoma with perineural involvement of the right inferior alveolar nerve.
a Axial FDG PET-CT.
b Sagittal FDG PET-CT. Marked linear increased uptake along the course of the right inferior alveolar nerve (slight misregistration artifact as well as CT beam-hardening is seen). Further incidental pleomorphic adenoma is noted in the left parotid gland.
c Axial contrast-enhanced CT demonstrates widening of the right mandibular canal.
d Orthopantomogram with clear asymmetry between the right and left.
e T2-weighted axial MRI of perineural spread in right inferior dental nerve with increased signal in the anterior mandible on the right.

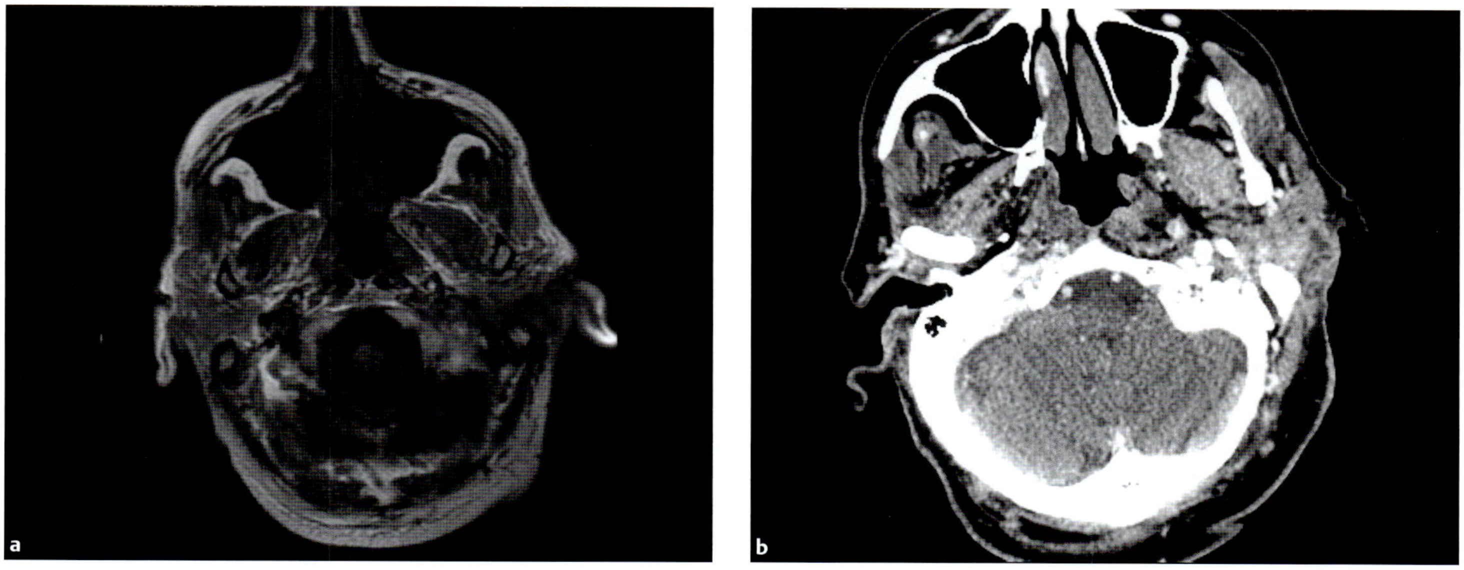

Fig. 3.49a, b Perineural spread from recurrent aggressive squamous cell carcinoma. Note the replacement of fat just inferior to the left stylomastoid foramen implying extension into the infratemporal segment of the left facial nerve. **a** Axial T1-weighted MR image. **b** Axial contrast-enhanced CT image.

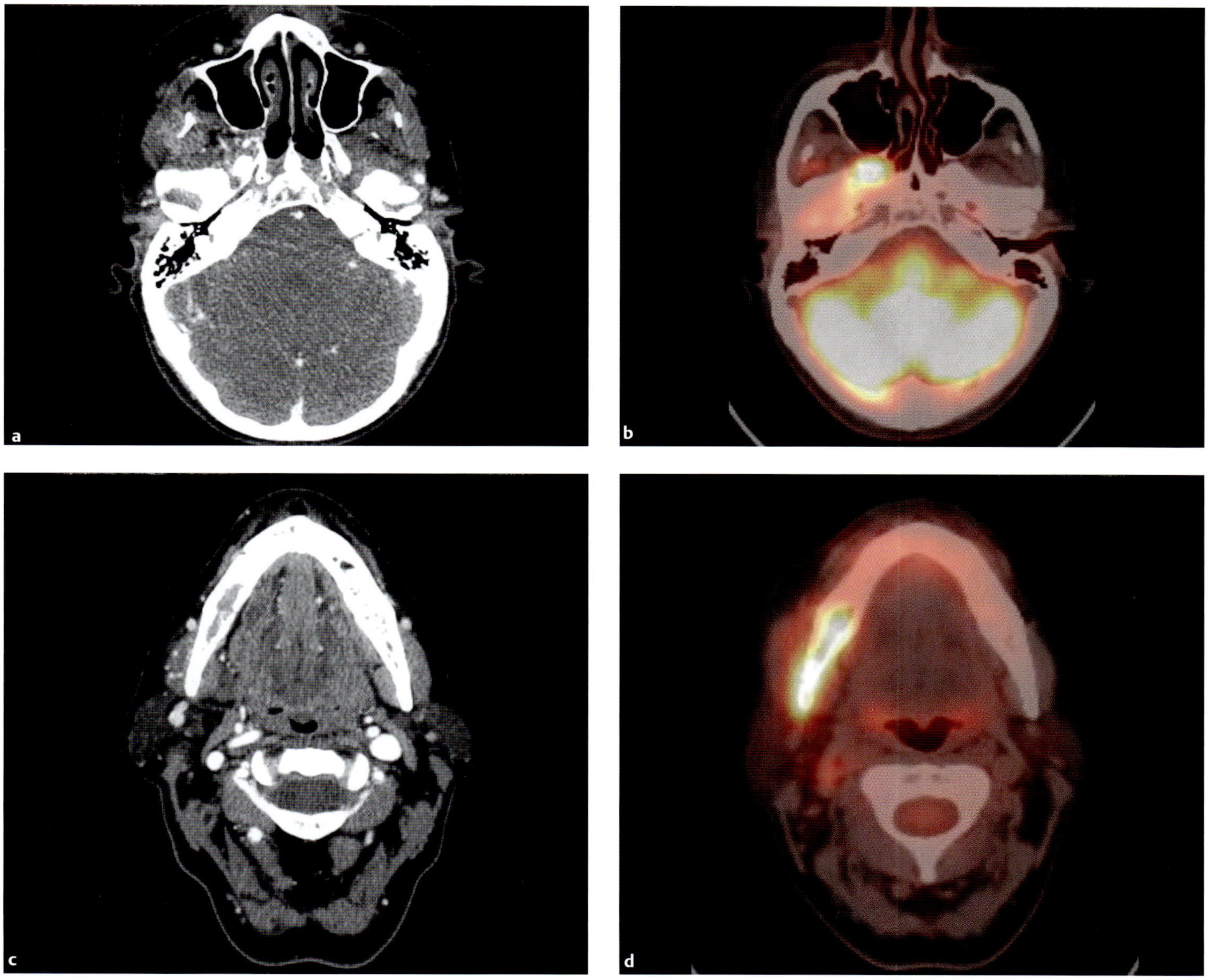

Fig. 3.50a–d A 58-year-old woman with advanced breast carcinoma with perineural spread. **a** Axial contrast-enhanced CT image with mandibular canal widening due to perineural spread into the right inferior dental nerve. **b** Axial FDG PET-CT image with marked linear uptake with perineural spread into the right inferior dental nerve. **c** Axial CT image demonstrates widening of the right pterygopalatine fossa due to perineural spread. **d** Axial FDG PET-CT image demonstrates marked uptake in the right pterygopalatine fossa due to perineural spread.

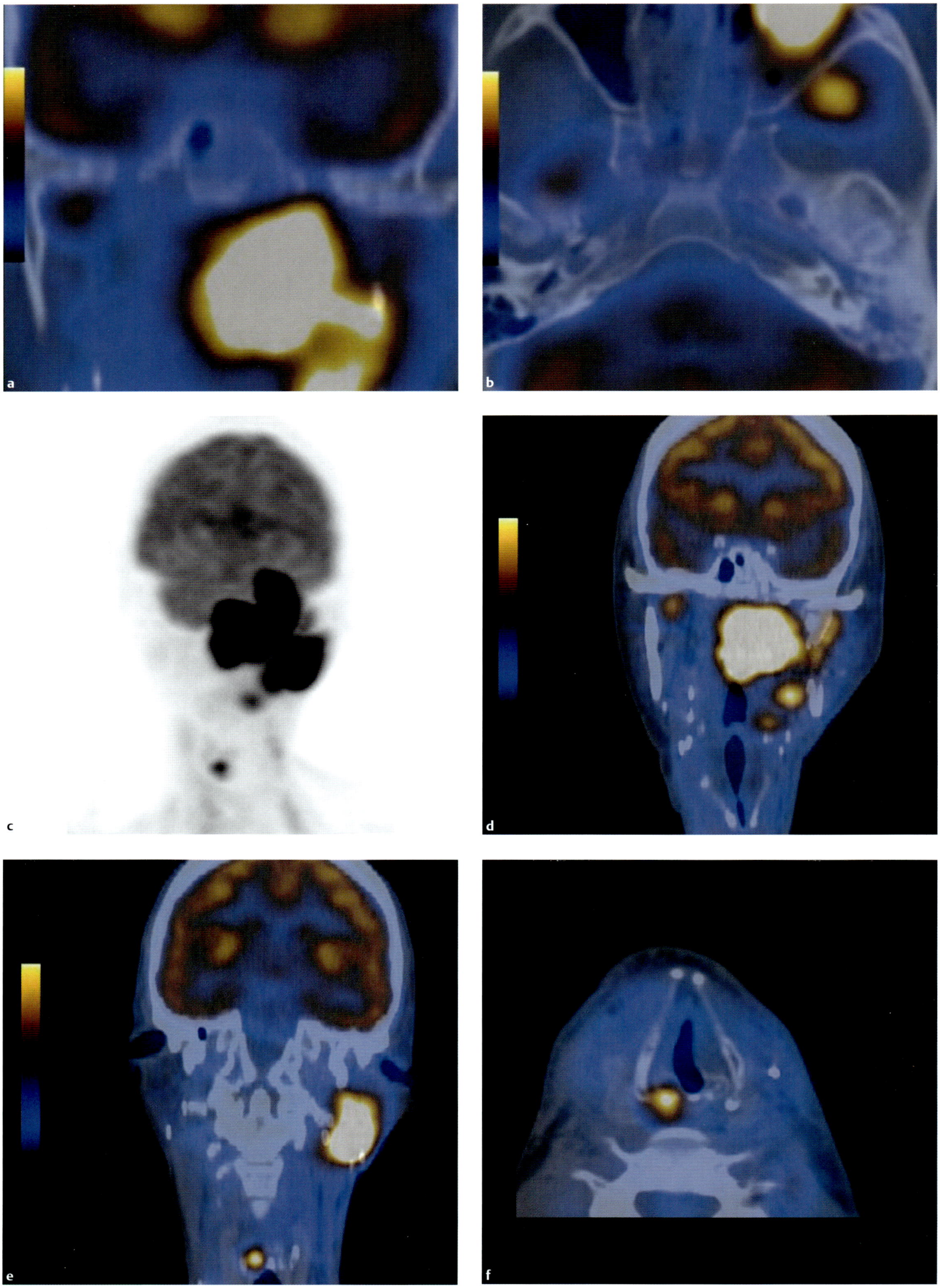

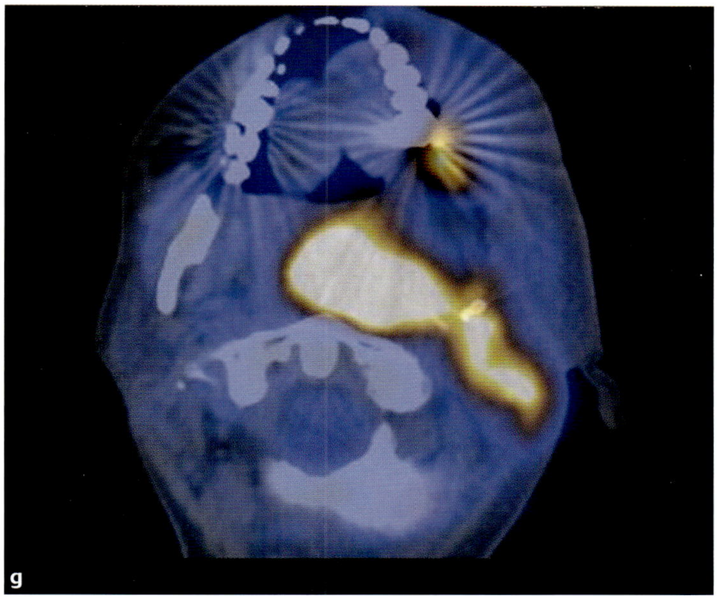

◂ **Fig. 3.51a–f** Previous T2N2 left tonsil SCC. Treated with surgical excision, neck dissection, free flap, as well as adjuvant chemoradiotherapy. Now presenting with left cranial nerve VII weakness and facial pain. FDG PET-CT demonstrating left maxillary recurrence with perineural spread toward foramen ovale as well as left parotid gland recurrence (auriculotemporal nerve).
a Coronal FDG PET-CT image.
b Axial FDG PET-CT image.
c, d Coronal FDG PET-CT images.
e, f Axial FDG PET-CT image.

▾ **Fig. 3.52a–d** A 54-year-old man with previous squamous cell carcinoma of the left parotid gland treated with resection, neck dissection, and free flap. He now has recurrence in the left lacrimal gland, which suggests perineural spread.
a Axial FDG PET-CT image.
b Axial contrast enhanced CT.
c Coronal FDG PET-CT image.
d Axial T2-weighted MR image with fat suppression.

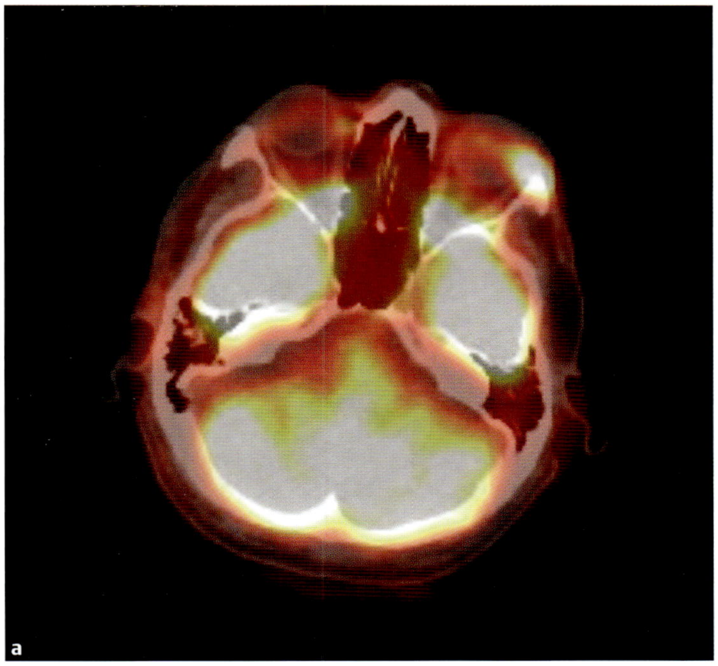

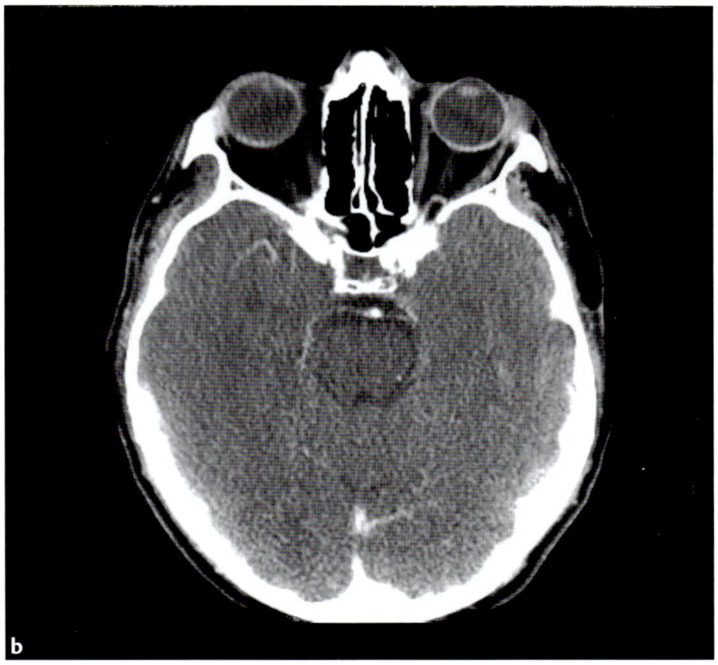

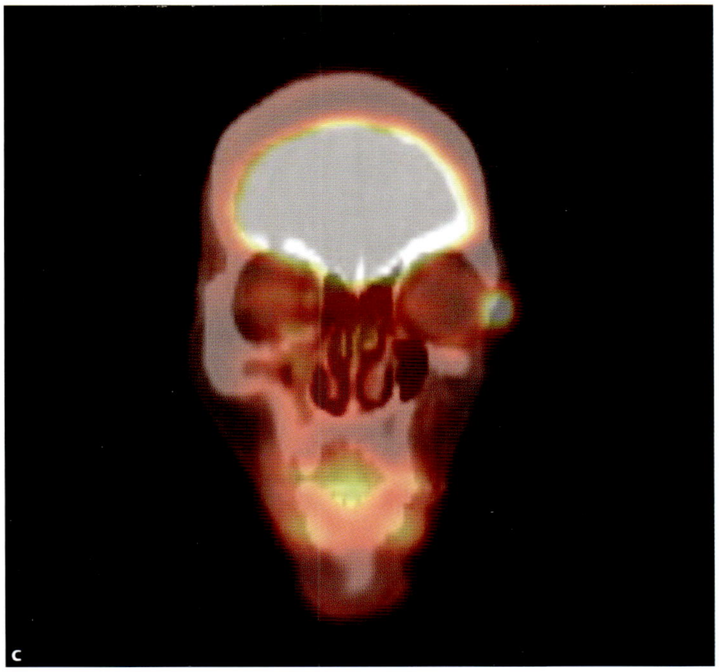

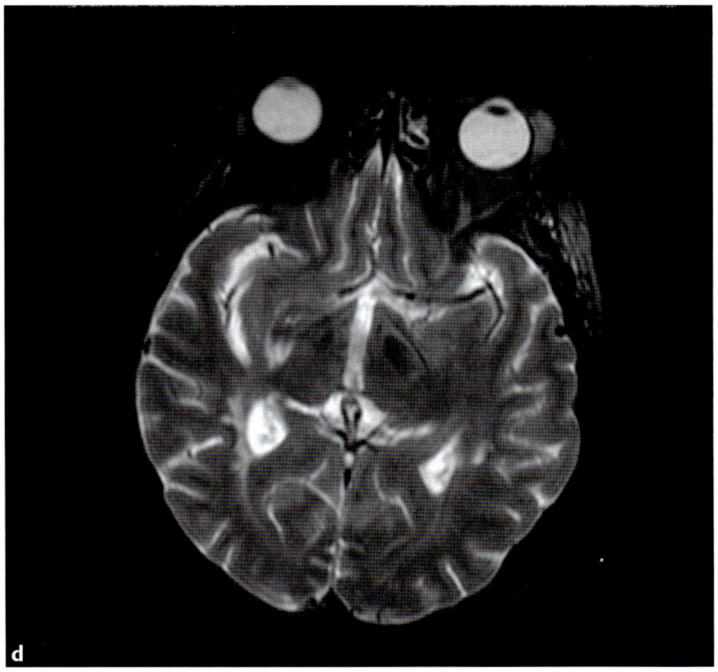

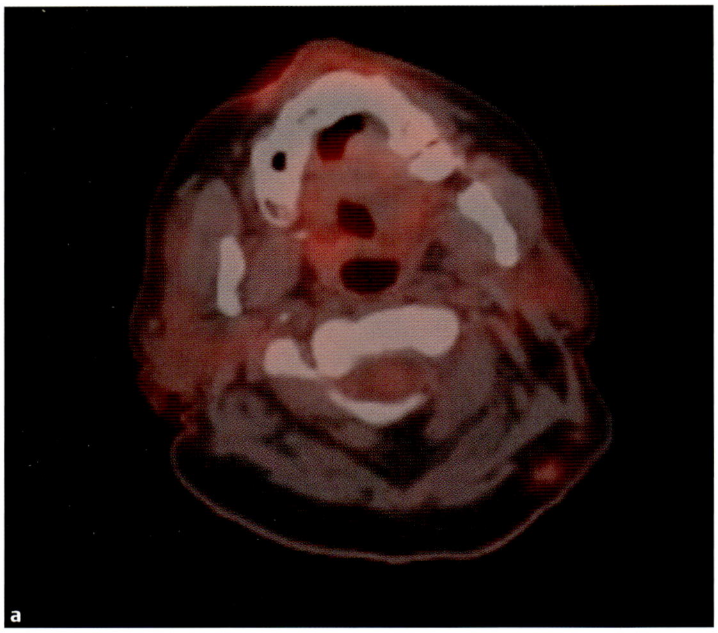

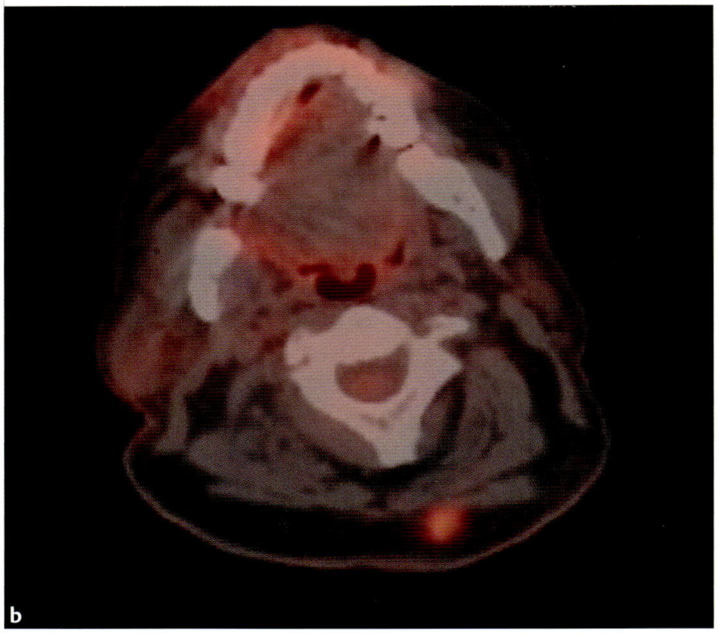

Fig. 3.53a, b History of clinically progressing, previously excised malignant melanoma of the back and left flank. Axial FDG PET-CT images demonstrate an FDG-avid posterior triangle subcutaneous metastasis and smaller in-transit metastatic deposits.

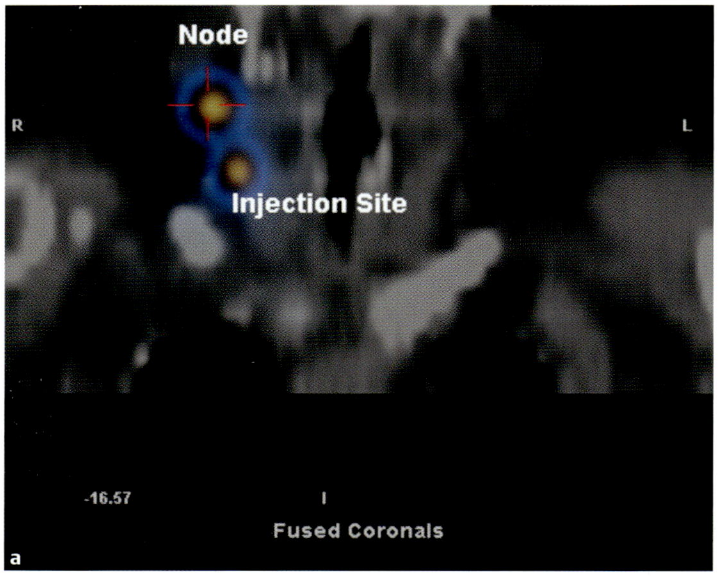

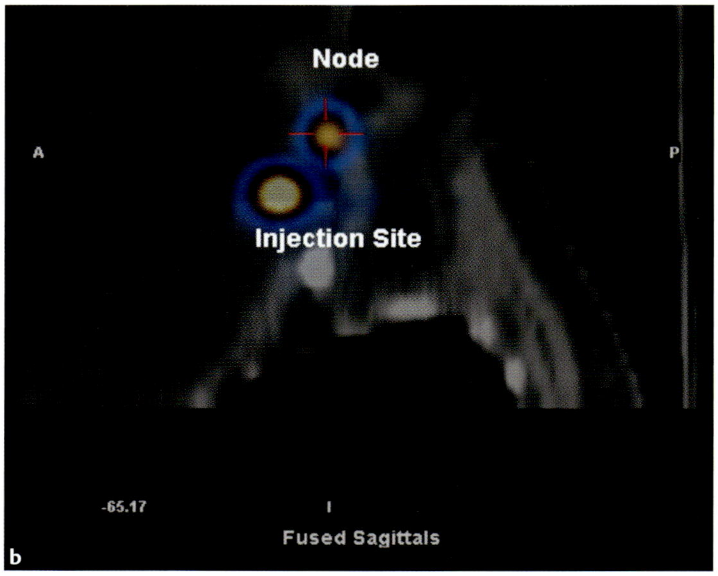

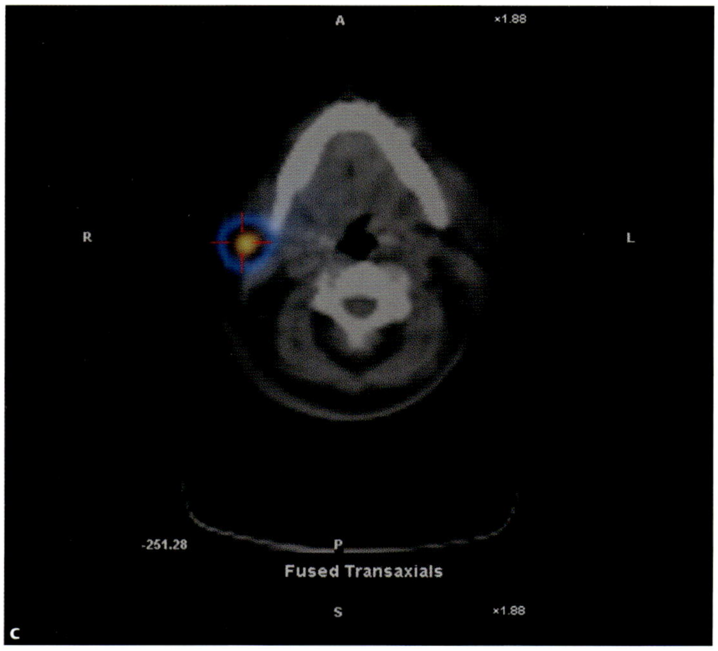

Fig. 3.54a–c Sentinel lymph node imaging with SPECT-CT for melanoma recurrence in the neck, following an intradermal injection of 20 MBq Tc-99 m nanocolloid in the vicinity of the tumor, demonstrates the injection site and sentinel node on the right (surgery was performed on the same day).
a Fused coronal SPECT-CT.
b Fused sagittal SPECT-CT.
c Fused axial SPECT-CT.

cells become dislodged from the skin primary and then become ensnared in dermal and subcutaneous lymphatics (**Fig. 3.53**).[94] Factors that result in an increased incidence of in-transit metastasis include mechanical disruption to lymphatic flow secondary to surgery or malignancy. Other authors suggest that adverse tumor biology such as high Breslow score, presence of angiolymphatic invasion, higher mitotic rate, and advanced age of the patient are more important risk factors.[28,93,95] Sentinel lymph node imaging with SPECT-CT (**Fig. 3.54**) is useful for detecting sentinel lymph nodes and in-transit metastasis in the head and neck region as well as the trunk.[96] Sentinel lymph node biopsy in head and neck carcinoma has been applied to those with node-negative necks, but its role still uncertain.[61] Furthermore, there is no direct evidence that it results in long-term clinical and survival improvement in patients with thyroid cancer.[97]

Future Research

- The role of sentinel node SPECT/CT imaging in the early stage neck cancers.
- The development of widely available but more specific PET tracers for malignancy and hypoxia.
- The role of PET-CT guided radiotherapy planning on long-term outcomes and complications.
- The role of gallium-68 PET in routine follow-up imaging of medullary thyroid carcinoma.
- Combined PET-MRI also with the use of DWI sequences in head and neck cancer recurrence.

Recommended Reading

- Offiah C, Hall E. Post-treatment imaging appearances in head and neck cancer patients. Clin Radiol 2011;66(1):13–24
- Ginsberg LE. Imaging of perineural tumor spread in head and neck cancer. In: Som PM, Hugh DC, eds. Head and Neck Imaging. 4th ed. St. Louis, MO: Mosby; 2003:865–886
- Luster M, Clarke SE, Dietlein M, et al. European Association of Nuclear Medicine (EANM). Guidelines for radioiodine therapy of differentiated thyroid cancer. Eur J Nucl Med Mol Imaging 2008;35(10):1941–1959
- von Schulthess GK. Molecular anatomic imaging: PET-CT and SPECT-CT Integrated Modality Imaging. 2nd ed. Lippincott, Williams & Wilkins 2006: 304–30
- Lonneux M, Lawson G, Ide C, Bausart R, Remacle M, Pauwels S. Positron emission tomography with fluorodeoxyglucose for suspected head and neck tumor recurrence in the symptomatic patient. Laryngoscope 2000;110(9):1493–1497
- Mukherji SK, Wolf GT. Evaluation of head and neck squamous cell carcinoma after treatment. AJNR Am J Neuroradiol 2003;24(9):1743–1746

References[1]

1. Kapoor V, Fukui MB, McCook BM. Role of 18FFDG PET/CT in the treatment of head and neck cancers: posttherapy evaluation and pitfalls. AJR Am J Roentgenol 2005;184(2):589–597
2. Vogl T, Bisdas S. Lymph node staging. Top Magn Reson Imaging 2007;18(4):303–316
3. Ronaghy A, Yaar R, Goldberg LJ, Mahalingam M, Bhawan J. Perineural involvement: what does it mean? Am J Dermatopathol 2010;32(5):469–476
4. Leiter U, Meier F, Schittek B, Garbe C. The natural course of cutaneous melanoma. J Surg Oncol 2004;86(4):172–178
5. American Head and Neck Society. Management of Cancer of the Head and Neck. Imaging: General Guidelines. http://www.ahns.info/clinicalresources/docs/imaginggeneral.php
6. Hudgins PA, Burson JG, Gussack GS, Grist WJ. CT and MR appearance of recurrent malignant head and neck neoplasms after resection and flap reconstruction. AJNR Am J Neuroradiol 1994;15(9):1689–1694
7. Vissink A, Jansma J, Spijkervet FK, Burlage FR, Coppes RP. Oral sequelae of head and neck radiotherapy. Crit Rev Oral Biol Med 2003;14(3):199–212
8. Offiah C, Hall E. Post-treatment imaging appearances in head and neck cancer patients. Clin Radiol 2011;66(1):13–24
9. Rabin BM, Meyer JR, Berlin JW, Marymount MH, Palka PS, Russell EJ. Radiation-induced changes in the central nervous system and head and neck. Radiographics 1996;16(5):1055–1072
10. Nabil S, Samman N. Incidence and prevention of osteoradionecrosis after dental extraction in irradiated patients: a systematic review. Int J Oral Maxillofac Surg 2011;40(3):229–243
11. Lim AA, Karakla DW, Watkins DV. Osteoradionecrosis of the cervical vertebrae and occipital bone: a case report and brief review of the literature. Am J Otolaryngol 1999;20(6):408–411
12. Yoo JS, Rosenthal DI, Mitchell K, Ginsberg LE. Osteoradionecrosis of the hyoid bone: imaging findings. AJNR Am J Neuroradiol 2010;31(4):761–766
13. Madrid C, Abarca M, Bouferrache K. Osteoradionecrosis: an update. Oral Oncol 2010;46(6):471–474
14. Arduino PG, Carrozzo M, Pentenero M, Bertolusso G, Gandolfo S. Non-neoplastic salivary gland diseases. Minerva Stomatol 2006;55(5):249–270
15. Leslie MD, Dische S. Parotid gland function following accelerated and conventionally fractionated radiotherapy. Radiother Oncol 1991;22(2):133–139
16. Menda Y, Graham MM. Update on ^{18}F-fluorodeoxyglucose/positron emission tomography and positron emission tomography/computed tomography imaging of squamous head and neck cancers. Semin Nucl Med 2005;35(4):214–219
17. Arduino PG, Carrozzo M, Pentenero M, Bertolusso G, Gandolfo S. Non-neoplastic salivary gland diseases. Minerva Stomatol 2006;55(5):249–270
18. Hermans R, Pameijer FA, Mancuso AA, Parsons JT, Mendenhall WM. CT findings in chondroradionecrosis of the larynx. AJNR Am J Neuroradiol 1998;19(4):711–718

1 References with asterisks indicate the most important reference articles on the topic.

19. Wu JC, Beale KK, Ma JD. Evaluation of current and upcoming therapies in oral mucositis prevention. Future Oncol 2010;6(11):1751–1770
20. Worthington HV, Clarkson JE, Eden OB. Interventions for preventing oral mucositis for patients with cancer receiving treatment. Cochrane Database Syst Rev 2006;(2):CD000 978
21. King AD, Ahuja AT, Yeung DK, et al. Delayed complications of radiotherapy treatment for nasopharyngeal carcinoma: imaging findings. Clin Radiol 2007;62(3):195–203
22. Bhargava P, Rahman S, Wendt J. Atlas of confounding factors in head and neck PET/CT imaging. Clin Nucl Med 2011;36(5):e20–e29
23. Engles JM, Quarless SA, Mambo E, Ishimori T, Cho SY, Wahl RL. Stunning and its effect on 3H-FDG uptake and key gene expression in breast cancer cells undergoing chemotherapy. J Nucl Med 2006;47(4):603–608
24. Kim SY, Kim JS, Yi JS, et al. Evaluation of ^{18}F-FDG PET/CT and CT/MRI with histopathologic correlation in patients undergoing salvage surgery for head and neck squamous cell carcinoma. Ann Surg Oncol 2011;18(9):2579–2584
25. Chong VFH. Post treatment imaging in head and neck tumours. Cancer Imaging 2005;5(1):8–10
26. Hervás I, Floria LM, Bello P, et al. Microvascularized fibular graft for mandibular reconstruction: detection of viability by bone scintigraphy and SPECT. Clin Nucl Med 2001;26(3):225–229
27. Streitz JM Jr, Shapshay SM. Airway injury after tracheotomy and endotracheal intubation. Surg Clin North Am 1991;71(6):1211–1230
28. Badellino F, Berrino P, Campora E, et al. Metastatic spread of floor of the mouth squamous cell carcinoma via pectoralis major myocutaneous flap. J Surg Oncol 1988;38(1):45–47
29. Schuepbach J, Dassonville O, Poissonnet G, Demard F. Early postoperative bone scintigraphy in the evaluation of microvascular bone grafts in head and neck reconstruction. Head Face Med 2007;3:20
30. Conway WC, Faries MB, Nicholl MB, et al. Age-related lymphatic dysfunction in melanoma patients. Ann Surg Oncol 2009;16(6):1548–1552
31. Goerres GW, Haenggeli CA, Allaoua M, et al. Direct comparison of F-18-FDG PET and ultrasound in the follow-up of patients with squamous cell cancer of the head and neck. Nucl Med (Stuttg) 2000;39(8):246–250
32. Ahuja A, Ying M. Sonography of neck lymph nodes. Part II: abnormal lymph nodes. Clin Radiol 2003; 58(5, Issue 5)359–366
33. van den Brekel MW, Castelijns JA. What the clinician wants to know: surgical perspective and ultrasound for lymph node imaging of the neck. Cancer Imaging 2005;5 Spec No A:S41–S49
34. van den Brekel MW, Reitsma LC, Quak JJ, et al. Sonographically guided aspiration cytology of neck nodes for selection of treatment and follow-up in patients with N0 head and neck cancer. AJNR Am J Neuroradiol 1999;20(9):1727–1731
35. Robitschek J, Straub M, Wirtz E, Klem C, Sniezek J. Diagnostic efficacy of surgeon-performed ultrasound-guided fine needle aspiration: a randomized controlled trial. Otolaryngol Head Neck Surg 2010;142(3):306–309
36. Eggers G, Rieker M, Kress B, Fiebach J, Dickhaus H, Hassfeld S. Artefacts in magnetic resonance imaging caused by dental material. MAGMA 2005;18(2):103–111
37. Mukherji SK, Isaacs DL, Creager A, Shockley W, Weissler M, Armao D. CT detection of mandibular invasion by squamous cell carcinoma of the oral cavity. AJR Am J Roentgenol 2001;177(1):237–243
38. Rankin S. CT and MRI. Surgery (Oxford) 2005 May 1;23(5):162–165
39. Rasheda L, Elwanb S, Abdurrahmanb L, El Fikyc L, Shehatac M, Basyounib R. The added value of DW-MRI in characterization of tissue in treated head and neck tumors. Egyptian J Ear Nose Throat Allied Sci 2010;(11):35–40.
40. Rivelli V, Luebbers HT, Weber FE, Cordella C, Grätz KW, Kruse AL. Screening recurrence and lymph node metastases in head and neck cancer: the role of computer tomography in follow-up. Head Neck Oncol 2011;3:18
41. Dill T. Contraindications to magnetic resonance imaging: non-invasive imaging. Heart 2008;94(7):943–948
42. Vandecaveye V, De Keyzer F, Dirix P, Lambrecht M, Nuyts S, Hermans R. Applications of diffusion-weighted magnetic resonance imaging in head and neck squamous cell carcinoma. Neuroradiology 2010;52(9):773–784
43. Vandecaveye V, De Keyzer F, Vander Poorten V, et al. Head and neck squamous cell carcinoma: value of diffusion-weighted MR imaging for nodal staging. Radiology 2009;251(1):134–146
44. Fukui MB, Blodgett TM, Meltzer CC. PET/CT imaging in recurrent head and neck cancer. Semin Ultrasound CT MR 2003;24(3):157–163
45. Isles MG, McConkey C, Mehanna HM. A systematic review and meta-analysis of the role of positron emission tomography in the follow up of head and neck squamous cell carcinoma following radiotherapy or chemoradiotherapy. Clin Otolaryngol 2008;33(3):210–222
46. Bongers V, Hobbelink MG, van Rijk PP, Hordijk GJ. Cost-effectiveness of dual-head ^{18}F-fluorodeoxyglucose PET for the detection of recurrent laryngeal cancer. Cancer Biother Radiopharm 2002;17(3):303–306
47. Lonneux M, Lawson G, Ide C, Bausart R, Remacle M, Pauwels S. Positron emission tomography with fluorodeoxyglucose for suspected head and neck tumor recurrence in the symptomatic patient. Laryngoscope 2000;110(9):1493–1497
48. Sherman SI. Thyroid carcinoma. Lancet 2003;361(9356):501–511
49. Iwano S, Kato K, Nihashi T, Ito S, Tachi Y, Naganawa S. Comparisons of I-123 diagnostic and I-131 post-treatment scans for detecting residual thyroid tissue and metastases of differentiated thyroid cancer. Ann Nucl Med 2009;23(9):777–782
50. Jarzab B, Handkiewicz-Junak D, Wloch J. Juvenile differentiated thyroid carcinoma and the role of radioiodine in its treatment: a qualitative review. Endocr Relat Cancer 2005;12(4):773–803
51. Luster M, Clarke SE, Dietlein M, et al.; European Association of Nuclear Medicine (EANM). Guidelines for radioiodine therapy of differentiated thyroid cancer. Eur J Nucl Med Mol Imaging 2008;35(10):1941–1959
52. James C, Starks M, MacGillivray DC, White J. The use of imaging studies in the diagnosis and management of thyroid cancer and hyperparathyroidism. Surg Oncol Clin N Am 1999;8(1):145–169
53. Klein HA, DiSibio KJ, Sims D, Singleton HC, Worthy LJ. I-123 whole body scanning: case report and discussion. Clin Nucl Med 2005;30(5):312–316
54. Bertagna F, Biasiotto G, Orlando E, Bosio G, Giubbini R. Role of ^{18}F-fluorodeoxyglucose positron emission tomography/computed tomography in patients affected by differentiated thyroid carcinoma, high thyroglobulin level, and negative ^{131}I scan: review of the literature. Jpn J Radiol 2010;28(9):629–636
55. Feine U, Lietzenmayer R, Hanke J-P, Held J, Wöhrle H, Müller-Schauenburg W. Fluorine-18-FDG and iodine-131-iodide uptake in thyroid cancer. J Nucl Med 1996;37(9):1468–1472

56. Khan N, Oriuchi N, Higuchi T, Zhang H, Endo K. PET in the follow-up of differentiated thyroid cancer. Br J Radiol 2003;76(910):690–695
57. Bozkurt MF, Uğur O, Banti E, Grassetto G, Rubello D. Functional nuclear medicine imaging of medullary thyroid cancer. Nucl Med Commun 2008;29(11):934–942
58. Krausz Y, Keidar Z, Kogan I, et al. SPECT/CT hybrid imaging with ^{111}In-pentetreotide in assessment of neuroendocrine tumours. Clin Endocrinol (Oxf) 2003;59(5):565–573
59. Harris L, Yoo J, Driedger A, et al. Accuracy of technetium-99 m SPECT-CT hybrid images in predicting the precise intraoperative anatomical location of parathyroid adenomas. Head Neck 2008;30(4):509–517
60. Frank-Raue K, Raue F, Buhr HJ, Baldauf G, Lorenz D, Ziegler R. Localization of occult persisting medullary thyroid carcinoma before microsurgical reoperation: high sensitivity of selective venous catheterization. Thyroid 1992;2(2):113–117
61. Seethala RR. Current state of neck dissection in the United States. Head Neck Pathol 2009;3(3):238–245
62. Ligey A, Gentil J, Créhange G, et al. Impact of target volumes and radiation technique on loco-regional control and survival for patients with unilateral cervical lymph node metastases from an unknown primary. Radiother Oncol 2009;93(3):483–487
63. Tartaglione T, Summaria V, Medoro A, Brunetti D, Di Lella GM, Zacchei P. Metastatic lymphadenopathy from ENT carcinoma: role of diagnostic imaging. Rays 2000;25(4):429–446
64. Chan JY, Chow VL, Mok VW, Ho AC, Wei WI. Prediction of surgical outcome using plasma Epstein–Barr virus DNA and ^{18}F-FDG PET-CT scan in recurrent nasopharyngeal carcinoma. Head Neck 2011: doi: 101 002/hed.21 768 [Epub ahead of print]
65. Liao CT, Chang JT, Wang HM, et al. Preoperative [^{18}F]fluorodeoxyglucose positron emission tomography standardized uptake value of neck lymph nodes predicts neck cancer control and survival rates in patients with oral cavity squamous cell carcinoma and pathologically positive lymph nodes. Int J Radiat Oncol Biol Phys 2009;74(4):1054–1061
66. Gor DM, Langer JE, Loevner LA. Imaging of cervical lymph nodes in head and neck cancer: the basics. Radiol Clin North Am 2006;44(1):101–110, viii.
67. Dirix P, Nuyts S, Bussels B, Hermans R, Van den Bogaert W. Prognostic influence of retropharyngeal lymph node metastasis in squamous cell carcinoma of the oropharynx. Int J Radiat Oncol Biol Phys 2006;65(3):739–744
68. Xie CM, Liang BL, Lin HG, Wu PH. [Assessment of retropharyngeal lymph node by comparing CT with MRI]. [Article in Chinese] Ai Zheng 2002;21(3):285–288
69. Su Y, Zhao C, Xie CM, et al. Evaluation of CT, MRI and PET-CT in detecting retropharyngeal lymph node metastasis in nasopharyngeal carcinoma. [Article in Chinese] Ai Zheng 2006;25(5):521–525
70. Zhang GY, Liu LZ, Wei WH, Deng YM, Li YZ, Liu XW. Radiologic criteria of retropharyngeal lymph node metastasis in nasopharyngeal carcinoma treated with radiation therapy. Radiology 2010;255(2):605–612
71. Donta TS, Smoker WR. Head and neck cancer: carcinoma of unknown primary. Top Magn Reson Imaging 2007;18(4):281–292
72. Subramaniam RM, Truong M, Peller P, Sakai O, Mercier G. Fluorodeoxyglucose-positron-emission tomography imaging of head and neck squamous cell cancer. AJNR Am J Neuroradiol 2010;31(4):598–604
73. Anzai Y, Brunberg JA, Lufkin RB. Imaging of nodal metastases in the head and neck. J Magn Reson Imaging 1997;7(5):774–783
74. Yousem DM, Gad K, Tufano RP. Resectability issues with head and neck cancer. AJNR Am J Neuroradiol 2006;27(10):2024–2036
75. Chong VF, Khoo JB, Fan YF. Imaging of the nasopharynx and skull base. Magn Reson Imaging Clin N Am 2002;10(4):547–571, v. *
76. Ginsberg LE. Imaging of perineural tumor spread in head and neck cancer. In: Som PM, Hugh DC, eds. Head and Neck Imaging. 4th ed. St Louis, MO: Mosby; 2003:865–886*
77. Nemec SF, Herneth AM, Czerny C. Perineural tumor spread in malignant head and neck tumors. Top Magn Reson Imaging 2007;18(6):467–471
78. Morris JGL, Joffe R. Perineural spread of cutaneous basal and squamous cell carcinomas. The clinical appearance of spread into the trigeminal and facial nerves. Arch Neurol 1983;40(7):424–429
79. Schmalfuss IM, Tart RP, Mukherji S, Mancuso AA. Perineural tumor spread along the auriculotemporal nerve. AJNR Am J Neuroradiol 2002;23(2):303–311
80. Chang PC, Fischbein NJ, McCalmont TH, et al. Perineural spread of malignant melanoma of the head and neck: clinical and imaging features. AJNR Am J Neuroradiol 2004;25(1):5–11
81. Blandino A, Gaeta M, Minutoli F, Pandolfo I. CT and MR findings in neoplastic perineural spread along the vidian nerve. Eur Radiol 2000;10(3):521–526
82. von Schulthess GK. Molecular anatomic imaging: PET-CT and SPECT-CT integrated modality imaging. 2nd ed. Lippincott, Williams & Wilkins; 2006:304–305
83. Fosko SW, Hu W, Cook TF, Lowe VJ. Positron emission tomography for basal cell carcinoma of the head and neck. Arch Dermatol 2003;139(9):1141–1146
84. Durden DD, Williams DW III. Radiology of skull base neoplasms. Otolaryngol Clin North Am 2001;34(6):1043–1064, vii vii
85. Lam KH, Lam LK, Ho CM, Wei WI. Mandibular invasion in carcinoma of the lower alveolus. Am J Otolaryngol 1999;20(5):267–272
86. Caldemeyer KS, Mathews VP, Righi PD, Smith RR. Imaging features and clinical significance of perineural spread or extension of head and neck tumors. Radiographics 1998;18(1):97–110, quiz 147
87. Lee TJ, Glastonbury CM, Buckley AF, Eisele DW, Hawkins RA. Perineural spread of melanoma demonstrated by F-18 FDG PET With MRI and pathologic correlation. Clin Nucl Med 2008;33(2):106–108
88. Nguyen BD, Roarke MC. Salivary duct carcinoma with perineural spread to facial canal: F-18 FDG PET/CT detection. Clin Nucl Med 2008;33(12):925–928
89. Standring S. Gray's Anatomy. 40th ed. Elsevier/Churchill Livingstone; 2008
90. Doyon D, Marsot-Dupuch K, Francke JP. The Cranial Nerves. Philadelphia: WB Saunders; 2004: 39–53
91. Dutton JJ. Radiology of the Orbit and Visual Pathways. 2nd ed. Elsevier; 2010
92. Lang PG. Current concepts in the management of patients with melanoma. Am J Clin Dermatol 2002;3(6):401–426
93. Pawlik TM, Ross MI, Thompson JF, Eggermont AMM, Gershenwald JE. The risk of in-transit melanoma metastasis depends on tumor biology and not the surgical approach to regional lymph nodes. J Clin Oncol 2005;23(21):4588–4590

94. Attie JN, Khafif RA. Melanotic Tumors: Biology, Pathology and Clinical Features. Springfield, IL: Charles C. Thomas; 1964:147–150
95. Stucky CC, Gray RJ, Dueck AC, et al. Risk factors associated with local and in-transit recurrence of cutaneous melanoma. Am J Surg 2010;200(6):770–774, discussion 774–775
96. Even-Sapir E, Lerman H, Lievshitz G, et al. Lymphoscintigraphy for sentinel node mapping using a hybrid SPECT/CT system. J Nucl Med 2003;44(9):1413–1420

4 Concurrent Chemotherapy and Re-irradiation for Recurrent Head and Neck Cancer

Kevin S. Choe, Joseph Kamel Salama, Ezra E.W. Cohen

Summary

- Recurrence of head and neck cancer or second primary tumors within a previously irradiated volume is a relatively common problem that is particularly challenging for oncologists.
- Concomitant chemotherapy with re-irradiation is a treatment option that offers a small but real chance of cure in select patients.
- Because of the risk of severe toxicity, appropriate patient selection is critical.
- Use of concomitant chemotherapy with re-irradiation should be limited to investigational protocols or be carried out only in experienced centers.

Introduction

Advances in all modalities to treat head and neck cancer (HNC)—surgery, radiotherapy (RT), chemotherapy—have led to significant improvements in treatment outcomes. Especially for patients with locoregionally advanced HNC, concurrent chemoradiotherapy, either definitively or postoperatively, has substantially improved locoregional control and overall survival.[1,2] However, even after optimal therapy, locoregional recurrence is still typically 20%–30%,[3–6] and constitutes the leading cause of mortality in HNC.[6–9] Furthermore, successfully treated HNC patients are at risk for developing second primary tumors, many of which are in the head and neck region.[10–13] For patients who develop a recurrence or second primary cancer in an area previously exposed to RT, therapeutic options are limited and survival is poor.[14]

When possible, the treatment of choice for recurrences that arise within a previously irradiated volume is surgical salvage.[15–17] However, only a small portion of patients with recurrent disease are candidates for surgical resection, due to tumor extent, medical comorbidities, or patient refusal.[18,19] Additionally, surgical salvage is associated with a reported major complication rate of 27% and operative mortality rate of 5%.[14] Furthermore, following surgery, adverse pathological features such as positive margins or extranodal extension are often found, raising the question of further adjuvant therapy.[14,20]

Systemic chemotherapy is the standard treatment for patients with an unresectable recurrence or second head and neck primary. However, despite the addition of targeted agents, response rates are ~30%, and the median survival is 6–10 months with almost no possibility of cure.[21–25] In addition, a pooled analysis demonstrated that a history of prior RT was a poor prognostic factor for patients receiving systemic therapy.[26] Therefore, the only curative therapeutic option for these patients is a second course of radiotherapy or re-irradiation (RRT). Although associated with substantial toxicity, RRT or combined chemotherapy and RRT (CRRT) has been shown to be feasible and offers a chance for long-term survival in a small group of patients.[27–30]

Reasons for Tumor Recurrence Following Definitive Therapy

To understand the current recommendation for combination systemic chemotherapy and RRT for recurrent HNC, we must first understand how recurrences occur within previously radiated fields. Then, we will discuss pathways of radioresistance and attempts to overcome them by the addition of systemic agents, targeted therapies, and alterations in the delivery of radiotherapy.

Radioresistance

A tumor may recur following a course of definitive radiotherapy for many reasons. First, persistence or recurrence of tumors despite an initial course of RT suggests the presence of radioresistant clonogens. Radioresistance is believed to be the primary cause of RT failure and tumor recurrence. Multiple pathways leading to radioresistance have been described, implicating mechanisms such as hypoxia, proficient DNA repair, activated oncogenic signaling, and radioresistant cancer stem cells.[31–34] Therefore, radioresistant tumor clonogens with such pathways activated are unlikely to respond well to a second course of radiotherapy. Several strategies have been developed to overcome radioresistance, including incorporation of radiation sensitizers and intensification of RT through dose escalation or altered fractionation.[35–37] Utilization of molecularly targeted agents that mitigate radioresistance (e.g., cetuximab) may also allow RRT to be more effective.

Radiation Coverage

A tumor may recur if the radiotherapy target did not include the entirety of the gross or microscopic tumor, constituting a "geographic miss." Improvements in tumor imaging with the increasing availability of multiplanar, high-resolution CT, MRI and FDG-PET certainly aid the clinician in accurately delineating target volumes. The use of advanced radiotherapy delivery techniques such as intensity-modulated radiation therapy (IMRT) allows the clinician to selectively not irradiate tissues that would have previously been irradiated with standard techniques. Although this tailored approach may reduce acute and late side-effects such as xerostomia, dermatitis, edema, and fibrosis, this technique also carries the risk of missing the microscopic cancer in the selectively unirradiated areas (geographic miss). In such cases, tumor recurrence may not represent radioresistance, and it may still be effectively treated with RT.

Field Cancerization

Previously irradiated patients may also develop second primary tumors. Head and neck cancer patients experience a potential 3% annual risk of developing second primary tumors.[10] This may be due to the effect of *field cancerization*, proposed by Slaughter, who suggested that patients who develop one tumor are at risk of developing a new second tumor in the same region, due to the exposure to carcinogens such as tobacco and alcohol.[38] Compared with recurrent tumors that may have proven radioresistance, second primary tumors may still be susceptible to cell killing by RT. Consistent with this hypothesis, there is clinical evidence that among patients treated with RRT, those with second primary malignancy have better survival than those with recurrent tumor.[37,39]

Regimens for Concurrent Chemotherapy with Re-irradiation

The most extensively utilized and studied CRRT regimen is the **FHX platform,** incorporating concomitant 5-fluorouracil (5-FU), hydroxyurea (HU), and RT. The rationale for this combination is based on the independent cytotoxic activity and radiosensitizing properties of 5-FU and HU.[40] Hydroxyurea is an antimetabolite thought to preferentially target cells within the most radioresistant phase of the cell cycle, S-phase, by inhibiting the conversion of ribonucleotides to deoxyribonucleotides.[41] 5-FU is a halogenated pyrimidine nucleoside analogue, commonly used in combination with RT. 5-FU is thought to contribute to radiosensitization by interfering with DNA damage repair after RT and also by cytotoxicity in the S-phase of the cell cycle.[42,43] In the FHX regimen, maximal radiosensitization is attempted by delivering 5-FU continuously for 5 days, along with hydroxyurea delivered orally 2 hours prior to each RT fraction. Each 14-day cycle consists of 5 days of concurrent chemotherapy and radiotherapy, followed by 9 days of no therapy. A complete course consists of 4 to 7 cycles based on the extent of pretreatment surgery as well as RRT fractionation (i.e., once daily versus twice daily).

Several studies investigating the FHX regimen observed long-term survivors,[27,44–46] and subsequently, the FHX regimen has served as a platform to which additional agents are combined. A series of third agents combined with FHX has been tested at the University of Chicago. Some agents, such as cisplatin and paclitaxel, were shown to improve locoregional control (LRC) and overall survival (OS), compared with FHX alone.[29] Another combination, gemcitabine, paclitaxel, 5-FU, and RT, led to impressive long-term LRC (5-year, 54.5%) and OS (5-year, 34.5%).[47] However, the favorable clinical outcomes were associated with severe acute toxicity, limiting the clinical applicability of this combination.[48] Another FHX-based regimen, consisting of paclitaxel, 5-FU, HU, and RT (TFHX), also demonstrated efficacy with 4-year LRC of 54% and OS of 22%,[49,50] and it was associated with a more tolerable toxicity profile. TFHX is a well-tested combination, and it is the recommended regimen for patients in the nonprotocol setting at the University of Chicago.

An **alternative** to the FHX-based regimens, developed at the Fox Chase Cancer Center and later adopted by the Radiation Therapy Oncology Group (RTOG), is a combination of paclitaxel (20 mg/m²) and cisplatin (15 mg/m²) administered in between twice-daily RT sessions.[28,51,52] Similarly to the FHX regimen, treatment is delivered for 5 days, followed by a 9-day break. A phase II study by RTOG (RTOG 9911), utilizing this regimen led to 2-year OS of 26%. There was also 28% grade 4–5 acute toxicity and 11% treatment-related deaths.[28]

Evidence for Concurrent Chemotherapy with Re-irradiation

Single-Institution Experiences

Large single-institution experiences with CRRT come primarily from the Institut Gustave-Roussy and the University of Chicago (**Table 4.1**). The Institut Gustave-Roussy series included 169 patients who presented with unresectable nonmetastatic HNC in a previously irradiated area.[27] One hundred and forty-two of the patients were treated with CRRT, most of them on the FHX regimen. The median cumulative RT dose was 120 Gy. With a median follow-up of 70 months, OS was 21% at 2 years and 9% at 5 years. Late toxicities were considerable, with 8% osteoradionecrosis and 21% mucosal necrosis. Five patients died of carotid hemorrhage while apparently in complete remission. Of the variables analyzed, only the volume of the second irradiation (≥650 cm³) was significantly associated with risk of death. Tumor site, interval between RT, and second primary versus recurrence were not significant.

The University of Chicago also reported the experience of CRRT in treatment of recurrent or second primary HNC.[29] One hundred and fifteen patients with squamous cell histology were included in this series. All patients were treated on FHX-based regimens with the median RRT dose of 64.5 Gy and cumulative dose of 131 Gy. Forty-nine of 115 patients (43%) had undergone surgical resection or debulking prior to CRRT. With the median follow-up of 67 months among surviving patients, the 3-year OS and LRC were 22% and 51%, respectively. The encouraging survival outcome is tempered by the 17% risk of treatment-related death. On multivariable analysis, good performance status, surgery prior to CRRT, RRT dose ≥58 Gy, and triple chemotherapy regimen were significantly associated with improved LRC and OS.

Prospective Cooperative Group Trials

Unresectable Second Primary and Recurrent Cancers

Encouraged by the early single-institution experiences which supported the feasibility and the potential of long-term survival with CRRT, the RTOG initiated a series of phase I/II trials for recurrent and second primary HNC. **RTOG 9610** was the first cooperative group trial of concurrent chemotherapy with RRT, investigating the FHX regimen in 86 patients with recurrent or second primary head and neck squamous cell carcinoma.[30,39] All patients had completed their initial RT course at least 6 months previously. Therapy consisted of concurrent 5-FU, hydroxyurea, and 60 Gy daily RRT. With the minimum follow-up of 5 years, the 2- and 5-year OS values were 15.2% and 3.8%, respectively. The longer interval between the initial RT and RRT was associated with improved survival. Of 81 analyzable patients, 6 died of hematological toxicity and 2 died of tumor hemorrhage. An additional 4 patients died during therapy of causes unrelated to treatment.[39]

Table 4.1 Selected studies of CRRT

Study (year)	No. of patients	RT median dose	Chemotherapy	Toxicity comments	Locoregional control	Overall survival
RTOG 96–10[30,39] (1996–1999)	79	60 Gy (b.i.d.) alternating weeks	5-FU and HU	63% acute grade 3+ toxicity 8% treatment-related deaths 8% unrelated deaths	–	15% (2-year) 4% (5-year)
RTOG 99–11[28] (2000–2003)	99	60 Gy (b.i.d.) alternating weeks	CDDP, paclitaxel, G-CSF	11% treatment-related deaths 50% grade 3–5 acute toxicity 4% osteoradionecrosis	–	26% (2-year)
De Crevoisier[27] (1988–1996)	106	60 Gy (daily), alternating weeks	5-FU and HU	21% mucosal necrosis 8% osteoradionecrosis 4% carotid hemorrhage	–	24% (2-year); 14% (5-year)
	36	60 Gy (BID), split course	5-FU, CDDP, and MMC			10% (2-year); 0% (5-year)
Salama[29] (1986–2001)	115	60–75 Gy (daily or b.i.d.) alternating weeks	5-FU, HU, and 3rd agent (gemcitabine, CPT-11, CDDP, paclitaxel)	4% carotid hemorrhage 11% osteoradionecrosis	51% (3-year)	22% (3-year)
Kramer[51] (1996–2002)	38	42–60 Gy (b.i.d.) alternating weeks	CDDP, paclitaxel, G-CSF	5% osteoradionecrosis 5% carotid hemorrhage 3% temporal lobe necrosis	37%	35% (2-year)
Spencer[46] (1992–1999)	52	50–60 Gy (daily or b.i.d.) split course	5-FU and HU	11% late complications, 4% soft tissue necrosis No treatment-related deaths	–	15% (2-year)

Subsequently, **RTOG 9911** tested the combination of cisplatin and paclitaxel with 60 Gy RRT.[28] Granulocyte colony-stimulating factor (G-CSF) was administered during off weeks. This study included 99 patients with comparable baseline characteristics to RTOG 9610. The toxicity was significant, with 85% of the patients experiencing grade 3–5 toxicity in the first 2 years, and the treatment-related mortality rate was 11%. However, with a median follow-up of 23.6 months, the 2-year OS was 25.9%. There are caveats associated with comparing phase II studies, but nevertheless, the survival rate from RTOG 9911 was significantly better than that from RTOG 9610 ($P = 0.0444$).

Resectable Second Primary and Recurrent Cancers

As previously mentioned, surgical salvage is the preferred treatment for patients with recurrent disease or second primary tumor in a previously irradiated field. However, recurrence is common even after surgery, and adjuvant therapy may be necessary.[19,53] The **Groupe d'Etude des Tumeurs de la Tête et du Cou (GETTEC)** and **Groupe d'Oncologie Radiotherapie Tête et Cou (GORTEC)** performed a randomized study to assess the efficacy of adjuvant CRRT after salvage surgery.[45] The randomized trial included 130 patients who had salvage surgery with no gross residual disease, a good performance status, and total wound healing within 4 weeks of surgery. Subjects were then assigned to either observation or postoperative CRRT (FHX regimen, daily radiation to 60 Gy). Patients in the postoperative CRRT arm had significantly improved LRC (49% versus 25%) and disease-free survival (hazard ratio = 1.68). However, there was no significant difference in OS ($P = 0.5$), perhaps due to the increased treatment-related deaths (5 versus 0) and second primary tumors (4 versus 1) in the CRRT arm. The toxicity associated with postoperative CRRT was comparable to that in other trials of CRRT. At 2 years, 40% of surviving patients experienced grade 3 or 4 late toxicity in the CRRT arm, compared with 10% in the observation arm.

Results from both cooperative group and large single-institution studies support the feasibility and the potential survival benefit of CRRT in HNC patients with locoregional recurrence in areas previously exposed to RT. However, as discussed below, CRRT is associated with substantial toxicity. A more effective strategy in patient selection and therapy intensification is needed.

■ Acute and Chronic Toxicities Associated with CRRT

For both physicians and patients, the risk of severe life-threatening toxicity tempers the enthusiasm for the small but real chance for cure with CRRT. The majority of severe toxicity is due to the cumulative impact of two full courses of radiotherapy on non–cancer containing head and neck organs, many of which have also been surgically manipulated. Unlike the primary treatment for HNC, in which significant effort is placed on sparing of normal tissues to maintain quality of life, in retreatment with RT it is often not possible to optimally spare normal tissues. Therefore, when discussing concurrent chemotherapy and re-irradiation, it is important to emphasize that the goal of therapy is life, not necessarily quality of life.

Acute Toxicities

Major acute toxicities associated with CRRT are similar to those with the initial course of chemoradiotherapy, including mucositis, dermatitis, pharyngitis, and hematological suppression. Although acute toxicities can lead to deterioration of general medical condition, sometimes necessitating unplanned treatment interruption and reduction in intensity of therapy, they generally resolve after the completion of therapy, and most patients recover with supportive measures. Compared with RRT alone, addition of concurrent chemotherapy significantly increases acute toxicities. The Institut Gustave-Roussy reported that grade 3 mucositis and dermatitis were less frequent in patients treated with RRT alone, compared with those who received concomitant chemotherapy, and the need for gastrostomy was also much less if radiotherapy alone was given (11% versus 40%).[27] Myelosuppression from systemic therapy is also a common acute toxicity from CRRT. The FHX regimen is usually associated with less myelosuppression, compared with regimens containing docetaxel and cisplatin or paclitaxel and cisplatin.[27,28,39,54]

With the FHX regimen, the type, time course, and intensity of acute toxicities are often predictable and therefore manageable in the setting of an experienced integrated team. It is also interesting to note that among patients treated with TFHX, severe acute mucositis (grade 4) was less common among patients undergoing RRT, compared with those receiving the first course of radiation (8% versus 28%).[49] This trend is observed in large cooperative group studies as well. Grade 3–4 mucositis rates are generally higher during the primary course of chemoradiation compared with CRRT (43%–71% versus 20%–28%).[5,39,45,55] The differences in irradiated field sizes (often smaller for CRRT) and scheduling of chemotherapy may contribute to these findings.

Chronic Toxicities

Interpretation of late toxicity data following CRRT is often complicated because it is difficult to discern which of many previous procedures, including the initial course of RT, is responsible for the complication. However, it is generally agreed that the risk of severe late toxicity from CRRT is substantial. In RTOG 9610, the cumulative incidence of grade 3+ late toxicity in patients surviving more than one year was 12.3%.[39] Common late toxicities are cervical fibrosis (5%–16%), osteoradionecrosis (5%–16%), trismus (9%–34%), and carotid hemorrhage (2%–5%).[36]

Neurological Toxicities

The most worrisome late complications are neurological toxicities (e.g., transverse myelitis or brainstem necrosis) as well as carotid rupture. Fortunately, these devastating complications occur rarely, even in patients who received lifetime radiation doses over 100 Gy. In the large series from the University of Chicago with 115 patients, after a median lifetime dose of 131 Gy, only one patient suffered spinal cord toxicity.[29] This patient had a recurrent tumor immediately adjacent to the spinal cord. In addition, no brachial plexopathy was observed, although the cumulative dose to the brachial plexus was not routinely monitored. Preclinical experiments with primates have suggested that the spinal cord has a substantial capacity to recover from radiation damage with time.[56] It is also suggested that in patients treated with RRT, the spinal cord may tolerate higher doses than previously believed if RT interval is greater than 6 months.[57] However, extreme caution should still be exercised. As the survival of these patients improves, there will be more opportunity for the late toxicity to manifest, and the true incidence may be higher.

Carotid Rupture

Another potential catastrophic late complication from CRRT is carotid rupture, which in almost all instances is associated with death.[58] Risk factors for carotid rupture include tumor recurrence, ongoing infection, presence of a pharyngocutaneous fistula, prior neck dissection, long-term tracheostomy or nasogastric tubes, and tumor adherence to the carotid fascia.[59] In patients with a high risk of carotid rupture, a preemptive intervention by surgical placement of fresh tissue overlying the vessel or endovascular stent-grafting may ameliorate the risk.[59–62] In addition, aggressive nutritional support and correction of hematological deficiencies may promote wound healing and lower the risk of carotid exposure and hemorrhage.[59]

> ! Compared with acute toxicities, late toxicities are generally less predictable and irreversible, and therefore more feared.

Brachytherapy for Recurrent Head and Neck Cancer

When the recurrence is limited and accessible, brachytherapy via interstitial catheters may be an effective treatment option. Because of the rapid fall-off of radiation dose beyond the implanted volume, this technique allows for focusing of high doses to the tumor and sparing of surrounding normal tissues. In addition, there is the benefit of short overall treatment time.

Several investigators have reported their experiences with brachytherapy in salvage RRT.[63–67] Puthawala and colleagues from the Long Beach Memorial Medical Center reported their experience of treating 220 patients with recurrent or second-primary HNC located within previously irradiated area.[67] A majority of the patients had undergone salvage surgery (52%), and 70% also received chemotherapy or interstitial hyperthermia treatments concomitantly with brachytherapy. Brachytherapy consisted of a low-dose-rate afterloading iridium-192 implant, which delivered a median tumor dose of 53 Gy (range 46–60 Gy). With a minimum follow-up of 6 months, local control was achieved in 77%. The 5-year OS was 22%. Moderate to severe late complications occurred in 27%, which included soft tissue necrosis, osteoradionecrosis, carotid ruptures, and hemorrhage.

Another group, from the Centre Alexis Vautrin in France, reported the long-term outcomes after interstitial brachytherapy alone, without any surgery.[63] The series included 84 patients with isolated neck recurrence, of whom 76 (90%) were previously treated with external beam RT. The mean dose of iridium-192 brachytherapy was 56.5 Gy (or 38 Gy if combined with external beam RT). The probability of neck control at 2 years was 31%. The 2-year OS was 13%. The treatment-related mortality was 7%, including 4 carotid ruptures.

For patients with limited recurrence that is not amenable to surgery, interstitial brachytherapy may offer durable local control and a chance of long-term survival. Encouraging outcomes have been reported but limited to few centers with considerable experiences in brachytherapy. At centers with the expertise, interstitial brachytherapy may be a valuable therapeutic option.

Patient Selection and Prognostic Factors

With the significant toxicity associated with CRRT, it is critical to identify patients who will potentially benefit the most from CRRT. Therefore, refinement of patient selection criteria that will

Table 4.2 Factors associated with improved survival after re-irradiation

Favorable prognostic factors	References
Second primary (versus recurrent tumors)	39, 37
Longer time interval to recurrence	30, 37, 72, 75, 80
Full dose re-irradiation (>50 Gy)	29, 69, 71, 73, 74, 77
No previous exposure to chemotherapy	68, 79
Surgical debulking	29, 74, 45, 71
Multiagent chemotherapy	29
Absence of medical comorbidities	81
Absence of feeding tube, tracheostomy, and/or soft tissue defect	81
Small tumor bulk (low rT-stage)	27, 81, 78
Primary site recurrence (versus neck recurrence)	71, 76

enhance the therapeutic benefit is of utmost interest. Several prognostic factors for survival have been proposed, and they are summarized in **Table 4.2**.[29,30,37,39,45,68–81]

As expected, tumors that are amenable to resection prior to CRRT and full dose re-irradiation fare better. In the series from the University of Chicago, patients who had surgical resection or debulking prior to CRRT had 3 year OS of 39%, compared with 11% if no surgery was performed.[29] Similarly, several reports have suggested that a full-dose RRT (generally >50 Gy) is associated with improved survival.[29,69,71,74,77] Second primary tumors and a longer interval from previous radiation are also favorable prognostic factors.[30,37,39,72,75,80] Presence of significant comorbidities and organ dysfunction (i.e., feeding tube dependency, tracheostomy, and osteonecrosis) confers distinctly worse prognosis. In a study from the Moffitt Cancer Center, patients with comorbidities and pre-existing organ dysfunctions had a median survival of 5.5 months, compared with 59.6 months in those who had neither.[81] For patients who are initially managed with salvage surgery, pathological findings may predict outcomes after CRRT.[82] Carotid sheath involvement was associated with poor local control and OS. Patients with soft tissue deposits were at increased risk for distant metastasis.

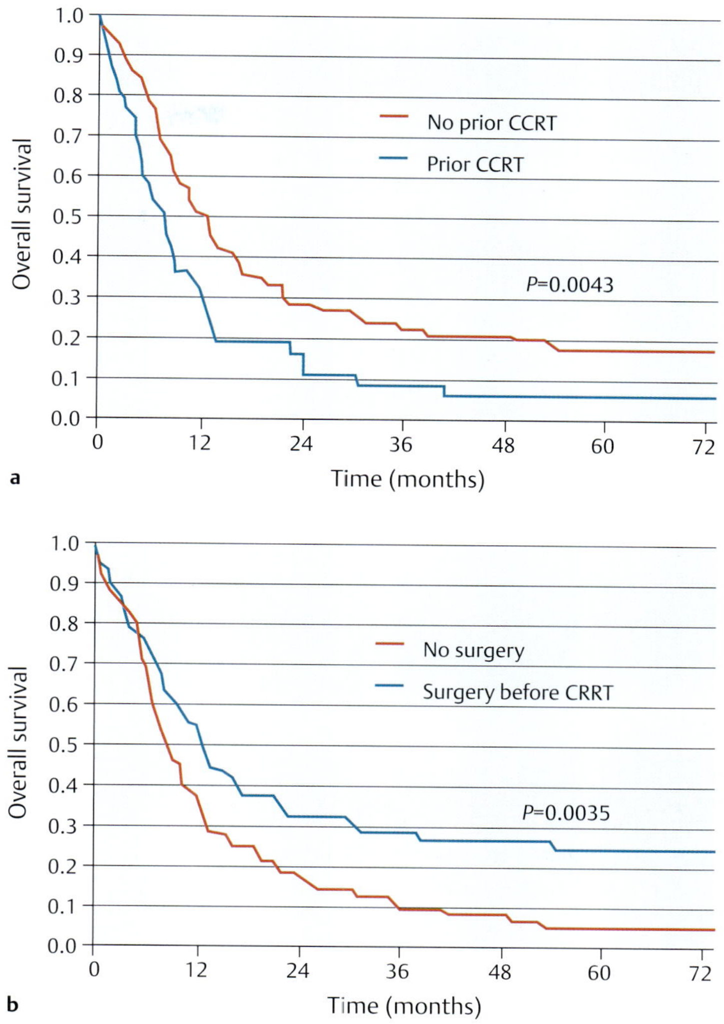

Fig. 4.1a, b Survival differences in patients dependent on therapy.
a Overall survival of patients receiving a second course of radiation concurrently with chemotherapy for recurrent or second primary head and neck cancer. The red line represents patients who were previously treated only with radiation. The blue line represents the survival of those who were previously treated with both chemotherapy and radiation.
b Overall survival of patients receiving a second course of radiation concurrently with chemotherapy for recurrent or second primary head and neck cancer by prior surgical resection. The blue line represents those that had an operation immediately before chemotherapy and re-irradiation. The red line represents no prior surgery before chemotherapy and re-irradiation.

Location of Recurrence

An important consideration regarding the potential effectiveness of CRRT is the location of recurrence with respect to the previous treatment field. For optimal analysis, detailed treatment plans from the initial course of radiation should be obtained and recreated on the current CT scan showing the areas of recurrence. Radiation coverage and dose distribution to critical normal structures should be evaluated, which will influence the feasibility and safety of RRT. Although no studies have evaluated the prognostic significance of the location of recurrence, intuitively, if the recurrence is in the low-dose region (e.g., electively treated neck) or the failure represents a geographic miss, the recurrence is less likely to be intrinsically radioresistant than those tumors that recur within the high-dose region.

Pre-recurrence Treatment

As concurrent chemoradiotherapy in the definitive or postoperative setting has become more common in recent years, the population of patients presenting with recurrent disease may have changed significantly.[83] It is reasonable to postulate that tumors that recur following concurrent chemoradiotherapy, as opposed to radiation alone, may be more aggressive and therapy-resistant. For these tumors, retreatment with CRRT may be less effective. Recent studies indeed suggest that previous exposure to concurrent chemoradiotherapy is associated with worse survival when treated with CRRT (**Fig. 4.1**).[68,79] Among patients treated with CRRT, those who failed initial concurrent chemoradiotherapy had 2-year OS of 11%, compared with 28% in those who were naive to concurrent chemoradiation.[68] These patients may require innovative treatment strategies, such as integration of novel agents and advanced radiation delivery techniques. The latest protocol at the University of Chicago incorporates cetuximab (epidermal growth factor receptor inhibitor) and sunitinib (multitargeted receptor tyrosine kinase inhibitor) with RRT.

Response to Induction

Another strategy to appropriately select patients for CRRT is to use the response to induction chemotherapy to choose candidates. In the definitive chemoradiation setting, response to induction chemotherapy can predict response to overall treatment and clinical outcome.[84–86] As a corollary, in recurrent tumors, those that respond poorly to induction chemotherapy may derive less benefit from CRRT. Based on this rationale, a protocol from the University of Chicago investigated induction chemotherapy with 2 monthly cycles of pemetrexed (500 mg/m²) and gemcitabine (1500 mg/m²), followed by CRRT (carboplatin AUC 5, pemetrexed 500 mg/m², and 63–70 Gy of RRT) and/or surgery.[87] After induction chemotherapy, radiographic and clinical response was determined. Analysis showed that disease progression during induction chemotherapy was a poor prognostic factor for progression-free survival and overall survival. The optimal choice of induction chemotherapy is difficult, as many patients have already been treated during their definitive course with the most active agents (e.g., cisplatin, carboplatin, 5-FU, and paclitaxel). Other approaches utilizing molecular profiling to predict therapy resistance and treatment response are under active investigation.[88,89]

Simulation and Planning for Re-irradiation

Positioning of the Patient

Due to the proximity to many critical organs that have already received a course of radiotherapy, precise delivery of radiation is particularly important in head and neck re-irradiation. Sharp dose gradients between targeted tumors and surrounding normal tissues are only possible when patients are positioned comfortably and reproducibly for each fraction of radiation. Swallowing, respiration, or coughing cause significant positional changes, and maintaining the position may be challenging in these patients, especially those with attached devices (e.g., tracheostomy and nasogastric tubes). Several immobilization devices are available to improve precision and comfort, and these include custom masks, foam casts, vacuum molds, and thermoplastic materials. For patients who require even more precise positioning (e.g., for stereotactic body radiotherapy), frames with fiducials are used.

> **!** Because of the large variations in tumor sites, patient anatomy, and patient cooperation, each case should be evaluated for the optimal positioning and required immobilization devices.

Typically, patients are positioned supine with the neck neutral or extended and shoulders pulled down. This position allows optimal exposure of the target area without unnecessarily treating the eyes or the arms. The head is then immobilized in this position by strips of radiolucent material or thermoplastic cast, which is fixed to the treatment table. It is critical that the immobilization device conforms tightly to the body and leaves no room for movement.

Appropriate use of bite blocks can aid in minimizing the volume of oral mucosa within the treatment field. For example, when the tongue or the floor of mouth is the target, the upper half of the mouth can be excluded from the high-dose irradiation by using a bite block to keep the mouth open. The bite block is created during the simulation procedure and used during each treatment.

Computed Tomography

Once properly immobilized, the patient undergoes planning CT. Contrast agents may be used to enhance visualization of the tumor and the normal tissues. The general recommendation is to scan at least 5 cm inferiorly and superiorly from the anticipated treatment volumes with the typical scan encompassing the area from the calvaria to the carina.[90]

Treatment planning requires accurate delineation of the target and normal tissues from the CT images. Other imaging studies (e.g., diagnostic CT, MRI, and FDG-PET) may be fused with the simulation CT to improve contouring. For postoperative cases, the images obtained prior to the surgery are useful to identify areas at risk for residual tumor. Areas of adverse pathological features (e.g., positive margin, perineural invasion, extracapsular extension) deserve particular attention.

Dose Calculation

The initial course of radiotherapy should be retrieved and evaluated, as discussed above. Critical structures, including the optic nerves, optic chiasm, brainstem, and spinal cord are also contoured, and dose distribution and maximal doses should be calculated. Evidence-based guidelines for maximally tolerated doses are not available in the setting of head and neck re-irradiation. Every effort is made to minimize doses to the above-mentioned critical structures. Although the risk of serious toxicities varies with the quality of radiation exposure from the initial course of radiation, the time interval between the two courses, and the proximity to the target area, the cumulative dose to the spinal cord is generally limited to 50 Gy. When the previous treatment plan is not available for a detailed review, it should be assumed that the surrounding critical organs have received the full tolerance doses.

Treatment Volume Definition

In the primary treatment of HNC, nodal regions potentially harboring occult metastasis are commonly included to minimize nodal recurrence. In re-irradiation, the potential benefit and toxicity of elective nodal irradiation need to be carefully considered, since the risk of toxicity is generally related to the volume of tissue irradiated.[78] Several studies have investigated the utility or futility of elective nodal irradiation in head and neck re-irradiation.[54,91,92] Results suggest that the overwhelming risk of recurrence is within the region of gross disease and that the probability of isolated failure in the electively treated areas is low. For example, a study from the University of Michigan reported on the pattern of recurrence after treating only the gross tumor with a tight margin to a median dose of 68 Gy.[92] After a median follow-up of 42 months, 47 of 66 patients (71%) developed locoregional failure (LRF). Of them, only 2 (4%) were in the neck outside the target area.

Although it should be evaluated on a case-by-case basis, treatment volume confined to the gross tumor expanded by a safety

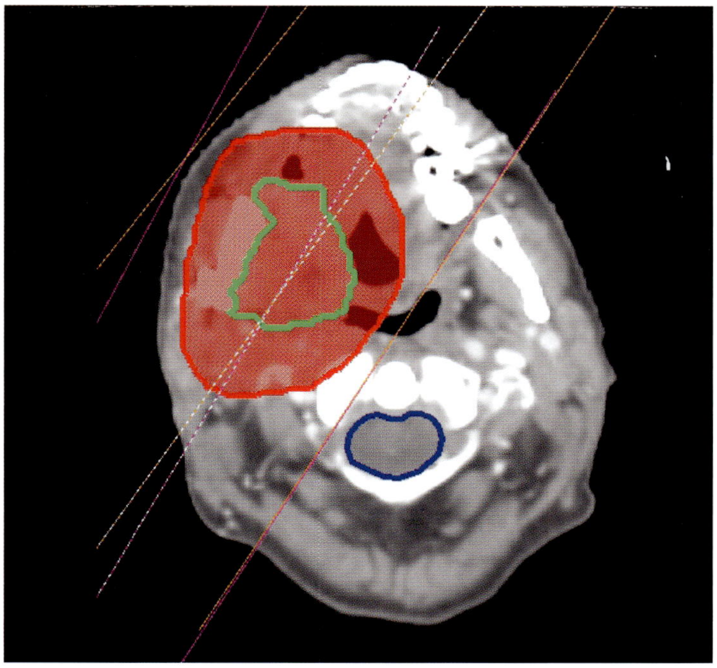

Fig. 4.2 Opposed oblique beam arrangement to treat a recurrent tumor from the floor of mouth. Gross tumor (green); planning target volume (red); spinal cord (blue).

margin of 1–1.5 cm appears to be appropriate. Prophylactic treatment of draining lymphatic regions is generally avoided. In areas closely abutting critical structures, the margin may be smaller to reduce the risk of complications. After surgical resection, only the tumor bed of the high-risk areas (e.g., positive margin and extracapsular extension) is typically targeted.

Beam Arrangement

Arrangement of the radiation beam is the next step in radiation planning. Optimal beam arrangements are designed using the beam's-eye-view display and adjusting the gantry angle, couch angle, and collimator shapes. When using conventional three-dimensional conformal techniques, the opposed oblique beam arrangement is commonly used in head and neck re-irradiation. This arrangement offers a relatively simple set-up, and the sharp dose fall-off at the beam edge can be exploited to spare critical organs, such as the spinal cord (**Fig. 4.2**). Compared with more advanced radiation techniques, such as IMRT, conventional radiation technique generally incorporates wider margins and is, therefore, less affected by organ motion and patient set-up uncertainties. In addition, the dose distribution is generally more uniform, and the areas of high dose (hot spots) are readily predictable and manipulated.

Because target shapes can be complex and critical organs are frequently in close proximity to the target volume, it is often difficult, if not impossible, to deliver curative doses of radiation to the target without exposing nearby organs to potentially damaging doses. Since intensification of RT and sparing of critical organs are particularly important in the setting of head and neck re-irradiation, the use of more advanced radiation delivery techniques may become necessary.

Advances in Delivery of Radiation

There have been significant improvements in delivery of radiation in recent years.

Intensity-Modulated Radiotherapy

Intensity-modulated radiotherapy (IMRT) is a form of three-dimensional conformal radiotherapy in which physician-defined target volumes, beam angles, and normal tissue tolerances are entered into complex computer algorithms, which in turn derive the optimal treatment plan. A high degree of dose conformity around irregularly shaped tumors can be achieved by dynamically controlling the intensity of the radiation beam. Use of IMRT may offer better sparing of the normal surrounding tissues and thus less morbidity in the setting of head and neck re-irradiation.

Figure 4.2 shows a case of recurrent oral cavity cancer with bilateral neck involvement. With conventional techniques, a large volume would receive the full dose of radiation, and it would be challenging to spare the spinal cord (in blue). With IMRT, multiple coplanar beams that converge on the target are used to generate a much more conformal dose distribution (**Fig. 4.3a, b**), and the surrounding normal tissues (including the spinal cord) can be spared from high doses of radiation.

A retrospective series from the MD Anderson Cancer Center showed that IMRT in CRRT is feasible and effective.[93] For 67 patients who were treated with curative intent, the median survival was an impressive 40 months. The 2-year OS and LRC were 61% and 67%, respectively. The rate of toxicity was similar to that in other studies, with 15 of the patients developing severe re-irradiation complications, including one treatment-related death. Another report from Memorial Sloan-Kettering Cancer Center also supported the efficacy of IMRT and suggested that the use of IMRT was associated with improved locoregional progression-free survival (but not overall survival) in multivariable analysis.[74] Although these results are encouraging, they are derived from carefully selected patients at institutions with a high level of expertise in IMRT and head and neck re-irradiation. Furthermore, although IMRT spares normal tissues from high doses of radiation, it may increase the areas receiving relatively low yet potentially damaging doses. Therefore, IMRT in re-irradiation should be utilized judiciously.

Stereotactic Body Radiotherapy

Hypofractionated image-guided radiotherapy that delivers high doses of radiation in a few fractions (generally 3–10 fractions), widely called stereotactic body radiotherapy (SBRT), has recently gained interest in head and neck re-irradiation.[94–96] This approach utilizes stereotactic localizers (radiological anatomical landmarks or surgically placed fiducials) to track target movement, and real-time images are used to guide highly focused radiation beams to the target. In a report from the Catholic University of Korea, 36 patients and 44 sites were treated with SBRT to a median dose of 30 Gy in 3–5 fractions.[95] No patients received concurrent chemotherapy. Major response (partial response or better) was obtained in 80% of the targeted sites, and with a median follow-up of 17 months the 2-year local recurrence free

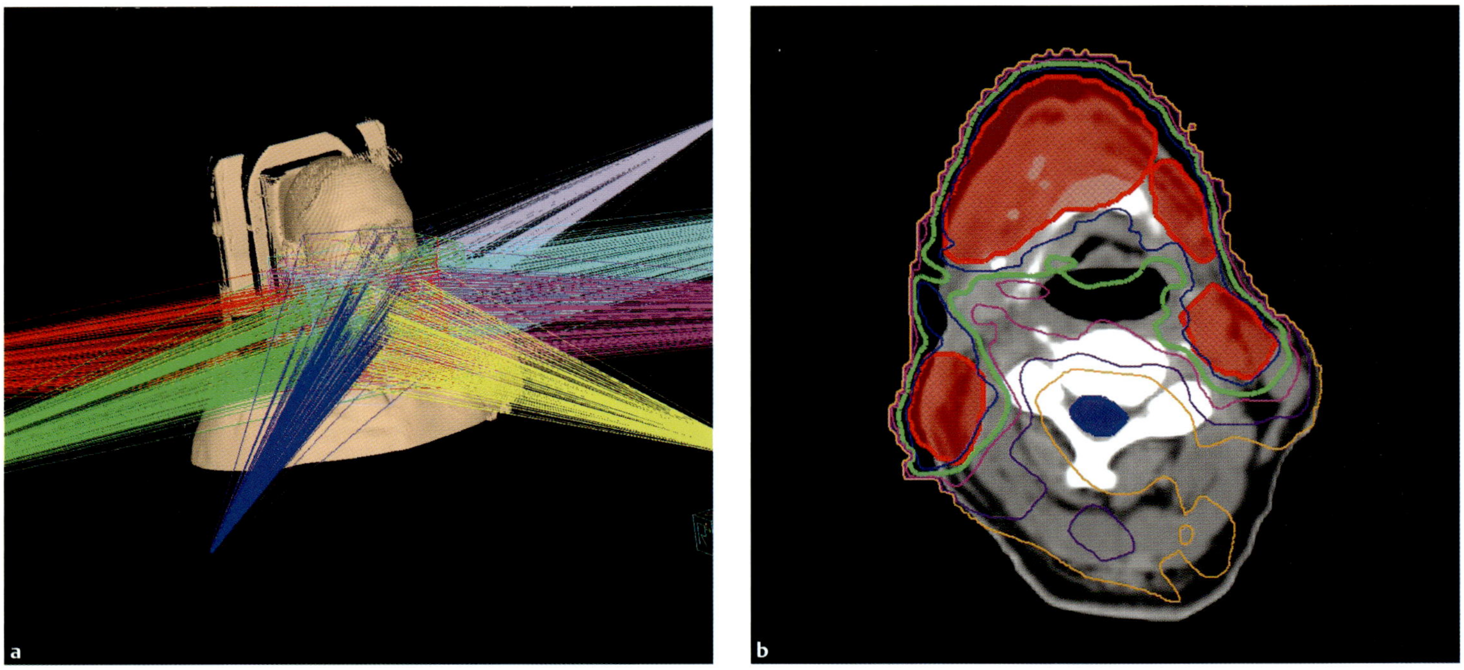

Fig. 4.3a, b Beam arrangement and dose distribution of an IMRT plan. **a** Multiple coplanar beams that converge on the target are shown. **b** The planning target volume is shown in red and the spinal cord in blue. Isodose lines: 110% (blue), 100% (green), 90% (magenta), 80% (purple), and 50% (orange).

survival was 52%. There was one case of intractable soft tissue necrosis, which eventually led to death. As more experience with SBRT is obtained, it may become an attractive alternative to or a new base for CRRT.

Charged Particles

Another possible approach to enhance the therapeutic ratio for patients with recurrent HNC is the use of charged particles. Compared with conventional photon therapy, charged particles—such as protons and carbon ions—offer different physical and biological properties that may be particularly useful in these patients who have previously been irradiated. Charged particles deposit a great deal of their energy at a given depth followed by a steep dose fall-off, with almost no dose deposition beyond what is called a Bragg peak. This property can be exploited to deliver higher doses to the target without exposing surrounding normal tissues to potentially damaging doses of radiation. In a report from the Loma Linda University Medical Center, re-irradiation with proton therapy was studied in 16 recurrent nasopharyngeal cancer patients who failed initial photon radiotherapy.[97] With a mean follow-up of 24 months, the 2-year OS was 50% and no central nervous system complications were reported. Another report from the Lawrence Berkeley Laboratory showed that the use of heavy ion particles in re-irradiation was associated with 59% 3-year OS and no fatal complications in 11 patients with recurrent nasopharyngeal carcinoma.[98] Although the technique is theoretically promising, the paucity of centers that offer this technology limits its widespread utility.

New Approaches to CRRT

Biologically Targeted Therapy

Despite the possibility of long-term survival after CRRT, cure is expected in a minority of patients, and there is a strong need for new strategies that can overcome therapeutic resistance without incurring more toxicity. One such strategy may be integration of **molecularly targeted agents** with CRRT. These agents may provide additional benefit to conventional therapy without intolerable toxicity. In the primary treatment of HNC, a randomized study demonstrated that combining cetuximab (an epidermal growth factor receptor inhibitor) and radiotherapy leads to improved locoregional control and overall survival, compared with radiotherapy alone.[99] Investigators from the Goethe University in Germany studied the feasibility of cetuximab in combination with re-irradiation for recurrent HNC.[100] Of the 7 patients in the series, 2 achieved complete response and another had stable disease. For toxicity, 2 developed grade 3 acneiform rash from cetuximab, but there was no acute grade 3+ RT-related toxicity. Interestingly, the two patients who developed moderate to severe acneiform rash were the ones who achieved complete response. Such a correlation was also observed in the primary therapy of HNC.[101]

Another method to overcome therapeutic resistance may be to target **vascular endothelial growth factor** (VEGF). VEGF is induced by radiation, and it is associated with tumor proliferation, metastasis, and therapeutic resistance.[102–104] The safety and efficacy of a VEGF inhibitor, bevacizumab combined with FHX regimen was investigated in a phase I trial from the University of Chicago.[105] The disease outcome was favorable, but the regimen was associated with a high rate of fistula formation and tissue necrosis (21%). Further characterization of bevacizumab toxicity in the setting of CRRT is needed.

A novel approach to locally intensify CRRT is the use of viral oncolytic therapy that can be injected into gross tumor. One such oncolytic virus that is currently being tested in a phase I/II trial is **TNFerade** (GenVec, Gaithersburg, MD, USA). TNFerade consists of replication-deficient adenovirus that contains the tumor necrosis factor-α (TNF-α) cDNA under the control of a radiation-inducible promoter, so that TNF-α expression is induced only when the injected area is irradiated. The protocol adds intratumoral injection of TNFerade to the FHX platform, and the preliminary results indicate feasibility.[106]

Hypoxic Tumor Sensitization

As tumors proliferate, they can outgrow the oxygen supply and tumor hypoxia ensues.[107] Since the biological effect of radiation is dependent on oxygenation, tumor hypoxia has important clinical implications, and several studies have shown that hypoxia is associated with poor locoregional control and survival in head and neck cancer patients treated with radiation.[108–110] One strategy to overcome radioresistant hypoxic cells may be to utilize tirapazamine (TPZ), which is a topoisomerase II inhibitor that becomes selectively active in hypoxic environment.[36]

To investigate the potential efficacy of a hypoxic cell sensitizer in recurrent HNC, Cohen and colleagues conducted a phase I trial that incorporated TPZ into CRRT.[111] Cisplatin (50 mg/m²) and TPZ (260 mg/m²) were administered with RT on weeks 1, 3, and 5. Tirapazamine alone (160 mg/m²) was added on days 1, 3, and 5 during week 2 of RT (initial cohort) or during weeks 2 and 4 of RT (cohort 2). With a median follow-up of 24 months, the 2-year OS was 27%. The response rate was an impressive 80% among evaluable patients, with 28% achieving a complete response. The toxicities were typical of other CRRT trials with two cases of fatal carotid artery rupture. The impact of hypoxia in these patients undergoing CRRT is unclear, but the therapeutic benefit may be further improved if the level of hypoxia is measured and used for patient selection.

Conclusion

Recurrence of head and neck cancer or second primary tumors within a previously irradiated volume is a relatively common problem that is particularly challenging for oncologists. Re-irradiation with concurrent chemotherapy can be effective, and cure is possible. However, because the associated toxicity is substantial, strategies to improve the therapeutic ratio are strongly needed. Incremental progress has been made with radiosensitizing chemotherapy, biologically targeted agents, and advances in the technology of radiotherapy delivery. Utilization of molecular profiling and further refinement of clinical prognostic factors may allow improved patient selection and therapeutic benefit.

Future Research

- Prognostic factors that will help identify appropriate patients for head and neck re-irradiation.
- Intensification of therapy with more targeted treatments that can overcome therapy resistance without increasing toxicity.
- Utilization of innovative radiation delivery techniques to improve quality-of-life after re-irradiation.

Recommended Reading

- De Crevoisier R, Bourhis J, Domenge C, et al. Full-dose re-irradiation for unresectable head and neck carcinoma: experience at the Gustave-Roussy Institute in a series of 169 patients. J Clin Oncol 1998;16(11):3556–3562 (One of the largest studies of head and neck re-irradiation.)
- Salama JK, Vokes EE, Chmura SJ, et al. Long-term outcome of concurrent chemotherapy and re-irradiation for recurrent and second primary head-and-neck squamous cell carcinoma. Int J Radiat Oncol Biol Phys 2006;64(2):382–391 (Comprehensive summary of seven phase II protocols investigating the toxicity and efficacy of head and neck re-irradiation with concurrent chemotherapy.)
- Spencer SA, Harris J, Wheeler RH, et al. Final report of RTOG 9610, a multi-institutional trial of re-irradiation and chemotherapy for unresectable recurrent squamous cell carcinoma of the head and neck. Head Neck 2008;30(3):281–288 (First cooperative group trial to show that long-term survival is possible with the concurrent chemo–re-irradiation approach.)
- Janot F, de Raucourt D, Benhamou E, et al. Randomized trial of postoperative re-irradiation combined with chemotherapy after salvage surgery compared with salvage surgery alone in head and neck carcinoma. J Clin Oncol 2008;26(34):5518–5523 (Multi-institution randomized study showing the benefit of concurrent chemo–re-irradiation after surgical resection.)

References

1. Bernier J, Cooper JS, Pajak TF, et al. Defining risk levels in locally advanced head and neck cancers: a comparative analysis of concurrent postoperative radiation plus chemotherapy trials of the EORTC (#22931) and RTOG (# 9501). Head Neck 2005;27(10):843–850
2. Pignon JP, Bourhis J, Domenge C, Designé L. Chemotherapy added to locoregional treatment for head and neck squamous-cell carcinoma: three meta-analyses of updated individual data. MACH-NC Collaborative Group. Meta-Analysis of Chemotherapy on Head and Neck Cancer. Lancet 2000;355(9208):949–955
3. Bernier J, Domenge C, Ozsahin M, et al. European Organization for Research and Treatment of Cancer Trial 22931. Postoperative irradiation with or without concomitant chemotherapy for locally advanced head and neck cancer. N Engl J Med 2004;350(19):1945–1952

4. Cooper JS, Pajak TF, Forastiere AA, et al. Radiation Therapy Oncology Group 9501/Intergroup. Postoperative concurrent radiotherapy and chemotherapy for high-risk squamous-cell carcinoma of the head and neck. N Engl J Med 2004;350(19):1937–1944
5. Forastiere AA, Goepfert H, Maor M, et al. Concurrent chemotherapy and radiotherapy for organ preservation in advanced laryngeal cancer. N Engl J Med 2003;349(22):2091–2098
6. Posner MR, Hershock DM, Blajman CR, et al. TAX 324 Study Group. Cisplatin and fluorouracil alone or with docetaxel in head and neck cancer. N Engl J Med 2007;357(17):1705–1715
7. Bourhis J, Le Maître A, Baujat B, Audry H, Pignon JP; Meta-Analysis of Chemotherapy in Head, Neck Cancer Collaborative Group; Meta-Analysis of Radiotherapy in Carcinoma of Head, Neck Collaborative Group; Meta-Analysis of Chemotherapy in Nasopharynx Carcinoma Collaborative Group. Individual patients' data meta-analyses in head and neck cancer. Curr Opin Oncol 2007;19(3):188–194
8. Brockstein B, Haraf DJ, Rademaker AW, et al. Patterns of failure, prognostic factors and survival in locoregionally advanced head and neck cancer treated with concomitant chemoradiotherapy: a 9-year, 337-patient, multi-institutional experience. Ann Oncol 2004;15(8):1179–1186
9. Salama JK, Seiwert TY, Vokes EE. Chemoradiotherapy for locally advanced head and neck cancer. J Clin Oncol 2007;25(26):4118–4126
10. Cooper JS, Pajak TF, Rubin P, et al. Second malignancies in patients who have head and neck cancer: incidence, effect on survival and implications based on the RTOG experience. Int J Radiat Oncol Biol Phys 1989;17(3):449–456
11. Lin K, Patel SG, Chu PY, et al. Second primary malignancy of the aerodigestive tract in patients treated for cancer of the oral cavity and larynx. Head Neck 2005;27(12):1042–1048
12. Spector JG, Sessions DG, Haughey BH, et al. Delayed regional metastases, distant metastases, and second primary malignancies in squamous cell carcinomas of the larynx and hypopharynx. Laryngoscope 2001;111(6):1079–1087
13. Vikram B, Strong EW, Shah JP, Spiro R. Second malignant neoplasms in patients successfully treated with multimodality treatment for advanced head and neck cancer. Head Neck Surg 1984;6(3):734–737
14. Goodwin WJ Jr. Salvage surgery for patients with recurrent squamous cell carcinoma of the upper aerodigestive tract: when do the ends justify the means? Laryngoscope 2000; 110(3 Pt 2, Suppl 93):1–18
15. Ganly I, Patel SG, Matsuo J, et al. Results of surgical salvage after failure of definitive radiation therapy for early-stage squamous cell carcinoma of the glottic larynx. Arch Otolaryngol Head Neck Surg 2006;132(1):59–66
16. McLaughlin MP, Parsons JT, Fein DA, et al. Salvage surgery after radiotherapy failure in T1–T2 squamous cell carcinoma of the glottic larynx. Head Neck 1996;18(3):229–235
17. Wong LY, Wei WI, Lam LK, Yuen AP. Salvage of recurrent head and neck squamous cell carcinoma after primary curative surgery. Head Neck 2003;25(11):953–959
18. Parsons JT, Mendenhall WM, Stringer SP, Cassisi NJ, Million RR. Salvage surgery following radiation failure in squamous cell carcinoma of the supraglottic larynx. Int J Radiat Oncol Biol Phys 1995;32(3):605–609
19. Taussky D, Dulguerov P, Allal AS. Salvage surgery after radical accelerated radiotherapy with concomitant boost technique for head and neck carcinomas. Head Neck 2005;27(3):182–186
20. Jones AS, Bin Hanafi Z, Nadapalan V, Roland NJ, Kinsella A, Helliwell TR. Do positive resection margins after ablative surgery for head and neck cancer adversely affect prognosis? A study of 352 patients with recurrent carcinoma following radiotherapy treated by salvage surgery. Br J Cancer 1996;74(1):128–132
21. Forastiere AA, Leong T, Rowinsky E, et al. Phase III comparison of high-dose paclitaxel + cisplatin + granulocyte colony-stimulating factor versus low-dose paclitaxel + cisplatin in advanced head and neck cancer: Eastern Cooperative Oncology Group Study E1393. J Clin Oncol 2001;19(4):1088–1095
22. Forastiere AA, Metch B, Schuller DE, et al. Randomized comparison of cisplatin plus fluorouracil and carboplatin plus fluorouracil versus methotrexate in advanced squamous-cell carcinoma of the head and neck: a Southwest Oncology Group study. J Clin Oncol 1992;10(8):1245–1251
23. Gibson MK, Li Y, Murphy B, et al.; Eastern Cooperative Oncology Group. Randomized phase III evaluation of cisplatin plus fluorouracil versus cisplatin plus paclitaxel in advanced head and neck cancer (E1395): an intergroup trial of the Eastern Cooperative Oncology Group. J Clin Oncol 2005;23(15):3562–3567
24. Soulieres D, Senzer NN, Vokes EE, Hidalgo M, Agarwala SS, Siu LL. Multicenter phase II study of erlotinib, an oral epidermal growth factor receptor tyrosine kinase inhibitor, in patients with recurrent or metastatic squamous cell cancer of the head and neck. J Clin Oncol 2004;22(1):77–85
25. Vermorken JB, Mesia R, Rivera F, et al. Platinum-based chemotherapy plus cetuximab in head and neck cancer. N Engl J Med 2008;359(11):1116–1127
26. Argiris A, Li Y, Forastiere A. Prognostic factors and long-term survivorship in patients with recurrent or metastatic carcinoma of the head and neck. Cancer 2004;101(10):2222–2229
27. De Crevoisier R, Bourhis J, Domenge C, et al. Full-dose re-irradiation for unresectable head and neck carcinoma: experience at the Gustave-Roussy Institute in a series of 169 patients. J Clin Oncol 1998;16(11):3556–3562
28. Langer CJ, Harris J, Horwitz EM, et al. Phase II study of low-dose paclitaxel and cisplatin in combination with split-course concomitant twice-daily re-irradiation in recurrent squamous cell carcinoma of the head and neck: results of Radiation Therapy Oncology Group Protocol 9911. J Clin Oncol 2007;25(30):4800–4805
29. Salama JK, Vokes EE, Chmura SJ, et al. Long-term outcome of concurrent chemotherapy and re-irradiation for recurrent and second primary head-and-neck squamous cell carcinoma. Int J Radiat Oncol Biol Phys 2006;64(2):382–391
30. Spencer SA, Harris J, Wheeler RH, et al. Final report of RTOG 9610, a multi-institutional trial of re-irradiation and chemotherapy for unresectable recurrent squamous cell carcinoma of the head and neck. Head Neck 2008;30(3):281–288
31. Baumann M, Krause M, Hill R. Exploring the role of cancer stem cells in radioresistance. Nat Rev Cancer 2008;8(7):545–554
32. Bussink J, van der Kogel AJ, Kaanders JH. Activation of the PI3-K/AKT pathway and implications for radioresistance mechanisms in head and neck cancer. Lancet Oncol 2008;9(3):288–296
33. Jorgensen TJ. Enhancing radiosensitivity: targeting the DNA repair pathways. Cancer Biol Ther 2009;8(8):665–670
34. Weinmann M, Welz S, Bamberg M. Hypoxic radiosensitizers and hypoxic cytotoxins in radiation oncology. Curr Med Chem Anticancer Agents 2003;3(5):364–374

35. Bentzen SM, Harari PM, Bernier J. Exploitable mechanisms for combining drugs with radiation: concepts, achievements and future directions. Nat Clin Pract Oncol 2007;4(3):172–180
36. Salama JK, Vokes EE. Concurrent chemotherapy and re-irradiation for locoregionally recurrent head and neck cancer. Semin Oncol 2008;35(3):251–261
37. Stevens KR Jr, Britsch A, Moss WT. High-dose re-irradiation of head and neck cancer with curative intent. Int J Radiat Oncol Biol Phys 1994;29(4):687–698
38. Slaughter DP, Southwick HW, Smejkal W. Field cancerization in oral stratified squamous epithelium; clinical implications of multicentric origin. Cancer 1953;6(5):963–968
39. Spencer SA, Harris J, Wheeler RH, et al. RTOG 96-10: re-irradiation with concurrent hydroxyurea and 5-fluorouracil in patients with squamous cell cancer of the head and neck. Int J Radiat Oncol Biol Phys 2001;51(5):1299–1304
40. Hong WK, Bromer R. Chemotherapy in head and neck cancer. N Engl J Med 1983;308(2):75–79
41. Seiwert TY, Salama JK, Vokes EE. The concurrent chemoradiation paradigm—general principles. Nat Clin Pract Oncol 2007;4(2):86–100
42. Lawrence TS, Tepper JE, Blackstock AW. Fluoropyrimidine–radiation interactions in cells and tumors. Semin Radiat Oncol 1997;7(4):260–266
43. McGinn CJ, Lawrence TS. Recent advances in the use of radiosensitizing nucleosides. Semin Radiat Oncol 2001;11(4):270–280
44. Haraf DJ, Weichselbaum RR, Vokes EE. Re-irradiation with concomitant chemotherapy of unresectable recurrent head and neck cancer: a potentially curable disease. Ann Oncol 1996;7(9):913–918
45. Janot F, de Raucourt D, Benhamou E, et al. Randomized trial of postoperative re-irradiation combined with chemotherapy after salvage surgery compared with salvage surgery alone in head and neck carcinoma. J Clin Oncol 2008;26(34):5518–5523
46. Spencer S, Wheeler R, Peters G, et al. Phase 1 trial of combined chemotherapy and re-irradiation for recurrent unresectable head and neck cancer. Head Neck 2003;25(2):118–122
47. Milano MT, Vokes EE, Salama JK, et al. Twice-daily re-irradiation for recurrent and second primary head-and-neck cancer with gemcitabine, paclitaxel, and 5-fluorouracil chemotherapy. Int J Radiat Oncol Biol Phys 2005;61(4):1096–1106
48. Milano MT, Haraf DJ, Stenson KM, et al. Phase I study of concomitant chemoradiotherapy with paclitaxel, fluorouracil, gemcitabine, and twice-daily radiation in patients with poor-prognosis cancer of the head and neck. Clin Cancer Res 2004;10(15):4922–4932
49. Brockstein B, Haraf DJ, Stenson K, et al. Phase I study of concomitant chemoradiotherapy with paclitaxel, fluorouracil, and hydroxyurea with granulocyte colony-stimulating factor support for patients with poor-prognosis cancer of the head and neck. J Clin Oncol 1998;16(2):735–744
50. Chmura SJ, Vokes EE, Garofalo MC, et al. Long-term outcome of re-irradiation with concomitant chemotherapy for locally recurrent squamous cell carcinoma of the head and neck. Int J Radiat Oncol Biol Phys 2003;57(2):S409–S410 Abstract
51. Kramer NM, Horwitz EM, Cheng J, et al. Toxicity and outcome analysis of patients with recurrent head and neck cancer treated with hyperfractionated split-course re-irradiation and concurrent cisplatin and paclitaxel chemotherapy from two prospective phase I and II studies. Head Neck 2005;27(5):406–414
52. Langer CJ, Duffy K, Horwitz EM, et al. Phase I trial of concurrent hyperfractionated split course radiotherapy (HFx RT), cisplatin (cDDP), and paclitaxel in patients with recurrent, previously irradiated, or treatment-naïve locally advanced upper aerodigestive malignancy. Cancer Invest 2006;24(2):164–173
53. Temam S, Koka V, Mamelle G, et al. Treatment of the N0 neck during salvage surgery after radiotherapy of head and neck squamous cell carcinoma. Head Neck 2005;27(8):653–658
54. Hehr T, Classen J, Belka C, et al. Re-irradiation alternating with docetaxel and cisplatin in inoperable recurrence of head-and-neck cancer: a prospective phase I/II trial. Int J Radiat Oncol Biol Phys 2005;61(5):1423–1431
55. Calais G, Alfonsi M, Bardet E, et al. Randomized trial of radiation therapy versus concomitant chemotherapy and radiation therapy for advanced-stage oropharynx carcinoma. J Natl Cancer Inst 1999;91(24):2081–2086
56. Ang KK, Jiang GL, Feng Y, Stephens LC, Tucker SL, Price RE. Extent and kinetics of recovery of occult spinal cord injury. Int J Radiat Oncol Biol Phys 2001;50(4):1013–1020
57. Nieder C, Grosu AL, Andratschke NH, Molls M. Update of human spinal cord re-irradiation tolerance based on additional data from 38 patients. Int J Radiat Oncol Biol Phys 2006;66(5):1446–1449
58. Wong SJ, Machtay M, Li Y. Locally recurrent, previously irradiated head and neck cancer: concurrent re-irradiation and chemotherapy, or chemotherapy alone? J Clin Oncol 2006;24(17):2653–2658
59. Upile T, Triaridis S, Kirkland P, et al. The management of carotid artery rupture. Eur Arch Otorhinolaryngol 2005;262(7):555–560
60. Chang FC, Lirng JF, Luo CB, et al. Patients with head and neck cancers and associated postirradiated carotid blowout syndrome: endovascular therapeutic methods and outcomes. J Vasc Surg 2008;47(5):936–945
61. Cohen J, Rad I. Contemporary management of carotid blowout. Curr Opin Otolaryngol Head Neck Surg 2004;12(2):110–115
62. Warren FM, Cohen JI, Nesbit GM, Barnwell SL, Wax MK, Andersen PE. Management of carotid 'blowout' with endovascular stent grafts. Laryngoscope 2002;112(3):428–433
63. Bollet MA, Lapeyre M, Marchal C, et al. Cervical lymph node relapses of head-and-neck squamous cell carcinoma: is brachytherapy a therapeutic option? Int J Radiat Oncol Biol Phys 2001;51(5):1305–1312
64. Fontanesi J, Hetzler D, Ross J. Effect of dose rate on local control and complications in the re-irradiation of head and neck tumors with interstitial iridium-192. Int J Radiat Oncol Biol Phys 1989;17(2):365–369
65. Peiffert D, Pernot M, Malissard L, et al. Salvage irradiation by brachytherapy of velotonsillar squamous cell carcinoma in a previously irradiated field: results in 73 cases. Int J Radiat Oncol Biol Phys 1994;29(4):681–686
66. Petrovich Z, Lam K, Langholz B, Astrahan M, Luxton G, Rice D. Interstitial thermoradiotherapy for recurrent head and neck cancer. Am J Otolaryngol 1989;10(4):257–260
67. Puthawala A, Nisar Syed AM, Gamie S, Chen YJ, Londrc A, Nixon V. Interstitial low-dose-rate brachytherapy as a salvage treatment for recurrent head-and-neck cancers: long-term results. Int J Radiat Oncol Biol Phys 2001;51(2):354–362
68. Choe KS, Solanki A, Haraf DJ, et al. Prior chemoradiotherapy adversely impacts outcomes of recurrent and second primary head and neck cancer treated with concurrent chemotherapy and re-irradiation. Cancer 2011 Jun 13. Epub ahead of print

69. Dawson LA, Myers LL, Bradford CR, et al. Conformal re-irradiation of recurrent and new primary head-and-neck cancer. Int J Radiat Oncol Biol Phys 2001;50(2):377–385
70. De Crevoisier R, Domenge C, Wibault P, et al. Full dose re-irradiation combined with chemotherapy after salvage surgery in head and neck carcinoma. Cancer 2001;91(11):2071–2076
71. Emami B, Bignardi M, Spector GJ, Devineni VR, Hederman MA. Re-irradiation of recurrent head and neck cancers. Laryngoscope 1987;97(1):85–88
72. Kowalski LP. Results of salvage treatment of the neck in patients with oral cancer. Arch Otolaryngol Head Neck Surg 2002;128(1):58–62
73. Langlois D, Eschwege F, Kramar A, Richard JM. Re-irradiation of head and neck cancers. Presentation of 35 cases treated at the Gustave Roussy Institute. Radiother Oncol 1985;3(1):27–33
74. Lee N, Chan K, Bekelman JE, et al. Salvage re-irradiation for recurrent head and neck cancer. Int J Radiat Oncol Biol Phys 2007;68(3):731–740
75. Levendag PC, Meeuwis CA, Visser AG. Re-irradiation of recurrent head and neck cancers: external and/or interstitial radiation therapy. Radiother Oncol 1992;23(1):6–15
76. Mabanta SR, Mendenhall WM, Stringer SP, Cassisi NJ. Salvage treatment for neck recurrence after irradiation alone for head and neck squamous cell carcinoma with clinically positive neck nodes. Head Neck 1999;21(7):591–594
77. Machtay M, Rosenthal DI, Chalian AA, et al. Pilot study of postoperative re-irradiation, chemotherapy, and amifostine after surgical salvage for recurrent head-and-neck cancer. Int J Radiat Oncol Biol Phys 2004;59(1):72–77
78. Mendenhall WM, Mendenhall CM, Malyapa RS, Palta JR, Mendenhall NP. Re-irradiation of head and neck carcinoma. Am J Clin Oncol 2008;31(4):393–398
79. Nagar YS, Singh S, Datta NR. Chemo-re-irradiation in persistent/recurrent head and neck cancers. Jpn J Clin Oncol 2004;34(2):61–68
80. Pomp J, Levendag PC, van Putten WL. Re-irradiation of recurrent tumors in the head and neck. Am J Clin Oncol 1988;11(5):543–549
81. Tanvetyanon T, Padhya T, McCaffrey J, et al. Prognostic factors for survival after salvage re-irradiation of head and neck cancer. J Clin Oncol 2009;27(12):1983–1991
82. Solanki A, Stenson K, Haraf DJ, et al. Pathologic predictors for outcome in recurrent and second primary head and neck cancer patients undergoing surgery followed by concurrent chemo-re-irradiation. Int J Radiat Oncol Biol Phys 2008;72(1):S402–S403 Abstract
83. Langendijk JA, Bourhis J. Re-irradiation in squamous cell head and neck cancer: recent developments and future directions. Curr Opin Oncol 2007;19(3):202–209
84. Haddad R, Tishler R, Wirth L, et al. Rate of pathologic complete responses to docetaxel, cisplatin, and fluorouracil induction chemotherapy in patients with squamous cell carcinoma of the head and neck. Arch Otolaryngol Head Neck Surg 2006;132(6):678–681
85. Salama JK, Stenson KM, Kistner EO, et al. Induction chemotherapy and concurrent chemoradiotherapy for locoregionally advanced head and neck cancer: a multi-institutional phase II trial investigating three radiotherapy dose levels. Ann Oncol 2008;19(10):1787–1794
86. Urba S, Wolf G, Eisbruch A, et al. Single-cycle induction chemotherapy selects patients with advanced laryngeal cancer for combined chemoradiation: a new treatment paradigm. J Clin Oncol 2006;24(4):593–598
87. Villaflor VM, Cohen EE, Haraf DJ, et al. Phase II trial pemetrexed-based induction chemotherapy followed by concomitant chemoradiotherapy in previously irradiated head and neck patients. J Clin Oncol 2008;26(15S): Abstract 6030
88. Khodarev NN, Beckett M, Labay E, Darga T, Roizman B, Weichselbaum RR. STAT1 is overexpressed in tumors selected for radioresistance and confers protection from radiation in transduced sensitive cells. Proc Natl Acad Sci U S A 2004;101(6):1714–1719
89. Weichselbaum RR, Ishwaran H, Yoon T, et al. An interferon-related gene signature for DNA damage resistance is a predictive marker for chemotherapy and radiation for breast cancer. Proc Natl Acad Sci U S A 2008;105(47):18 490–18 495
90. Mutic S, Palta JR, Butker EK, et al. AAPM Radiation Therapy Committee Task Group No. 66. Quality assurance for computed-tomography simulators and the computed-tomography-simulation process: report of the AAPM Radiation Therapy Committee Task Group No. 66. Med Phys 2003;30(10):2762–2792
91. Kasperts N, Slotman BJ, Leemans CR, de Bree R, Doornaert P, Langendijk JA. Results of postoperative re-irradiation for recurrent or second primary head and neck carcinoma. Cancer 2006;106(7):1536–1547
92. Popovtzer A, Gluck I, Chepeha DB, et al. The pattern of failure after re-irradiation of recurrent squamous cell head and neck cancer: implications for defining the targets. Int J Radiat Oncol Biol Phys 2009;74(5):1342–1347
93. Sulman EP, Schwartz DL, Le TT, et al. IMRT re-irradiation of head and neck cancer-disease control and morbidity outcomes. Int J Radiat Oncol Biol Phys 2009;73(2):399–409
94. Heron DE, Ferris RL, Karamouzis M, et al. Stereotactic body radiotherapy for recurrent squamous cell carcinoma of the head and neck: results of a phase I dose-escalation trial. Int J Radiat Oncol Biol Phys 2009;75(5):1493–1500
95. Roh KW, Jang JS, Kim MS, et al. Fractionated stereotactic radiotherapy as re-irradiation for locally recurrent head and neck cancer. Int J Radiat Oncol Biol Phys 2009;74(5):1348–1355
96. Truong MT, Grillone G, Tschoe C, Chin L, Kachnic LA, Jalisi S. Emerging applications of stereotactic radiotherapy in head and neck cancer. Neurosurg Focus 2009;27(6):E11
97. Lin R, Slater JD, Yonemoto LT, et al. Nasopharyngeal carcinoma: repeat treatment with conformal proton therapy—dose–volume histogram analysis. Radiology 1999;213(2):489–494
98. Feehan PE, Castro JR, Phillips TL, et al. Recurrent locally advanced nasopharyngeal carcinoma treated with heavy charged particle irradiation. Int J Radiat Oncol Biol Phys 1992;23(4):881–884
99. Bonner JA, Harari PM, Giralt J, et al. Radiotherapy plus cetuximab for squamous-cell carcinoma of the head and neck. N Engl J Med 2006;354(6):567–578
100. Balermpas P, Hambek M, Seitz O, Rödel C, Weiss C. Combined cetuximab and re-irradiation for locoregional recurrent and inoperable squamous cell carcinoma of the head and neck. Strahlenther Onkol 2009;185(12):775–781
101. Cohen EE, Halpern AB, Kasza K, Kocherginsky M, Williams R, Vokes EE. Factors associated with clinical benefit from epidermal growth factor receptor inhibitors in recurrent and metastatic squamous cell carcinoma of the head and neck. Oral Oncol 2009;45(10):e155–e160
102. Artman T, Schilling D, Gnann J, Molls M, Multhoff G, Bayer C. Irradiation-induced regulation of plasminogen activator inhibitor type-1 and vascular endothelial growth factor in six human squamous cell carcinoma lines of the head and neck. Int J Radiat Oncol Biol Phys 2010;76(2):574–582

103. Sauter ER, Nesbit M, Watson JC, Klein-Szanto A, Litwin S, Herlyn M. Vascular endothelial growth factor is a marker of tumor invasion and metastasis in squamous cell carcinomas of the head and neck. Clin Cancer Res 1999;5(4):775–782
104. Smith BD, Smith GL, Carter D, Sasaki CT, Haffty BG. Prognostic significance of vascular endothelial growth factor protein levels in oral and oropharyngeal squamous cell carcinoma. J Clin Oncol 2000;18(10):2046–2052
105. Seiwert TY, Haraf DJ, Cohen EE, et al. Phase I study of bevacizumab added to fluorouracil- and hydroxyurea-based concomitant chemoradiotherapy for poor-prognosis head and neck cancer. J Clin Oncol 2008;26(10):1732–1741
106. Vokes EE, Seiwert TY, Blair EE, et al. A phase I dose escalation study of Ad Gv.EGR.TNF.11D (TNFerade) with concurrent chemoradiotherapy in patients with recurrent head and neck cancer (HNC). J Clin Oncol 2008;26(15S): Abstract 6067
107. Isa AY, Ward TH, West CM, Slevin NJ, Homer JJ. Hypoxia in head and neck cancer. Br J Radiol 2006;79(946):791–798
108. Brizel DM, Dodge RK, Clough RW, Dewhirst MW. Oxygenation of head and neck cancer: changes during radiotherapy and impact on treatment outcome. Radiother Oncol 1999;53(2):113–117
109. Nordsmark M, Bentzen SM, Rudat V, et al. Prognostic value of tumor oxygenation in 397 head and neck tumors after primary radiation therapy. An international multi-center study. Radiother Oncol 2005;77(1):18–24
110. Nordsmark M, Overgaard M, Overgaard J. Pretreatment oxygenation predicts radiation response in advanced squamous cell carcinoma of the head and neck. Radiother Oncol 1996;41(1):31–39
111. Cohen EE, Rosine D, Haraf DJ, et al. Phase I trial of tirapazamine, cisplatin, and concurrent accelerated boost re-irradiation in patients with recurrent head and neck cancer. Int J Radiat Oncol Biol Phys 2007;67(3):678–684

5 Systemic Therapy in the Treatment of Recurrent and Metastatic Head and Neck Carcinoma

Lisa Licitra, Jan B. Vermorken, Pol Specenier, Augusto Caraceni

Summary

- Recurrent head and neck carcinoma, particularly locoregional relapse, usually causes severe morbidity and therefore requires a well-organized management plan.
- Only a small fraction of patient with locoregional tumor relapse can be salvaged.
- Clinical decision making should take into account treatment-induced morbidity.
- Risk versus benefit of cancer treatment should be assessed by a multidisciplinary team.
- No progress was made in systemic therapy until recent integration of a biologic agent with chemotherapy.
- The management algorithm should include end-of-life supportive care.

Causes of treatment failure are locoregional recurrence (60%), followed by metastatic disease (up to 30%) and by second primaries.[1] Ten percent of patients have metastatic disease at initial presentation.[2] An individual patient's prognosis depends on the tumor's site, its extension, nodal involvement, and grading.[3] Treatments of these diverse groups of cancers include surgery, radiotherapy, chemotherapy, and their combinations. Due to the patterns of disease recurrence as well as to the adverse effects of previous treatments, patients with recurrent HNSCC often have a relatively prolonged course of disease marked by serious illness, debility, and several physical and psychological symptoms that include pain, weight loss, dysphagia, disfigurement, depression, and infections. These features pose unique challenges to the caregivers, particularly those providing palliative management. One of the fundamental principles of palliative care is that it should be practiced within a multidisciplinary team that includes head and neck surgeons, radiation and medical oncologists, nutritionists, dedicated nurses, social workers, and palliative care clinicians. It is advisable that such a team starts to integrate palliative care into the care plan earlier in the course of disease, thus reinforcing the idea both for patients and clinicians that palliation is not equal to end-of-life care. The interdisciplinary team also helps sole caregivers to share their personal burdens in caring for seriously ill patients.

End-of-life care of these patients also poses unique issues. It can be particularly difficult to predict time of survival. For example, sudden major bleeding or dyspnea due to laryngeal edema can lead to catastrophic events in few minutes. Accordingly, a timely and accurate expert assessment is needed to prevent such events happening at home because this can be exceedingly disruptive for the family.[4]

! The prognosis of patients with head and neck squamous cell carcinoma (HNSCC) remains relatively poor. The 5-year survival rates in Europe were 40%, 49%, and 63% for patients diagnosed with HNSCC located the pharynx, oral cavity, and larynx, respectively, in the period 1995–1999.[5] Interestingly a recent paper reported improvement in the survival of patients with head and neck cancers in Europe from years 1990–1994 to 1995–99.[6]

Patient's Clinical Profile and Assessment

On the basis of a specific clinical profile, the assessment of patients with recurrent and metastatic (R/M) HNSCC needs a multidimensional approach. Typically such patients are elderly, have comorbidities, are malnourished, have been previously treated with extensive surgery and/or radiation with or without chemotherapy, have poor immunocompetence, are symptomatic, and have specific sociodemographic features. Individual patients often have most or all of these characteristics, which have to be taken into consideration before therapeutic decisions are made. Currently, available treatments have a wide spectrum of acute toxicity so that appropriate assessment of a patient is mandatory to try to individualize palliative treatment. Careful assessment followed by an expert clinical judgment is highly recommended. Unfortunately, expertise in the management of head and neck cancer patients takes time to build. This is mainly due to the relative low number of patients who seek medical oncological care, along with the complexity of dealing with patients so severely ill.

Sociodemographic Status

Studies have shown that patients who are uninsured or are insured by Medicaid are more likely to present with advanced cancer. After adjusting for known risk factors, the risk of death from recurrence or other reasons in this patient subset was significantly increased relative to patients having private insurance.[7] In another study, pretreatment cognitive functional status and to a lesser extent marital status was significantly associated with recurrence.[8]

Disfigurement

Patients may suffer great physical and psychological distress due to debilitating effect of a fungating, function limiting, often malodorant tumor. Care of such wounds is often complicated, which requires interdisciplinary management.

Depression

Several studies have reported that depression is significantly associated with the cancer population.[9] Patients with HNSCC, similarly to those with pancreatic, breast, and lung cancer, are associated with one of the highest rate of depression, which ranges between 20% and 57%. Depression and mental distress were linked to poor performance status (PS) and advanced disease. Moreover, individuals suffering depression at any time are at higher risk of dying.[10]

Advanced age

It has been estimated that as many as 25% of patients diagnosed with HNSCC are older than 70 years. This proportion is likely to increase as a result of increasing population life expectancy. Elderly patients usually have carcinoma of the larynx, oral cavity, and oropharynx. The male-to-female ratio in elderly patients differs from that of younger cohorts with a relatively higher proportion of females. In general, elderly patients tend to present with more locally advanced disease (T4 disease) but fewer neck nodes.

Although palliative chemotherapy has been shown to have a similar response rate and a similar *progression-free survival* (PFS) in older compared with younger patients, the median survival was shorter. It is noteworthy that elderly patients had a significantly higher toxicity (nephrotoxicity, thrombocytopenia, and diarrhea).[11] A higher rate of toxic death was reported, but it does not reach statistical significance (13% vs. 8%). In general, this is a high price to pay for a palliative treatment that stresses the importance of a careful risk versus benefit analysis before prescribing therapy. Age is associated with pharmacokinetic and pharmacodynamic changes, with an increased susceptibility to toxic complications. Moreover, multiple medications for intercurrent ailments and comorbidity may interfere with antineoplastic treatment, increasing the risks.

Nutrition

Nutritional assessment and intervention before antineoplastic treatment is started have proven to be critical in improving a patient's prognosis. In particular, maintaining adequate nutrient intake and avoiding deterioration in body weight and strength allows patients to better tolerate treatment provided. Although nutrition therapy might not result in weight gain or reversal of malnutrition,[12,13] such support is helpful in lessening side effects, reducing risk of infection (if given enterally), reducing asthenia, and improving well-being. In individuals with advanced cancer, the main goal of nutrition therapy is to improve comfort and symptom relief.[14]

Clinical Decision Making

Treatment Aims

Depending on the extent and primary tumor site, a few patients with locoregional relapse can be salvaged with surgery, re-irradiation with chemotherapy, or their combinations, particularly when the recurrences are detected early. The indications and strategies for re-treatment are site specific and are presented in Chapter 4 and treatment of individual sites in this book. Unfortunately, most patients with R/M-HNSCC are only eligible for palliative treatment. Treatment options in these patients include supportive care only, or supportive care plus single-agent chemotherapy, combination chemotherapy, or targeted therapies, either alone or in combination with cytotoxic agents. Treatment choices are based on factors such as the extent of disease, performance status, comorbidity, prior treatment, symptoms, patient preference, and logistics.[15] Goals of treatments in these circumstances are mainly symptom control and prevention of new cancer-related symptoms, and improvement in quality of life (QoL). However, if applicable, objective tumor response (OR), disease stabilization (SD), or both combined (disease control; DC), and prolongation of overall survival (OS) and progression-free survival (PFS) can also be taken into account. Unfortunately, correlation between objective tumor regression (or DC) and subjective benefit (symptom control and QoL) has not been adequately studied, underscoring the importance of clinical trials in this patient group.[16]

Prognostic Factors

Several clinical prognostic factors have been proposed to define patients who are most likely to benefit from palliative systemic therapy and these can be categorized as patient-, tumor- and treatment-related. Performance status is one of the most important prognostic factors that not only influences the rate of response to chemotherapy but also effects the overall survival of these patients regardless of the response to the agents used.[17] Patients with only local recurrence with or without regional lymph node involvement and no bony erosion after definitive treatment have a better chance of responding to chemotherapy than do patients with systemic and visceral metastases. Other factors that have been reported to influence outcome are a good response to prior induction (adjuvant) chemotherapy or radiotherapy, a long interval between primary and recurrence, good organ functions, poorly differentiated histological type, and the response to palliative treatment.[18–21]

Data from two more recently conducted US trials in R/M-HNSCC (E1395 and E1393) were combined and analyzed to identify prognostic factors for response and survival.[22] The median follow-up of the patients in these two trials was 4.7 years with overall survival (OS) rates at 1, 2, 3, and 5 years of 32%, 12%, 7%, and 3.6%, respectively, and a median overall survival of 7.8 months. The overall response (OR) rate was 32%. On multivariate analysis, the investigators were able to identify one pathological feature (tumor cell differentiation) and four clinical baseline characteristics (ECOG performance status, weight loss, location of the primary tumor, and prior radiotherapy) as independent predictors of OS. They constructed a prognostic model for OS based on the presence of these five independent prognostic factors and were able to categorize the patients into two groups with significant differences in outcome, i.e., one in which patients had only 0–2 adverse prognostic factors and another in which patients had ≥3 poor prognostic factors. The median survival of the first group was nearly twice that of the second group (0.98 years versus 0.52 years). In this study, 283 of the 399 patients included in the analysis had three or more adverse factors, explaining the median survival of only 7.8 months. The authors also identified that the same variables and the presence of residual tumor at the primary site were independent predictors of response to chemotherapy.[22] In fact, response to chemotherapy was found to be of prognostic significance. When the investigators added response to chemotherapy to the model, the location of the primary tumor lost its prognostic significance, but all other parameters, including tumor cell differentiation, retained their significance as independent predictors of survival. Predictors of better 2-year survivorship were complete or partial response to chemotherapy (CR/PR vs. no response), white ethnicity (vs. others), ECOG performance status of 0 (vs. 1), poor cell differentiation (vs. good/moderate) and no prior radiotherapy. Interestingly, all long-term survivors had locally recurrent disease at entry into the study. The findings in this study suggested that (1) there is an urgent need of better therapy for this category of patients; (2) response to systemic therapy has a major impact on survival; (3) patients with locally recurrent disease, but not the patients with distant metastases, who are primarily treated with chemotherapy, will rarely be cured of their disease; and (4) future trials in patients with R/M-SCCHN should take the five adverse prognostic factors into consideration.

R/M-HNSCC patients who fail platinum-based first-line therapy do very poorly; they have a very low likelihood of responding to second-line chemotherapy and have an extremely poor survival.[23,24] Leon et al., in a retrospective analysis of the outcome of patients with R/M-HNSCC who were progressing while on platinum-based palliative chemotherapy, reported no responses using traditional chemotherapeutic agents and a median OS of 3.4 months.[23] Specenier et al. more recently reported that in these unfavorable conditions a taxane (docetaxel) in a weekly dose regimen induced response in only 6.7% of patients and reported a median OS of 17.9 weeks.[24] This is a practical problem in evaluating the effectiveness of new agent(s), which very often are tested in previously treated patients.

Risk/Benefit Ratio

There has been only one small study in the past testing whether the systemic chemotherapy had any impact on survival when compared with best supportive care (BSC) alone, using randomized controlled trial methodology. In that trial, 31 patients treated with single-agent cisplatin demonstrated prolonged survival compared with 26 patients treated with supportive measures only.[25] A study from the same Liverpool Head and Neck Oncology Group suggested that cisplatin was leading to a better survival than methotrexate alone, but at the cost of more toxicity at that time.[26] However, later randomized studies on single agents did not confirm superiority of any single drug or even platinum-based combination chemotherapy over methotrexate alone in terms of overall survival (see later). In recent randomized trials of the anti-epidermal growth factor receptor (EGFR) antibody cetuximab plus cytotoxic chemotherapy versus cytotoxic chemotherapy alone, an improvement in PFS has become noticeable[27–29] and in one study there was even a significant OS benefit reported.[27] However, irrespective of any survival benefit, tumor response may be of benefit to the patient. A placebo-controlled study of intratumoral cisplatin/epinephrine, using a validated new instrument for measuring benefit associated with local tumor response, has shown a positive correlation between patient benefit and target tumor response.[30]

If indeed palliation is the main goal, and if palliation is synonymous with response, then only one out of 4–6 patients is expected to achieve palliation with single-agent chemotherapy.[20,21,31–35] Although weekly standard-dosed methotrexate is considered a standard palliative measure, about 10% of patients may suffer from severe stomatitis, which can have a negative effect on patients' well-being. With the use of platinum-based combinations, frequently used nowadays with or without cetuximab, twice the number of patients can expected to respond, and thus perhaps be palliated. This must be balanced against the greater toxicity observed with these more aggressive combination regimens. Treatment-related mortality with these platinum-based combinations varies from 1% to 7% in different randomized studies[21,27,31,36,37] and the addition of cetuximab to these regimens did not seem to increase this rate, despite the fact that more infectious complications are being observed with this combined approach.[27] In the National Comprehensive Cancer Network (NCCN) guidelines there is a clear advice for R/M-HNSCC patients who are not candidates for surgery or re-irradiation to be treated with systemic chemotherapy, unless they are of ECOG performance status 3 and some patients with ECOG performance status 2, who might be better candidates for BSC.[38] NCCN guidelines also recommend participation in clinical trials at all times.

Medical Treatment

Cytotoxic Chemotherapy

HNSCC is a chemosensitive disease as is evident from responses observed with various drugs of different classes of cytotoxic agents.[39] The four most extensively studied single cytotoxic agents in advanced or recurrent disease are bleomycin, methotrexate, 5-fluo-

Table 5.1 Randomized single agent trials in recurrent/metastatic HNSCC

Author	No. of patients	Drugs randomized	Respiration rate (%)	Median OS (months)
Grose[40]	100	Methotrexate	16	4.6
		Cisplatin	8	4.1
Hong[41]	38	Methotrexate	23	6.1
		Cisplatin	29	6.3
Schornagel[32]	264	Methotrexate	16	6.0
		Edetrexate	21	6.0
Vermorken[33]	95	Methotrexate	16	6.8
		Paclitaxel 3 h (vs. 24 h)	11 (–23)	6.5
Pivot[34]	139[a]	Methotrexate	11	3.5
		Nolatrexed	3	3.7
Guardiola[42]	57	Methotrexate	15[b]	3.9
		Docetaxel	27	3.7

[a]62% had failed first-line chemotherapy for R/M SCCHN.
[b]$P < 0.05$.

Table 5.2 Cisplatin/5-fluorouracil (PF) versus single agents or other platinum-containing regimens: randomized trials

Reference	No. of patients	Agents	RR (%)	MS (months)
Jacobs et al.[21]	249	PF	32[a]	5.5
		P	17	5.0
		F	13	6.1
Forastiere et al.[20]	277	PF	32[b]	6.6
		CF	21	5.0
		M	10	5.6
Clavel et al.[31]	382	CABO	34[b]	
		PF	31[c]	7.0
		P	15	
Gibson et al.[37]	218	PF	27	8.7
		PT	26	8.1

[a]$P = 0.035$; [b]$P < 0.001$; [c]$P = 0.003$.
P = cisplatin; C = carboplatin; M = methotrexate; B = bleomycin; V = vincristine; T = paclitaxel; CABO=P+M+B+V.

rouracil, and cisplatin. Response rates with these agents, but also with several other conventional agents of different classes (the platinum analog carboplatin, the alkylating agents ifosfamide and cyclophosphamide, the anthracycline doxorubicin, and the vinca alkaloid vinblastine), are generally in the 15%–30% range, while response duration is generally between 3 and 5 months. Similar response rates, mostly observed in phase II studies, were observed with newer agents such as paclitaxel, docetaxel, vinorelbine, irinotecan, edetrexate, nolatrexed, pemetrexed, capecitabine, orzel, and S-1. The taxanes paclitaxel and docetaxel are among those with the highest in activity in this disease setting, but data in nonrandomized trials are extremely variable due to variations in patient characteristics. Data from randomized studies are therefore more reliable (**Table 5.1**), and do not indicate superiority of one drug over another, although the taxanes might need some further testing.

No progress had been made since the first studies with cisplatin in patients with R/M-HNSCC were reported in the 1970s until recently. Platinum-based combination chemotherapy regimens were compared with single agent chemotherapy with the hope of obtaining survival benefit. All randomized trials of cytotoxic therapies with a reasonable sample size failed to show an improvement in survival (**Table 5.2**). However, they did show a significant increase in response rate, which may be of benefit for the patient with symptomatic disease, as described earlier in the chapter on risk–benefit ratio. Although on the basis of these reference studies we might expect an overall response rate of 30%, a median survival of approximately 6 months and a 1-year survival of 20%–40%, these figures might be slightly different in more recent trials, depending on patient selection characteristics and improved supportive care.

■ Targeted Therapy

Several biological therapies have been studied in HNSCC patients because of their different mechanism of action, the greater selectivity (target of action is overexpressed as compared with normal tissue), the different toxicity profiles, or because they play a role in carcinogenesis.[15,43] These include drugs that target growth factors and their receptors, signal transduction, cell cycle control, prostaglandin synthesis, protein degradation, hypoxia, or angiogenesis.[44] As randomized trials leading to a further improvement in outcome in this disease setting have only been performed with drugs targeting the growth factors and/or growth factor receptors, in particular those of the HER family, these randomized trials will be the main focus of this part of the chapter.

Epidermal Growth Factor Inhibitors

The epidermal growth factor receptor (EGFR) inhibitors are of particular interest, because EGFR and its ligand TGF-α are overexpressed in the vast majority of HNSCC. In contrast, erbB2 expression in HNSCC ranges between 40% and 60%.[45] Although EGFR overexpression and increased EGFR copy number have been related to poor prognosis in patients with HNSCC[46,47] the prognostic role of EGFR is more specifically related to the treatment received, such as radiotherapy[46] and chemotherapy.[48] Two EGFR targeting strategies are currently in clinical use, i.e., monoclonal antibodies (MAbs) directed at the extracellular domain of the receptor, and the small molecule and ATP-competitive tyrosine kinase inhibitors (TKIs). **Table 5.3** summarizes some important EGFR inhibitors under clinical investigation in R/M-HNSCC.

Mode of Action

EGFR-activated signaling pathways and the effect of activation on cell proliferation and survival are well documented.[49] Ligand binding to the EGFR is followed by stimulation of several different signal transduction cascades, including the mitogen-activated protein kinase (MAPK) pathway and the phosphatidylinositol 3-kinase (PI3K)-Akt pathway. The MAbs and TKIs act at different points on the pathway to disrupt signaling. However, it is likely that the effects of these agents are not mediated by disruption of EGFR signaling pathways alone. Also, antibody-dependent cellular

Table 5.3 Selection of relevant EGFR-targeting agents under clinical investigation in SCCHN

Monoclonal antibodies				Toxicity
Cetuximab	IMC225	Chimeric human/ murine	IgG1	Skin
Matuzumab	EMD72000	Humanized mouse	IgG1	Skin
Nimotu-zumab	h-R3	Humanized mouse	IgG1	Systemic/ hemodynamic
Zalutu-mumab	2F8	Human	IgG1	Skin
Panitu-mumab	ABX-EGF	Human	IgG2	Skin
Tyrosine kinase inhibitors				
Gefitinib	ZD1839	Reversible	EGFR	Skin/gastrointestinal (GI)
Erlotinib Lapatinib	OSI-774 G-572016	Reversible Reversible	EGFR EGFR/erbB2	Skin/GI Skin/GI/systemic
Afatinib	BIBW2992	Reversible	EGFR/erbB2	Skin/GI/systemic
Canertinib	CI-0033	Irreversible	EGFR	Skin/oral/GI/systemic

cytotoxicity (ADCC) is thought to be an important mechanism of action, but for a long time it was thought that this only referred to IgG1 MAbs.[50,51] However, very recently it was discovered that also human IgG2 MAbs against EGFR effectively trigger ADCC but, in contrast to IgG1, only by cells of the myeloid lineage.[52] The ability of many EGFR inhibitors to enhance the effects of radiation and/or chemotherapy has been demonstrated both in vitro and in vivo.[53]

Cetuximab

In patients with R/M-HNSCC, both anti-EGFR MAbs and TKIs have shown antitumor effects, in both the second-line and the first-line settings.[39] However, as yet only cetuximab is approved for the treatment of patients with R/M-HNSCC, both in the second-line setting after failing platinum treatment (USA only) and in the first-line setting, i.e., in patients who were never treated earlier with chemotherapy for their R/M-HNSCC. For the approval in the second-line setting, the single-drug phase II study in platinum-refractory R/M-HNSCC patients has been instrumental.[54]

Single-agent cetuximab induced a response in 13% of the 103 treated patients, disease control (CR+PR+NC) in 46% of the patients, a median time to progression of 2.3 months, and a median survival of 5.9 months. Similar data were observed in two other studies, in which in addition to cetuximab the platinum was reintroduced,[55,56] suggesting that in that setting the reintroduction of platinum will only lead to additional toxicity for the patient and will not add to further symptom control.

EXTREME Study

The approval of cetuximab in the first-line R/M-HNSCC disease setting is based on the EXTREME study.[27] In that study 442 patients were randomized to receive either platinum-infusional fluorouracil (PF) alone (cisplatin 100 mg/m² or carboplatin AUC 5 on day 1 followed by 5-fluorouracil 1000 mg/m²/day for 4 days) or the same PF regimen combined with weekly cetuximab (initial loading dose of 400 mg/m² followed by weekly doses of 250 mg/m²). Cycles were repeated every 3 weeks for a maximum of 6 cycles. Thereafter, in the combined arm, cetuximab was continued as a single agent until disease progression or unacceptable toxicity, whichever came first. No crossover was permitted in this study. Excluded were patients who had received prior chemotherapy except when this had been part of their primary treatment, provided this chemotherapy was discontinued at least 6 months before inclusion into the study. The primary end point was overall survival, defined as the time from randomization to death. Secondary end points were PFS, best overall response, disease control, time to treatment failure, duration of response, and safety.

With the combined use of PF and cetuximab the median OS was 10.1 months (95% confidence interval [CI], 8.6 to 11.2) versus 7.4 months (95% CI, 6.4 to 8.3) with PF alone (hazard ratio for death, 0.80; 95% CI, 0.64 to 0.99; *P* = 0.04) (**Fig. 5.1**). Median PFS was 5.6 months in the PF plus cetuximab group and 3.3 months in the PF alone group (hazard ratio for progression, 0.54; 95% CI, 043 to 0.67; *P* < 0001). The addition of cetuximab to PF chemotherapy was also associated with significant increases in the overall response rate (36% vs. 20%, *P* < 0001) (see **Fig. 5.1**), disease-control rate (81% vs. 60%, *P* < 0001) and time to treatment failure (4.8 vs. 3.0 months). The duration of response in the two groups did not differ significantly (5.6 vs. 4.7 months, *P* = 0.21). The beneficial effect was evident both in patients treated with cisplatin/5-FU and

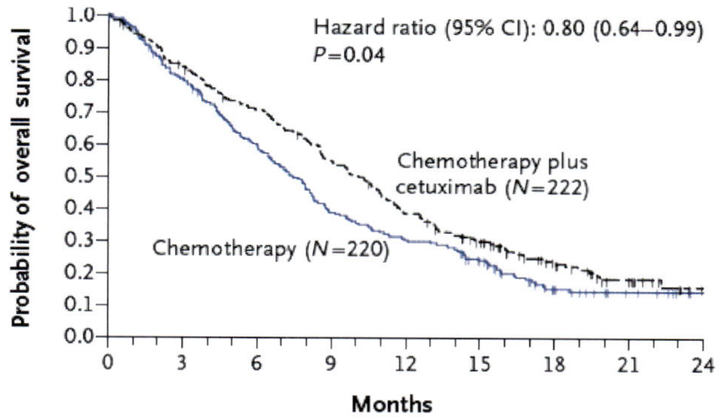

No. at risk									
Chemotherapy	220	173	127	83	65	47	19	8	1
Chemotherapy plus cetuximab	222	184	153	118	82	57	30	15	3

Fig. 5.1 Overall survival with platinum/5-FU combination chemotherapy with or without cetuximab. (From Vermorken JB, Mesia R, Rivera F, et al. Platinum-based chemotherapy plus cetuximab in head and neck cancer. NEJM 2008;359(11):1116–1127; with permission of Massachusetts Medical Society.)

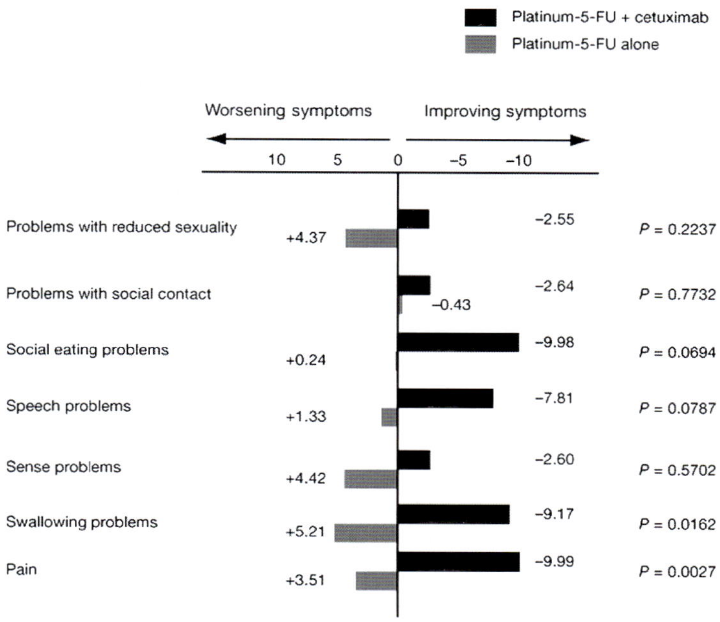

Fig. 5.2 Symptom control in the EXTREME study (Mesìa R, Rivera F, Kawecki A, et al. Quality of life of patients receiving platinum-based chemotherapy plus cetuxiamb first line for recurrent and/or metastatic squamous cell carcinoma of the head and neck. Annals of Oncology 2010;21(10):1967–73; with permission of Oxford University Press on behalf of European Society for Medical Oncology.)

those treated with carboplatin/5-FU, although also in this study response rates with carboplatin/5-FU were below those obtained with cisplatin/5-FU, independently of the treatment arm. Protocol-defined subgroup analyses showed that the beneficial effects of adding cetuximab to PF chemotherapy on OS and PFS were evident in nearly all subgroups analyzed.

The most common grade 3 or 4 adverse events in the chemotherapy-alone and cetuximab groups were anemia (19% and 13%, respectively), neutropenia (23% and 22%), and thrombocytopenia (11% in both groups). Sepsis occurred in 9 patients in the cetuximab group and in 1 patient in the chemotherapy-alone group (*P* = 0.02). There were 11 cases of grade 3 or 4 hypomagnesemia in the cetuximab group, compared with 3 cases in the chemotherapy-alone group (*P* = 0.05). Of the 219 patients receiving cetuximab, 9% had grade 3 skin reactions and 3% had grade 3 or 4 infusion-related reactions. Ten deaths (3 in the cetuximab group and 7 in the PF-alone group) were considered to be treatment related. There were no cetuximab-related deaths.

A very important aspect of the trial was the evaluation of quality of life and symptom control (**Fig. 5.2**). A recent update indicated that for QLQ-H&N35, the mean score for the cetuximab arm was not significantly worse than that for the chemotherapy-alone arm for all symptom scales at all postbaseline visits. In that analysis the improvement in symptom scores was even more significant than in the first analysis and showed significance at cycle 3 for pain, swallowing, speech problems, and social eating.[57] This is the first time in over 30 years that superiority (in terms of survival) of a new regimen over standard platinum-based combination chemotherapy has been observed. Platinum-based combination chemotherapy plus cetuximab is now considered as a new standard for the treatment of R/M-HNSCC for those who are able to tolerate platinum-based combination chemotherapy regimens.[58,59]

Case Study

Figure 5.3 shows a patient with regional recurrence after surgery and postoperative radiation. He received three cycles of platinum-based chemotherapy combined with monoclonal antibody against epidermal growth factor receptor with a favorable response.

Other Studies with Cetuximab or Panitumumab

Although the EXTREME study is so far the only study in which a significant benefit in OS has been observed, other randomized studies with cetuximab or panitumumab (a fully human IgG2 MAb against EGFR) are clearly in support of these data[28,60]; **Table 5.4**).

In **ECOG 5397**[60] 117 patients were assigned to cisplatin 100 mg/m² every 4 weeks either with weekly cetuximab or with weekly placebo. The primary end point of this study was progression-free survival. The study was designed to detect a difference in median PFS of 2 months, i.e., 2 months with cisplatin plus placebo and 4 months with the experimental arm. However, the observed median PFS in the control arm was longer than expected (2.7 months). The median PFS in the cetuximab arm was 4.2 months and that difference did not reach statistical significance ($P = 0.09$). In fact, the actual power to detect a 2 months difference in this situation was only 50%. However, the objective response rate was 26% in the experimental arm versus 10% in the control arm ($P = 0.03$). Median overall survival was not significantly different (9.2 months versus 8 months, $P = 0.21$). Interestingly, development of cetuximab-related skin toxicity was associated with an improved overall survival (hazard ration 0.42, $P = 0.01$).

The **SPECTRUM study** is a large phase III trial, in which panitumumab was evaluated in the first-line setting. Panitumumab is a fully human IgG2 antibody with very strong binding to the receptor.[43,61] It blocks ligand binding and induces internalization of the receptor but does not induce receptor degradation. The side effects that can be observed with this compound include pruritus, skin rash, dyspnea, fatigue, abdominal pain, asthenia, and diarrhea. In the SPECTRUM study, 657 patients with R/M-HNSCC in first line were randomized to receive cisplatin/5-fluorouracil alone or with panitumumab. The patient population differed slightly from that in the EXTREME study in that only patients with performance status 0 and 1 were eligible for the trial. The trial differed from EXTREME also in that all patients started on cisplatin/5-FU (and were not allowed to start with carbloplatin/5-FU) and in that maintenance with single-agent panitumumab (once the chemotherapy was stopped) was optional, while in EXTREME it was mandatory to

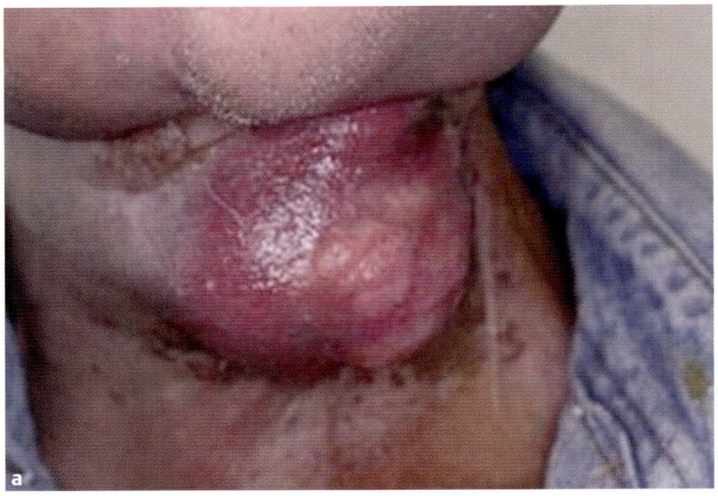

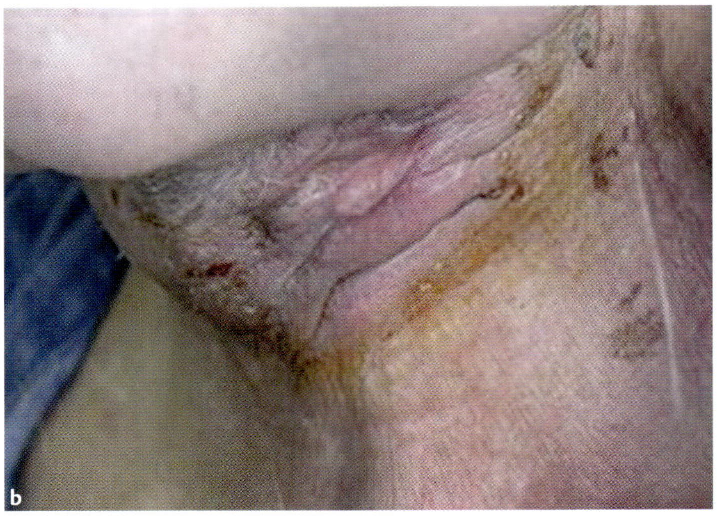

Fig. 5.3 A patient with regional recurrence after surgery and postoperative radiation.

Table 5.4 Completed randomized trials in first-line recurrent/metastatic SCCHN

Study/ reference	*N*	Regimen	RR (%)	PFS (months)	OS (months)
ECOG 5397/ Burtness et al.[60]	117	Cisplatin + cetuximab	26	4.2	9.2
		Cisplatin + placebo	10	2.7	8.0
EXTREME/Vermorken et al.[27]	442	PF + cetuximab	36	5.6	10.1
		PF	20	3.3	7.4
SPECTRUM/Vermorken et al.[28]	657	PF + panitumumab	36	5.8	11.1
		PF	25	4.6	9.0

continue with cetuximab. Unfortunately, the primary end point (a significant increase in OS) was not reached, but benefit in terms of a significant improvement in PFS and an increase in response rate was observed. The trial was presented at ESMO 2010 and results of further analyses of the data are expected.

Other Studies

Three randomized phase III trials have been completed in the second-line R/M-HNSCC disease setting: two studies that evaluated the value of the TKI gefitinib (see **Fig. 5.2**) and one study that evaluated the value of the fully human MAb zalutumumab in this setting (**Table 5.5**). In general, EGFR TKIs have a somewhat less favorable outcome. Single-arm trials with gefitinib, erlotinib, and lapatinib (an inhibitor of EGFR and erbB2) showed response rates ranging from 0% to 15% and a median PFS of approximately 3.5 months (summarized in papers by Specenier and Vermorken in 2007 and 2010[43,62]). Drug toxicity was generally mild, consisting of skin rash and diarrhea, which were more frequent at higher dosages. Cohen et al. reviewed individual patient data from five clinical trials of gefitinib, erlotinib, or lapatinib to determine whether there are clinical characteristics that are associated with clinical benefit. Performance status (PS) ($P = 0.04$), older age ($P = 0.02$), and development of rash ($P < 0.01$), diarrhea ($P = 0.03$), or oral side effects ($P = 0.02$) were independently associated with clinical benefit. Older age, better PS, and development of rash were associated with longer PFS and OS. EGFR mechanistic toxicities that developed during therapy were also highly associated with benefit and suggested a relationship between drug exposure and outcome.[63]

Gefitinib

The suggestion that outcome might be related also to the dose used was tested in a large phase III trial (1839 IL/0704; IMEX, **Table 5.5**) in which 482 patients with R/M-HNSCC, unresponsive to platinum or unfit for platinum, were randomized in a 3-armed study to receive one of gefitinib 250 mg/day or gefitinib 500 mg/day or methotrexate 40 mg/m² IV weekly.[64] Neither gefitinib 250 mg/day nor gefitinib 500 mg/day improved survival compared with single agent methotrexate. Overall response rates were 2.7%, 7.6%, and 3.9%, respectively, and median overall survival was 5.6, 6.0, and 6.7 months, respectively. An interesting aspect in the trial was the observation that in the cohort of patients with platinum-refractory R/M-HNSCC the use of methotrexate resulted in a better survival than the two gefitinib dose regimens, illustrating the potential of this cytotoxic agent in R/M-HNSCC patients in less favorable conditions.

ECOG conducted a randomized, placebo-controlled trial of docetaxel 35 mg/m² on days 1, 8, and 15 every 28 days, with or without gefitinib 250 mg/day in recurrent or metastatic SCCHN patients. The combination was well tolerated and improved the time to progression from 2.0 to 3.5 months ($P = 0.03$). However, this did not translate into an improved overall survival (**Table 5.5**). This study (ECOG 1302) was reported at ASCO in 2009.[65]

Table 5.5 Completed randomized trials in second-line recurrent/metastatic SCCHN

Study/ reference	N	Regimen	RR (%)	PFS (months)	OS (months)
IMEX/Stewart et al.[64]	486	Gefitinib (250 mg)	2.7	ND	5.6
		Gefitinib (500 mg)	7.6	ND	6.0
		Methotrexate	3.9	ND	6.7
ECOG 1302/ Argiris et al.[65]	270	D + Gefitinib	12	3.3	6.8
		D + placebo	6	2.2	6.2
Zalute/ Machiels et al.[29]	286	Z + BSC (−MTX)	6	2.3[a]	6.7[b]
		BSC (optional MTX)	1	1.9*	5.2[b]

BSC = best supportive care; Z = zalutumumab; MTX = methotrexate; ND = no data. [a]HR (95% CI): 0.62 (0.47–0.83), $P = 0.0012$. [b]HR (95% CI): 0.77 (0.57–1.05), $P = 0.0649$.

> **Case Study**
>
> A patient presented with lung metastases after treatment of a locally advanced head and neck carcinoma. The disease responded well to treatment with gefitinib for 3 months (**Fig. 5.4**).

Zalutumumab

Zalutumumab is a fully human IgG1 EGFR directed MAb.[43] The frequency of acneiform rash with this compound increases with the dose. This MAb has been studied in a phase III trial versus best supportive care in second-line in patients who failed standard platinum-based chemotherapy.[29] However, in this so-called ZALUTE trial the great majority of patients (78%) in the BSC alone arm received weekly methotrexate as allowed by the protocol. The primary end point in this study was again overall survival. There was a strong trend in favor of the zalutumumab arm for overall survival, but it did not reach statistical significance (median 6.7 vs. 5.2 months, $P = 0.0649$). However, there was a statistically highly significant difference in progression free survival in favor of the experimental arm (median 9.9 vs. 8.4 weeks; $P = 0.0010$), and nearly double the number of patients were alive and progression-free at the tail of each of the two survival curves. The disease control with zalutumumab was 48% (quite similar to the 46% observed with cetuximab in the single-arm phase II study, mentioned earlier). The most common serious adverse events were tumor hemorrhage (28 [15%] patients given zalutumumab vs. 13 [14%] controls), pneumonia (13 [7%] vs. 3 [3%]), and dysphagia (11 [6%] vs. 2 [2%]). The results of this trial give further support to reported activity of cetuximab in this platinum-refractory disease setting.[66]

Afatinib

Although the data on EGFR or EGFR/erbB2 TKIs so far were not as promising observations with the monoclonal antibodies targeting EGFR, one study has to be mentioned separately. This concerns a study with afatinib (BIBW 2992), a highly potent inhibitor of EGFR and erbB2.[67,68] This compound retains activity for EGFRvIII mutation and provides a sustained blockage of the receptor and inhibition of tumor cell proliferation. Seiwert presented early results at ASCO 2010 of a randomized, open-label, phase II study of afatinib versus cetuximab in R/M-HNSCC patients who had failed platinum-containing therapy.[69] The primary end point of that study was shrinkage of target tumors before any crossover. Diarrhea, dehydration, epistaxis, and asthenia occurred more frequently with afatinib, but tumor shrinkage also occurred more frequently with afatinib than with cetuximab (objective response 21.7% vs. 13.3%).

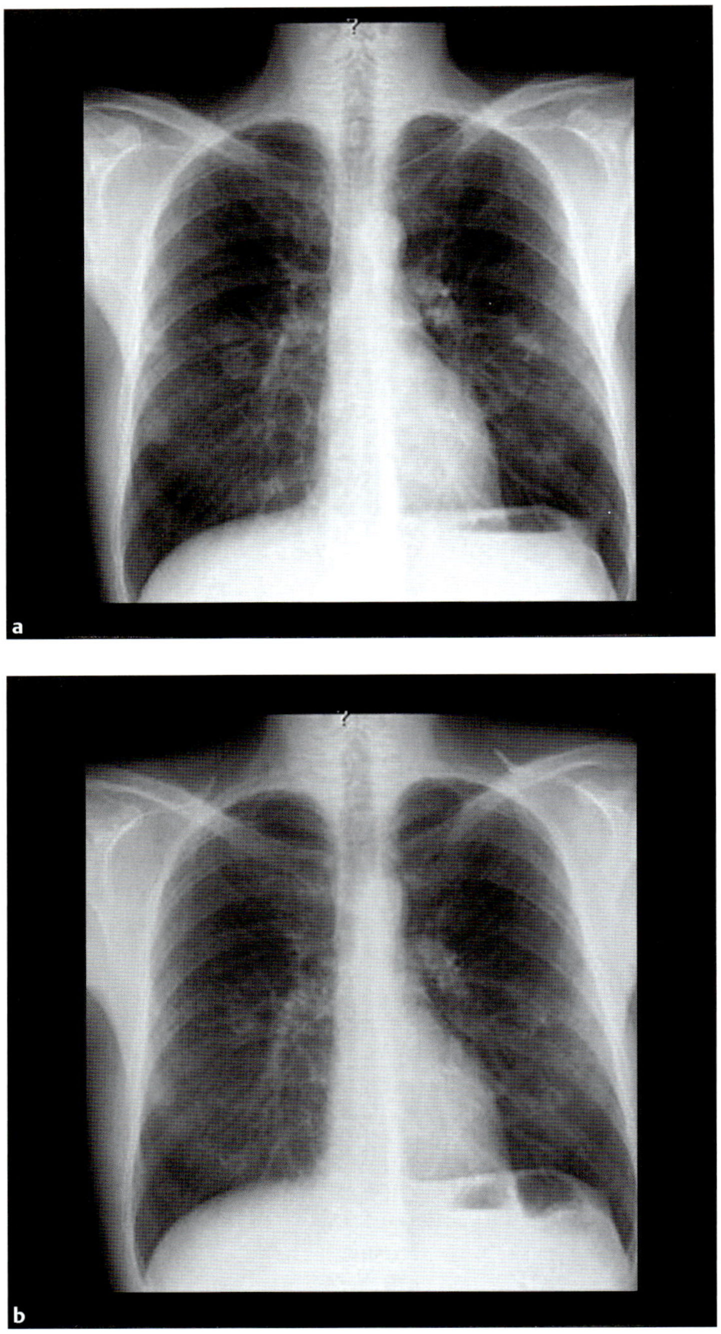

Fig. 5.4a, b A patient who presented with lung metastases after treatment of a locally advanced head and neck carcinoma.

The disease control was comparable (56.7% vs. 61.7%) as was the progression-free survival (median 16 weeks with afatinib [95% CI, 10–19] and 10 weeks with cetuximab [95% CI, 8–17]). Afatinib is the first TKI to demonstrate antitumor activity in SCCHN that appears to be at least comparable to that of cetuximab.

■ Other Therapies

Boron Neutron Capture Therapy

Boron neutron capture therapy (BNCT) is a tumor cell–targeted radiotherapy. It is a binary cancer treatment modality that involves the selective accumulation of boron-10 (^{10}B) carriers in tumors followed by irradiation with a neutron beam.[70,71] The high energy transfers α particles and recoiling ^{7}Li nuclei. These \u03b1 particles and recoiling ^{7}Li nuclei are emitted during the capture of a thermal neutron in the ^{10}B (η,α) ^{7}Li reaction which carry an average total kinetic energy of 2.34 MeV, and have a short range (4–9 mm) of approximately one cell diameter. The result is an induction of a large relative biological effectiveness and selective destruction of tumor cells containing ^{10}B.[70,71] Selective delivery of boron compounds into tumor tissues and high accumulation in the tissues are crucial to avoiding damage of adjacent healthy cells and achieving effective BNCT.[70,71] Two boron drugs have been used clinically: sodium borocaptate and a dihydroxyboryl derivative of phenylalanine called boronophenylalanine.[70–72] Several key issues still have to be solved. There is a clear need for better boron delivery agents. Much attention has been focused on the liposomal drug delivery system as an attractive, intelligent technology for targeting and controlled release of ^{10}B compounds.[73] Dosimetry for BNCT is still imprecise and is based on treating to normal tissue tolerance, based on blood boron values, rather than any real-time information on the boron content of the residual tumor that is to be irradiated.[70,71] Another major problem has been the total dependence on nuclear reactors as neutron sources for BNCT, which limits its use to a few centers worldwide.[70,71] In small single-center studies, BNCT of HNSCC was associated with similar toxicities as conventional photon radiation therapy. The data suggest that the technique is safe and promising enough to proceed to larger studies.[74–78] The availability of compact accelerator-based neutron generators, compatible with installment in hospital environments, should facilitate such trials.

Hyperthermia

Hyperthermia (HT) is a type of cancer treatment in which body tissue is exposed to high temperatures (around 42–43°C during 1 hour) to damage and kill cancer cells.[79] This temperature in itself is able to kill tumor cells under certain conditions and also increases the lethal effect of radiation on tumor cells. Hyperthermia is an appealing complementary therapy to radiation.[79] Cancer cells most resistant to radiation are precisely those most sensitive to heat. Cells that are resistant to radiation include those that are hypoxic, at low pH, nutritionally deprived, or in S phase of the cell cycle. All of these characteristics make cells particularly sensitive to heat.[79] Hyperthermia also has been shown to increase perfusion, resulting in improved tumor oxygenation for subsequent radiation treatments. Therefore, HT is usually combined with radiotherapy.[79] The combination improves local control and overall survival when compared with radiotherapy alone in locoregionally advanced cervical cancer.[80] The results in rectal cancer were less compelling.[81] The head and neck region is characterized by many tissue transitions, large cooling vessels, and the presence of critical tissue very nearby. Applying good HT treatment to this region is therefore a challenging task and requires sophisticated and expensive equipment. Until recently, the application of HT in the head and neck region was limited to superficial tumors, mostly lymph nodes. Two small randomized trials suggested improved local control with the addition of HT to conventionally fractionated irradiation.[82,83] The technology to apply deep heating to the head and neck region became available very recently.[84] Thus far, this technique has been applied in a very limited number of centers worldwide and in a limited number of highly selected patients. This precludes any conclusions about optimal patient selection and efficacy.

Electrochemotherapy–Electroporation

Electrochemotherapy (ECT) is the local application of pulses of electric current to tumor tissue to render the cell membranes permeable to otherwise nonpermeant or poorly permeant anticancer drugs, thereby facilitating a potent localized cytotoxic effect.[85] Among several drugs tested in preclinical studies, the hydrophilic bleomycin and cisplatin have been found to be the most suitable agents for ECT.[85–87] Electroporation does not enhance the therapeutic potential of lipophilic agents. The appropriate electric pulses (short and intense square-wave electric pulses) have no apparent cytotoxic or systemic effects. They transiently and reversibly permeabilize the affected cells and consequently facilitate a passive increase in the delivery of nonpermeant drugs within the tumor cell. In preclinical studies, a 300- to 700-fold enhancement in the cytotoxicity of bleomycin has been demonstrated when used in combination with electropermeabilization.[85] The bleomycin electroporation therapy technique consists of injections of bleomycin directly into the tumor under local or general anesthesia, after which the 4–6 needle-electrodes of a disposable applicator are inserted into the tumor.[88] Following insertion, voltage pulses are delivered to the tumor, while the polarity between opposite needles continually switches.[88] The technique is easy to perform, safe, and well tolerated. However, efficacy data are limited to a few phase II studies which demonstrated encouraging local tumor control rates in heavily pretreated patients.[85–88]

Photodynamic Therapy

Photodynamic therapy (PDT) involves the use of a light-sensitive drug or photosensitizer, in combination with light of a visible wavelength, to destroy target cells (e.g., cancerous or precancerous cells).[89] Photosensitizers can be administered systemically or topically, which targeted cells then preferentially absorb. A period of time is required to permit photosensitizer uptake, after which light is directed at the area to be treated.[89] The photochemical reaction resulting from excitation of the photosensitizer produces singlet oxygen, which is highly toxic and can directly kill tumor cells by apoptosis or necrosis.[89] It also damages the tumor vasculature, resulting in indirect tumor cell kill via hypoxia and starvation.[89] Singlet oxygen is highly reactive and can only diffuse a distance of 0.02 µm. Tissue damage is therefore restricted to the penetration depth of the light used to activate the photosensitizer. Some of the light absorbed by photosensitizers is re-emitted at a different wavelength, a process known as fluorescence; this can be used as a means of detecting the presence and location of tumors. This technique may be used alongside PDT.[89] Major disadvantages of the first generation photosensitizers, such as the purified commercially available Photofrin, are the prolonged skin photosensitivity for 4–12 weeks and the requirement of a prolonged illumination time.[89] *meta*-Tetrahydroxyphenylchlorin (mTHPC; Foscan) has a much stronger absorption peak at 652 nm than the absorption peak for Photophrin at 630 nm.[89] Longer wavelengths of light penetrate deeper in tissue, leading to more effective tumor treatment. Therefore, mTHPC is much more potent than the first-generation photosensitizers, requiring light doses of only 10–20 J/cm². In addition, patients can tolerate subdued indoor light 4 or 5 days after injection, and the period of photosensitivity persists for only 3 weeks after mTHPC compared with 6–12 weeks after photophrin.[89] Lasers are the preferred sources of light for PDT. Because they emit coherent monochromatic light, the power is greater than can be achieved with broadband lamps and can be channeled down a single fiber.[89] Photodynamic therapy has been studied in multicenter phase II trials in patients with early-stage cancers or early recurrences in the oral cavity, nasopharynx, and larynx.[90–94] Durable complete responses have been observed in about 90% of the patients with Cis, T1, or T2 tumors [90–94]. Interstitial photodynamic therapy is a technique for applying photodynamic therapy to internal tumors using light delivered via fibers inserted percutaneously. It can provide worthwhile palliation with few complications for otherwise untreatable advanced head and neck cancers.[95]

Special Issues in End-of-Life Supportive Care

The advanced phase of incurable head and neck cancer is characterized by special therapeutic and care needs demanding a particular effort on the side of professionals, health care services, and social support. Appropriate access to active treatment could change the disease trajectory, but many patients, their family members, and caregivers are confronted with lack of available efficacious treatment. The occurrence of incurable illness can arise suddenly at any time during the course of one individual history or can be foreseen as an actual relevant risk by the oncologist.

Accordingly, integration of palliative care services into the multidisciplinary care is paramount in the overall therapeutic strategy. The shift of therapeutic goals from cure to care and from quantity to quality of life has to happen smoothly and with the least psychological distress to the patient.[96]

Head and neck cancer progression causes significant and difficult symptoms. Pain, odor, dysphagia, disfigurement, psychological distress, depression, and social isolation increase the complexity of the clinical presentation. These conditions require appropriate assessment, interventions, and monitoring to improve symptom control. Skilled professionals and high-level palliative care services may be needed to manage difficult medications, complication of tracheostomy, enteral or parenteral nutrition, and pain. Psychological, social, and spiritual support are also a good example of the concepts embodied in the definition of "total pain," which summarizes how palliative care interventions, in their own disciplinary approach, cannot be limited to the domain of physical medical interventions. This approach can be implemented according to patients' needs, independently of prognosis, as early as felt useful in the course of incurable diseases.

For these very reasons, a global approach to care is based on actively sharing a common care plan between professionals from different disciplines, together with an efficient communication process with the patient and the family.

Communication and information about the implications of advanced disease are necessary to enable the patient to make informed choices about critical aspects of managing complications and symptoms, and deciding the place of care and of death. Information and communication with incurable patients are within the goals of palliative care and should be viewed as a process not as a procedure. A process in which patient preferences can change in time, patient awareness can fluctuate, rational and irrational hopes can be present at the same time, and the amount of truth that the patient is able and willing to bear can differ according to the stage and prognosis.[97] Communication with the patient and family, if available, is part of therapy and requires time and coordination between different disciplines and professions.

Local progression of head and neck cancer can pose significant clinical challenges, to make decisions first about the palliative surgical treatment of upper airways and digestive tract obstruction and subsequently about the management of the end-of-life course of symptoms such as pain, breathing difficulty, and massive bleeding. Ethical dilemmas can arise in managing critical decisions such as the recourse to palliative tracheostomy or parenteral nutrition in patients who may want to refuse them. The therapeutic choices need to be discussed thoroughly within the caring team, with the patient, and if possible with the family early in the course of the advanced illness. Advance directives or advance care plans are useful to inform and ease the decision process but are not a substitute for a direct personal relationship with the patient. The attempt in palliative care to offer to such frail and suffering patients a chance to be cared for in a "safe" environment can only be helped by coordination of care with all oncological disciplines and continuous interprofessional communication to avoid the risk of deteriorating quality of life for the patient and of perceived therapeutic abandonment.

Future Research

- Discovery of biomarkers that can predict likelihood of tumor response to various cytotoxic or biologic agents is paramount for customizing therapy.
- Systematic studies of mechanisms of drug resistance will help in development of more effective agents.
- More effort should be devoted to address recording and reporting of quality of life.
- Guidelines for supportive care should be developed and disseminated.

Recommended Reading

- Argiris A, Li Y, Forastiere A. Prognostic factors and long-term survivorship in patients with recurrent or metastatic carcinoma of the head and neck. Cancer 2004;101(10):2222–2229 (This work presents a prognostic model for overall survival base on one pathological feature and four clinical baseline characteristics (performance status, weight loss, primary tumor site, and prior radiotherapy.)
- Vermorken JB, Mesia R, Rivera F, et al. Platinum-based chemotherapy plus cetuximab in head and neck cancer. N Engl J Med 2008;359(11):1116–1127 (The only phase III trial in three decades that demonstrated an improvement in overall survival in patients with recurrent-metastatic head and neck carcinoma.)
- Stewart JS, Cohen EE, Licitra L, et al. Phase III study of gefitinib compared with intravenous methotrexate for recurrent squamous cell carcinoma of the head and neck [corrected]. J Clin Oncol 2009;27(11):1864–1871 (This phase III trial shows that gefitinib is not better than methotrexate for the treatment of recurrent or metastatic head and neck carcinoma refractory to platinum.)

References[1]

1. Vokes EE, Weichselbaum RR. Measurable impact: multimodality therapy of head and neck cancer. Int J Radiat Oncol Biol Phys 1993;27(2):481–482
2. Argiris A, Eng C. Epidemiology, staging, and screening of head and neck cancer. Cancer Treat Res 2003;114:15–60
3. Fortin A, Couture C, Doucet R, Albert M, Allard J, Tetu B. Does histologic grade have a role in the management of head and neck cancers? J Clin Oncol 2001;19(21):4107–4116
4. Goldstein NE, Genden E, Morrison RS. Palliative care for patients with head and neck cancer: "I would like a quick return to a normal lifestyle". JAMA 2008;299(15):1818–1825
5. Berrino F, De Angelis R, Sant M, et al. EUROCARE Working group. Survival for eight major cancers and all cancers combined for European adults diagnosed in 1995–99: results of the EUROCARE-4 study. Lancet Oncol 2007;8(9):773–783
6. Zigon G, Berrino F, Gatta G, et al. EUROCARE Working Group. Prognoses for head and neck cancers in Europe diagnosed in 1995–1999: a population-based study. Ann Oncol 2011;22(1):165–174
7. Kwok J, Langevin SM, Argiris A, Grandis JR, Gooding WE, Taioli E. The impact of health insurance status on the survival of patients with head and neck cancer. Cancer 2010;116(2):476–485
8. de Graeff A, de Leeuw JR, Ros WJ, Hordijk GJ, Blijham GH, Winnubst JA. Sociodemographic factors and quality of life as prognostic indicators in head and neck cancer. Eur J Cancer 2001;37(3):332–339
9. Massie MJ. Prevalence of depression in patients with cancer. J Natl Cancer Inst Monogr 2004;32(32):57–71
10. Lazure KE, Lydiatt WM, Denman D, Burke WJ. Association between depression and survival or disease recurrence in patients with head and neck cancer enrolled in a depression prevention trial. Head Neck 2009;31(7):888–892
11. Argiris A, Li Y, Murphy BA, Langer CJ, Forastiere AA. Outcome of elderly patients with recurrent or metastatic head and neck cancer treated with cisplatin-based chemotherapy. J Clin Oncol 2004;22(2):262–268
12. Zeman FJ. Nutrition and cancer. In: Zeman FJ, ed. Clinical Nutrition and Dietetics. 2nd ed. New York: Macmillan; 1991: 571–598
13. Albrecht JT, Canada TW. Cachexia and anorexia in malignancy. Hematol Oncol Clin North Am 1996;10(4):791–800
14. American Cancer Society. Nutrition for the Person with Cancer: A Guide for Patients and Families. Atlanta, GA: American Cancer Society, Inc.; 2000
15. Vermorken JB. Medical treatment in head and neck cancer. Ann Oncol 2005;16(Suppl 2):ii258–ii264
16. Colevas AD. Chemotherapy options for patients with metastatic or recurrent squamous cell carcinoma of the head and neck. J Clin Oncol 2006;24(17):2644–2652
17. Amer MH, Al-Sarraf M, Vaitkevicius VK. Factors that effect response to chemotherapy and survival of patients with advanced head and neck cancer. Cancer 1979;43(6):: 2202–2206
18. Stell PM, McCormick MS. The design of phase III palliative chemotherapy trials in head and neck cancer. Clin Otolaryngol Allied Sci 1986;11(1):21–29
19. Al-Sarraf M. Head and neck cancer: chemotherapy concepts. Semin Oncol 1988;15(1):70–85

1 References with asterisks indicate the most important reference articles on the topic.

20. Forastiere AA, Metch B, Schuller DE, et al. Randomized comparison of cisplatin plus fluorouracil and carboplatin plus fluorouracil versus methotrexate in advanced squamous-cell carcinoma of the head and neck: a Southwest Oncology Group study. J Clin Oncol 1992;10(8):1245–1251
21. Jacobs C, Lyman G, Velez-García E, et al. A phase III randomized study comparing cisplatin and fluorouracil as single agents and in combination for advanced squamous cell carcinoma of the head and neck. J Clin Oncol 1992;10(2):257–263
22. Argiris A, Li Y, Forastiere A. Prognostic factors and long-term survivorship in patients with recurrent or metastatic carcinoma of the head and neck. Cancer 2004;101(10):2222–2229
23. León X, Hitt R, Constenla M, et al. A retrospective analysis of the outcome of patients with recurrent and/or metastatic squamous cell carcinoma of the head and neck refractory to a platinum-based chemotherapy. Clin Oncol (R Coll Radiol) 2005;17(6):418–424
24. Specenier P, Rasschaert M, Vroman Ph, et al. Weekly docetaxel in patients with recurrent and-or metastatic squamous cell carcinoma of the head and neck. Am J Clin Oncol 2011;34(5):472–477
25. Morton RP, Rugman F, Dorman EB, et al. Cisplatinum and bleomycin for advanced or recurrent squamous cell carcinoma of the head and neck: a randomised factorial phase III controlled trial. Cancer Chemother Pharmacol 1985;15(3):283–289
26. Liverpool Head and Neck Oncology Group. A phase III randomised trial of cisplatinum, methotrextate, cisplatinum + methotrexate and cisplatinum + 5-FU in end stage squamous carcinoma of the head and neck. Br J Cancer 1990;61(2):311–315
27. Vermorken JB, Mesia R, Rivera F, et al. Platinum-based chemotherapy plus cetuximab in head and neck cancer. N Engl J Med 2008;359(11):1116–1127
28. Vermorken JB, Stöhlmacher J, Davidenko I, et al. Primary efficacy and safety results of SPECTRUM, a phase 3 trial in patients (PTS) with recurrent and/or metastatic (R/M) squamous cell carcinoma of the head and (SCCHN) receiving chemotherapy with or without panitumumab (PMAB). Ann Oncol 2010; 21(Suppl 8): viii12
29. Machiels JP, Subramanian S, Ruzsa A, et al. Zalutumumab plus best supportive care versus best supportive care alone in patients with recurrent or metastatic squamous-cell carcinoma of the head and neck after failure of platinum-based chemotherapy: an open-label, randomised phase 3 trial. Lancet Oncol 2011;12(4):333–343
30. Werner JA, Kehrl W, Pluzanska A, et al. A phase III placebo-controlled study in advanced head and neck cancer using intratumoural cisplatin/epinephrine gel. Br J Cancer 2002;87(9):938–944
31. Clavel M, Vermorken J,Cognetti F, et al. Randomized comparison of cisplatin, methotrexate, bleomycin and vincristine (CABO) versus cisplatin and 5-fluorouracil (CF) versus cisplatin (C) in recurrent or metastatic squamous cell carcinoma of the head and neck A phase III study of the EORTC Head and Neck Cancer Cooperative Group Ann Oncol (1994) 5(6): 521–526.
32. Schornagel JH, Verweij J, de Mulder PH, et al. Randomized phase III trial of edatrexate versus methotrexate in patients with metastatic and/or recurrent squamous cell carcinoma of the head and neck: a European Organization for Research and Treatment of Cancer Head and Neck Cancer Cooperative Group study. J Clin Oncol 1995;13(7):1649–1655
33. Vermorken JB, Catimel G, de Mulder P, et al. Randomized phase II trial of weekly methotrexate versus two schedules of three-weekly paclitaxel in patients with metastatic or recurrent squamous cell carcinoma of the head and neck. Proc Am Soc Clin Oncol 1999;18:395a (Abstract 1527)
34. Pivot X, Wadler S, Kelly C, et al. Result of two randomized trials comparing nolatrexed (Thymitaq) versus methotrexate in patients with recurrent head and neck cancer. Ann Oncol 2001;12(11):1595–1599
35. Pivot X, Awada A, Gedouin D, et al. Results of randomised phase II studies comparing S16020 with methotrexate in patients with recurrent head and neck cancer. Ann Oncol 2003;14(3):373–377
36. Schrijvers D, Johnson J, Jiminez U, et al. Head and Neck Interferon Cooperative Study Group. Phase III trial of modulation of cisplatin/fluorouracil chemotherapy by interferon alfa-2b in patients with recurrent or metastatic head and neck cancer. J Clin Oncol 1998;16(3):1054–1059
37. Gibson MK, Li Y, Murphy B, et al. Eastern Cooperative Oncology Group. Randomized phase III evaluation of cisplatin plus fluorouracil versus cisplatin plus paclitaxel in advanced head and neck cancer (E1395): an intergroup trial of the Eastern Cooperative Oncology Group. J Clin Oncol 2005;23(15):3562–3567
38. National Comprehensive Cancer Network. www.nccn.org (accessed April 14, 2011) *
39. Vermorken JB, Specenier P. Optimal treatment for recurrent/metastatic head and neck cancer. Ann Oncol 2010;21(Suppl 7):vii252–261
40. Grose WE, Lehane DE, Dixon DO, Fletcher WS, Stuckey WJ. Comparison of methotrexate and cisplatin for patients with advanced squamous cell carcinoma of the head and neck region: a Southwest Oncology Group Study. Cancer Treat Rep 1985;69(6):577–581
41. Hong WK, Schaefer S, Issell B, et al. A prospective randomized trial of methotrexate versus cisplatin in the treatment of recurrent squamous cell carcinoma of the head and neck. Cancer 1983;52(2):206–210
42. Guardiola E, Peyrade F, Chaigneau L, et al. Results of a randomised phase II study comparing docetaxel with methotrexate in patients with recurrent head and neck cancer. Eur J Cancer 2004;40(14):2071–2076
43. Specenier P, Vermorken JB. Targeted therapies in head and neck cancer. Target Oncol 2007;2(2):73–78
44. Cohen EEW. Novel therapeutic targets in squamous cell carcinoma of the head and neck. Semin Oncol 2004;31(6):755–768
45. Xia W, Lau YK, Zhang HZ, et al. Combination of EGFR, HER-2/neu, and HER-3 is a stronger predictor for the outcome of oral squamous cell carcinoma than any individual family members. Clin Cancer Res 1999;5(12):4164–4174
46. Ang KK, Berkey BA, Tu X, et al. Impact of epidermal growth factor receptor expression on survival and pattern of relapse in patients with advanced head and neck carcinoma. Cancer Res 2002;62(24):7350–7356
47. Chung CH, Ely K, McGavran L, et al. Increased epidermal growth factor receptor gene copy number is associated with poor prognosis in head and neck squamous cell carcinomas. J Clin Oncol 2006;24(25):4170–4176
48. Santini J, Formento JL, Francoual M, et al. Characterization, quantification, and potential clinical value of the epidermal growth factor receptor in head and neck squamous cell carcinomas. Head Neck 1991;13(2):132–139
49. Scaltriti M, Baselga J. The epidermal growth factor receptor pathway: a model for targeted therapy. Clin Cancer Res 2006;12(18):5268–5272

50. Kimura H, Sakai K, Arao T, Shimoyama T, Tamura T, Nishio K. Antibody-dependent cellular cytotoxicity of cetuximab against tumor cells with wild-type or mutant epidermal growth factor receptor. Cancer Sci 2007;98(8):1275–1280
51. Bleeker WK, Lammerts van Bueren JJ, van Ojik HH, et al. Dual mode of action of a human anti-epidermal growth factor receptor monoclonal antibody for cancer therapy. J Immunol 2004;173(7):4699–4707
52. Schneider-Merck T, Lammerts van Bueren JJ, Berger S, et al. Human IgG2 antibodies against epidermal growth factor receptor effectively trigger antibody-dependent cellular cytotoxicity but, in contrast to IgG1, only by cells of myeloid lineage. J Immunol 2010;184(1):512–520
53. Rapidis AD, Vermorken JB, Bourhis J. Targeted therapies in head and neck cancer: past, present and future. Rev Recent Clin Trials 2008;3(3):156–166
54. Vermorken JB, Trigo J, Hitt R, et al. Open-label, uncontrolled, multicenter phase II study to evaluate the efficacy and toxicity of cetuximab as a single agent in patients with recurrent and/or metastatic squamous cell carcinoma of the head and neck who failed to respond to platinum-based therapy. J Clin Oncol 2007;25(16):2171–2177
55. Baselga J, Trigo JM, Bourhis J, et al. Phase II multicenter study of the antiepidermal growth factor receptor monoclonal antibody cetuximab in combination with platinum-based chemotherapy in patients with platinum-refractory metastatic and/or recurrent squamous cell carcinoma of the head and neck. J Clin Oncol 2005;23(24):5568–5577
56. Herbst RS, Arquette M, Shin DM, et al. Phase II multicenter study of the epidermal growth factor receptor antibody cetuximab and cisplatin for recurrent and refractory squamous cell carcinoma of the head and neck. J Clin Oncol 2005;23(24):5578–5587
57. Mesía R, Rivera F, Kawecki A, et al. Quality of life of patients receiving platinum-based chemotherapy plus cetuximab first line for recurrent and/or metastatic squamous cell carcinoma of the head and neck. Ann Oncol 2010;21(10):1967–1973
58. Petrelli NJ, Winer EP, Brahmer J, et al. Clinical Cancer Advances 2009: major research advances in cancer treatment, prevention, and screening—a report from the American Society of Clinical Oncology. J Clin Oncol 2009;27(35):6052–6069
59. Gregoire V, Lefebvre J-L, Licitra L, Felip E. Squamous cell carcinoma of the head and neck: EHNS-ESMO-ESTRO clinical practice guidelines for diagnosis, treatment and follow-up. Ann Oncol 2010;21(suppl 5):v184–186
60. Burtness B, Goldwasser MA, Flood W, Mattar B, Forastiere AA; Eastern Cooperative Oncology Group. Phase III randomized trial of cisplatin plus placebo compared with cisplatin plus cetuximab in metastatic/recurrent head and neck cancer: an Eastern Cooperative Oncology Group study. J Clin Oncol 2005;23(34):8646–8654
61. Cartenì G, Fiorentino R, Vecchione L, Chiurazzi B, Battista C. Panitumumab a novel drug in cancer treatment. Ann Oncol 2007;18(Suppl 6):vi16–vi21
62. Specenier P, Vermorken JB. Advances in the systemic treatment of head and neck cancers. Curr Opin Oncol 2010;22(3):200–205
63. Cohen EE, Halpern AB, Kasza K, Kocherginsky M, Williams R, Vokes EE. Factors associated with clinical benefit from epidermal growth factor receptor inhibitors in recurrent and metastatic squamous cell carcinoma of the head and neck. Oral Oncol 2009;45(10):e155–e160
64. Stewart JS, Cohen EE, Licitra L, et al. Phase III study of gefitinib compared with intravenous methotrexate for recurrent squamous cell carcinoma of the head and neck [corrected]. J Clin Oncol 2009;27(11):1864–1871
65. Argiris A, Ghebremichael M, Gilbert J, et al. A phase III randomized, placebo-controlled trial of docetaxel with or without gefitinib in recurrent or metastatic squamous cell carcinoma of the head and neck: A trial of the Eastern Cooperative Oncology Group (ECOG). J Clin Oncol 2009; 27(15 Suppl): 303s (Abstr 6011)
66. Vermorken JB, Herbst RS, Leon X, Amellal N, Baselga J. Overview of the efficacy of cetuximab in recurrent and/or metastatic squamous cell carcinoma of the head and neck in patients who previously failed platinum-based therapies. Cancer 2008;112(12):2710–2719
67. Eskens FA, Mom CH, Planting AS, et al. A phase I dose escalation study of BIBW 2992, an irreversible dual inhibitor of epidermal growth factor receptor 1 (EGFR) and 2 (HER2) tyrosine kinase in a 2-week on, 2-week off schedule in patients with advanced solid tumours. Br J Cancer 2008;98(1):80–85
68. Li D, Ambrogio L, Shimamura T, et al. BIBW2992, an irreversible EGFR/HER2 inhibitor highly effective in preclinical lung cancer models. Oncogene 2008;27(34):4702–4711
69. Seiwert TY, Haraf DJ, Cohen EEW, et al. Phase I study of bevacizumab added to fluorouracil- and hydroxyurea-based concomitant chemoradiotherapy for poor-prognosis head and neck cancer. J Clin Oncol 2008;26(10):1732–1741
70. Barth RF, Coderre JA, Vicente MG, Blue TE. Boron neutron capture therapy of cancer: current status and future prospects. Clin Cancer Res 2005;11(11):3987–4002
71. Barth RF. Boron neutron capture therapy at the crossroads: challenges and opportunities. Appl Radiat Isot 2009; 67(7–8, Suppl) S3–S6
72. Wittig A, Collette L, Appelman K, et al. EORTC trial 11001: distribution of two 10B-compounds in patients with squamous cell carcinoma of head and neck, a translational research/phase 1 trial. J Cell Mol Med 2009;13(8B):1653–1665
73. Nakamura H. Liposomal boron delivery for neutron capture therapy. Methods Enzymol 2009;465:179–208
74. Kato I, Fujita Y, Maruhashi A, et al. Effectiveness of boron neutron capture therapy for recurrent head and neck malignancies. Appl Radiat Isot 2009; 67(7–8, Suppl)S37–S42 Epub2009Apr2.
75. Kimura Y, Ariyoshi Y, Shimahara M, et al. Boron neutron capture therapy for recurrent oral cancer and metastasis of cervical lymph node. Appl Radiat Isot 2009; 67(7–8, Suppl)S47–S49.
76. Fuwa N, Suzuki M, Sakurai Y, et al. Treatment results of boron neutron capture therapy using intra-arterial administration of boron compounds for recurrent head and neck cancer. Br J Radiol 2008;81(969):749–752
77. Kankaanranta L, Seppälä T, Koivunoro H, et al. Boron neutron capture therapy in the treatment of locally recurred head and neck cancer. Int J Radiat Oncol Biol Phys 2007;69(2):475–482
78. Kato I, Ono K, Sakurai Y, et al. Effectiveness of BNCT for recurrent head and neck malignancies. Appl Radiat Isot 2004;61(5):1069–1073
79. Hurwitz MD. Today's thermal therapy: not your father's hyperthermia: challenges and opportunities in application of hyperthermia for the 21st century cancer patient. Am J Clin Oncol 2010;33(1):96–100

80. Lutgens L, van der Zee J, Pijls-Johannesma M, et al. Combined use of hyperthermia and radiation therapy for treating locally advanced cervix carcinoma. Cochrane Database Syst Rev 2010;3(3):CD006377 101002/14651858.CD006377.pub3
81. De Haas-Kock DFM, Buijsen J, Pijls-Johannesma M, et al. Concomitant hyperthermia and radiation therapy for treating locally advanced rectal cancer. Cochrane Database Syst Rev 2009;3(3):CD006269 101002/14651858.CD006269.pub2
82. Valdagni R, Amichetti M. Report of long-term follow-up in a randomized trial comparing radiation therapy and radiation therapy plus hyperthermia to metastatic lymph nodes in stage IV head and neck patients. Int J Radiat Oncol Biol Phys 1994;28(1):163–169
83. Datta NR, Bose AK, Kapoor HK, Gupta S. Head and neck cancers: results of thermoradiotherapy versus radiotherapy. Int J Hyperthermia 1990;6(3):479–486
84. Paulides MM, Bakker JF, Linthorst M, et al. The clinical feasibility of deep hyperthermia treatment in the head and neck: new challenges for positioning and temperature measurement. Phys Med Biol 2010;55(9):2465–2480
85. Gargiulo M, Moio M, Monda G, Parascandolo S, Cubicciotti G. Electrochemotherapy: actual considerations and clinical experience in head and neck cancers. Ann Surg 2010;251(4):773
86. Campana LG, Mocellin S, Basso M, et al. Bleomycin-based electrochemotherapy: clinical outcome from a single institution's experience with 52 patients. Ann Surg Oncol 2009;16(1):191–199
87. Bloom DC, Goldfarb PM. The role of intratumour therapy with electroporation and bleomycin in the management of advanced squamous cell carcinoma of the head and neck. Eur J Surg Oncol 2005;31(9):1029–1035
88. Tijink BM, De Bree R, Van Dongen GA, Leemans CR. How we do it: Chemo-electroporation in the head and neck for otherwise untreatable patients. Clin Otolaryngol 2006;31(5):447–451
89. Fayter D, Corbett M, Heirs M, Fox D, Eastwood A. A systematic review of photodynamic therapy in the treatment of pre-cancerous skin conditions, Barrett's oesophagus and cancers of the biliary tract, brain, head and neck, lung, oesophagus and skin. Health Technol Assess 2010;14(37):1–288
90. Karakullukcu B, van Oudenaarde K, Copper MP, et al. Photodynamic therapy of early stage oral cavity and oropharynx neoplasms: an outcome analysis of 170 patients. Eur Arch Otorhinolaryngol 2011;268(2):281–288
91. Jerjes W, Upile T, Akram S, Hopper C. The surgical palliation of advanced head and neck cancer using photodynamic therapy. Clin Oncol (R Coll Radiol) 2010;22(9):785–791
92. Wildeman MA, Nyst HJ, Karakullukcu B, Tan BI. Photodynamic therapy in the therapy for recurrent/persistent nasopharyngeal cancer. Head Neck Oncol 2009;1:40
93. Nyst HJ, Tan IB, Stewart FA, Balm AJ. Is photodynamic therapy a good alternative to surgery and radiotherapy in the treatment of head and neck cancer? Photodiagn Photodyn Ther 2009;6(1):3–11
94. D'Cruz AK, Robinson MH, Biel MA. mTHPC-mediated photodynamic therapy in patients with advanced, incurable head and neck cancer: a multicenter study of 128 patients. Head Neck 2004;26(3):232–240
95. Lou PJ, Jäger HR, Jones L, Theodossy T, Bown SG, Hopper C. Interstitial photodynamic therapy as salvage treatment for recurrent head and neck cancer. Br J Cancer 2004;91(3):441–446
96. Goldstein NE, Genden E, Morrison RS. Palliative care for patients with head and neck cancer: "I would like a quick return to a normal lifestyle". JAMA 2008;299(15):1818–1825
97. Hancock K, Clayton JM, Parker SM, et al. Truth-telling in discussing prognosis in advanced life-limiting illnesses: a systematic review. Palliat Med 2007;21(6):507–517

6 Principles and Concepts of Reconstruction in the Recurrent Setting

Ralph Gilbert

Summary

- Treatment of the patient failing nonsurgical organ preservation therapy represents a major challenge for the reconstructive surgeon.
- Liberal use of free tissue transfer and regional myocutaneous flaps provides patients with the best probability of high-quality functional and complication-free perioperative course.
- The surgeon contemplating operative procedures on this group of patients needs to have the full repertoire of reconstructive options for recipient vessels, including recipient sites outside the neck.
- Patients being considered for salvage surgery should be managed in centers with tertiary/quaternary expertise and strong multidisciplinary programs.

Introduction

Reconstruction of a patient following salvage surgery for failure of previous treatment represents a daunting challenge for the head and neck surgeon. Patients for the most part will have been treated with organ-preserving approaches, radiation or chemoradiation, or will have been previously treated with surgery and have received adjuvant radiation or chemoradiation. The surgical management of these patients from the ablative perspective is complex and often requires radical surgical approaches leaving little in the way of local options or vasculature for the reconstructive head and neck surgeon. In addition, patients being treated for salvage of prior treatment have a low probability of long-term survival and can least afford a long hospital stay as a result of surgical complications. This reality adds a significant degree of pressure and responsibility on the reconstructive surgeon to provide the highest degree of functional rehabilitation and the lowest probability of perioperative complications.

Issues in Surgical Approach—Impact of Previous Treatment

Prior Radical Radiotherapy or Chemoradiation

The vast majority of patients presenting with advanced oropharyngeal, laryngeal or hypopharyngeal mucosal malignancies are currently considered for and treated with altered fractionation radiotherapy or some combination of concomitant chemotherapy and radiation. The treatment may also include induction chemotherapy, usually including a taxane and cisplatinum. For patients treated with radiation alone for organ preservation there is historical literature that addresses the risks of perioperative fistula and wound healing problems in patients undergoing surgical salvage. Fundamentally, these reports have demonstrated higher fistula rates and delayed wound healing.[1–3] The clear etiology of these problems is based on the effect of radiation on the residual local tissue, with injuries to the microvasculature delaying the normal wound healing response and the ability of the local tissues to respond to any bacterial or salivary contamination. In patients treated with chemoradiation this local wound injury is enhanced with more severe fibrosis within the microvasculature and little in the way of an early wound healing response (**Fig. 6.1**). The literature reviewing the complications associated with salvage procedures in this group of patients has demonstrated higher complications than in the radiation-alone group of patients.[4,5] Experienced surgeons salvaging this group of patients strongly endorse the liberal use of either local myocutaneous or free tissue transfer to support the repair of pharyngeal defects.

The literature on the impact of radiation or chemoradiation on the potential recipient vessels for free flap reconstruction of the head and neck suggests that on a biological level the intima of these vessels is more fragile and the media of the larger arterial vessels is usually replaced by fibrous tissue. Technically, however, there appears to be little in the way of a major impact of previous treatment on the risk of perioperative thrombosis compared with the primary surgery setting.[6]

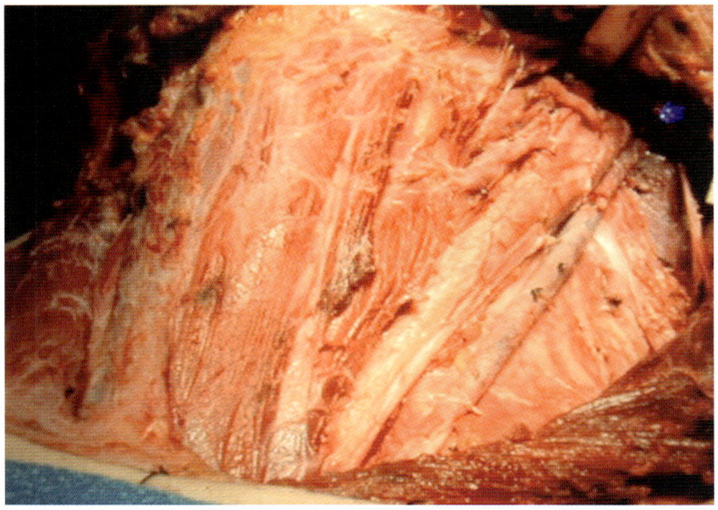

Fig. 6.1 Clinical photograph of bilateral neck dissection following chemoradiation. Note the absence of bleeding and level of fibrosis.

Previous Surgery

Patients undergoing salvage following previous surgery or following surgery and adjuvant radiation or chemoradiation have some additional challenges to those undergoing salvage surgery following failure of organ preservation approaches. The majority of patients have previously undergone either unilateral or bilateral neck dissection and so have had the majority of veins and arteries previously dissected, in addition to the impact of radiation This fact obviously reduces the number of recipient vessels available in the head and neck. Patients who have previously had surgical manipulation of the potential recipient vessels and adjuvant treatment represent a major surgical challenge in terms of identification and dissection of potential recipient vessels. The usual landmarks for identifying recipient vessels are absent and critical structures such as the hypoglossal, accessory, or vagus nerves may be injured in the approaches to potential recipient vessels.

One factor often overlooked in discussions of salvage surgery following previous surgical approaches is the condition of the overlying skin of the neck or face. Often the skin is extremely precarious and reconstructive techniques may require an element of neck or facial resurfacing to allow uncomplicated wound healing.

Management of the Vessel-depleted Neck

As mentioned previously, the greatest challenge for the reconstructive surgeon performing salvage surgery, particularly following previous neck dissection, is the identification of appropriate recipient vessels. Several general principles apply to managing this situation.

Consider a Myocutaneous Flap

In patients undergoing salvage procedures, reconstructive surgeons often consider free tissue transfer where a regional myocutaneous flap would produce an equivalent result. While the donor site defect might be problematic, a regional flap will be the simplest and most appropriate technique, particularly for defects of the pharynx.

Consider the Opposite Neck

While relatively obvious, identifying vessels in the unoperated neck provides a highly reliable recipient vessel source.[7] The facial artery and superior thyroid artery, if of appropriate size and caliber, can be mobilized close to the midline. Alternatively, flaps with long vascular pedicles can be tunneled to easily reach these vessels in the unoperated neck.

Consider Vessels Low in the Neck

With the increasing use of selective neck dissection, radical clearance of low level Vb nodes is infrequently performed in the modern era. This fact often means that the transverse cervical vessels—artery and vein—are often in good condition and relatively easily dissected. The transverse cervical vessels when fully mobilized will often reach at least to the mid-neck in the majority of patients.

Consider Vessels Outside the Neck

In many salvage situations, there will be no vessels available in the neck, or accessing these vessels will be associated with an increased risk of injury to critical nerves or vasculature. The options below the clavicle include the internal mammary vessels, accessed by removing the medial portions of the second, third, or fourth ribs. In addition, the thoracoacromial vessels or the subscapular system of vessels in the axilla may be considered.[8] The thoracoacromial, or TAC, system of vessels that supply the pectoralis major and minor can be used. However, the venae comitantes with this artery may be small. The thoracodorsal branch of the subscapular system supplying the latissimus dorsi and serratus anterior may be used and will reach up to the deltopectoral groove.

Cephalic Vein Transfer or Vein Loop

In many revision scenarios, the surgeon will have access to a recipient artery but the jugular vein and external jugular veins will be absent. One option that is well described is turning the cephalic vein from the arm up into the neck.[9] The vessel may be dissected from the antecubital fossa to its origin in the deltopectoral groove and rotated into the ipsilateral neck. This vessel, in most patients, is of large caliber and will reach to the upper neck. Great care must be taken with geometry to avoid twisting or kinking of the cephalic vein.

The other option in this scenario is to consider a vein loop.[10] In this technique, the short or long saphenous vein or cephalic vein is harvested. One end is then anastomosed to the recipient artery within or outside the neck and the other end is anastomosed to a large available vein within or outside the neck (proximal jugular or subclavian). The loop is allowed to perfuse as an arteriovenous shunt for 30–40 minutes to ensure patency and then used as an arterial and venous source for the flap. The surgeon contemplating these approaches with vein grafting must be aware that the risks of venous and arterial thrombosis are higher than with direct repair to local recipient vessels; however, in many vessel-depleted necks this may be the only available option.

Site-specific Defect Considerations

Larynx

Partial Laryngectomy

Early staged laryngeal cancer (T1 and T2) that fails radiation or chemoradiation is often amenable to partial salvage procedures including supracricoid partial laryngectomy with cricohyoidoepiglottopexy or cricohyoidopexy horizontal supraglottic laryngectomy and vertical frontolateral procedures. These procedures are often not considered because of the belief that the local wound healing will preclude an adequate functional result in radiation failure patients and so many surgeons opt instead for a total laryngectomy and tracheoesophageal puncture (TEP).

The vertical procedures are often not considered in radiation failure because of the absence of well-vascularized localized tissue to reconstruct the hemilaryngeal defect. Delaerre[11] has described the concept of vascularized carriers, which incorporates cartilage and mucosa with a free fascial flap to provide blood supply. In Delaerre's approach to the vertical defect he performs a two-stage procedure, wrapping the distal trachea with a forearm flap and then moving the vascularized trachea in a second stage to recreate the hemi- or extended hemilaryngeal defect.[12] We have described

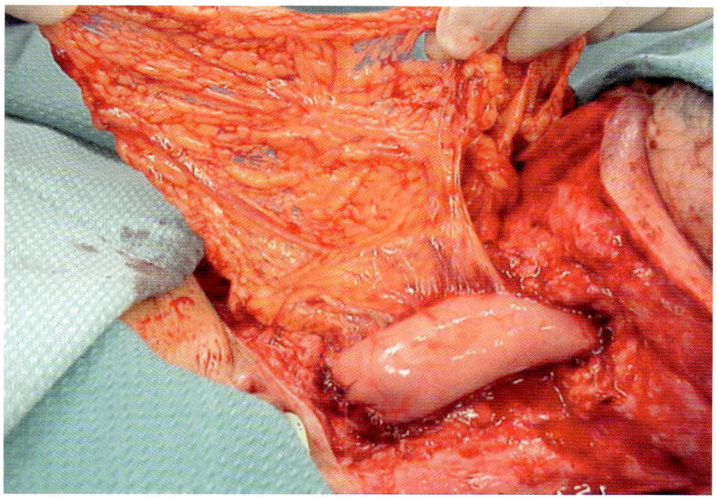

Fig. 6.2 The free gastro-omental flap inset into a total pharyngectomy defect. Note the attached omentum to provide vascular protection.

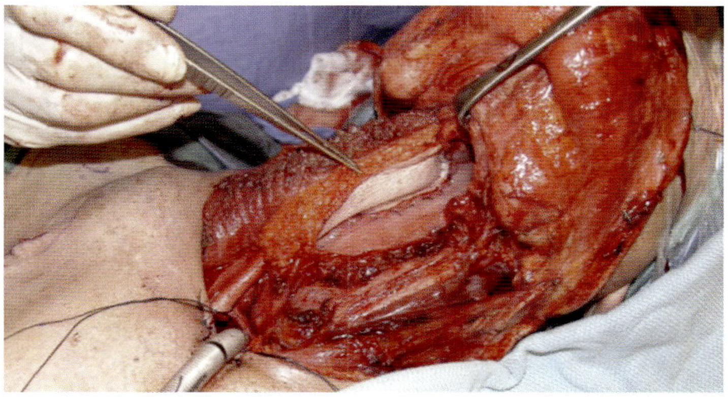

Fig. 6.3 Inset of pectoralis major myocutaneous flap for pharyngeal reconstruction.

a one-stage approach that incorporates the free temporoparietal flap as a one-stage reconstruction of the vertical hemilaryngeal defect.[13] This approach provides a reliable reconstruction of the hemilaryngectomy defect following radiation failure and requires a single open operative procedure.

Case Study

A 68-year-old man treated previously for extensive postcricoid carcinoma (T4aN2b) with chemoradiation (platinum/RT 70 Gy in 35 fractions). Recurrent lesion noted in postcricoid region with laryngeal extension. CT and MRI demonstrate recurrent resectable lesion with persisting neck disease. Planned bilateral neck dissection with laryngopharyngectomy, and planned reconstruction with gastro-omental free flap and omentum (see **Fig. 6.2**). Omentum provides vascular protection and wound healing promotion.

Laryngectomy or Partial Laryngopharyngectomy

Patients not amenable to partial procedures or patients with advanced recurrent laryngeal carcinoma or early-stage recurrent hypopharyngeal carcinoma are often considered for laryngopharyngectomy. In patients treated with standard or altered radiotherapy fractionation, there is certainly a higher fistula rate associated with primary closure. In this subset of patients considered for primary closure, some centers offer some type of supporting vascularized tissue. The majority of patients are undergoing a pectoralis major myogenous (muscle only) flap to support the primary repair . Some centers, however, offer free fascial flaps such as the forearm or temporoparietal flap reconstruction. The evidentiary basis for these approaches is weak and the use of these techniques is based on the view that anything that can reduce the incidence of fistula and promote rapid healing should be considered. Our approach is to consider the use of these techniques in selected high risk patients with vascular comorbidities, diabetes, malnutrition, or immunosuppression.

In patients failing chemoradiation, the approach needs to be more aggressive. In spite of the equivocal literature from the chemoradiation trials, most experienced surgeons advocate the routine use of some type of supporting vascular tissue in this subset of patients. The rationale is similar: the use of supporting vascular tissue may reduce the rate of fistula; and if a fistula occurs it will promote the local wound healing response, allowing for rapid wound healing.

In patients undergoing partial pharyngectomy one of the important questions is when to use a cutaneous or enteric flap incorporated into the pharyngeal repair. There is no literature pertaining specifically to this question, but most experienced surgeons would advocate the use of a cutaneous or myocutaneous flap if there is any suggestion of a tight closure. Current options include the pectoralis major myocutaneous flap (**Fig. 6.3**), with the free flap options including the free forearm flap and the anterolateral thigh flap. In our practice, we prefer to use the free flap option in women where the pectoralis major flap would result in a secondary breast deformity and in patients without significant comorbidity as presented earlier. Where possible, based on body habitus, we prefer the anterolateral thigh flap based on the limited donor site morbidity and that the incorporated fascia lata provides a second layer for closure reducing the risk of perioperative fistula.

Circumferential Pharyngeal Defects

Considerable controversy exists regarding the optimal reconstruction of the total pharyngectomy defect. The goals of reconstruction of this defect are to provide a high-quality swallowing result, with the potential for tracheoesophageal speech with the least morbidity using the simplest technique. The gastric transposition has been widely used and advocated particularly for patients who require upper esophageal resections along with pharyngectomy. The gastric transposition provides high-quality swallowing, but it does not allow high-quality TEP speech and has a very high perioperative mortality.[14] For these reasons, many centers offer tube reconstructions either with cutaneous or enteric free tissue transfers. The relative advantages and disadvantages of each technique are summarized in **Table 6.1**.

In our opinion, the free jejuna flap, which we have used extensively, is problematic because of the poor swallowing results and the poor TEP voice results. Currently, if we are going to consider an enteric reconstruction, we prefer the gastro-omental flap.[15,16] This flap has the advantages of a customizable tube size, excellent TEP speech, and the attached omentum, which can protect major vessels and promote wound healing. It has the same major disadvantage as the jejunum—the need for an abdominal harvest. We use this reconstruction selectively in patients with a good performance status who we feel would benefit from the omental transfer.

Table 6.1 Outcomes of flaps for pharyngolaryngectomy

Flap	Swallowing	TEP speech	Morbidity
Gastric transposition	++++	+	++++
Free jejunal transfer	++	+	++
Free gastro-omental flap	++++	+++	++
Tubed forearm flap	+++	++++	+
Anterolateral thigh flap	+++	++++	+

+ = Poor (for swallowing and TEP speech), Lowest (for morbidity); ++++ = Best (for swallowing and TEP speech), Highest (for morbidity).

In the majority of patients, we prefer the anterolateral or forearm flaps. We prefer skin tubes because of the minimal donor site morbidity and the excellent functional results. The one major disadvantage of tube skin flaps is the high distal stricture rate. We have overcome this problem by routinely using slapstick salivary stents, e.g., the Montgomery salivary bypass tube[17] (**Fig. 6.4**).

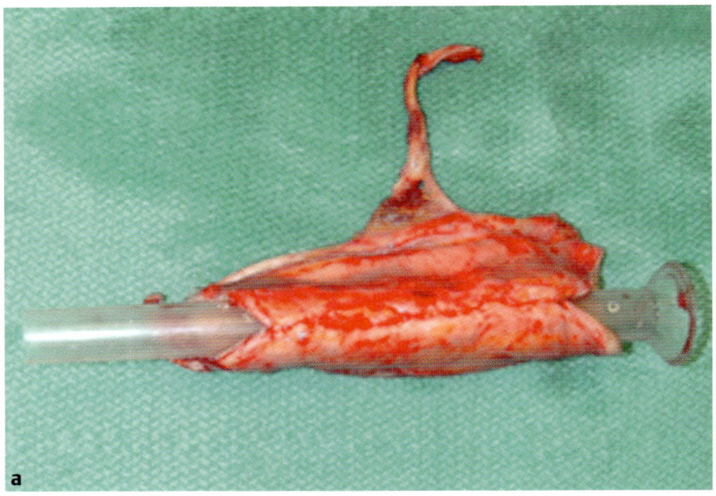

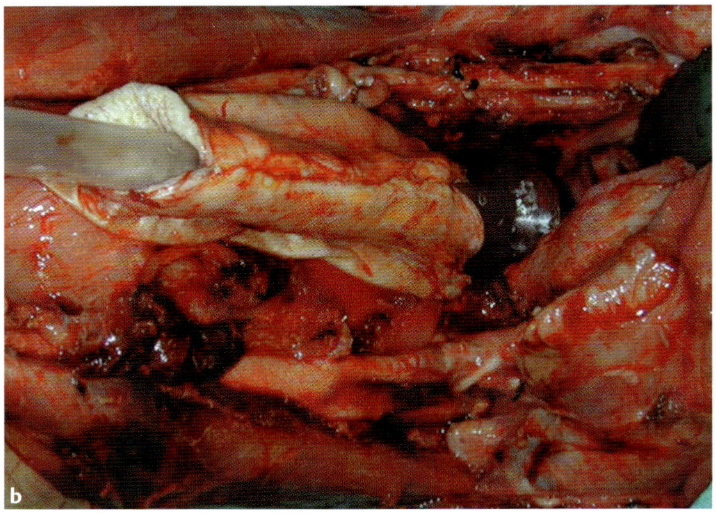

Fig. 6.4a, b Stents and bypass tubes.
a Tubed anterolateral thigh flap tube with salivary bypass tube.
b Tubed anterolateral thigh flap being prepared for inset.

■ Oral Cavity and Oropharynx

The reconstructive considerations in oral and oropharyngeal malignancies undergoing salvage procedures are similar to those in the primary setting. The principles of closure are the same, with a focus on volume replacement and maintaining the movement of the residual tongue. In patients undergoing mandibular reconstruction, attention to the patient's residual occlusion and the position of the condyle for optimizing mouth opening are critical. In the reoperative setting, two additional considerations are often present: recipient vessels absent or at a distance, and the presence of a composite defect (oral lining and external skin).

In addition, in the reoperative setting, the access approaches to the oral cavity (transoral, mandibular swing, lingual release) need to be carefully considered.

In the patient with recipient vessels at a distance, the reconstructive surgeon needs to consider flaps with a long vascular pedicle. Included among these are the forearm flap, the latissimus dorsi flap, and its perforator-based flap the thoradorsal artery perforator flap (TDAP). In patients undergoing bone reconstruction, the only flap with a long vascular pedicle is the angular tip of scapular flap based on the angular branch of the thoradorsal artery.[18] However, the maximum bone length with this flap is 10–12 cm, limiting its use in patients with extensive mandibular defects.

In patients requiring composite reconstruction of the oral lining and external skin, the options are two flaps (osseocutaneous for oral, second cutaneous flap for cover) or a single osseocutaneous flap with a large skin paddle. The options in the latter situation are the free fibular donor site with a large skin island and the scapular system of flaps. The fibular pedicle may be short, particularly with large defects. We prefer the angular tip of scapula flap, providing bone lengths of up to 12 cm with an incorporated latissimus dorsi flap or TDAP flap. The advantages of this flap are its long vascular pedicle (>10 cm), a cutaneous or myocutaneous island that can rotate independently of the bone, and the limited donor site morbidity (**Fig. 6.5**). An additional consideration in such patients is the issue of the vessel-depleted neck. In this group of patients there may be a limited number of recipient vessel options, making a single composite flap a more attractive option.

In accessing the oral cavity or oropharynx in the recurrent setting, we tend to prefer the mandibular swing approach over other degloving or release techniques. The mandibular swing offers limited dissection of the overlying skin and retains the majority of mucosal attachments. The one problem with this approach is the osteotomy. In revision cases or salvage cases we carefully plan the location of the osteotomy to avoid placing it in the previous high-dose planned treatment volume (PTV). This requires a review of the radiation treatment record and usually means that the osteotomy is moved from the paramedian location to the midline.

■ Maxillary Reconstruction

Reconstruction of the maxilla is one of the new frontiers of reconstructive head and neck surgery. Techniques incorporating the use of myo-osseous flaps or osseocutaneous flaps have been described and are increasingly being used in the primary surgery setting. The majority of these techniques (iliac crest and internal oblique,[19] angular tip of scapula with serratus anterior[20]) require neomucosalization of the muscle flap for wound healing. In the radiation

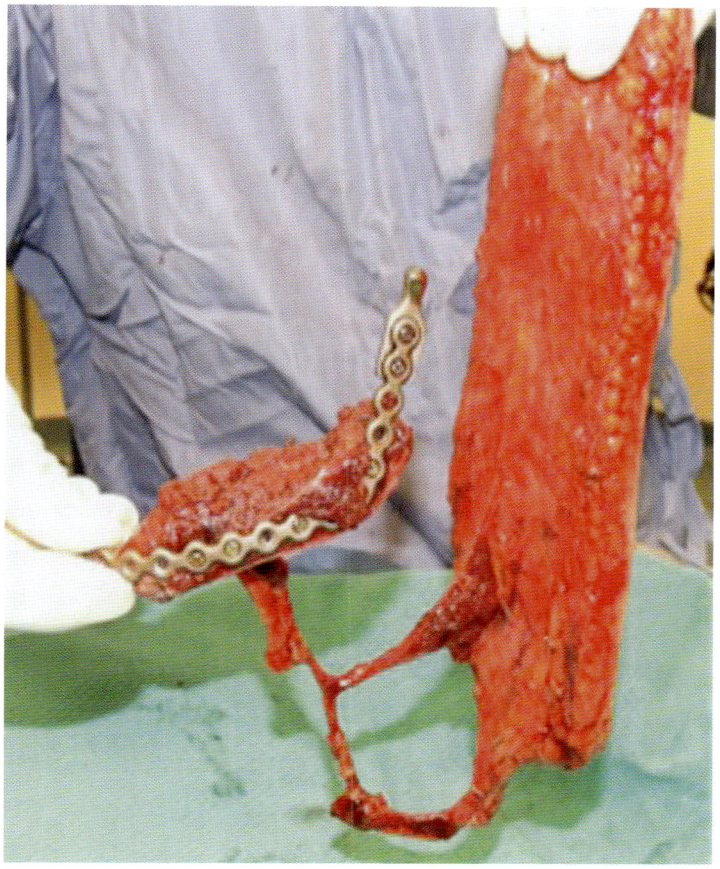

Fig. 6.5 Angular tip of scapular flap based on the angular artery with the latissimus dorsi flap.

or chemoradiation failure setting, this would be compromised. There is no published experience with these approaches in the salvage group of patients. Currently the majority of experienced reconstructive surgeons reserve these reconstructive approaches to the primary surgery setting, and use obturation in the recurrent setting. The exceptions to this might be the patient undergoing resection of the orbital floor or requiring some type of obliterative procedure of the orbit combined with a craniofacial resection where free tissue transfer represents the only reconstructive option and the patient with a total or near total palate defect where a maxillary obturator will not function effectively.

Skull Base

Open craniofacial procedures in the primary or salvage setting rarely require complex reconstruction. The vast majority of anterior craniofacial resections are simply reconstructed with a pericranial flap with duraplasty either with alloplastic dura or fascia lata. As indicated in the section on maxilla, free tissue transfer may be required for defects that include orbital exenteration and craniofacial resection to provide a safe separation of the intracranial contents from the nose or external skin. The favored flaps in this scenario are the rectus abdominus myocutaneous or myogenous flaps or the latissimus dorsi myogenous or myocutaneous flaps.[21] We prefer the rectus flap because we do not have to consider patient positioning. In the recurrent setting with reoperation the pericranial flap may not be available and in this scenario we would use a fasciocutaneous or fascia-only forearm flap or anterolateral thigh flap for reconstruction of the anterior skull base. The major issue in this group of patients is usually the availability of recipient vessels and vein loops may be required to the facial artery and branches of the internal jugular vein.

Resurfacing the Neck

Frequently, salvage surgery following either failure of organ preservation procedures or previous surgery incorporates the resection of the overlying neck skin. The reconstructive requirement in this clinical scenario is the provision of well-vascularized covering tissue that will protect the underlying vasculature and that can tolerate adjuvant irradiation or re-irradiation. The options in this situation include regional myogenous flaps with skin grafting, regional myocutaneous flaps, or free cutaneous flaps. If adjuvant therapy is being considered, muscle flaps with skin grafts should not be considered as the muscular atrophy will essentially leave the patient with a skin graft sitting on the carotid. We prefer the regional myocutaneous flaps, pectoralis major or latissimus dorsi, or a free cutaneous flap (parascapular, anterolateral thigh, and others). In the vessel-depleted neck or in the patient with significant comorbidity, regional flaps represent the best initial choice.

Conclusion

Salvage of the patient for whom primary organ preservation strategies or previous surgery and adjuvant therapy has failed, represent the ultimate challenge for the head and neck surgeon. Of all the patients we treat surgically, this group of patients requires complex ablative and reconstructive procedures and has the greatest requirement for a rapid recovery and good functional outcomes in terms of speech, swallowing, and facial aesthetics, given the low probability of locoregional control and survival.

These patients have high-risk wounds in terms of delayed and compromised wound healing requiring a liberal use of complex reconstructive techniques. In many scenarios, the simplest option will be the best, given the absence of local recipient vessels and the comorbidities that are associated with many of these patients. Patients of this group are best managed in high-volume centers with strong multidisciplinary programs incorporating tertiary/quaternary head and neck oncological and reconstructive surgery, speech pathology, social work, and specialized oncology nursing.

Future Research

- New techniques to improve local vascularization and reverse the effects of radiation and chemoradiation.
- Innovation in cell therapy and tissue engineering to reverse radiation injuries.
- Long-term reports of outcomes of salvage surgery, both locoregional control and survival and functional outcome.
- Improved documentation of QoL outcomes for patients undergoing salvage surgery.

Recommended Reading

- Clark JR, de Almeida J, Gilbert R, et al. Primary and salvage (hypo)pharyngectomy: Analysis and outcome. Head Neck 2006;28(8):671–677 (Review of a large series of laryngopharyngectomy patients reconstructed with regional and free tissue flaps; focus on complications.)
- Weber RS, Berkey BA, Forastiere A, et al. Outcome of salvage total laryngectomy following organ preservation therapy: the Radiation Therapy Oncology Group trial 91–11. Arch Otolaryngol Head Neck Surg. 2003;129(1):44–49. (Review of the complications of surgical salvage from RTOG-9111 for treatment of laryngeal cancer.)
- Delaere PR, Hermans R. Tracheal autotransplantation as a new and reliable technique for the functional treatment of advanced laryngeal cancer. Laryngoscope 2003;113(7):1244–1251 (Description of new technique for laryngeal reconstruction after radiation failure.)
- Patel RS, Makitie AA, Goldstein DP, et al. Morbidity and functional outcomes following gastro-omental free flap reconstruction of circumferential pharyngeal defects. Head Neck 2009;31(5):655–663 (Largest series of gastro-omental flaps reported in the literature.)
- Brown JS. Deep circumflex iliac artery free flap with internal oblique muscle as a new method of immediate reconstruction of maxillectomy defect. Head Neck 1996;18(5):412–421 (First description of the myo-osseous free flap option for maxilla reconstruction.)

References

1. Clark JR, de Almeida J, Gilbert R, et al. Primary and salvage (hypo)pharyngectomy: Analysis and outcome. Head Neck 2006;28(8):671–677
2. Parikh SR, Irish JC, Curran AJ, Gullane PJ, Brown DH, Rotstein LE. Pharyngocutaneous fistulae in laryngectomy patients: the Toronto Hospital experience. J Otolaryngol 1998;27(3):136–140
3. Sassler AM, Esclamado RM, Wolf GT. Surgery after organ preservation therapy. Analysis of wound complications. Arch Otolaryngol Head Neck Surg 1995;121(2):162–165
4. Chepeha DB, Annich G, Pynnonen MA, et al. Pectoralis major myocutaneous flap vs revascularized free tissue transfer: complications, gastrostomy tube dependence, and hospitalization. Arch Otolaryngol Head Neck Surg 2004;130(2):181–186
5. Weber RS, Berkey BA, Forastiere A, et al. Outcome of salvage total laryngectomy following organ preservation therapy: the Radiation Therapy Oncology Group trial 91–11. Arch Otolaryngol Head Neck Surg 2003;129(1):44–49
6. Aitasalo K, Relander M, Virolainen E. Microvascular free tissue transfers after preoperative irradiation in head and neck reconstructions. Acta Otolaryngol Suppl 1997;529:247–250
7. Head C, Sercarz JA, Abemayor E, Calcaterra TC, Rawnsley JD, Blackwell KE. Microvascular reconstruction after previous neck dissection. Arch Otolaryngol Head Neck Surg 2002;128(3):328–331
8. Harris JR, Lueg E, Genden E, Urken ML. The thoracoacromial/cephalic vascular system for microvascular anastomoses in the vessel-depleted neck. Arch Otolaryngol Head Neck Surg 2002;128(3):319–323
9. Kim KA, Chandrasekhar BS. Cephalic vein in salvage microsurgical reconstruction in the head and neck. Br J Plast Surg 1998;51(1):2–7
10. Lin CH, Mardini S, Lin YT, Yeh JT, Wei FC, Chen HC. Sixty-five clinical cases of free tissue transfer using long arteriovenous fistulas or vein grafts. J Trauma 2004;56(5):1107–1117
11. Delaere PR, Liu ZY, Hermans R, Sciot R, Feenstra L. Experimental tracheal allograft revascularization and transplantation. J Thorac Cardiovasc Surg 1995;110(3):728–737
12. Delaere PR, Hermans R. Tracheal autotransplantation as a new and reliable technique for the functional treatment of advanced laryngeal cancer. Laryngoscope 2003;113(7):1244–1251
13. Gilbert RW, Neligan PC. Microsurgical laryngotracheal reconstruction. Clin Plast Surg 2005;32(3):293–301, v
14. Spiro RH, Shah JP, Strong EW, Gerold FP, Bains MS. Gastric transposition in head and neck surgery. Indications, complications, and expectations. Am J Surg 1983;146(4):483–487
15. Genden EM, Kaufman MR, Katz B, Vine A, Urken ML. Tubed gastro-omental free flap for pharyngoesophageal reconstruction. Arch Otolaryngol Head Neck Surg 2001;127(7):847–853
16. Patel RS, Makitie AA, Goldstein DP, et al. Morbidity and functional outcomes following gastro-omental free flap reconstruction of circumferential pharyngeal defects. Head Neck 2009;31(5):655–663
17. Mäkitie AA, Beasley NJ, Neligan PC, Lipa J, Gullane PJ, Gilbert RW. Head and neck reconstruction with anterolateral thigh flap. Otolaryngol Head Neck Surg 2003;129(5):547–555
18. Coleman JJ III, Sultan MR. The bipedicled osteocutaneous scapula flap: a new subscapular system free flap. Plast Reconstr Surg 1991;87(4):682–692
19. Brown JS. Deep circumflex iliac artery free flap with internal oblique muscle as a new method of immediate reconstruction of maxillectomy defect. Head Neck 1996;18(5):412–421
20. Clark JR, Vesely M, Gilbert R. Scapular angle osteomyogenous flap in postmaxillectomy reconstruction: defect, reconstruction, shoulder function, and harvest technique. Head Neck 2008;30(1):10–20
21. Neligan PC, Mulholland S, Irish J, et al. Flap selection in cranial base reconstruction. Plast Reconstr Surg 1996;98(7):1159–1166, discussion 1167–1168

7 Patient Selection for Treatment

Vinidh Paleri, Charles G. Kelly

Summary

- The decision-making process for treatment selection in recurrent cancer is one of the most difficult areas in head and neck oncology practice.
- Detailed information about previous treatments received is essential to ensure the formulation of a comprehensive management plan for the recurrent tumor.
- Apart from tumor factors and patient factors, the management should be equally driven by patient expectations and a detailed discussion of the impact on function and quality of life.
- Treatment of recurrent cancers should not be undertaken lightly and optimal outcomes are achieved at centers with experienced teams managing high case volumes.

Introduction

Recurrent head and neck cancer is a complex clinical problem for several reasons. A recurrence usually develops within 2 years of the previous treatment, a time when the patient has often become reconciled to and adapted to the functional implications of the previous treatment. This is also the time when the organ function and quality of life can begin to approach pretreatment levels. The news of recurrence of tumor takes a significant emotional toll on the patient and carers. Being fully aware of the poor prognosis in recurrent tumors and the limited literature on which treatment recommendations are based, the clinician's dilemma is to formulate an optimal management plan that takes into consideration the extent of the recurrent tumor, the previous treatment modalities, and the patient's performance status and comorbidities, while also ensuring that the treatment does not have a further detrimental effect on the quality of life, given that life expectancy may be shortened. It must be recognized that in many clinical scenarios there is very often a fine line in the decision-making process between a second attempt at curative treatment and providing best supportive care, which may include palliative surgery, radiotherapy, or chemotherapy. Thus, appropriate patient selection is of paramount importance in formulating a management plan that will strike a balance between oncological control and quality of life.

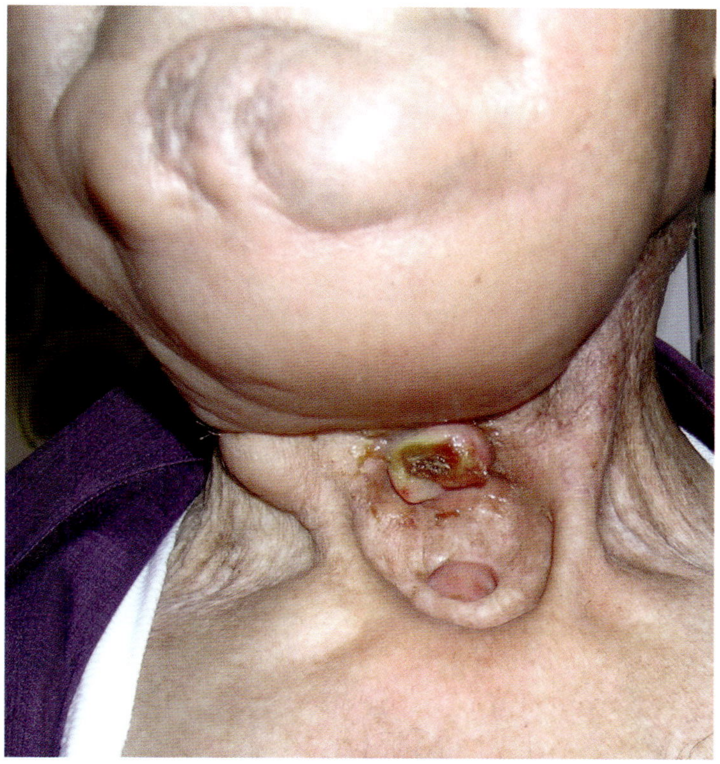

Fig. 7.1 Recurrent tumor occurring 18 months after previous total laryngectomy and neck dissection. Clinical examination suggests that this recurrence is localized in the midline and may be resectable completely, with several reconstructive options. Despite this, the patient will need comprehensive assessment prior to planning treatment, including cross-sectional imaging to stage locoregional disease and look for distant metastases, endoscopic assessment, and re-biopsy.

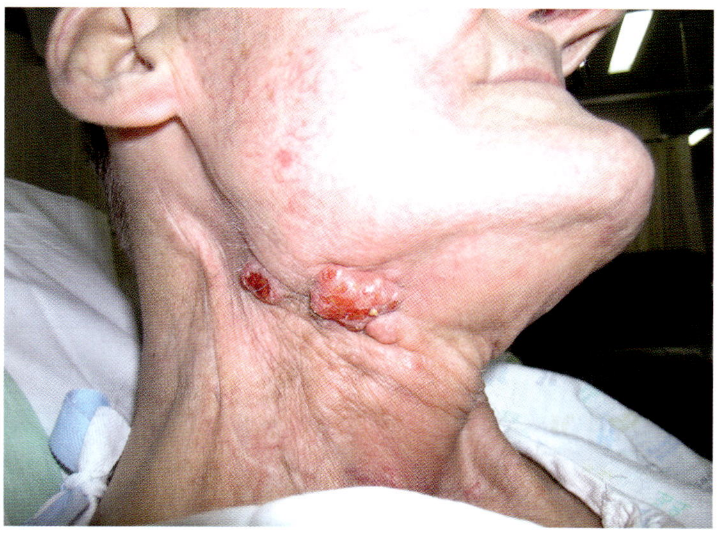

Fig. 7.2 Recurrent metastatic tumor in the neck occurring 9 months after neck dissection and resection of primary tumor in the oral cavity. This patient refused to receive postoperative concurrent chemoradiation for extracapsular disease. Note the multiple areas of recurrence, several involving the skin.

Assessment of the Recurrent Cancer

In addition to a comprehensive clinical examination, the newly diagnosed recurrent tumor needs a complete staging work-up akin to that for a new tumor before a treatment decision is made. This should include clinical examination, radiological assessment, and re-biopsy of the tumor, and in most instances an assessment under anesthesia is required (**Fig. 7.1**). In our practice, an ^{18}FDG PET-CT fusion scan is often performed as these patients are more often prone to distant metastases than at primary presentation. It must be recognized that recurrent tumors do not follow the relatively predictable patterns of lymphatic drainage seen with primary cancers (**Fig. 7.2**). This is especially the case when the patient has had a neck dissection or has received radiation to the neck. An exception can be made in certain instances where a residual tumor has been diagnosed at an early stage in a site that has been under close supervision and the risk of lymphatic spread is considered to be negligible, for example, the glottis. Another example is where early residual tumor presents soon after resection at a site where resection margins were close, for example, the oral tongue.

Factors Involved in Treatment Selection

A complex interplay of several factors will influence both the clinician and the patient in the selection of the most appropriate treatment. These are guided by the trade-off between treatment morbidity and the potential for cure (**Fig. 7.3**).

Nearly 60% of patients with head and neck cancer have concurrent medical disease (comorbidity) at presentation, one of the highest figures seen in any tumor site.[1] The burden of comorbidity has a high likelihood of increasing following treatment.[2] Where there is not considered to be enough physiological reserve for the patient to tolerate re-treatment, this will affect the subsequent management decisions. Age by itself would not be a contraindication; the patient's performance status and physiological reserve would be considered more important than chronological age. For instance, a patient in his or her sixth decade with small-volume radiorecurrent glottic cancer that is deemed to be salvageable by partial laryngectomy may not be a suitable candidate for this procedure in the presence of significant pulmonary function deficit that may not tolerate potential aspiration; the patient will require a total laryngectomy instead.

In addition, comorbidity has been shown to have a significant adverse effect on the outcome of treatment, at least as much as the TNM stage. This is probably mediated by modifying the host response to disease.[1] Thus, a comprehensive medical assessment is mandatory before arriving at a management decision, as concurrent medical illnesses are very likely to influence the choice of treatment.

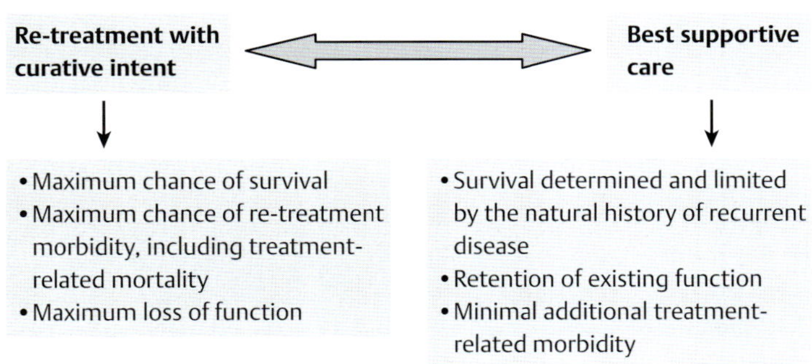

Fig. 7.3 The trade-off continuum on which the management of recurrent head and neck cancer is based.

Tumor Factors

From a strategic management viewpoint, the first question to ask is if this is a recurrence or a new primary cancer. This can be difficult to answer, but if there is a period of several years before the second tumor appears, then this might be a new primary tumor and therefore potentially curable with appropriate radical treatment. It is well recognized that there is often an alteration in tumor behavior in recurrence, often for the worse. Recurrence is associated with specific genetic aberrations.[3] As discussed below, re-assessment should include imaging to identify the extent of local, regional, and distant disease. The presence of certain findings often constitutes a contraindication to further treatment, but the decision needs to be individualized to each case.

Considerations for Revision Surgery

The same tumor factors that preclude curative surgical resection in the previously untreated patient will also play a role in recurrent disease. Invasion of the prevertebral muscles, brachial plexus, and skull base are absolute contraindications for attempting resection of neck disease, as clear macroscopic margins will not be obtained. In highly selected cases, tumor encasement of the carotid artery may be resectable[4] (**Fig. 7.4**). In carefully selected cases, surgery may be appropriate for symptom control, such as pain, mass effect, or fungating lesions. Often, in scenarios where curative resection can be accomplished, but where there is an unacceptably high sacrifice of function and quality of life (e.g., glossolaryngectomy for radiorecurrent tongue base cancer; **Fig. 7.5**), only supportive care may be appropriate.

Considerations for Re-irradiation

If the patient develops what is thought to be recurrent disease relatively early after the first treatment (within the first 12–24 months), then the site of recurrence should be reviewed with the original radiotherapy plan to see whether recurrence was due to "geographic miss"—that is, did the original radiotherapy field exclude some part of the tumor that subsequently did not receive the full radiotherapy dose. If this is the case, then in theory further radical treatment can be undertaken and a new radiotherapy volume can be matched onto the previous volume. In practice this is often very difficult to do because of the dose/volume compromises required in matching onto the previous radiotherapy to avoid overdose of organs at risk.

Previous Treatment and Sequelae

Previous treatment morbidity will play a major role in dictating treatment offered for disease recurrence. All efforts must be made to secure as much information as possible regarding the results of previous investigations, the pathology, and the treatment process. Patients with recurrent cancer are also more likely to seek a second opinion. Their previous experience with the treatment processes including the toxicity, any complications, and current quality of life all dictate how satisfied they are with the care that they receive. This can cause real or perceived apprehension leading to loss of confidence in the treating team. In these instances,

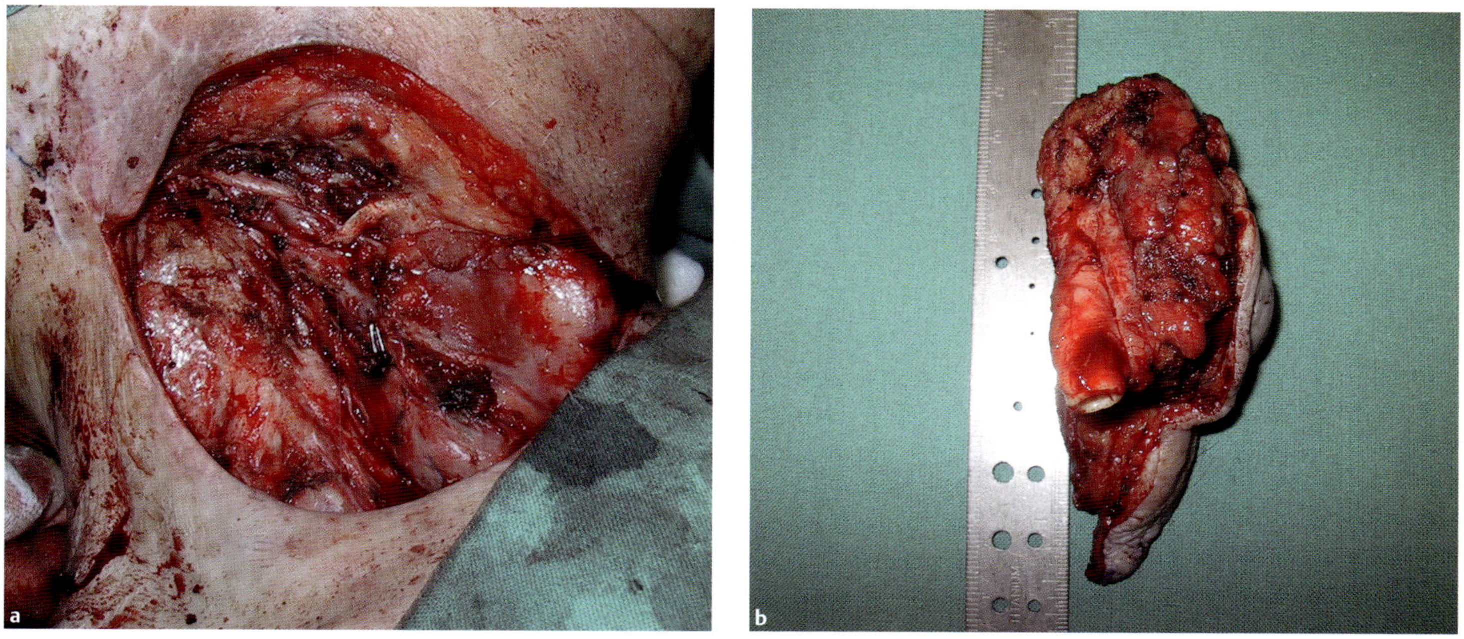

Fig. 7.4a, b Residual metastatic tumor in the neck after chemoradiation for an oropharyngeal primary. The primary site responded completely. The residual neck node invaded the common carotid artery, necessitating its sacrifice. Note the surgical field devoid of the carotid artery and the arterial lumen in the resected specimen. (Photograph courtesy of Suren Krishnan, Adelaide.)

the referring team must ensure that a comprehensive summary of the previous treatment accompanies the patient to their team of choice to expedite further care. In the absence of local expertise to manage disease recurrence, appropriate advice must be sought. The dictum *primum non nocere* (first do no harm) is very relevant in this setting.

The role of previous treatment in determining the choice of the treatment modality for the recurrent cancer is discussed below with examples.

Previous Radiation Therapy

As a rule of thumb, where feasible, radiorecurrent cases are best dealt with by surgical resection, owing to the significant increase in morbidity and relatively poor control rates with re-irradiation. The surgical procedure may need to be modified to take into consideration poor healing following previous irradiation. This will include counseling patients regarding a higher risk of complications, poorer functional outcome, a lower threshold for reconstruction, and longer postoperative stay.

Several variables regarding the previous treatment need to be carefully considered before embarking on re-irradiation. These include the total dose and dose per fraction to organs at risk, including the spinal cord, the brainstem, the brain itself, the eyes, optic nerves and optic chiasm, and the interval since previous treatment (see below). However, certain types of post-treatment morbidity may demand significant changes to the treatment plan. For example, even small tonsil recurrences may not be amenable to excision by endoscopic approaches owing to trismus and a stiff neck caused by previous treatment. In some scenarios, the suspicion of recurrent tumor can be difficult to ascertain owing to persistent postradiation side effects. This is typically seen in cases of advanced laryngeal tumors, where persistent local pain, laryngeal edema and chondronecrosis raise suspicion of residual/recurrent tumor and surgical clearance is needed.

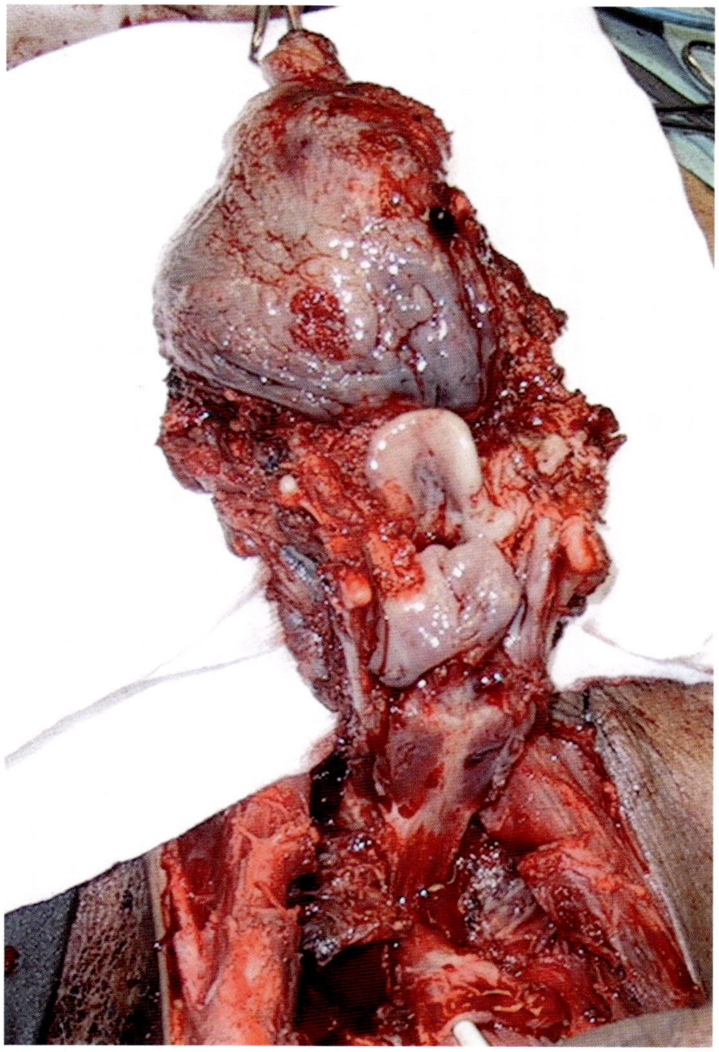

Fig. 7.5 Total glossolaryngectomy performed in a 43-year-old patient with a base of tongue tumor that did not respond to concurrent chemoradiation. She underwent extensive assessment and was counseled by surgeons, oncologists, speech and language therapists, dieticians, and psychologists prior to the procedure. Unfortunately, despite histological evidence of clear margins, local recurrence occurred within 16 weeks.

Previous Surgery

The previous surgical notes should be reviewed to correlate the site of recurrent tumor with the histological margins. Tumor recurring in the early months (<12 months) at sites where margins were "close" may indicate residual tumor. In these instances, where access is easy and tumor is not "buried," revision surgery may be the best way to deal with the disease. Recurrence following previous surgical resection alone does not necessarily rule out further surgery in many instances. For instance, recurrent tumors of the laryngeal glottis following previous endoscopic surgical resection, picked up during close follow-up, may be resectable by the same technique. Other options in this setting may include open partial laryngectomy and total laryngectomy. Large neck recurrences occurring after previous neck dissection are best controlled by wider surgical resections followed by adjuvant radiation. The extent of previous surgery and the reconstruction will also dictate treatment choice. Recurrent tumor under a bulky flap will pose a difficult surgical exercise, with poor chance of achieving clear margins. For instance, recurrence in a previously radiated total maxillectomy cavity that has been reconstructed with a flap is best dealt with by re-irradiation as the new tissue in the cavity will permit adequate and appropriate re-irradiation doses to be delivered. If the tumor is confirmed to be resectable, careful attention should be paid to the extent of functional impairment after revision surgery.

Long-term Morbidity and Functional Status

The current functional status and the presence of severe residual symptoms from previous treatment may make the patient reluctant to consider further treatment. The effect that any further treatment will have on function needs to be very carefully considered before embarking on a treatment process. Active osteoradionecrosis or chondronecrosis can contraindicate further radiation and make surgery a more appropriate option. Counterintuitively, xerostomia is not usually a contraindication to retreatment as it has often been maximally induced by the initial course of radiotherapy and further treatment does not usually make it much worse. Often, obstructive dysphagia seen with recurrent cancer is likely to worsen following irradiation, especially if the pharyngeal constrictor muscles are in the re-irradiation volume and surgical resection and reconstruction is preferred where feasible.

■ Interval following Previous Treatment

Patients with recurrent head and neck cancer fall into one of two broad groups. The favorable group presents with recurrent tumor following a period of remission that sees them recover some function and quality of life (QoL). These patients usually are very aware of their baseline symptoms and will seek help when any change is detected. The second group experiences persisting symptoms and disability following treatment that does not improve with time in the expected fashion. Patients in this group have residual tumor that is likely to be a result of repopulation by a radioresistant clone or have had an incomplete resection at the time of surgery. A widely used custom is to use a 12-month cut-off point to distinguish between residual (<12 months) and recurrent tumor (>12 months), but there can be an overlap between the two groups.

If geographic miss (see above) has not occurred and residual tumor persists within the high-dose volume, re-irradiation is often inappropriate because tumor persistence in itself would suggest that this cancer is a relatively radioresistant. It has already survived one course of radiotherapy and the surviving clonal populations may be even more radioresistant than in the original tumor. In this situation, surgery is usually a more appropriate form of salvage after radiotherapy failure. With increasing time since radiotherapy, normal tissue recovery does occur and even neurological tissue, previously thought to undergo permanent change after radiotherapy, demonstrates some recovery.[5] A longer gap between the first radiation course and re-irradiation for recurrence reduces risk of complications.

From a surgical perspective, the timing of recurrence is not as crucial to planning as long as the tumor is deemed resectable. Where surgery is undertaken within 3 months of radiation, long-term effects of radiation (primarily fibrosis) may not be present. With increasing delay after radiation, surgical dissection may be more difficult due to fibrosis.

■ Family and Psychosocial Support

There is no body of research in the medical literature dealing with social support and the retreatment of head and neck cancer, despite head and neck cancer patients having some of the highest rates of depression among all cancer patients.[6] There are inevitable changes to lifestyle patterns following a diagnosis of head and neck cancer.[7] However, most of the findings regarding social support in primary cancer will be applicable in this scenario.

Many head and neck cancer patients have limited family and social support due to their poorer socio-economic status, physical and psychological comorbidities including those produced by nicotine and alcohol dependence and their life choices. Following primary treatment of head and neck cancer, higher social support is usually related to higher quality of life scores,[8,9] but there have been some exceptions,[10] which may reflect the complexity and multiplicity of factors that affect quality of life in head and neck cancer. Social support seeking behaviors, for example, increased social contact and widening of social networks, have been shown to be very important coping mechanisms in patients awaiting initial treatment for head and neck cancer. It must be recognized that physicians are poor at identifying patient distress and the need for increased social support in their patients.

It may be possible to predict which patients are at greater risk of developing depression after treatment by the use of pretreatment assessment of their physical and depressive symptoms, the extent of their emotional and social support and their level of avoidance coping (mentally or physically avoiding something that causes distress).[11] There were fewer depressive symptoms in head and neck cancer patients where social support was available, whether they received it or not.[12]

Marital status has been shown to be an independent predictor for recurrence and survival in head and neck cancer.[13] Having a partner is associated with a decreased risk of recurrence.[13] Patients' partners may know little about the patient's own experience, attitudes or anxieties about the head and neck cancer, but this has been shown to be improved by better patient cancer education, which stimulates improved communication within the family.[14] Treatment survivors with a lack of adequate family support have decreased life satisfaction scores, which usually improve over time.[15] Improved communication between clinicians and the family regarding social support has been shown to improve long-term rehabilitation outcomes.[16,17]

It is feasible that increased family support can lead to demands for more aggressive treatment with curative intent.

> ! It is important that robust mechanisms are in place for social and psychological support for all patients with recurrent cancer, and especially for those planned for re-treatment.

Faith, Religion, and Spirituality

Although religion and spirituality are independent constructs with overlap, when discussed in the context of health, they can be treated as synonymous.[18] For the purpose of this discussion, these terms will be used interchangeably. There are no studies that deal exclusively with the issue of spirituality and religion in head and neck cancer. However, several lessons can be learnt from the oncological literature that will be applicable to this scenario.

Spirituality influences all aspects of the cancer experience. Studies of cancer patients across different cultures suggest that those who rely on spiritual and religious beliefs use an active coping style, dealing with their illness in a positive way, thus significantly contributing to psychosocial adjustment to cancer.[19–21] Spirituality may even be the primary source of psychological support among some religious groups,[22] and the availability of spiritual support is associated with better QoL.[23]

Refusal of treatment with either chemotherapy or radiotherapy on grounds of religious or ethical belief is unusual. In patients receiving end-of-life support, several studies have shown that religious individuals more frequently want aggressive measures to extend life.[23,24] The exact reasons for this association are less well understood, but this has significant relevance within the setting of recurrent head and neck cancer.

Some patients who will not accept blood transfusions, such as Jehovah's Witnesses, need to be informed that in normal practice blood transfusion is sometimes indicated for patients who experienced chemotherapy-induced anemia. This can usually be managed in other ways, thereby avoiding transfusion, but the potential risk of further bone marrow damage may curtail any more chemotherapy being given. Similarly, with careful preoperative planning, major head and neck resections and reconstructions are feasible in this religious group.[25]

The many spiritual needs of patients with advanced cancer may not be met by the community or the medical system. Despite this, most physicians agree that they should be aware of a patient's religious beliefs and accommodate those beliefs in devising treatment plans.[26] Validated tools exist to measure spiritual needs.

Involving the Patient in the Decision-making Process

Unlike with cancer at first presentation, the evidence base in the literature from which to choose appropriate treatment for recurrent or residual cancer is significantly limited. Consequently, decisions are made on the basis of personal experience of the treating team and philosophy of care at the treating institution. The management will understandably vary among centers, as will the results. It is of paramount importance that patients are actively involved in the decision-making process for recurrent cancer, as much as at initial presentation. In many instances, having gone through previous treatment, patients with recurrent cancer will be better informed and have more concrete ideas and expectations of the treatment process. This section will discuss some of the key concepts that help in deciding upon management plans that are appropriate and lead to optimal patient satisfaction, illustrated by clinical examples.

Strategies for Good Decision Making in Oncological Practice

Within oncological practice, a systematic review showed that the primary determinant of satisfaction with care is that the need for information about the disease and its treatment and the requirement for treatment with respect and empathy are fully met.[27] Interestingly, subjective perception of a high level of caring attention and physician empathy seems to be predictive of patients reporting that their information needs were fully met.[28]

There is good evidence to show that communication of the risks of treatments during consultation is associated with high levels of satisfaction.[29] While it is feasible that the risk communication and decision making may make only small differences to the outcome of the consultation, the increase in patient participation that leads to greater satisfaction justifies these measures. Within oncological practice, Gattellari et al.[30] showed that any perceived role that patients took in shared decision making significantly and independently predicted satisfaction with the consultation and with the perceived amount of information and emotional support received from the physician. Patients who were least satisfied included those who reported that the decision was exclusively made by themselves alone or by the consulting physician alone. In the arena of head and neck cancer, it has been demonstrated that information needs vary greatly and may need to be individualized.[31] Tailoring of information has an impact on long-term satisfaction with care[32] and it must be noted that patients and nonpatients will not always make the same decisions given the same information,[33] nor do they necessarily have the same objectives.[34]

The authors believe that in the setting of recurrent cancer, where treatment decisions are constrained by the lack of high-level evidence and where the stakes are high, shared decision making should form a cornerstone in the consultation process. Physician counseling may be greatly enhanced by the use of patient decision aids. These are tools developed to help in the decision-making process by providing information about management options and outcomes and clarifying personal values.

There are some caveats to this approach that need to be kept in mind: it is very likely that some patients, especially elderly, may not prefer to participate[35] and patient preferences may also change during the course of the illness.[36] Treatment refusal, when it occurs, is on grounds that additional treatment toxicity is likely to be unacceptable when weighed against a relatively low chance of substantial clinical improvement. This is to be welcomed if it shows that patients are being given more information about potential outcomes and that shared decision making is actively being practiced.

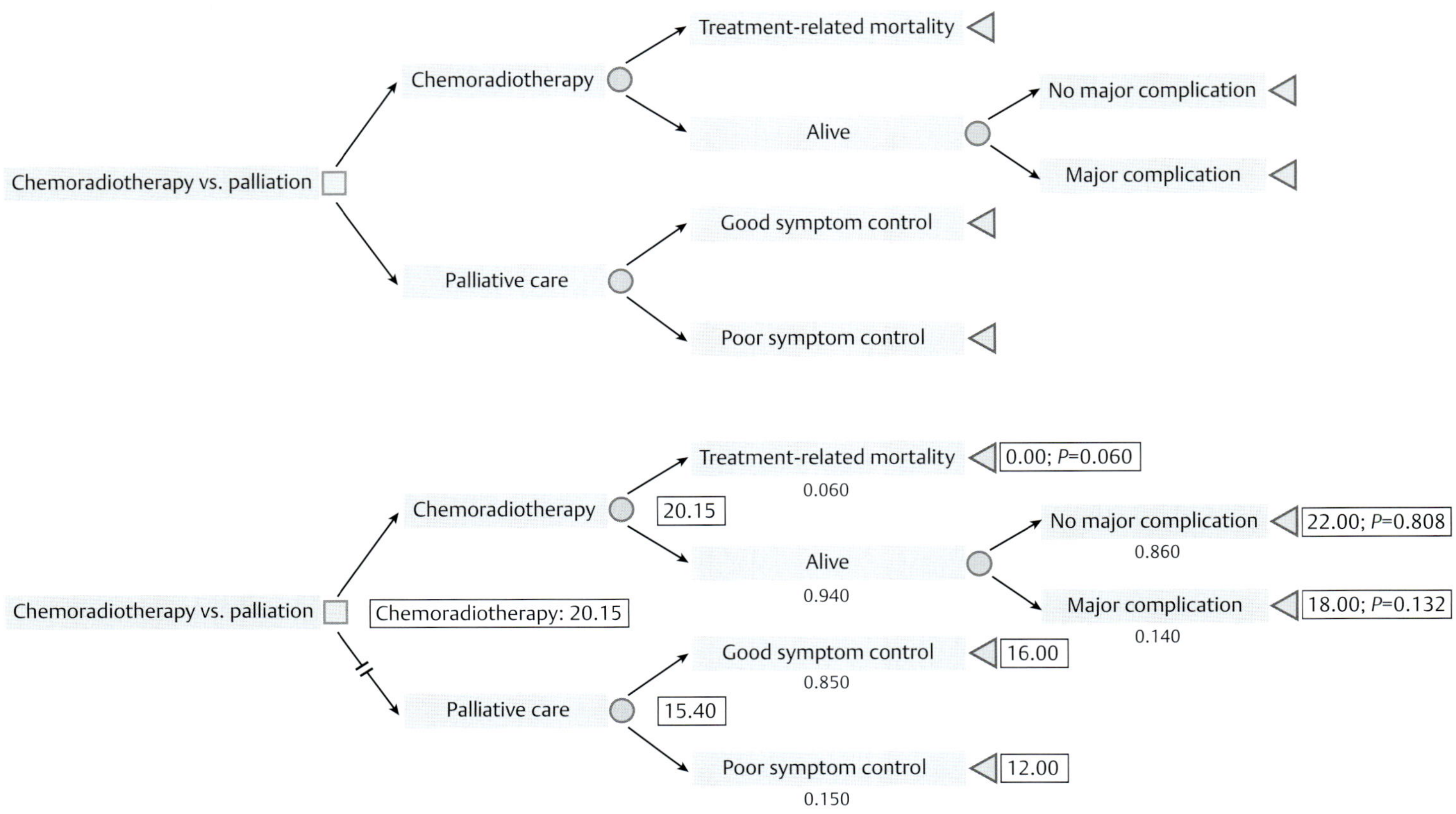

Fig. 7.6 A decision analysis model comparing quality-adjusted life years (QALYs; boxed numbers on the left side between arrows) between patients undergoing concurrent chemotherapy with re-irradiation (CTReRT) and best supportive care for radiorecurrent head and neck squamous cancer was generated. Survival data from recent reviews on the topic were used. An expert panel arrived at a consensus to assign utility values for the various health state outcomes when CTReRT is administered for recurrent cancer, or in the setting of palliative care for these patients. Utility values range between 0 and 1, with 1.0 equating to perfect health and 0 to death. Patients who do not suffer a severe complication following CTReRT were assigned by the expert panel to have a utility value of 0.7, and those who suffered one, a utility value of 0.6. The utility value assigned in the setting of good palliation was 0.8, with 0.6 given when symptom control was less than optimal. The model showed superior QALYs for the CTReRT arm of approximately 5 weeks (20 weeks vs. 15 weeks for palliation).

Theories of Decision Making

It is appropriate at this point to introduce the three theories that underpin the interventions in use to improve patient decision making.

Descriptive Theories

The descriptive theories of decision making suggest that individuals rely on and prefer heuristic processing strategies (subconscious, intuitive) to make decisions as opposed to systematic processing (conscious, analytic), primarily due to finite cognitive resources. While heuristic processing leads to satisfactory decisions being made most of the time, the disadvantage is that these may not necessarily lead to good decisions. In recurrent disease scenarios where the chance of a good outcome with curative treatment is very small, patients may choose intuitively to receive best supportive care (see the box). Conversely, patients may intuitively choose "treatments" where there is only a 1%–2% chance of clinical improvement at the cost of considerable morbidity because they wish to have treatment, whatever it is, at any cost.

Case Study

Mr. J.R. was a 68-year-old man with a squamous cell cancer of the supraglottis, treated by radiation therapy 3 years previously. The recurrent cancer, following investigations, was judged to be endolaryngeal and resectable and, given his good general health, he was offered a total laryngectomy. His father had died following throat surgery for cancer in the 1950s. Mr. J.R. was steadfast in his refusal of any active intervention. He was offered social and psychological support and lived for 8 months until he died of a chest infection.

Normative Theories

Normative theories provide frameworks for reaching the optimal choice, based on mathematical axioms. Various forms of decision aids can be developed based on the criteria that guide the available choices. Decision analysis models are a form of decision aid based on the expected utility theory. A utility is a measure of a decision maker's relative preference for an outcome or health state, and is expressed as a single value between 0 and 1. Utilities for outcomes in health care are usually assessed relative to two extremes, referred to as anchor states. The commonly used anchor states are "death," assigned a value of 0, and "full health," assigned a value of 1. Utility measures provide summary scores that aggregate the positive and negative aspects of quality of life, and can incorporate attitudes toward risk and length of life.

Utility values for health states are best estimated directly in appropriate subjects, using reliable and valid methods or indirectly using preference-based, health-related quality of life instruments

(Health Utilities Index, EuroQoL-5D). In the absence of this data, they can be estimated in several ways:

- Arbitrarily assign values based on the judgment of the assessor.
- Have a group of experts reach a consensus on the estimates for the utility values.
- Search for relevant, published utility values in the literature.

In recurrent, unresectable head and neck cancer, decision analysis models informed by results from systematic reviews and expert panel–generated utility values showed that concurrent chemotherapy and re-irradiation offers an improvement in QALYs for patients of approximately 5 weeks compared with best supportive care (**Fig. 7.6**).[37] The disadvantage of expected utility theory is that patients asked to make choices with specific criteria may make decisions with which they are less satisfied.

Prescriptive Approaches

Prescriptive approaches recommend a range of techniques to encourage the individual's better thinking about a decision. Decision aid interventions informed by the prescriptive approach will encourage individuals to better consider the decision. Advantages of this approach are that it is responsive to the different needs of the decision context and the individual. However, given that there are many techniques to support decision making, the precise components that facilitate decision making can vary between contexts. No research has focused on applying the prescriptive technique in head and neck cancer (see box).

Case Study

D.W. was a fit 71-year-old widower with three grown children, who was still actively running a medium-sized family business. He developed a recurrent carcinoma of the lateral margin and base of the tongue, 2 years after surgical resection and reconstruction of a T2N0M0 lateral tongue cancer. The current recurrence was staged rT4aN0M0. He was seen in the multidisciplinary clinic and the diagnosis was discussed with him and the family. He expressed the desire to be actively involved in the decision-making process for the treatment of his cancer.

Following a discussion of the treatment options available to him (best supportive care, palliative chemotherapy, palliative or radical courses of radiotherapy, or combined treatment), he was sent a brochure on the natural history of untreated cancer. This brochure had been developed 2 years before by a patient group following publication of a large cohort study. He was offered a half-day educational program designed for patients with head and neck cancer, which he declined. He was also given written information about a range of chemotherapy agents used for palliation. He received a video about radiation therapy that explained to him the preparatory steps, the procedure, the side effects, and the recovery process, which he viewed with his family. The proportional benefits, risks and survival of each treatment scenario were communicated to him using pictograms of 100 human subjects, the data for which was derived from the local head and neck cancer database. Previous research on risk communication to head and neck cancer patients had identified formats that patients find acceptable when communicating survival data. He decided that his optimal objectives would be:

- To live long enough to ensure full transfer of his business interests to his children.
- To retain maximal tongue function because his business dealings were predominantly telephone-based.
- To try to minimize pain and loss of tongue function from tumor progression.

After considering all of his options and their consequences and trade-offs, he accepted the course of external beam radiation using an intensity-modulated radiotherapy technique, to reduce radiation dose to the parotids and mandible. Following treatment there was considerable tumor reduction and D.W. died 24 months later from myocardial infarction, having maintained a functional telephone voice and ability to eat and swallow and having successfully transferred all this business assets to his family.

Decision Aids

Kassirer[38] set out in 1994 the indications for explicitly listing patients' preferences in clinical practice. These are set out in the box below. It is impressive that many patients with recurrent head and neck cancer will satisfy almost all of the seven criteria. A systematic review[39] showed that patients exposed to decision aids are more likely to participate in decision making and achieve higher-quality decisions.

Indications for Using Decision Aids

- There are major differences in the kinds of possible outcomes (e.g., death versus disability).
- There are major differences between treatments in the likelihood and impact of complications.
- The choices involve trade-offs between near-term and long-term outcomes.
- One of the choices can result in a small chance of a grave outcome.
- The apparent difference between options is marginal.
- The patient is particularly averse to taking risks.
- The patient attaches unusual importance to certain possible outcomes.

Treatment Options

When counseling patients with recurrent head and neck cancer, clinicians should provide realistic expectations of the outcomes of the possible management plans based on tumor stage and site. The complications and side effects of treatment and the functional outcome should be clearly identified. The paucity of data in this setting needs to be emphasized.

Best Supportive Care

Patients receiving supportive care alone have a poor median survival, between 3 months[40] and 5 months[41]. The objective of supportive care is not primarily to prolong life but to improve the quality of life for whatever time remains by managing and minimizing new symptoms. Treatments may have a secondary effect of prolonging life, but this is an incidental effect.

Surgical Resection with Curative Intent

Patients who have recurred following previous surgery alone will need to be assessed on an individual basis. Small recurrent tumors that occur in the surgical bed that have not been reconstructed may present early and may be re-resected with little additional morbidity. Large-volume recurrences following primary surgery may also be suitable for resection based on the extent of local invasion and if no contraindications exist. Favorable outcomes are usually seen in organs where the tumor is well confined to the site of recurrence, e.g., the larynx.

Recurrence in the neck that has been previously treated by neck dissection is often associated with fixity to deeper structures. Often, disruption of tissue planes will make the true extent of the tumor difficult to assess and the additional morbidity of revision surgery must be balanced against the probability of tumor control. It is likely that most patients in this group will also need adjuvant radiation, if possible.

Recurrences occurring in a previously irradiated field provide unique challenges. As a general rule, where possible, radiorecurrent tumors that are deemed to be resectable with acceptable morbidity are best managed by surgical excision. Radiation-induced fibrosis and disruption of normal lymphatic pathways can make for some of the most complex management decisions encountered. Surgery in the irradiated field is technically more difficult, especially when fibrosis and other late complications set in. These procedures are best performed by experienced surgeons. Postoperative complications are also more frequent, with a greater chance of infection, wound dehiscence, failure of microvascular anastamosis, and delayed healing.[42,43] For instance, the incidence of pharyngocutaneous fistula is higher (30%) following laryngectomy for radiorecurrent tumors as opposed to a 15% incidence for primary laryngectomy. Meticulous surgical technique is needed and there should be a lower threshold for bringing in new nonirradiated tissue that will help with the healing.

Case Study

Mr. S.W. is a 69-year-old man who underwent concurrent chemoradiation for an endolaryngeal squamous cell cancer staged T3N0M0. Within 18 months of treatment, he developed a recurrence at the primary site. This was salvaged by a total laryngectomy, selective neck dissection levels II, III, and IV, and augmentation of the pharyngeal circumference by a radial forearm free flap. Speech rehabilitation was performed using a speech valve inserted 6 months later. He remains disease free more than 24 months after his surgical resection.

Surgical Debulking

Surgical debulking may have a role in selected scenarios. There is a limited evidence base from prospective studies to suggest that debulking surgery prior to concurrent chemotherapy with re-irradiation[44–48] or brachytherapy leads to better local control.[49,50]

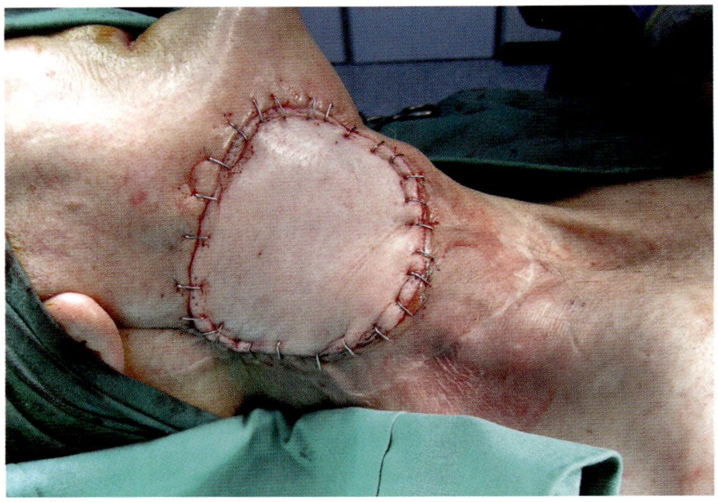

Fig. 7.7 Extended radical neck dissection with sacrifice of the overlying skin and reconstruction of the defect with a bulky pectoralis major myocutaneous flap.

Case Study

Mr. J.W. is a 62-year-old man who underwent neck dissection followed by concurrent chemoradiation for an oropharyngeal squamous cell cancer staged T2N2aM0, with clinical and radiological complete response. A year and half after treatment, he developed a recurrence in his ipsilateral neck. The neck lump measured 4 cm × 6 cm extending over levels II and III. He underwent an extended radical neck dissection with sacrifice of the overlying skin and reconstruction of the defect with a bulky pectoralis major myocutaneous flap (**Fig. 7.7**). The margins of the resection were not free and the gross tumor was left behind at the skull base. Following this, he underwent chemoradiation to his neck. He remains disease free 36 months later.

Palliative Radiation

Indications for palliative radiotherapy are not well defined in recurrent disease. If the recurrence has occurred shortly after previous irradiation then further palliative radiotherapy may be inappropriate as it will inevitably lead to increased morbidity with little chance of response if we assume that radioresistance is proven by its early recurrence. In this situation the use of palliative chemotherapy, especially if the patient is chemotherapy naive, or the use of best supportive care may well be more appropriate.

If palliative radiotherapy is to be used in patients with recurrence who have had or not had radiotherapy before, there is no agreed schedule or regimen, and widely differing treatment schedules have been tried.

Re-irradiation with Curative Intent

Re-irradiation can take the form of external beam treatment, brachytherapy, or concomitant chemoradiotherapy, delivered using conventional techniques or other advanced planning techniques (e.g., intensity-modulated radiotherapy, IMRT). Although cure may be achieved in a very few individual patients, long-term

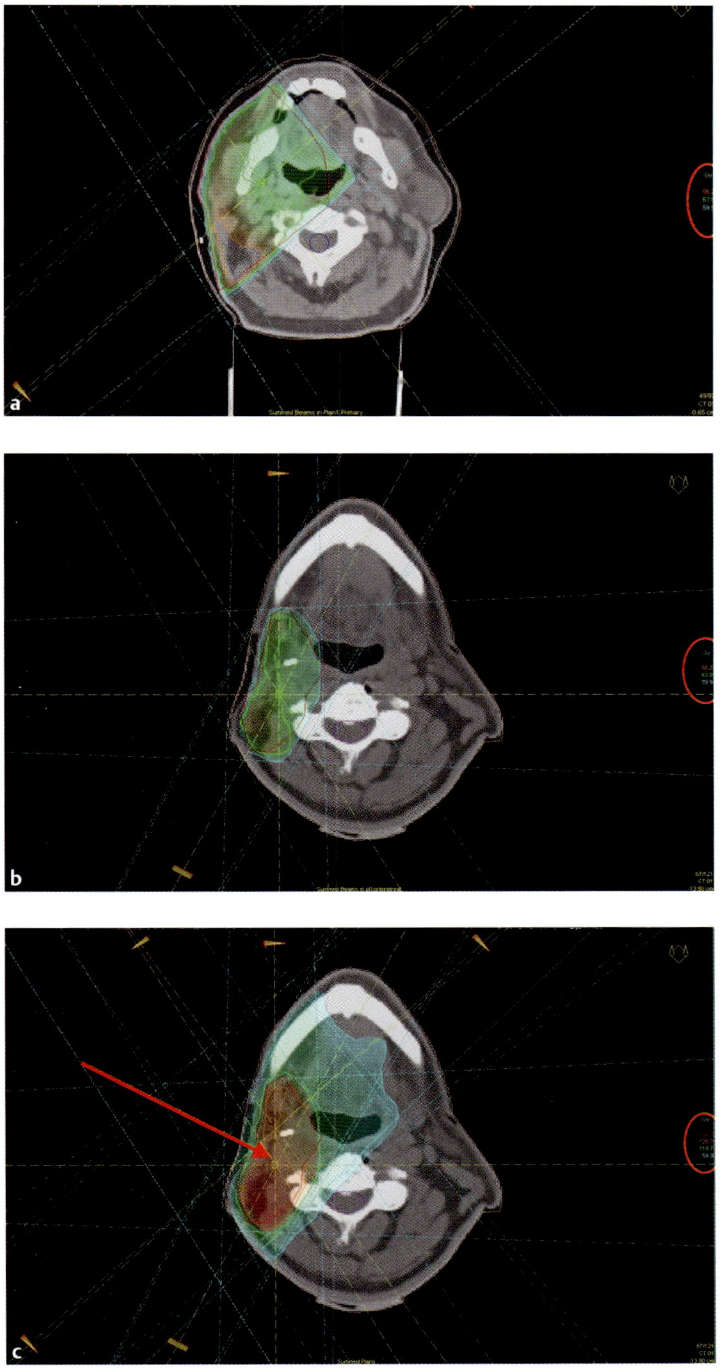

Fig. 7.8 a–c Patient with oropharyngeal cancer who received 63 Gy in 30 fractions in 2006 (**a**) was diagnosed with a recurrent tumor in 2011. The tumor was planned for re-irradiation (**b**) with 63 Gy in 30 fractions. The summated plan (**c**) shows complete overlap of the treated area superiorly (arrow), but the spinal cord dose remaining within tolerance.

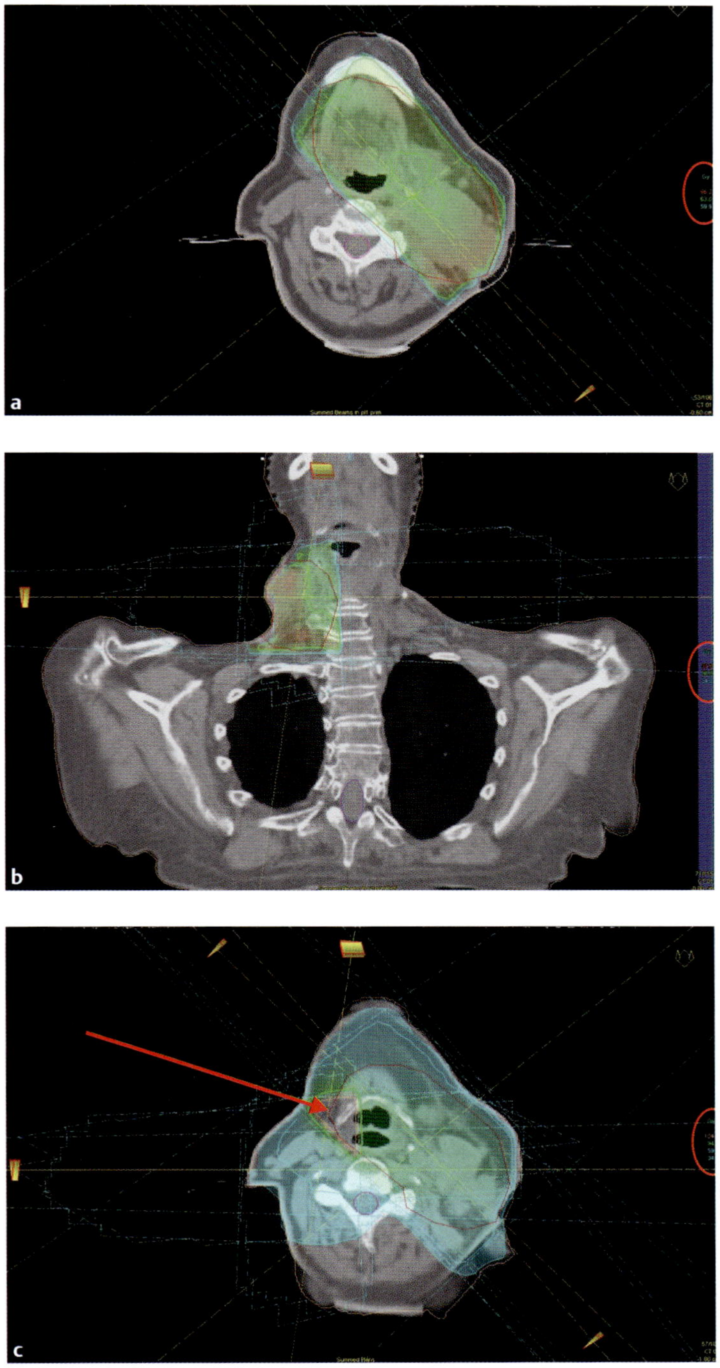

Fig. 7.9 a–c Patient with advanced oropharyngeal cancer who received 63 Gy in 30 fractions in 2009 (**a**), returned with a contralateral node 2 years later. The patient's position was vastly different and thus it was difficult to fully assess overlap of fields (**b**). The summated plan (**c**) shows complete overlap of the treated area superiorly (arrow), but the total planned dose to the spinal cord was 57.06 Gy, exceeding the spinal cord tolerance. This required re-planning.

palliation may be achieved in a greater number. At present there is no accurate way of identifying those few patients who will do exceptionally well and who will essentially be cured. These include the following scenarios: (1) primary sites such as nasopharynx and larynx have higher control rates than other subsites; (2) the longer interval between the first treatment and re-irradiation, the better the response with less additional morbidity; and (3) second primaries respond better than recurrences.

Since re-irradiation is palliative for the majority of the treated patients, the balance of potential benefit versus potential toxicity is the most important factor to be considered. Choosing the correct dose and fractionation regimen and tailoring it appropriately for the individual patient can be very difficult. Re-irradiation giving full radical dose for a second time may give the best chance of cure or long-term palliation but at the expense of maximal accumulated tissue damage from both courses of treatment, especially to connective tissue and the microvasculature, leading to irreparable tissue necrosis and nonhealing ulceration. Since late radiation damage is secondary to microvascular damage, from both radiotherapy treatments, re-irradiation can be given after salvage surgery where microvascular free flap reconstruction has taken place without detriment to the free flap.[51] Re-irradiation dose and fractionation regimens are based on other factors such as the patient's functional age and performance status, the tumor bulk, the size of the volume that has to be re-irradiated, the amount of overlap with the initial radiotherapy volume, and probably most importantly the time since previous irradiation.[52] Where possible, patients undergoing re-irradiation for head and neck cancer should do so within clinical trials.[48]

Recent technological advances using IMRT or tomotherapy permit construction of complicated three-dimensional dose distribution volumes with high doses of radiation delivered within the tumor volume, and much lower doses delivered to surrounding normal structures or organs at risk than could be achieved with previous techniques. This is especially useful as tissues and organs which had previously had high-dose treatment can be outlined and designated as particularly low-dose areas in the re-treatment volumes, thus keeping the cumulative total dose to these organs below tissue tolerance dose (**Figs. 7.8 and 7.9**).

Clinical Trials

Several ethical issues come to the fore when dealing with recurrent tumors. In scenarios where there is no consensus on the treatment intent (curative vs. palliative), what should be the optimal management strategy? Among patients with recurrent cancer and those who approach the end of life, there is greater inclination to accept higher treatment-related risk and be willing to participate in experimental treatments.[53] Inclusion into trial protocols that have undergone rigorous peer and ethical assessment may be appropriate if selection criteria are met. Although the primary aim in phase I trials is to determine toxicity and dosing of experimental therapies, studies in the phase I clinical trial population show that a significant proportion enrolled in phase I trials expect therapeutic benefit and even cure.[53,54]

Future Research

- Analyze the factors that dictate choice of treatment options for patients with recurrent head and neck cancer.
- Studies on the oncological efficacy of the available treatment options.
- Assess quality of life for patients with recurrent head and neck cancer before and following treatment.
- Identify optimal methods of communicating risks associated with treatment or best supportive care.
- Identify factors that help the decision-making process in patients with recurrent head and neck cancer.

Recommended Reading

- National Comprehensive Cancer Network. Clinical Practice Guidelines in Oncology (www.nccn.org) and Scottish Intercollegiate Guidelines Network (www.sign.ac.uk/pdf/sign90.pdf). (These two evidence-based guidelines, although not helpful in patient selection, provide an excellent overview of the poor evidence base on which current treatment for recurrent head and neck cancer is provided.)
- Edwards A, Glyn Elwyn G, eds. Shared Decision-Making in Health Care: Achieving Evidence-Based Patient Choice. 2nd ed. Oxford: Oxford University Press; 2009 (An excellent primer to the principles of decision making discussed in this chapter.)

References

1. Paleri V, Wight RG, Silver CE, et al. Comorbidity in head and neck cancer: A critical appraisal and recommendations for practice. Oral Oncol 2010;46(10):712–719
2. Yung KC, Piccirillo JF. The incidence and impact of comorbidity diagnosed after the onset of head and neck cancer. Arch Otolaryngol Head Neck Surg 2008;134(10):1045–1049
3. Agada FO, Patmore H, Alhamarneh O, Stafford ND, Greenman J. Genetic profile of head and neck squamous cell carcinoma: clinical implications. J Laryngol Otol 2009;123(3):266–272
4. Freeman SB. Advanced cervical metastasis involving the carotid artery. Curr Opin Otolaryngol Head Neck Surg 2005;13(2):107–111
5. Supe SS, Ganesh KM, Naveen T, Jacob S, Sankar BN. Spinal cord response to altered fractionation and re-irradiation: radiobiological considerations and role of bioeffect models. J Cancer Res Ther 2006;2(3):105–118
6. Lydiatt WM, Moran J, Burke WJ. A review of depression in the head and neck cancer patient. Clin Adv Hematol Oncol 2009;7(6):397–403
7. Semple CJ, Dunwoody L, George Kernohan W, McCaughan E, Sullivan K. Changes and challenges to patients' lifestyle patterns following treatment for head and neck cancer. J Adv Nurs 2008;63(1):85–93
8. Karnell LH, Christensen AJ, Rosenthal EL, Magnuson JS, Funk GF. Influence of social support on health-related quality of life outcomes in head and neck cancer. Head Neck 2007;29(2):143–146
9. Vakharia KT, Ali MJ, Wang SJ. Quality-of-life impact of participation in a head and neck cancer support group. Otolaryngol Head Neck Surg 2007;136(3):405–410
10. Petruson KM, Silander EM, Hammerlid EB. Effects of psychosocial intervention on quality of life in patients with head and neck cancer. Head Neck 2003;25(7):576–584
11. de Leeuw JR, de Graeff A, Ros WJ, Blijham GH, Hordijk GJ, Winnubst JA. Prediction of depressive symptomatology after treatment of head and neck cancer: the influence of pre-treatment physical and depressive symptoms, coping, and social support. Head Neck 2000;22(8):799–807
12. De Leeuw JR, De Graeff A, Ros WJ, Hordijk GJ, Blijham GH, Winnubst JA. Negative and positive influences of social support on depression in patients with head and neck cancer: a prospective study. Psychooncology 2000;9(1):20–28
13. de Graeff A, de Leeuw JR, Ros WJ, Hordijk GJ, Blijham GH, Winnubst JA. Sociodemographic factors and quality of life as prognostic indicators in head and neck cancer. Eur J Cancer 2001;37(3):332–339
14. Chaitchik S, Kreitler S, Rapoport Y, Algor R. What do cancer patients' spouses know about the patients? Cancer Nurs 1992;15(5):353–362
15. Morton RP. Life-satisfaction in patients with head and neck cancer. Clin Otolaryngol Allied Sci 1995;20(6):499–503

16. de Boer MF, Pruyn JF, van den Borne B, Knegt PP, Ryckman RM, Verwoerd CD. Rehabilitation outcomes of long-term survivors treated for head and neck cancer. Head Neck 1995;17(6):503–515
17. Baker CA. Factors associated with rehabilitation in head and neck cancer. Cancer Nurs 1992;15(6):395–400
18. Miller WR, Thoresen CE. Spirituality, religion, and health. An emerging research field. Am Psychol 2003;58(1):24–35
19. Weaver AJ, Flannelly KJ. The role of religion/spirituality for cancer patients and their caregivers. South Med J 2004; 97(12):1210–1214
20. Crane JN. Religion and cancer: examining the possible connections. J Psychosoc Oncol 2009;27(4):469–486
21. Howsepian BA, Merluzzi TV. Religious beliefs, social support, self-efficacy and adjustment to cancer. Psychooncology 2009;18(10):1069–1079
22. Harandy TF, Ghofranipour F, Montazeri A, et al. Muslim breast cancer survivor spirituality: coping strategy or health seeking behavior hindrance? Health Care Women Int. 2010;31(1):88–98.
23. Balboni TA, Vanderwerker LC, Block SD, et al. Religiousness and spiritual support among advanced cancer patients and associations with end-of-life treatment preferences and quality of life. J Clin Oncol 2007;25(5):555–560
24. Phelps AC, Maciejewski PK, Nilsson M, et al. Religious coping and use of intensive life-prolonging care near death in patients with advanced cancer. JAMA 2009;301(11):1140–1147
25. Skoner JM, Wax MK. Microvascular free-tissue transfer for head and neck reconstruction in Jehovah's Witness patients. Head Neck 2008;30(4):455–460
26. Handzo G, Koenig HG. Spiritual care: whose job is it anyway? South Med J 2004;97(12):1242–1244
27. Lis CG, Rodeghier M, Gupta D. Distribution and determinants of patient satisfaction in oncology: A review of the literature. Patient Prefer Adherence 2009;3:287–304
28. Neumann M, Wirtz M, Ernstmann N, et al. Identifying and predicting subgroups of information needs among cancer patients: an initial study using latent class analysis. Support Care Cancer 2011;19(8):1197–1209
29. Davis RE, Dolan G, Thomas S, et al. Exploring doctor and patient views about risk communication and shared decision-making in the consultation. Health Expect 2003;6(3):198–207
30. Gattellari M, Butow PN, Tattersall MH. Sharing decisions in cancer care. Soc Sci Med 2001;52(12):1865–1878
31. Newell R, Ziegler L, Stafford N, Lewin RJ. The information needs of head and neck cancer patients prior to surgery. Ann R Coll Surg Engl 2004;86(6):407–410
32. Llewellyn CD, McGurk M, Weinman J. How satisfied are head and neck cancer (HNC) patients with the information they receive pre-treatment? Results from the satisfaction with cancer information profile (SCIP). Oral Oncol 2006;42(7):726–734
33. List MA, Rutherford JL, Stracks J, et al. Prioritizing treatment outcomes: head and neck cancer patients versus nonpatients. Head Neck 2004;26(2):163–170
34. Sharp HM, List M, MacCracken E, Stenson K, Stocking C, Siegler M. Patients' priorities among treatment effects in head and neck cancer: evaluation of a new assessment tool. Head Neck 1999;21(6):538–546
35. Pinquart M, Duberstein PR. Information needs and decision-making processes in older cancer patients. Crit Rev Oncol Hematol 2004;51(1):69–80
36. Say R, Murtagh M, Thomson R. Patients' preference for involvement in medical decision making: a narrative review. Patient Educ Couns 2006;60(2):102–114
37. Paleri V, Kelly CG. Re-irradiation with concurrent chemotherapy in recurrent head and neck cancer: a decision analysis model based on a systematic review. Clin Otolaryngol 2008;33(4):331–337
38. Kassirer JP. Incorporating patients' preferences into medical decisions. N Engl J Med 1994;330(26):1895–1896
39. Stacey D, Samant R, Bennett C. Decision making in oncology: a review of patient decision aids to support patient participation. CA Cancer J Clin 2008;58(5):293–304
40. León X, Hitt R, Constenla M, et al. A retrospective analysis of the outcome of patients with recurrent and/or metastatic squamous cell carcinoma of the head and neck refractory to a platinum-based chemotherapy. Clin Oncol (R Coll Radiol) 2005;17(6):418–424
41. Jones AS. The untreated patient with squamous carcinoma of the head and neck. Am J Clin Oncol 1995;18(4):363–368
42. Kruse AL, Luebbers HT, Grätz KW, Obwegeser JA. Factors influencing survival of free-flap in reconstruction for cancer of the head and neck: a literature review. Microsurgery 2010;30(3):242–248
43. Schultze-Mosgau S, Grabenbauer GG, Radespiel-Tröger M, et al. Vascularization in the transition area between free grafted soft tissues and pre-irradiated graft bed tissues following preoperative radiotherapy in the head and neck region. Head Neck 2002;24(1):42–51
44. Dawson LA, Myers LL, Bradford CR, et al. Conformal re-irradiation of recurrent and new primary head-and-neck cancer. Int J Radiat Oncol Biol Phys 2001;50(2):377–385
45. De Crevoisier R, Bourhis J, Domenge C, et al. Full-dose reirradiation for unresectable head and neck carcinoma: experience at the Gustave-Roussy Institute in a series of 169 patients. J Clin Oncol 1998;16(11):3556–3562
46. De Crevoisier R, Domenge C, Wibault P, et al. Full dose reirradiation combined with chemotherapy after salvage surgery in head and neck carcinoma. Cancer 2001;91(11):2071–2076
47. Machtay M, Rosenthal DI, Chalian AA, et al. Pilot study of postoperative reirradiation, chemotherapy, and amifostine after surgical salvage for recurrent head-and-neck cancer. Int J Radiat Oncol Biol Phys 2004;59(1):72–77
48. Salama JK, Vokes EE, Chmura SJ, et al. Long-term outcome of concurrent chemotherapy and reirradiation for recurrent and second primary head-and-neck squamous cell carcinoma. Int J Radiat Oncol Biol Phys 2006;64(2):382–391
49. Nutting C, Horlock N, A'Hern R, et al. Manually after-loaded 192Ir low-dose rate brachytherapy after subtotal excision and flap reconstruction of recurrent cervical lymphadenopathy from head and neck cancer. Radiother Oncol 2006;80(1):39–42
50. Narayana A, Cohen GN, Zaider M, et al. High-dose-rate interstitial brachytherapy in recurrent and previously irradiated head and neck cancers—preliminary results. Brachytherapy 2007;6(2):157–163
51. Suh JD, Kim BP, Abemayor E, et al. Reirradiation after salvage surgery and microvascular free flap reconstruction for recurrent head and neck carcinoma. Otolaryngol Head Neck Surg 2008;139(6):781–786
52. Tanvetyanon T, Padhya T, McCaffrey J, et al. Prognostic factors for survival after salvage reirradiation of head and neck cancer. J Clin Oncol 2009;27(12):1983–1991

53. Meropol NJ, Weinfurt KP, Burnett CB, et al. Perceptions of patients and physicians regarding phase I cancer clinical trials: implications for physician-patient communication. J Clin Oncol 2003;21(13):2589–2596

54. Sulmasy DP, Astrow AB, He MK, et al. The culture of faith and hope: patients' justifications for their high estimations of expected therapeutic benefit when enrolling in early phase oncology trials. Cancer 2010;116(15):3702–3711

8 Recurrent Laryngeal Cancer

Marc A. Cohen, Ramez Nassif, David P. Goldstein, Ralph Gilbert, Patrick Gullane

Summary

- Predictors of primary failure for laryngeal malignancies include advanced tumor stage, extensive thyroid cartilage destruction, extralaryngeal spread, poor differentiation, advanced nodal stage, and presence of extracapsular extension.
- Patients with signs or symptoms suggestive of recurrence require evaluation including imaging (CT, MRI, or PET) and direct visualization with biopsy as necessary.
- The management approach for patients with recurrent laryngeal cancer must balance cure with quality of life.
- The optimal salvage treatment depends on patient factors (age, comorbidities, performance status, and wishes), tumor factors (stage and site of disease), and treatment modalities used earlier (surgery, radiation, and/or chemotherapy).
- Transoral laser microsurgery and other conservation laryngeal surgery procedures are indicated for treatment of rT1 and some rT2/T3 lesions.
- Total laryngectomy remains the gold standard salvage procedure against which all others are measured; the procedure is versatile and can be used in cases of nonsurgical and surgical primary treatment failure.

Introduction

Laryngeal carcinomas comprises 0.8% of all malignancies diagnosed in the United States, with squamous cell carcinoma accounting for approximately 95% of all larynx carcinoma cases.[1] The primary management options for laryngeal cancer are radiation (with or without chemotherapy) and surgery (with or without adjuvant treatment). The choice of primary management depends upon the disease site and stage, and patient comorbidities and preferences. The goal of management is to maintain a functioning larynx, while achieving maximum control and survival rates. Despite effective management strategies, recurrence is observed after curative treatment, despite complete clinical, radiographic, and pathological responses.

Management of recurrent laryngeal cancer poses a therapeutic challenge, particularly with regard to oncological efficacy as well as preservation of organ function. The primary objective of this chapter is to describe an approach for diagnosing and managing early and late locally recurrent laryngeal squamous cell carcinoma that develops after primary surgery or radiation (with or without chemoradiation). For the purpose of this chapter, early laryngeal carcinomas are defined as T1 and T2 carcinomas without nodal metastases, and advanced laryngeal carcinomas are defined as either local early stage cancers (T1 and T2) with nodal metastases or locally advanced cancers (T3 and T4) with or without nodal metastases. This chapter is focused on the surgical management of recurrent glottic and supraglottic cancers. Subglottic cancers are rare and comprise only 1% of laryngeal malignancies; therefore, they have not been included in this chapter. Management of recurrent cancers with either re-irradiation and/or chemotherapy is discussed in Chapters 4 and 5.

Epidemiology

The control rates for laryngeal cancer differ depending upon tumor stage, tumor site, and primary modality of therapy. The literature on this issue is varied in terms of reported outcomes, and interpretation is difficult because of small sample sizes, varying follow-up periods (years), different outcomes measured, nonuniform treatment approaches used within series and between centers, and inclusion of patients with tumors from the different laryngeal subsites, as well as hypopharyngeal cancers, all of which have different outcomes independent of treatment.

The local control rates for early glottic and supraglottic cancers treated with primary surgery have been reported to range from 60% to 100%, with most studies reporting control rates greater than 90%.[1–6] The recurrence rates for glottic and supraglottic lesions appear to be independent of the type of primary surgery performed, with reported control rates for transoral laser (TOL) microsurgery and open partial laryngectomy ranging from 60% to 100% and from 92% to 100%, respectively.[7–10]

Several clinicopathological factors have been shown to predict failure after surgical intervention for early laryngeal squamous cell carcinoma. Patients with supraglottic lesions are reported to have significantly worse outcomes than do patients with glottic lesions.[1,11] Furthermore, patients with T2 lesions have higher recurrence rates than do those with T1 lesions.[8,11] Anatomical factors that are associated with higher failure rates include vocalis muscle invasion and inferior extension broaching the subglottis.[12,13] The literature regarding the prognostic implications of anterior commissure involvement is inconclusive.[12,13] While positive margin status increases the risk of local recurrence, there are mixed reports regarding the importance of margin status after TOL microsurgery compared with open surgery techniques.[9,14]

The reported control rates after primary radiation for early stage cancers also vary widely and range between 68% and 93%.[8,15,16] In a literature review by Mendenhall et al., the recurrence rates for T1 and T2 laryngeal carcinomas managed using primary radiation were reported to be approximately 10% (range, 7%–20%) and 30% (range, 11%–73%), respectively.[8] Predictors of failure after management with radiation alone for early tumors include high T category, bulky tumors, endophytic growth pattern,[8,15] poorly differentiated tumors,[17] and involvement of the anterior commissure.[18] Other factors associated with higher recurrence rates after radiation include low pretreatment hemoglobin levels and the use of radiation doses less than 66 Gy.[19,20]

The recurrence rates of advanced-stage cancers are higher than those of early-stage cancers. Radiation, which is most commonly used in conjunction with chemotherapy, is the primary modality for the management of advanced-stage disease. Local control rates after concurrent chemoradiation are reported to be approximately 50%–75%.[21,22,23] The negative prognostic factors with respect to recurrence in patients undergoing radiation or chemoradiation for advanced laryngeal cancer include advanced T category (T4 vs. T3), vocal cord fixation, airway compromise, advanced nodal stage, and extracapsular extension.[24–26] Poor patient performance status is also a negative prognostic marker in patients undergoing chemoradiation for advanced head and neck malignancies.[27]

In centers with experience in conservation laryngeal surgery, surgery may be the primary management option of choice for advanced disease. Local control rates after supraglottic laryngectomy (neck dissection with or without adjuvant radiation or chemoradiation) for advanced stage supraglottic lesions range from 41% to 100%,[28–31] while control rates after supracricoid partial laryngectomy (neck dissection with or without adjuvant therapy) have been reported to range between 79% and 96% in selected patients.[6,28,32–34] Control rates after total laryngectomy are reported to be 53%–83%.[35–37] Compared with regional and distant failure, local recurrence after total laryngectomy is relatively uncommon (~5%).[38,39] The fact that higher control rates are obtained after conservation surgery than after total laryngectomy reflects a more highly selected patient population with lower burden of disease being eligible for conservation surgery. The clinicopathological factors associated with locoregional recurrence after surgery for advanced malignancies of the larynx include locally advanced tumor stage, nodal metastases (particularly in the paratracheal or pretracheal nodes), extracapsular nodal extension, subglottic extension, extralaryngeal spread, and extensive thyroid cartilage destruction.[24,28,40–42] Positive surgical margins have repeatedly been shown to be a negative prognostic indicator.[42–44]

Smoking during and after treatment is an important prognostic factor for local or regional recurrence—independent of the treatment modality—with an odds ratio of recurrence as high as 5.75.[45–47] An early series reported an increased recurrence rate associated with preoperative tracheostomy,[48] which was thought to be caused by direct tumor implantation in the stomal area.[48,49] However, the current literature suggests that preoperative tracheostomy is usually required in cases involving more extensive disease, which in turn is associated with recurrence.[50]

Diagnosis of Recurrent Laryngeal Cancer

After primary treatment for laryngeal cancer, patients should be regularly followed up for detection of persistent disease, recurrence, or a second primary tumor. A detailed history should be elicited and complete head and neck examination together with fiber-optic examination of the larynx performed at each follow-up visit. The signs and symptoms that may be indicative of recurrent disease include hoarseness, pain, dysphagia, odynophagia, otalgia, weight loss, and node enlargement.[51,52] Persistent edema of the larynx after radiation has been noted as a potential manifestation of disease recurrence[52]. Patients should be counseled on the symptoms of recurrence and instructed to seek early medical attention on development of any of these symptoms.

Although computed tomography (CT) and magnetic resonance imaging (MRI) are frequently used for assessment after treatment, there are no recognized standards for surveillance imaging of patients treated for laryngeal cancer. A review that appraised studies conducted to determine the diagnostic accuracy of CT or MRI imaging in laryngeal cancer recurrence after radiation found that these studies did not meet the Cochrane Collaboration criteria.[53] The results of recent studies suggest that positron emission tomography (PET) scans may be better than CT and MRI scans for identifying recurrent laryngeal cancer in asymptomatic patients as well as in those at a high risk of recurrence.[54,55] However, further research is required to evaluate the efficacy of CT, MRI, and PET scans as part of the routine surveillance strategy used for patients treated for laryngeal cancers.

In patients with signs or symptoms suggestive of recurrence, further work-up with imaging techniques (such as CT, MRI, or PET) and direct laryngeal evaluation are required. Histopathological confirmation of recurrence is also required and can be obtained by performing biopsies in the surgeon's office by using biopsy forceps through the side channel of a flexible laryngoscope. More frequently, the patient requires an examination under general anesthesia (EUA), which provides the surgeon an opportunity to obtain superficial and deep specimens, as well as to assess the extent of recurrence to plan treatment modality. EUA should be performed to rule out recurrence for cases in which recurrence is suspected but is not evident through the flexible laryngoscope.

One of the great challenges involved in the diagnosis of recurrent laryngeal cancer after primary radiotherapy is the development of treatment-related chondronecrosis. Patients with chondronecrosis typically present with signs and symptoms similar to those of recurrence—pain, hoarseness, dysphagia, and edema—with or without tissue ulceration. Although data suggest that PET scans may help differentiate chondronecrosis from recurrence, histopathological analysis is required for definitive diagnosis of recurrence.[56]

Imaging tests (usually CT or MRI) should evaluate the extent of recurrence as well as the presence of regional and distant nodal metastases. Imaging tests—together with clinical evaluation under anesthesia—are integral in treatment planning, particularly when the clinician is considering partial laryngeal salvage surgery. However, both CT and MRI can underestimate the extent of recurrence.[56] Since the lungs are the most common site of distant metastases, chest CT should be performed because it has higher sensitivity than does chest radiography in detecting metastases.[57,58] A fusion PET-CT scan may also help in detecting distant metastases in the case of recurrent tumors.[59]

Staging of Recurrent Laryngeal Cancer

The International Union against Cancer (UICC) and American Joint Committee on Cancer (AJCC) classification criteria for laryngeal cancer recurrence are identical to those used for untreated primary tumors, except that the prefix "r" is added to the tumor-node-metastasis (TNM) categories (rTNM). The composite laryngeal recurrence staging system (CLRSS) was developed for the

Table 8.1 CLRSS tumor classification

	CLRSS original	CLRSS-2
Stage I	Patients with initial TNM stage I tumors with local or regional recurrence	Patients with initial TNM I with local recurrence
Stage II	Patients with initial TNM II or III with local recurrence	Patients with initial TNM II or III with local recurrence
Stage III	Patients with initial TNM II or III with regional recurrence	Initial TNM I, II, or III with regional recurrence
Stage IV	Patients with initial TNM IV or those with distant recurrence	Patients with TNM IV or any TNM with distant recurrence

staging of recurrent laryngeal cancers because TNM staging may be inadequate for staging in a subset of patients who may have undergone prior surgical intervention, precluding the evaluation of vocal cord function and the presence of neck disease.[60] The CLRSS, which is presented in **Table 8.1**, has been validated and found to be more specific and to have greater prognostic value than the TNM system for recurrent laryngeal cancer.[61] The CLRSS was modified on the basis of the finding that patients who initially have TNM stage I cancer and develop regional recurrence (CLRSS stage I) have worse outcomes than do patients who initially have TNM stage II or III cancer and develop only local recurrence (CLRSS stage II).[62] This staging system was designated CLRSS-2 and is also presented in **Table 8.1**. Despite the greater prognostic value of this system, neither version has yet been widely adopted.

Principles of Management

The management approach used for patients with recurrent laryngeal cancer must balance cure rates with the effect of the management approach on the patient's quality of life. Input from a multidisciplinary tumor board involving individuals from surgical oncology, radiation oncology, medical oncology, speech therapy, and other paramedical specialties is essential to determine the most appropriate management approach for patients with recurrent laryngeal cancer. This choice involves determination of the potential curability of recurrent disease in a patient, i.e., the possibility of treating recurrent cancer with no subsequent local, regional, or metastatic disease. Local or regionally recurrent disease that develops after radiation is usually considered incurable if (1) negative margins cannot be obtained with salvage surgery, (2) if the tumor encases the internal carotid artery, or (3) the tumor extends to involve the prevertebral fascia or skull base. However, there are exceptions to these criteria for determining incurability; for example, some groups consider carotid sacrifice and reconstruction despite 5-year survival rates of only around 10% for those with recurrent disease.[63]

Palliative Treatment

A palliative approach is recommended for patients considered incurable or for patients in whom treatment would result in high morbidity rates, for example, total laryngectomy and total glossectomy for disease extension to the tongue base. In the latter case, the patient should be provided with detailed information focused on the subsequent devastating changes in the quality of life and the expected poor prognosis.[64] The goals of palliative treatment are to reduce pain, manage tumor bleeding, provide nutritional support (with or without a gastrostomy tube), and prevent airway obstruction. The palliative approach may involve the use of radiation or chemotherapy for controlling pain and bleeding or for attempting to slow the progression of the disease. The extent of treatment will depend upon prior treatment received and must be balanced with the patient's quality of life. Surgery is mainly used for cases of incurable recurrent laryngeal cancer for preventing airway obstruction by performing a tracheotomy or for life-threatening bleeding that cannot be controlled using a nonsurgical approach.

Salvage Treatment

The optimal salvage treatment for patients who have recurrent laryngeal cancer and are undergoing potentially curative treatment depends upon several factors: patient factors (age, medical comorbidities, performance status, and the patient's wishes), tumor factors (stage and site of disease), treatment modalities used earlier (surgery, radiation, and/or chemotherapy), and physician or institutional factors (experience with conservation laryngeal surgery and reconstruction or managing the complexity of re-irradiation and its potential side effects). Other factors that should be considered include the patient's profession, support system, and wishes regarding treatment and quality of life, particularly in those undergoing organ sacrifice (i.e., laryngectomy) or high-risk interventions such as re-irradiation. If treatment involves total laryngectomy, consultation with a speech and language pathologist is vital for helping the patient understand the rehabilitation options for speech and swallowing after treatment.

Choice of Treatment Modalities

The treatment modalities used in the initial management of laryngeal cancer dictate the options that can be used for managing the recurrence. If the patient had initially undergone radiation (with or without chemotherapy), then surgery is considered the primary salvage modality when complete resection with negative margins is considered possible. Re-irradiation after surgery may be considered in selected cases with positive microscopic margins after salvage surgery, when acceptable levels of morbidity are anticipated. Patients who have resectable recurrent tumors for which they have undergone surgery earlier may often be able undergo further salvage surgery. Laryngeal conservation surgery—with or without postoperative radiation therapy—may be considered in cases of small recurrent tumors. In the case of recurrent tumors with greater local extension, total laryngectomy is frequently required, particularly if patients have undergone radiation therapy earlier. If radiation (with or without chemotherapy) has not been used initially, it can be used for management of recurrent tumors—

either as sole therapy if salvage surgery would entail a total laryngectomy or as adjuvant therapy after salvage surgery.

If surgery or radiation is chosen for the management of recurrence, the extent of resection or fields of radiation, respectively, should involve not just the tumor visualized on clinical or radiographic examination but also the original extent of the primary tumor. As with all head and neck squamous cell carcinomas, if there is clinical or radiographic evidence of nodal disease, the neck is usually managed using the same modality used to treat the recurrent primary tumor. Management of the neck in patients with recurrent laryngeal cancer and no clinical or radiographic evidence of nodal metastases depends upon the stage and site of the primary tumor and the management approach used earlier for the neck. The incidence of occult nodal disease for patients with a primary glottic lesion is lower than that for patients with a primary supraglottic or subglottic lesion. Early-stage lesions, particularly glottic carcinomas, have a lower propensity to metastasize than do locally advanced tumors.[65] Therefore, elective neck management is typically not required for early recurrent lesions of the true glottis (rT1/rT2) but should be considered for early-stage supraglottic tumors. With locally advanced tumors the neck nodes at risk should be considered for management. One study reported a 20% incidence of occult regional disease in rT3 tumors.[66] In a study on the treatment of recurrent laryngeal malignancies after primary radiotherapy Farrag et al. reported that the likelihood of occult nodal metastases in such cases was similar to that expected for the primary lesion.[67] Importantly they found the likelihood of nodal metastases after salvage was 3% in patients whose initial tumors had been staged as N0 clinically and radiographically. Other studies have reported that performing neck dissection does not provide any advantage in patients who develop recurrent laryngeal cancer without clinical evidence of nodal metastases after radiation.[68]

Surgical Management of Recurrent Disease

Transoral laser (TOL) microsurgery or open conservation surgery procedures may be used for rT1 and rT2 glottic and supraglottic tumors. Total laryngectomy is the standard surgical treatment option for more advanced tumors (rT3 or rT4); however, centers that have experience with conservation surgery may offer patients more extended conservation procedures, such as extended TOL procedures or supracricoid partial laryngectomy. In patients without clinical evidence of nodal metastases, management of the neck depends on the stage and site of the recurrent laryngeal tumor. If the neck is being accessed for either open laryngeal procedures or for reconstruction, limited node dissection can be performed with limited morbidity. In patients with extensive local disease, particularly those undergoing total laryngectomy, paratracheal and upper mediastinal node dissection should be performed. While good outcomes are obtained with many of the larynx preservation surgeries in the primary setting, the literature on outcomes for recurrent setting after radiation is very limited, with most of these studies reporting good efficacy in appropriately selected patients (see data below). These procedures are potentially associated with a higher risk of wound complications in the recurrent setting after radiation than in the case of conservation surgery in the primary setting; however, there does not seem to be any significant literature on this issue.

Open Salvage Conservation Laryngeal Surgery: General Principles

! Goals of Conservation Laryngectomy

- Local control with survival rates equivalent to those of total laryngectomy
- Absence of a permanent tracheostomy
- Effective swallowing
- Satisfactory voice intelligibility

Indications

Conservation laryngeal surgery in the recurrent setting is usually limited to early-stage local recurrences and is used in more advanced local recurrences only under selective conditions. Vertical hemilaryngectomy or supracricoid laryngectomy (SCPL) with cricohyoidoepiglottopexy (CHEP) are the primary forms of open conservation laryngeal surgery for recurrent tumors originating in the glottis. Recurrent supraglottic tumors can be treated using SCPL; if the tumor extends to the glottis, then SCPL with cricohyoidopexy (CHP) can be performed. By definition, all of the conservation laryngeal procedures allow for extirpation of the tumor together with preservation of function of the larynx.

Outcomes

Conservation laryngeal surgery has varying oncological outcomes, with organ preservation rates ranging from 65% to 90% in different clinical series that evaluated both primary and recurrent tumors (see data below). The speech and swallowing outcomes, particularly those of salvage surgery, have yet to be properly evaluated. Some studies involving voice quality analysis have reported that the speech of patients who undergo partial laryngectomy (SCPL and VPL) is not superior to that of patients who undergo total laryngectomy and surgical voice rehabilitation.[69] However, use of conservation surgery avoids the laryngectomy stoma and the stigma associated with it.

Appropriate staging and assessment of the extent of the tumor is critical for conservation laryngeal surgery, especially after radiation failure. The full extent of the tumor, particularly submucosal extension, may not be clinically evident before surgery. It may be difficult to distinguish between the tumor and normal tissue interface after irradiation, even in tumors that have been appropriately evaluated. Therefore, frozen section assessment of margins is vitally important, and if the margins are positive, then conversion to total laryngectomy is essential. Patients undergoing conservation laryngeal surgery must have adequate cardiopulmonary reserve as all patients have some degree of pulmonary aspiration. Reserve pulmonary function tests should be performed to assess pulmonary function; however, the results of some studies suggest that the ability to climb two flights of stairs is sufficient for patients undergoing such surgery.[70]

The following sections outline different open laryngeal conservation procedures together with their indications, contraindications, technical nuances, and outcomes. The literature on the outcomes of each of these procedures, particularly the conservation procedures, needs to be interpreted with caution as there are only a

Table 8.2 Indications and contraindications

Procedure	Main indications	Contraindications
Transoral laser microsurgery	Mainly used for T1/T2 tumors of the glottis and supraglottis; centers with significant experience use for more advanced tumors	Patient anatomical factors such as neck stiffness, prominent teeth, and anteriorly placed glottis; impaired vocal cord mobility, involvement of: extensive subglottis, thyroid cartilage, cricoid cartilage, or extralaryngeal spread
Vertical hemilaryngectomy	T1 and T2 glottic tumors that may or may not extend to the supraglottis or minimal amount of subglottis	Involvement of: preepiglottic space, cricoid cartilage, thyroid cartilage, interarytenoid area; fixation of: vocal cord, arytenoid
Supraglottic laryngectomy	T1, T2, and some T3 tumors of the supraglottis with some preepiglottic space involvement	Involvement of: true vocal cords, thyroid cartilage, paraglottic space, postcricoid region, interarytenoid area, and arytenoid
Supracricoid partial laryngectomy	Supraglottic tumors that extend to the glottis or transglottic tumors that originate at the true glottis (T1, T2, and some T3)	Involvement of: extensive preepiglottic space, extensive thyroid cartilage, cricoid cartilage (or >1 cm of subglottic extension), bilateral arytenoid involvement, vallecula, base of tongue, posterior pharyngeal wall, postcricoid region, and fixation of: arytenoid
Total laryngectomy	All stage disease that is not amenable to conservation procedures. Specifically, large tumors with thyroid cartilage invasion and extralaryngeal spread, tumors causing laryngeal dysfunction, bilateral arytenoid involvement, cricoid cartilage invasion, postcricoid involvement, intractable aspiration after conservation larynx surgery	Involvement of: prevertebral fascia, carotid artery, great vessels in mediastinum, skull base; distant metastases

limited number of publications on these techniques that are used to manage recurrent laryngeal cancers and, of those published, many have small sample sizes and a heterogeneous sample of patients.

Vertical Partial Laryngectomy

Indications

Vertical partial laryngectomy (VPL) or frontolateral VPL is indicated in patients with rT1 and rT2 tumors of the glottis that may or may not extend to involve the supraglottis. The contraindications for salvage VPL are listed in **Table 8.2**. Both preoperative endoscopy and imaging are critical for determining the extent of disease, as inaccurate assessment can lead to over-resection (necessitating tracheostomy dependence; total laryngectomy) or under-resection, leading to local failure.

Technique

A VPL is performed by making vertical cuts through the anterior and posterior laryngeal cartilage on the side ipsilateral to the tumor. With a VPL, the ipsilateral vocal cord, with or without the anterior commissure, the ipsilateral arytenoids, and up to 75% of the thyroid cartilage may be resected. The resection can be extended across the anterior commissure to resect the anterior one-third portion of the contralateral cord (**Fig. 8.1**).

Various reconstructive techniques have been described for the primary setting; however, in the recurrent setting, many patients receive radiation therapy, which interferes with wound healing. Imbrication laryngoplasty, which is frequently performed in the primary setting, involves inferior advancement of the false vocal fold mucosal flap into a superomedially displaced segment of the thyroid cartilage. This allows synchronous correction of the glottic defect, producing voice quality comparable to a medialized paralyzed true vocal cord.[71,72] Free tissue reconstruction is the primary reconstructive method used at the Princess Margaret Hospital following VPL for recurrent glottic tumors after radiation. Reconstruction of the endolarynx is performed using a temporoparietal fascial free flap that serves as the vascularized carrier for a cartilage strip used to recreate the vocal fold and for a buccal mucosa-free graft sutured onto the free flap to reconstitute the mucosal defect. The neo-larynx is then stented with a Montgomery stent and tracheotomy placed for approximately 14 days.

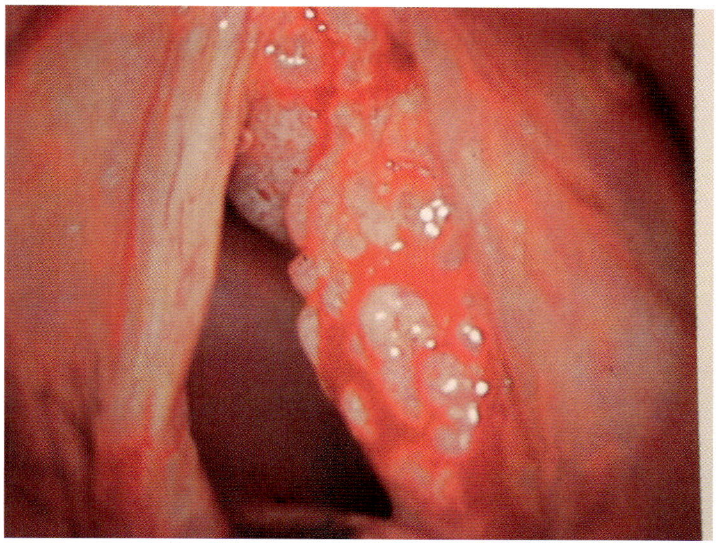

Fig. 8.1 Typical recurrent glottic malignancy suitable for vertical partial laryngectomy. This T2 right true glottic primary failed radical radiation and desired organ-preservation therapy.

Complications

Early complications include wound complications, such as a hematoma or seroma. Aspiration is a complication of VPL, especially in cases where adequate reconstruction has not been performed.

Late complications include: delay in decannulation or permanent tracheostomy; continued aspiration, requiring a gastrostomy tube; and laryngeal stenosis. Other rare complications include subcutaneous emphysema, laryngeal chondritis, and laryngocele formation.

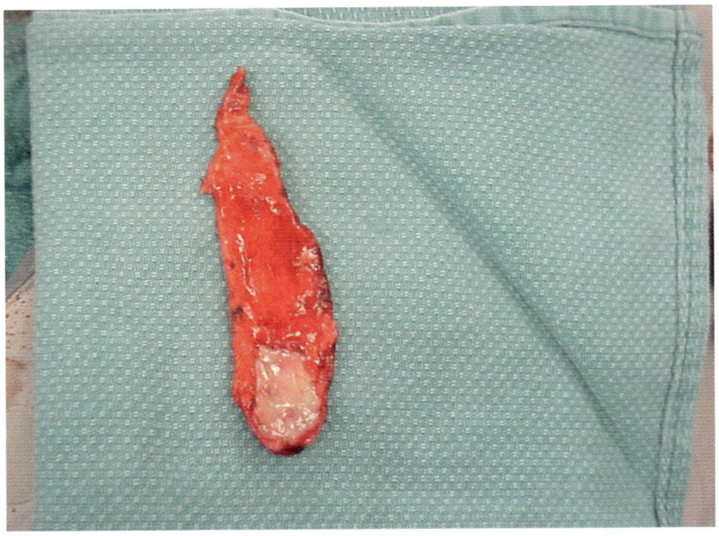

Fig. 8.2 Demonstration of the temporoparietal free flap with buccal mucosa for the endolaryngeal surface of the reconstruction.

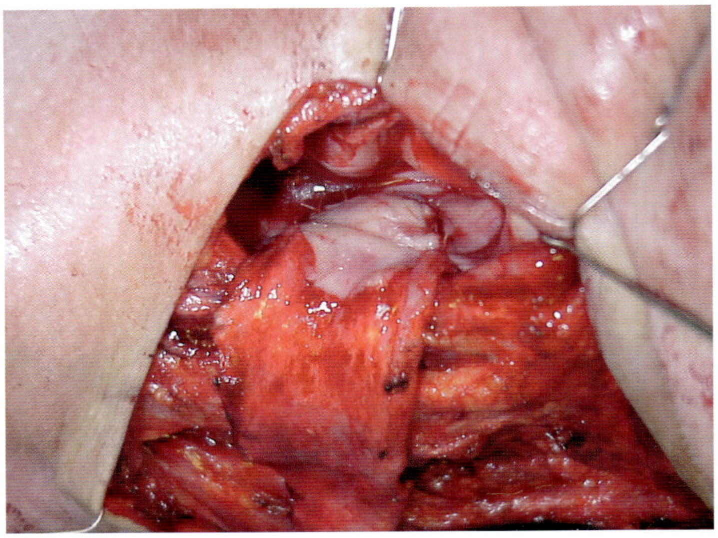

Fig. 8.3 Demonstration of the inset of the temporoparietal fascial free flap with the overlying buccal mucosa in place for reconstruction of the left true vocal cord.

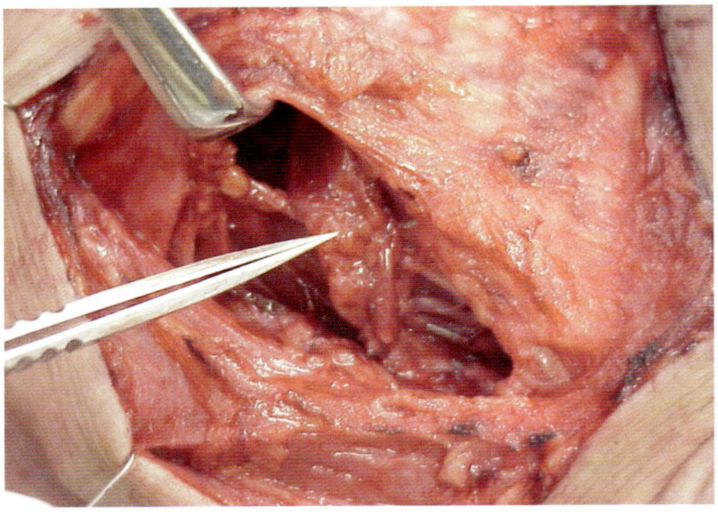

Fig. 8.4 The location of the vascular pedicle following the reconstruction.

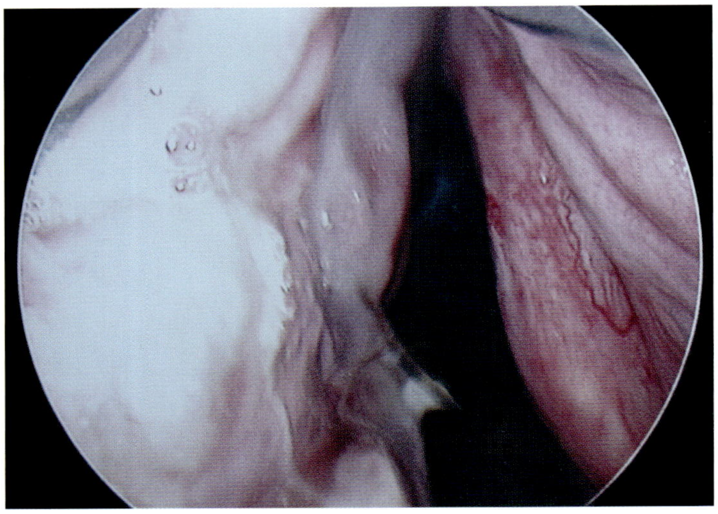

Fig. 8.5 Appearance of the larynx immediately after stent removal on postoperative day 14.

Outcomes

A systematic review of the literature by Motamed et al. evaluated studies assessing a total of 407 patients who had undergone partial laryngeal surgery (including VPL and supracricoid partial laryngectomy) for recurrent laryngeal carcinoma. Patients were only included if they had been followed-up for more than 24 months.[73] They reported a local control rate of 56%–100%, with a weighted average of 77%. A further systematic review and meta-analysis by Paleri et al. found that local control rate at 24 months after open partial laryngectomy was 86.9% (84%–89.5%) for 560 patients, and overall survival was 83.1% (79.1%–86.7%) from 360 patients.[99] Total laryngectomy performed in patients with recurrence after salvage VPL, led to an ultimate local control rate of 77%–100%, with a weighted average of 90%. This highlights the fact that VPL and SCPL provide an alternative to total laryngectomy for carefully selected patients with recurrent laryngeal cancers after radiation. Furthermore, in the event of failure of salvage VPL, total laryngectomy remains a reasonable option, without compromising ultimate local control.

Case Study

A 62-year-old construction worker with a 40 pack a year smoking history presented with a T2N0 squamous cell carcinoma of the left vocal cord that was managed with primary radiotherapy (64 Gy in 40 fractions). He had a complete response after radiation, and was seen at 3-month intervals.

Examination at 9 months following radiotherapy revealed a thickened lesion of the entirety of the left true cord with extension into the subglottis. CT of the head and neck revealed thickening of the left glottis with extension into the immediate subglottis and no evidence of lymphadenopathy. There was no evidence of paraglottic space involvement, cartilage invasion, or extralaryngeal spread. A panendoscopy was performed to determine the extent of disease, as well as feasibility of resection with a conservation laryngeal procedure.

The patient underwent a tracheotomy, left vertical hemilaryngectomy, and left selective neck dissection. Reconstruction was performed by harvesting a temporoparietal free flap that was lined with a buccal mucosa graft for the mucosal reconstruction of the larynx (**Fig. 8.2**). A strip of cartilage was harvested from the superior aspect of the contralateral thyroid cartilage to recreate a vocal cord. It was secured to the remaining posterior one-third of the ipsilateral thyroid cartilage and covered by the temporoparietal free flap. The flap was secured anteriorly to the contralateral thyroid cartilage and the microvascular anastomosis was performed to the superior thyroid artery and internal jugular vein (**Figs. 8.3 and 8.4**). A female Montgomery stent was placed with the tracheotomy kept in place. A nasogastric tube was placed for feeding. At 14 days postoperatively the patient returned to the operating room to have the stent removed (**Fig. 8.5**). The patient was decannulated approximately 2 weeks later and was discharged tolerating a normal diet. He is currently without evidence of disease recurrence at 3 years of follow up.

Horizontal Partial Laryngectomy

Horizontal partial laryngectomy is a term used to define several different surgical procedures used for tumors arising from both the glottis and supraglottis.

Supraglottic Laryngectomy

Supraglottic laryngectomy (SGL) involves resection of the entire supraglottic larynx—with or without the hyoid bone—in continuity with the superior portion of the thyroid cartilage. Reconstruction entails approximation of the remaining larynx with the tongue base or hyoid (if present). This procedure is ideal for recurrent small tumors of the supraglottis (T1/T2) that do not invade the thyroid cartilage, paraglottic space, postcricoid or interarytenoid region, and arytenoids. The procedure can be extended to include resection of the base of the tongue, the arytenoid mucosa, or superior lesions of the pyriform sinus. It has also been used to resect small T3 tumors where preepiglottic space involvement was observed but normal vocal cord function was maintained. These extended approaches are typically used for primary tumors rather than for recurrent tumors after radiation failure.

Supracricoid Partial Laryngectomy with Cricohyoidopexy

Supracricoid partial laryngectomy (SCPL) with cricohyoidopexy (CHP)[74,75] is indicated in patients with supraglottic lesions that have extended to involve the glottis (with or without decreased vocal cord mobility, but without arytenoid fixation), preepiglottic space (nonextensive involvement), and limited thyroid cartilage invasion. It can also be used for transglottic tumors that originate in the glottis. The surgery involves en bloc resection of the epiglottis; thyrohyoid membrane; preepiglottic space; paraglottic spaces; and the entire thyroid cartilage, with cuts just superior to the cricoid cartilage, anterior to the arytenoids (with the possibility of resecting one arytenoid, if required), and inferior to the hyoid. Reconstruction is performed by approximating the hyoid bone to the cricoid cartilage, and requires at least one functional cricoarytenoid unit.

SCPL-cricohyoidoepiglottopexy (CHEP) can also be used for glottic tumors, and this combined procedure is mainly used in selected rT1b tumors with involvement of the anterior commissure and more than one-third of the contralateral cord, and in selected rT2 and rT3 tumors. SCPL-CHEP involves resection of the thyroid cartilage, true vocal cords, the petiole of the epiglottis, paraglottic spaces bilaterally, and one arytenoid (if required), with reconstruction via approximation of the cricoid to the epiglottis and hyoid.

Contraindications to SCPL include subglottic extension greater than 5 mm posteriorly and 10 mm anteriorly; cricoid cartilage invasion; extensive thyroid cartilage invasion; bilateral arytenoid involvement; and extension to the vallecula, base of the tongue, postcricoid region, or posterior pharyngeal wall. To achieve appropriate function, the superior laryngeal nerve and recurrent laryngeal nerve must be spared during horizontal partial laryngeal surgery. Furthermore, in SCPL, excess mucosa must be removed to prevent obstruction. The impaction sutures used for reconstruction must be placed firmly in the appropriate location. The use of low tracheostomy (i.e., between the fifth and sixth tracheal rings) separates the repair site from the tracheostomy site, and it has been hypothesized that use of this procedure allows for quicker swallowing rehabilitation.[76] Swallowing improves after decannulation in the case of SGL and SCPL. Immediately after SCPL, the patient should expectorate into a basin as this assists with deglutition rehabilitation.

Complications

Early complications following SGL and SCPL include: wound complications; aspiration pneumonia; and the rupture of the suture line of the CHP or cricohyoidoepiglottopexy, which is very rare. In the case of radiation failure, the surgeons must be cognizant of the complications that may arise because of poor wound healing associated with radiation.

Late complications include permanent tracheostomy or permanent gastrostomy and glottic stenosis. A zero to 12.5% risk of fistula development has been reported for supraglottic laryngectomy.[77]

Outcomes

Several studies have reported the oncological efficacy of horizontal partial laryngectomy in the primary setting. Excellent local control rates have been reported for T1 and T2 lesions (87%–100%) with supraglottic laryngectomy[29,78,79] and for T1, T2, and T3 lesions (93%–100%) with SCPL.[32,74,75,80,81] Some studies involving a smaller number of patients have reported the oncological efficacy of horizontal partial laryngectomy for salvage treatment that mainly involved SCPL, although standard supraglottic laryngectomy was used for some patients.[82–84] A recent review of the literature reported local control after SCPL for recurrent disease to be 84.5%.[85] The authors found that 67% of the patients with local failure were successfully treated using total laryngectomy.

■ Transoral Laser Microsurgery

Indications and Contraindications

Over the past 30 years, a significant number of studies have reported the efficacy of transoral laser (TOL) microsurgery for laryngeal cancer, including recurrent cancers. TOL surgery is most efficacious for early malignancies of the glottis and supraglottis; however, its indications have been extended to include advanced laryngeal lesions.[86] Contraindications include impaired vocal cord mobility, extensive subglottic extension, thyroid or cricoid cartilage invasion, and extralaryngeal spread. Extension to the anterior commissure is considered a relative contraindication mainly because of the difficulty in its exposure, and therefore in complete eradication of the tumor. However, in centers with vast experience in TOL microsurgery, anterior commissure involvement is not a contraindication for surgery. For TOL microsurgery, adequate exposure of the tumor and the larynx under the microscope is essential. Neck stiffness, prominent teeth, and an anteriorly placed larynx may make access difficult, rendering TOL microsurgery infeasible.

Technique

Surgery is performed through a laryngoscope, using a microscope and carbon dioxide (CO_2) laser with a micromanipulator. Most surgeons use the laser in the continuous mode, with the power setting ranging from 1 to 6 W. This setting ensures excellent hemostasis and does not interfere with pathological interpretation. Compared with the use of TOL microsurgery in the primary setting, recurrent lesions of the larynx after radiation often provide technical challenges as exposure of the tumor and determination of the tumor margins can be difficult in such cases. Use of local flaps for reconstruction is not required, and healing is achieved by secondary intention. Decisions regarding the placement of a tracheostomy tube or nasogastric tube are made on the basis of the size of the defect, the patient's age, and the patient's performance status (particularly with respect to aspiration risk). TOL microsurgery allows for the resection of tumors with clear margins, while potentially avoiding tracheostomy and other sequelae of open surgery. Laryngeal function is minimally disrupted because the laryngeal framework is preserved. Understanding the concept of transection of the tumor, which was popularized by Steiner and Motta[87,88] and which allows for appropriate assessment of the depth required to be resected, is critical to the use of TOL microsurgery. Intraoperative frozen sections should be obtained where there is expertise for that, together with detailed descriptions of the orientation of the specimens.

In cases where the tumor crosses the anterior commissure to involve the contralateral cord, staged resection can be performed to decrease the risk of webbing. The more extensive side is resected first, followed by resection of the second side four weeks later.

Complications

Severe bleeding is a potentially life-threatening complication that arises after TOL microsurgery, particularly after resection of advanced tumors. A center with experience in TOL surgery reported a 0.4% risk of catastrophic hemorrhage in a large cohort of patients.[89] Chondritis and possibly chondronecrosis, is also a potential risk because of exposure of the cartilage due to surgery. The risk may potentially be lowered by perioperative use of antibiotic in resections where the cartilage is exposed. Postoperative granulomas, glottic synechiae, and stenosis after TOL microsurgery have also been reported. While the risks associated with TOL microsurgery in the primary setting are relatively rare, the risks associated with this procedure in the recurrent setting have yet to be determined. The greatest concern after extensive salvage TOL procedures following prior radiation is the ability of the larynx to heal by secondary intention.

Outcomes

Many retrospective studies on TOL microsurgery have reported excellent local control rates and disease-free survival rates for patients undergoing surgery for primary lesions. Only a very limited number of studies have evaluated this technique in the recurrent setting. Grant et al. evaluated TOL microsurgery in a cohort of patients with recurrent disease (supraglottic and glottic) and reported a locoregional control rate of 88% at 2 years.[90] Furthermore, Steiner et al. reported local control in 74% of patients with glottic recurrences undergoing TOL microsurgery.[91] This series included patients with early and locally advanced stage recurrences. Furthermore, most of the clinical series have not provided data regarding functional outcomes. This is possibly due to the lack of uniformity with respect to reporting both speech and swallowing handicaps.

■ Salvage Total Laryngectomy

Total laryngectomy remains the gold-standard salvage procedure against which all other surgical techniques are judged. The procedure is versatile and can be used in cases where nonsurgical or surgical primary treatment has failed. While the technique has evolved over 140 years, the principles have remained unchanged since Billroth performed the first total laryngectomy.[92] This procedure involves the extirpation of the entire larynx with the hyoid, thyroid, and cricoid cartilages en bloc.

Indications

Total laryngectomy is indicated in patients with locally recurrent tumors that are not amenable to salvage conservation procedures because of advanced disease or poor cardiopulmonary function. It is specifically indicated in the following cases:

- Large recurrent tumors with thyroid cartilage invasion and/or extralaryngeal spread
- Tumors causing severe dysfunction of the larynx, whereby any laryngeal conservation procedures would only result in preservation of a nonfunctioning larynx and a requirement for tracheotomy and a gastrostomy-tube
- Bilateral arytenoid involvement
- Extensive submucosal disease
- Cricoid cartilage invasion
- Postcricoid involvement
- Unresponsive osteoradionecrosis of the larynx or intractable aspiration after larynx-preserving surgeries

The contraindications for this procedure are similar to those for any surgical intervention, such as prevertebral fascia involvement, carotid artery involvement, extension through the skull base, extension to the great vessels in the mediastinum, and distant metastases.

Technique

Salvage total laryngectomy poses an operative challenge when performed in patients who have had prior surgery or chemoradiation. Perioperative antibiotic therapy is important for limiting the risk of wound infections. There is debate about whether the stoma should be incorporated into the neck incision or should be brought out through the lower skin flap. In the latter situation, it is felt that the stoma is less likely to be involved if a pharyngocutaneous fistula develops. The extent of thyroidectomy is dictated by the extent and location of the recurrence. Creating a tracheoesophageal puncture (TEP) after laryngectomy is essential to vocal rehabilitation after total laryngectomy; however, perspectives differ on whether a primary a secondary TEP should be performed. Some studies suggest that secondary TEP is associated with a lower incidence of pharyngocutaneous fistula. Emerick et al. reported a 50% (10/20) and 0% (0/10) incidence of fistulas in those who had undergone primary TEP and in those who had undergone secondary TEP, respectively, after salvage laryngectomy.[93] However, these data are observational retrospective data that involve only a relatively small number of patients. Secondary TEP is usually the best option in cases when there may be poor wound healing, particularly in patients with chemoradiation failure and patients in whom reconstruction is performed using free flaps.

Complications and Sequelae

Pharyngocutaneous fistula is one of the most significant sequelae of total laryngectomy. The risk factors for pharyngocutaneous fistulas include diabetes, hypothyroidism, and poor nutritional status.[94] Patients undergoing total laryngectomy after receiving radiation therapy have a significantly increased risk of fistulae, approximately 30%; the risk is highest in patients who undergo concurrent chemoradiation.[94,95] Usually, pharyngocutaneous fistulas are initially treated conservatively, i.e., by packing of the wound and maintaining the nil-by-mouth (NPO) status, unless the carotid artery and internal jugular vein are exposed and are therefore at risk of rupture. If there are exposed vessels or persistent fistulas despite conservative measures being followed, the fistula can be diverted or a regional flap, such as the pectoralis major muscle or latissimus dorsi muscle flap, can be used to help seal the fistula.

Hypoparathyroidism is also a potential risk depending upon the extent of thyroidectomy and central compartment neck dissection. Late complications include stomal stenosis and pharyngoesophageal stricture. Patients who are at risk for pharyngoesophageal stricture include those who have received radiation therapy before or after surgery and those who have undergone significant pharynx resection without adequate reconstruction.

Patients undergoing salvage laryngectomy are also at risk for posttreatment hypothyroidism, even with preservation of part of the thyroid gland; therefore, thyroid function should be assessed routinely in this patient population.

Outcomes

Local and regional control for patients undergoing total laryngectomy has been reported to range between 50% and 80%. Studies evaluating only salvage total laryngectomy have reported overall survival rates as low as 15%[96] and as high as 72%.[95] McLaughlin et al. reported an initial salvage rate of approximately 64% in T1 and T2 radiation failure patients undergoing salvage total laryngectomy, with an 80% risk of locoregional failure in cases where salvage surgery was performed.[97] Furthermore, multiple studies from Washington University have reported a 0%–42% ultimate control rate for recurrent advanced-stage glottic malignancies.[42,44,98] Given the increase in use of conservation strategies in the past 20 years, it is likely that further studies will be performed on the efficacy of salvage total laryngectomy.

Reconstruction Procedure

Primary closure of the pharyngeal mucosa is the reconstruction procedure most commonly used for defects caused by total laryngectomy. An optimal amount of mucosa must be preserved for tension-free closure. Suturing techniques that invert the mucosa, such as the Connell suture technique, are recommended in straight-line closures and T-type closures (closure in the horizontal and vertical planes). In the case of heavily irradiated or chemoirradiated tissue, the suture line and neopharynx can be bolstered using well-vascularized tissue, such as a muscle-only regional flap (pectoralis major flap or latissimus dorsi flap) or fascial free flap (temporoparietal flap or deepithelized fasciocutaneous free flap). For defects caused by total laryngectomy and partial pharyngectomy where primary closure is not possible, a regional or free flap is required for reconstructing the pharynx. The benefits of using the pectoralis major flap or latissimus dorsi flap for a partial pharyngeal defect are the ease of harvest, the lack of requirement for microvascular anastomosis, and the additional muscle that provides a large amount of well-vascularized tissue that is of significant benefit in a poorly vascularized radiated bed. The drawback to using the latissimus dorsi flap is the positioning of the patient; and the drawbacks to using the pectoralis major muscle are the effect on the appearance of the donor site as well as a 10% rate of distal flap necrosis that leads to pharyngocutaneous fistulas. Reconstruction with a fasciocutaneous flap, such as the radial forearm flap (RFFF) or anterolateral thigh flap (ALT), avoids issues regarding donor site appearance and ensures a lower rate of partial flap necrosis. The disadvantage is a potential increase in the complexity of the surgery and the limited amount of vascularized tissue available to cover the great vessels and radiated bed. Regional flaps are not now usually used for reconstruction in the case of defects caused by total laryngopharyngectomy because of the difficulty in tubing a bulky flap. Possible free tissue transfer options include enteric flaps (jejunal free flap or gastro-omental free flap) and fasciocutaneous flaps (RFFF or ALT flap). At the Princess Margaret Hospital, the ALT flap is the preferred reconstruction modality for circumferential defects in cases of laryngeal cancer with radiation failure, whereas the gastro-omental flap is the preferred modality for the chemoradiated neck because of the large amount of well-vascularized omentum that bolsters the reconstruction and covers the great vessels.

Future Research

- Further research should focus on assessment of the utility of PET-CT and other imaging modalities for the early detection of recurrent and residual disease.
- The oncological efficacy of minimally invasive transoral surgical interventions, such as use of the operative robot, should be investigated within prospective protocols for recurrent laryngeal tumors.
- Both basic and translational research is underway investigating various targeted molecular techniques in the treatment of head and neck squamous cell carcinoma; these techniques include tumor vaccination, monoclonal antibodies, and gene therapy and should focus on patients with recurrent malignancies.

Recommended Reading[1]

- Mendenhall WM, Werning JW, Hinerman RW, Amdur RJ, Villaret DB. Management of T1-T2 glottic carcinomas. Cancer 2004;100(9):1786–1792 (Thorough review of the literature assessing both radiation and surgical management of early glottic malignancies.)
- Gourin CG, Conger BT, Sheils WC, Bilodeau PA, Coleman TA, Porubsky ES. The effect of treatment on survival in patients with advanced laryngeal carcinoma. Laryngoscope 2009;119(7):1312–1317. (Analysis of survival based on treatment modality for 451 patients treated for laryngeal lesions; this review revealed significantly improved survival for patients with T4 lesions treated surgically.)**
- Kao J, Vu HL, Genden EM, et al. The diagnostic and prognostic utility of positron emission tomography/computed tomography-based follow-up after radiotherapy for head and neck cancer. Cancer 2009;115(19):4586–4594. (On evaluation of 240 PET/CT scans in 80 patients treated with radiation, the authors demonstrated PET/CT to be a sensitive technique for recurrent disease detection.)**
- Motamed M, Laccourreye O, Bradley PJ. Salvage conservation laryngeal surgery after irradiation failure for early laryngeal cancer. Laryngoscope 2006;116(3):451–455. (Review article that revealed conservation surgery is efficacious for early laryngeal lesions that fail radiation therapy; larynx preservation for external conservation and laser strategies was 77% and 65%, respectively.)**
- Steiner W, Vogt P, Ambrosch P, Kron M. Transoral carbon dioxide laser microsurgery for recurrent glottic carcinoma after radiotherapy. Head Neck 2004;26(6):477–484. (Retrospective evaluation that showed 24 of 34 patients (71%) with all-stage recurrent tumors were treated successfully with transoral laser microsurgery.)**

References

1. Armstrong WBVD, Maisel RH. Malignant tumors of the larynx. In: Flint PW, Haughey BH, Lund VJ, et al., eds. Cummings Otolaryngology: Head and Neck Surgery. Philadelphia: Mosby; 2010
2. Ambrosch P, Kron M, Steiner W. Carbon dioxide laser microsurgery for early supraglottic carcinoma. Ann Otol Rhinol Laryngol 1998;107(8):680–688
3. Grant DG, Salassa JR, Hinni ML, Pearson BW, Hayden RE, Perry WC. Transoral laser microsurgery for carcinoma of the supraglottic larynx. Otolaryngol Head Neck Surg 2007;136(6):900–906
4. Laccourreye O, Brasnu D, Merite-Drancy A, et al. Cricohyoidopexy in selected infrahyoid epiglottic carcinomas presenting with pathological preepiglottic space invasion. Arch Otolaryngol Head Neck Surg 1993;119(8):881–886
5. Rodrigo JP, Suárez C, Silver CE, et al. Transoral laser surgery for supraglottic cancer. Head Neck 2008;30(5):658–666
6. Schwaab G, Kolb F, Julieron M, et al. Subtotal laryngectomy with cricohyoidopexy as first treatment procedure for supraglottic carcinoma: Institut Gustave-Roussy experience (146 cases, 1974–1997). Eur Arch Otorhinolaryngol 2001;258(5):246–249
7. Gallo A, de Vincentiis M, Manciocco V, Simonelli M, Fiorella ML, Shah JP. CO_2 laser cordectomy for early-stage glottic carcinoma: a long-term follow-up of 156 cases. Laryngoscope 2002;112(2):370–374
8. Mendenhall WM, Werning JW, Hinerman RW, Amdur RJ, Villaret DB. Management of T1-T2 glottic carcinomas. Cancer 2004;100(9):1786–1792
9. Spector JG, Sessions DG, Chao KS, Hanson JM, Simpson JR, Perez CA. Management of stage II (T2N0M0) glottic carcinoma by radiotherapy and conservation surgery. Head Neck 1999;21(2):116–123
10. Thomas JV, Olsen KD, Neel HB III, DeSanto LW, Suman VJ. Early glottic carcinoma treated with open laryngeal procedures. Arch Otolaryngol Head Neck Surg 1994;120(3):264–268
11. Jones AS, Fish B, Fenton JE, Husband DJ. The treatment of early laryngeal cancers (T1-T2 N0): surgery or irradiation? Head Neck 2004;26(2):127–135
12. Mortuaire G, Francois J, Wiel E, Chevalier D. Local recurrence after CO2 laser cordectomy for early glottic carcinoma. Laryngoscope 2006;116(1):101–105
13. Peretti G, Nicolai P, Redaelli De Zinis LO, et al. Endoscopic CO2 laser excision for tis, T1, and T2 glottic carcinomas: cure rate and prognostic factors. Otolaryngol Head Neck Surg 2000;123(1 Pt 1):124–131
14. Blanch JL, Vilaseca I, Bernal-Sprekelsen M, et al. Prognostic significance of surgical margins in transoral CO2 laser microsurgery for T1-T4 pharyngo-laryngeal cancers. Eur Arch Otorhinolaryngol 2007;264(9):1045–1051
15. Franchin G, Minatel E, Gobitti C, et al. Radiotherapy for patients with early-stage glottic carcinoma: univariate and multivariate analyses in a group of consecutive, unselected patients. Cancer 2003;98(4):765–772
16. Hoffman HTIT, Karnell LH, et al. Management of early glottic cancer. Flint PW, Haughey BH, Lund VJ, et al., eds. Cummings Otolaryngology: Head and Neck Surgery. Philadelphia: Mosby; 2010
17. Mendenhall WM, Amdur RJ, Morris CG, Hinerman RW. T1-T2N0 squamous cell carcinoma of the glottic larynx treated with radiation therapy. J Clin Oncol 2001;19(20):4029–4036
18. Chen MF, Chang JT, Tsang NM, Liao CT, Chen WC. Radiotherapy of early-stage glottic cancer: analysis of factors affecting prognosis. Ann Otol Rhinol Laryngol 2003;112(10):904–911
19. Cho EI, Sasaki CT, Haffty BG. Prognostic significance of pretreatment hemoglobin for local control and overall survival in T1-T2N0 larynx cancer treated with external beam radiotherapy. Int J Radiat Oncol Biol Phys 2004;58(4):1135–1140
20. Warde P, O'Sullivan B, Bristow RG, et al. T1/T2 glottic cancer managed by external beam radiotherapy: the influence of pretreatment hemoglobin on local control. Int J Radiat Oncol Biol Phys 1998;41(2):347–353
21. Lambert L, Fortin B, Soulières D, et al. Organ preservation with concurrent chemoradiation for advanced laryngeal cancer: are we succeeding? Int J Radiat Oncol Biol Phys 2010;76(2):398–402

1 References with asterisks indicate the most important reference articles on the topic.

22. Pfister DG, Laurie SA, Weinstein GS, et al. American Society of Clinical Oncology. American Society of Clinical Oncology clinical practice guideline for the use of larynx-preservation strategies in the treatment of laryngeal cancer. J Clin Oncol 2006;24(22):3693–3704
23. Rodriguez CP, Adelstein DJ, Rybicki LA, et al. Clinical predictors of larynx preservation after multiagent concurrent chemoradiotherapy. Head Neck 2008;30(12):1535–1542
24. Gourin CG, Conger BT, Sheils WC, Bilodeau PA, Coleman TA, Porubsky ES. The effect of treatment on survival in patients with advanced laryngeal carcinoma. Laryngoscope 2009;119(7):1312–1317
25. Hirabayashi H, Koshii K, Uno K, et al. Extracapsular spread of squamous cell carcinoma in neck lymph nodes: prognostic factor of laryngeal cancer. Laryngoscope 1991;101(5):502–506
26. Mendenhall WM, Parsons JT, Stringer SP, Cassisi NJ. Radiotherapy for carcinoma of the supraglottis. Otolaryngol Clin North Am 1997;30(1):145–161
27. Gasparini G, Bevilacqua P, Bonoldi E, et al. Predictive and prognostic markers in a series of patients with head and neck squamous cell invasive carcinoma treated with concurrent chemoradiation therapy. Clin Cancer Res 1995;1(11):1375–1383
28. Dias FL, Lima RA, Kligerman J, Cernea CR. Therapeutic options in advanced laryngeal cancer: an overview. ORL J Otorhinolaryngol Relat Spec 2005;67(6):311–318
29. Lee NK, Goepfert H, Wendt CD. Supraglottic laryngectomy for intermediate-stage cancer: U.T.M.D. Anderson Cancer Center experience with combined therapy. Laryngoscope 1990;100(8):831–836
30. Myers EN, Alvi A. Management of carcinoma of the supraglottic larynx: evolution, current concepts, and future trends. Laryngoscope 1996;106(5 Pt 1):559–567
31. Scola B, Fernández-Vega M, Martínez T, Fernández-Vega S, Ramirez C. Management of cancer of the supraglottis. Otolaryngol Head Neck Surg 2001;124(2):195–198
32. Chevalier D, Piquet JJ. Subtotal laryngectomy with cricohyoidopexy for supraglottic carcinoma: review of 61 cases. Am J Surg 1994;168(5):472–473
33. de Vincentiis M, Minni A, Gallo A, Di Nardo A. Supracricoid partial laryngectomies: oncologic and functional results. Head Neck 1998;20(6):504–509
34. Naudo P, Laccourreye O, Weinstein G, Hans S, Laccourreye H, Brasnu D. Functional outcome and prognosis factors after supracricoid partial laryngectomy with cricohyoidopexy. Ann Otol Rhinol Laryngol 1997;106(4):291–296
35. Mendenhall WM, Parsons JT, Stringer SP, Cassisi NJ, Million RR. Stage T3 squamous cell carcinoma of the glottic larynx: a comparison of laryngectomy and irradiation. Int J Radiat Oncol Biol Phys 1992;23(4):725–732
36. Razack MS, Maipang T, Sako K, Bakamjian V, Shedd DP. Management of advanced glottic carcinomas. Am J Surg 1989;158(4):318–320
37. Yuen A, Medina JE, Goepfert H, Fletcher G. Management of stage T3 and T4 glottic carcinomas. Am J Surg 1984;148(4):467–472
38. DeSanto LW. T3 glottic cancer: options and consequences of the options. Laryngoscope 1984;94(10):1311–1315
39. Yuen AP, Ho CM, Wei WI, Lam LK. Analysis of recurrence after surgical treatment of advanced laryngeal carcinoma. J Laryngol Otol 1995;109(11):1063–1067
40. Oosterkamp S, de Jong JM, Van den Ende PL, Manni JJ, Dehing-Oberije C, Kremer B. Predictive value of lymph node metastases and extracapsular extension for the risk of distant metastases in laryngeal carcinoma. Laryngoscope 2006;116(11):2067–2070
41. Shikama N, Sasaki S, Nishikawa A, et al. Risk factors for local-regional recurrence following preoperative radiation therapy and surgery for head and neck cancer (stage II-IVB). Radiology 2003;228(3):789–794
42. Spector GJ, Sessions DG, Lenox J, Newland D, Simpson J, Haughey BH. Management of stage IV glottic carcinoma: therapeutic outcomes. Laryngoscope 2004;114(8):1438–1446
43. Sessions DG, Lenox J, Spector GJ. Supraglottic laryngeal cancer: analysis of treatment results. Laryngoscope 2005;115(8):1402–1410
44. Spector JG, Sessions DG, Lenox J, Simpson J. Management of T3N1 glottic carcinoma: therapeutic outcomes. Laryngoscope 2006;116(1):106–110
45. Benninger MS, Gillen J, Thieme P, Jacobson B, Dragovich J. Factors associated with recurrence and voice quality following radiation therapy for T1 and T2 glottic carcinomas. Laryngoscope 1994;104(3 Pt 1):294–298
46. Ritoe SC, Verbeek AL, Krabbe PF, Kaanders JH, van den Hoogen FJ, Marres HA. Screening for local and regional cancer recurrence in patients curatively treated for laryngeal cancer: definition of a high-risk group and estimation of the lead time. Head Neck 2007;29(5):431–438
47. Terhaard CH, Snippe K, Ravasz LA, van der Tweel I, Hordijk GJ. Radiotherapy in T1 laryngeal cancer: prognostic factors for locoregional control and survival, uni- and multivariate analysis. Int J Radiat Oncol Biol Phys 1991;21(5):1179–1186
48. Keim WF, Shapiro MJ, Rosin HD. Study of postlaryngectomy stomal recurrence. Arch Otolaryngol 1965;81:183–186
49. Schneider JJ, Lindberg RD, Jesse RH. Prevention of tracheal stoma recurrences after total laryngectomy by postoperative irradiation. J Surg Oncol 1975;7(3):187–190
50. Imauchi Y, Ito K, Takasago E, Nibu K, Sugasawa M, Ichimura K. Stomal recurrence after total laryngectomy for squamous cell carcinoma of the larynx. Otolaryngol Head Neck Surg 2002;126(1):63–66
51. Paniello RC, Virgo KS, Johnson MH, Clemente MF, Johnson FE. Practice patterns and clinical guidelines for posttreatment follow-up of head and neck cancers: a comparison of 2 professional societies. Arch Otolaryngol Head Neck Surg 1999;125(3):309–313
52. Ward PH, Calcaterra TC, Kagan AR. The enigma of post-radiation edema and recurrent or residual carcinoma of the larynx. Laryngoscope 1975;85(3):522–529
53. Brouwer J, Hooft L, Hoekstra OS, et al. Systematic review: accuracy of imaging tests in the diagnosis of recurrent laryngeal carcinoma after radiotherapy. Head Neck 2008;30(7):889–897
54. Brouwer J, de Bree R, Comans EF, et al. Improved detection of recurrent laryngeal tumor after radiotherapy using 18FDG-PET as initial method. Radiother Oncol 2008;87(2):217–220
55. Kao J, Vu HL, Genden EM, et al. The diagnostic and prognostic utility of positron emission tomography/computed tomography-based follow-up after radiotherapy for head and neck cancer. Cancer 2009;115(19):4586–4594

56. Zbären P, Christe A, Caversaccio MD, Stauffer E, Thoeny HC. Pretherapeutic staging of recurrent laryngeal carcinoma: clinical findings and imaging studies compared with histopathology. Otolaryngol Head Neck Surg 2007;137(3):487–491
57. Ghosh SK, Roland NJ, Kumar A, et al. Detection of synchronous lung tumors in patients presenting with squamous cell carcinoma of the head and neck. Head Neck 2009;31(12):1563–1570
58. Jäckel MC, Reischl A, Huppert P. Efficacy of radiologic screening for distant metastases and second primaries in newly diagnosed patients with head and neck cancer. Laryngoscope 2007;117(2):242–247
59. Senft A, de Bree R, Hoekstra OS, et al. Screening for distant metastases in head and neck cancer patients by chest CT or whole body FDG-PET: a prospective multicenter trial. Radiother Oncol 2008;87(2):221–229
60. Lacy PD, Piccirillo JF. Development of a new staging system for patients with recurrent laryngeal squamous cell carcinoma. Cancer 1998;83(5):910–917
61. Lacy PD, Kennedy JT, Piccirillo JF. Validation of the composite laryngeal recurrence staging system. Cancer 2004;101(4):761–767
62. León X, López M, García J, Viza I, Gich I, Quer M. Recurrent laryngeal squamous cell carcinoma: rTNM versus composite laryngeal recurrence staging system. Proposal for a modification of the CLRSS to improve patient classification. Head Neck 2008;30(7):939–945
63. Ozer E, Agrawal A, Ozer HG, Schuller DE. The impact of surgery in the management of the head and neck carcinoma involving the carotid artery. Laryngoscope 2008;118(10):1771–1774
64. Harrison D. The questionable value of total glossectomy. Head Neck Surg 1983;6(2):632–638
65. Mukherji SK, Armao D, Joshi VM. Cervical nodal metastases in squamous cell carcinoma of the head and neck: what to expect. Head Neck 2001;23(11):995–1005
66. Yao M, Roebuck JC, Holsinger FC, Myers JN. Elective neck dissection during salvage laryngectomy. Am J Otolaryngol 2005;26(6):388–392
67. Farrag TY, Lin FR, Cummings CW, et al. Neck management in patients undergoing postradiotherapy salvage laryngeal surgery for recurrent/persistent laryngeal cancer. Laryngoscope 2006;116(10):1864–1866
68. Bohannon IA, Desmond RA, Clemons L, Magnuson JS, Carroll WR, Rosenthal EL. Management of the N0 neck in recurrent laryngeal squamous cell carcinoma. Laryngoscope 2010;120(1):58–61
69. So YK, Yun YS, Baek CH, Jeong HS, Son YI. Speech outcome of supracricoid partial laryngectomy: comparison with total laryngectomy and anatomic considerations. Otolaryngol Head Neck Surg 2009;141(6):770–775
70. Beckhardt RN, Murray JG, Ford CN, Grossman JE, Brandenburg JH. Factors influencing functional outcome in supraglottic laryngectomy. Head Neck 1994;16(3):232–239
71. Liu C, Ward PH, Pleet L. Imbrication reconstruction following partial laryngectomy. Ann Otol Rhinol Laryngol 1986;95(6 Pt 1):567–571
72. Har-El G, Paniello RC, Abemayor E, Rice DH, Rassekh C. Partial laryngectomy with imbrication laryngoplasty for glottic carcinoma. Arch Otolaryngol Head Neck Surg 2003;129(1):66–71
73. Motamed M, Laccourreye O, Bradley PJ. Salvage conservation laryngeal surgery after irradiation failure for early laryngeal cancer. Laryngoscope 2006;116(3):451–455
74. Laccourreye H, Laccourreye O, Weinstein G, Menard M, Brasnu D. Supracricoid laryngectomy with cricohyoidopexy: a partial laryngeal procedure for selected supraglottic and transglottic carcinomas. Laryngoscope 1990;100(7):735–741
75. Laccourreye H, Laccourreye O, Weinstein G, Menard M, Brasnu D. Supracricoid laryngectomy with cricohyoidoepiglottopexy: a partial laryngeal procedure for glottic carcinoma. Ann Otol Rhinol Laryngol 1990;99(6 Pt 1):421–426
76. Bron L, Brossard E, Monnier P, Pasche P. Supracricoid partial laryngectomy with cricohyoidoepiglottopexy and cricohyoidopexy for glottic and supraglottic carcinomas. Laryngoscope 2000;110(4):627–634
77. Burstein FD, Calcaterra TC. Supraglottic laryngectomy: series report and analysis of results. Laryngoscope 1985;95(7 Pt 1):833–836
78. Bocca E, Pignataro O, Oldini C, Sambataro G, Cappa C. Extended supraglottic laryngectomy. Review of 84 cases. Ann Otol Rhinol Laryngol 1987;96(4):384–386
79. Herranz-González J, Gavilán J, Martínez-Vidal J, Gavilán C. Supraglottic laryngectomy: functional and oncologic results. Ann Otol Rhinol Laryngol 1996;105(1):18–22
80. Laccourreye O, Salzer SJ, Brasnu D, Shen W, Laccourreye H, Weinstein GS. Glottic carcinoma with a fixed true vocal cord: outcomes after neoadjuvant chemotherapy and supracricoid partial laryngectomy with cricohyoidoepiglottopexy. Otolaryngol Head Neck Surg 1996;114(3):400–406
81. Piquet JJ, Chevalier D. Subtotal laryngectomy with crico-hyoido-epiglotto-pexy for the treatment of extended glottic carcinomas. Am J Surg 1991;162(4):357–361
82. Deganello A, Gallo O, De Cesare JM, et al. Supracricoid partial laryngectomy as salvage surgery for radiation therapy failure. Head Neck 2008;30(8):1064–1071
83. Pellini R, Pichi B, Ruscito P, et al. Supracricoid partial laryngectomies after radiation failure: a multi-institutional series. Head Neck 2008;30(3):372–379
84. Yiotakis J, Stavroulaki P, Nikolopoulos T, et al. Partial laryngectomy after irradiation failure. Otolaryngol Head Neck Surg 2003;128(2):200–209
85. Marioni G, Marchese-Ragona R, Pastore A, Staffieri A. The role of supracricoid laryngectomy for glottic carcinoma recurrence after radiotherapy failure: a critical review. Acta Otolaryngol 2006;126(12):1245–1251
86. Steiner WAP. Martin A, et al. Results of transoral laser microsurgery of laryngeal cancer European Congress of the European Federation of Oto-Rhino-Laryngological Societies. Budapest: Bologna Monduzzi Editore; 1996
87. Motta G, Villari G, Motta G Jr, Ripa G, Salerno G. The CO2 laser in the laryngeal microsurgery. Acta Otolaryngol Suppl 1986;433:1–30
88. W.p. Endoscopic therapy of early laryngeal cancer. Indications and results. In: Wigand ME, Steiner W, Stell PM, ed. Functional Partial Laryngectomy. New York: Springer; 1984:163–170
89. Salassa JR, Hinni ML, Grant DG, Hayden RE. Postoperative bleeding in transoral laser microsurgery for upper aerodigestive tract tumors. Otolaryngol Head Neck Surg 2008;139(3):453–459
90. Grant DG, Salassa JR, Hinni ML, Pearson BW, Hayden RE, Perry WC. Transoral laser microsurgery for recurrent laryngeal and pharyngeal cancer. Otolaryngol Head Neck Surg 2008;138(5):606–613

91. Steiner W, Vogt P, Ambrosch P, Kron M. Transoral carbon dioxide laser microsurgery for recurrent glottic carcinoma after radiotherapy. Head Neck 2004;26(6):477–484
92. Weir NF. Theodore Billroth: the first laryngectomy for cancer. J Laryngol Otol 1973;87(12):1161–1169
93. Emerick KS, Tomycz L, Bradford CR, et al. Primary versus secondary tracheoesophageal puncture in salvage total laryngectomy following chemoradiation. Otolaryngol Head Neck Surg 2009;140(3):386–390
94. Thawley SE. Complications of combined radiation therapy and surgery for carcinoma of the larynx and inferior hypopharynx. Laryngoscope 1981;91(5):677–700
95. Weber RS, Berkey BA, Forastiere A, et al. Outcome of salvage total laryngectomy following organ preservation therapy: the Radiation Therapy Oncology Group trial 91–11. Arch Otolaryngol Head Neck Surg 2003;129(1):44–49
96. Young VN, Mangus BD, Bumpous JM. Salvage laryngectomy for failed conservative treatment of laryngeal cancer. Laryngoscope 2008;118(9):1561–1568
97. McLaughlin MP, Parsons JT, Fein DA, et al. Salvage surgery after radiotherapy failure in T1-T2 squamous cell carcinoma of the glottic larynx. Head Neck 1996;18(3):229–235
98. Sessions DG, Lenox J, Spector GJ, et al. Management of T3N0M0 glottic carcinoma: therapeutic outcomes. Laryngoscope 2002;112(7 Pt 1):1281–1288
99. Paleri V, Thomas L, Basavaiah N, Drinnan M, Mehanna H, Jones T. Oncological outcomes of open conservation laryngectomy for radiorecurrent laryngeal carcinoma: a systematic review and meta-analysis of English-language literature. Cancer 2011;117(12):2668–2760

9 Management of Recurrent Hypopharyngeal Cancer

Jarrod Homer, Nick Slevin, Priyamal Silva

Summary

- The increasing trend for organ preservation strategies is resulting in treatment by chemoradiation for most hypopharyngeal cancers, with surgery being reserved for salvage cases.
- Careful follow-up is required to detect early recurrence, to improve patients' chances of successful surgical salvage.
- Only a relatively small proportion of patients treated initially with chemoradiation will be suitable candidates for salvage treatment.
- Salvage surgery after chemoradiation is associated with good locoregional disease control and overall survival rates comparable to primary disease treated by surgery.
- The morbidity of salvage surgery is significantly increased, particularly with respect to poor wound healing and fistula formation.
- This risk can be mitigated to a certain extent through preoperative optimization, and careful choice of flap in reconstruction.
- If salvage surgery is performed, then treatment should be radical, without compromise, as this usually represents the last chance of at least locoregional cure.
- Accordingly, pharyngectomy should be circumferential in most cases; and there should be a low threshold to perform total thyroidectomy and mediastinal dissection/manubriumectomy.
- For recurrences after primary surgery with postoperative (chemo)radiotherapy, selected cases of peristomal recurrence may be suitable for further salvage surgery.

Incidence and Patterns of Recurrence in Hypopharyngeal Cancer

Hypopharyngeal cancers, by virtue of the anatomy and clinical presentation, often present at an advanced stage (~75% stage III/IV) and consequently are associated with an unfavorable and poor prognosis. The overall incidence of recurrence in hypopharyngeal cancer is around 40%–50%, with the commonest type of recurrence being distant metastasis. Although it is generally accepted that overall survival rates are similar when comparing primary surgery and primary chemoradiotherapy for cancer of the hypopharynx, there is a higher local recurrence rate (around 40%) with chemoradioradiotherapy as primary treatment,[1] compared with primary surgery (around 15%).[2]

Outcome after Treatment for Recurrence

There is a paucity of data on prognostic factors after treatment for recurrence. In a recent series of hypopharyngeal cancers treated with salvage surgery by subsite, salvage was most successful in postcricoid recurrences (40%), and lowest in the posterior pharyngeal wall.[1] In a series of 72 patients who underwent salvage surgery for recurrent disease, the 5-year overall and disease specific rates were 31% and 40%, with the following patterns of recurrence after salvage surgery: local in 14 patients, regional in 13, and distant in 11 patients. Disease recurrence (after salvage surgery) was treated with curative intent by further surgical salvage in two patients. On multivariate analysis, tumor grade was a major predictor of local control.[3] In a similar series of patients surgically salvaged after chemoradiotherapy failure, Kadota et al. reported a 5-year disease-free survival of 57.1% and local control rate of 92.9%. Of the six patients with a further recurrence in the salvage-surgery group, recurrences were local in one, regional in two, and distant in three patients.[4] To put the outcome data into perspective, of patients who are suitable for salvage surgery after chemoradiation failure, their overall survival after salvage surgery is similar to that achieved by patients who undergo primary surgery for cancer of the hypopharynx.[1,3]

Detection of Recurrent Disease

Following successful primary treatment of hypopharyngeal tumors, careful attention in follow-up may help earlier detection of recurrent disease. Careful history taking, examination and fiberoptic examination may help in the early identification of recurrence. New symptoms such as dysphagia, odynophagia, or localized pain should be sought in the history. Significant signs include hypopharyngeal ulceration, persistent vocal cord fixation, and persistent edema. PET-CT may be of value in detecting early recurrence or predicting failure after chemoradiotherapy.[5]

Investigations

Investigations for recurrent hypopharyngeal cancer are similar to those for primary disease, that is locoregional imaging, imaging for distant metastases and second primaries, cytology of neck disease, and biopsy with panendoscopy of the local site and upper aerodigestive tract. Contrast swallow may also be useful in the determination of the distal extent of recurrence (see Chapter 1 for more detail). A significant problem in imaging is the differentiation between tumor recurrence and treatment effect.[6]

Locoregional imaging is best performed with MRI. PET-CT may also help differentiate between the two, as well as serving as an imaging modality to detect distant metastases, including bone[7] and second primaries.[8] The rate of second primaries and distant metastases is significantly higher in this patient group, approaching 25% and 30% respectively.[9,10]

In case of palpable or radiological evidence of neck disease, fine-needle aspiration cytology can be performed with ultrasound guidance. This may be useful when there is some doubt on axial imaging about the nature of neck disease when primary recurrence has been proven.

Principles of Management

Recurrence after Radiotherapy and Chemoradiotherapy

Due to the fact that chemoradiotherapy regimens can be used to successfully preserve laryngeal structure without compromising survival, patients are increasingly being treated in this manner as their primary treatment, with salvage surgery (pharyngolaryngectomy) reserved for local recurrence.[11] However, fewer than half of such recurrent cases are considered suitable for salvage surgery, either because the patient is unfit for major surgery or because of the extent of disease recurrence.[1] Of those that can be salvaged surgically, major complication rates are high, with fistula and wound breakdown rates of 40%–50%.[1,3] Thus, the guiding principles for selection of patients for salvage surgery are:

- The proven absence of distant metastases and second primaries
- The locoregional recurrent disease being operable
- The candidacy of the patient for high-risk salvage surgery

For patients in whom salvage surgery is not possible, a plan of best supportive care and palliation (See Chapter 21 for more detail) should be instigated. Re-irradiation may also be an option in selected patients not suitable for surgery (see below).

Lymph Node Recurrence after Primary Chemoradiotherapy

In situations where there is regional disease in the absence of any primary disease recurrence, then treatment of the neck mandates a comprehensive neck dissection. Nearly all patients, even those originally staged N0 before treatment, will have had neck lymph node irradiation. There are no significant differences in the salvage of neck recurrence in hypopharyngeal cancer compared with other upper aerodigestive tract cancers. The surgical salvage of the neck recurrence is covered in Chapter 12.

Attention should, however, be paid to the fact that many patients after chemoradiation will have some sort of swallowing dysfunction; and the additional impact of salvage neck dissection may tip the balance in some patients toward aspiration. It should also be emphasized that it is paramount, using the investigations above, also to exclude the possibility of primary recurrence in these patients.

Recurrence after Primary Surgery

In patients who have had initial conservation surgery to the primary, there may rarely be an option for further conservation or transoral surgery, if the recurrence is small and well localized. This may be influenced in part by whether the patient was given adjuvant radiotherapy at the time, and also depends on existing and predicted function in terms of swallow, voice, and airway.

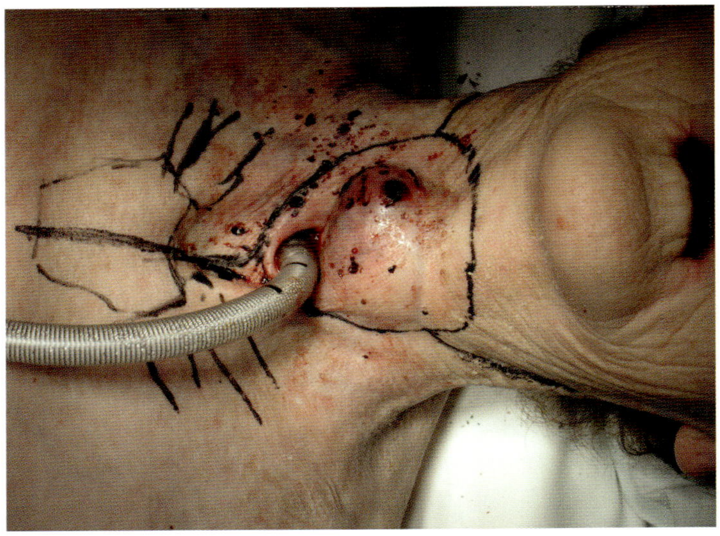

Fig. 9.1 Sisson grade II peristomal recurrence.

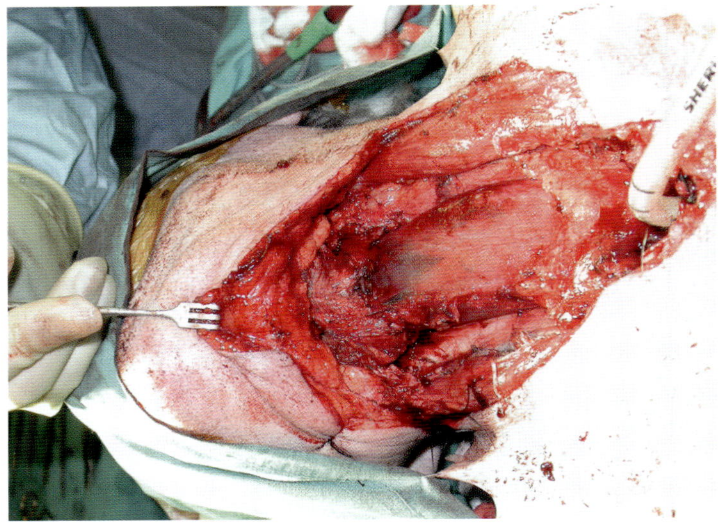

Fig. 9.2 Salvage surgery with manubriumectomy and mediastinal dissection, with reconstruction with gastric transposition. Note the bulk of the flap helping to fill mediastinal dead space.

For most patents with a recurrence, salvage pharyngolaryngectomy remains the most suitable option if the recurrence is salvageable. The vast majority of patients who have undergone pharyngolaryngectomy as primary treatment will have received postoperative radiotherapy or chemoradiotherapy. Of those that go on to recur locally after surgery, it is exceptional for a patient to be eligible for further surgery.

Further surgical salvage might be possible in a small proportion that recur with a peristomal recurrence of Sisson grade I or II (superior half of stoma with or without esophageal involvement) (**Fig. 9.1**).[12] Despite the poor prognosis of peristomal recurrence, a valid argument for surgical salvage is to improve the course of death, which otherwise is characterized by progressive tracheostomal obstruction or hemorrhage over a period of a few months. In the series of peristomal recurrences reported by Gluckman and colleagues, there was a 45% 2-year survival with relatively low morbidity and mortality. Those patients who failed to survive 2 years were still considered to have good palliation. This contrasts with a 2-year survival for Sisson grade III and IV of 9%, and with high peri- and postoperative morbidity and mortality.[13]

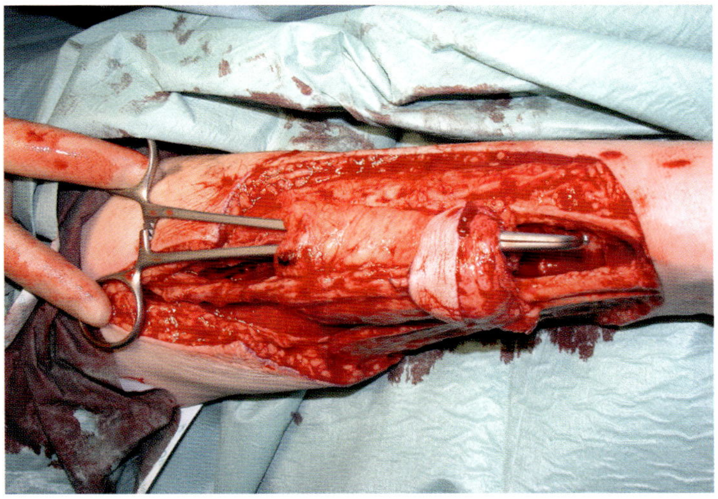

Fig. 9.3 Radial artery forearm flap, tubed. Note the monitoring paddle.

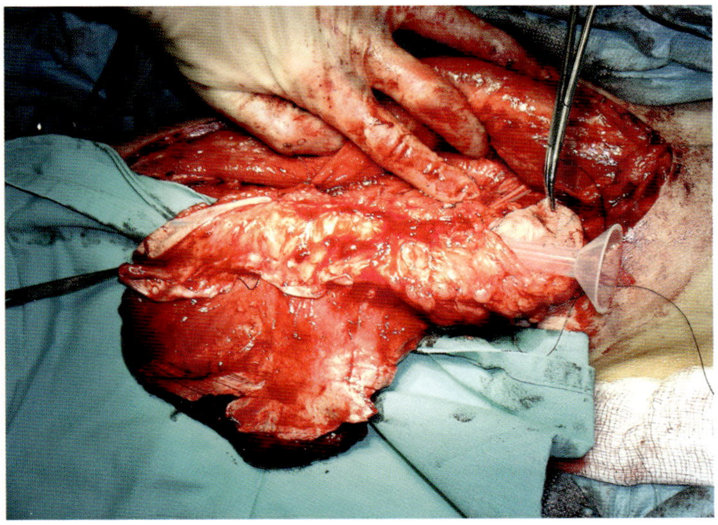

Fig. 9.4 Anterolateral thigh flap, tubed around the salivary bypass tube.

Surgical salvage of peristomal recurrence, popularized by Sisson,[12] primarily involves removal of the tracheostoma and the surrounding skin, mediastinal dissection with removal of the manubrium and the heads of the clavicles, and resection of involved pharyngoesophageal segments (**Fig. 9.2**). Reconstruction is required of the resected pharynx/esophagus; dead space around major vessels, and skin. This is best achieved using a bulky flap, such as an anterolateral thigh (ALT) flap with some vastus lateralis; gastric transposition (**Fig. 9.2**) or gastro-omental free flap (see below). It should be noted that many patients with hypopharyngeal cancer treated with primary surgery, will have had pharyngolaryngectomy with flap reconstruction, and salvage for peristomal recurrence will involve resection of previously reconstructed pharynx. A further option for peristomal recurrence is re-irradiation (see below).

In patients who develop neck disease without local recurrence following a pharyngolarygectomy, it is likely they would have already had bilateral neck dissections at their initial surgery; and, in most cases, postoperative radiotherapy or chemoradiotherapy. Thus, the salvage options are very limited. In patients who develop a neck recurrence in a previously unoperated neck, such as the contralateral side, then a salvage neck dissection offers the patients a reasonable chance of chance of disease control. The issues around neck regional recurrence are further discussed in Chapter 12.

Surgical Techniques of Salvage Pharyngolaryngectomy

It is important to remember that salvage pharyngolaryngectomy represents the patient's last chance of a potential cure. Circumferential (rather than noncircumferential) pharyngolaryngectomy should be the preferable option. For patients after (chemo)radiotherapy, the margins are more difficult to judge and leaving an irradiated pharyngeal strip serves little purpose.

As part of salvage pharyngolaryngectomy, there should be a low threshold for inclusion of a total thyroidectomy, as disease recurrence is often extensive. It is possible that prior radiotherapy or chemoradiotherapy disrupts normal tissue properties and barriers that prevent direct extension of carcinoma.[14] While thyroxine replacement is not a particular issue, control of calcium due to hypoparathyroidism can be troublesome, particularly for patients who undergo gastric transposition, who may have problems with vitamin D absorption.

Reconstruction Options

There is a choice of reconstruction options appropriate for such a defect. Microvascular reconstruction is preferred and the main options include free jejunal graft, tubed anterolateral thigh flap, tubed radial forearm flap, or gastro-omental flap. Arguments for each flap can be made, and there are certain circumstances that might favor a particular flap. In general, surgical teams will favor the flap that gives good consistent results for them.

Radial Forearm Flap

The radial forearm flap is easily tubed (**Fig. 9.3**); however, it is thin.

Tubed Anterolateral Thigh Flap

The ALT flap (**Fig. 9.4**) is arguably the cutaneous free flap of choice. It can be relatively easily tubed in most patients, has minimal donor site morbidity, possesses two genuine layers (important in this group of patients at higher risk of fistula), and can be used to reconstruct defects of considerable length.[15] Because it can be raised with muscle, this can provide cover for a skin defect, for example, if there is skin involvement by recurrent tumor or preoperative tracheostomy. Both of these cutaneous flaps can be used for circumferential or noncircumferential defects.

Case Study

A 68-year-old man was originally staged T3N1 SCC of the left piriform fossa. He was treated with synchronous chemoradiotherapy 18 months previously. He was an ex-smoker of 20 cigarettes a day and previously alcoholic. His comorbidities included hypertension; and well controlled COPD. The patient presented in follow-up clinic with left odynophagia. On examination, he had a fixed left hemilarynx; with edema of the left aryepiglottic fold and pooling in piriform fossae.

MRI of the neck showed recurrent disease within left piriform fossa with esophageal thickening (circumferential) within the cervical esophagus with no lymphadenopathy. CT of thorax was clear. Rigid endoscopy showed a poorly defined tumor within the left piriform fossa, extending to the postcricoid area. All the hypopharynx and the cervical esophagus appeared irregular. Biopsies showed recurrent SCC of the piriform fossa and postcricoid area; other biopsies from posterior pharyngeal wall and cervical esophagus showed radiotherapy change with some atypia.

After discussion in MDM, the proposed treatment plan was salvage circumferential pharyngolaryngectomy with manubriumectomy, superior mediastinal dissection, total thyroidectomy, and bilateral comprehensive neck dissections. Reconstruction was planned with a tubed ALT free flap around a salivary bypass tube.

The key points in the decision-making process are that:

- The patient was fit enough for salvage surgery.
- It can be argued that, for most patients with recurrent hypopharyngeal cancer, the pharyngectomy should be circumferential; in this case, there is disease involving the postcricoid area and also concerns of field change of the posterior pharyngeal wall, thus making a circumferential resection mandatory.
- The combination of factors of recurrent disease, ill-defined margins, and possible field recurrence meant that resection should include the cervical esophagus. To facilitate the access required both for resection and reconstruction, as well as to perform a true en-bloc resection of paratracheal tissue, manubriumectomy and superior mediastinal resection was performed.
- The use of the ALT flap for reconstruction means that the reasonably long length of defect is not a problem, as well as providing two genuine layers for reconstruction.

Free Jejunal Grafts

Free jejunal grafts (**Fig. 9.5**) obviously do not require tubing, and can be used for longer defects into the esophagus. There is less ischemic time than other flaps and postoperative monitoring is vital. Good functional results with low morbidity are reported by teams who regularly use this flap.[16] One essential pitfall to avoid is using too much length, which is easily done as the flap will concertina to appear much shorter than it actually is stretched out when the patient is operated on in a position of neck extension.

Tubed Gastro-omental Free Flap

A tubed gastro-omental free flap has been specifically proposed for this situation, and especially useful for coverage of vessel and mediastinal dead space if mediastinal dissection and manubrial resection is performed.[17]

Gastric Transposition

For cases in a vessel-depleted neck, or when microvascular anastamosis may be high risk, gastric transposition may be the next best option.[18] For cases when significant esophageal resection is required, it may be the preferred reconstruction technique. The problems associated with gastric transposition include significant peri- and postoperative mortality and morbidity (and some variability in swallow function) and dumping syndrome in some

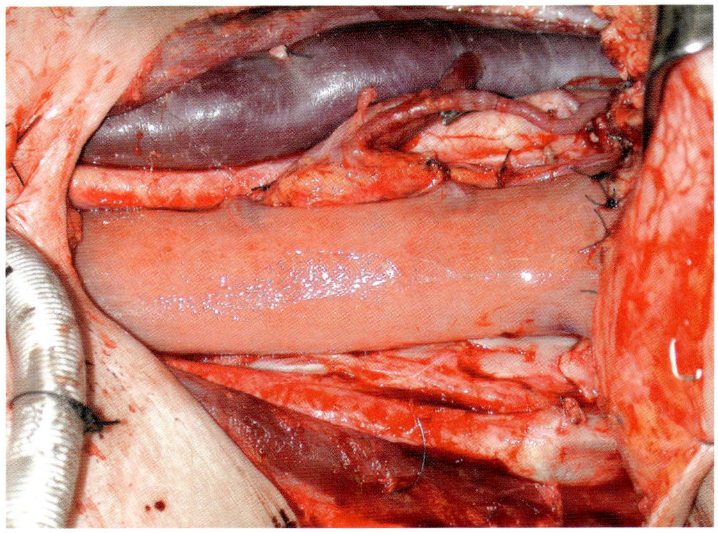

Fig. 9.5 Jejunal flap in situ. Note the "stretch" in the flap: essential for good swallowing function.

patients.[19] The stomach's thickness means that it can be used to help fill dead space and can be skin grafted if necessary, making it useful for peristomal recurrence reconstruction (see **Fig. 9.2**).

Other nonmicrovascular flap options are much less ideal. A pectoralis major myocutaneous flap can occasionally be tubed[20]; or can be employed as a 270° flap onto prevertebral fascia.[21]

Manubriumectomy and Mediastinal Dissection

These maneuvers are a crucial component of the salvage for peristomal recurrence, as discussed above. It has been argued that, even for primary surgery, there should be a low threshold for performing manubiumectomy and mediastinal dissection[22] to prevent peristomal recurrence in at-risk patients. However, it can be argued that effective paratracheal lymph node dissection can be achieved transcervically.[23]

In salvage pharyngolaryngectomy, the same applies but with a much lower threshold, and there is greater emphasis on achieving a true en-bloc resection of the paratracheal and superior mediastinal lymph nodes. Again, the principle is that this is the last reasonable attempt at cure, and the additional morbidity relating to these maneuvers is small. Thus, for advanced recurrent disease with soft tissue involvement, tracheal invasion, bilateral piriform fossa apical involvement, preoperative tracheostomy, and cervical esophageal or postcricoid involvement, manubriumectomy and mediastinal dissection should be considered. The additional access this affords also makes it technically easier to perform the lower anastamosis for cases in which the resection includes the cervical esophagus.

Specific Measures to Prevent Fistula

Complication rates for salvage surgery after chemoradiotherapy are considerably higher than after radiotherapy[24]; and, of these, pharyngeal fistula is the commonest serious complication.

There is a general consensus that salvage pharyngolaryngectomy fistula rates are around double that of primary surgery.[3,24,25]

Now that the standard of care for most patients with hypopharyngeal cancer treated initially nonsurgically is chemoradiotherapy, it is generally accepted that the fistula rate in salvage surgery increases further, compared with initial radiotherapy alone.[26,27] However, much of this data includes laryngectomy (and pharyngolaryngectomy with primary closure), i.e., using irradiatied tissue for pharyngeal repair, and it is not known just how much this applies for salvage pharyngolaryngectomy, especially when circumferential,. While Clark et al. reported increased fistula rates of 38% compared with 24% in salvage surgery, most salvage pharyngolaryngectomies were noncircumferential.[3]

Additionally the time interval from primary radiotherapy to salvage surgery has been found to influence fistula rates, with fistula rates as high as 75% in the first 4 months post radiotherapy, dropping to 25% after 4 months and dropping to near zero after 12 months in one series.[24]

The use of a salivary bypass tube (see **Fig. 9.4**) may well reduce fistula rates.[28] It protects the healing suture line from salivary contamination; and may permit minor dehiscence of a flap, allowing healing to take place without disastrous effects. In the situation of flap loss and fistula formation, it may mitigate neck tissue breakdown, facilitating the possibility of salvaging the situation with a second flap. Our protocol is to leave the bypass tube in situ for 2 weeks postoperatively.

It is important to ensure that all patient morbidities are optimized as much as possible. Immunosuppression caused by conditions such as diabetes or relative malnutrition should be optimized since they predispose to complications including wound infection and wound breakdown. There has been interest in the use of perioperative enteral immunoenhanced feeding in head and neck cancer patients undergoing major surgery, which may influence the postoperative outcomes by reducing the frequency rate of infections and wound complications. On a more basic level, the use of preoperative gastrostomy feeding helps optimize nutrition of patients, many of whom have weight loss due to poor swallowing and/or pain. Bearing in mind the significant rate of fistulization in the patient group, having a gastrostomy in situ is advantageous in managing any postoperative fistula if a period of no oral feeding is anticipated.

The early identification of flap problems is essential to possibly salvage a failing flap, or to use a new flap before gross tissue breakdown occurs. As all flaps employed in pharyolaryngectomy reconstruction are buried, monitoring using implantable Doppler probes or exteriorized flap segments (see **Fig. 9.3**) is recommended.[29]

Function

Most patients undergoing salvage surgery will have surgical voice restoration. There is an argument to perform this as a secondary procedure in salvage cases, but there is no clear consensus. Most data regarding function (voice, swallow) after salvage surgery pertains to total laryngectomy for laryngeal cancer, and that shows poorer function after salvage surgery[30]. This may, at least in part, be related to the higher incidence of fistula, and one assumes that it applies to salvage pharyngolaryngectomy in the same way.

Re-irradiation for Recurrent Hypopharyngeal Cancer

Re-irradiation is accepted as a potentially curative option for recurrent hypopharyngeal cancer, whether recurrence is primary, nodal, or peristomal. The chance of disease control is related to tumor bulk, whether disease is radiorecurrent, geographic "miss," or second primary as well as being influenced by the retreatment schedule used.

The specific experience of re-irradiation for hypopharyngeal cancer is subsumed in the general reported experience of head and neck re-irradiation, detailed in Chapter 4. Of particular relevance to the hypopharynx as a site are the concerns of potential devastating toxicity in terms of carotid rupture, myelopathy, and chondronecrosis if the larynx has not been surgically removed. To optimize the conformality of re-irradiation to gross disease, it is attractive to adopt modalities such as charged particles, brachytherapy, and stereotactic techniques. If conventional photon therapy is used, a small fraction size (2 Gy or less) approach to 60 Gy may be recommended; as synchronous chemotherapy will increase late normal tissue effects, it is attractive to use biological response modifiers as an alternative. In the exceptional circumstances of the patient being of good performance status, unsuitable for surgery, with localized recurrence, induction chemotherapy should be considered.

For parastomal recurrence, there is better conformality of dose with IMRT compared with 3D conformal radiotherapy due to the change in patient contour from neck to chest; although it is not normal IMRT practice, it may well be advisable to consider the use of bolus to overlie the tumor. For primary and nodal recurrences, there may be added value to using PET-CT to distinguish tumor from treatment effect; for well-defined recurrence a margin of 1–1.5 cm is adequate.

Recommended Reading

- Hall SF, Groome PA, Irish J, O'Sullivan B. Radiotherapy or surgery for head and neck squamous cell cancer: establishing the baseline for hypopharyngeal carcinoma? Cancer 2009;115(24):5711–5722 (This paper provides the context of the treatment of primary disease of the hypopharynx and demonstrates no difference in survival between the two modalities of primary treatment.)
- Taki S, Homma A, Oridate N, et al. Salvage surgery for local recurrence after chemoradiotherapy or radiotherapy in hypopharyngeal cancer patients. Eur Arch Otorhinolaryngol 2010;267(11):1765–1769 (This paper shows similar survival rates comparing primary and salvage surgery, but with greatly increased morbidity in salvage surgery.)
- Theile DR, Robinson DW, Theile DE, Coman WB. Free jejunal interposition reconstruction after pharyngolaryngectomy: 201 consecutive cases. Head Neck 1995;17(2):83–88
- Yu P, Hanasono MM, Skoracki RJ, et al. Pharyngoesophageal reconstruction with the anterolateral thigh flap after total laryngopharyngectomy. Cancer 2010;116(7):1718–1724
- Shuangba H, Jingwu S, Yinfeng W, et al. Complication following gastric pull-up reconstruction for advanced hypopharyngeal or cervical esophageal carcinoma: a 20-year review in a Chinese institute. Am J Otolaryngol 2010;32(4):275–278 (These three papers are the largest series for free jejunal, ALT, and gastric transposition flaps, respectively)

- Patel RS, Goldstein DP, Brown D, Irish J, Gullane PJ, Gilbert RW. Circumferential pharyngeal reconstruction: History, critical analysis of techniques, and current therapeutic recommendations. Head Neck 2010;32(1):109–120 (Summary of different flaps and issues in circumferential reconstruction.)

References

1. Taki S, Homma A, Oridate N, et al. Salvage surgery for local recurrence after chemoradiotherapy or radiotherapy in hypopharyngeal cancer patients. Eur Arch Otorhinolaryngol 2010;267(11):1765–1769
2. Mochiki M, Sugasawa M, Nibu K, Asai M, Nakao K, Asakage T. Prognostic factors for hypopharyngeal cancer: a univariate and multivariate study of 142 cases. Acta Otolaryngol Suppl 2007;(559):136–144
3. Clark JR, de Almeida J, Gilbert R, et al. Primary and salvage (hypo)pharyngectomy: Analysis and outcome. Head Neck 2006;28(8):671–677
4. Kadota H, Fukushima J, Nakashima T, et al. Comparison of salvage and planned pharyngolaryngectomy with jejunal transfer for hypopharyngeal carcinoma after chemoradiotherapy. Laryngoscope 2010;120(6):1103–1108
5. Passero VA, Branstetter BF, Shuai Y, et al. Response assessment by combined PET-CT scan versus CT scan alone using RECIST in patients with locally advanced head and neck cancer treated with chemoradiotherapy. Ann Oncol 2010;21(11):2278–2283
6. Wycliffe ND, Grover RS, Kim PD, Simental A Jr. Hypopharyngeal cancer. Top Magn Reson Imaging 2007;18(4):243–258
7. Basu D, Siegel BA, McDonald DJ, Nussenbaum B. Detection of occult bone metastases from head and neck squamous cell carcinoma: impact of positron emission tomography computed tomography with fluorodeoxyglucose F 18. Arch Otolaryngol Head Neck Surg 2007;133(8):801–805
8. Haerle SK, Strobel K, Hany TF, Sidler D, Stoeckli SJ. 18F-FDG-PET/CT versus panendoscopy for the detection of synchronous second primary tumors in patients with head and neck squamous cell carcinoma. Head Neck 2010;32(3):319–325
9. Spector JG, Sessions DG, Haughey BH, et al. Delayed regional metastases, distant metastases, and second primary malignancies in squamous cell carcinomas of the larynx and hypopharynx. Laryngoscope 2001;111(6):1079–1087
10. Perlow A, Bui C, Shreve P, Sundgren PC, Teknos TN, Mukherji SK. High incidence of chest malignancy detected by FDG PET in patients suspected of recurrent squamous cell carcinoma of the upper aerodigestive tract. J Comput Assist Tomogr 2004;28(5):704–709
11. Hall SF, Groome PA, Irish J, O'Sullivan B. Radiotherapy or surgery for head and neck squamous cell cancer: establishing the baseline for hypopharyngeal carcinoma? Cancer 2009;115(24):5711–5722
12. Sisson GA, Bytell DE, Edison BD, Yeh S Jr. Transsternal radical neck dissection for control of stomal recurrences—end results. Laryngoscope 1975;85(9):1504–1510
13. Gluckman JL, Hamaker RC, Schuller DE, Weissler MC, Charles GA. Surgical salvage for stomal recurrence: a multi-institutional experience. Laryngoscope 1987;97(9):1025–1029
14. Elliott MS, Odell EW, Tysome JR, et al. Role of thyroidectomy in advanced laryngeal and pharyngolaryngeal carcinoma. Otolaryngol Head Neck Surg 2010;142(6):851–855
15. Yu P, Hanasono MM, Skoracki RJ, et al. Pharyngoesophageal reconstruction with the anterolateral thigh flap after total laryngopharyngectomy. Cancer 2010;116(7):1718–1724
16. Theile DR, Robinson DW, Theile DE, Coman WB. Free jejunal interposition reconstruction after pharyngolaryngectomy: 201 consecutive cases. Head Neck 1995;17(2):83–88
17. Genden EM, Kaufman MR, Katz B, Vine A, Urken ML. Tubed gastro-omental free flap for pharyngoesophageal reconstruction. Arch Otolaryngol Head Neck Surg 2001;127(7):847–853
18. Shuangba H, Jingwu S, Yinfeng W, et al. Complication following gastric pull-up reconstruction for advanced hypopharyngeal or cervical esophageal carcinoma: a 20-year review in a Chinese institute. Am J Otolaryngol 2011;32(4):275–278
19. Harrison DF, Thompson AE. Pharyngolaryngoesophagectomy with pharyngogastric anastomosis for cancer of the hypopharynx: review of 101 operations. Head Neck Surg 1986;8(6):418–428
20. Shektman A, Silver C, Strauch B. A re-evaluation of hypopharyngeal reconstruction: pedicled flaps versus microvascular free flaps. Plast Reconstr Surg 1997;100(7):1691–1696
21. Spriano G, Pellini R, Roselli R. Pectoralis major myocutaneous flap for hypopharyngeal reconstruction. Plast Reconstr Surg 2002;110(6):1408–1413; discussion 1414–1416
22. Harrison DF. Surgical management of cancer of the hypopharynx and cervical oesophagus. Br J Surg 1969;56(2):95–103
23. Timon CV, Toner M, Conlon BJ. Paratracheal lymph node involvement in advanced cancer of the larynx, hypopharynx, and cervical esophagus. Laryngoscope 2003;113(9):1595–1599
24. Dirven R, Swinson BD, Gao K, Clark JR. The assessment of pharyngocutaneous fistula rate in patients treated primarily with definitive radiotherapy followed by salvage surgery of the larynx and hypopharynx. Laryngoscope 2009;119(9):1691–1695
25. Tsou Y-A, Hua C-H, Lin M-H, Tseng H-C, Tsai M-H, Shaha A. Comparison of pharyngocutaneous fistula between patients followed by primary laryngopharyngectomy and salvage laryngopharyngectomy for advanced hypopharyngeal cancer. Head Neck 2010;32(11):1494–1500
26. Ganly I, Patel S, Matsuo J, et al. Postoperative complications of salvage total laryngectomy. Cancer 2005;103(10):2073–2081
27. Furuta Y, Homma A, Oridate N, et al. Surgical complications of salvage total laryngectomy following concurrent chemoradiotherapy. Int J Clin Oncol 2008;13(6):521–527
28. Varvares MA, Cheney ML, Gliklich RE, et al. Use of the radial forearm fasciocutaneous free flap and montgomery salivary bypass tube for pharyngoesophageal reconstruction. Head Neck 2000;22(5):463–468
29. Disa JJ, Cordeiro PG, Hidalgo DA. Efficacy of conventional monitoring techniques in free tissue transfer: an 11-year experience in 750 consecutive cases. Plast Reconstr Surg 1999;104(1):97–101
30. de Casso C, Slevin NJ, Homer JJ. The impact of radiotherapy on swallowing and speech in patients who undergo total laryngectomy. Otolaryngol Head Neck Surg 2008;139(6):792–797

10 Carcinoma of the Oral Cavity

Alexander D. Rapidis, Hisham M. Mehanna, K. Kian Ang

Summary

- The recurrence rates of squamous cell carcinoma (SCC) of the oral cavity treated with surgery, alone or with postoperative radiotherapy exceeds 35%.
- The recurrence rates of advanced SCC treated with chemoradiation approaches 50%.
- Early detection of local recurrence remains the most important prognostic factor for patients' survival after salvage surgery.
- Clinical examination remains the most useful method of early detection of recurrent cancer of the oral cavity.
- Patients treated for oral cancer should be followed up for locoregional recurrences for the first 3 years after treatment. Further follow-up does not provide any additional benefit.
- Recurrent cancer of the oral cavity carries the gravest prognosis from recurrent cancer in all other subsites of the head and neck area.

Introduction

Local failure remains a significant problem for patients with oral cavity squamous cell carcinoma (SCC), particularly those with locoregionally advanced disease. Recurrence of cancer at the primary site is relatively common compared with recurrence in the neck and metastasis at distant sites. Despite all the advances of modern multidisciplinary care and treatment, a recurrence at the primary site occurs in approximately 30% to 50% of oral cancer patients and remains the primary cause of treatment failure.[1–3] Recurrent disease also contributes to the majority of oral cancer–related deaths. Patients who have completed treatment for oral SCC should undergo follow-up examinations at regular intervals. Follow-up programs in patients with cancer in general are based on the assumption that patients whose recurrence is detected at an asymptomatic or earlier stage have better therapeutic options, higher chance for salvage, and decreased cancer-specific morbidity. About 90% of patients who develop recurrence after treatment of oral SCC do so within 2 years. The mean time of detection of recurrence from the date of the initial curative treatment is less than 12 months.[4]

! In locoregionally advanced cancers of the oral cavity, several risk features affect outcome. Positive surgical margins and extracapsular extension (ECE) from neck nodes have consistently been associated with higher rates of locoregional relapse and distant metastasis and are so far the most significant unfavorable prognostic factors in locally advanced oral cancer.[5–7] Other less prominent risk features include involvement of two or more nodes without ECE, depth of invasion above 5 mm, perineural infiltration, and level IV–V nodal involvement.[8–10]

Posttreatment Surveillance

Objectives

The objectives of posttreatment surveillance are manifold. First, it is essential to evaluate the therapeutic efficacy for endpoint reporting and, when applicable, management of functional impairments that may result from the tumor or its treatment. Second, initiation of psychosocial rehabilitation and reintegration can improve the quality of life. Third, early detection of locoregional relapse can increase the potential for successful salvage.[11] For example, among 377 patients with recurrent SCC, the mean time of detection of recurrence from the date of the initial curative treatment was 11 months and 90% of the recurrences were detected within 25 months after the primary curative operation.[12] Finally, early detection of new primary tumor manifestations may maximize the likelihood for curative therapy. Patients cured of a head and neck carcinoma are more likely to develop second primary cancers than patients with other neoplasms. The late development of second primary tumors is the most common cause of posttreatment "failure" after 36 months. The reported incidence is approximately 10% to 15% overall (2%–4% per year), and highest for current smokers, followed by former smokers, and then nonsmokers.[13–15]

Evidence

Despite the widespread use of posttreatment surveillance in the clinical setting, surprisingly few data are available to support its value, particularly in terms of improving survival.[16] There are very few prospective data, none of them demonstrating a survival benefit for any follow-up strategy in patients treated for oral SCC, and available retrospective data are conflicting.[17,18] Guidelines for posttreatment surveillance from the American Head and Neck Society were initially published in 1996 as collaboration between the American Society for Head and Neck Surgery and the Society for Head and Neck Surgeons.[19] The 2002 update, adopted by the National Comprehensive Cancer Network (NCCN), recommends continued follow-up evaluation consisting of history, physical examination, and head and neck imaging at regular, progressively longer, intervals and annual chest radiographs.[20–23] Similar guidelines regarding posttreatment surveillance have been recommended by several European Institutions.[18,24–26]

Boysen et al.[27] have prospectively studied the value of regular follow-up in a group of 661 consecutive patients treated curatively for head and neck SCC. Patients were seen at 2- to 3-monthly intervals in the first 2 years, and every 3–4 months in the following 3 years. After 5 years, follow-up was usually discontinued. A total of 220 patients (33%) developed recurrences and 76% of these were diagnosed during the first 2 years and 11% in the third year following the completion of primary treatment. The first recurrence was at the primary tumor site in 131 (20%), in the regional nodes in 54 (8%), and at distant sites in 35 (5%). Recurrences were diagnosed through symptoms and signs presented by the patients in 61% and by follow-up physical examination in 39%. Surprisingly, only 22% of regional recurrences were detected through physical examination.[27,28] Visscher and Manni found that the mean survival of patients with recurrences detected on routine follow-up was nearly double that of patients detected after self-referral. This group also pointed out the psychological value of reassuring patients of normal results of a follow-up examination.[13]

Diagnosis of Recurrence

When a relapse is suspected from physical examination, staging work-up, including endoscopy and diagnostic imaging such as computed tomography (CT), magnetic resonance imaging (MRI), and/or positron emission tomography (PET) using ^{18}F-fluorodeoxyglucose (FDG) as a metabolic tracer, should be completed to establish the extent of the locoregional recurrence, its relationship to critical structures, and whether metastatic disease is present. All of these findings determine the prognosis and the therapeutic strategy, e.g., recommending potentially curative therapy versus palliative care.[29–34] A biopsy specimen or at least an ultrasound-guided fine-needle aspiration must also be obtained for histopathological confirmation. More details on this are provided in Chapter 1.

Principles of Management

Tumor-related factors and the general condition of patients who seek treatment for a recurrent oral cavity SCC influence treatment recommendation and the expected prognosis. The site and stage of the recurrent cancer as well as the modality and magnitude of the initial therapy are important factors in choosing treatment. In addition, the time elapsed from the initial therapy to first recurrence may represent indirect evidence of tumor virulence and/or host resistance. The general health and activity level of the patient reflected by the performance status, along with the presence or absence of specific comorbidities, may impact both host resistance and the capability of the patient to complete therapy for recurrence.

Early-stage Recurrent Tumors of the Oral Cavity

Patients with early-stage recurrent tumors of the oral cavity appear to be more likely to benefit from salvage, with a 70% chance of living at least 2 years without recurrence.[35] Patients with recurrent T1 and T2 oral SCC who are former smokers or nonsmokers were the best candidates for salvage surgery and microvascular free flap reconstruction.[35] Primary TNM classification before initial treatment, the extent of recurrence, and the recurrent tumor size appear to be the independent prognostic factors for patients with recurrent oral SCC, as demonstrated by Pearlman's study[36] and that of Yueh et al.[37] The recurrent cases with primary TNM stage III or IV before initial treatment had a significantly worse survival outcome compared with cases with primary TNM stage I.[38] Favorable surgical salvage candidates are younger, have a disease-free interval after receiving definitive therapy, have small recurrent tumors for which it is possible to obtain negative surgical margins, and have no recurrent neck disease.[39] If salvage surgery had been limited to patients who had had a disease-free interval and small recurrent tumors, then the 3- and 5-year overall survival rates would have been 74% and 44%, respectively.[38]

Advanced-staged Recurrent Oral SCC

Advanced-staged recurrent oral SCC is arguably the greatest challenge faced by the multidisciplinary teams of physicians and surgeons who treat these patients. This group of patients presents a unique set of dilemmas with regard to treatment because the chance for a cure is low, and prior treatment generally has a negative impact on all current therapeutic options. For example, salvage surgery is more difficult in the face of scarring from prior surgery and/or the tissue changes caused by radiation therapy. In addition, unwanted side effects of therapy are often cumulative, further reducing quality of life through loss of speech and swallowing function and changes in appearance. Finally, the already marginal therapeutic index defined by the previously mentioned considerations may be further reduced by the presence of comorbidities, reduced performance status, and advanced age.

Treatment of Relapse after Surgery or Local Radiation Alone

Patients who develop isolated resectable nodal recurrence after prior surgery alone can be treated with neck dissection, followed in the presence of adverse features by adjuvant radiotherapy to the neck alone when recurrent disease manifests more than 1 year after initial operation, or to the neck and the primary tumor bed when relapse occurs in less than 1 year.[40] In the presence of extranodal extension (ECE+) or positive margins, radiation with concurrent cisplatin is the current standard of care if there are no contraindications for chemotherapy.[6,8] More information is presented in Chapter 12 on the management of nodal recurrence.

Patients presenting with local recurrence, whether with or without nodal relapse, are more challenging to manage.[41] The main limitation of salvage surgery of recurrence at the primary site in the past was the limited possibility for reconstruction. The advent of microvascular free tissue transfer has greatly expanded the potential population of patients with recurrent head and neck cancer who might be considered candidates for salvage surgery.[42] Although wound healing complications are more common after prior cancer treatment, free flaps have proven to be reliable in this setting. With the proven efficacy of free flaps, the patient selection criteria for salvage surgery now focuses on issues related to tumor resectability, patient comorbidity, quality of life outcome, and cancer prognosis.[43]

When the volume and location of recurrent disease are amenable to resection and the patient is considered medically operable, surgical salvage, usually followed by radiotherapy or chemoradiotherapy, provides the best opportunity for long-term survival.[44] Salvage surgery generally consists of wide local resection with neck dissection and reconstruction.[12,45] Adjuvant radiotherapy with or without concurrent cisplatin, depending on the surgical pathological findings, is generally indicated in such patients. Unfortunately, the potential for salvage is often limited by extensive tumor involvement, difficult resection and reconstruction after previous surgery or radiotherapy, poor candidacy for radiotherapy, and poor general health of the patients at the time of recurrence. In such cases, radiotherapy combined with chemotherapy can be attempted but the outcome is generally poor.

Treatment of Relapse after Combined Therapy

Management of recurrence in patients who had prior surgery and radiation (± chemotherapy) or chemoradiation is a very challenging clinical situation. Selected patients may be suitable for surgical salvage, and a few cases may be eligible for re-irradiation combined with chemotherapy—as adjuvant therapy or as primary treatment for the recurrence (see Chapter 4). However, the majority are offered palliative chemotherapy (see Chapter 5) or supportive care (see Chapter 21).

Surgical Approaches and Techniques

Indications

The advent of microvascular free tissue transfer has greatly expanded the potential population of patients with recurrent head and neck cancer who might be considered candidates for salvage surgery. Unfortunately, the outcome of patients undergoing salvage surgery with microvascular free tissue transfer for recurrent oral SCC is rarely reported in the literature. It remains unknown whether the availability of microvascular surgery allows more curative procedures to be performed or whether the ability to reconstruct extensive defects has simply increased the number of poor-prognosis patients undergoing surgery.

The lack of potentially suitable cervical recipient blood vessels, for example, because of previous selective or modified radical neck dissection performed as a part of the initial surgical treatment, does increase the complexity of achieving successful free flap perfusion and thereby may increase the risk of free flap thrombosis and failure. However, neck dissection or prior radiotherapy are not contraindications for microvascular free flap reconstruction in suitable patients scheduled for salvage surgery. In a study of 59 patients who underwent free flap reconstruction following previous neck dissection, a flap success rate of 100% was achieved.[46] About 15% of the neck dissections were contralateral to the defect site. Prior radiation therapy did not appear to have a negative impact on flap survival since 71% of these patients had preoperative radiation therapy. Although the flaps proved reliable, 61% of patients required use of cervical recipient blood vessels in the contralateral neck, reflecting an increased complexity of reconstruction. Indeed, all patients who had had modified radical or radical neck dissection required use of cervical recipient blood vessels in the opposite side of the neck.[47,48]

If a suitable recipient vein cannot be found or accessed in the contralateral neck, cephalic vein transposition can be performed. This involves transposing the cephalic vein from the ipsilateral arm to the neck to serve as a recipient vein for free flap perfusion.[35,49] Advantages of this technique include the fact that only one microvenous anastomosis is required, and the high-flow, low-pressure cephalic–subclavian system may be resistant to stasis and thrombosis. The primary disadvantage of this technique arises from the increased potential of kinking or extrinsic compression of the venous pedicle within its long subcutaneous course, particularly where the cephalic vein crosses over the clavicle.[35,46]

Limitations

It is important to understand the specific limits of surgical resection as they exist today. Although technically feasible, the value of resecting the common or internal carotid artery, distal trachea, esophagus, and prevertebral soft tissue is controversial. The possibility of cure is small when these structures are involved, and each of these maneuvers greatly increases operative risk.[45] The patient and family rely on the surgeon's judgment, and the crucial question becomes whether the surgery is more likely to help or harm the patient. Although there have been limited reports of success with resection and replacement of the internal carotid artery, this should be viewed as high risk, especially in patients who have failed prior irradiation.[50] Biller et al.[51] showed that carotid resection was technically feasible in a series of 26 patients. Only 7% of this group suffered neurological complications when arterial bypass was used as part of the surgical technique. Despite their ability to technically perform the procedure with acceptable morbidity, 12-month disease free survival was only 25%. Miao et al. used an expanded PTFE arterial graft to reconstruct the internal carotid artery after its en-bloc resection with recurrent tumor of the neck in a cohort of 13 patients. All patients survived the operation and the disease-free survival was 40% at 2 years.[52]

Carotid Artery Involvement

Rupture

Carotid artery rupture, also referred to as "carotid blow-out" as a complication of head and neck cancer treatment is a catastrophic life-threatening emergency. It has been reported to occur in 3%–5% of patients who undergo major head and neck resections, but may also occur in cases where radiotherapy was the only treatment modality.[53]

Hemorrhage from the common, internal or external carotid arteries is usually controlled by direct pressure and arterial ligation. The reported mortality varies from 3% to over 50%, with acute rupture and severe neurological deficits from 16% to over 50% in those who initially survive.[54]

Carotid artery rupture is proceeded by "herald bleed," which almost invariably occurs as the initial manifestation as the artery becomes eroded, leaks, and clots until a major bleed occurs with cardiovascular manifestations necessitating operative intervention. Major postoperative complications (pharyngocutaneous fistulas, tumor recurrence, infection, and local flap failure) almost always precede and are the most common contributing factors to wound breakdown, necrosis, and fistula formation and carotid artery exposure with eventual artery rupture.[53]

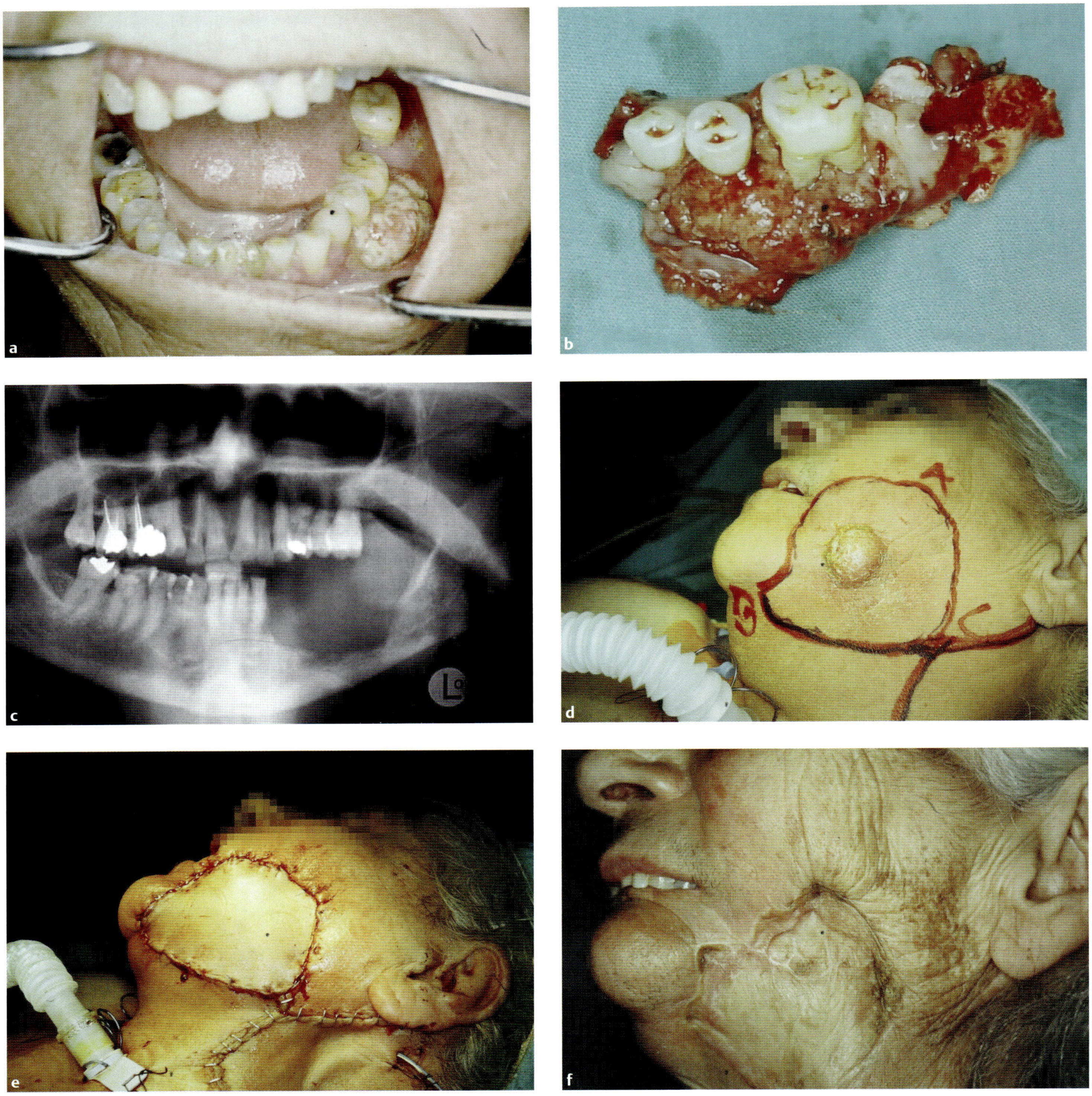

Fig. 10.1a–f Exophytic T2N0M0 squamous cell carcinoma of the mandibular alveolus with no radiographic evidence of mandibular bone involvement.
a Clinical presentation.
b Specimen.
c Postoperative OPG.
d, e En bloc resection of the mandible, skin of the submandibular area, and radical neck dissection and reconstruction of the created defect with a pectoralis major myocutaneous flap.
f Postoperative radiotherapy.

Infection

Infection plays an extremely important role in predisposing to arterial rupture. In the neck, infection may be manifested either by disrupted skin flaps or by a pharyngocutaneous fistula. Another important consideration predisposing to poor wound healing is the long-term presence of mobile foreign bodies (tracheostomy and nasogastric tubes) potentially causing irritation and a chronic inflammatory response.[55] These foreign bodies may cause continued postoperative irritation and, in the case of cuffed tracheostomy tubes, pressure on compromised tissue, occasionally leading to tissue necrosis and fistula formation.[56] After head and neck surgery with radical neck dissection and tracheostomy, the common carotid artery lies unprotected under the skin. Radical neck dissection exposing the carotid artery considerably compromises the nutrition of the artery, independently of irradiation, because the artery derives 80% of its blood supply from its adventitia, which is often injured during the dissection, especially in node stripping.[57] Carotid artery stripping of nodal metastasis is reported to be associated with up to 25% rupture rates in nonirradiated patients. This is because simple stripping has been associated with residual disease in the arterial wall in up to 42% of cases.[53,56]

Arterial Disease

Radiation injury can result in clinically significant arterial disease of large arteries, including occlusive disease. Injury to the vasa vasorum after irradiation may account for an increased incidence of rupture of the carotid vessels.[58,59] Signs of imminent rupture include oozing from the tumor mass, skin necrosis, an exposed artery, hemoptysis, hematemesis, and frank bleeding.[60] These herald bleeds must raise one's clinical suspicion sufficiently to impose a "lead time" during which appropriate investigations and management can be instituted. The issue of whether to resect and reconstruct or ligate the artery is compounded in the emergency setting of carotid artery rupture. Recently, endovascular embolization has been successfully employed as an alternative to surgical ligation. Whether endovascular embolization or stenting would be applicable in all cases is an unresolved issue.[61] An endovascular approach would not allow the treatment of the underlying causes of the arterial bleed nor would it allow the opportunity for adjunctive surgical therapy, for example, insertion of afterloading catheters for later brachytherapy to residual tumor if necessary. In summary, resection of the carotid artery is technically feasible, but there is little support for this high-risk maneuver in terms of its providing improved survival. It is therefore reserved and indicated as a treatment option only in a select group of highly motivated and otherwise healthy patients.[62]

Pitfalls and Limitations of Salvage Surgery

The results of salvage surgery clearly justify its use in around 70% of the patients who are treated for an early-stage (stage I/II) recurrence and in 25%–30% of the patients who have surgery for a late-stage (stage III/IV) resectable recurrence. Many patients, though, are subjected to salvage surgery only to see no real or lasting benefits. Frequently, the recurrent tumor in the oral cavity will be submucosal and will not be evident on clinical examination and not detected until imaging is performed or the tumor mass becomes large enough to become evident due to mass effect. We must therefore improve our diagnostic efficacy in the initial posttreatment surveillance period to better identify recurrences at an early stage to improve the overall therapeutic results.

It is still unclear what the extent of resection in salvage surgery should be. The question whether the resection should be confined to the pretreatment tumor extent or only to the residual tumor is a difficult to answer, especially when initial treatment was chemoradiation. It is not clearly understood whether chemoradiation kills tumor concentrically, leaving a central residual mass of viable tumor, or whether the tumor death is diffuse, leaving small pockets of viable tumor throughout the extent of the pretreatment tissue.[63,64] A recent study shed some light on these questions and suggested that the latter is the case.[65] The same dilemma exists for patients who show partial response after chemoradiotherapy.[66–68]

While salvage surgery has significant risks after concurrent chemoradiotherapy, it is usually the only potential curative option available to patients who fail this aggressive primary treatment regimen. Currently, data are sparse on the efficacy of salvage after concomitant chemoradiotherapy in oral SCC, but when stage of disease is taken into consideration it appears to be similar to that of salvage after radiotherapy.[63] It is important as the treatment regimens continue to evolve that we continue to gather data on efficacy and morbidity of salvage surgery to better direct patient care.

The expected efficacy of salvage surgery is strongly correlated with the stage of the recurrent disease, but only weakly correlated with the site of the recurrent cancer, and not at all correlated with time to presalvage recurrence.[44] Survival and disease-free survival correlate best with the recurrent stage, and improvement in quality of life (QoL) correlates with both recurrent stage and with the site of recurrence. The cost of salvage surgery for the patients in terms of complications, surgical mortality, length of hospital stay, and reduction in QoL also correlates best with recurrent stage.

As mentioned before, the advent of free flap reconstruction has expanded the range of salvage surgery that was previously constrained by limited reconstructive options. Also, the ability to bring nonirradiated vascularized tissue into the wound has decreased the incidence of local wound complications. Free flap reconstruction is not a panacea, however, and carries its own set of disadvantages: prolonged surgical time in patients who are typically in poor general health, significantly increased cost, creation of a second wound and associated donor site morbidity, and increased postoperative monitoring.

Locoregional Recurrent Cancers of the Oral Cavity

Locoregional recurrent cancers of the oral cavity pose several distinct problems in the salvage surgical treatment and the reconstruction of the surgical defects. Many of these are attributed to the anatomical subsites of the oral cavity and whether local recurrence involves soft tissues only or extends to osseous parts of the facial skeleton. SCC of the mandibular alveolus that invades the mandibular bone above the inferior dental canal may be treated with marginal resection of the mandible instead of segmental mandibulectomy. However, marginal mandibulectomies, although they are considered oncologically safe procedures, carry a higher rate of recurrences than segmental mandibular resections.[69–72] The subsequent surgical salvage requires extensive procedures and complex reconstructions with either locoregional pedicled flaps or free tissue transfer (see **Fig. 10.1**).[73]

Case Study

An 82-year-old white woman with an exophytic T2N0M0 squamous cell carcinoma of the mandibular alveolus with no radiographic evidence of mandibular bone involvement (**Fig. 10.1a**). The patient had a CT scan that confirmed the absence of regional neck metastasis and orthopantomogram (OPG) that showed no bony involvement.

Figure 10.1d: Twelve months after a marginal mandibulectomy via the intraoral route. The patient developed recurrence in the area of previous resection with involvement of the skin of the cheek area. Salvage surgical treatment included en-bloc resection of the mandible, the skin of the submandibular area, and radical neck dissection. The created defect was reconstructed with the use of a pectoralis major myocutaneous flap (**Fig. 10.1e**). The patient received postoperative radiotherapy and remained free of recurrence (**Fig. 10.1f**). She died from other causes 5 years postoperatively.

Carcinoma of the Tongue

Carcinoma of the tongue represents the most common intraoral malignancy. It is also the most common oral site for local recurrence. Detection of early recurrence is usually easy and salvage surgery can be offered to the patient with good therapeutic results. The surgical treatment of tongue recurrences usually requires resections of large segments of the tongue. These extended, subtotal, near-total, or total glossectomies, will leave the patient unable to speak or swallow, unless the surgical defect is reconstructed intraoperatively.[74] Before the introduction of free tissue transfer and the development of free flaps with microvascular anastomoses, this was an especially difficult task because reconstruction had to be performed with pedicled flaps, the workhorse of which was, and in many instances still is, the pectoralis major myocutaneous flap.[75,76] Among the free flaps, the radial forearm fasciocutaneous flap is the most commonly used, although other types such as the anterolateral thigh, fasciocutaneous flaps, the latissimus dorsi muscle flap and the rectus abdominis flap have all been used with good functional and esthetic results (see box and **Fig. 10.2**).

Case Study

A 56-year-old white man with a T1N0M0 squamous cell carcinoma of the left lateral border of the tongue presented with a local recurrence 1 year after a local excision via intraoral route (**Fig. 10.2a**). The neck was negative to palpation.

The patient had a CT scan that confirmed the absence of regional neck metastasis.

Treatment was scheduled for extended hemiglossectomy with suprahomohyoid neck dissection (**Fig. 10.2b**) and immediate reconstruction of the created defect with the use of a radial forearm fasciocutaneous flap. The patient received postoperative radiotherapy and is free of disease 8 years postoperatively (**Fig. 10.2c**).

Carcinoma of the Nasal Cavity

The middle third of the face and especially the maxilla and the maxillary sinus are poor candidates for surgical salvage. Recurrences from SCC or glandular cell carcinomas in these sites have the tendency to spread toward the anterior and middle cranial

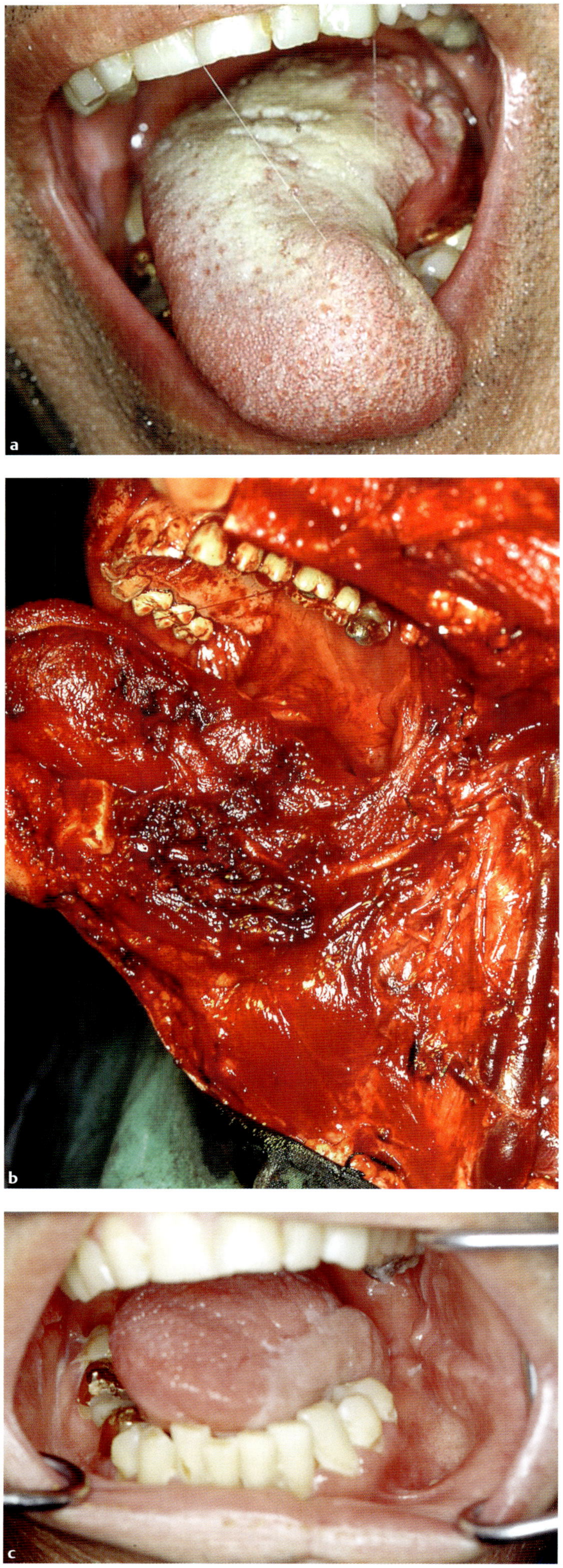

Fig. 10.2a–c T1 N0 M0 squamous cell carcinoma of the left lateral border of the tongue
a Clinical presentation.
b Extended hemiglossectomy with suprahomohyoid neck dissection and immediate reconstruction of the created defect with the use of a radial forearm fasciocutaneous flap.
c Postoperative radiotherapy.

fossa, making surgical extirpation with disease-free margins impossible. The same clinical behavior is seen in tumors of the ethmoids, which have a tendency as recurrent tumors to invade the base of the skull. In cases where surgical salvage is possible, the resection of large segments of the middle third of the face leaves considerable functional and esthetic impairment to the patient despite reconstructive techniques with either local and locoregional flaps, free tissue transfer, the use of prosthetic appliances in the form of obturators, or combinations of the above (see **Fig. 10.3**).

Case Study

A 76-year-old white woman with a recurrent squamous cell carcinoma of the lateral aspect of the anterior nasal cavity extending to the left maxillary sinus invading the left orbital cavity. The patient has had several surgical operations and postoperative radiotherapy which failed to eradicate disease (**Fig. 10.3a**). A CT scan confirmed that the tumor extended to the entire left lateral part of the middle third of the face.

Figure 10.3b: Resection en bloc of the left lateral part of the middle third of the face including the orbit, nose, nasal cavity, maxillary antrum, and ethmoids. The created defect was reconstructed with a latissimus dorsi muscle free flap covered with split-thickness skin graft (**Fig. 10.3c**). The patient remains disease free 3 years postoperatively although the aesthetic results are suboptimal (**Fig. 10.3d**).

Postoperative Complications

It is clear that salvage surgery after chemoradiotherapy carries significant risk to the patient with serious complications occurring in a quarter to a third of all patients undergoing the procedure.[63] This complication rate is higher than in primary surgery or in salvage surgery after radiotherapy without chemotherapy.[77] Many of the associated complications are thought to be a result of the poor quality of tissue in the local surgical site resulting in less than optimal wound healing and postoperative function.

A distinction should be made between neck dissection alone and surgery that breaches a mucosal barrier (e.g., resection of a primary cancer plus neck dissection in continuity) in a previously irradiated field.[78] Most cases of recurrent oral SCC fall into this latter category. Surgery that breaches a mucosal barrier in an area that has been previously irradiated is more frequently accompanied by complications, particularly fistula formation.[79] For patients undergoing neck dissection alone, free tissue transfer is not usually necessary, and coverage of any skin defect or area of exposed carotid artery is easily accomplished with a pectoralis myofascial flap.[35,80]

! Because most patients undergoing surgical salvage have previously undergone surgery and/or radiation therapy, complication rates can be significant.[44]

In a study of 124 patients undergoing salvage surgery after locoregional recurrence of head and neck cancer, the overall rate of postoperative complications was 53.2% (66 of 124 patients).[50] Complications were minor in 53 patients (42.7%) and major in 23 (18.5%). Thirty patients (24.2%) had more than one complication, most commonly fistulas, infections, and wound dehiscence. Ten patients (8.1%) had both minor and major complications. The length of hospital stay ranged from 1 to 90 days (mean 11.2 days). The mean length of stay was 7.4 days for patients without surgical complications, compared with 14.5 days for those with complications. The most frequent surgical complications were wound infections in 31 patients (25.0%), salivary fistulas in 28 (22.6%), wound dehiscence in 14 (11.3%), and partial flap necrosis in 12 (9.7%). Neither age nor sex correlated with the development of minor or major surgical complications. The site of the primary tumor, which indirectly reflects the type of surgery, was also not associated with a risk of postoperative complications. Patients with advanced clinical stage recurrences (stages III and IV) showed higher overall rates of postoperative complications, 58.4% and 30.4%, respectively. On multivariate analysis, an independent risk factor for overall postoperative complications was advanced clinical stage (stages III and IV) of the recurrent tumor. Patients with longer than 1 year between initial treatment and salvage surgery were at increased risk of major complications. Advanced clinical stage was also an independent risk factor for minor postoperative complications, as was the previous site treated (local tumor plus the neck).

Outcomes

Survival and Locoregional Control

Notwithstanding that salvage surgery offers the only realistic chance of survival for patients with recurrent oral cavity cancer, few studies have evaluated outcome after salvage surgery. Even within these studies, it is difficult to discern whether those patients with initial advanced disease, who are most likely to have a recurrence, could be salvaged. Surgical salvage of local recurrence can achieve 5-year disease-free survival in 35% of the patients. However, only 30% of patients with local recurrence are feasible for surgical salvage. The overall salvage rate of local recurrence is only about 10%.[12,35,44] In a series of 377 patients with recurrent head and neck cancer, 102 patients (27%) had surgical salvage, 49 (13%) had radiotherapy as salvage treatment, 96 (25%) had chemotherapy alone, and 130 (35%) had only supportive care.[12] Only patients who were salvaged by surgery achieved 5-year disease-free survival. The mean survival of patients without surgical salvage was 6 months. The mean survival of patients treated with radiotherapy and chemotherapy was 7 months. The mean survival of patients who received supportive care was 5 months, and the mean improvement of survival was only 2 months with radiotherapy and chemotherapy compared with supportive care. Local recurrence of oral cavity and laryngeal carcinoma had a tendency for higher surgical salvage rates compared with that of the oropharynx and hypopharynx. The median disease-free interval for the group as a whole was 17.9 months after salvage surgery, and the overall 2-year disease-free survival was 44%. Significant operative complications occurred in 22 patients (20.2%), and 2 patients (1.8%) died within 30 days of surgery. In an article reporting on 24 patients who underwent salvage surgery and reconstruction of head and neck defects due to recurrent oral cancers, the 1-, 3-, and 5-year overall survival rates were 72.8%, 30.9%, and 20.6%, respectively.[38,81] Agra et al.[50] reported a 5-year survival rate of 32.5%

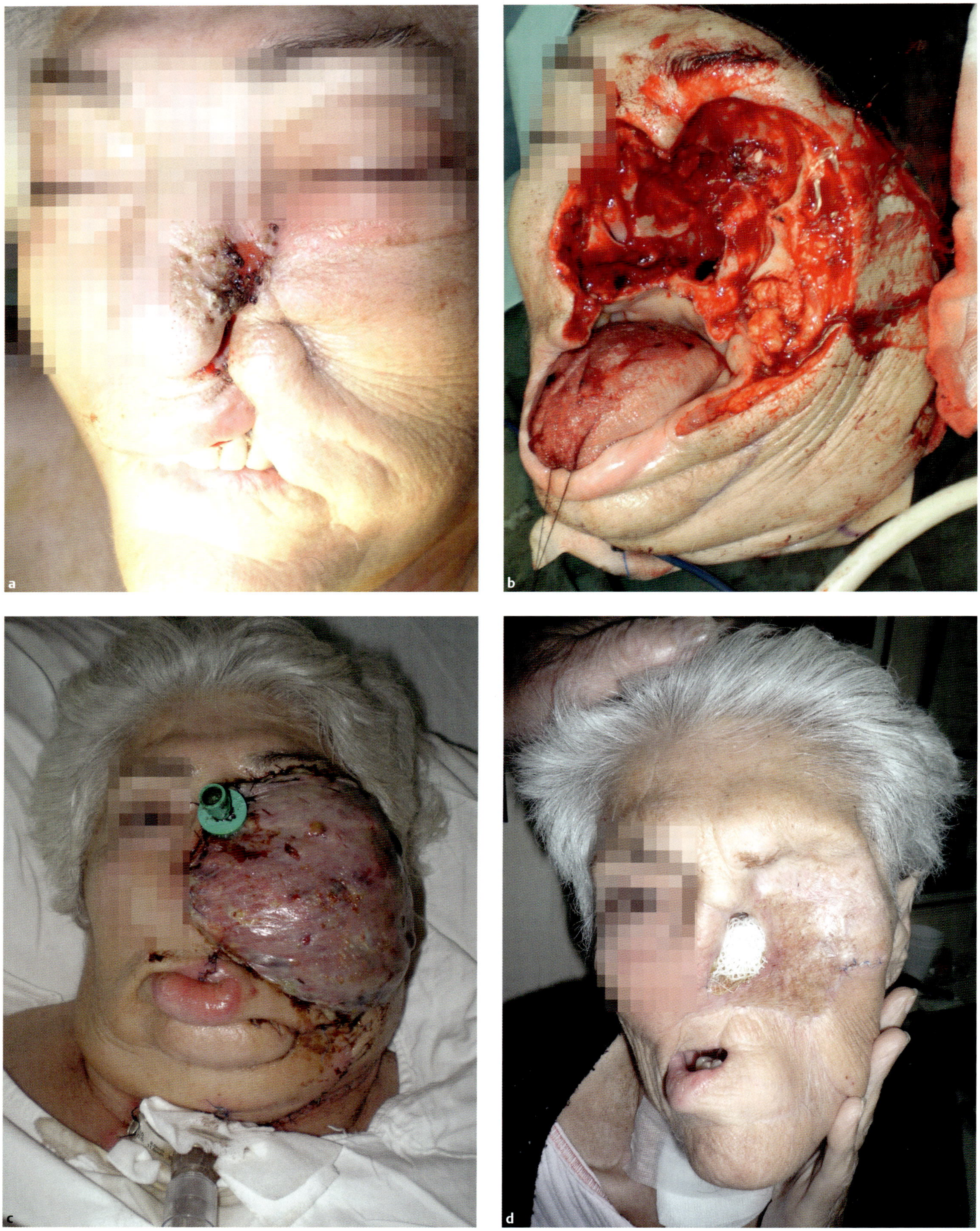

Fig. 10.3a–d Recurrent squamous cell carcinoma of the lateral aspect of the anterior nasal cavity extending to the left maxillary sinus invading the left orbital cavity.
a Clinical presentation. **b** Resection en bloc of the left lateral part of the middle third of the face including the orbit, nose, nasal cavity, maxillary antrum, and ethmoids. **c** The created defect was reconstructed with a latissimus dorsi muscle free flap covered with split thickness skin graft. **d** The patient remains disease free 3 years postoperatively although the aesthetic results are suboptimal.

among 246 patients treated with salvage surgery for recurrent oral and oropharyngeal cancer, with prognosis being associated with recurrent tumor stage and disease-free interval between initial cancer treatment and recurrence. Another study of 68 patients with recurrent oral SCC submitted to salvage surgical treatment with curative intent yielded 1-, 3-, and 5-year disease-free survival rates of 38.1%, 16.3%, and 10.9%, respectively.[38,81] The poorer prognosis of oral cavity and oropharynx recurrences was again confirmed in a study of 96 patients who had recurrence after radiotherapy with a 5-year survival of 25.3% after salvage surgery.[82]

> ! The likelihood of cure for patients who have a recurrence after therapy for T3 and T4 head and neck cancer is low, even with aggressive salvage surgery.

Goodwin's study[44] assessed the value of salvage surgical procedures in the treatment of local and regional recurrence of SCC of the upper aerodigestive tract (UAT). He used two complementary methods of investigation, a meta-analysis of the published literature and a prospective observational study of patients undergoing salvage surgery for recurrent cancer of the UAT. The meta-analysis combined 32 published reports to obtain an estimate of average treatment effect for salvage surgery, whereas the prospective observational study included detailed data in 109 patients who underwent salvage surgery. The meta-analysis comprised 1080 patients from 28 different institutions. The 5-year survival in this group of patients was 39%. In the prospective study of the 109 patients the median disease-free survival was 17.9 months and this correlated strongly with recurrent stage of disease. The stage of the original cancer bore no relationship to survival following salvage surgery. The results observed for the analysis by original site of SCC of the UAT revealed significant differences in median cancer-specific survival. The oral cavity had a 10.4 months survival whereas the larynx had a 30.8 months survival ($P = 0.43$). Survival was also related to whether a patient had received chemotherapy at some point before salvage surgery but not to whether they had received previous radiotherapy or surgery. Patients who had received chemotherapy had a median survival of 8.8 months compared with 26.9 months for those who had not received chemotherapy ($P = 0.0007$).

In the cohort of the 109 observational patients who had salvage surgery for advanced-stage recurrent disease, there was a 40% chance of improvement in quality of life and approximately a 50% chance of living 14 months without recurrence.[44] The rate of complications in later-stage recurrences was above 30%.

In another study, the likelihood of cure for patients who have a recurrence after therapy for T3 and T4 oral cancer is remote, even with aggressive salvage surgery.[83] While the majority of surgically salvaged patients had another recurrence within 1 year, there were occasional patients in whom surgery did lead to prolonged survival. Only one patient out of 48 who had recurrences and underwent treatment for cure was successfully salvaged.[83] Analysis of these patients showed that neither the time to the original recurrence nor the stage of the recurrent tumor was important. Contrary to the results presented by Goodwin[44] that radiotherapy was not associated with low survival, successful salvage was very unlikely if the patient had initially been treated with a combination of surgical resection and postoperative radiation therapy.

Quality of Life

With regard to the overall impact on survival and resulting quality of life (QoL), it is critically important to identify patients with the best prognosis to respond to salvage surgery before such treatment is undertaken. QoL declines immediately after major surgery for treatment of head and neck cancer, and it may take a full year after surgery for QoL to recover to the preoperative level.[44] Patients who underwent salvage surgery and experienced cancer re-recurrence had a mean disease-free interval of only 9 months. It is likely therefore that few of these patients experienced a significant palliative benefit from salvage surgery, on the basis of the short average time course to cancer re-recurrence.

Despite the substantial complications associated with salvage surgery, there is some evidence that patients report an improvement in QoL following salvage surgery. A prospective observational study of 107 patients measured baseline and after-surgery QoL data with two measures, the Functional Living Index for Cancer (FLIC), which is a general measure of QoL, and the Performance Status Scale (PSS) for Head and Neck Cancer Patients, which includes subscales that measure normalcy of diet, understandability of speech, and eating in public.[44] After surgery, 51% of patients showed improvement in FLIC, with a 16% average increase in FLIC score over baseline, achieved over a mean of 4.8 months. The percentages of patients who reached or exceeded their presurgery baseline PSS score for normalcy of diet, understandability of speech, and public eating behavior were 47%, 41%, and 50% with average improvement of 2%–30% over baseline.

Future Research

- To identify the histopathological and molecular parameters that affect the clinical course of patients with oral cancer especially those who have aggressive locoregional disease despite diagnosis at an early stage.
- To classify, evaluate, and introduce into every day clinical practice the prognostic markers that have been generated for predicting the outcome of disease.
- To identify the clinical and biological parameters that can predict response or resistance to specific therapies so that the patients receive appropriate treatment.
- To identify the molecular markers of early recurrence and to incorporate them in the radiographic and radionuclide diagnostic procedures.

Recommended Reading

- Manikantan K, Khode S, Dwivedi RC, et al. Making sense of post-treatment surveillance in head and neck cancer: when and what of follow-up. Cancer Treat Rev 2009;35(8):744–753. (A comprehensive review summarizing the strategies for follow-up, imaging modalities and key investigations in the literature published between 1980 and 2009.)
- de Visscher AV, Manni JJ. Routine long-term follow-up in patients treated with curative intent for squamous cell carcinoma of the larynx, pharynx, and oral cavity. Does it make sense? Arch Otolaryngol Head Neck Surg 1994;120(9):934–939

(A well-designed study that evaluated whether additional curative treatment was possible in patients for whom routine long-term follow-up had led to the early detection of locoregional recurrence, distant metastases, and second primary tumors.)

- Agrawal A, Hammond TH, Young GS, Avon AL, Ozer E, Schuller DE. Factors affecting long-term survival in patients with recurrent head and neck cancer may help define the role of post-treatment surveillance. Laryngoscope 2009;119(11):2135–2140 (The authors found that despite the high compliance with recommended surveillance, survival remains extremely poor for patients with recurrent disease previously treated for advanced stage disease or with those with regional recurrence.)
- Joshi A, Calman F, O'Connell M, Jeannon JP, Pracy P, Simo R. Current trends in the follow-up of head and neck cancer patients in the UK. Clin Oncol (R Coll Radiol) 2010;22(2):114–118. (Despite the fact that there is little benefit after 3-year follow up, most of the clinicians follow up their patients up to a minimum of 5 years, with a significant minority who followed up the patients treated for cancers of the head and neck for longer periods.)
- Kim AJ, Suh JD, Sercarz JA, et al. Salvage surgery with free flap reconstruction: factors affecting outcome after treatment of recurrent head and neck squamous carcinoma. Laryngoscope 2007;117(6):1019–1023. (Patients with recurrent T1 and T2 tumors are the best candidates for salvage surgery and microvascular flap reconstruction for treatment of recurrent SCC of the head and neck.)
- Ang KK, Harris J, Garden AS, et al. Concomitant boost radiation plus concurrent cisplatin for advanced head and neck carcinomas: radiation therapy oncology group phase II trial 99–14. J Clin Oncol 2005;23(13):3008–3015. (Despite the intensification of the treatment, the estimated 2-year locoregional relapse and distant metastasis rates were 34.7% and 16.1%, respectively. The estimated 2-year overall survival and disease-free survival rates were 71.6% and 53.5%, respectively.)
- Goodwin WJ Jr. Salvage surgery for patients with recurrent squamous cell carcinoma of the upper aerodigestive tract: when do the ends justify the means? Laryngoscope 2000; 110(3 Pt 2, Suppl 93)1–18. (The only study with two complimentary methods of investigation: a meta-analysis of the published literature and a prospective observational study of patients undergoing salvage surgery for recurrent cancer of the upper aerodigestive tract.)

References

1. Genden EM, Ferlito A, Silver CE, et al. Contemporary management of cancer of the oral cavity. Eur Arch Otorhinolaryngol 2010;267(7):1001–1017
2. Rapidis AD, Gullane P, Langdon JD, Lefebvre JL, Scully C, Shah JP. Major advances in the knowledge and understanding of the epidemiology, aetiopathogenesis, diagnosis, management and prognosis of oral cancer. Oral Oncol 2009;45(4–5):299–300
3. Andry G, Hamoir M, Leemans CR. The evolving role of surgery in the management of head and neck tumors. Curr Opin Oncol 2005;17(3):241–248
4. Argiris A, Li Y, Forastiere A. Prognostic factors and long-term survivorship in patients with recurrent or metastatic carcinoma of the head and neck. Cancer 2004;101(10):2222–2229
5. Bernier J. Chemoradiation in locally advanced head and neck cancer: new evidence, new challenges. Expert Rev Anticancer Ther 2004;4(3):335–339
6. Cooper JS, Pajak TF, Forastiere AA, et al.; Radiation Therapy Oncology Group 9501/Intergroup. Postoperative concurrent radiotherapy and chemotherapy for high-risk squamous-cell carcinoma of the head and neck. N Engl J Med 2004;350(19):1937–1944
7. Sklenicka S, Gardiner S, Dierks EJ, Potter BE, Bell RB. Survival analysis and risk factors for recurrence in oral squamous cell carcinoma: does surgical salvage affect outcome? J Oral Maxillofac Surg 2010;68(6):1270–1275
8. Bernier J, Domenge C, Ozsahin M, et al. European Organization for Research and Treatment of Cancer Trial 22931. Postoperative irradiation with or without concomitant chemotherapy for locally advanced head and neck cancer. N Engl J Med 2004;350(19):1945–1952
9. Garden AS, Harris J, Vokes EE, et al. Preliminary results of Radiation Therapy Oncology Group 97–03: a randomized phase II trial of concurrent radiation and chemotherapy for advanced squamous cell carcinomas of the head and neck. J Clin Oncol 2004;22(14):2856–2864
10. Bourhis J, Le Maître A, Baujat B, Audry H, Pignon JP. Meta-Analysis of Chemotherapy in Head, Neck Cancer Collaborative Group; Meta-Analysis of Radiotherapy in Carcinoma of Head, Neck Collaborative Group; Meta-Analysis of Chemotherapy in Nasopharynx Carcinoma Collaborative Group. Individual patients' data meta-analyses in head and neck cancer. Curr Opin Oncol 2007;19(3):188–194
11. Manikantan K, Khode S, Dwivedi RC, et al. Making sense of post-treatment surveillance in head and neck cancer: when and what of follow-up. Cancer Treat Rev 2009;35(8):744–753
12. Wong LY, Wei WI, Lam LK, Yuen AP. Salvage of recurrent head and neck squamous cell carcinoma after primary curative surgery. Head Neck 2003;25(11):953–959
13. de Visscher AV, Manni JJ. Routine long-term follow-up in patients treated with curative intent for squamous cell carcinoma of the larynx, pharynx, and oral cavity. Does it make sense? Arch Otolaryngol Head Neck Surg 1994;120(9):934–939
14. Fortin A, Wang CS, Vigneault E. Influence of smoking and alcohol drinking behaviors on treatment outcomes of patients with squamous cell carcinomas of the head and neck. Int J Radiat Oncol Biol Phys 2009;74(4):1062–1069
15. Browman GP, Wong G, Hodson I, et al. Influence of cigarette smoking on the efficacy of radiation therapy in head and neck cancer. N Engl J Med 1993;328(3):159–163
16. Agrawal A, Hammond TH, Young GS, Avon AL, Ozer E, Schuller DE. Factors affecting long-term survival in patients with recurrent head and neck cancer may help define the role of post-treatment surveillance. Laryngoscope 2009;119(11):2135–2140
17. Brockstein B, Haraf DJ, Rademaker AW, et al. Patterns of failure, prognostic factors and survival in locoregionally advanced head and neck cancer treated with concomitant chemoradiotherapy: a 9-year, 337-patient, multi-institutional experience. Ann Oncol 2004;15(8):1179–1186

18. Grégoire V, Lefebvre JL, Licitra L, Felip E; EHNS-ESMO-ESTRO Guidelines Working Group. Squamous cell carcinoma of the head and neck: EHNS-ESMO-ESTRO Clinical Practice Guidelines for diagnosis, treatment and follow-up. Ann Oncol 2010;21(Suppl 5):v184–v186
19. Paniello RC, Virgo KS, Johnson MH, Clemente MF, Johnson FE. Practice patterns and clinical guidelines for posttreatment follow-up of head and neck cancers: a comparison of 2 professional societies. Arch Otolaryngol Head Neck Surg 1999;125(3):309–313
20. Haas I, Hauser U, Ganzer U. The dilemma of follow-up in head and neck cancer patients. Eur Arch Otorhinolaryngol 2001;258(4):177–183
21. Hsu YB, Chu PY, Liu JC, et al. Role of chest computed tomography in head and neck cancer. Arch Otolaryngol Head Neck Surg 2008;134(10):1050–1054
22. Hujala K, Sipilä J, Grenman R. Panendoscopy and synchronous second primary tumors in head and neck cancer patients. Eur Arch Otorhinolaryngol 2005;262(1):17–20
23. Warner GC, Cox GJ. Evaluation of chest radiography versus chest computed tomography in screening for pulmonary malignancy in advanced head and neck cancer. J Otolaryngol 2003;32(2):107–109
24. Joshi A, Calman F, O'Connell M, Jeannon JP, Pracy P, Simo R. Current trends in the follow-up of head and neck cancer patients in the UK. Clin Oncol (R Coll Radiol) 2010;22(2):114–118
25. British Association of Head and Neck Oncologists. Practice care guidance for clinicians participating in the management of head and neck cancer patients in the UK. Drawn up by a Consensus Group of Practising Clinicians. Eur J Surg Oncol. 2001(Suppl A):S1–17
26. [No authors listed] The development of quality of care measures for oral cavity cancer. Arch Otolaryngol Head Neck Surg 2008;134(6):672
27. Boysen M, Lövdal O, Tausjö J, Winther F. The value of follow-up in patients treated for squamous cell carcinoma of the head and neck. Eur J Cancer 1992;28(2–3):426–430
28. Snow GB. Follow-up in patients treated for head and neck cancer: how frequent, how thorough and for how long? Eur J Cancer 1992;28(2–3):315–316
29. Cohan DM, Popat S, Kaplan SE, Rigual N, Loree T, Hicks WL Jr. Oropharyngeal cancer: current understanding and management. Curr Opin Otolaryngol Head Neck Surg 2009;17(2):88–94
30. Gourin CG, Watts T, Williams HT, Patel VS, Bilodeau PA, Coleman TA. Identification of distant metastases with PET-CT in patients with suspected recurrent head and neck cancer. Laryngoscope 2009;119(4):703–706
31. Greven KM, Williams DW III, McGuirt WF Sr, et al. Serial positron emission tomography scans following radiation therapy of patients with head and neck cancer. Head Neck 2001;23(11):942–946
32. Hany TF, Steinert HC, Goerres GW, Buck A, von Schulthess GK. PET diagnostic accuracy: improvement with in-line PET-CT system: initial results. Radiology 2002;225(2):575–581
33. Kao J, Vu HL, Genden EM, et al. The diagnostic and prognostic utility of positron emission tomography/computed tomography-based follow-up after radiotherapy for head and neck cancer. Cancer 2009;115(19):4586–4594
34. Lowe VJ, Boyd JH, Dunphy FR, et al. Surveillance for recurrent head and neck cancer using positron emission tomography. J Clin Oncol 2000;18(3):651–658
35. Kim AJ, Suh JD, Sercarz JA, et al. Salvage surgery with free flap reconstruction: factors affecting outcome after treatment of recurrent head and neck squamous carcinoma. Laryngoscope 2007;117(6):1019–1023
36. Pearlman NW. Treatment outcome in recurrent head and neck cancer. Arch Surg 1979;114(1):39–42
37. Yueh B, Feinstein AR, Weaver EM, Sasaki CT, Concato J. Prognostic staging system for recurrent, persistent, and second primary cancers of the oral cavity and oropharynx. Arch Otolaryngol Head Neck Surg 1998;124(9):975–981
38. Sun GW, Tang EY, Yang XD, Hu QG. Salvage treatment for recurrent oral squamous cell carcinoma. J Craniofac Surg 2009;20(4):1093–1096
39. Liauw SL, Amdur RJ, Morris CG, Werning JW, Villaret DB, Mendenhall WM. Isolated neck recurrence after definitive radiotherapy for node-positive head and neck cancer: salvage in the dissected or undissected neck. Head Neck 2007;29(8):715–719
40. Kowalski LP. Results of salvage treatment of the neck in patients with oral cancer. Arch Otolaryngol Head Neck Surg 2002;128(1):58–62
41. Merkx MA, van Gulick JJ, Marres HA, et al. Effectiveness of routine follow-up of patients treated for T1-2N0 oral squamous cell carcinomas of the floor of mouth and tongue. Head Neck 2006;28(1):1–7
42. Jones AS, Tandon S, Helliwell TR, Husband DJ, Jones TM. Survival of patients with neck recurrence following radical neck dissection: utility of a second neck dissection? Head Neck 2008;30(11):1514–1522
43. Janot F, de Raucourt D, Benhamou E, et al. Randomized trial of postoperative reirradiation combined with chemotherapy after salvage surgery compared with salvage surgery alone in head and neck carcinoma. J Clin Oncol 2008;26(34):5518–5523
44. Goodwin WJ Jr. Salvage surgery for patients with recurrent squamous cell carcinoma of the upper aerodigestive tract: when do the ends justify the means? Laryngoscope 2000; 110(3 Pt 2, Suppl 93)1–18
45. Arnold DJ, Goodwin WJ, Weed DT, Civantos FJ. Treatment of recurrent and advanced stage squamous cell carcinoma of the head and neck. Semin Radiat Oncol 2004;14(2):190–195
46. Head C, Sercarz JA, Abemayor E, Calcaterra TC, Rawnsley JD, Blackwell KE. Microvascular reconstruction after previous neck dissection. Arch Otolaryngol Head Neck Surg 2002;128(3):328–331
47. Singh B, Cordeiro PG, Santamaria E, Shaha AR, Pfister DG, Shah JP. Factors associated with complications in microvascular reconstruction of head and neck defects. Plast Reconstr Surg 1999;103(2):403–411
48. Schusterman MA, Miller MJ, Reece GP, Kroll SS, Marchi M, Goepfert H. A single center's experience with 308 free flaps for repair of head and neck cancer defects. Plast Reconstr Surg 1994;93(3):472–478, discussion 479–480
49. Kim KA, Chandrasekhar BS. Cephalic vein in salvage microsurgical reconstruction in the head and neck. Br J Plast Surg 1998;51(1):2–7
50. Agra IM, Carvalho AL, Pontes E, et al. Postoperative complications after en bloc salvage surgery for head and neck cancer. Arch Otolaryngol Head Neck Surg 2003;129(12):1317–1321
51. Biller HF, Urken M, Lawson W, Haimov M. Carotid artery resection and bypass for neck carcinoma. Laryngoscope 1988;98(2):181–183

52. Miao B, Lu Y, Pan X, Liu D. Carotid artery resection and reconstruction with expanded polytetrafluoroethylene for head and neck cancer. Laryngoscope 2008;118(12):2135–2138
53. Upile T, Triaridis S, Kirkland P, et al. The management of carotid artery rupture. Eur Arch Otorhinolaryngol 2005;262(7):555–560
54. Witz M, Korzets Z, Shnaker A, Lehmann JM, Ophir D. Delayed carotid artery rupture in advanced cervical cancer—a dilemma in emergency management. Eur Arch Otorhinolaryngol 2002;259(1):37–39
55. Skoner JM, Andersen PE, Cohen JI, Holland JJ, Hansen E, Wax MK. Swallowing function and tracheotomy dependence after combined-modality treatment including free tissue transfer for advanced-stage oropharyngeal cancer. Laryngoscope 2003;113(8):1294–1298
56. Huvos AG, Leaming RH, Moore OS. Clinicopathologic study of the resected carotid artery. Analysis of sixty-four cases. Am J Surg 1973;126(4):570–574
57. Ladas G, Rhys-Evans PH, Goldstraw P. Anterior cervical-transsternal approach for resection of benign tumors at the thoracic inlet. Ann Thorac Surg 1999;67(3):785–789
58. Ang KK, Harris J, Garden AS, et al. Concomitant boost radiation plus concurrent cisplatin for advanced head and neck carcinomas: radiation therapy oncology group phase II trial 99–14. J Clin Oncol 2005;23(13):3008–3015
59. Friedlander AH, Federico M, Yueh R, Norman KM, Chin EE. Radiation-associated carotid artery atherosclerosis: case report and review of contemporaneous literature. Spec Care Dentist 2009;29(2):75–79
60. Lango MN, Myers JN, Garden AS. Controversies in surgical management of the node-positive neck after chemoradiation. Semin Radiat Oncol 2009;19(1):24–28
61. Morrissey DD, Andersen PE, Nesbit GM, Barnwell SL, Everts EC, Cohen JI. Endovascular management of hemorrhage in patients with head and neck cancer. Arch Otolaryngol Head Neck Surg 1997;123(1):15–19
62. Ozer E, Agrawal A, Ozer HG, Schuller DE. The impact of surgery in the management of the head and neck carcinoma involving the carotid artery. Laryngoscope 2008;118(10):1771–1774
63. Lee SC, Shores CG, Weissler MC. Salvage surgery after failed primary concomitant chemoradiation. Curr Opin Otolaryngol Head Neck Surg 2008;16(2):135–140
64. Simon C, Goepfert H, Rosenthal DI, et al. Presence of malignant tumor cells in persistent neck disease after radiotherapy for advanced squamous cell carcinoma of the oropharynx is associated with poor survival. Eur Arch Otorhinolaryngol 2006;263(4):313–318
65. Zbären P, Nuyens M, Curschmann J, Stauffer E. Histologic characteristics and tumor spread of recurrent glottic carcinoma: analysis on whole-organ sections and comparison with tumor spread of primary glottic carcinomas. Head Neck 2007;29(1):26–32
66. Shaha AR. Preoperative evaluation of the mandible in patients with carcinoma of the floor of mouth. Head Neck 1991;13(5):398–402
67. Brown JS, Lowe D, Kalavrezos N, D'Souza J, Magennis P, Woolgar J. Patterns of invasion and routes of tumor entry into the mandible by oral squamous cell carcinoma. Head Neck 2002;24(4):370–383
68. Söderholm AL. Oral carcinoma of the mandibular region. Br J Oral Maxillofac Surg 1990;28(6):383–389
69. De Vicente JC, Recio OR, Pendás SL, López-Arranz JS. Oral squamous cell carcinoma of the mandibular region: A survival study. Head Neck 2001;23(7):536–543
70. Ord RA, Sarmadi M, Papadimitrou J. A comparison of segmental and marginal bony resection for oral squamous cell carcinoma involving the mandible. J Oral Maxillofac Surg 1997;55(5):470–477, discussion 477–478
71. Song CS, Har-El G. Marginal mandibulectomy: Oncologic and non-oncologic outcome. Am J Otolaryngol 2003;24(1):61–63
72. Dubner S, Heller KS. Local control of squamous cell carcinoma following marginal and segmental mandibulectomy. Head Neck 1993;15(1):29–32
73. Gulllane PJN, Novak PC. C.B. Management of the mandible in cancer of the oral cavity. Operative Techniques in Otolaryngology 2004;15(4):256–263
74. Archontaki M, Athanasiou A, Stavrianos SD, et al. Functional results of speech and swallowing after oral microvascular free flap reconstruction. Eur Arch Otorhinolaryngol 2010;267(11):1771–1777
75. Dubsky PC, Stift A, Rath T, Kornfehl J. Salvage surgery for recurrent carcinoma of the hypopharynx and reconstruction using jejunal free tissue transfer and pectoralis major muscle pedicled flap. Arch Otolaryngol Head Neck Surg 2007;133(6):551–555
76. Zou H, Zhang WF, Han QB, Zhao YF. Salvage reconstruction of extensive recurrent oral cancer defects with the pectoralis major myocutaneous flap. J Oral Maxillofac Surg 2007;65(10):1935–1939
77. Richey LM, Shores CG, George J, et al. The effectiveness of salvage surgery after the failure of primary concomitant chemoradiation in head and neck cancer. Otolaryngol Head Neck Surg 2007;136(1):98–103
78. Morgan JE, Breau RL, Suen JY, Hanna EY. Surgical wound complications after intensive chemoradiotherapy for advanced squamous cell carcinoma of the head and neck. Arch Otolaryngol Head Neck Surg 2007;133(1):10–14
79. van der Putten L, van den Broek GB, de Bree R, et al. Effectiveness of salvage selective and modified radical neck dissection for regional pathologic lymphadenopathy after chemoradiation. Head Neck 2009;31(5):593–603
80. Agra IM, Carvalho AL, Ulbrich FS, et al. Prognostic factors in salvage surgery for recurrent oral and oropharyngeal cancer. Head Neck 2006;28(2):107–113
81. Lung T, Tăşcău OC, Almăşan HA, Mureşan O. Head and neck cancer, treatment, evolution and post therapeutic survival – Part 2: a decade's results 1993–2002. J Craniomaxillofac Surg 2007;35(2):126–131
82. Netscher DT, Meade RA, Goodman CM, Alford EL, Stewart MG. Quality of life and disease-specific functional status following microvascular reconstruction for advanced (T3 and T4) oropharyngeal cancers. Plast Reconstr Surg 2000;105(5):1628–1634
83. Gleich LL, Ryzenman J, Gluckman JL, Wilson KM, Barrett WL, Redmond KP. Recurrent advanced (T3 or T4) head and neck squamous cell carcinoma: is salvage possible? Arch Otolaryngol Head Neck Surg 2004;130(1):35–38

11 Carcinoma of the Oropharynx

Mark E. Zafereo, Beth M. Beadle, Randal S. Weber

Summary

- Important epidemiological considerations are increasing incidence of oropharyngeal cancer, younger patient population, fewer locoregional recurrences, and increased incidence of distant failure.
- Patients must be carefully selected for salvage surgery, and salvage surgery should be presented to patients within the full context of treatment options, including re-irradiation, palliative chemotherapy, and supportive care.
- Clinical factors most important in salvage surgery selection include recurrent tumor size (T stage), disease-free interval, recurrent overall stage (which takes into account recurrent neck disease), and smoking status.
- With microvascular reconstruction and postoperative ancillary services, patients can achieve baseline quality of life and functional outcomes if they survive their disease. However, many may not survive long enough to achieve this.
- Biomarkers, including human papillomavirus, will likely become important prognostic factors for selecting patients for salvage surgery and represent an exciting area of research.

Epidemiology

Data from the United States National Cancer Institute Surveillance, Epidemiology, and End Results database reveals that over the last two decades oropharyngeal and tongue cancer absolute numbers have increased, while other oral cavity sites and larynx are declining. This trend of increased incidence of primary squamous cell carcinoma of the oropharynx (SCCOP) has largely been reported among nonsmokers and young patients, and has been linked to human papillomavirus (HPV) exposure.[1] Coupled with improvements in multimodality therapy, the changing demographics of patients with SCCOP have led to decreased incidence of locoregional failure and improved overall and disease-specific survival. Drs. H. Gilbert and A.R. Kagan performed a meta-analysis in 1974, reporting 10%–40% disease-free survival for SCCOP.[2] In a recent study of 107 patients with SCCOP treated with chemotherapy and intensity-modulated radiation therapy (IMRT), overall and disease-free survivals were 83% and 81%, respectively, at 3 years.[3]

While SCCOP locoregional failures have decreased, distant failures have potentially increased. In a study of 280 oral cavity and oropharyngeal cancers in Boston, locoregional failure decreased, from 26% between 1988 and 1993 to 16% between 1994 and 1999. Conversely, distant failures increased significantly from 3% to 8% during the same time periods.[4] Similarly, Yao and colleagues studied 66 patients with SCCOP between 2000 and 2004, reporting only 4 patients who developed locoregional recurrence but 15 patients who developed either distant metastases or distant second primary tumors.[5] Prevention, detection, and control of distant metastases and second primary malignancies will therefore become progressively more critical in improving overall patient survival after successful locoregional treatment of SCCOP.

Prognostic Factors

The clinical and biological profile of patients at increased risk for recurrence following treatment for SCCOP has become increasingly important for determining prognosis, identifying tumors for target-specific therapies, and developing treatment alternatives and algorithms. Over the last decade, as the role of HPV in many patients with SCCOP has become gradually more clear, two distinct pathways for development of SCCOP have emerged: the classic alcohol- and tobacco-induced SCCOP, and an alternate pathway for SCCOP development related to HPV.[6] Improved survival for nonsmokers with HPV type 16 (HPV-16)-positive tumors has been consistently demonstrated.[7–10] Higher HPV-16 viral load and higher p16 expression, which may represent a surrogate marker for HPV-16, have also been linked to improved survival in patients with SCCOP.[11–13] Other tumor biological markers that have recently been associated with improved survival for SCCOP patients include lower epidermal growth factor receptor (EGFR) expression and low p53 expression coupled with low Bcl-xL expression (Bcl-xL is an apoptotis-blocking protein that inhibits apoptosis in tumors with wild-type p53).[13] Clinical markers associated with increased risk of locoregional failure in chemoradiation protocols

Table 11.1 Factors that predict locoregional failure in chemoradiation of oropharyngeal squamous cell carcinoma

Factor	Status
T stage	High, especially T4
Sex	Female > male
HPV 16	Negative
HPV viral load/titers	Low
p16 expression	Low (may be surrogate for HPV status)
p53 tumor suppressor gene	Low
Bcl-xL gene expression	High
Pretreatment FDG-PET	SUV > 6
Body mass index	< 25

FDG-PET, ^{18}F-fluorodeoxyglucose positron emission tomography; HPV, human papillomavirus; SUV, standardized uptake value; T, tumor.
From: Current Oncology Reports, Surgical salvage of cancer of the oropharynx after chemoradiation, vol. 11, Jan 1, 2009, p. 152, Bumpous Jeffrey M., table 1, with kind permission from Springer Science +Business Media.

for SCCOP include advanced T-stage,[14] female sex,[15] pretreatment ^{18}F-fluorodeoxyglucose positron emission topography (FDG-PET) SUV greater than 6,[16] and body mass index (BMI) less than 25[17] (**Table 11.1**).[18]

Investigations

Modalities and Timing

Patients are routinely evaluated approximately 6–12 weeks following treatment for SCCOP to assess for locoregional residual disease. Earlier evaluation (6–8 weeks) offers the advantage of early detection of residual disease so that salvage treatment can be initiated quickly before proliferation of resistant tumor cells and extensive fibrosis and scar tissue that develop after treatment. However, later assessment (10–12 weeks) may allow a more accurate assessment of response, as posttreatment inflammation, edema, and tissue distortion from radiation and surgery can limit early detection of recurrence after treatment. Clinical examination alone is generally inadequate to assess treatment response, providing less than 50% accuracy in diagnosing residual disease.[19,20] Posttreatment evaluation should be accompanied by computed tomography (CT) or FDG-PET imaging, but distinguishing viable tumor from tumor necrosis and posttreatment changes with CT or FDG-PET imaging represents a significant challenge after chemoradiotherapy. Direct laryngoscopy with biopsies remains the gold standard for diagnosing locally residual/recurrent disease.

FDG-PET imaging has been increasingly studied over the last decade for monitoring treatment response and assessing residual or recurrent disease after treatment for SCCOP. The negative predictive value of FDG-PET following radiotherapy is generally very high and is associated with a good prognosis,[21–23] whereas the positive predictive value at the primary site is only approximately 50%–75%.[24,25] As FDG-PET positivity is associated with both posttreatment inflammation and residual/recurrent disease, a positive FDG-PET result after chemoradiotherapy must be correlated with the clinical scenario and a biopsy.

PET may be superior in some cases to clinical examination or conventional CT or MRI imaging.[21,26,27] In an Australian study of 78 patients, Martin and others demonstrated PET as significantly better than clinical assessment and conventional imaging ($P < 0.002$, $P < 0.001$, respectively) in restaging patients after chemoradiotherapy.[21] Other studies have shown conventional CT to be equivalent to FDG-PET in evaluating residual or recurrent disease.[28,29] In a large recent prospective trial of 98 patients undergoing FDG-PET 8 weeks after chemoradiation therapy, the authors found that the positive and negative predictive values of FDG-PET-CT were similar to those for CT alone in an unselected study population. However, FDG-PET outperformed conventional CT in assessing selected high-risk HPV-negative patients with tobacco history.[28]

The timing of FDG-PET following completion of chemoradiation is also a subject of controversy. While some authors have suggested accuracy of FDG-PET scanning may increase with longer (10–12 weeks) postradiotherapy intervals,[24,25,30–32] others have described 6–8 weeks as appropriate for posttreatment imaging.[28,33–37] Proponents of earlier imaging contend that earlier detection allows timely initiation of potential salvage therapy before postradiation fibrotic changes and tumor growth, while advocates of later imaging argue that both false positives and false negatives decline with increasing interval between end of therapy and PET imaging. The emerging consensus suggests that waiting 3 months after irradiation offers the best sensitivity and specificity. Early imaging may be considered for selected patients with high risk for residual disease, but PET-FDG positivity must be interpreted cautiously and in combination with the clinical scenario and biopsy results. An algorithm proposed by the Memorial Sloan-Kettering Cancer Center suggests a routine PET-CT at 10–12 weeks post treatment, but a CT or MRI at 4–8 weeks if disease progression is suspected.[24]

Controversies in Postradiation Planned Neck Dissections and FDG-PET Imaging

Planned neck dissections have traditionally been the gold standard for both diagnosing and treating regionally residual disease following chemoradiation therapy, as discrepancies between imaging findings, fine-needle aspiration biopsies, and pathology in neck dissection specimens have led to an argument for planned neck dissections for patients with N2 and N3 neck disease. While planned postradiation neck dissections performed 4–12 weeks after completion of radiotherapy were initially shown to have better outcomes,[38–40] more recent improved locoregional control rates following chemoradiation therapy have called into question the necessity for planned neck dissections in all patients with N2 and N3 disease. Some centers continue to offer planned neck dissections for patients with N2 and N3 disease,[41–44] but others have adopted a more conservative approach, arguing for a more selective approach of planned neck dissection only for patients with N3 disease,[45,46] or electing to observe all patients with a complete radiographic response to therapy, regardless of initial nodal stage.[38,47,48]

Studies have looked at the utility of ultrasound-guided fine-needle aspiration biopsy, CT imaging, and FDG-PET imaging in evaluating patients with neck disease who are observed following chemoradiation therapy. Putten et al. recently found the sensitivity and specificity of ultrasound-guided fine-needle aspiration in postirrradiation patients with suspicion for recurrent/residual neck disease to be only 80% and 42%, respectively, when compared with neck dissection specimens.[49] Several institutions have reported CT imaging to be highly sensitive for posttreatment residual neck disease, allowing good neck control rates in observed patients.[29,38,39,45,48] However, other studies have shown significantly higher regional recurrence rates despite complete responses on CT imaging.[50] Recent discussion and controversy in the literature have focused on the role of FDG-PET imaging in evaluating patients for residual disease after chemoradiation therapy.

FDG-PET scans have been shown in multiple recent retrospective studies to have a very high negative predictive value in evaluating residual lymphadenopathy, and therefore may be a valuable tool in avoiding unnecessary postradiation neck dissections in patients with oropharyngeal lymph node metastases.[21–23,30,35,51–53] A pooled meta-analysis of 13 studies evaluating persistent nodal disease after chemoradiation has reported a pooled mean negative predictive value of 96% for FDG-PET.[25] However, some have expressed concern about the timely identification of patients who will benefit from postradiotherapy neck dissection using

FDG-PET imaging.[54] Several studies have shown FDG-PET to be have a significantly lower sensitivity for detecting residual neck disease 1 month after radiation therapy.[31,55] FDG-PET may be inadequately sensitive to assess treatment response during the early postradiation period (4–6 weeks) when the timing is optimal for a postradiation planned neck dissection.[54] Prospective clinical trials including RTOG 0522.[56] the Ontario Clinical Oncology Group PET PREVENT trial,[57] and the UK PET NECK trial[58] are currently evaluating the role of postchemoradiotherapy FDG-PET in determining the population of patients who benefit from planned neck dissection. Chapter 12 discusses the management of regional recurrence in greater detail.

Principles of Management

Options with Treatment Failure

Patients with distant metastasis are generally treated with chemotherapy and potentially with targeted radiotherapy, depending on the distant site. Treatment options for locally recurrent SCCOP differ depending on the extent of disease and previous treatment.

Options for local SCCOP recurrences following chemoradiation include:

- Surgical salvage
- Re-irradiation with or without chemotherapy
- Palliative chemotherapy
- Supportive care

Options for patients who have local recurrence after treatment of SCCOP with single-modality therapy consisting of surgery alone include:

- Second surgery with postoperative chemoradiation therapy
- Chemoradiation therapy

Patients with regional failure that is surgically resectable should undergo salvage neck dissection. Most patients will have had previous radiotherapy to the neck as part of their primary treatment, and re-irradiation is often not an option due to high associated morbidity and mortality. (Chapter 4 discusses details of the indications and risks of re-irradiation.)

Some institutions advocate interstitial brachytherapy as adjuvant therapy with salvage neck dissections. A recent retrospective case series from MD Anderson Cancer Center reported 67% 2-year disease-free survival and few complications with salvage neck dissection and brachytherapy.[59] For patients with recurrent neck disease who undergo salvage neck dissection, adjuvant chemotherapy should be considered to reduce the risk of distant metastases. Chapter 12 discusses management of isolated regional recurrence in greater detail.

Minimally Invasive Surgical Techniques

In current practice, the vast majority of patients with SCCOP recurrence undergoing treatment will have a traditional, open, en bloc surgical resection with wide margins, with or without regional pedicled or microvascular free flap reconstruction.[60–64]

Transoral Laser Microsurgery

A handful of case series in the recent literature describe transoral laser microsurgery (TLM) resection for recurrent SCCOP, following the principles popularized by Steiner et al.[65] In contrast to the traditional en bloc oncological resection, an incisional resection technique is performed under microscopic guidance, dividing and resecting the tumor piecemeal. TLM proponents argue that in selected patients this technique offers equivalent survival outcomes with lower rates of morbidity and mortality and shortened hospitalizations compared with conventional open surgical resection.[65–68] Several case series have reported TLM in the treatment of recurrent SCCOP, generally in patients who had been previously treated with surgery alone,[65,66] but the inclusion of heterogeneous patient groups with tumors of the oral cavity, larynx, and hypopharynx in these studies makes it difficult to draw any specific conclusions for recurrent SCCOP. Grant et al. published a series including 15 patients with recurrent or persistent tongue base squamous cell carcinoma, approximately half of whom had previously been treated with chemoradiation therapy, reporting 2- and 5-year survivals of 68% and 46%, respectively.[67]

Transoral Robotic Surgery

A second minimally invasive surgical technique, transoral robotic surgery (TORS), has been recently been reported in several case series as a surgical alternative for primary SCCOP,[69,70] but there are only case reports[71] in the literature describing TORS for recurrent SCCOP.

> **!** There is very limited evidence in the literature to make an argument for any minimally invasive surgical resection in the treatment of recurrent SCCOP, even in a patient with limited, early-stage disease without previous chemoradiotherapy. The treatment of recurrent SCCOP with minimally invasive surgical techniques should therefore be reserved for patients enrolled in clinical trials by head and neck surgeons experienced in these techniques.

Patient Selection for Salvage Surgery: Tips and Pitfalls

Clinical Factors

Patient selection is arguably the most challenging aspect of salvage surgery for SCCOP, and the decision process requires the expertise of a multidisciplinary head and neck oncology team as well as medical and surgical intensivists with expertise in preoperative assessment and optimization of medical comorbidities. Patients with distant metastases, carotid artery encasement, prevertebral fascia involvement, or extension to the skull base are very rarely candidates for salvage surgery. In addition to these contraindications for surgery, several other prognostic factors have been shown to influence the effectiveness of salvage surgery for SCCOP. Kim et al. studied factors that influence re-recurrence and survival in 109 patients with predominately oral cavity and oropharyngeal SCC who underwent surgical salvage and free flap reconstruction.[62]

They found that advanced T stage, advanced overall stage, and smoking status were associated with re-recurrence after salvage surgery. On multivariate analysis, smoking status at the time of diagnosis of recurrence was the best predictor of re-recurrence following salvage surgery, with 95% of current smokers developing re-recurrence. Agra et al. also studied prognostic factors for 246 patients who underwent salvage surgery for oropharyngeal and oral cavity SCC and found advanced recurrent overall stage and disease-free interval to be most predictive of re-recurrence.[60]

In the experience of MD Anderson Cancer Center with salvage surgery for 41 patients with recurrent SCCOP, disease-free interval, recurrent T stage, and recurrent neck disease significantly influenced re-recurrence and survival. Patients with a disease-free interval following initial therapy for their tumor who underwent salvage surgery had 3-year overall survival of almost 60%, while those who did not have a disease-free interval had a 3-year overall survival of less than 20%.[63] Even for patients who underwent nonsurgical treatment, the presence of a disease-free interval significantly influenced their life expectancy. Of patients with a disease-free interval who underwent re-irradiation and/or chemotherapy, 80% were alive at 1 year. In contrast, only 30% of these patients were alive at 1 year if they had no disease-free interval. Recurrent tumor (T) stage was another variable predictive of survival in this study. At 3 years, over 60% of surgical salvage patients with recurrent stage T1 and T2 disease were alive, as compared with a little over 20% of surgical salvage patients with recurrent T3 and T4 disease. Examining a subset of 14 salvage surgery patients with both a disease-free interval and small tumors for which it was possible to obtain negative surgical margins, over 70% were alive at 3 years and 45% alive at 5 years. However, this was a highly selected subset of 14 patients, constituting only 3% of the initial 434 patients in the study who presented with locally recurrent oropharyngeal cancer. It should also be noted that only 10% of the cohort of patients presenting with recurrent SCCOP were found to be suitable for salvage surgery in this study.

> **!** The most important clinical factors when considering salvage surgery in a patient with recurrent SCCOP are:
> - Disease-free interval
> - Recurrent T stage
> - Recurrent overall stage (which takes into account whether or not the patient has recurrent neck disease)
> - Smoking status

Patients with distant metastases are very rarely considered candidates for salvage surgery. As illustrated with the MD Anderson experience, few patients will be considered favorable salvage candidates. However, careful selection coupled with comprehensive surgical and reconstructive planning can lead to long-term disease control and survival.

Biological Markers

Looking to the future, perhaps biological markers more than clinical factors will likely help determine which patients are the best candidates for salvage surgery and which patients would be better suited to re-irradiation and/or chemotherapy, or supportive care. Agra et al. retrospectively studied over 100 patients who underwent salvage surgery for recurrent oropharyngeal and oral cavity squamous cell carcinoma, examining both clinical factors and biological markers in association with disease-free survival after salvage surgery.[72] Patients who had a disease-free interval of greater than 1 year and tumors that were epidermal growth factor receptor–negative had an 80% 3-year disease-free survival, while patients who both had a disease-free interval of less than 1 year and EGFR-positive tumors had a 3-year disease-free survival of only 20%. The authors also found that advanced-stage recurrent tumors had a poorer prognosis, and they developed an algorithm for treatment of recurrent squamous cell carcinoma of the oral cavity and oropharynx using all three of these prognostic factors (**Fig. 11.1**). On the basis of their findings, patients without a significant disease-free interval who have a large recurrent tumor that is also EGFR-positive are recommended for nonsurgical treatment. The remainder of the patients are recommended for salvage surgery.

In conclusion, while clinical factors have been well studied in association with prognosis following surgical salvage, biological markers such as EGFR, HPV status, and p16 status represent exciting and promising areas of research in identifying patients best suited for salvage surgery.

> **!** Treatment algorithms incorporating both clinical and biological markers will potentially be used in the future to select the best patients for salvage surgery.

■ Patient Selection for Re-irradiation: Tips and Pitfalls

Although there are promising results that describe long-term survivors of re-irradiation for recurrent head and neck cancers, many of which are oropharynx cancers, these reflect a highly selected group of patients. Choosing which patients will benefit from re-irradiation with a good chance of long-term survival, and acceptable toxicity, becomes challenging. Each patient should be discussed in a multidisciplinary forum to characterize the recurrence, review the prior treatment plan and delivery, and discuss multimodality management. Overall, re-irradiation is never routine and must be respected as a promising but high-risk treatment modality for selected patients.

Importance of Prior Treatment Records and Characterization of Disease with Respect to Prior Treatment

In all cases in which re-irradiation is being considered, the original treatment plan should be obtained from the treating physician. For patients who were treated prior to CT-based planning, the original simulation films should be reviewed, and the integral dose calculated. For those patients treated since 3-D planning became customary, it is important to obtain color images of dose distributions. This will provide the most comprehensive appreciation of the original treatment plan. In addition, the physician's notes during treatment, and ideally a treatment summary, provide further understanding of the course of primary treatment. In addition to the propriety of the dose and volumes in the initial treatment plan, these records will provide information regarding treatment breaks, toxicities experienced during treatment, and general tolerance to radiation during the first course.

The records of the initial definitive radiation treatment will answer questions regarding: (a) whether the original treatment was adequate and well-designed for the initial tumor and (b) whether the treatment delivery was compromised. This will help to define the characteristics of the recurrent disease; recurrence may reflect growth of the tumor despite adequate initial treatment or, alternatively, a failure of the initial treatment due to inadequate targeting (missing the tumor), inadequate dose (marginal miss, design of substandard dose volumes), or inadequate delivery (excessive treatment breaks, poor management of toxicities). As well as assessing the recurrent disease with regard to the original plan, the doses given to adjacent normal tissues need to be assessed. Although it is believed that there is some recovery of radiation tolerance with time, it is unclear to what extent normal tissues "forgive" the prior radiation therapy that they receive. It is therefore crucial that the nominal delivered doses be ascertained from the original treatment plan and taken into consideration for salvage re-irradiation. With the original treatment records at hand, the recurrent disease should be characterized with regard to initial treatment fields. Using physical examination and imaging (including CT, MRI, PET, or a combination), the recurrent disease should be described with regard to the original treatment volumes and doses. Normal tissues should also be assessed using the same modalities. The findings of significant radiation toxicity from the initial treatment, such as neck fibrosis, telangiectasias, or necrosis, should be taken into consideration and weighed carefully when planning salvage radiation therapy.

In general, re-irradiation is limited to patients with isolated local recurrences. However, this is defined differently in different studies, variously based on volume measurements, overlap with prior fields, or general gestalt regarding the size of the recurrence and chance of control with salvage radiation. In general, extensive disease recurrences, for instance those that span several levels of the upper aerodigestive tract or involve disparate lesions, are largely avoided in selecting patients for re-irradiation. This is because the extent of irradiation that would be needed to control such substantial burdens of disease would risk significant treatment-related toxicity, and potentially death.

> ! Re-irradiation is limited to patients with isolated local recurrences.

Importance of Duration of the Recurrence-free Interval

There has been some data suggesting that the longer the interval between initial treatment and recurrence, the better the expectations for re-irradiation. Data from the RTOG 9610 collaborative trial suggested that patients who experience relapse more than 1 year after the initial radiation therapy treatment had better survival than those who were less than 1 year from the prior treatment; the median survival was 9.8 versus 5.8 months, respectively ($P = 0.036$).[73] However, the subsequent study, RTOG 9911, failed to reproduce these results.[74] In this study, patients who had a disease-free interval of more than 36 months prior to relapse had no better outcome than those that relapsed in 36 months or less; the 1-year OS rates were 56.3% vs. 44.6% (P = NS). Similar results were seen in single-institution studies, including recent analysis of the experiences at MDACC[75] and MSKCC.[76] In both cases, the duration of the relapse-free interval did not impact the outcomes of salvage re-irradiation treatment. Of note, the majority of trials, both single-institution and the two large RTOG trials, exclude patients who experience recurrence within 6 months of their initial treatment. It is believed that these patients may have persistent disease and hence should not be considered in the same group as those with a notable disease-free interval.

Although the data have not consistently supported a superior outcome in patients who have been disease-free for a longer period, it is conceptually appealing to believe that patients who had more time between their initial diagnosis/treatment and a recurrence are at an advantage over those patients with less time. In fact, patients with a more remote history of their initial disease and radiation therapy have had more time to heal from the effects of the prior radiation therapy, which may provide increased tolerance to re-irradiation, even if it does not provide a benefit in terms of tumor control.

Overall Guide for Patient Selection

The appropriate selection of patients for re-irradiation is crucial for optimal outcomes. Both the retrospective and the prospective studies have been criticized for having a limited, highly selected pool of patients for enrollment. While the entrance criteria were relatively broad, inherent biases were recognized for enrollment and treatment with re-irradiation. Physicians are more likely to offer the potential risks of re-irradiation in patients with smaller recurrences, who have less toxicity from their original radiation, and who are able to tolerate multimodality salvage therapy with good performance status. In all cases, patients should be discussed in a multidisciplinary forum to create a comprehensive plan for salvage therapy.

Performance Status and Comorbidities

The majority of trials and practice patterns captured in retrospective reviews require candidates for re-irradiation to have good performance status and minimal comorbidities. This makes intuitive sense; patients who are in the best general health are more likely to tolerate re-irradiation, and hence to benefit from it.

Minimal Toxicities from the First Treatment

In addition, multiple studies have required that the patients have minimal toxicity from their original radiation therapy. As enumerated by Puthawala et al., requirements such as intact skin, no deep ulcerations that expose bone or blood vessels, and no hard fibrosis are often implemented to select a group of patients who are less likely to have significant treatment-related toxicity from re-irradiation.[77] Such criteria are important; re-irradiation is likely to be more problematic in patients who have notable residual effects from their first course of radiation.

Tumor Bulk

In addition to general performance status and minimal toxicities from the first treatment, ideal candidates for re-irradiation have limited disease. Although some studies have enumerated specific size limitations for eligibility for re-irradiation, for instance a maximum tumor dimension of 5 cm in Puthawala et al.,[77] others have simply noted that smaller, more confined recurrences are more appropriate for re-irradiation. In the MD Anderson IMRT experience, the recurrences selected for re-irradiation tended to be located in the pharynx (57%) with a median volume of just under 65 cm^3.[75] Although size criteria are not agreed upon, in general, recurrences should be limited in size and be isolated. Extensive disease that involves multiple levels of the pharyngeal axis or with concurrent neck recurrence makes salvage treatment more difficult due to the significantly larger volume that will need to be subjected to re-irradiation. In these settings, it is difficult to spare normal tissues while treating the full extent of disease. For these reasons, extensive or multifocal recurrences are often not ideal candidates for re-irradiation.

Recurrence-free Interval

Finally, the duration of a recurrence-free interval is a controversial topic in the consideration of re-irradiation. Although there are no firm data, it is more attractive to offer re-irradiation to patients with a longer disease-free interval. In fact, the retrospective and prospective studies have specifically excluded patients who have recurred within 6 months since completing their initial definitive treatment. This is appropriate because a recurrence in this time frame would suggest disease persistence or resistance to therapy; in either case, a course of re-irradiation would not be indicated. After 6 months, the longer the interval between initial therapy and recurrence, the more attractive is re-irradiation as a salvage option. A longer interval suggests a better response to the initial treatment and provides a greater opportunity for the normal tissues to heal from the effects of the prior radiation; however, the data do not suggest that this confers a clear benefit in terms of outcome.

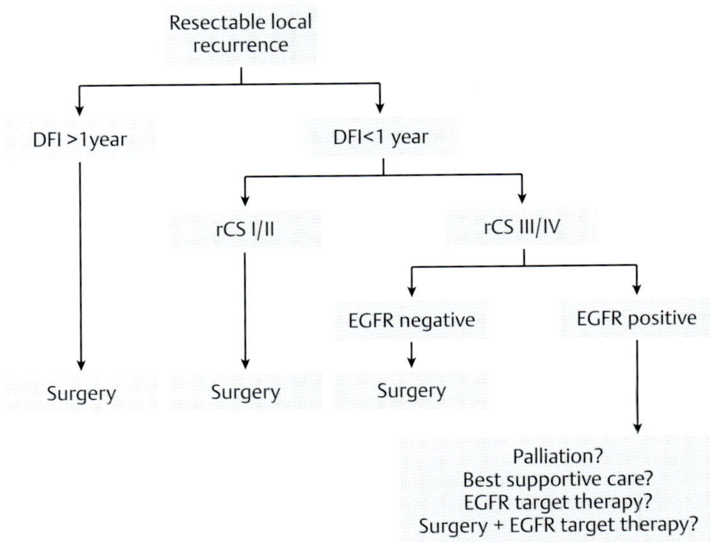

Fig. 11.1 Treatment algorithm for locally recurrent oral and oropharyngeal carcinomas. DFI indicates disease-free interval; EGFR, epidermal growth factor receptor; and rCS, clinical stage of recurrence. (From Agra IMG, Carcalho AL, Pinto CAL, et al. Biological markers and prognosis in recurrent oral cancer after salvage surgery. Arch Otolaryngol Head Neck Surg 2008;134:743–749, with permission from AMA.)

■ Techniques

> ! As transoral robotic surgery and endoscopic transoral laser surgery have yet to be well studied and validated for recurrent SCCOP, almost all cases of recurrent SCCOP are treated with open surgical approaches.

Surgery and Reconstructive Techniques: Tips and Pitfalls

Resection Margins

Resecting pretreatment surgical margins and obtaining negative surgical margins is paramount. In a recent survey of American Head and Neck Society members, around 25% of respondents reported that they resect tumors to the visible recurrence only, rather than to the pretreatment margin, in patients who receive chemotherapy and/or radiotherapy.[78] However, evidence from both clinical and biological studies suggests that resecting pretreatment tumor margins in patients with recurrent SCCOP is essential to achieving long-term local disease control. In the MD Anderson study, all 7 patients who had close or positive surgical margins developed a second recurrence.[63] Histological studies of primary and recurrent laryngeal tumors have suggested that recurrent disease often presents with multicentric tumor foci, dissociated malignant cells in surrounding tissue, and an increased propensity for perineural invasion.[79]

When recurrent SCCOP involves the tongue base and the oral tongue, aggressive margins (generally 2–3 cm) are essential due to the propensity for submucosal tumor spread and the lack of barrier to tumor spread within the tongue musculature. When recurrent SCCOP extends to the posterior base of tongue and vallecula, total laryngectomy is generally necessary to obtain adequate margins. Patients with recurrent SCCOP extending to the midline oral or base of the tongue will require total glossectomy to obtain adequate margins. While total glossectomy does not absolutely necessitate total laryngectomy, laryngeal preservation with total glossectomy has been associated with significant postoperative morbidity and poor survival.[80]

Mandibulotomy and Mandibulectomy

Most salvage surgical oropharyngeal resections require either a mandibulotomy or mandibulectomy. Mandibulectomy is indicated if the tumor invades the periosteum of the mandible or extends to the pterygoid musculature. For patients who do not require a mandibulectomy, a mandibulotomy is usually necessary to allow adequate exposure for wide surgical margins. If postoperative re-irradiation is expected, care should be taken to perform the mandibulotomy anterior to the expected radiation field. In rare cases in which pretreatment margins and recurrent tumor involve only small lesions of the midline base of tongue or oropharyngeal wall (i.e., do not extend laterally to the tonsillar fossa, retromolar trigone, or lateral oropharyngeal wall), a lateral pharyngotomy or lingual-mandibular release (tongue pull-through) approach can be considered. However, since recurrent SCCOP has propensity for

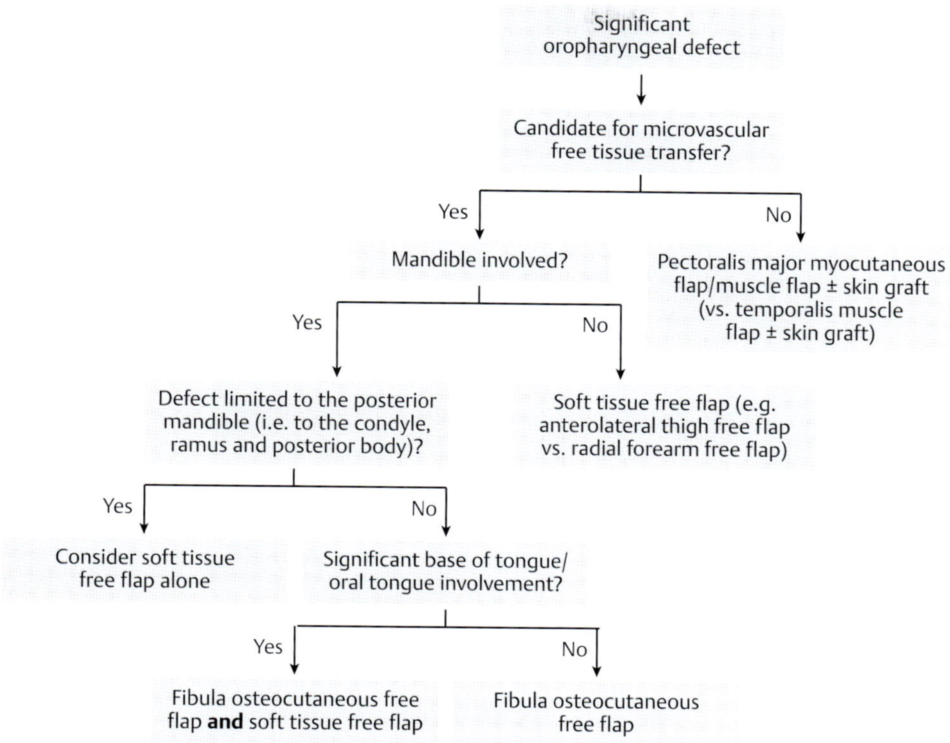

Fig. 11.2 Institutional treatment algorithm for oropharyngeal reconstruction after oncological resection of advanced cancer. (From Zafereo ME, Weber RS, Lewin JS, Roberts DB, Hanasono MM. Complications and functional outcomes following complex oropharyngeal reconstruction. Head Neck 2010;32(8):1003–1011, with permission from John Wiley.)

submucosal tumor spread and tumor islands that often cannot be appreciated on physical examination and preoperative imaging, these approaches are generally not recommended.

Reconstruction and Rehabilitation

Equally important as the decision whether or not to attempt surgical salvage is the choice of reconstruction and rehabilitation following the ablative procedure. Because of large surgical defects in a bed of often previously irradiated tissue, oropharyngeal reconstruction and rehabilitation following salvage surgery represents one of the greatest challenges in the treatment of head and neck cancer. Reconstruction with regional pedicled or microvascular free flaps is preferred over healing by secondary intention, skin grafting, or reconstruction with local flaps because of concerns of insufficient tissue to close large defects, poor healing in previously irradiated tissues, and the development of scar contracture that limits the chance of any postoperative speech and swallowing rehabilitation.[81–83]

Zafereo and others described an MD Anderson Cancer Center institutional treatment algorithm for oropharyngeal reconstruction after oncological resection of advanced cancer (**Fig. 11.2**).[84]

- **Pectoralis major pedicled flaps** are often the best reconstructive option for patients with limited defects, poor-quality recipient vessels (either because of neck dissection or radiation history), significant medical comorbidities, or a poor oncological prognosis.[84–87]
- **Temporalis muscle pedicled flaps** are an alternative regional pedicled flap for patients with limited superior defects, such as of the tonsillar fossa or palate.[88,89]
- **Radial forearm fasciocutaneous free flaps** offer good functional outcomes for limited defects, when the mandible is not involved and the surgical defect is primarily mucosal.[84,90–94]
- **Anterolateral thigh (ALT)**[84,95] or **rectus abdominis**[96–98] **free flaps** offer better coverage for larger defects because they provide more soft tissue bulk to reconstruct the base of tongue, reducing the risk of long-term aspiration.
- **Rectus abdominis flaps** have fallen out of favor at some centers because of increased donor site morbidity including pain limiting deep breathing and clearance of tracheal secretions, risk of abdominal hernia or bulge, difficult primary closure of large donor site wounds, greater propensity for the rectus abdominis muscle to undergo atrophy after free tissue transfer, and difficulty with simultaneous resection and flap harvest with two surgical teams because of the closer proximity of the primary and donor sites.[84]
- **Fibula free flaps** are the most commonly utilized reconstructive option for tumors involving the mandible with extension anteriorly to the body.[84,93,97,98]

> **!** Patients with more extensive defects, adequate recipient vessels, favorable medical status, and an acceptable prognosis have good functional outcomes, and no increased cost or morbidity, with free flap reconstruction.[64,84,87,90–93]

Soft tissue reconstruction alone with an ALT, rectus, or radial forearm free flap is favored for patients with defects limited to the posterior mandible (extending no farther anteriorly than the mid-body) and condyle, as tongue and pharyngeal reconstruction is simplified, trismus is rare, and dental occlusion is comparable to that with bony reconstruction when the condyle is not preserved.[84,96,99] Patients with tumors that involve significant anterior and posterior mandible as well as substantial amounts of tongue and pharyngeal mucosa often undergo reconstruction with simultaneous free flaps, such as a fibula and a radial forearm for smaller tongue defects, or a fibula and an ALT for larger defects involving substantial amounts of the oral tongue or base of tongue.[84,100]

Patients should receive broad-spectrum IV antibiotics (e.g., ampicillin/sulbactam or clindamycin plus levofloxacin) perioperatively and postoperatively during their hospital course. A nasogastric or percutaneous gastrostomy tube is always secured in the operating room if the patient does not have prior enteral feeding access. Uncomplicated patients are generally weaned from the ventilator on the morning following surgery, transferred to the ward on postoperative day 1, and kept in the hospital for approximately 1 week. Smokers and patients with pulmonary disease may require longer intensive care and hospital stays,[84] and aggressive pulmonary management by a critical care team that includes respiratory therapists is essential for these patients. Since most patients have had previous radiation therapy, they remain on enteral tube feeds at home for 4–6 weeks before undergoing a modified barium swallow as outpatients. Most patients have their tracheostomy tube removed during a follow-up visit in clinic 1 week after discharge from the hospital, although some patients are able to be decannulated prior to discharge, and a small minority require a tracheostomy tube for an extended period.

Re-irradiation Techniques: Tips and Pitfalls

When patients are found to be appropriate candidates for re-irradiation after multidisciplinary evaluation, the technical aspects of treatment planning are crucial for good outcomes. The data on re-irradiation involve several different approaches in terms of dose, fractionation, concurrent therapy and technique; many of which have produced promising results.

Dose and Fractionation

There have been several strategies for dose and fractionation in the treatment of patients with salvage re-irradiation. The two large RTOG trials (RTOG 9610 and 9911) and the pioneering work at the University of Chicago have utilized a twice-daily fractionation scheme with a week-on/week-off schedule.[73,74101] In these studies, the prescribed radiation dose was 60 Gy to the gross tumor with margin delivered as two 1.5 Gy fractions each day with at least a 6-hour interval between treatments. Radiation was delivered for 5 days with concurrent chemotherapy followed by a 9-day break; this cycle was repeated four times, for a total dose of 60 Gy. Given that the median dose of prior radiation was 65.2 Gy (range 45–73.8 Gy) in RTOG 9610 and 65.4 Gy (range 45–75 Gy) in RTOG 9911, these patients received a total lifetime dose of radiation in excess of 125 Gy.

More recent retrospective studies, which have employed more modern techniques such as IMRT, have largely treated patients with once-daily re-irradiation. Within the published MSKCC re-irradiation experience of 105 patients, 91 patients received once-daily fractionation and 14 received altered fractionation; a total of 74 out of 105 patients were treated with IMRT.[76] In this series, the median salvage re-irradiation dose was 59.4 Gy (range 30–70 Gy), and the median prior radiation dose was 62 Gy (range 28–78 Gy). In the MD Anderson experience of re-irradiation using exclusively IMRT, 73 out of 74 patients were treated with once-daily radiation therapy in 2 Gy daily fractions.[75] The median radiation dose of retreatment was 60 Gy; the median dose of initial treatment was also 60 Gy. In multivariate analysis, a higher cumulative lifetime radiation dose was associated with improved locoregional control (HR = 0.56). In the majority of cases in both of these studies, treatment with IMRT was given continuously, with once-a-day fractionation of 2 Gy.

In the design of re-irradiation treatment, it is necessary to deliver a curative dose to the recurrent tumor and also to protect normal tissues. The recovery of normal tissues from radiation therapy is not completely understood. While it is believed that there is some degree of forgiveness of prior radiation dose with time, and preclinical studies support this,[102,103] caution must be used in the delivery of additional dose to normal tissues, especially the spinal cord, brainstem, brain, and carotid artery. Without rigorous data regarding the tolerance of human tissues to additional radiation, conservative limits need to be put on normal tissues when planning re-irradiation. In the RTOG trials, the spinal cord was limited to a total lifetime dose of 50 Gy.[73,74] A similar constraint was used in the MSKCC and MD Anderson retrospective series; in addition, the MSKCC group limited the cumulative dose to the brainstem to 60 Gy.[75,76] Although definitive constraints were not elucidated for other normal tissues, in general, care should be taken to limit the doses to normal tissues as much as possible. At times, compromises may need to be made to respect normal tissues and optimize coverage of the target.

Delineation of Treatment Targets

The delineation of targets for re-irradiation requires careful attention to the extent of recurrence, prior fields, and normal tissue. In studies that have utilized conventional fields, including the original University of Chicago studies, RTOG 9610, and some patients on RTOG 9911, the targets were gross disease with a minimum of a 2 cm margin.[73,74101] In general, elective irradiation, including adjacent nodal basins, was not performed. Simulation and some mechanism of immobilization were required on the RTOG studies; however, CT simulation and 3D planning were not mandated. Since these studies spanned several years and mechanisms of immobilization, the planning target volume (PTV) margins varied widely.

When IMRT was integrated into the algorithm for re-irradiation, target delineation became more specific. In the MD Anderson series, the gross tumor volume (GTV) was delineated based on 3D planning.[75] In some cases, additional clinical target volumes (CTVs) were used to cover high-risk areas adjacent to a subclinical dose. Overall, however, elective nodal radiation was avoided. A PTV of 3–5 mm was used to account for set-up error; however, compromises were made close to critical structures, such as the spinal cord. In the MSKCC series, a similar set of criteria was used.[76] The GTV was identified as any visible disease on physical examination or any imaging modality, and the CTV included at least the GTV. PTVs ranged from 1 to 2 cm, and these were also adjusted to account for nearby critical structures.

Given the complexity and risks inherent in re-irradiation, significant care should be taken in the design and implementation of treatment for these patients. With our current standards of technological advancement, patients should be planned using CT simulation with careful immobilization. Although it has not been implemented in prior studies, daily imaging guidance may offer additional comfort in treating these patients by ensuring precise set-up prior to daily treatment delivery. When treatment is being planned, all methods of visualizing the tumor should be integrated, including physical examination and radiography. The GTV should be delineated on the planning scans. A margin of approximately 8 mm to 2 cm, depending on clinical judgment, may be added to account for adjacent subclinical disease. Finally, a PTV should be added that reflects the proven set-up error for a given immobilization at a given treatment facility, as this will vary. Generally, elective nodal irradiation has not been implemented in re-irradiation cases. Gross disease, with a margin for subclinical extent, has typically been the target of interest for curative doses, allowing maximal sparing of adjacent normal tissues.

Utilization of Concurrent or Adjuvant Treatments

Re-irradiation has been used as salvage therapy as a single modality with promising results; however, the use of re-irradiation in conjunction with other treatments has shown even better outcomes. Overall, multidisciplinary evaluation is necessary to decide on the best combination of treatments for a given patient.

The use of concurrent chemotherapy with re-irradiation is largely based on extrapolated data from studies of definitive radiation. The two large RTOG trials (RTOG 9610 and 9911) have both involved the use of concurrent chemoradiation as salvage therapy. In RTOG 9610, the patients were treated with concurrent 5-fluorouracil and hydroxyurea.[73] In RTOG 9911, the patients were treated with concurrent cisplatin and paclitaxel.[74] The smaller retrospective studies have included populations that are treated with and without concurrent chemotherapy. In the MD Anderson experience, 49% of patients received chemotherapy with their salvage re-irradiation; there was no impact on locoregional control or overall survival comparing those patients treated with chemotherapy and those that were not.[75] In the MSKCC experience, 71% of patients received chemotherapy as part of their salvage treatment.[76] There was no statistically significant association with longer progression-free survival in these patients treated with chemotherapy. It is difficult, however, to use the retrospective data to support or refute the use of chemotherapy as part of salvage re-irradiation, due to a clear selection bias. Although a rigorous investigation of the additional benefit of chemotherapy versus radiation alone has not been performed in the salvage setting, data showing the benefit of concurrent treatment in definitive cases is compelling.[104] In patients in whom concurrent chemotherapy is possible, from a toxicity and performance status perspective, its use is often favored. Chapter 4 discusses in greater detail the role of chemotherapy in the management of recurrence.

Multiple studies of re-irradiation for recurrent head and neck cancer have looked at the impact of surgical resection as part of multidisciplinary management. Within the compiled University of Chicago experience of 115 patients, 49 underwent salvage surgery as part of their treatment, followed by concurrent chemo–re-irradiation.[101] Those patients who were treated with surgery had significantly improved overall survival, progression-free survival, and locoregional control compared with those who did not. In the MSKCC experience of 105 patients with recurrent head and neck cancers treated with re-irradiation, 36 patients (34%) had surgery immediately prior to re-irradiation; of these, 25 had gross total resection of their recurrent disease.[76] There was a trend toward better locoregional progression-free survival in patients who underwent surgical resection (HR = 0.61; P = 0.088). In the MD Anderson experience of 78 patients treated with IMRT for salvage re-irradiation, 20 patients (27%) received salvage surgery[75]; there was no correlation in this retrospective series between salvage surgery and improved outcome. Although there is some discrepancy, patients who are candidates for surgical resection of their recurrent oropharyngeal disease should have this performed, if it can be done with minimal morbidity.

Outcomes

Salvage Surgery

Survival

Reviews of the effectiveness of salvage surgery for patients with locoregionally recurrent SCCOP are rare in the literature. Because of small patient populations and ethical considerations, there are no randomized or prospective studies in the literature directly comparing salvage surgery with nonsurgical treatment for recurrent SCCOP. Most often, recurrent SCCOP is analyzed retrospectively in conjunction with advanced primary SCCOP or recurrences at other head and neck sites, most of which have better survival than recurrent SCCOP.

In the 1970s, Gilbert and Kagan reported that fewer than 10% of recurrent tonsillar SCC were successfully surgically salvaged.[2] Although surgical reconstruction of large oropharyngeal defects has become increasingly possible over the past several decades because of advances in microvascular reconstructive techniques, rates of successful surgical salvage for SCCOP have only slightly increased. In a meta-analysis published in 2000, Goodwin reviewed patients with recurrent pharyngeal cancer previously treated definitively with radiation, reporting only 25% recurrence-free survival at 2 years and 26% overall survival at 5 years.[61] Patients with recurrent pharyngeal cancer who underwent surgical salvage had higher recurrence and lower survival than similar patients with recurrent oral cavity or larynx cancer. Similarly, in a recent cohort of 106 patients with predominately recurrent oral cavity and oropharyngeal carcinoma who underwent surgical salvage with microvascular reconstruction, Kim et al. reported that 74% of patients developed a second recurrence an average of only 9 months after undergoing salvage surgery.[62]

In a recent comprehensive review of salvage surgery for SCCOP at MD Anderson Cancer Center, 3-year overall and recurrence-free survivals after salvage surgery were 42% and 26%, respectively.[63] Additionally, the authors compared overall survival after salvage surgery with overall survival after other treatment options (re-irradiation, palliative chemotherapy, or supportive care only). While these treatment groups were not directly comparable, as this was a retrospective study with inherent selection bias, the study places salvage surgery within the context of other treatment options. There was no statistically significant difference in survival among patients who had salvage surgery versus those who were re-irradiated, and 3-year overall survival was less than 10% for patients who had palliative chemotherapy or supportive care only (**Fig. 11.3**).

Quality of Life and Functional Outcomes

Quality of life and functional outcomes are closely tied to the ability to perform an adequate reconstruction, and there is evidence that, while re-recurrence and survival are important when evaluating the effectiveness of salvage surgery, quality of life may be

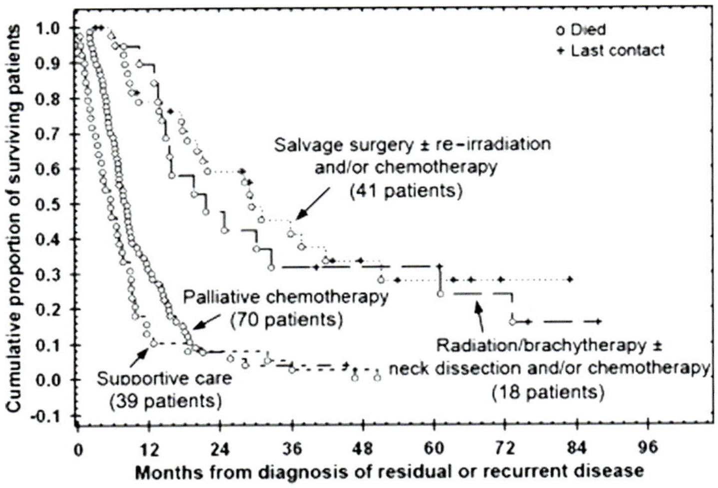

Fig. 11.3 Overall survival illustrated for 168 patients with recurrent squamous cell carcinoma of the oropharynx stratified by treatment type: salvage surgery versus re-irradiation ($P = 0.59$), salvage surgery versus palliative chemotherapy or supportive care ($P < 0.001$), re-irradiation versus palliative chemotherapy or supportive care ($P < 0.001$), and palliative chemotherapy versus supportive care ($P = 0.10$). ± Indicates "with or without." (From Zafereo ME, Hanasono MM, Rosenthal DI, Sturgis EM, Lewin JS, Roberts DB, Weber RS. The Role of Salvage Surgery in Recurrent Oropharyngeal Squamous Cell Carcinoma. Cancer 2009;115(24):5723–5733, with permission from John Wiley.)

an even more important concern. List et al. presented a study of principal concerns of head and neck cancer patients at the time of *initial* diagnosis, finding that survival far outweighed other considerations, including functional concerns such as speech and swallowing.[105] However, it has been suggested that this balance of patient concerns shifts with recurrent disease such that pain and overall quality of life become the most important considerations, as patients perhaps become more realistic about chances of long-term survival.[106] This may be especially true for recurrent SCCOP, which has a poorer prognosis for cure than recurrence at other head and neck cancer sites such as the oral cavity or larynx.

For recurrent SCCOP, it is therefore important to evaluate functional outcomes in the context of survival. Netscher et al. studied quality of life and disease-specific functional status following microvascular reconstruction in 34 patients with advanced primary pharyngeal cancer and found that most patients return to baseline functional status by 6 months after extensive surgery and surpass pretreatment thresholds by 1 year.[64] In comparison, median time to re-recurrence after salvage surgery for recurrent SCCOP is approximately 8 months.[62,63,105] Therefore, many patients will develop recurrent disease before they achieve or surpass their baseline functional status.

In a prospective observational study, Goodwin specifically studied the percentage of patients who were able to achieve a return to their baseline function following salvage surgery.[61] He utilized the Functional Living Index for Cancer (FLIC), a commonly used quality of life assessment, as well as performance scales for normalcy of diet, intelligibility of speech, and eating in public. For recurrent pharyngeal cancer, while half of patients were able to achieve return to their baseline FLIC score, only one-third were able to achieve a return to their baseline diet, speech, and public eating scores.

Zafereo et al. retrospectively studied functional outcomes in 41 SCCOP salvage surgery patients at MD Anderson Cancer Center.[63] Approximately 80% of patients were able to continue oral speech following surgical salvage, while 20% used an electrolarynx, tracheoesophageal prosthesis, or writing. About one-third of patients tolerated oral feeding without a feeding tube, another one-third remained partially dependent on their feeding tube, and one-third were completely feeding tube dependent. Of patients who had a tracheotomy, almost 90% were decannulated. While these are acceptable functional outcomes following large surgical resection and reconstruction, they must be considered in context of a 67% re-recurrence rate at a median of 8 months following surgical salvage. In this light, for most of the patients who had re-recurrence following surgical salvage, either they did not achieve their baseline functional status or the achievement of baseline functional status quickly deteriorated due to recurrent disease.

Case Study

A 65-year-old woman with a history of chemoradiation therapy 2 years previously for a T3N2b SCC of the right tonsillar fossa presented with new right otalgia and odynophagia.

Physical examination and CT scan revealed recurrent cancer involving the tonsillar fossa, soft palate, lateral maxilla, retromolar trigone, and posterior mandible.

She underwent a right oropharyngeal composite resection that included a right infrastructure maxillectomy and a right segmental mandibulectomy (**Fig. 11.4**) and was reconstructed with an anterolateral thigh microvascular free flap (**Fig. 11.5**). The lower lip-splitting incision was necessary for adequate exposure. Reconstructive considerations in this case included the patient's age and a history of significant peripheral vascular disease which precluded harvest of a free fibula flap. Elderly patients, or those patients with poor performance status or peripheral vascular disease, often undergo soft tissue reconstruction alone, even for defects that extend to the anterior mandible. Patients who undergo vascularized soft tissue reconstruction often have functional outcomes equivalent to patients with vascularized bony reconstruction.[107] However, for defects that extend to the anterior mandible in young patients with good performance status, vascularized bony reconstruction remains the standard of care.

The patient's Dobhoff tube was removed 3 weeks following surgery after a modified barium swallow indicated no leak. She takes all of her nutrition orally with a 40 mm interincisor mouth opening and a 10 mm crossbite.

At 3 years following surgery, she remains without evidence of disease. **Figure 11.6** illustrates the postoperative result 1 month after surgery.

Complications

Postoperative complications are common in patients undergoing salvage surgery for SCCOP, occurring in about 50% of patients. Perioperative deaths have been reported in 0%–3% of patients, related to pneumonia, stroke, infection, and carotid artery blowout. For patients who undergo microvascular free flap reconstruction, total flap loss is rare, occurring in 0%–7% of patients. Most common postoperative complications include wound infection/dehiscence, fistula, and pneumonia.[63,84,108–110]

Cost

In Goodwin's meta-analysis, surgical salvage of recurrent pharyngeal cancer was more costly than surgical salvage of other

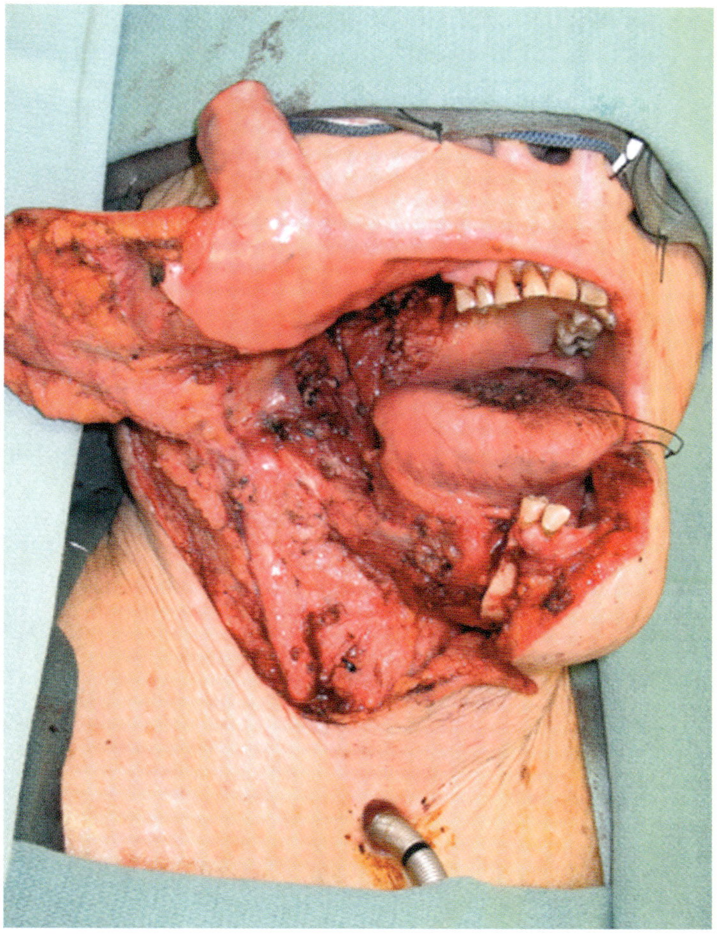

Fig. 11.4 Surgical defect in a 65-year-old woman with recurrent right tonsil squamous cell carcinoma involving the tonsillar fossa, base of tongue, and posterior mandible. The oropharyngeal composite resection included a right infrastructure maxillectomy and a right segmental mandibulectomy. (Photograph courtesy of Dr. Matthew Hanasono, The University of Texas MD Anderson Cancer Center.)

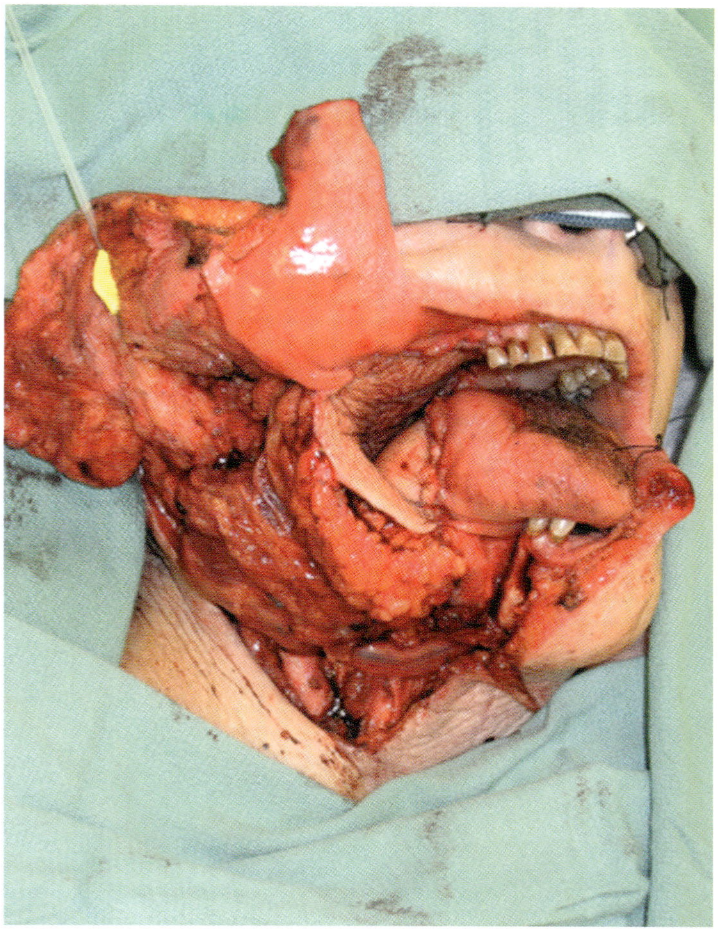

Fig. 11.5 Anterolateral thigh free flap reconstruction of a right oropharyngeal defect in a 65-year-old woman who underwent oropharyngeal composite resection for recurrent tonsil squamous cell carcinoma. (Photograph courtesy of Dr. Matthew Hanasono, The University of Texas MD Anderson Cancer Center.)

head and neck sites, with average hospital and physician charges of $86 000 per patient.[61] Similarly, in the MD Anderson Cancer Center study of recurrent oropharyngeal cancer, average hospital and physician charges during the first 30 days averaged $82 500 per patient.[63] While economic factors do not take priority when considering the individual patient, societal expenditures for expensive interventions with unproven benefit will likely become increasingly scrutinized with rising costs of health care and limited private and government health-care dollars.

External Beam Re-irradiation with Chemotherapy: Survival Outcomes and Complication Rates

Five-year overall survival rates as high as 20% have been reported for re-irradiation in the setting of recurrent head and neck cancer, although up to one-third of patients can experience severe or fatal complications.[111] Almost all studies in the literature include multiple head and neck sites, including two recent Radiation Therapy Oncology Group trials that included 40%–50% recurrent oropharyngeal cancer patients.[73,74] RTOG 9610 was the first prospective multi-institutional trial evaluating re-irradiation combined with chemotherapy consisting of 5-fluorouracil and hydroxyurea for recurrent squamous cell carcinoma of the head and neck.[73] With 79 patients, 2- and 5-year survivals were 15% and 4%, respectively. Twenty-five percent of patients experienced at least grade 4 acute toxicity, and there were six (8%) treatment-related deaths. A second phase II prospective, multi-institutional study, RTOG 9911, accrued 105 patients who underwent re-irradiation combined with cisplatin and paclitaxel.[74] Median survival was 1 year and 25% of patients were alive at 2 years. Grade 4 or higher treatment toxicity occurred in 28% of patients, and over 10% of patients had fatal treatment-related complications.

More recent technological improvements in radiation delivery, namely IMRT, have been implemented in single-institution series of salvage re-irradiation. IMRT allows the delivery of high doses to target volumes and attempts to minimize doses to adjacent normal tissues by utilizing multiple beams that are individually adjusted through the treatment delivery. The use of IMRT for the treatment of recurrent head and neck cancers at Memorial Sloan-Kettering Cancer Center (MSKCC) was reviewed in 2007; in a series of 105 patients with recurrent disease, 21 of these patients had oropharynx cancers.[76] A total of 74 patients (70%) were treated with IMRT for salvage, with a median re-irradiation dose of 59.4 Gy; a total of 75 patients were treated with concurrent chemotherapy as well (largely platinum-based). The 2-year overall survival rate was 37%. Patients treated with IMRT had a better 2-year locoregional progression-free survival (20% vs. 52%; $P < 0.001$), and patients without locoregional failure had better overall survival. This study

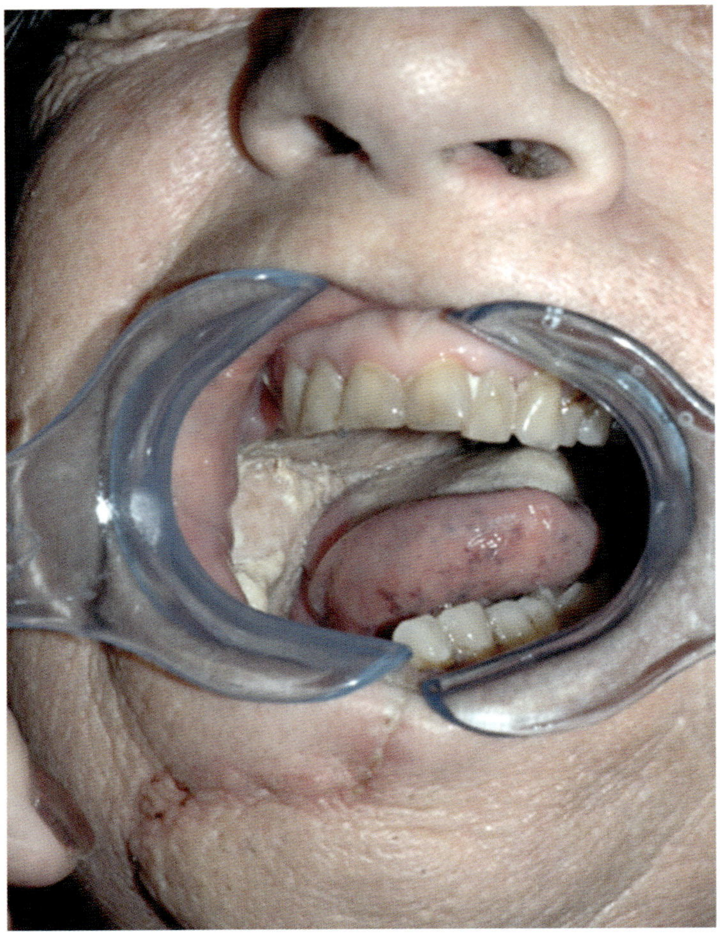

Fig. 11.6 Postoperative result 1 month after right oropharyngeal composite resection and anterolateral thigh free flap reconstruction for a 65-year old woman with recurrent tonsil squamous cell carcinoma. (Photograph courtesy of Dr. Matthew Hanasono, The University of Texas MD Anderson Cancer Center.)

suggested that IMRT was not only feasible, but beneficial, in the setting of re-irradiation.

The experience at the MD Anderson Cancer Center described a series of 74 patients treated with salvage IMRT.[75] Of these, 41% of patients had oropharynx cancers. Twenty-seven percent of patients received surgical salvage as well, and 49% received chemotherapy. The median re-irradiation dose was 60 Gy. With a median follow-up of 25 months, the 2-year overall survival and locoregional control rates were 58% and 64%, respectively. Twenty percent of patients had severe treatment-related toxicities. On both univariate and multivariate analyses, there was no correlation with the site of the primary tumor and outcomes.

Overall, external beam radiation therapy, typically with concurrent chemotherapy, has been implemented as salvage therapy for recurrent oropharynx cancers with some degree of success. The single-institution and collaborative studies suggest that toxicities are high; however, there is a potential for long-term disease control in carefully selected patients who understand the risks and benefits of this approach.

■ Brachytherapy

Interstitial brachytherapy using a catheter-based technique has also been studied for treatment of recurrent oropharyngeal cancers in previously irradiated tissues. Brachytherapy offers a significant theoretical benefit over external beam radiation therapy in the setting of re-irradiation; the implantation of radioactive wires directly into the tissue allows for the delivery of high doses of radiation in a localized area, while the rapid dose fall-off minimizes the dose delivered to nearby (previously irradiated) normal tissues.

Several single-institution experiences using brachytherapy for re-irradiation of head and neck cancers have been published.[77,112,113] Peiffert and associates described the use of salvage brachytherapy in the treatment of velotonsillar cancers in previously radiated fields.[113] A total of 73 patients were treated with iridium-192 interstitial implants alone to a dose of 60 Gy as salvage treatment. The 5-year local control was 80% for T1 tumors and 67% for T2 tumors; the 5-year overall survival was 30%. There were no grade 3 or 4 complications reported; 42% of patients died of other cancers. The authors conclude that brachytherapy is an optimal treatment for tonsillar cancers that develop in prior radiation fields and caution that these patients are at high risk for subsequent malignancies.

In another single-institution experience, Puthawala and colleagues described their use of brachytherapy as salvage treatment for 220 patients with recurrent head and neck cancers.[77] Of these patients, 104 patients (47%) had disease in the oropharynx. The salvage treatment consisted of a low–dose rate afterloading iridium-192 implant; the median minimum tumor dose was 53 Gy. Forty percent of patients received concurrent chemotherapy, and 60% received interstitial hyperthermia. Overall, the 5-year overall survival rate was 21.7%; moderate to severe late toxicities occurred in 27% of patients. Local control at 5 years was 51%. Looking at the local control by subsite, local control was achieved in 2/2 patients with soft-palate recurrences (100%), 13/20 tonsillar recurrences (65%), and 39/45 base of tongue recurrences (87%).

In a more modern series, MSKCC has reported the use of high-dose rate brachytherapy (HDR) in the treatment of recurrent and previously irradiated head and neck cancers.[114] In this study, 30 patients were treated with HDR, with or without external beam radiation; 5 patients had oropharynx tumors. The 2-year local control (LC) for the entire group was 71%, with a 2-year OS of 63%. Patients treated with surgical resection and HDR had better local control than those who did not receive surgery. A total of six grade 2 and four grade 3 complications were observed. The authors conclude that HDR provides promising local control for patients with recurrent head and neck cancers along with acceptable toxicities; they also note that surgical resection, if possible, improves outcomes.

Brachytherapy is a feasible method of delivering salvage radiation in the setting of recurrent oropharyngeal cancers, but its adoption has been limited. Although it is theoretically appealing, and individual institutions have perfected its implementation, treatment delivery is technically challenging and heavily dependent on the skills of the treating physician. In addition, like external beam radiation therapy for salvage, the selection of patients who will benefit from this technique is crucial to long-term outcomes.

■ Survival Outcomes with Palliative Chemotherapy and Supportive Care

Although chemotherapy alone can provide palliation in patients with recurrent SCCOP, it is not a curative option. Approximately one-third of patients with recurrent squamous cell carcinoma of the oropharynx have a partial response to platinum-based chemotherapy regimens.[115] For recurrent SCCOP treated with chemotherapy, median survival ranges from 4 to 6 months, and 2-year overall survival is 5%–10%.[115] A recent, multicenter, randomized, prospective clinical trial of 442 patients with untreated recurrent or metastatic squamous cell carcinoma of the head and neck in the *New England Journal of Medicine* indicated that patients who received cetuximab plus platinum–fluorouracil chemotherapy had almost 3 months survival benefit (11.1 months vs. 7.4 months) compared with patients who received platinum–fluorouracil chemotherapy alone, with no increase in toxicity.[116]

For patients who forego any treatment for recurrent SCCOP, the median survival can be estimated at 3–4 months. Kowalski et al. studied almost 200 patients with advanced or recurrent oropharyngeal cancer in Brazil who were given supportive care but no oncological treatment secondary to advanced tumor stage, poor performance status, or patient refusal of treatment. Median survival was 4 months, and only 2% of patients were alive at 1 year.[117] Stell reported median survival of approximately 3 months in a case series of over 4000 untreated head and neck cancer patients in Liverpool over a 25-year period.[118] In both the Brazil and Liverpool studies, performance status was the best indicator of survival time.[117,118]

Future Research

- Human papillomavirus status as a prognostic indicator for success of salvage treatments.
- Molecular markers for predicting favorable salvage treatment candidates and selection strategies for salvage treatment based on tumor biology.
- Utility, timing, and cost-effectiveness of PET-CT in monitoring response to chemoradiation therapy and in predicting favorable surgical salvage candidates.
- Advances in chemotherapy and radiotherapy regimens to reduce toxicity and increase effectiveness of treatment.

Recommended Reading

- Kumar B, Cordell KG, Lee JS, et al. EGFR, p16, HPV Titer, Bcl-xL and p53, sex, and smoking as indicators of response to therapy and survival in oropharyngeal cancer. J Clin Oncol 2008;26(19):3128–3137. (A prospective analysis of HPV and other clinical and biological prognostic factors predicting recurrence and survival following chemoradiation therapy for SCCOP.)
- Goodwin WJ Jr. Salvage surgery for patients with recurrent squamous cell carcinoma of the upper aerodigestive tract: when do the ends justify the means? Laryngoscope 2000; 110(3 Pt 2, Suppl 93)1–18. (A prospective observational study and meta-analysis of salvage surgery for head and neck SCC. Includes recurrence and survival outcomes and quality of life and cost comparisons among recurrences at different head and neck sites.)
- Zafereo ME, Hanasono MM, Rosenthal DI, et al. The role of salvage surgery in patients with recurrent squamous cell carcinoma of the oropharynx. Cancer 2009;115(24):5723–5733. (A comprehensive retrospective review of salvage surgery for recurrent SCCOP, with a comparative review of patients undergoing nonsurgical treatment modalities and supportive care.)
- Zafereo ME, Weber RS, Lewin JS, Roberts DB, Hanasono MM. Complications and functional outcomes following complex oropharyngeal reconstruction. Head Neck 2010;32(8):1003–1011 (A comprehensive retrospective review of microvascular free flap and pectoralis muscle flap reconstruction of oropharyngeal defects. Includes a treatment algorithm for complex oropharyngeal reconstruction.)
- Agra IMG, Carvalho AL, Pinto CAL, et al. Biological markers and prognosis in recurrent oral cancer after salvage surgery. Arch Otolaryngol Head Neck Surg 2008;134(7):743–749 (A retrospective cohort study analyzing prognostic markers for recurrence and survival after treatment for recurrent SCCOP. Includes a treatment algorithm combining biological and clinical prognostic factors.)
- Langer CJ, Harris J, Horwitz EM, et al. Phase II study of low-dose paclitaxel and cisplatin in combination with split-course concomitant twice-daily reirradiation in recurrent squamous cell carcinoma of the head and neck: Results of Radiation Therapy Oncology Group Protocol 9911. J Clin Oncol. 2007;25(30):4800–4805 (An RTOG prospective phase II study of chemoradiation for recurrent head and neck cancer, including 40% with recurrent SCCOP.)

References

1. Sturgis EM, Cinciripini PM. Trends in head and neck cancer incidence in relation to smoking prevalence: an emerging epidemic of human papillomavirus-associated cancers? Cancer 2007;110(7):1429–1435
2. Gilbert H, Kagan AR. Recurrence patterns in squamous cell carcinoma of the oral cavity, pharynx, and larynx. J Surg Oncol 1974;6(5):357–380
3. Daly ME, Le QT, Maxim PG, et al. Intensity-modulated radiotherapy in the treatment of oropharyngeal cancer: clinical outcomes and patterns of failure. Int J Radiat Oncol Biol Phys 2010;76(5):1339–1346
4. Taneja C, Allen H, Koness RJ, Radie-Keane K, Wanebo HJ. Changing patterns of failure of head and neck cancer. Arch Otolaryngol Head Neck Surg 2002;128(3):324–327
5. Yao M, Nguyen T, Buatti JM, et al. Changing failure patterns in oropharyngeal squamous cell carcinoma treated with intensity modulated radiotherapy and implications for future research. Am J Clin Oncol 2006;29(6):606–612
6. D'Souza G, Kreimer AR, Viscidi R, et al. Case-control study of human papillomavirus and oropharyngeal cancer. N Engl J Med 2007;356(19):1944–1956
7. Gillison ML, Koch WM, Capone RB, et al. Evidence for a causal association between human papillomavirus and a subset of head and neck cancers. J Natl Cancer Inst 2000;92(9):709–720
8. Licitra L, Perrone F, Bossi P, et al. High-risk human papillomavirus affects prognosis in patients with surgically treated oropharyngeal squamous cell carcinoma. J Clin Oncol 2006;24(36):5630–5636
9. Mellin H, Friesland S, Lewensohn R, Dalianis T, Munck-Wikland E. Human papillomavirus (HPV) DNA in tonsillar cancer: clinical correlates, risk of relapse, and survival. Int J Cancer 2000;89(3):300–304

10. Lindel K, Beer KT, Laissue J, Greiner RH, Aebersold DM. Human papillomavirus positive squamous cell carcinoma of the oropharynx: a radiosensitive subgroup of head and neck carcinoma. Cancer 2001;92(4):805–813
11. Worden FP, Kumar B, Lee JS, et al. Chemoselection as a strategy for organ preservation in advanced oropharynx cancer: response and survival positively associated with HPV16 copy number. J Clin Oncol 2008;26(19):3138–3146
12. Cohen MA, Basha SR, Reichenbach DK, Robertson E, Sewell DA. Increased viral load correlates with improved survival in HPV-16-associated tonsil carcinoma patients. Acta Otolaryngol 2008;128(5):583–589
13. Kumar B, Cordell KG, Lee JS, et al. EGFR, p16, HPV Titer, Bcl-xL and p53, sex, and smoking as indicators of response to therapy and survival in oropharyngeal cancer. J Clin Oncol 2008;26(19):3128–3137
14. Been MJ, Watkins J, Manz RM, et al. Tumor volume as a prognostic factor in oropharyngeal squamous cell carcinoma treated with primary radiotherapy. Laryngoscope 2008;118(8):1377–1382
15. Kumar B, Cordell KG, Lee JS, et al. Response to therapy and outcomes in oropharyngeal cancer are associated with biomarkers including human papillomavirus, epidermal growth factor receptor, gender, and smoking. Int J Radiat Oncol Biol Phys 2007; 69(2, Suppl)S109–S111
16. Kim SY, Roh JL, Kim MR, et al. Use of ^{18}F-FDG PET for primary treatment strategy in patients with squamous cell carcinoma of the oropharynx. J Nucl Med 2007;48(5):752–757
17. McRackan TR, Watkins JM, Herrin AE, et al. Effect of body mass index on chemoradiation outcomes in head and neck cancer. Laryngoscope 2008;118(7):1180–1185
18. Bumpous JM. Surgical salvage of cancer of the oropharynx after chemoradiation. Curr Oncol Rep 2009;11(2):151–155
19. McHam SA, Adelstein DJ, Rybicki LA, et al. Who merits a neck dissection after definitive chemoradiotherapy for N2-N3 squamous cell head and neck cancer? Head Neck 2003;25(10):791–798
20. Peters LJ, Weber RS, Morrison WH, Byers RM, Garden AS, Goepfert H. Neck surgery in patients with primary oropharyngeal cancer treated by radiotherapy. Head Neck 1996;18(6):552–559
21. Martin RC, Fulham M, Shannon KF, et al. Accuracy of positron emission tomography in the evaluation of patients treated with chemoradiotherapy for mucosal head and neck cancer. Head Neck 2009;31(2):244–250
22. Abgral R, Querellou S, Potard G, et al. Does ^{18}F-FDG PET/CT improve the detection of posttreatment recurrence of head and neck squamous cell carcinoma in patients negative for disease on clinical follow-up? J Nucl Med 2009;50(1):24–29
23. Malone JP, Gerberi MAT, Vasireddy S, et al. Early prediction of response to chemoradiotherapy for head and neck cancer: reliability of restaging with combined positron emission tomography and computed tomography. Arch Otolaryngol Head Neck Surg 2009;135(11):1119–1125
24. Schöder H, Fury M, Lee N, Kraus D. PET monitoring of therapy response in head and neck squamous cell carcinoma. J Nucl Med 2009;50(Suppl 1):74S–88S
25. Isles MG, McConkey C, Mehanna HM. A systematic review and meta-analysis of the role of positron emission tomography in the follow up of head and neck squamous cell carcinoma following radiotherapy or chemoradiotherapy. Clin Otolaryngol 2008;33(3):210–222
26. Wang YF, Liu RS, Chu PY, et al. Positron emission tomography in surveillance of head and neck squamous cell carcinoma after definitive chemoradiotherapy. Head Neck 2009;31(4):442–451
27. Kubota K, Yokoyama J, Yamaguchi K, et al. FDG-PET delayed imaging for the detection of head and neck cancer recurrence after radio-chemotherapy: comparison with MRI/CT. Eur J Nucl Med Mol Imaging 2004;31(4):590–595
28. Moeller BJ, Rana V, Cannon BA, et al. Prospective risk-adjusted [18F]Fluorodeoxyglucose positron emission tomography and computed tomography assessment of radiation response in head and neck cancer. J Clin Oncol 2009;27(15):2509–2515
29. Tan A, Adelstein DJ, Rybicki LA, et al. Ability of positron emission tomography to detect residual neck node disease in patients with head and neck squamous cell carcinoma after definitive chemoradiotherapy. Arch Otolaryngol Head Neck Surg 2007;133(5):435–440
30. Porceddu SV, Jarmolowski E, Hicks RJ, et al. Utility of positron emission tomography for the detection of disease in residual neck nodes after (chemo)radiotherapy in head and neck cancer. Head Neck 2005;27(3):175–181
31. Greven KM, Williams DW III, McGuirt WF Sr, et al. Serial positron emission tomography scans following radiation therapy of patients with head and neck cancer. Head Neck 2001;23(11):942–946
32. Yao M, Smith RB, Graham MM, et al. The role of FDG PET in management of neck metastasis from head-and-neck cancer after definitive radiation treatment. Int J Radiat Oncol Biol Phys 2005;63(4):991–999
33. Andrade RS, Heron DE, Degirmenci B, et al. Posttreatment assessment of response using FDG-PET/CT for patients treated with definitive radiation therapy for head and neck cancers. Int J Radiat Oncol Biol Phys 2006;65(5):1315–1322
34. Goerres GW, Schmid DT, Bandhauer F, et al. Positron emission tomography in the early follow-up of advanced head and neck cancer. Arch Otolaryngol Head Neck Surg 2004;130(1):105–109, discussion 120–121
35. Kim SY, Lee SW, Nam SY, et al. The feasibility of ^{18}F-FDG PET scans 1 month after completing radiotherapy of squamous cell carcinoma of the head and neck. J Nucl Med 2007;48(3):373–378
36. Delbeke D, Martin WH. Positron emission tomography imaging in oncology. Radiol Clin North Am 2001;39(5):883–917
37. Kostakoglu L, Goldsmith SJ. PET in the assessment of therapy response in patients with carcinoma of the head and neck and of the esophagus. J Nucl Med 2004;45(1):56–68
38. Liauw SL, Mancuso AA, Amdur RJ, et al. Postradiotherapy neck dissection for lymph node-positive head and neck cancer: the use of computed tomography to manage the neck. J Clin Oncol 2006;24(9):1421–1427
39. Clayman GL, Johnson CJ II, Morrison W, Ginsberg L, Lippman SM. The role of neck dissection after chemoradiotherapy for oropharyngeal cancer with advanced nodal disease. Arch Otolaryngol Head Neck Surg 2001;127(2):135–139
40. Brizel DM, Esclamado R. Concurrent chemoradiotherapy for locally advanced, nonmetastatic, squamous carcinoma of the head and neck: consensus, controversy, and conundrum. J Clin Oncol 2006;24(17):2612–2617
41. McHam SA, Adelstein DJ, Rybicki LA, et al. Who merits a neck dissection after definitive chemoradiotherapy for N2-N3 squamous cell head and neck cancer? Head Neck 2003;25(10):791–798

42. Brizel DM, Prosnitz RG, Hunter S, et al. Necessity for adjuvant neck dissection in setting of concurrent chemoradiation for advanced head-and-neck cancer. Int J Radiat Oncol Biol Phys 2004;58(5):1418–1423
43. Frank DK, Hu KS, Culliney BE, et al. Planned neck dissection after concomitant radiochemotherapy for advanced head and neck cancer. Laryngoscope 2005;115(6):1015–1020
44. Velázquez RA, McGuff HS, Sycamore D, Miller FR. The role of computed tomographic scans in the management of the N-positive neck in head and neck squamous cell carcinoma after chemoradiotherapy. Arch Otolaryngol Head Neck Surg 2004;130(1):74–77
45. Argiris A, Stenson KM, Brockstein BE, et al. Neck dissection in the combined-modality therapy of patients with locoregionally advanced head and neck cancer. Head Neck 2004;26(5):447–455
46. Goguen LA, Posner MR, Tishler RB, et al. Examining the need for neck dissection in the era of chemoradiation therapy for advanced head and neck cancer. Arch Otolaryngol Head Neck Surg 2006;132(5):526–531
47. Robbins KT, Doweck I, Samant S, Vieira F. Effectiveness of superselective and selective neck dissection for advanced nodal metastases after chemoradiation. Arch Otolaryngol Head Neck Surg 2005;131(11):965–969
48. Corry J, Peters L, Fisher R, et al. N2-N3 neck nodal control without planned neck dissection for clinical/radiologic complete responders—results of Trans Tasman Radiation Oncology Group Study 98.02. Head Neck 2008;30(6):737–742
49. van der Putten L, van den Broek GB, de Bree R, et al. Effectiveness of salvage selective and modified radical neck dissection for regional pathologic lymphadenopathy after chemoradiation. Head Neck 2009;31(5):593–603
50. Adelstein DJ, Saxton JP, Rybicki LA, et al. Multiagent concurrent chemoradiotherapy for locoregionally advanced squamous cell head and neck cancer: mature results from a single institution. J Clin Oncol 2006;24(7):1064–1071
51. Brkovich VS, Miller FR, Karnad AB, Hussey DH, McGuff HS, Otto RA. The role of positron emission tomography scans in the management of the N-positive neck in head and neck squamous cell carcinoma after chemoradiotherapy. Laryngoscope 2006;116(6):855–858
52. Ong SC, Schöder H, Lee NY, et al. Clinical utility of 18F-FDG PET/CT in assessing the neck after concurrent chemoradiotherapy for locoregional advanced head and neck cancer. J Nucl Med 2008;49(4):532–540
53. Cho AH, Shah S, Ampil F, Bhartur S, Nathan CO. N2 disease in patients with head and neck squamous cell cancer treated with chemoradiotherapy: is there a role for posttreatment neck dissection? Arch Otolaryngol Head Neck Surg 2009;135(11):1112–1118
54. Lango MN, Myers JN, Garden AS. Controversies in surgical management of the node-positive neck after chemoradiation. Semin Radiat Oncol 2009;19(1):24–28
55. Rogers JW, Greven KM, McGuirt WF, et al. Can post-RT neck dissection be omitted for patients with head-and-neck cancer who have a negative PET scan after definitive radiation therapy? Int J Radiat Oncol Biol Phys 2004;58(3):694–697
56. Clinical Trials.gov. Radiation Therapy and Cisplatin With or Without Cetuximab in Treating Patients With Stage III or Stage IV Head and Neck Cancer. Clinical Trials.gov identifier NCT00265941. Available at: http://clinicaltrials.gov/ct2/show/NCT0026594. (Accessed July 4, 2010)
57. Clinical Trials.gov. Positronic Emission Tomography (PET) Imaging in Post Radiation Evaluation of Head and Neck Tumours (PET PREVENT Trial). Clinical Trials.gov identifier NCT00147472. Available at: http://clinicaltrials.gov/ct2/show/NCT00147472. (Accessed July 4, 2010)
58. Clinical Trials.gov. PET/CT Scan-Guided Watchful Waiting or Neck Dissection of Locally Advanced Lymph Node Metastases in Treating Patients Undergoing Chemotherapy and Radiation Therapy for Primary Head and Neck Cancer. Clinical Trials.gov identifier NCT00720070. Available at: http://clinicaltrials.gov/ct2/show/NCT00720070. (Accessed July 4, 2010)
59. Kupferman ME, Morrison WH, Santillan AA, et al. The role of interstitial brachytherapy with salvage surgery for the management of recurrent head and neck cancers. Cancer 2007;109(10):2052–2057
60. Agra IMG, Carvalho AL, Ulbrich FS, et al. Prognostic factors in salvage surgery for recurrent oral and oropharyngeal cancer. Head Neck 2006;28(2):107–113
61. Goodwin WJ Jr. Salvage surgery for patients with recurrent squamous cell carcinoma of the upper aerodigestive tract: when do the ends justify the means? Laryngoscope 2000; 110(3 Pt 2, Suppl 93)1–18
62. Kim AJ, Suh JD, Sercarz JA, et al. Salvage surgery with free flap reconstruction: factors affecting outcome after treatment of recurrent head and neck squamous carcinoma. Laryngoscope 2007;117(6):1019–1023
63. Zafereo ME, Hanasono MM, Rosenthal DI, et al. The role of salvage surgery in patients with recurrent squamous cell carcinoma of the oropharynx. Cancer 2009;115(24):5723–5733
64. Netscher DT, Meade RA, Goodman CM, Alford EL, Stewart MG. Quality of life and disease-specific functional status following microvascular reconstruction for advanced (T3 and T4) oropharyngeal cancers. Plast Reconstr Surg 2000;105(5):1628–1634
65. Steiner W, Ambrosch P. Endoscopic Laser Surgery of the Upper Aerodigestive Tract. With Special Emphasis on Cancer Surgery. Stuttgart: Thieme; 2000
66. Christiansen H, Hermann RM, Martin A, et al. Long-term follow-up after transoral laser microsurgery and adjuvant radiotherapy for advanced recurrent squamous cell carcinoma of the head and neck. Int J Radiat Oncol Biol Phys 2006;65(4):1067–1074
67. Grant DG, Salassa JR, Hinni ML, Pearson BW, Hayden RE, Perry WC. Transoral laser microsurgery for recurrent laryngeal and pharyngeal cancer. Otolaryngol Head Neck Surg 2008;138(5):606–613
68. Grant DG, Salassa JR, Hinni ML, Pearson BW, Perry WC. Carcinoma of the tongue base treated by transoral laser microsurgery, Part Two: Persistent, recurrent and second primary tumors. Laryngoscope 2006;116(12):2156–2161
69. O'Malley BW Jr, Weinstein GS, Snyder W, Hockstein NG. Transoral robotic surgery (TORS) for base of tongue neoplasms. Laryngoscope 2006;116(8):1465–1472
70. Moore EJ, Olsen KD, Kasperbauer JL. Transoral robotic surgery for oropharyngeal squamous cell carcinoma: a prospective study of feasibility and functional outcomes. Laryngoscope 2009;119(11):2156–2164
71. Iseli TA, Kulbersh BD, Iseli CE, Carroll WR, Rosenthal EL, Magnuson JS. Functional outcomes after transoral robotic surgery for head and neck cancer. Otolaryngol Head Neck Surg 2009;141(2):166–171

72. Agra IMG, Carvalho AL, Pinto CAL, et al. Biological markers and prognosis in recurrent oral cancer after salvage surgery. Arch Otolaryngol Head Neck Surg 2008;134(7):743–749
73. Spencer SA, Harris J, Wheeler RH, et al. Final report of RTOG 9610, a multi-institutional trial of reirradiation and chemotherapy for unresectable recurrent squamous cell carcinoma of the head and neck. Head Neck 2008;30(3):281–288
74. Langer CJ, Harris J, Horwitz EM, et al. Phase II study of low-dose paclitaxel and cisplatin in combination with split-course concomitant twice-daily reirradiation in recurrent squamous cell carcinoma of the head and neck: results of Radiation Therapy Oncology Group Protocol 9911. J Clin Oncol 2007;25(30):4800–4805
75. Sulman EP, Schwartz DL, Le TT, et al. IMRT reirradiation of head and neck cancer-disease control and morbidity outcomes. Int J Radiat Oncol Biol Phys 2009;73(2):399–409
76. Lee N, Chan K, Bekelman JE, et al. Salvage re-irradiation for recurrent head and neck cancer. Int J Radiat Oncol Biol Phys 2007;68(3):731–740
77. Puthawala A, Nisar Syed AM, Gamie S, Chen YJ, Londrc A, Nixon V. Interstitial low-dose-rate brachytherapy as a salvage treatment for recurrent head-and-neck cancers: long-term results. Int J Radiat Oncol Biol Phys 2001;51(2):354–362
78. Meier JD, Oliver DA, Varvares MA. Surgical margin determination in head and neck oncology: current clinical practice. The results of an International American Head and Neck Society Member Survey. Head Neck 2005;27(11):952–958
79. Zbären P, Nuyens M, Curschmann J, Stauffer E. Histologic characteristics and tumor spread of recurrent glottic carcinoma: analysis on whole-organ sections and comparison with tumor spread of primary glottic carcinomas. Head Neck 2007;29(1):26–32
80. Barry B, Baujat B, Albert S, et al. Total glossectomy without laryngectomy as first-line or salvage therapy. Laryngoscope 2003;113(2):373–376
81. Smith RB, Sniezek JC, Weed DT, Wax MK; Microvascular Surgery Subcommittee of American Academy of Otolaryngology--Head and Neck Surgery. Utilization of free tissue transfer in head and neck surgery. Otolaryngol Head Neck Surg 2007;137(2):182–191
82. Abemayor E, Blackwell KE. Reconstruction of soft tissue defects in the oral cavity and oropharynx. Arch Otolaryngol Head Neck Surg 2000;126(7):909–912
83. Gullane PJ. Changing concepts in soft tissue repair of oral and oropharyngeal defects. Arch Otolaryngol Head Neck Surg 2000;126(7):912–913
84. Zafereo ME, Weber RS, Lewin JS, Roberts DB, Hanasono MM. Complications and functional outcomes following complex oropharyngeal reconstruction. Head Neck 2010;32(8):1003–1011
85. Liu R, Gullane P, Brown D, Irish J. Pectoralis major myocutaneous pedicled flap in head and neck reconstruction: retrospective review of indications and results in 244 consecutive cases at the Toronto General Hospital. J Otolaryngol 2001;30(1):34–40
86. Vartanian JG, Carvalho AL, Carvalho SM, Mizobe L, Magrin J, Kowalski LP. Pectoralis major and other myofascial/myocutaneous flaps in head and neck cancer reconstruction: experience with 437 cases at a single institution. Head Neck 2004;26(12):1018–1023
87. Sabri A. Oropharyngeal reconstruction: current state of the art. Curr Opin Otolaryngol Head Neck Surg 2003;11(4):251–254
88. Hanasono MM, Utley DS, Goode RL. The temporalis muscle flap for reconstruction after head and neck oncologic surgery. Laryngoscope 2001;111(10):1719–1725
89. Smith JE, Ducic Y, Adelson R. The utility of the temporalis muscle flap for oropharyngeal, base of tongue, and nasopharyngeal reconstruction. Otolaryngol Head Neck Surg 2005;132(3):373–380
90. de Bree R, Reith R, Quak JJ, Uyl-de Groot CA, van Agthoven M, Leemans CR. Free radial forearm flap versus pectoralis major myocutaneous flap reconstruction of oral and oropharyngeal defects: a cost analysis. Clin Otolaryngol 2007;32(4):275–282
91. Smeele LE, Goldstein D, Tsai V, et al. Morbidity and cost differences between free flap reconstruction and pedicled flap reconstruction in oral and oropharyngeal cancer: matched control study. J Otolaryngol 2006;35(2):102–107
92. Rieger JM, Zalmanowitz JG, Li SY, et al. Functional outcomes after surgical reconstruction of the base of tongue using the radial forearm free flap in patients with oropharyngeal carcinoma. Head Neck 2007;29(11):1024–1032
93. Seikaly H, Maharaj M, Rieger J, Harris J. Functional outcomes after primary mandibular resection and reconstruction with the fibular free flap. J Otolaryngol 2005;34(1):25–28
94. Bozec A, Poissonnet G, Chamorey E, et al. Quality of life after oral and oropharyngeal reconstruction with a radial forearm free flap: prospective study. J Otolaryngol Head Neck Surg 2009;38(3):401–408
95. Lin DT, Coppit GL, Burkey BB. Use of the anterolateral thigh flap for reconstruction of the head and neck. Curr Opin Otolaryngol Head Neck Surg 2004;12(4):300–304
96. Kroll SS, Robb GL, Miller MJ, Reese GP, Evans GR. Reconstruction of posterior mandibular defects with soft tissue using the rectus abdominis free flap. Br J Plast Surg 1998;51(7):503–507
97. Deleyiannis FW, Rogers C, Lee E, et al. Reconstruction of the lateral mandibulectomy defect: management based on prognosis and location and volume of soft tissue resection. Laryngoscope 2006;116(11):2071–2080
98. Rosenthal E, Carroll W, Dobbs M, Scott Magnuson J, Wax M, Peters G. Simplifying head and neck microvascular reconstruction. Head Neck 2004;26(11):930–936
99. Butler CE, Lewin JS. Reconstruction of large composite oromandibulomaxillary defects with free vertical rectus abdominis myocutaneous flaps. Plast Reconstr Surg 2004;113(2):499–507
100. Hanasono MM, Weinstock YE, Yu P. Reconstruction of extensive head and neck defects with multiple simultaneous free flaps. Plast Reconstr Surg 2008;122(6):1739–1746
101. Salama JK, Vokes EE, Chmura SJ, et al. Long-term outcome of concurrent chemotherapy and reirradiation for recurrent and second primary head-and-neck squamous cell carcinoma. Int J Radiat Oncol Biol Phys 2006;64(2):382–391
102. Ang KK, Jiang GL, Feng Y, Stephens LC, Tucker SL, Price RE. Extent and kinetics of recovery of occult spinal cord injury. Int J Radiat Oncol Biol Phys 2001;50(4):1013–1020
103. Ang KK, Price RE, Stephens LC, et al. The tolerance of primate spinal cord to re-irradiation. Int J Radiat Oncol Biol Phys 1993;25(3):459–464
104. Pignon JP, le Maître A, Maillard E, Bourhis J; MACH-NC Collaborative Group. Meta-analysis of chemotherapy in head and neck cancer (MACH-NC): an update on 93 randomised trials and 17 346 patients. Radiother Oncol 2009;92(1):4–14
105. List MA, Butler P, Vokes EE, et al. Head neck cancer patients: How do patients prioritize potential treatment outcomes. American Society for Clinical Oncology, Los Angeles, CA, May 16–19, 1998 (abstr 1472)

106. Arnold DJ, Goodwin WJ, Weed DT, Civantos FJ. Treatment of recurrent and advanced stage squamous cell carcinoma of the head and neck. Semin Radiat Oncol 2004;14(2):190–195
107. Hanasono MM, Zevallos JP, Skoracki RJ, Yu P. A prospective analysis of bony versus soft-tissue reconstruction for posterior mandibular defects. Plast Reconstr Surg 2010;125(5):1413–1421
108. Agra IMG, Carvalho AL, Pontes E, et al. Postoperative complications after en bloc salvage surgery for head and neck cancer. Arch Otolaryngol Head Neck Surg 2003;129(12):1317–1321
109. Lavertu PL, Bonafede JP, Adelstein DJ, et al. Comparison of surgical complications after organ-preservation therapy in patients with stage III or IV squamous cell head and neck cancer. Arch Otolaryngol Head Neck Surg 1998;124(4):401–406
110. Klug C, Berzaczy D, Voracek M, et al. Experience with microvascular free flaps in preoperatively irradiated tissue of the oral cavity and oropharynx in 303 patients. Oral Oncol 2005;41(7):738–746
111. Garofalo MC, Haraf DJ. Reirradiation: a potentially curative approach to locally or regionally recurrent head and neck cancer. Curr Opin Oncol 2002;14(3):330–333
112. Fontanesi J, Hetzler D, Ross J. Effect of dose rate on local control and complications in the reirradiation of head and neck tumors with interstitial iridium-192. Int J Radiat Oncol Biol Phys 1989;17(2):365–369
113. Peiffert D, Pernot M, Malissard L, et al. Salvage irradiation by brachytherapy of velotonsillar squamous cell carcinoma in a previously irradiated field: results in 73 cases. Int J Radiat Oncol Biol Phys 1994;29(4):681–686
114. Narayana A, Cohen GN, Zaider M, et al. High-dose-rate interstitial brachytherapy in recurrent and previously irradiated head and neck cancers—preliminary results. Brachytherapy 2007;6(2):157–163
115. Forastiere AA, Metch B, Schuller DE, et al. Randomized comparison of cisplatin plus fluorouracil and carboplatin plus fluorouracil versus methotrexate in advanced squamous-cell carcinoma of the head and neck: a Southwest Oncology Group study. J Clin Oncol 1992;10(8):1245–1251
116. Vermorken JB, Mesia R, Rivera F, et al. Platinum-based chemotherapy plus cetuximab in head and neck cancer. N Engl J Med 2008;359(11):1116–1127
117. Kowalski LP, Carvalho AL. Natural history of untreated head and neck cancer. Eur J Cancer 2000;36(8):1032–1037
118. Stell PM. Survival times in end-stage head and neck cancer. Eur J Surg Oncol 1989;15(5):407–410

12 Management of Nodal Recurrence

Hisham M. Mehanna, Miroslav Tedla, K. Kian Ang, Christopher M. Nutting

Summary

- Nodal recurrence can be treated successfully in approximately 50% of patients.
- Careful evaluation is necessary to exclude a recurrence at the primary site. PET-CT scanning is the most practical imaging modality for detection of recurrence.
- For the previously untreated neck, treatment of recurrence is by surgery, followed by radiotherapy ± chemotherapy if poor prognostic features are present.
- For previously treated neck, treatment is by surgery + chemotherapy and re-irradiation if possible. Patients should be counseled regarding potential benefits versus late complications.
- Poor prognostic factors include recurrence more than 3 cm in size, recurrence in a previously dissected neck, history of a previous local recurrence before the regional recurrence, extranodal extension, and surgery alone without re-irradiation.

Introduction

Nodal recurrence is the most common type of treatment failure in head and neck cancer.[1] This is often considered to be a very poor prognostic indicator. Many studies report poor outcome of salvage treatments, which are often technically challenging.[2] Furthermore, morbidity from treatment is considerable, posing further dilemmas to patients and clinicians alike. In this chapter, we consider the epidemiology of nodal recurrence in head and neck cancer, current and new investigation modalities, the evidence for the different treatment options available, the outcomes and morbidity associated with these treatments, and special considerations in the management of nodal recurrence.

Incidence and Distribution of Nodal Recurrence

Reported nodal recurrence rates vary according to the site of the primary cancer. Nutting et al. reported a retrospective series of 72 patients presenting with regional recurrence, of whom two-thirds had had previous surgery and all had had previous radiotherapy or chemoradiotherapy. The primary sites were as follows: salivary gland 8%, ear 8%, nasal cavity 1.5%, nasopharynx 4%, oral cavity 24%, oropharynx 22%, larynx 19%, hypopharynx 7%, thyroid 1.5%, occult 6%.[3]

Reported regional recurrence rates vary considerably for the same primary site. This is partly a reflection of the case and stage mix. Ord reported a regional recurrence rate of 8.5% in a retrospective cohort of 349 patients with oral squamous cell carcinoma (SCC) treated surgically by one surgeon.[2] On the other hand, Sun et al. reported a regional recurrence of 19.3% in 233 patients with tongue cancer.[2] Jeong et al. reported an overall regional recurrence of 5.4% in a retrospective study of 436 patients treated for SCC of the larynx;[4] 74% of these recurrences were confined to the neck nodes. Recurrence rates varied by primary site: 4.8% of glottic lesions had a regional recurrence, 6% of supraglottic lesions, and 8.6% of sub/transglottic lesions.[4]

The nodal recurrence rate may also vary according to the type of initial treatment. A systematic review and meta-analysis performed by our group found a nodal recurrence rate of 1.6% in patients who had a neck dissection following complete response to primary radical chemoradiotherapy. In contrast, patients who achieved a complete response but did not have a neck dissection demonstrated 8.2% nodal recurrence rate. The meta-analysis also demonstrated that patients who did not achieve complete response to chemoradiotherapy and therefore had a neck dissection had a nodal recurrence rate of 5.2% following that. These differences were not statistically significant, however (D. Howe, c.c. McConkey, H. Mehanna, unpublished data). The role of PET-CT in the detection of persistent nodal disease after chemoradiotherapy may decrease later recurrence rates due to better detection and earlier management of persistent disease.

Little information is available about the distribution of nodal recurrence. Nutting et al. reported that, in their series of 72 patients, 31% had recurrence in two nodal levels, and 5% in 3 or more levels. Level II was involved in 44 patients, level III in 19 patients, and level IV in 13 patients.[3]

Evaluation of Nodal Recurrence

! Careful assessment of patients who present with nodal recurrence is mandatory, as it is important to answer the following questions as comprehensively as possible, through a combination of investigations, for formulation of a treatment plan:

- What was the previous treatment?
- Is there recurrence at the primary site, too?
- Is there any evidence of distant metastases?
- What is the distribution of the nodal recurrence?
- Is there evidence of nodal extracapsular extension by physical examination and on imaging?
- Is there evidence of involvement and extent of involvement of the carotid arteries, brachial plexus, and prevertebral muscles?
- Can the recurrence be removed surgically with no gross tumor left behind?

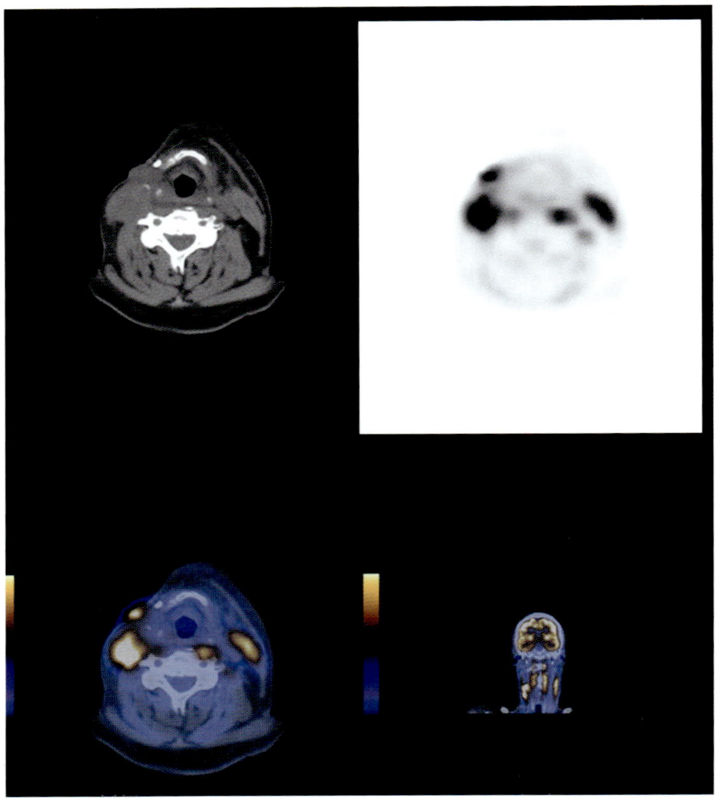

Fig. 12.1 PET-CT scan showing nodal recurrence. (With permission from Dr. Olu Adesanya, consultant radiologist, University Hospital Coventry and Warwickshire, UK.)

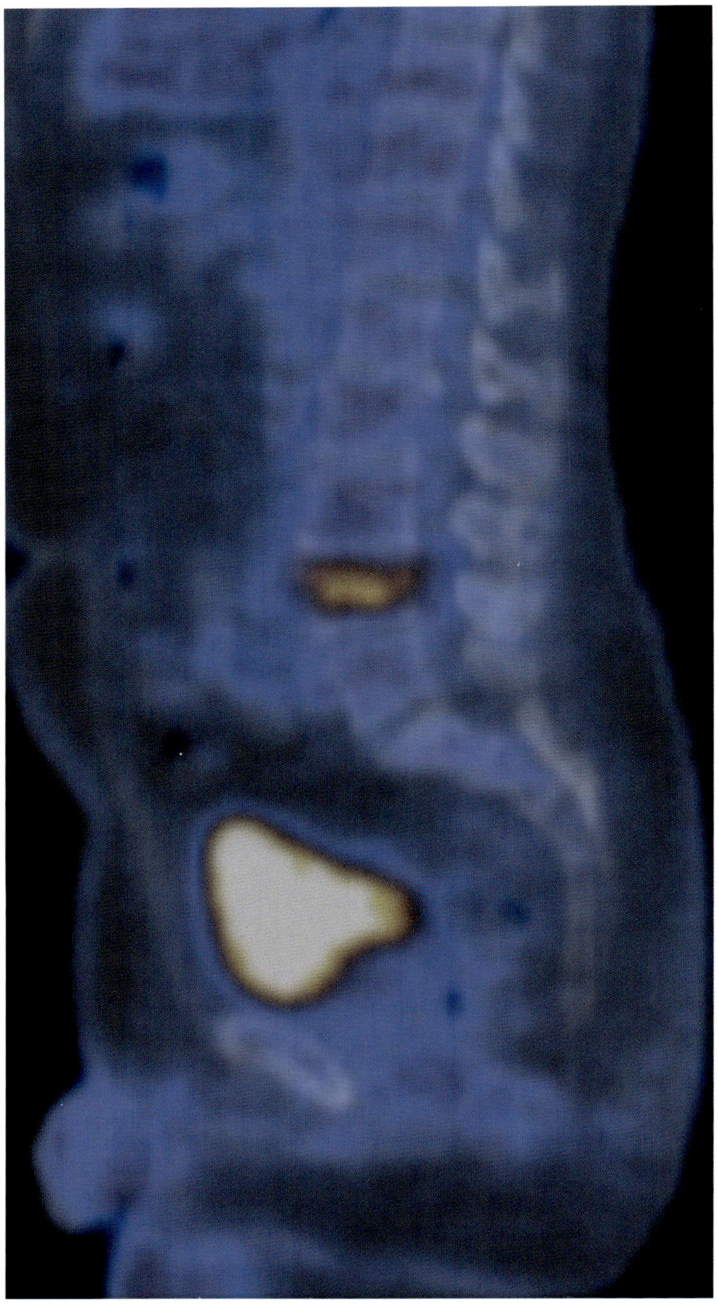

Fig. 12.2 PET-CT showing distant metastasis. (With permission from Dr. Olu Adesanya, consultant radiologist, University Hospital Coventry and Warwickshire, UK.)

■ History and Examination

The history should elicit the duration of any symptoms suggestive of recurrence. It should also elicit previous treatments in as much detail as possible. The patient's current medical history and performance status should be assessed, as that is often one of the main determinants of eligibility for surgical and nonsurgical treatments. Risk factors such as continuing smoking should also be ascertained.

On examination, fixity of the nodal recurrence should be assessed, as well as the number and distribution of the nodal metastases. A full clinical examination of the primary site and the rest of the upper aerodigestive tract should be undertaken to exclude primary site recurrence and second primaries, respectively.

■ Previous Treatment Records

It is important to attempt to obtain the patient's previous treatment records, including details of their operations, radiotherapy plans, all chemotherapy given, any documentation of toxicity, complications and compliance with the treatments. Relapse within high radiation dose regions, for example, indicates that the tumor may be relatively radioresistant, which decreases the expectation for successful outcome with re-irradiation. It is also important to obtain the original diagnostic and resection histopathology specimens, and submit them for review by a pathologist specializing in head and neck cancer to confirm the initial histological diagnosis and identify any poor prognostic factors that the patient may have had that predisposed them to developing recurrence, for example, poor tumor differentiation, vascular and perineural invasion, extranodal extension, and involved resection margins.

■ Imaging

Computed tomography (CT) or magnetic resonance imaging (MRI) with contrast are appropriate first-line investigations. These allow assessment of the recurrence in the neck, and its relations to the vital structures, especially the carotid artery. It can also allow assessment of the likelihood of extranodal extension. In patients who have had previous surgery, the extent of the previous operations, as well as sacrificed and preserved structures, should be carefully assessed. For example, it should be ascertained whether both internal jugular veins are present and patent.

However, neither of these imaging modalities may be able to accurately assess recurrence at the primary site in some cases. We therefore recommend that additional assessments of the primary site should be undertaken. If available, PET-CT scanning would be the preferred diagnostic modality, as it has been shown to be the

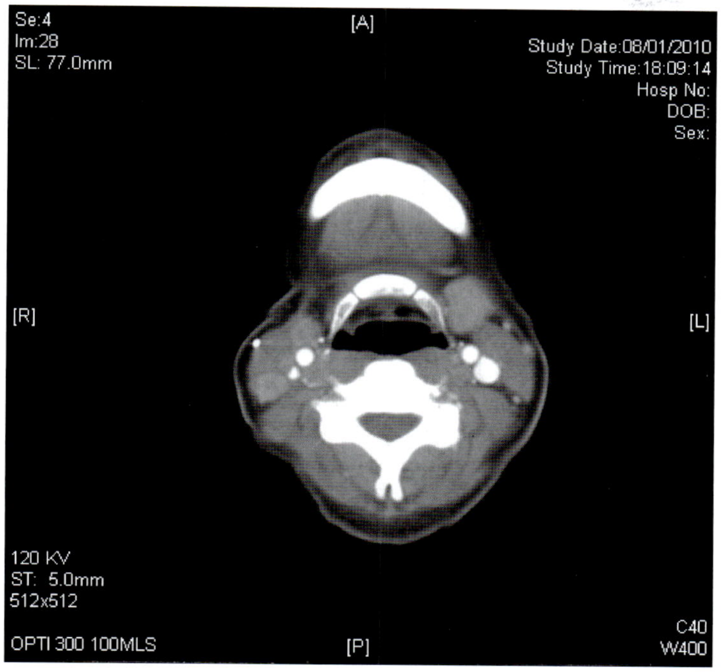

Fig. 12.3 CT of nodal recurrence in the right neck.

most accurate method for assessment of nodal recurrence, exceeding that of CT or MRI. A systematic review and meta-analysis by our group examined 1871 papers and found 27, mainly reporting retrospective cohorts, that were eligible for inclusion.[5] Most studies reported on a combination of patients with persistent nodal disease and patients with recurrent disease. The mean sensitivity of detection of nodal recurrence by PET scanning was 74% (95% CI, 50%–89%), and the mean specificity was 88% (95% CI, 74%–95%). The pooled mean positive and negative predictive values for the detection of recurrent disease in the neck were 49% (95% CI, 29%–70%), and 96% (95% CI, 84%–99%), respectively. Importantly, the sensitivity of the PET-CT scan was significantly higher for scans performed more than 10 weeks after treatment ($P = 0.002$).

A further important advantage of PET-CT is that it may detect distant metastases (**Figs. 12.1 and 12.2**) that are not detected by other modalities, as its sensitivity and specificity for this are very high (92% and 82%, respectively). Importantly, its negative predictive value has been reported to be up to 98% in a follow-up cohort of 80 patients with head and neck cancer.[7] Therefore, if there are no distant metastases on PET-CT scan, then it is extremely likely that there is no current distant metastasis. It is essential to rule out distant metastases before embarking on potentially morbid treatments.

If PET-CT scanning is not readily available, then, in addition to an examination under anesthetic, the assessment may include serial CT (**Fig. 12.3**) or MRI, comparing the posttreatment scan with the pretreatment scan and/or a baseline posttreatment scan of the primary site.[7,8] This has been shown to improve the accuracy of the detection of primary site recurrences. Further details are provided in Chapter 1.

■ Examination under Anesthetic

Examination under anesthetic (EUA) is not necessary if the patient has isolated nodal metastases that have been confirmed on needle biopsy and where the primary site has been assessed carefully by clinical examination and detailed imaging, as described above. However, EUA is recommended if only limited assessment of the primary site has been possible, since clinical examination has a low sensitivity in previously treated regions. EUA is also recommended if there is a confirmed primary site recurrence on clinical examination or cross-sectional imaging, as it allows accurate assessment of the primary site extent and potential resectability, and allows samples to be obtained for histological confirmation of the diagnosis.

■ Needle or Open Biopsy

It is important to obtain a cytological or histological diagnosis of recurrence, as diagnostic imaging investigations often have a low specificity. If a primary site recurrence is present, then histological confirmation can be obtained by biopsy during the examination under anesthetic. Diagnosis in the case of isolated nodal metastases can be obtained by fine-needle biopsy or core biopsy of the neck nodes. It is important that the cytology is examined by head and neck pathologists to decrease the risk of false positives and negatives. If a result cannot be confirmed on needle biopsy, then a diagnosis can be obtained by open biopsy or frozen section. Care should be taken when undertaking the biopsy to plan incisions with potential further surgical treatments in mind.

Management

■ Recurrence in the Untreated Neck

Surgery with or without Adjuvant Therapy

In patients whose previous treatment did not include neck dissection, the treatment options for nodal recurrence depend predominantly on whether there is also a recurrence at the primary site.

The preferred treatment of an isolated nodal recurrence, if operable, is by a neck dissection.[2] Histopathological examination of the specimens will yield information for making an informed decision on whether adjuvant therapy is necessary in the form of postoperative radiotherapy or chemoradiotherapy.

A recent combined analysis of the results of two large randomized controlled trials examining the efficacy of chemoradiotherapy in the postoperative setting demonstrated that patients with nodal extracapsular extension or involved resection margins were most likely to benefit from the addition of concomitant cisplatin to postoperative radiotherapy. Patients with multiple nodes, lymphovascular invasion, or perineural invasion did not clearly benefit from adding cisplatin to postoperative radiotherapy.[9–11]

Radiotherapy with or without Chemotherapy

In some situations where surgery is not possible, radiotherapy or chemoradiation to the nodal recurrence can be an effective option, particularly when the nodal recurrence is less than 3 cm in maximum size.[12] In modern clinical practice this approach is therefore usually limited to patients of poor performance status or those who are medically inoperable. Brachytherapy, which generally requires anesthesia, is not an option for such patients.

When radiotherapy is given in this context, external beam photon radiation to doses of 65–70 Gy over 6–7 weeks is preferred as it will allow the irradiation of the whole hemi-neck, which is almost always at risk. The indication for elective irradiation of the contralateral neck nodes depends on the site of the primary tumor and the relapse-free interval from previous treatment. Mid-line primary tumors and short relapse-free intervals are generally indications for bilateral radiation.

■ Recurrence in the Previously Treated Neck

Salvage Surgery for Recurrence following Chemoradiotherapy

There is evidence in the literature that surgical salvage of nodal recurrence following radiotherapy or chemoradiotherapy is feasible in a significant number of patients. Overall, it is only successful in controlling the regional disease in approximately 50% of cases. For example, Ord reported a salvage rate of 50% for regional recurrence in their retrospective cohort of 349 oral cancer patients.[2] Homma et al.[13] reported on 27 patients who had persistent or recurrent nodal disease following chemoradiotherapy. Twenty-one patients proceeded to neck dissection, 16 of whom had nodal control. Of the 27 patients, seven had a recurrence after initial remission of N2-N3 nodal disease with chemoradiotherapy. Four of these patients had neck dissection, two of whom achieved regional control. The other three patients refused neck dissection, two of whom died. The remainder of the patients had N1 disease (7 patients) or N2 disease (13 patients) that did not achieve complete response to chemoradiotherapy in the neck. Neck dissection yielded nodal control 4 of the 7 with persistent N1 disease and in 10 of the 13 with persistent N2 nodal disease.

In a series of 65 patients treated with chemoradiotherapy reported by Rengan,[14] nine had nodal recurrence. Neck dissection was performed in four patients and yielded nodal control. Two patients refused further treatment and the remaining three did not undergo salvage because of poor performance status. Lavertu et al. analyzed the results of a phase III trial that randomized 100 patients to radiotherapy or chemoradiotherapy. Of the 50 patients who showed complete response following treatment, 7 had nodal recurrence, of whom 4 had N1 disease and 3 had N2/N3 disease. Long-term salvage was only achieved in one patient who had initial N1 disease.[15]

Salvage Surgery for Recurrence following Previous Neck Dissection

Surgical salvage of nodal recurrence in a previously dissected neck is difficult and less likely to succeed than in a neck previously treated with chemoradiotherapy.[16] This is related to a variety of factors, most importantly the proximity and attachment of recurrent tumor to critical tissues (vessels and nerves) in a fibrotic neck and patients' unwillingness to pursue further salvage surgery with its increased morbidities and functional deficits. Krol et al. found that a previous neck dissection was a negative predictive factor for survival after salvage of nodal recurrence.[16] Wong et al. reported a salvage rate of 56% and 5-year tumor free rate of 32% for unilateral nodal recurrence in a previously undissected neck. In contrast, these rates fell to 32% and 18%, respectively, for nodal recurrence in a previously dissected neck.[17] Jeong et al. also found trends for poorer salvage rates in patients with a recurrence in a previously dissected neck.[4] Unfortunately, there is little data reported on the complication rates of surgical salvage in this setting.

Re-irradiation and Chemotherapy following Surgical Salvage

Intuitively, re-irradiation following failure due to previous radiotherapy is a difficult concept to accept. This is because there is evidence that clonogens surviving initial radiation are likely to be radioresistant.[18] It thus raises the question whether the resultant considerable late complications within the normal tissues can be justified by the potential survival benefit of adding re-irradiation. However, recurrent tumors may still be radiosensitive for a variety of reasons. First, they may represent second primary tumors that were not exposed to previous radiation, and so may be expected still to be sensitive to it. Second, recurrences, especially those at the penumbra of treatment fields, may represent geographic misses of treatment. Finally, some cytotoxic agents may increase radiosensitivity of tumors. In addition, resection or maximal debulking may decrease radioresistant clonogens to a minimum.[18] These issues are discussed in more detail in Chapters 4 and 5.

Re-irradiation and chemotherapy appear to confer a survival and control advantage when given to patients who have undergone macroscopically complete resections of nodal recurrence in a previously treated field. However, selection criteria vary among centers, series are usually small, and reported outcomes are inconsistent. Ord et al. reported achieving the highest salvage rate (70.6%–100%) of regional recurrence in patients who had surgery followed by radiotherapy or chemoradiotherapy compared with surgery alone (28.5%). De Crevoisier et al. reported a pilot study of 25 patients with positive margins or nodal extracapsular extension following macroscopically complete resections for recurrence.[19] The patients received re-irradiation of 60 Gy in alternating weeks and concomitant 5-fluorouracil and hydroxyurea. They reported a 64% 6-month locoregional control and a 36% disease-free survival rate at 2 years. Machtay et al. reported a similar pilot study in 16 patients with locally advanced rT3 or T4 or N+ recurrent disease. Patients received 54–60 Gy split-course radiotherapy and cisplatin, 5-fluorouracil, and amifostine. They reported 2- and 3-year locoregional control rates of 100% and 81%, respectively.[20] The GETTEC and GORTEC groups in France then conducted a randomized trial of 65 patients with recurrence treated with salvage surgery with macroscopic complete resection. Patients were randomized to surveillance or radiotherapy (60 Gy over 11 weeks) with concomitant fluorouracil and hydroxyurea. Disease-free survival was improved in the chemo-re-irradiation arm (odds ratio, 1.68; 95% CI, 1.13–2.50) but there was no statistically significant difference in overall survival. Thus re-irradiation with concomitant chemotherapy appears to confer a locoregional control and disease-specific survival advantage when given to patients who have undergone macroscopically complete resections of nodal recurrence in a previously treated field.

One of the main reasons for the low acceptance of re-irradiation is the concern over acute and late toxicity, which is often considered to be a high price to pay for the relatively low potential cure or benefit. The GETTEC/GORTEC study reported increased acute and late toxicities in the chemoirradiation arm compared with the surveillance-only arm.[22] However, other studies have not shown increased acute toxicity rates.[20,21] The late toxicity may be considerable and can include cervical fibrosis (up to 44%), soft tissue complications (up to 38%), mucosal necrosis (up to 20%), osteoradionecrosis (up to 16%), and pharyngeal complications and dysphagia (up to 38%). Thus, re-irradiation with chemotherapy should only be offered to carefully selected patients, usually those who have had complete macroscopic resection, after weighing the potential benefit against risks. Patients should be counseled carefully and consent obtained regarding the potential severe complications and the relatively low cure rates.

Unresectable Recurrences

The published series using brachytherapy only for salvage of recurrent neck nodes report a 25% local control rate at 3 months.[22] Bollet et al.[23] report a 31% local control rate at 2 years and only 1% at 5 years, at the risk of a 35% complication rate and a 7% rate of toxic death.

Techniques involving surgical excision and brachytherapy are reported by several authors.[24–26] Punthwala et al.[25] report local control rates of 74% at 6 months and 23% disease-free survival at 5 years with a 27% late complication rate from radiotherapy. Zelefsky et al.[26] report a local control rate of 65% at 1 year, 26% at 2 years, and 20% overall survival at 2 years. A 6% severe complication rate was reported, including a 3% carotid blowout rate. Park et al.[24] reported a disease-free survival rate of 41% at 5 years and a 36% significant complication rate with iodine-125 seed implantation.

Nutting et al. reported in-field local control rates of 40%–62% at 2 years and 40%–58% at 5 years. This figure is higher than that of Zelefsky et al.,[26] which may be due to improved techniques or to more stringent definition of what represents in-field local control versus locoregional control. One of the problems is the difficulty of determining the exact site of recurrence in relation to the brachytherapy dose distribution. Our data show that these local control figures can be maintained out to 5 years, a previously unpublished observation.[3] The data from Park et al.[24] appear to show a much higher rate of disease-free survival than other series. This is probably due to patient selection; in particular not all patients in that series had previously undergone radiation therapy. Furthermore, the lack of pathological data as to the incidence of macroscopic residual disease after resection makes comparison between series difficult.

In our series of 72 patients, we have demonstrated that surgical excision (even if subtotal), reconstruction, and low-dose-rate brachytherapy to the tumor bed offers a reasonable chance of achieving local control and even prolonged disease-free interval in the absence of a significant risk of serious toxicity. The overall major complication rates compares favorably with other series, and is a reflection of the degree of previous therapy received by this patient group.

Initial experiences with direct insertion of brachytherapy wires into bulky residual tumor masses without attempting tumor debulking were disappointing, with no patient achieving locoregional control at 2 years. Potential explanations for this finding include the suboptimal radiation dosimetry achieved with this approach, the failure to reduce the density of radiation-resistant clonogens, and the toxicity of treatment to normal tissues.

■ Patient Selection and Risk Factors for Poor Outcomes after Salvage

Patient and Tumor Features

The number and size of the nodal recurrence (larger than 3 cm) may predispose to a higher failure rate.[4] Recurrence in a previously dissected neck is associated with a poorer treatment outcome,[2,4] as is a history of a previous local recurrence before the regional recurrence.[4] Furthermore, some studies appear to suggest that initial N1 disease may be more amenable to control if the nodal disease fails to respond,[16] while others do not show the same finding.[15]

Treatment Factors

Combined treatment of the nodal recurrence by surgery and radiotherapy, with or without chemotherapy, results in better control rates.[2,20,21] It should also be noted that patients with extranodal extension or positive margins after neck dissection have a higher risk of failure after neck dissection.[15,27]

Special Considerations

■ Surgery

Type of Neck Dissection

Traditionally, surgical treatment of nodal recurrence was considered to necessitate a radical neck dissection, or at least a modified radical neck dissection. This would include all five nodal levels, even if they were not all involved by recurrence. However, the morbidity of a level V neck dissection has encouraged further examination of this principle. Level V nodal involvement is uncommon even in the recurrent situation. More recently, a more selective approach to neck dissection for nodal recurrence has emerged. A prospective study showed that in persistent nodal disease following chemoradiotherapy setting, only 2 out 54 necks had disease in more than one nodal level.[28] Another study from the same group prospectively examined the nodal recurrence rates following 106 neck dissections in 84 patients with bulky nodal recurrence after chemoradiotherapy. They reported a 17% (2 of 17) regional failure rate in patients who had modified radical neck dissections, compared with 5% (3 of 65) regional failure rate in patients having selective neck dissection. They also reported on a small series of 7 superselective neck dissections—where only the nodal levels that were involved and those that were immediately next to them were removed. There were no recurrences in that group.[29]

Van der Putten et al.[30] reported on a series of 68 neck dissections in 61 patients with suspected nodal recurrence after chemoradiotherapy, 26 of whom had confirmed tumor on neck dissection. Half of the patients had a selective neck dissection and half had a modified radical neck dissection. Four developed regional recurrence in the dissected neck, with no difference in incidence between patients who had selective and modified neck dissections.

Stenson reported on a retrospective cohort of 69 patients with advanced stage III and IV head and neck cancer who received chemoradiotherapy and had posttreatment selective neck dis-

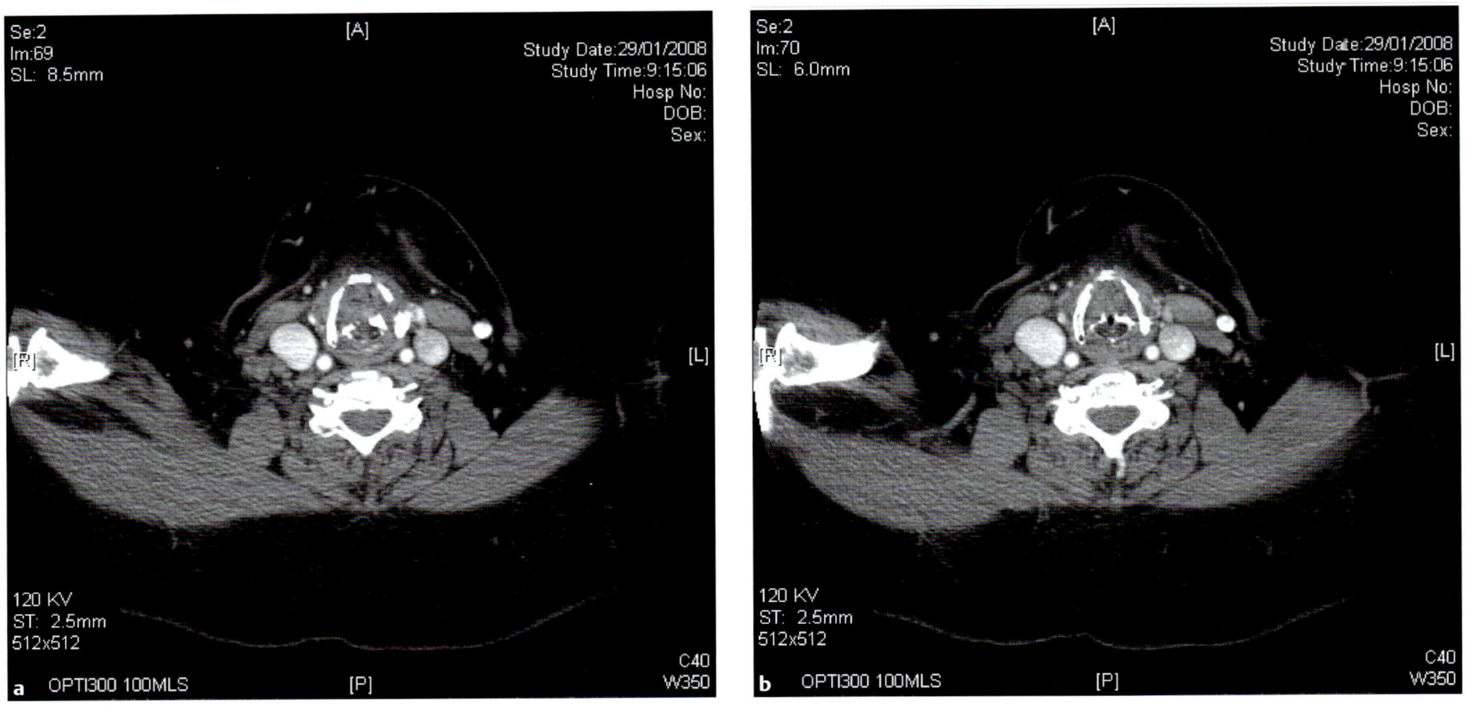

Fig. 12.4a, b Nodal recurrence behind the jugular vein following treatment for supraglottic carcinoma.

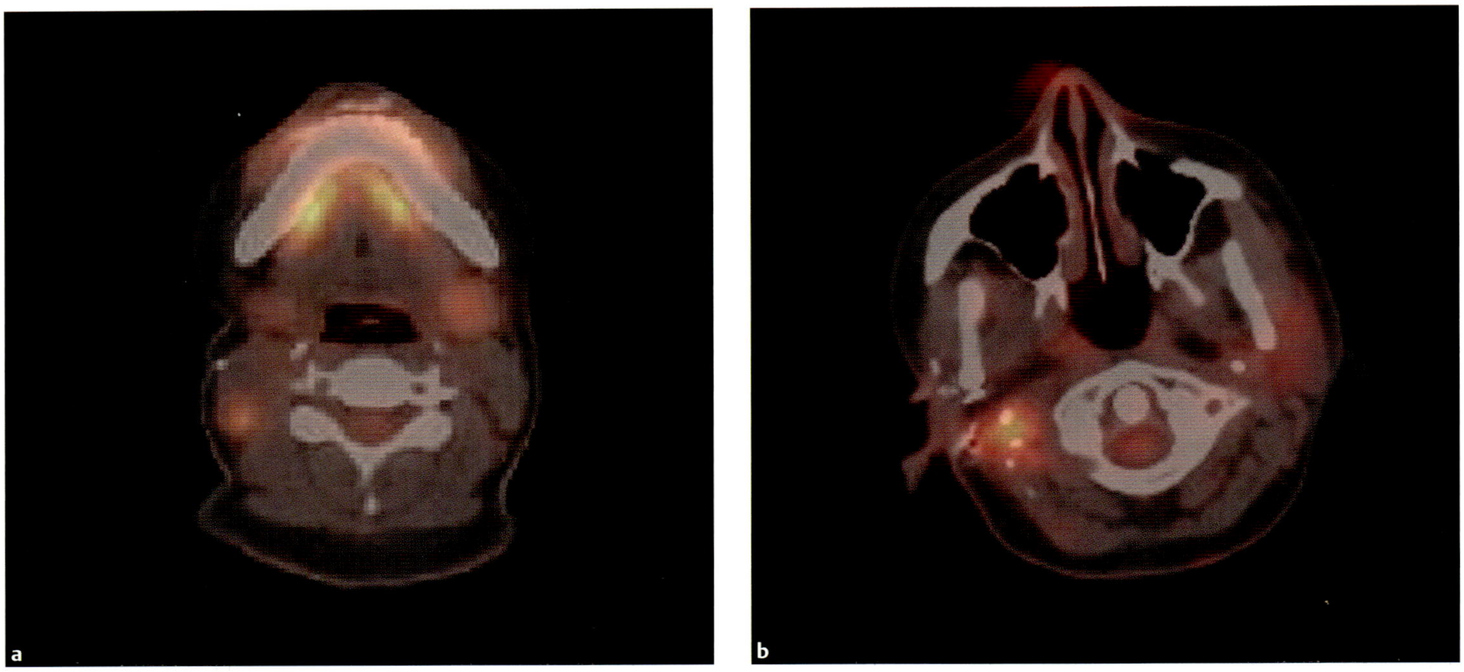

Fig. 12.5a, b PET-CT scans showing multiple recurrent nodes in the neck (**a**) and in the parotid bed (**b**).

sections. Of those, only one recurred in the neck.[31] These studies therefore support selective neck dissection as a viable option for the treatment of nodal recurrence. Care should be exercised in extrapolating these data as the studies are mainly retrospective cohort studies, and therefore patient selection criteria might affect the overall outcome.

Case Study

A 69-year-old woman presented with hoarseness. She was found to have a T3N1 supraglottic squamous cell carcinoma, with a metastatic lymph node in level III on the right (1.5 cm in cross-sectional diameter with suspicious features on contrast CT scanning). She received primary radical concomitant chemoradiotherapy—70 Gy in 35 fractions with two doses of concomitant cisplatin (100 mg/m^2). Three months after the end of chemoradiotherapy, the patient had a PET-CT scan that showed no evidence of persistent disease. The patient received out-patient monthly follow-up according to the institution's protocol. Eighteen months later, the patient complained of increased breathlessness. Flexible nasendoscopy showed edema of the supraglottis but no evidence of local recurrence.

A contrast CT scan confirmed supraglottic edema, but also detected two suspicious lymph nodes (12 mm and 8 mm in cross-sectional diameter) in level III on the right side (**Fig. 12.4**). The CT scan of her chest was clear. US-guided needle aspiration was performed, which confirmed metastatic squamous carcinoma. A panendoscopy confirmed that there was no recurrence in the larynx.

We recommended that the patient have a selective right neck dissection (levels II–V). Seventeen nodes were identified on histopathological examination of the specimen, of which one (20 mm maximum diameter) was involved with metastatic tumor, with extranodal extension. Adjuvant chemo–re-irradiation was discussed with the patient, who declined the treatment. Disease control was achieved in the neck for a further 20 months, when the patient developed a second primary non–small cell lung carcinoma with metastasis. She is undergoing palliative treatment and is still alive.

Special Considerations

- If this patient presented now, we would perform a PET-CT scan to exclude locoregional and distant metastasis, instead of a CT scan.
- The patient is also counseled about the higher risk of spinal accessory nerve sacrifice during her operation, as well as the usual risks of the operation.
- The patient was offered chemo–re-irradiation of the neck following surgery. She was counseled about the possible complications, including late complications of irradiation. She declined.

Case Study

A 28-year-old patient presents with parotid lump which is removed in a local hospital. The histology is an epithelial-myoepithelial carcinoma of parotid. She has no clinically evident nodal disease on examination or contrast CT scan or MRI. A local recurrence is identified 18 months after her first operation, with no evidence of regional recurrence. She undergoes a further MRI scan of the head and neck, as well as CT scan of the neck and chest. This confirms a local recurrence in the parotid with extraparotid extension and no nodal or distant metastases. Fine-needle aspiration confirms recurrent carcinoma. We review her initial histology and confirm the diagnosis. She therefore undergoes a second operation to have a total parotidectomy, and resection of the mastoid tip and sampling of the level II nodes—which were clear on frozen section. On histological examination, she has a large recurrence with extraparotid extension with clear margins and grade 2 facial nerve function. The seven level II nodes were clear on histology. Due to the size of the recurrence, extraparotid spread, and the intermediate histology with rapid recurrence suggesting an aggressive course, she has radiotherapy of 55 Gy to the parotid bed including some of level II of the neck.

She undergoes a further MRI scan of the head and neck, as well as CT scan of the neck and chest. This confirmed many abnormal lymph nodes in the neck in all five levels. There is no recurrence at the primary site. She also has a PET-CT scan which shows no distant metastases (**Fig. 12.5**).

We recommended that the patient have a completion neck dissection ± re-irradiation. We explained to the patient that she would have a modified radical neck dissection with likely sacrifice of the internal jugular vein and sternomastoid muscle. We also explained that it is highly likely that we may need to convert the procedure to a radical neck dissection with sacrifice of the spinal accessory nerve, and its resultant morbidities.

At the operation, the spinal accessory nerve was preserved, but the sternomastoid muscle and internal jugular vein were sacrificed. Fifty-eight nodes were removed, of which 48 are involved with metastatic tumor, with extranodal extension and soft tissue deposits. We have recommended that she has postoperative irradiation to the nodal bed, which would include re-irradiation of level II nodes. As the histology was epithelial carcinoma of the parotid, there is no evidence to support the addition of chemotherapy. The patient has recently undergone re-irradiation, and experienced acute skin toxicities. This has settled, leaving her with pigmentation of her skin, but no other side-effects.

Special Considerations

- The patient was counseled about the higher risk of spinal accessory nerve sacrifice during her operation, as well as the usual risks of the operation.
- The patient is 30 years old. As she was going to have re-irradiation of the neck she was counseled about the possible complications, including late complications of irradiation. She was also counseled about the small risk of secondary sarcomas in future.

Incisions

Due to the poor vascularity of the skin in patients following chemoradiotherapy, one should consider avoiding any three-point junctions, especially over the carotid sheath and level V. The use of single mid-neck horizontal incision or the McFee incisions provides more than adequate exposure if a neck dissection is required. It can also be extended medially into a lip split incision if required. For the combined surgical treatment of laryngeal and nodal recurrences, a U-shaped utility incision is usually adequate.

In situations where there is difficulty closing the skin following surgery, consideration should be given to the use of a pedicled flap, such as a pectoralis major myocutaneous flap with skin paddle, or a fasciocutaneous free flap, such as free radial forearm flap. This reduces the tension on the skin flaps and is likely to decrease the risk of devascularization and wound dehiscence.

Carotid Encasement

Resection of the tumor may be difficult in situations where the carotid is in contact with the recurrent tumor. This is especially the situation when there has been previous surgery or radiotherapy, due to reactive fibrosis, which causes obliteration and loss of the natural planes. In these cases, it is wise to secure control of the carotid vessels above and below the area concerned so that if there is a breach of the vessel wall, control of the hemorrhage can be achieved while repair can be performed.

Gross complete resection of the tumor becomes increasingly difficult when the tumor is in contact with the carotid artery over more than 180° of its circumference. It is widely accepted that when the tumor is in contact over 270° of the circumference, removal

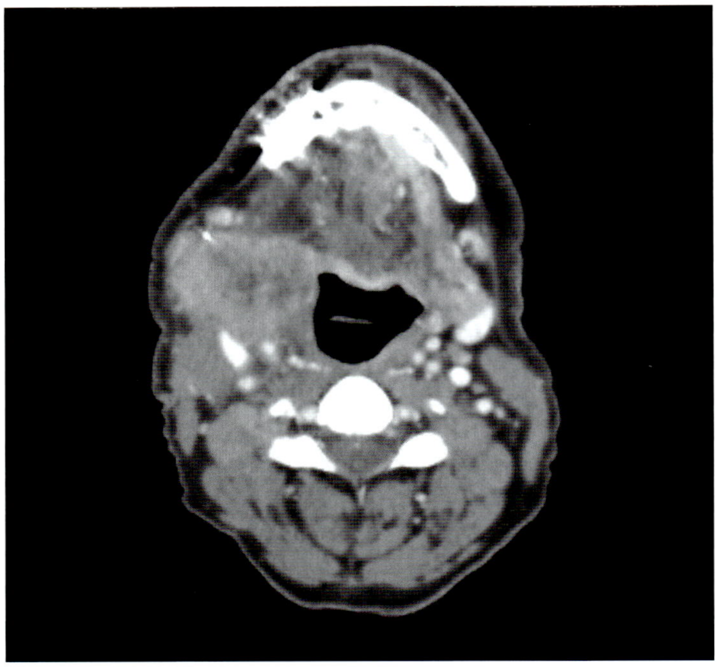

Fig. 12.6 Carotid encasement by massive lymphadenopathy.

without breaching the tumor is not usually possible (**Fig. 12.6**). In that case, the only other option is ligation and resection of the carotid, with either no reconstruction or reconstruction using an interposition graft (usually either saphenous vein or a synthetic graft). This procedure requires the input of a vascular surgeon and can carry significant potential morbidity in the form of cerebrovascular accidents and death. Furthermore, outcomes of tumor control and survival following carotid resection are very poor.

A meta-analysis of carotid resection for head and neck cancers, including 158 patients, from 22 articles, revealed that 35% of patients had ligation and 65% had reconstruction, mainly with autologous vein. The overall rate of neurological complications was 26%, of which 16.7% were major cerebrovascular accidents and 10.7% were mild pareses. There was no difference in the risk of cerebrovascular accident between the patients who had a ligation and those who had reconstruction of the carotid. The overall 2-year recurrence rate was 74%: 32% local, 47% regional, and 21% distant recurrence. The overall 2-year disease-free survival rate was 22%, which was lower than in a control group that did not have carotid artery resection. It should be noted that these outcomes included both primary and recurrent patient groups.[32] Biller et al. reported on 25 patients with recurrent head and neck cancer treated with carotid resection and reconstruction. Neurological sequelae were seen in 7% of patients and the 1-year disease-free survival rate was only 25%.[33] Therefore, carotid artery resection and reconstruction in the recurrent setting should only be performed in highly selected patients, with careful assessment and counseling on potential complications and on possible benefits and outcomes.

Assessment Prior to Carotid Resection

Initial assessment is by magnetic resonance angiography (MRA) of the cerebral circulation to see whether there are any collaterals between the two circulations. Importantly, conventional angiography with awake temporary balloon occlusion should be performed to assess the patient's cognitive and neurological function while the balloon is occluded for 10 minutes. In addition, distal carotid stump pressure measurements can be made. High stump pressures during occlusion signify a good collateral circulation and a low risk of neurological sequelae. Finally some centers perform single-photon emission computed tomography (SPECT) during balloon occlusion, which demonstrates the cerebral function during occlusion (**Fig. 12.7**). Others use intraoperative transcranial Doppler to monitor cerebral circulation intraoperatively in response to temporary clamping of the carotid artery.

Radiation with or without Chemotherapy

Patients who have not received previous neck irradiation presenting with isolated recurrence in a single node, measuring less than 3 cm without extranodal extension, can be observed after neck dissection. Adjuvant radiotherapy is only indicated when multiple nodes are involved and, in patient who are medically fit, concurrent cisplatin is recommended in the presence of extranodal extension or positive margins. The radiation doses are typically 60–66 Gy to the positive nodal basin and 50–54 Gy to the remaining uninvolved ipsilateral lymphatics given in single daily fractions of 2 Gy over 6–6.5 weeks. When nodal relapse occurs in less than 1 year from initial treatment of the primary tumor, it might be reasonable to include the primary tumor bed and, when the index cancer is situated at or near mid-line, and also to include the uninvolved contralateral neck nodes.

The indications and technique of radiotherapy for patients who have recurrence after previous radiation with or without chemotherapy are presented in more detail in Chapter 4. Briefly, postoperative re-irradiation can yield long-term disease control and survival in carefully select patients. The target volume should be kept as small as possible, for example, only ipsilateral lymphatics for those with isolated nodal recurrence, to minimize complications. The radiation dose is limited to 56–60 Gy in daily 2 Gy fractions and cisplatin is added concurrently in patients with high-risk pathological features such as extracapsular spread or positive margins. The use of intensity-modulated radiation therapy is beneficial for conforming radiation to the high-risk tissues while sparing as much of normal organs as possible. Re-irradiation with intraoperative brachytherapy can be considered in very selected cases but this should be performed by an experienced radiation oncologist.

Selected nodal relapse that is not amenable to neck dissection can be treated with re-irradiation combined with chemotherapy. In the re-irradiation setting, the dose is generally kept at 60 Gy in 30 fractions.

Outcomes

Salvage surgery following recurrence after radiotherapy and chemoradiotherapy is successful in approximately 50% of patients, as reported by several studies detailed above. There is, however, little data on the actual survival outcomes of such patients. Wong for example reported a 5-year tumor-free rate of 32%.[17] Overall survival is often much lower than successful salvage rates due to

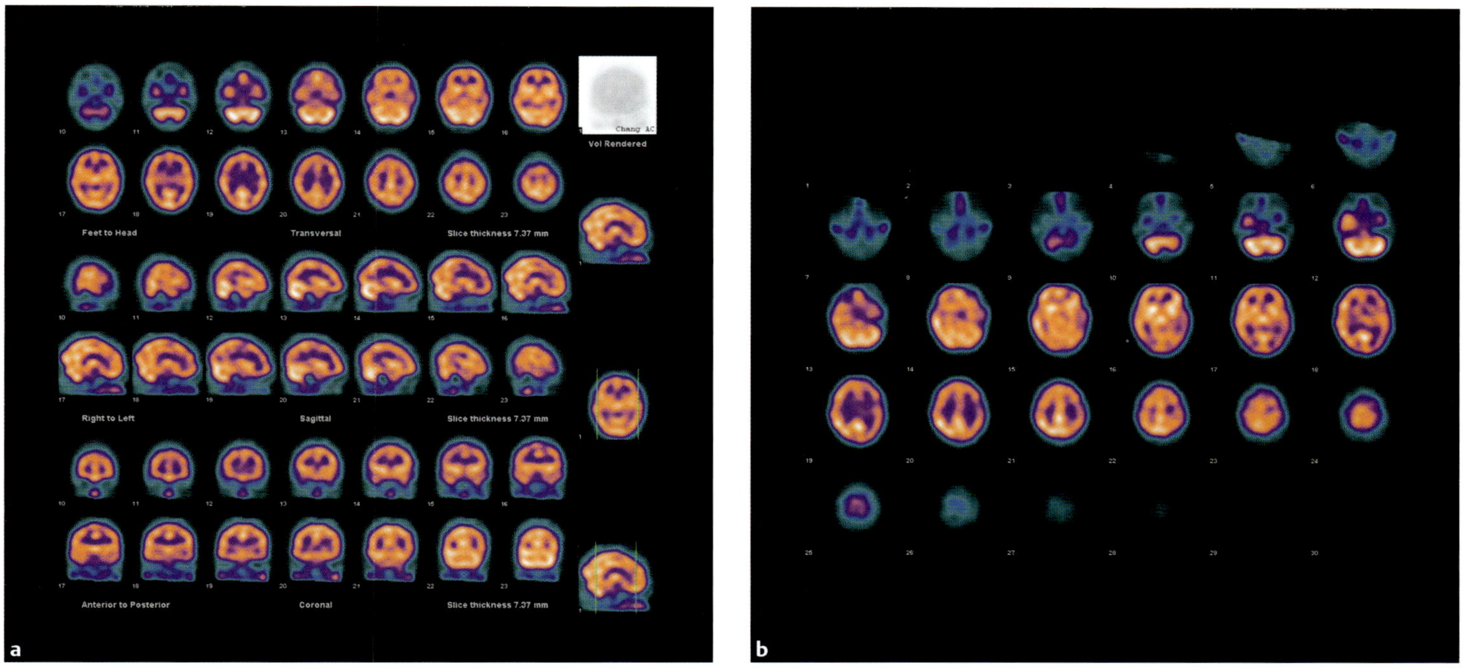

Fig. 12.7a, b Normal (**a**) and abnormal SPECT activity (**b**) in the brain.

death from primary recurrence, distant metastases, and other intercurrent illnesses.

Recurrence following previous neck dissection carries a poor prognosis whether patients were also treated with chemoradiotherapy or not (**Fig. 12.8**). Krol et al. found that a previous neck dissection was a negative predictive factor for survival after salvage of nodal recurrence.[16] In the series reported by Wong, 5-year tumor-free survival fell to 18% for nodal recurrence in a previously dissected neck.[17]

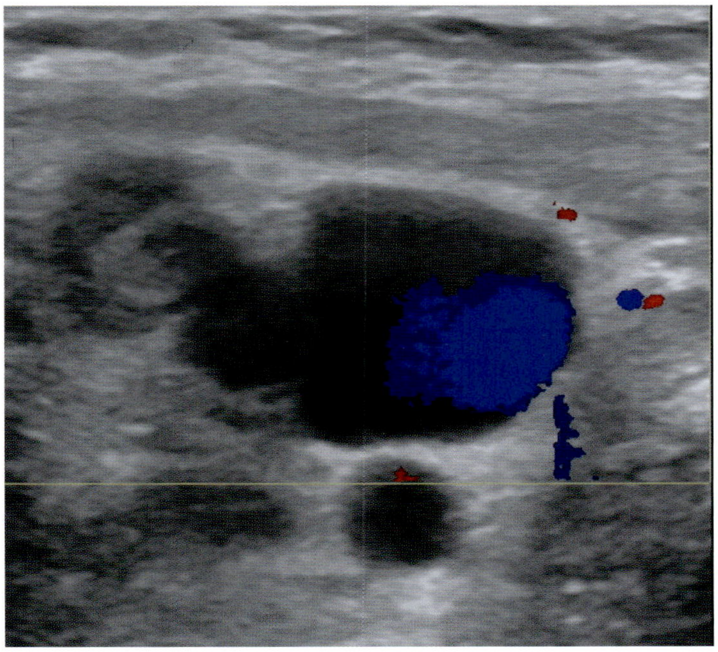

Fig. 12.8 Nodal recurrence—enhancing on scan—in a previously dissected neck carries a poor prognosis.

Complication Rates

Surgery

Complication rates for neck dissection in the recurrent setting are very poorly reported. Intuitively, however, it is likely that complication rates following salvage surgery may be higher if previous treatment had taken place. Indeed, Lin et al. found that the 53 patients treated for recurrence had higher rate of complications (60.7%) compared with 135 previously untreated patients (30.4%). However, they found no difference in *major* complication rates between the two groups.[34] Lavertu reported retrospectively on a cohort of 30 patients who had salvage neck dissection for recurrence after radiotherapy or chemoradiotherapy compared with 29 who had planned neck dissections. There was a significantly increased complication rate in patients who had salvage procedures compared with those who had planned neck dissections (60% vs. 31%, $P = 0.04$). Overall, 60% of patients having salvage neck dissection had complications. Of those, 6 (20%) had a major complication including carotid artery rupture, pharyngocutaneous fistula, sepsis, cerebrovascular accident, bleeding duodenal ulcer, and pharyngeal stenosis; 12 (40%) had minor complications including skin incision breakdown, partial small-bowel obstruction, and granulation at tracheostomy. There were no differences in either major or minor complication rates between patients who had radiotherapy and those who had chemradiotherapy.[35]

Re-irradiation

Patients treated successfully with re-irradiation risk long-term permanent side effects. Late complications can affect any of the tissues in the neck including skin, subcutaneous tissues, muscle, nerves, bone, thyroid gland, and spinal cord. Overall, severe late radiation complications are seen in approximately 25.7% of patients who are treated by re-irradiation. Higher rates of normal tissue damage are seen in patients treated with chemoradiation.

Radionecrosis of the skin is occasionally seen and is usually precipitated by trauma. Late radiotherapy effects of the skin, muscles, and other tissues leads to scarring, fibrosis, and stiffness of the neck. Hypothyroidism is common after re-irradiation of the low neck and should be biochemically screened for in this patient group. Clinically, damage to the phrenic, vagus, and hypoglossal nerves is rare. Avoidance of re-irradiation of the spinal cord and the mandible is critical to avoid damage to these organs. Lethal carotid hemorrhage is seen in 3%.[36] Refer to Chapter 4 for more details.

Future Research

- Predictive biomarker for propensity of nodal spread to identify patients for aggressive elective therapy to minimize nodal relapse.
- Role of surgical debulking before chemotherapy and re-irradiation in patients where resection cannot achieve complete gross clearance.
- Functional and quality of life outcomes following the different treatments for recurrent nodal disease.
- The role of targeted agents in the treatment of nodal recurrence to improve therapeutic ratio.

Recommended Reading

- Creak AL, Harrington K, Nutting C. Treatment of recurrent head and neck cancer: re-irradiation or chemotherapy? Clin Oncol (R Coll Radiol) 2005;17(3):138–147. (Good review on treatment of recurrent head and neck cancer by re-irradiation.)
- Ord RA, Kolokythas A, Reynolds MA. Surgical salvage for local and regional recurrence in oral cancer. J Oral Maxillofac Surg 2006;64(9):1409–1414. (Good study on surgical salvage in local and regional recurrence in oral cancer.)
- Salama JK, Vokes EE. Concurrent chemotherapy and re-irradiation for locoregionally recurrent head and neck cancer. Semin Oncol 2008;35(3):251–261. (Good review on treatment of recurrent head and neck cancer by re-irradiation and chemotherapy.)
- Isles MG, McConkey C, Mehanna HM. A systematic review and meta-analysis of the role of positron emission tomography in the follow up of head and neck squamous cell carcinoma following radiotherapy or chemoradiotherapy. Clin Otolaryngol 2008;33(3):210–222. (Review of accuracy of PET-CT in the detection of regional recurrence.)

References

1. Ridge JA. Squamous cancer of the head and neck: surgical treatment of local and regional recurrence. Semin Oncol 1993;20(5):419–429
2. Ord RA, Kolokythas A, Reynolds MA. Surgical salvage for local and regional recurrence in oral cancer. J Oral Maxillofac Surg 2006;64(9):1409–1414
3. Nutting C, Horlock N, A'Hern R, et al. Manually after-loaded ^{192}Ir low-dose rate brachytherapy after subtotal excision and flap reconstruction of recurrent cervical lymphadenopathy from head and neck cancer. Radiother Oncol 2006;80(1):39–42
4. Jeong WJ, Jung YH, Kwon SK, et al. Role of surgical salvage for regional recurrence in laryngeal cancer. Laryngoscope 2007;117(1):74–77
5. Isles MG, McConkey C, Mehanna HM. A systematic review and meta-analysis of the role of positron emission tomography in the follow up of head and neck squamous cell carcinoma following radiotherapy or chemoradiotherapy. Clin Otolaryngol 2008;33(3):210–222
6. Kao J, Vu HL, Genden EM, et al. The diagnostic and prognostic utility of positron emission tomography/computed tomography-based follow-up after radiotherapy for head and neck cancer. Cancer 2009;115(19):4586–4594
7. van den Broek GB, Rasch CR, Pameijer FA, Peter E, van den Brekel MW, Balm AJ. Response measurement after intraarterial chemoradiation in advanced head and neck carcinoma: magnetic resonance imaging and evaluation under general anesthesia? Cancer 2006;106(8):1722–1729
8. Hermans R, Pameijer FA, Mancuso AA, Parsons JT, Mendenhall WM. Laryngeal or hypopharyngeal squamous cell carcinoma: can follow-up CT after definitive radiation therapy be used to detect local failure earlier than clinical examination alone? Radiology 2000;214(3):683–687
9. Bernier J, Domenge C, Ozsahin M, et al. European Organization for Research and Treatment of Cancer Trial 22931. Postoperative irradiation with or without concomitant chemotherapy for locally advanced head and neck cancer. N Engl J Med 2004;350(19):1945–1952
10. Cooper JS, Pajak TF, Forastiere AA, et al. Radiation Therapy Oncology Group 9501/Intergroup. Postoperative concurrent radiotherapy and chemotherapy for high-risk squamous-cell carcinoma of the head and neck. N Engl J Med 2004;350(19):1937–1944
11. Bernier J, Cooper JS, Pajak TF, et al. Defining risk levels in locally advanced head and neck cancers: a comparative analysis of concurrent postoperative radiation plus chemotherapy trials of the EORTC (#22931) and RTOG (# 9501). Head Neck 2005;27(10):843–850
12. Brizel DM, Prosnitz RG, Hunter S, et al. Necessity for adjuvant neck dissection in setting of concurrent chemoradiation for advanced head-and-neck cancer. Int J Radiat Oncol Biol Phys 2004;58(5):1418–1423
13. Homma A, Furuta Y, Oridate N, et al. "Watch-and-see" policy for the clinically positive neck in head and neck cancer treated with chemoradiotherapy. Int J Clin Oncol 2006;11(6):441–448
14. Rengan R, Pfister DG, Lee NY, et al. Long-term neck control rates after complete response to chemoradiation in patients with advanced head and neck cancer. Am J Clin Oncol 2008;31(5):465–469
15. Lavertu P, Adelstein DJ, Saxton JP, et al. Management of the neck in a randomized trial comparing concurrent chemotherapy and radiotherapy with radiotherapy alone in resectable stage III and IV squamous cell head and neck cancer. Head Neck 1997;19(7):559–566
16. Krol BJ, Righi PD, Paydarfar JA, et al. Factors related to outcome of salvage therapy for isolated cervical recurrence of squamous cell carcinoma in the previously treated neck: a multi-institutional study. Otolaryngol Head Neck Surg 2000;123(4):368–376

17. Wong LY, Wei WI, Lam LK, Yuen AP. Salvage of recurrent head and neck squamous cell carcinoma after primary curative surgery. Head Neck 2003;25(11):953–959
18. Creak AL, Harrington K, Nutting C. Treatment of recurrent head and neck cancer: re-irradiation or chemotherapy? Clin Oncol (R Coll Radiol) 2005;17(3):138–147
19. De Crevoisier R, Domenge C, Wibault P, et al. Full dose reirradiation combined with chemotherapy after salvage surgery in head and neck carcinoma. Cancer 2001;91(11):2071–2076
20. Machtay M, Rosenthal DI, Chalian AA, et al. Pilot study of postoperative reirradiation, chemotherapy, and amifostine after surgical salvage for recurrent head-and-neck cancer. Int J Radiat Oncol Biol Phys 2004;59(1):72–77
21. Janot F, de Raucourt D, Benhamou E, et al. Randomized trial of postoperative reirradiation combined with chemotherapy after salvage surgery compared with salvage surgery alone in head and neck carcinoma. J Clin Oncol 2008;26(34):5518–5523
22. Pierquin B, Raventos A, Chassagne D. Endocurietherapy of malignant cervical adenopathy by iridium-192 (124 cases treated at the Institut Gustave-Roussy). [Article in French] J Radiol Electrol Med Nucl 1970;51(5):237–240
23. Bollet MA, Lapeyre M, Marchal C, et al. Cervical lymph node relapses of head-and-neck squamous cell carcinoma: is brachytherapy a therapeutic option? Int J Radiat Oncol Biol Phys 2001;51(5):1305–1312
24. Park RI, Liberman FZ, Lee DJ, Goldsmith MM, Price JC. Iodine-125 seed implantation as an adjunct to surgery in advanced recurrent squamous cell cancer of the head and neck. Laryngoscope 1991;101(4 Pt 1):405–410
25. Puthawala A, Nisar Syed AM, Gamie S, Chen YJ, Londrc A, Nixon V. Interstitial low-dose-rate brachytherapy as a salvage treatment for recurrent head-and-neck cancers: long-term results. Int J Radiat Oncol Biol Phys 2001;51(2):354–362
26. Zelefsky MJ, Zimberg SH, Raben A, et al. Brachytherapy for locally advanced and recurrent lymph node metastases. J Brachytherapy Int 1998;14:123–130
27. Pellizzon ACA, Salvajoli JV, Kowalski LP, Carvalho AL. Salvage for cervical recurrences of head and neck cancer with dissection and interstitial high dose rate brachytherapy. Radiat Oncol 2006;1:27
28. Robbins KT, Shannon K, Vieira F. Superselective neck dissection after chemoradiation: feasibility based on clinical and pathologic comparisons. Arch Otolaryngol Head Neck Surg 2007;133(5):486–489
29. Robbins KT, Doweck I, Samant S, Vieira F. Effectiveness of superselective and selective neck dissection for advanced nodal metastases after chemoradiation. Arch Otolaryngol Head Neck Surg 2005;131(11):965–969
30. van der Putten L, van den Broek GB, de Bree R, et al. Effectiveness of salvage selective and modified radical neck dissection for regional pathologic lymphadenopathy after chemoradiation. Head Neck 2009;31(5):593–603
31. Stenson KM, Haraf DJ, Pelzer H, et al. The role of cervical lymphadenectomy after aggressive concomitant chemoradiotherapy: the feasibility of selective neck dissection. Arch Otolaryngol Head Neck Surg 2000;126(8):950–956
32. Snyderman CH, D'Amico F. Outcome of carotid artery resection for neoplastic disease: a meta-analysis. Am J Otolaryngol 1992;13(6):373–380
33. Biller HF, Urken M, Lawson W, Haimov M. Carotid artery resection and bypass for neck carcinoma. Laryngoscope 1988;98(2):181–183
34. Lin YC, Hsiao JR, Tsai ST. Salvage surgery as the primary treatment for recurrent oral squamous cell carcinoma. Oral Oncol 2004;40(2):183–189
35. Lavertu P, Bonafede JP, Adelstein DJ, et al. Comparison of surgical complications after organ-preservation therapy in patients with stage III or IV squamous cell head and neck cancer. Arch Otolaryngol Head Neck Surg 1998;124(4):401–406
36. Schleicher UM, Phonias C, Spaeth J, Schlöndorff G, Ammon J, Andreopoulos D. Intraoperative radiotherapy for pre-irradiated head and neck cancer. Radiother Oncol 2001;58(1):77–81

13 Carcinoma of the Nasopharynx

William I. Wei, Lai Wan Dora Kwong

Summary

- Early detection of recurrence is essential for a successful salvage and this can be achieved with checking of circulating Epstein–Barr viral DNA and endoscopic examination.
- For recurrence in the nasopharynx, imaging studies should be performed to ascertain the extent of tumor. The appropriate approach to remove the tumor adequately should then be selected.
- Local recurrence of nasopharyngeal carcinoma is amenable to salvage surgery or re-irradiation. In general, rT1–T2 diseases are best treated with surgery or brachytherapy while rT3–T4 disease require external re-irradiation with a contemporary precise radiation technique such as stereotactic radiation or intensity-modulated radiotherapy.
- For recurrence in the neck, the salvage procedure is radical neck dissection.
- Late toxicity from re-irradiation is significant and dose limiting.
- Treatment for distant metastases is palliative. First-line chemotherapy is usually platinum based. Recent studies using targeted therapy and immunotherapy for recurrent nasopharyngeal carcinoma has shown limited efficacy.

Epidemiology

Nasopharyngeal carcinoma (NPC) is endemic in China and in the South-East Asian region. The histology is non-keratinizing or undifferentiated carcinoma (World Health Organization [WHO] type 2 or 3) in 98.5% of cases and virtually all are associated with the Epstein–Barr virus. NPC is sensitive to radiotherapy (RT) and chemotherapy. The primary treatment of all stages of NPC without distant metastases at diagnosis is RT with or without chemotherapy. Local failure of NPC is potentially salvageable with surgery and re-irradiation. However, distant failure is only amenable to palliative treatment.

In a population-based analysis by the Hong Kong NPC Study group reviewing treatment outcome of NPC treated from 1996 to 2000, the 5-year local, nodal, and distant failure-free rates were 85%, 94%, and 81%, respectively.[1] Thus, distant metastasis has become the predominant mode of failure and occurred in 11% for stage I–II and 25% for stage III–IVB disease after primary treatment. The most common sites of distant metastasis from NPC were bone, liver, and lung metastases in that order.[2] Multiple organ involvement is common at relapse (36.7%). Combined locoregional failure and distant failures occurred in 3% of patients.

The reported rates of local failure after primary treatment for NPC ranged from 9% to 40%. Local failure of NPC can be categorized as persistent disease or local recurrence. Persistent disease refers to detectable residual disease in the nasopharynx (NP) after primary RT. Recurrence is the reappearance of disease after a period of remission. The definition of persistent disease varies in different reported series, from disease noted 4 weeks to 6 months after primary RT. Some have defined persistent disease as any suspicious lesion noted on post-RT endoscopic examination and would not require histological confirmation of positive carcinoma in all cases. Even histological confirmation of residual carcinoma is not always definitive evidence of persistent disease. Kwong et al. reported the time course of histological remission after RT for 803 NPC patients,[3] which showed that 16.3% of patients who had initial positive histology in post-RT biopsies had no detectable tumor in subsequent repeat biopsy within 12 weeks of completion of RT. By 12 weeks post-RT, only 6.9% patients still had positive biopsy and were considered persistent disease. Thus, a high proportion of patients with early positive histology underwent spontaneous remission. This group with delayed remission did not have worse outcome. Therefore, for series that gave brachytherapy treatment for residual disease within 12 weeks from primary external RT, the improved local control over external RT alone may be due to a combination of factors: dose escalation from brachytherapy boost as well as salvage for persistent disease.

Most reported series on local failures are from single-center experience with small numbers of patients. The Hong Kong NPC Group reported a comprehensive review of local failure of NPC after primary treatment in the modern era of RT with CT or MRI staging.[4] In a multicenter review of all cases treated in five public oncology centers in Hong Kong, there were 319 local failures as the first site of relapse in 2915 patients treated between 1996 and 2000. Primary treatment consisted of radical RT with a median dose of 66 Gy with standard fractionation of 2 Gy daily in most cases (87%). The majority were treated with two-dimensional planning using Ho's technique but some were treated with three-dimensional conformal radiotherapy. Chemotherapy, mostly cisplatin based, was given in neoadjuvant, concurrent, or adjuvant setting to 23% of locally advanced cases. The T classification distribution of the local failure was 21% rT1 to T2a, 29% rT2b, 26% rT3, and 24% rT4. Among these 319 patients with local failure, 275 patients (86%) had isolated local failure, of whom only 200 patients (73%) had salvage treatment. (84% of these patients did not have any distant metastases or regional failure.) One hundred and fifty-nine patients (80%) received re-irradiation (108 external beam RT, 44 brachytherapy, and 7 external RT and brachytherapy), 22 patients (11%) underwent nasopharyngectomy with or without postoperative RT, and 19 patients (9%) were treated with chemotherapy alone. The 3-year actuarial overall survival was 74% for the whole group of 275 patients with isolated local failure.

Clinical Features

Symptoms and signs of early recurrent tumor in the nasopharynx are usually trivial. Patients might complain of repeated attacks of episodes of minor epistaxis or decreased hearing on one side due to the development of serous otitis media. Nasal obstruction, persistent headache, and cranial nerve palsies are signs of advanced recurrence. Whenever a recurrence is suspected, investigation is indicated.

The first sign of recurrence in the neck is usually the reappearance of a neck mass. This might be at the site of the initial lymph node that had disappeared after the primary treatment, or it might occur at a different site in the neck. The neck recurrence in the early phase is usually not obvious clinically as the fibrosis of the neck tissue after the primary radiotherapy frequently affects the accuracy of palpation. This fibrosis also affects the accurate assessment of the mobility of the neck node. Information from imaging studies would be useful to determine the presence or degree of deep infiltration. When the neck lymph node has ulcerated through the neck skin, or when the skin on the node was fixed to the lymph node, the skin has to be removed during salvage surgery.

Investigations

Viral Serology

Epstein–Barr (EB) viral serology might be useful in the diagnosis of a new patient suffering from nasopharyngeal carcinoma. However, it is not sensitive enough to detect any recurrence. The more sensitive marker in the detection of recurrent nasopharyngeal carcinoma both in the neck and in the nasopharynx is serum EB viral DNA copies. It has been reported that copies of EB viral DNA can be detected even before macroscopic appearance of the recurrence.[5]

Imaging

The extent of recurrence in the neck lymph node and that in the nasopharynx can both be determined by sectional imaging.

Magnetic resonance imaging (MRI) reveals the extent of soft tissue involvement and sometimes might differentiate between tumor and inflammation, especially in the sphenoid sinus. It might sometimes also demonstrate perineural tumor infiltration along the cranial nerves and this might extend into the foramina at the skull base and beyond. MRI with contrast is useful to show the relationship of recurrent tumor to major vessels both in the neck and at the skull base. This information is mandatory before radical salvage procedure is planned.

Although **computed tomography** (CT) has lower resolution than MRI for the imaging of soft tissue, it is useful in the visualization of the integrity of bony structures, both in the neck and at the skull base. Tumor erosion of bone can frequently be detected with bone window images on fine-cut CT. The depth of tumor in the soft tissue above the bone can be determined and this factor provides a three-dimensional assessment of the size of the tumor.

Positron emission tomography (PET) is useful in the detection of sizable local recurrence and distant metastases. Its sensitivity depends on the metabolic activities of the recurrent tumor. It might not be able to differentiate a small, slow-growing tumor from the surrounding inflammatory tissue, especially when there is associated osteoradionecrosis in the region. However, it should be done to rule out distant disease before a major salvage procedure is planned. A PET scan should be done when indicated, before fine-needle aspiration or biopsy, as otherwise a false-positive result might follow these procedures.

Fine-needle Aspiration

Recurrent disease should be confirmed before any salvage procedure. Fine-needle aspiration under ultrasound guidance should be performed for suspected recurrence in the neck. The yield is not high, however—overall, fine-needle aspiration will be able to obtain unequivocal malignant cells in only around 50% of tumor-containing neck nodes. This is because many of these nodes contain a significant portion of fibrous tissue and the needle might not accurately aspirate the malignant cells.

Endoscopy

When recurrent disease in the nasopharynx is suspected, endoscopic examination of the nasopharynx is essential. Suspected lesions seen in the nasopharynx should be biopsied for histological confirmation of recurrence. Sometimes the disease might be submucosal in location and a deep biopsy should be performed to obtain adequate tissue for histological evaluation. Endoscopic examination also determines the extent of the recurrence in the nasopharynx and this contributes to the planning of the salvage procedure.

> **!** When tissue diagnosis, either by cytology or by histology, cannot be obtained from suspected recurrence, then it might not be appropriate to proceed with radical salvage procedure. The patient would then be seen again after an interval for repetition of the investigations. Progression of disease shown on imaging or PET scan might be considered an indication for exploration and salvage.

Principles of Management

The salvage of recurrent nasopharyngeal carcinoma depends on the location of the recurrence. Relapse in the neck and nasopharynx is considered extensive disease. Evaluation of the possibility of distant metastasis and disease in the paranasopharyngeal space should be done before definitive salvage procedure. In general, one form of salvage procedure, either surgery or radiation is used for both the neck and the primary recurrence. When the patient's condition is satisfactory, the salvage procedure is performed for both sites at the same time. Alternatively, the salvage treatment can be performed in stages, usually with 6 weeks between the two procedures.

Recurrence in the Neck Lymph Node

When the disease is only in the neck lymph node, salvage with further external radiotherapy will lead to significant side effects and the outcome has not been satisfactory. Surgery is the optimal salvage if the disease is amenable to resection. The salvage procedure is radical neck dissection that includes removal of the sternomastoid muscle, the internal jugular vein, and the spinal accessory nerve together with all the lymph nodes in the neck. Studies on serial sectioning of specimens of radical neck dissection performed for these patients showed that the neck harbored five times more tumor-bearing lymph nodes than were clinically evident. These nodes exhibited extracapsular spread in over 70% of the specimens; they were in the muscle and lying close to the accessory nerve in over 30% of the specimens.[6] Thus, radical neck dissection is the recommended salvage procedure for recurrent neck node in nasopharyngeal carcinoma.

■ Infiltration of Overlying Neck Skin or Deeper Tissues

When the tumor-bearing node infiltrates the overlying neck skin or the deeper tissue in the neck, then the tissue margins achieved even with radical neck dissection might be close. To give additional control of tumor at the margin, after-loading brachytherapy with iridium wires has been used. Our study results showed that for patients with advanced neck disease, the control of tumor with this technique is similar to that in those patients who have less advanced disease and undergo radical neck dissection alone. Accordingly, this procedure is recommended for extensive recurrent disease in the neck.[7]

■ Recurrence in the Nasopharynx

For recurrence in the nasopharynx, following the appropriate evaluation, the optimal choice of therapy should be given:

- For a small tumor mainly confined to nasopharynx, brachytherapy or surgery should be considered.
- For tumor involving skull base or too extensive for surgery or brachytherapy, external beam re-irradiation with stereotactic radiation or intensity-modulated radiotherapy would be required.

Most recurrent tumor in the nasopharynx, however, is located on the lateral wall of the nasopharynx and surgical resection of the tumor offers a high chance of eradication. A wide exposure of the tumor is essential for an oncological resection of the recurrence in the nasopharynx.

> **!** The nasopharynx is located in the center of the head; at a distance of more than 10 cm from the skin surface on all sides.

Surgical Approaches to the Nasopharynx

Lateral Approach

The approach to the nasopharynx through the infratemporal fossa from the lateral aspect was described over two decades ago.[8] This procedure is technically demanding, as it requires radical mastoidectomy and mobilization of the cranial nerve and floor of the middle cranial fossa; associated morbidities were not negligible. In addition, it mainly exposes the lateral wall of the nasopharynx on the side of the surgery and it is difficult to remove the lesion that has extended across the midline to the contralateral side.

Inferior Approach

The nasopharynx can also be approached from the inferior aspect employing the transpalatal, transmaxillary, and transcervical approach.[9,10] These approaches are useful for tumors located in the central part of the nasopharynx. For tumors extending to the lateral wall, the dissection of the paranasopharyngeal space is difficult from below. With the inferior approaches, the internal carotid artery has to be protected and it is not easy to control the superolateral margin of resection.

Anterolateral Approach

The anterolateral or the maxillary swing approach adequately exposes the nasopharynx and its vicinity; radical resection of the recurrent tumor is possible. The procedure has limited morbidity and allows identification of the internal carotid artery, thus preventing injury to it. This is the appropriate surgical salvage procedure for most recurrent tumor in the nasopharynx.

Endoscopic Approach

For a small but thick tumor located in the posterior wall of the nasopharynx, surgical salvage can be done with the endoscopic approach; adequate tumor removal can be achieved with the endoscope inserted through the nasal and oral cavities. However, the endoscopic rigid instruments are unable to remove laterally situated tumor.

Resection and Outcome

A small tumor located in the lateral wall might be resected using the Da Vinci Robot applied through a split-palate approach. The versatile robotic endowrist allows resection of a small laterally situated tumor in the nasopharynx.

For more advanced local recurrences, extending into the paranasopharyngeal space, then with the maxillary swing approach nasopharyngectomy, the carotid artery might be exposed at the end of the operation. To prevent subsequent dehydration and possible carotid artery rupture, a microvascular muscle flap might be used to reconstruct the defect in the nasopharynx, covering the carotid artery and improving healing.

The success of surgical salvage depends on whether the tumor can be adequately removed to achieve a negative resection margin. During tumor resection, the margins are examined with frozen section and efforts are made to remove all tumor. Resection is limited, however, when tumor cells are found to involve the internal carotid artery and infiltrate the clivus and skull base bone.

> **!** When the recurrences in the neck or in the nasopharynx, because of their location or extensive involvement, preclude curative surgical salvage, they are usually considered for palliative management. This is usually through radiation or chemora-

diation or palliative surgical intervention. In general, more focused therapy would be delivered to the affected region; the aim would be to control symptoms such as bleeding or pain.

Case Study

A southern Chinese woman, 43 years of age, suffered from nasopharyngeal carcinoma (T2bN2N0) with the main bulk of the tumor located in the right nasopharynx. She was managed with concurrent chemoradiation at another institute and at completion of treatment the primary tumor and the cervical lymph node regressed completely.

At 20 months after treatment, she developed a 2 cm diameter left upper neck lymph node, which was mobile. Fine-needle aspiration of the lymph node yielded carcinoma cells. Investigation of the nasopharynx and rest of the body showed no evidence of disease. A left radical neck dissection was performed with McFee neck incision and she recovered smoothly from the operation. Pathological study of the resected specimen revealed a total of 32 lymph nodes; 2 in level I, 16 in level II, 7 in level III, 3 in level IV, and 4 in level V. Two lymph nodes in level II were infiltrated by undifferentiated carcinoma cells and there was extranodal extension. No further treatment was given.

Ten months later, serum EB viral DNA testing showed an elevation from zero to 231 copies. Endoscopic examination showed a polypoid lesion in the right nasopharynx and biopsy showed nasopharyngeal carcinoma. Imaging study revealed that the recurrence in the nasopharynx was confined to the nasopharynx (**Fig. 13.1a**) and PET showed increased FDG uptake in the nasopharynx only. There was no evidence of distant metastasis. Surgical salvage was performed; this included a nasopharyngectomy with right maxillary swing approach. The tumor was removed en bloc and the resection margins were free of disease (**Fig. 13.1b, c**). A Weber–Ferguson facial incision was used for the right maxillary swing. The patient recovered well from the operation, and there was no palatal fistula. She resumed a normal diet and was discharged from the hospital on the 10th postoperative day.

When she was seen at 14 months after the operation, the facial and neck wounds had healed completely. However, she experiences some degree of trismus (**Fig. 13.1d–f**).

Surgical Techniques

Salvage Surgery for the Neck

Radical Neck Dissection

Radical neck dissection is performed with the patient in supine position; a support is placed behind the shoulders to keep the neck extended. As the neck has been included in the radiation field, the McFee incision is frequently employed for the radical neck dissection. The parallel incision in the neck reduces the incidence of skin necrosis and eliminates the possibility of carotid artery exposure and rupture. After lifting the skin flap with the platysma muscle, the neck dissection starts from the area where there is less pathological lymph node. The sternomastoid muscle, the accessory nerve, the internal jugular vein, and all the associated lymphatic tissue and nodes are removed en bloc. When the radical neck dissection is performed on the left side, attention should be paid to the thoracic duct; when it is encountered, it should be ligated to prevent postoperative chyle leakage.

Extended Radical Neck Dissection

When the recurrent or persistent lymph node has infiltrated the skin or floor of the posterior triangle, the skin overlying the pathological node has to be excised and removed together with the radical neck dissection. The area of close resection margins is identified and a hollow plastic tube is placed on this area at the time of the operation; the tubes have to be 1 cm apart and fixed to the underlying tissue. This allows the insertion of a radiation source such as iridium wire as a form of afterloading brachytherapy to improve the local disease control. The skin defect in the neck should be reconstructed with a pedicled flap. This can be either a deltopectoral flap or a pectoralis major myocutaneous flap. The flap brings vascular and nonirradiated tissue into the area so that they can stand further afterloading brachytherapy.

Complications

The early complications of radical neck dissection include bleeding and seroma formation and these can be eliminated with careful hemostasis at the time of the operation. The late complications are relatively mild. The removal of the sternomastoid muscle and soft tissue in the neck leads to depressive deformity of neck and mild facial edema. Sacrificing the accessory nerve causes atrophy of the trapezius and sometimes this leads to pain and limitation of movement of the shoulder. These symptoms in general improve with physiotherapy and exercise.[11]

Salvage Surgery for Recurrence at the Primary Site

Endoscopic Nasopharyngectomy

Endoscopic nasopharyngectomy is performed when the tumor is located in the central part of the posterior wall of the nasopharynx. An endoscope is introduced through one nasal passage and the diathermy is inserted through the other nasal cavity. The diathermy cuts into the mucosa of nasopharyngeal wall around the tumor to ensure an adequate resection margin. The superior incision should include the mucosa over the vomer. Laterally, the incision might include a portion of the eustachian tube cushion cartilage. The incision cuts through the mucosa as well as the muscle layer of the nasopharyngeal wall. Then a grasping forceps replaces the diathermy in the nasal cavity and holds up the edge of the incised nasopharyngeal wall. The tip of the diathermy is bent and introduced behind the soft palate into the nasopharynx and cuts the tissue between the prevertebral tissue and the nasopharyngeal wall with the tumor. En bloc resection of the tumor with adequate resection margin can be achieved. However, with limitation by the curvature of the endoscopic instruments, it is difficult to remove the entire crura of the auditory-tympanic tube with this endoscopic technique. Improved exposure of the region can

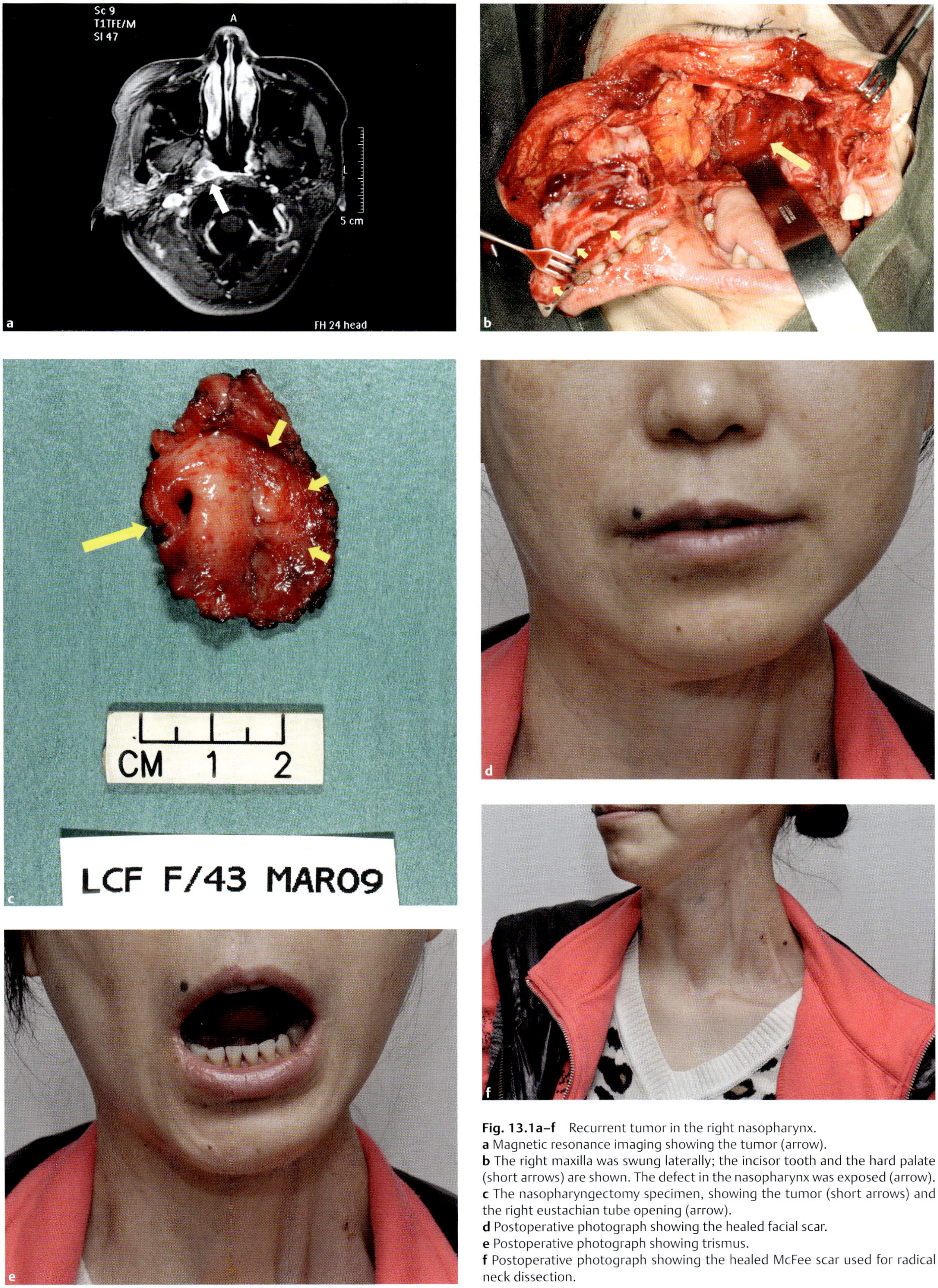

Fig. 13.1a–f Recurrent tumor in the right nasopharynx.
a Magnetic resonance imaging showing the tumor (arrow).
b The right maxilla was swung laterally; the incisor tooth and the hard palate (short arrows) are shown. The defect in the nasopharynx was exposed (arrow).
c The nasopharyngectomy specimen, showing the tumor (short arrows) and the right eustachian tube opening (arrow).
d Postoperative photograph showing the healed facial scar.
e Postoperative photograph showing trismus.
f Postoperative photograph showing the healed McFee scar used for radical neck dissection.

be achieved by removing the posterior part of the maxilla. Good results can be achieved with this approach in selected patients.[12]

Robotic Nasopharyngectomy

In recent years, transoral robotic surgery has been used to resect lesions at the tonsil and the tongue base. The three-dimensional endoscope coupled with the versatile robotic wrist allows good visualization of the pathology and adequate removal of the tumor with good margin. Through a split-palate approach, removal of a recurrent tumor in the fossa of Rosenmüller, together with crura of the eustachian tube has been reported. The morbidity associated with the operation is not significant. With the development of more appropriate instruments for working at the skull base, this might become one of the approaches for resection of localized lesions in the nasopharynx.[13]

Nasopharyngectomy via the Maxillary Swing Approach

The nasopharynx is located in the center of the head; it is therefore difficult to get adequate exposure of the region for an oncological resection. The anterolateral or the maxillary swing approach exposes the nasopharynx and its vicinity adequately for a salvage nasopharyngectomy.

This is performed with the patient in supine position. A tracheotomy is performed to allow free access to the mouth and the nasal cavities. Tarsorraphy is performed for the eye on the side of the swing and ointment is placed in the contralateral eye, which is draped off the operative field. Weber–Ferguson facial incision as for maxillectomy is performed on the side of the swing. The skin incision goes through skin, the subcutaneous tissue, and the orbicularis oris muscle. The facial skin is lifted until the orbital rim is reached. A limited amount of soft tissue over the anterior wall of the maxilla is elevated to expose a strip of anterior maxilla bone for osteotomy.

The palatal wound is a curved incision, starting at 0.5 mm from the opposite lateral incisor; it is continued along the margin of the teeth starting until the last molar tooth. It is then curved laterally behind the molar tooth toward the buccal mucosa. The mucoperiosteum over the hard palate is lifted off the bony hard palate as far as the soft palate, which is detached from its attachment on the posterior edge of the hard palate.

The osteotomy over the anterior wall of the maxilla is placed at 0.5 cm below the orbital rim and extends laterally to the zygomatic arch and then turned downward through the lower edge of the arch. Thus, only the lower part of the zygomatic arch is divided and the inferior orbital rim remains attached to the zygoma.

A curved osteotome is placed into the groove between the maxillary tuberosity and the pterygoid plates. Driving it with the mallet separates the maxillary antrum from the pterygoid plates.

The midline osteotomy goes between the two central incisors, the hard palate, and lower part of the nasal septum. The last osteotomy goes through the medial wall of the antrum; it is placed above the inferior turbinate and below the middle turbinate.

After the completion of the four osteotomies, the maxilla bone drops down, but remains attached to the anterior cheek flap. The maxilla can be swung laterally to expose the nasopharynx and the paranasopharyngeal space. Pathologies in the region with its surrounding tissue are adequately exposed and can be removed with conventional instruments under direct vision.

En bloc resection of the nasopharyngeal carcinoma can be performed and the resection includes the eustachian tube crura.

After tumor resection and adequate hemostasis, the maxilla is then returned to its original position. The soft palate is reattached to the hard palate and two titanium plates are used to fix the maxilla to the rest of the facial skeleton, one over the zygoma, one over the midline. The palatal flap is returned and a few sutures are used to fix the posterior part of the flap to the alveolar margin. The nasal cavity is packed and the facial wound is closed in layers. A nasogastric tube is inserted for postoperative feeding.

Special Considerations

- The horizontal limb of the Weber–Ferguson facial incision limb is placed approximately 5 mm below and parallel to the lower eyelid margin to avoid ectropion.
- The infraorbital nerve is identified while raising the facial flap and is divided between clamps; this maneuver reduces blood loss during the osteotomy over the anterior wall of the maxilla.
- Before the osteotomy, holes for the titanium plate are drilled and screws are inserted and then removed. These holes will ensure accurate repositioning of the maxilla when it is returned.
- After the maxilla is swung laterally, the posterior part of the nasal septum is removed to improve the visualization of the contralateral nasopharynx.
- The inferior turbinate on the side of the swing is resected; its mucosa is taken off. This is laid onto the raw area in the nasopharynx as a free graft or temporary dressing.
- A prefabricated dental plate ensures accurate repositioning of the maxilla on its return and also holds the palatal flap in position.

Complications

Palatal fistula was a common complication when the incision of the palate was in the midline as originally described.[14] This could be managed conservatively with a dental plate or closed surgically with a palatal flap. In recent years, we have modified the palatal incision and this has eliminated the palatal fistula problem.[15] Many patients experienced some degree of trismus after the operation and most of them responded to conservative treatment. The development of ectropion was infrequent and problems associated with the titanium plates were also uncommon.

Nasopharyngectomy with Microvascular Free Flap Reconstruction

For patients in whom, following adequate tumor resection, the carotid artery remains exposed at the end of the surgery, some vascularized tissue should be used to cover the vessel and the vicinity. This will promote healing and also allow further radiation to the region if indicated. The vascularized tissue frequently employed is the rectus abdominis or the vastus lateralis muscle. The free muscle with its vascular pedicle is taken from the abdomen or the thigh and transferred to the nasopharynx. The pedicle is passed through a tunnel in the lateral pharyngeal wall at the level of the soft palate. The pedicle delivered to the neck is anastomosed to the facial vessels with microvascular technique.

Outcome

When radical neck dissection was performed for the neck recurrences, the 5-year local control of disease was 66% and the 5-year survival of was 37%.[16] When maxillary swing salvage nasopharyngectomy was performed for 246 patients with localized disease in the nasopharynx, the 5-year local control of disease was 74% and the 5-year disease-free survival was 56%.[17] We have also analyzed the quality of life of those patients who underwent the maxillary swing approach for salvage nasopharyngectomy and the survey showed satisfactory results. A total of 41 patients who had nasopharyngectomy with the maxillary swing approach participated in the Quality of Life study. When the EORTC QLQ-C30 questionnaire was used, the global score was 68.7 ± 24.2, suggesting that the quality of life in general was satisfactory. When specific domains were examined employing the QLQ-H&N35 questionnaire, trismus less than 2.5 cm and palatal fistula were found to affect social eating and this led to weight loss.[18]

Radiation Techniques

Radiotherapy (RT) for recurrent NPC always involves re-irradiation as patients would have been treated with radiation after initial diagnosis. Due to the intricate location of NPC, re-irradiation for NPC carries significant risk of severe radiation complications. Critical organs at risk (OARs), such as brainstem, spinal cord, and sometimes the optic pathway, may have received near tolerance dose from the first RT course. Thus, in considering re-irradiation for NPC, the dose, extent, and technique of radiotherapy in first course RT should be reviewed.

If the patient has been treated with three-dimensional conformal radiotherapy or intensity-modulated radiotherapy, reviewing the isodose distribution and dose volume histogram will be very useful to indicate what dose OARs have received.

For patients treated with conventional two-dimensional radiotherapy, structures that have been shielded throughout the course of RT are assumed not to have been irradiated; for example, the median lower anterior cervical shield would have protected the lower cervical spinal cord and a pituitary shield would have protected the optic chiasm from radiation. These shielded structures can be assumed to have received minimal radiation. It is also useful to fuse the recurrence images with the primary RT plan to see whether tumor recurrence is due to marginal miss or whether recurrence is in the underdosed area. If so, the chance of salvage with re-irradiation may be better since the tumor is assumed to be less radioresistant than that recurring in the high-dose region.

Re-irradiation for NPC involves either external radiotherapy such as second course radiotherapy with intensity-modulated radiotherapy or stereotactic radiation, or brachytherapy using different techniques such as intracavity intubation, gold grain implantation, or iridium mold. Brachytherapy is preferred over external radiotherapy for small superficial mucosal lesions mainly localized in the nasopharynx, i.e., rT1 or early rT2a/b disease. High dose can be delivered to superficial tumor with brachytherapy while the rapid dose fall-off will minimize radiation dose to critical OARs. However, for extensive, deep-sited infiltrative tumors or tumors with skull base erosion (i.e., rT3/rT4 disease), brachytherapy sources cannot be placed in close proximity to tumor, and so external radiotherapy will be required. External RT can cover larger extent of disease but the dose will be limited by tolerance of adjacent OARs. **Table 13.1** summarizes the results of re-irradiation with different radiation techniques.

Brachytherapy

Radioactive Gold Grain Implantation

The nasopharynx can be accessed by a split-palate approach, which offers a better view and more room for manipulation than an endoscopic approach. This is done under general anesthesia with the patient in supine position; an oral nonkinking tube is inserted. A Dingman mouth gag is used to expose the hard and soft palate. The incision starts at the base of the uvula, and then extends superiorly along the midline of the soft palate onto the hard palate to stop at approximately 2 cm from the incisors. The soft palate together with the mucoperiosteum of the hard palate is lifted and retracted laterally. Following the retraction of the palatal flaps, the tumor in the nasopharynx is exposed.

Radioactive gold-198 grains are inserted into the recurrent tumor under direct vision with help of a specialized gold grain gun (Royal Marsden Gold Grain Implantation Gun MKIII). The gold grain implant is a permanent interstitial implant. A template may be used to guide the implant to ensure the geometry of gold grain distribution. The aim is to deliver 60 Gy at 0.5 cm from the plane of implantation. After implantation of the radioactive gold grains, the palatal wound is repaired in three layers. The surgical procedure is simple and the morbidity related to surgery is low.[19] Gold implantation is an effective salvage treatment for recurrent NPC that is confined to the nasopharynx. A report of the long-term results of 106 patients treated with gold grain implantation showed 5-year local control rates of 87.2%, 62.7%, and 23.4% for patients implanted for persistent disease and first and second recurrence in nasopharynx, respectively.[20]

Special Considerations

- Precautionary steps are necessary to reduce radiation exposure of medical personnel in the operating room after implantation of the radioactive gold grains. A small piece of lead shield is placed in the nasopharynx over the area of the gold grain implant and a lead shield trolley is moved in to surround the head of the patient. The surgeon stands behind the shield, observing the operative field through a lead glass to repair the palatal wound with long instruments. All instruments for the palatal repair should be prepared and ready, so that the surgery can be completed as soon as possible to reduce the time of radiation exposure.
- Patient selection is important for the success of gold grain implantation. Because of its short treatment distance, a gold grain implant is most suitable for well-defined nasopharyngeal mucosal lesions without extension outside the nasopharynx. Patients with imaging evidence of disease extension outside the nasopharynx were found to have a lower local control than those with lesions confined to the nasopharynx (5-year local control rate of 52% vs. 72.3%). Also, lesions near the choana or over the eustachian cushion are not suitable for gold grain

Table 13.1 Comparison of contemporary results of re-irradiation with different radiation techniques for local recurrence of NPC

Author (year)	RT	Dose (Gy)	Disease (rT stage)	No. of cases	Median follow-up (months)	Local control (%)	Complications
Kwong (2001)[20]	GG implant	60	P	45	49	87.2 [5 years]	Headache 28.3%
			1st R	53	45	62.7	Palatal fistula 18.9%
			2nd R (rT1–3)	8	27	23.4	NP necrosis 16%
Law (2002)[21]	Ir mold ± ERT	40	P	23	79	90 [5 years]	NP necrosis 33%
		50–55	1st R	78	77	89	Atlantoaxial instability 11%
			2nd R (rT1–2a)	6	44	33	Temporal lobe necrosis 8% Cranial nerve palsy 22%
Leung (2000)[22]	ICBT	22.5–24	P (rT1–3)	87	64	85 [5 years]	Cranial neuropathy 1% Endocrine dysfunction 9% Ulcer of NP/nasal septum 4% Epistaxis 2.5%
Leung (2000)[30]	ICBT	24–45	R (rT1–3)	8	27–55	50 [crude]	26% (cumulative incidence of neuroendocrine complications)
	ERT + ICBT	50 +14.8		42		57	71%
	ERT	57.3		41		39	46%
Chua (2009)[24]	SRS SRT	8–18 20–49	P+R (rT1; rT2–4)	25;18 23;20	40 24	69;28 [3 years] 88;78	SRS vs. SRT Severe complication: 33% vs. 21% Brain necrosis: 16% vs. 12 Massive bleeding: 2% vs. 4%
Chua (2005)[33]	IMRT ± SRS ± C	50–60	R(rT1–3; rT4)	17;14	11	100;35 [1 year]	1-year rate of grade 3 late toxicity, mostly ototoxicity/cranial neuropathy 25%
Lu (2004)[33]	IMRT	68–70	R(rT1–4)	49	9	100	Acute toxicity acceptable, late toxicity not reported

GG, interstitial gold-198 grain implantation; Ir, iridium-192; ICBT, intracavitary brachytherapy; ERT, external radiotherapy, 2-dimensional conventional radiotherapy; SRS, stereotactic radiosurgery (single fraction); SRT, stereotactic radiotherapy (multiple fractions); IMRT, intensity-modulated radiotherapy; C, chemotherapy; P, persistent disease; R, recurrence

implantation because the irregular surface and the thin mucosa over these sites will not hold the implanted grains. Well-defined superficial mucosal lesions may now be treated with endoscopic resection, and thus the indication for gold grain implantation may decrease. However, gold grain implantation still offers the additional advantage of treating 0.5 mm beyond the mucosa and can be considered in combination with endoscopic resection for treatment of exophytic recurrence.

Complications

Complications attributable to gold grain implants included headache, palatal fistula, and mucosal radiation necrosis at the implant site, which occurred in 28.3%, 18.9%, and 16% of patients, respectively. The incidence of palatal fistula can be reduced by closing the palatal wound in two layers instead of in one layer.

Case Study

A 55-year-old woman was referred to our center for treatment of local recurrence of NPC. She had NPC diagnosed 2 years before, presenting with neck node enlargement. She had had RT in another city. However, the initial disease stage and details of the first course of RT were unknown to us. This lack of information of the previous RT was of concern because the dose given to critical OARs will limit the tolerance of further radiation.

Endoscopy showed a 1 cm slightly elevated mass over the roof and posterior wall of the right nasopharynx. The left side of nasopharynx and recesses were clear. Biopsy of the right roof lesion showed undifferentiated carcinoma. Multiple biopsies were also taken from the periphery of the lesion for mapping out the extent of disease and were negative for malignancy. The tumor was small and mucosal, and suitable for gold grain implantation. Three gold grains were inserted with the split-palate approach. **Figure 13.2a** shows the post-implantation check film with the location of gold grains in the nasopharynx. **Figure 13.2b** shows the isodose distribution of the gold grain implant. The rapid dose fall-off from the plane of the implant would cause minimal radiation to brainstem and spinal cord.

The palatal wound was well healed after surgery. Endoscopy and repeat nasopharyngeal biopsies at 8 weeks post implantation showed no malignancy. The patient was well with no disease at 6 months after implantation and subsequently returned to her home town.

Iridium Mold

Preloaded or manually afterloaded iridium-192 molds have been used to treat mucosal recurrence of the nasopharynx. Tumors suitable for mold brachytherapy include those confined to the nasopharynx (rT1) or involving the upper choana with less than 5 mm

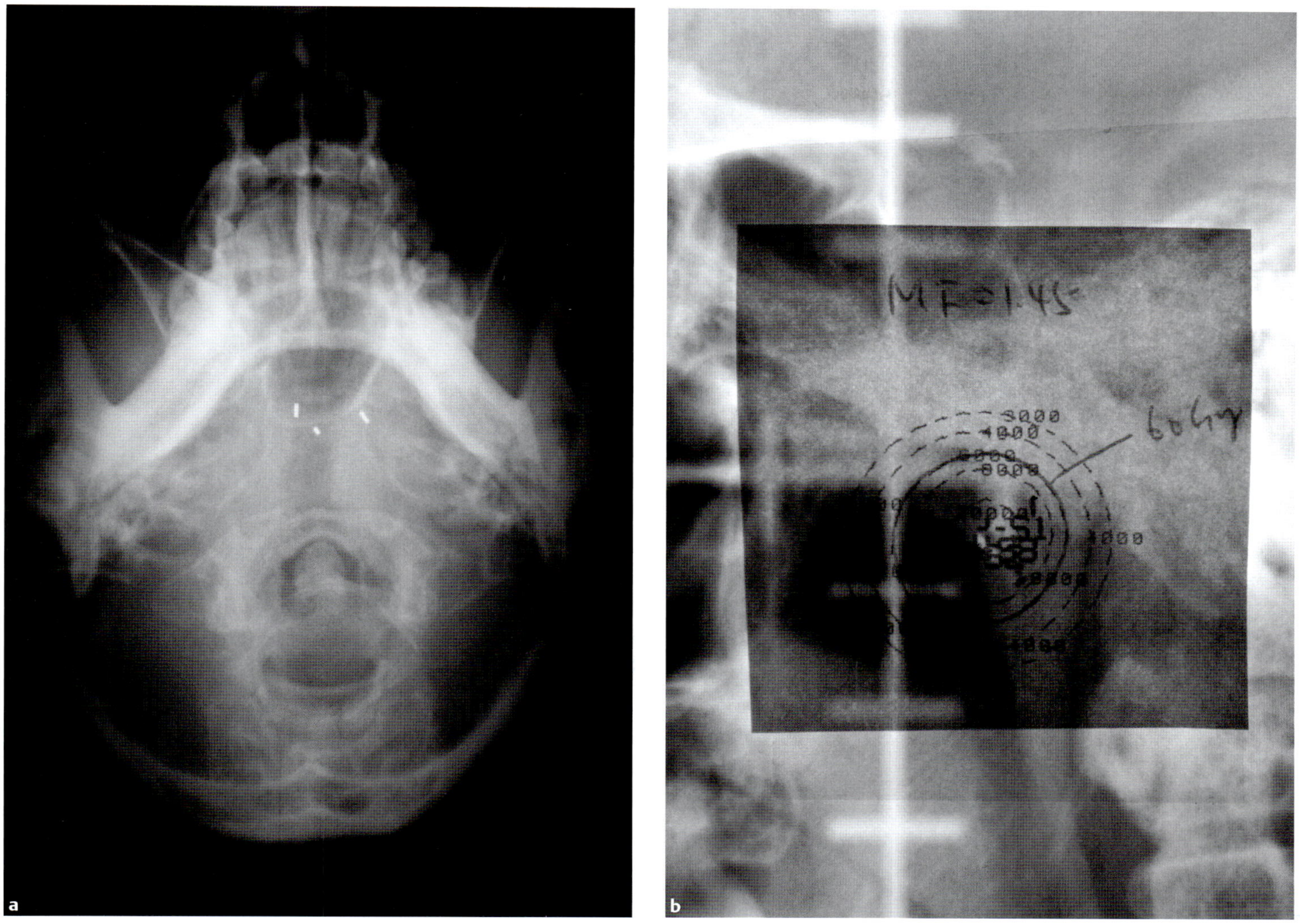

Fig. 13.2a, b Gold grain implant.
a Check film showing the gold grains in the nasopharynx after implantation.
b Isodose distribution superimposed on the lateral skull radiograph in centigrays (cGy) at the level of clivus and C1/2. The prescribed dose was 6000 cGy.

nasal extension (rT2a). Lesions that involve the following sites are considered too distant from the radioactive sources and should be excluded: the anterior lip of the eustachian cushion; the middle and lower third of the nasal septum; or an extension to >1 cm depth from the recess base.

To deliver adequate dose to the tumor, the mold must conform to and rest close to the mucosa of the nasopharynx. An individual tailor-made mold conforming to the contour of the nasopharynx surface is constructed. The tumor extent is mapped and the nasopharynx cavity dimensions are measured to make the mold. Insertion of the mold starts with recess dissection under local anesthetic. This will open up the recess and allows access to the depth of the recess by the peripheral sources of the mold. Better dosing to the recess and the medial part of paranasopharyngeal space can thus be achieved. Tumor debulking is performed as necessary to reduce tumor load and to facilitate positioning of the mold, and thus to improve the dose conformity.

Under local anesthesia, the mold is inserted through the mouth and pulled by catheters in the nasal fossa through the pharyngeal passage at the level of the soft palate to be lodged in lateral recesses of the nasopharynx. Catheters are placed on the surface of the mold for manual afterloading. The prescribed dose is 50–55 Gy in 4–7 days for recurrence and 40 Gy for persistent disease. The dose is prescribed empirically at 1 cm perpendicular to the source plane at the level of the pharyngeal recess. The mold is removed after 5 days when the prescribed dose has been delivered. The reported overall complete remission rate was 97% and the 5-year local control rate was 85% in selected series of patients.[21]

Special Considerations

- Compared with gold grain implantation, mold therapy can treat diffuse, superficial lesions that involve the whole nasopharynx and those with choanal involvement. Expertise is required in the making of the mold and its insertion. The completed mold is flexible and can be bent not only longitudinally to fit the angular junction between the roof and the posterior wall of the nasopharynx but also laterally for ease of insertion through the pharyngeal passage (**Fig. 13.3**). There are four catheters in the mold for housing manually afterloaded iridium-192 wires: two lateral sources for treating disease at the pharyngeal recess and two inner sources for disease in the central nasopharynx and choanal region. Since the central sources are close to each other, they have to be differentially loaded with three to four times less activity than the outer sources to achieve a more uniform dose distribution. When inserted into the nasopharynx, the separation between the source plane of the mold and the mucosal surface is around 3–4 mm.

- Mold brachytherapy is falling out of favor now because new precise external radiotherapy techniques such as stereotactic radiotherapy or intensity-modulated radiotherapy can give similar and more homogenous dose distribution and are less dependent on expertise. The sharp bending of the lateral sources at the junction of the roof and posterior wall of nasopharynx makes negotiation of sources difficult and the technique cannot be adapted for remote afterloading systems. Therefore, as with gold grain implantation, there is also radiation exposure to operator.

Complications

The reported 5-year major complication rate was 46.9%. Major complications included nasopharynx necrosis with headache, necrosis of cervical vertebrae with atlantoaxial instability, temporal lobe necrosis, and cranial nerve palsy. Due to the high dose delivered to the whole nasopharyngeal mucosa, acute confluent mucositis was universal and followed by persistent nasopharyngeal necrosis in 33% of patients, of whom 64% required analgesics for headache for a median duration of 6 months. One peculiar complication associated with mold therapy is necrosis of the arch of the atlas and the odontoid process. In a series of 118 patients reported by Law et al., this complication was observed after mold therapy in 13 patients, associated in all of them with extensive necrosis of nasopharynx. Five patients had atlantoaxial dislocation and two died with quadriparesis subsequently. The cumulative risk of developing this complication was 11%. The high surface dose to the posterior pharyngeal wall overlying the arch of the atlas was considered the culprit, as subsequent mucosal necrosis would erode into the underlying bone. Thus, in planning for radiation dose distribution, the arch of the atlas should be considered one of the OARs.

Intracavitary Brachytherapy by Intubation

Intracavitary brachytherapy of the nasopharynx has a long history and has been reported since the 1920s. Radioactive sources were put into the nasopharynx cavity through the nasal fossa to deliver a high dose to the whole nasopharynx mucosa. The sources used in the past included radium and cesium and were manually loaded. With the advance of high-dose-rate afterloading, intracavitary brachytherapy can be performed with more comfort and less radiation exposure to the operator. A 6F bronchial applicator is placed inside a 3.2 mm diameter nylon tube and is used as a nasopharyngeal applicator (microSelectron nylon tube nasal technique). Two applicators are positioned under topical anesthesia with fiberoptic endoscopic guidance. Afterloading is performed with an iridium-192 source (microSelectron; Nucletron, Veenendaal, The Netherlands), giving 10–12 Gy in two weekly fractions as boost after external RT or 22.5–24 Gy in three weekly sessions for recurrence. The dose is prescribed at a distance of 1 cm from the center of the surface defined by the sources. The long-term local control rate for persistent disease is 85%[22] and recurrent disease ranges from 45%–67%.[23,24]

Special Considerations

Intracavitary therapy is perhaps the most commonly used brachytherapy technique. It has the advantage of being easy to apply, without the need for general anesthesia and surgical exposure. The technique can be adapted from most remote afterloading facilities

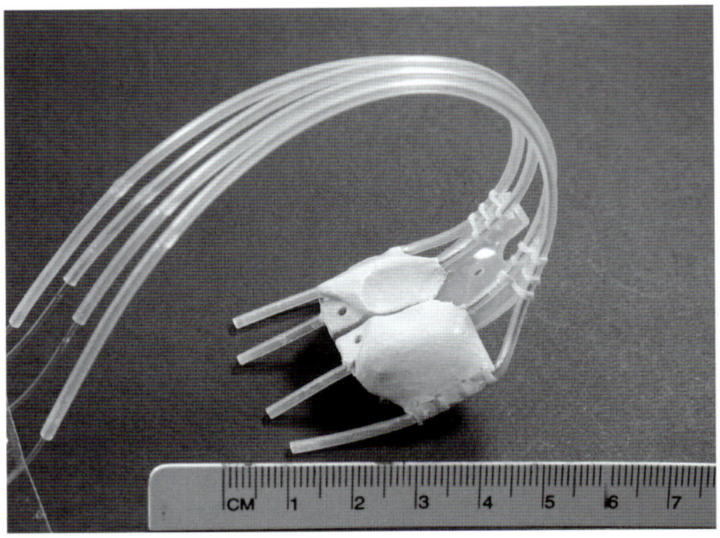

Fig. 13.3 The afterloaded mold showing its bending flexibility in the longitudinal plan. The polyform-made body is divided into two symmetrical halves to allow lateral folding to facilitate insertion. (Courtesy of Dr. S.C.K. Law, Department of Clinical Oncology, Queen Elizabeth Hospital, Hong Kong.)

and thus avoids radiation exposure to the operator. It is also less dependent on expertise and is widely applicable to most patients and in most radiotherapy centers. Intracavitary brachytherapy can be used for T1and T2a/b disease as a boost after external RT, or used with or without additional external RT for persistent or recurrent NP disease. It can be used for diffuse disease involving the nasopharynx bilaterally, which would not be suitable for gold grain implantation. In placing the catheter applicators, it is important to get the applicators positioned close to the roof of the nasopharynx, with two catheters each placed near to one of the lateral recesses (**Fig. 13.4**). This will allow the catheters to get close to the mucosal surface, provide adequate dose to lateral wall of the nasopharynx, and avoid overcrowding of sources and hot spot. With the catheters in place, the afterloading facility can allow three-dimensional reconstruction and optimization of the radiation plan.

Complications

Reported complications include soft tissue necrosis of the nasopharynx, perforation of the nasal septum, epistaxis, cranial neuropathy, temporal lobe necrosis, and endocrine disturbances. The 5-year major and central nervous system complication-free rates were 26.7% and 47.8% for patients with local recurrence treated with intracavitary brachytherapy with or without two-dimensional external re-irradiation.

■ External Radiotherapy

Stereotactic Radiation

Stereotactic radiation is the technique in which a small target is stereotactically localized and irradiated with multiple convergent beams. By combining treatment precision and rapid dose fall-off beyond the isocenter, a high radiation dose can be delivered to the target while sparing the adjacent critical structures. The margin around tumor is tight, usually around 2–3 mm. The radiation can be delivered as a large single dose (**Fig. 13.5**) or in multiple

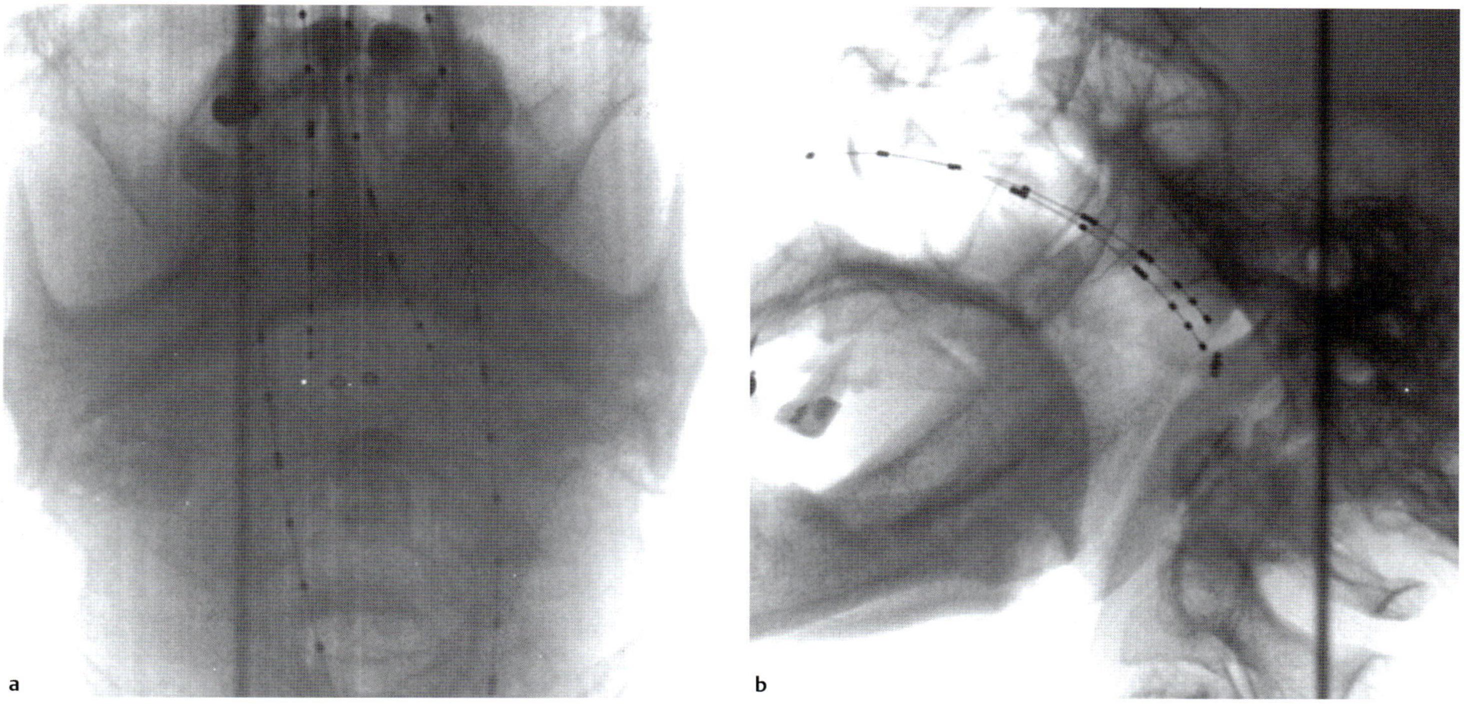

Fig. 13.4a, b Anterior (**a**) and lateral (**b**) check films showing the nasal tubes inserted for intracavitary radiation with radiopaque dummies in situ.

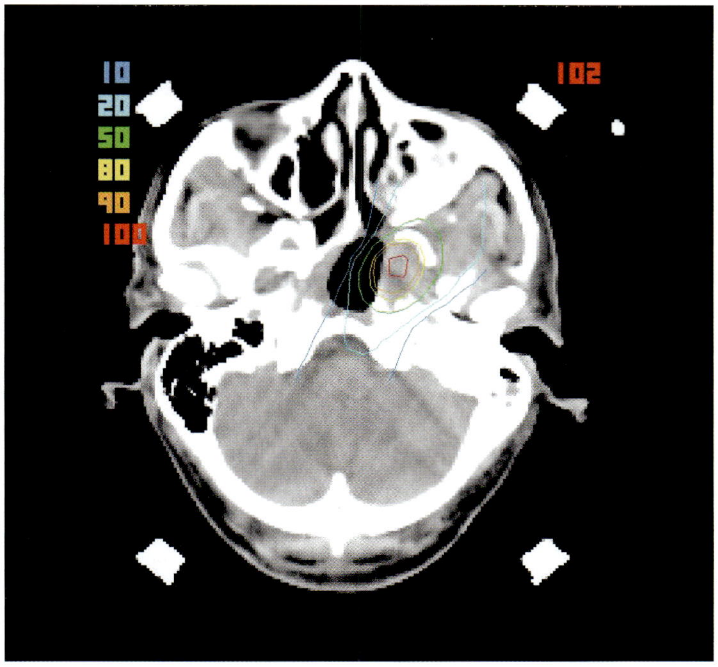

Fig. 13.5 Isodose distribution of stereotactic radiosurgery for recurrent nasopharyngeal carcinoma. Isodose lines are in percentage dose. A dose of 12 Gy was prescribed to the 80% isodose.

fractions (stereotactic radiotherapy). Due to the small volume of irradiation, hypofractionation can be employed.

Stereotactic radiation has been used in treatment of recurrent nasopharyngeal carcinoma, particularly for rT3–T4 disease when surgery and brachytherapy is not possible or for rT1–T2 disease when the patient is not suitable for brachytherapy or refuses surgery. Single doses of 8–18 Gy and fractionated doses of 14–65 Gy have been employed. Series are generally small (<100 patients) but have reported 3-year local control rates of 31%–100%. In a case-matched cohort study comparing a single fraction with median dose of 12.5 Gy with multiple fraction of stereotactic radiation with a median dose of 34 Gy in 2–6 fractions, the 3-year local control rate was found to be better with fractionated sterotactic radiotherapy (83% vs. 51%, $P = 0.003$).[25,26] Complication rates were also lower in the fractionated stereotactic radiotherapy. Thus, fractionated treatment is preferred. In another cohort, comparison of patients treated with gold grain implantation or stereotactic radiosurgery, 3-year local control was better with gold grain implantation, although the difference was not statistically significant (77.9% vs. 68.3%).[27]

Special Considerations

- Most modern linear accelerators allow adaptation for stereotactic treatment with multiple-arc photon beams. Thus, stereotactic radiation can be performed in most modern radiotherapy centers.
- Head immobilization and target localization are achieved with a fixed stereotactic device for a single fraction or using relocatable devices for fractionated stereotactic radiotherapy.
- Chua et al. have devised a prognostic score for selecting patients for stereotactic radiosurgery for local failure of nasopharyngeal carcinoma. The scores incorporate five factors for considerations: age (>45 years), time interval from primary radiotherapy (>6 months), rT4 disease, tumor volume (10 cm^3 or more), and prior local failure. Using a combined prognostic score, patients are grouped into good, intermediate and poor prognostic groups. Those with poor prognostic score are not recommended for radiosurgery.[28] The applicability of this prognostic score needs to be validated in further studies.

Complications

There is a 2%–5% incidence of severe hemorrhage, which can be potentially fatal, after stereotactic radiation. Severe hemorrhage after re-irradiation can be due to mucosal necrosis, tumor regrowth, and carotid rupture due to aneurysm. To avoid carotid rupture,

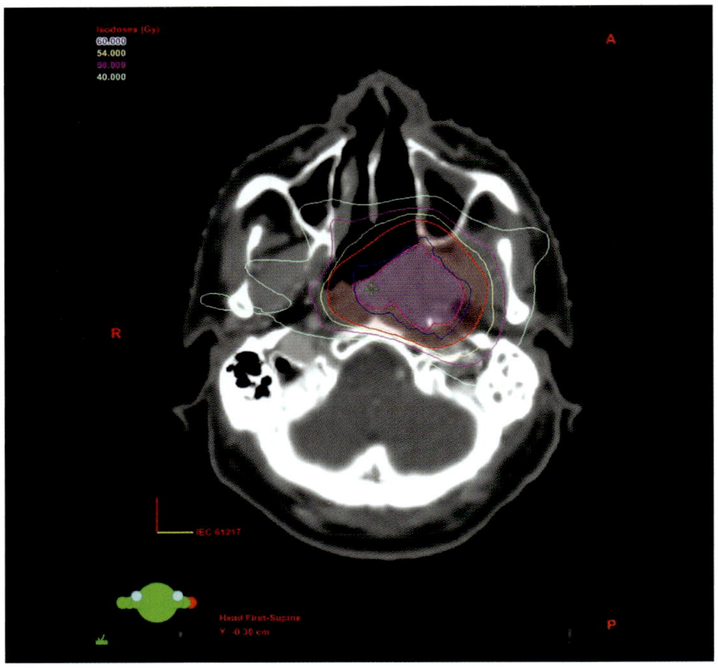

Fig. 13.6 Isodose distribution of intensity-modulated radiotherapy treatment for left side recurrent nasopharyngeal carcinoma. The planning target volume (red filled area) receives 50 Gy while the gross tumor volume (magenta outline) receives 60 Gy in 30 fractions. Isodose lines are absolute dose in grays.

patients with direct tumor encasement of cavernous sinus and internal carotid artery should not be treated by single-dose stereotactic radiation. The fractional dose in stereotactic radiotherapy is also important, as large fractional doses are also prone to causing carotid rupture. In patients with tumor encasement of the carotid artery, a small fractional dose, not exceeding 6 Gy, is recommended. Neuroendocrine complications are also common after stereotactic radiation and include 12%–16% brain necrosis.

Intensity Modulated Radiotherapy

For patients with extensive local recurrence not amenable to brachytherapy, surgery, or stereotactic radiation, external re-irradiation remains the only option. With conventional two-dimensional re-irradiation, the rate of successful local salvage ranged from 21% to 41% with formidable late complications. A dose of 60 Gy or above is found to be necessary for local salvage.[29] The advance of three-dimensional conformal RT and intensity-modulated radiotherapy (IMRT) improved re-irradiation by giving a more precise high dose to tumor and a limited dose to critical OARs that have already received a high radiation dose in the primary treatment. Compared with three-dimensional conformal RT, IMRT has improved tumor dose homogeneity and lower normal tissue doses, and is thus the preferred technique for modern external beam re-irradiation.[30]

With IMRT, a re-irradiaton dose of 50–70 Gy can be achieved in tumor without overdosing critical OARs (**Fig. 13.6**). Chemotherapy is generally used in combination with IMRT. Induction chemotherapy is used in some case to reduce tumor bulk before re-irradiation, and concurrent chemotherapy can be used with IMRT re-irradiation. Brachytherapy boost can be added to external re-irradiation and has been found to improve local control.[31]

Koutcher et al. reported 29 patients treated with external beam RT with or without brachytherapy.[32] Thirteen patients received intracavitary brachytherapy boost, 85% received IMRT, and 93% received chemotherapy, which was platinum-based for 85% of patients. The 5-year local control rate was 52%. In another study reported by Chua et al., the 1-year locoregional control was 56% for 31 patients re-irradiated with IMRT.[33] Some patients also had chemotherapy and radiosurgery boost in addition to IMRT. Lu et al. reported 100% local control at a median follow-up of 9 months after re-irradiation with IMRT.[34] Thus, the early result of IMRT re-irradiation appears to be favorable compared with historical series using two-dimensional conventional RT for re-irradiation. Patients with positive resection margins after surgery for local recurrence may also be considered for postoperative IMRT.

Special Considerations

As most cases treated by IMRT are rT3 or rT4 disease with skull base or intracranial extension, the most important function of IMRT is to achieve a high dose in tumor while keeping down the dose to critical OARs such as brainstem, spinal cord, and sometimes the optic pathway in re-irradiation. If there is a long interval between primary RT and recurrence, some degree of recovery has taken place, even for neural tissue.

High doses to the temporal lobe are common as the tumor often invades the cavernous sinus and/or skull base. However, the volume of temporal lobes that receives 60 Gy or more should be minimized. The re-irradiation dose to recurrent tumor is often limited by tolerance of the OARs. Woo et al. compared treatment plans of IMRT and stereotactic radiosurgery for the treatment of intracranial lesions. They found the IMRT treatment plan to be superior to the radiosurgery plan using multiple isocenters for a large (>4 cm) irregularly shaped intracranial target. To have meaningful local control, a tumor dose of 50 Gy or more is required. Patients treated with 60 Gy or higher had better local control.

For a tumor that is too extensive to be irradiated, chemotherapy can be given to reduce tumor load and the feasibility of re-irradiation should be reassessed after 3–4 cycles.[35] Brachytherapy or stereotactic radiation can be used to supplement the dose to tumor.

Complications

Documenting late complications of external re-irradiation is difficult as most patients already have a degree of late radiation toxicities from the first RT course. These are most commonly xerostomia, hearing loss, and neck fibrosis. New toxicities may arise after a second course of RT, but it can be difficult to differentiate re-irradiation complications from tumor progression. The reported severe (grade 3 or more) late complications after external re-irradiation range from 6% to 73%. Most of the complications are soft tissue fibrosis and neurological complications including ototoxicity, cranial neuropathy, and brain necrosis. Brain necrosis, especially temporal lobe necrosis, occurs in 2%–27% after re-irradiation. Radionecrosis of nasopharyngeal mucosa was observed in patients treated with more than 68 Gy to tumor. The late complication rates of IMRT appear to be less than with conventional two-dimensional re-irradiation, but the follow-up periods of IMRT series were still short.

Chemotherapy

As mentioned above, chemotherapy is frequently given before or during re-irradiation for salvage of local failure. For patients with distant metastases, chemotherapy is mainly for palliation.

Cisplatin-based combination regimens are the most commonly used in the metastatic setting, with an overall response rate (ORR) of 50%–70% and median survival (MS) of approximately 11 months. Cisplatin and 5-fluorouracil (5-FU) is the standard combination. However, as more and more patients are exposed to cisplatin and 5-FU in primary treatment, novel chemotherapeutic agents are required for treatment of recurrence. Used as first-line chemotherapy, the cisplatin and capecitabine combination has a reported ORR of 62.5% and MS of 13.3 months.[36]

Taxanes are useful in squamous cell head and neck cancers and have been assessed in nasopharyngeal carcinoma also. The combination of docetaxel and cisplatin as first-line treatment showed an ORR of 62.6% and MS of 12.4 months.[37] Paclitaxel and carboplatin showed an ORR of 59%.[38]

Gemcitabine is active in nasopharyngeal carcinoma. In a phase II study of 44 patients with metastatic or recurrent nasopharyngeal carcinoma, more than half of the patients had previous exposure to platinum-based chemotherapy. In that study, the combination of gemcitabine and cisplatin achieved an ORR of 73% and 1-year survival of 62%.[39] In another study using gemcitabine and oxaliplatin as first-line treatment of recurrent or metastatic nasopharyngeal carcinoma, the ORR was 56.1% and MS was 19.6 months.[40] Gemcitabine alone had an ORR of 28% for chemo-naive and 48% for previously treated patients.[41] Treatment was well tolerated.

For platinum-resistant patients, the combination of ifosfamide, 5-FU and leucovorin achieved an ORR of 56% and 1-year overall survival of 51%.[42] Airoldi et al. reported partial response in 3 out of 12 patients using carboplatin plus taxol for recurrent nasopharyngeal carcinoma after failure of platinum and 5-FU. Median survival was 9.5 months.[43] The combination of gemcitabine and vinorelbine showed ORR of 36% and median survival of 11.9 months with significant toxicities.[44] Oral capecitabine achieved an ORR of 23.5% and MS was 7.6 months.[45] Irinotecan had an ORR of 14% and MS of 11.4 months with moderate toxicity.[46]

Targeted Therapy

Epidermal growth factor receptor (EGFR) is frequently overexpressed in nasopharyngeal carcinoma. However, attempts at targeted therapy on the EGFR pathway have not met with much success. Chan et al. reported combining carboplatin with cetuximab, a monoclonal antibody against EGFR, in the treatment of 60 patients with platinum-resistant recurrent or metastatic NPC.[47] Overall response rate was 11.7% with no complete response and median survival was 233 days.

Gefitinib, an oral EGFR-specific tyrosine kinase inhibitor, showed no objective response in two phase II trials in patients pretreated with platinum-based chemotherapy.[48,49]

Sorafenib is an oral inhibitor of the serine/threonine kinases C-raf and B-raf and of the receptor tyrosine kinases of vascular endothelial growth factor. A phase II trial of sorafenib in patients with recurrent/metastatic squamous cell head and neck cancers and nasopharyngeal carcinoma yielded negative results. In the seven patients with nasopharyngeal carcinoma, the time to progression was 3.2 months and median survival was 7.7 months.[50]

Immunotherapy

As virtually all undifferentiated and poorly differentiated NPCs harbor latent EBV, the viral antigens expressed by tumor cells are potential targets for immunotherapy. Nasopharyngeal carcinoma expresses a restricted set of immunogenic viral antigens, namely Epstein–Barr nuclear antigen 1 (EBNA-1) and latent membrane proteins 1 and 2 (LMP-1 and 2). LMP-1 and LMP-2 are immunogenic and detectable in approximately 50% of nasopharyngeal carcinoma. These antigens are able to elicit an immune cytotoxic T-lymphocyte (CTL, particularly $CD8^+$ T cells)-mediated response directed against nasopharyngeal carcinoma cells. Two immunotherapy approaches used are adoptive immunotherapy and active immunotherapy.

Adoptive Immunotherapy

Adoptive immunotherapy involves the adoptive transfer of cytotoxic T-lymphocytes specific for EBV antigens. A pilot study was reported in 2001.[51] Autologous EBV-transformed B-lymphoblastoid cell line reactivated T cells were generated in vitro and infused back to four patients with advanced nasopharyngeal carcinoma. The treatment was found to be safe, with no inflammatory or other complications, but with no reduction of tumor bulk. Two subsequent clinical trials have evaluated the use of autologous EBV-specific cytotoxic T-lymphocytes for nasopharyngeal carcinoma. Comoli et al. reported 60% disease control and two partial responses in 10 patients with stage IV nasopharyngeal carcinoma showing progression after conventional RT and chemotherapy.[52] In another study, 10 patients were treated: 4 of the patients had been in complete remission after treatment and 6 patients had recurrent/metastatic disease.[53] All 4 patients who were in complete remission remained disease free with a follow-up of approximately 27 months. For the 6 patients with refractory disease, 2 had complete response for 11 to 23 months, 1 had partial response that persisted for 12 months, 1 had stable disease for more than 14 months, and 2 had no response. Toxicity reported in both trials was mild.

Active Immunotherapy

Active immunotherapy consists of delivering selected tumor-associated antigens to patients with the aim of inducing an immune response that may result in the eradication of malignant cells. A vaccine consisting of dendritic cells pulsed with peptides derived from LMP-2 has been evaluated in 16 patients with recurrent or metastatic disease.[54] Epitope-specific T cell responses were elicited or boosted in 9 patients and partial response was observed in 2 patients. Another strategy is to develop an epitope-based vaccination by using a recombinant poxvirus vaccine that encodes a polyepitope protein comprising epitopes derived from LMP-1.[55]

Future Research

- Determining the exact extent of tumor by new imaging technique and biological behavior so that surgical salvage can be performed effectively.
- Identifying a method for accurate assessment of the resection margin at the time of surgery to ensure that all disease is removed.
- Continued research on pathways accounting for radio- and chemoresistance of NPC is important for personalized treatment and predicting patients at high risk of recurrence after primary treatment.
- Novel pathways for biological/targeted therapy should be explored to develop more effective systemic treatment other than chemotherapy.

Recommended Reading

- Wei WI, Sham JS. Nasopharyngeal carcinoma. Lancet 2005;365(9476):2041–2054
- Wei WI, Ho CM, Wong MP, Ng WF, Lau SK, Lam KH. Pathological basis of surgery in the management of postradiotherapy cervical metastasis in nasopharyngeal carcinoma. Arch Otolaryngol Head Neck Surg 1992;118(9):923–929, discussion 930
- Wei WI, Chan JY, Ng RW, Ho WK. Surgical salvage of persistent or recurrent nasopharyngeal carcinoma with maxillary swing approach—critical appraisal after 2 decades. Head Neck 2011;33(7):969–975
- Wei WI. Cancer of the nasopharynx: functional surgical salvage. World J Surg 2003;27(7):844–848

Essential Reading for Clinical Oncologists

- Kwong DL, Wei WI, Cheng AC, et al. Long term results of radioactive gold grain implantation for the treatment of persistent and recurrent nasopharyngeal carcinoma. Cancer 2001;91(6):1105–1113
- Law SC, Lam WK, Ng MF, Au SK, Mak WT, Lau WH. Reirradiation of nasopharyngeal carcinoma with intracavitary mold brachytherapy: an effective means of local salvage. Int J Radiat Oncol Biol Phys 2002;54(4):1095–1113
- Leung TW, Tung SY, Sze WK, et al. Salvage radiation therapy for locally recurrent nasopharyngeal carcinoma. Int J Radiat Oncol Biol Phys 2000;48(5):1331–1338
- Chua DT, Wu SX, Lee V, Tsang J. Comparison of single versus fractionated dose of stereotactic radiotherapy for salvaging local failures of nasopharyngeal carcinoma: a matched-cohort analysis. Head Neck Oncol 2009;1:13

References

1. Lee AW, Sze WM, Au JS, et al. Treatment results for nasopharyngeal carcinoma in the modern era: the Hong Kong experience. Int J Radiat Oncol Biol Phys 2005;61(4):1107–1116
2. Hui EP, Leung SF, Au JS, et al. Lung metastasis alone in nasopharyngeal carcinoma: a relatively favorable prognostic group. A study by the Hong Kong Nasopharyngeal Carcinoma Study Group. Cancer 2004;101(2):300–306
3. Kwong DL, Nicholls J, Wei WI, et al. The time course of histologic remission after treatment of patients with nasopharyngeal carcinoma. Cancer 1999;85(7):1446–1453
4. Yu KH, Leung SF, Tung SY, et al. Hong Kong Nasopharyngeal Carcinoma Study Group. Survival outcome of patients with nasopharyngeal carcinoma with first local failure: a study by the Hong Kong Nasopharyngeal Carcinoma Study Group. Head Neck 2005;27(5):397–405
5. Lo YM, Chan LY, Chan AT, et al. Quantitative and temporal correlation between circulating cell-free Epstein–Barr virus DNA and tumor recurrence in nasopharyngeal carcinoma. Cancer Res 1999;59(21):5452–5455
6. Wei WI, Ho CM, Wong MP, Ng WF, Lau SK, Lam KH. Pathological basis of surgery in the management of postradiotherapy cervical metastasis in nasopharyngeal carcinoma. Arch Otolaryngol Head Neck Surg 1992;118(9):923–929, discussion 930
7. Wei WI, Ho WK, Cheng AC, et al. Management of extensive cervical nodal metastasis in nasopharyngeal carcinoma after radiotherapy: a clinicopathological study. Arch Otolaryngol Head Neck Surg 2001;127(12):1457–1462
8. Fisch U. The infratemporal fossa approach for nasopharyngeal tumors. Laryngoscope 1983;93(1):36–44
9. Fee WE Jr, Roberson JB Jr, Goffinet DR. Long-term survival after surgical resection for recurrent nasopharyngeal cancer after radiotherapy failure. Arch Otolaryngol Head Neck Surg 1991;117(11):1233–1236
10. Morton RP, Liavaag PG, McLean M, Freeman JL. Transcervico-mandibulo-palatal approach for surgical salvage of recurrent nasopharyngeal cancer. Head Neck 1996;18(4):352–358
11. Wei WI. Salvage neck dissection after radiation and/or chemotherapy. Operative Techniques in Otolaryngology 2004;15:269–272
12. Chen MK, Lai JC, Chang CC, Liu MT. Minimally invasive endoscopic nasopharyngectomy in the treatment of recurrent T1-2a nasopharyngeal carcinoma. Laryngoscope 2007;117(5):894–896
13. Wei WI, Ho WK. Transoral robotic resection of recurrent nasopharyngeal carcinoma. Laryngoscope 2010;120(10):2011–2014
14. Wei WI, Lam KH, Sham JS. New approach to the nasopharynx: the maxillary swing approach. Head Neck 1991;13(3):200–207
15. Ng RW, Wei WI. Elimination of palatal fistula after the maxillary swing procedure. Head Neck 2005;27(7):608–612
16. Wei WI, Lam KH, Ho CM, Sham JS, Lau SK. Efficacy of radical neck dissection for the control of cervical metastasis after radiotherapy for nasopharyngeal carcinoma. Am J Surg 1990;160(4):439–442
17. Wei WI, Chan JYW, Ng RW, Ho WK. Surgical salvage of persistent or recurrent nasopharyngeal carcinoma with maxillary swing approach—critical appraisal after 2 decades. Head Neck 2011;33(7):969–975
18. Ng RW, Wei WI. Quality of life of patients with recurrent nasopharyngeal carcinoma treated with nasopharyngectomy using the maxillary swing approach. Arch Otolaryngol Head Neck Surg 2006;132(3):309–316
19. Wei WI, Sham JS, Choy D, Ho CM, Lam KH. Split-palate approach for gold grain implantation in nasopharyngeal carcinoma. Arch Otolaryngol Head Neck Surg 1990;116(5):578–582
20. Kwong DL, Wei WI, Cheng AC, et al. Long term results of radioactive gold grain implantation for the treatment of persistent and recurrent nasopharyngeal carcinoma. Cancer 2001;91(6):1105–1113
21. Law SC, Lam WK, Ng MF, Au SK, Mak WT, Lau WH. Reirradiation of nasopharyngeal carcinoma with intracavitary mold brachytherapy: an effective means of local salvage. Int J Radiat Oncol Biol Phys 2002;54(4):1095–1113

22. Leung TW, Tung SY, Sze WK, Sze WM, Wong VY, O SK. Salvage brachytherapy for patients with locally persistent nasopharyngeal carcinoma. Int J Radiat Oncol Biol Phys 2000;47(2):405–412
23. Zhang YW, Liu TF, Fi CX. Intracavitary radiation treatment of nasopharyngeal carcinoma by the high dose rate afterloading technique. Int J Radiat Oncol Biol Phys 1989;16(2):315–318
24. Wang CC. Re-irradiation of recurrent nasopharyngeal carcinoma—treatment techniques and results. Int J Radiat Oncol Biol Phys 1987;13(7):953–956
25. Chua DT, Wu SX, Lee V, Tsang J. Comparison of single versus fractionated dose of stereotactic radiotherapy for salvaging local failures of nasopharyngeal carcinoma: a matched-cohort analysis. Head Neck Oncol 2009;1:13
26. Wu SX, Chua DT, Deng ML, et al. Outcome of fractionated stereotactic radiotherapy for 90 patients with locally persistent and recurrent nasopharyngeal carcinoma. Int J Radiat Oncol Biol Phys 2007;69(3):761–769
27. Chua DT, Wei WI, Sham JS, Hung KN, Au GK. Stereotactic radiosurgery versus gold grain implantation in salvaging local failures of nasopharyngeal carcinoma. Int J Radiat Oncol Biol Phys 2007;69(2):469–474
28. Chua DT, Sham JS, Hung KN, Leung LH, Au GK. Predictive factors of tumor control and survival after radiosurgery for local failures of nasopharyngeal carcinoma. Int J Radiat Oncol Biol Phys 2006;66(5):1415–1421
29. Lee AW, Law SC, Foo W, et al. Retrospective analysis of patients with nasopharyngeal carcinoma treated during 1976–1985: survival after local recurrence. Int J Radiat Oncol Biol Phys 1993;26(5):773–782
30. Hsiung CY, Yorke ED, Chui CS, et al. Intensity-modulated radiotherapy versus conventional three-dimensional conformal radiotherapy for boost or salvage treatment of nasopharyngeal carcinoma. Int J Radiat Oncol Biol Phys 2002;53(3):638–647
31. Leung TW, Tung SY, Sze WK, et al. Salvage radiation therapy for locally recurrent nasopharyngeal carcinoma. Int J Radiat Oncol Biol Phys 2000;48(5):1331–1338
32. Koutcher L, Lee N, Zelefsky M, et al. Reirradiation of locally recurrent nasopharynx cancer with external beam radiotherapy with or without brachytherapy. Int J Radiat Oncol Biol Phys 2010;76(1):130–137
33. Chua DT, Sham JS, Leung LH, Au GK. Re-irradiation of nasopharyngeal carcinoma with intensity-modulated radiotherapy. Radiother Oncol 2005;77(3):290–294
34. Lu TX, Mai WY, Teh BS, et al. Initial experience using intensity-modulated radiotherapy for recurrent nasopharyngeal carcinoma. Int J Radiat Oncol Biol Phys 2004;58(3):682–687
35. Chua DT, Sham JS, Au GK. Induction chemotherapy with cisplatin and gemcitabine followed by reirradiation for locally recurrent nasopharyngeal carcinoma. Am J Clin Oncol 2005;28(5):464–471
36. Li YH, Wang FH, Jiang WQ, et al. Phase II study of capecitabine and cisplatin combination as first-line chemotherapy in Chinese patients with metastatic nasopharyngeal carcinoma. Cancer Chemother Pharmacol 2008;62(3):539–544
37. Chua DT, Sham JS, Au GK. A phase II study of docetaxel and cisplatin as first-line chemotherapy in patients with metastatic nasopharyngeal carcinoma. Oral Oncol 2005;41(6):589–595
38. Yeo W, Leung TW, Chan AT, et al. A phase II study of combination paclitaxel and carboplatin in advanced nasopharyngeal carcinoma. Eur J Cancer 1998;34(13):2027–2031
39. Ngan RK, Yiu HH, Lau WH, et al. Combination gemcitabine and cisplatin chemotherapy for metastatic or recurrent nasopharyngeal carcinoma: report of a phase II study. Ann Oncol 2002;13(8):1252–1258
40. Ma BB, Hui EP, Wong SC, et al. Multicenter phase II study of gemcitabine and oxaliplatin in advanced nasopharyngeal carcinoma—correlation with excision repair cross-complementing-1 polymorphisms. Ann Oncol 2009;20(11):1854–1859
41. Foo KF, Tan EH, Leong SS, et al. Gemcitabine in metastatic nasopharyngeal carcinoma of the undifferentiated type. Ann Oncol 2002;13(1):150–156
42. Chua DT, Kwong DL, Sham JS, Au GK, Choy D. A phase II study of ifosfamide, 5-fluorouracil and leucovorin in patients with recurrent nasopharyngeal carcinoma previously treated with platinum chemotherapy. Eur J Cancer 2000;36(6):736–741
43. Airoldi M, Pedani F, Marchionatti S, et al. Carboplatin plus taxol is an effective third-line regimen in recurrent undifferentiated nasopharyngeal carcinoma. Tumori 2002;88(4):273–276
44. Wang CC, Chang JY, Liu TW, Lin CY, Yu YC, Hong RL. Phase II study of gemcitabine plus vinorelbine in the treatment of cisplatin-resistant nasopharyngeal carcinoma. Head Neck 2006;28(1):74–80
45. Chua D, Wei WI, Sham JS, Au GK. Capecitabine monotherapy for recurrent and metastatic nasopharyngeal cancer. Jpn J Clin Oncol 2008;38(4):244–249
46. Poon D, Chowbay B, Cheung YB, Leong SS, Tan EH. Phase II study of irinotecan (CPT-11) as salvage therapy for advanced nasopharyngeal carcinoma. Cancer 2005;103(3):576–581
47. Chan AT, Hsu MM, Goh BC, et al. Multicenter, phase II study of cetuximab in combination with carboplatin in patients with recurrent or metastatic nasopharyngeal carcinoma. J Clin Oncol 2005;23(15):3568–3576
48. Chua DT, Wei WI, Wong MP, Sham JS, Nicholls J, Au GK. Phase II study of gefitinib for the treatment of recurrent and metastatic nasopharyngeal carcinoma. Head Neck 2008;30(7):863–867
49. Ma B, Hui EP, King A, et al. A phase II study of patients with metastatic or locoregionally recurrent nasopharyngeal carcinoma and evaluation of plasma Epstein–Barr virus DNA as a biomarker of efficacy. Cancer Chemother Pharmacol 2008;62(1):59–64
50. Elser C, Siu LL, Winquist E, et al. Phase II trial of sorafenib in patients with recurrent or metastatic squamous cell carcinoma of the head and neck or nasopharyngeal carcinoma. J Clin Oncol 2007;25(24):3766–3773
51. Chua D, Huang J, Zheng B, et al. Adoptive transfer of autologous Epstein–Barr virus-specific cytotoxic T cells for nasopharyngeal carcinoma. Int J Cancer 2001;94(1):73–80
52. Comoli P, Pedrazzoli P, Maccario R, et al. Cell therapy of stage IV nasopharyngeal carcinoma with autologous Epstein–Barr virus-targeted cytotoxic T lymphocytes. J Clin Oncol 2005;23(35):8942–8949
53. Straathof KC, Bollard CM, Popat U, et al. Treatment of nasopharyngeal carcinoma with Epstein–Barr virus-specific T lymphocytes. Blood 2005;105(5):1898–1904
54. Lin CL, Lo WF, Lee TH, et al. Immunization with Epstein–Barr virus (EBV) peptide-pulsed dendritic cells induces functional CD8+ T-cell immunity and may lead to tumor regression in patients with EBV-positive nasopharyngeal carcinoma. Cancer Res 2002;62(23):6952–6958
55. Duraiswamy J, Sherritt M, Thomson S, et al. Therapeutic LMP1 polyepitope vaccine for EBV-associated Hodgkin disease and nasopharyngeal carcinoma. Blood 2003;101(8):3150–3156

14 Skull Base and Sinonasal Cancer

Claudio R. Cernea, Lenine Garcia Brandão, Eduardo Weltman

Summary

- It is important to establish the diagnosis of a recurrent skull base tumor with a positive biopsy before considering therapeutic options.
- Radiological findings of inoperability include gross invasion of vital parts of the CNS and bilateral gross orbital invasion in a nonblind patient.
- You should try to obtain data concerning the previous treatment, including initial biopsies, radiological findings, and, when applicable, radiation treatment.
- In surgical cases, meticulously close any dural defect and carefully reconstruct the craniofacial diaphragm, to avoid CSF leak and meningitis.

Introduction

The treatment of recurrent skull base tumors (RSBTs) represents a formidable challenge. Early detection of tumor relapse may be very difficult, due to distortion of anatomical landmarks and presence of fibrosis/gliosis, as well as reconstructive flaps used at the previous operation. Recurrence may involve vital areas of the central nervous system, precluding radical resection with a reasonable chance of cure, while preserving life quality at a functional level. On the other hand, significant long-term palliation may be obtained, especially with slow-growing tumors.

Radiation therapy (RT) can play an important role in salvaging patients with recurrent skull base and sinonasal cancer, after either primary surgery or initial chemoradiotherapy. In these cases, it is mandatory to perform a careful local and systemic staging, assessing the locoregional tumor extension and distant disease, and also to assess general clinical condition before recommending an extremely aggressive treatment.

Since there has not been any randomized study on this subject, due to rarity of the disease, all evidence presented in this chapter is level 4 or 5.

Prevalence and Prognostic Factors

Since the popularization of oncological skull base surgery, especially after the landmark papers published by Ketcham et al.[1] and Janecka et al.,[2] many patients with advanced skull base tumors have been submitted to very extensive operations. As increasing number of patients with locally advanced tumors underwent surgical resection, the prevalence of recurrent lesions also increased, leading to some very difficult situations. It is difficult to estimate properly the prevalence of these recurrent skull base tumors after treatment with curative intent, but in some series it may be as high as 50%.[3]

Prognostic factors identified in recurrent skull base tumors include histology, invasion of some structures (bone, dura mater, brain, venous sinuses, etc.), and type and extent of the previous treatment. In terms of radiation therapy (RT), the presence of sensitive tissues, such as brain and nerves, adjacent to or inside the target poses an additional challenge to the radiation oncology team in delivering tumoricidal doses of generally more than 60 Gy. RT of the skull base region carries the risks of temporal lobe necrosis, cranial nerve damage, and glandular dysfunction. Lee et al.[4] reviewed outcomes of 1008 patients treated for a T1 nasopharyngeal carcinoma at Queen Elizabeth Hospital (Hong Kong) between 1976 and 1985 using conventional RT. Seventy-four patients (7.3%) developed temporal lobe necrosis. Multivariate analyses showed that in a series of patients receiving total dose ranging from 45.6 to 60 Gy, the dose per fraction (from 2.5 to 4.2 Gy) was the most significant radiation factor for inducing necrosis ($P = 0.022$). Thus, in addition to the total dose, the dose per fraction should be carefully planned in a second series of RT.

The general guideline for normal tissue dose constraints for treating skull base cancer with fractionated RT up front is to limit the maximum point doses to brainstem and spinal cord to less than 60 Gy and 50 Gy, respectively, while keeping the maximum dose encompassing 1 cm^3 of the brainstem and spinal cord to below 54 Gy and 45 Gy, respectively. The maximum dose to the optic chiasm and optic nerves is usually kept to less than 54 Gy and the dose to the temporomandibular joints and mandible to below 70 Gy.[5] These constraints should be applied in the treatment of RSBTs after surgery but cannot be met in patients who develop recurrence after prior RT. Therefore, the risk of severe normal tissue complication should be weighed against the potential benefit of re-treatment in individual cases. The use of high-precision conformal RT, such as intensity-modulated radiotherapy and stereotactic radiosurgery, allows improvement of dose distribution inside the target and around the sensitive tissues. The steep dose fall-off outside the target volume allows appropriate protection of sensitive structures while treating the tumor with radical doses.

Clinical Assessment and Work-up

The diagnosis of a recurrent skull base tumor may be established on the basis of clinical or radiological findings.

- **Clinical findings:** Clinical findings depend on the location of the recurrence and of the involved structures. Usually, invasion of a branch of the trigeminal nerve causes pain, extension into orbit induces visual changes, and central relapse causes epistaxis.

- **Radiological findings:** The most used imaging methods for detection of a RSBT are computed tomography, magnetic resonance imaging, and PET-CT. Any mass in the skull base detected by one of these methods, especially PET-CT, must be considered a recurrence, unless proven otherwise.

Principles of Management

Management of Failure after Surgery

Patients with RSBT must undergo multidisciplinary evaluation, and imaging studies adequate to determine the extent of the lesion and to establish operability. If it is operable then wide resection, with watertight closure of dural defects if applicable, and microvascular flap reconstruction of large defects should be considered as this therapy provides the best chance for salvage. Postoperative adjuvant RT is indicated in such cases, especially for patients presenting recurrent meningiomas, where the actuarial second local recurrence rate at 10 years decreases from 70% for patients treated with surgery alone to 11% for patients receiving postoperative radiation therapy.[6]

In selected cases, focused RT such as radiosurgery can be of value. For example, Kocher et al.[7] reported a small series of 13 patients with RSBT, who had had single or multiple tumor resections or RT and were not considered for further conventional fractionated RT or surgery. These patients were treated with a single fraction of radiosurgery to a median dose of 15 Gy (range 9–24 Gy). The median survival time of eight patients with recurrent nasopharyngeal carcinomas was 9 months but three patients who had complete or partial remission survived 1.5–3.5 years. All five patients with sarcoma responded to radiosurgery and four were alive after a follow-up of 28–67 months. The authors concluded that radiosurgery was an effective tool for palliative treatment of extensively treated RSBT.

Series of conventional adjuvant RT usually included some patients who had been treated after resection of RSBT. It is therefore difficult to tease out the outcome of patients with RSBT. Since patients have not received RT, it is straightforward to follow the conventional recommendations in terms of dose and fractions as well as normal tissue dose limits. Although the role of chemotherapy is not clear in these rare tumors, taking in account the benefit demonstrated in other head and neck squamous cell carcinomas, neoadjuvant or concomitant chemotherapy can be considered because the overall prognosis is very poor.

Management of Failure after Radiotherapy

Patients presenting with local recurrence after full-dose RT have extremely poor prognosis as relapse usually occurs intracranially, outside the radiation portal, thus making it unresectable. Chemotherapy yielded response rates ranging from 10% to 40%[8] and a median survival between 6 and 9 months.[9] Although re-irradiation may be considered for few patients, this treatment must be decided upon very carefully and discussed on a case-by-case basis because it carries a high morbidity rate.[10,11]

Re-irradiation poses a major challenge to the radiation oncology team, and the goal of protecting the normal tissue by restricting the dose-volume needs sharp target definition, precise set-up during the treatment, and a steep dose fall-off outside the target volume. Intensity-modulated radiation therapy (IMRT) and stereotactic radiosurgery (single dose, hypofractionated, or with multiple fractions) are fundamental technical strategies for achieving success in these clinical situations.

Tanvetyanon et al.[12] reviewed the records of 103 patients reirradiated at H. Lee Moffitt Cancer Center between 1993 and 2008. They found that comorbidity and preexisting organ dysfunction were the most important prognostic factors for these patients. Other independent prognostic factors were interval from previous radiation, extent of recurrent tumor (stage and bulk) at reirradiation and re-irradiation dose. These results suggest that reirradiation could be considered more enthusiastically in patients with minimal comorbidity and presenting with relatively small tumors long after previous RT. To achieve this goal, it is fundamental to know the pattern of failure after re-irradiation and to better define the targets.[13]

In the series of Sulman et al.,[9] 31of the 74 evaluable patients (42%) had relapse near or at skull base (including sinonasal tumors). With a median re-irradiation dose of 60 Gy (median lifetime irradiation dose of 116.1 Gy), the 2-year overall survival and locoregional control rates were 58% and 64%, respectively. Severe related toxicity occurred in 15 patients (20%) and one treatment-related death was observed.

Roh et al.[8] re-irradiated 36 patients presenting with recurrent head and neck tumors with fractionated CyberKnife radiosurgery. The treatment volume in 29 of these patients (81%) included the skull base or maxillary sinus. Overall, 15 patients (42.9%) showed complete tumor regression and 13 patients (37.1%) had partial tumor regression. The 1- and 2-year local recurrence-free survival rates were 61.0% and 52.2%, respectively. Long-term adverse events were noted in three patients, two of them with nasopharyngeal cancer, presenting with trismus, soft tissue necrosis, and skull base bone necrosis. These three patients received 30–33 Gy in three fractions, which led the authors to change the dose-fractionation to 25–40 Gy in five fractions over five consecutive days. There was one treatment-related death due to progressive soft tissue necrosis and skull-base bone necrosis at 5 months after retreatment.

Tokuuye et al.[14] re-irradiated with stereotactic fractionated radiotherapy (median dose of 42 Gy in 7 fractions over 2.3 weeks) 19 patients with brain and base of skull tumors after conventional radiotherapy (mean total dose of 50 Gy in 5 weeks). Three of these patients presented with metastatic tumor for skull base. Fifteen of these patients achieved local control 5–51 months after re-irradiation, and only one patient with a history of extensive radiotherapy developed progressive radionecrosis 9 months after re-irradiation.

Selected recurrent, unresectable vestibular schwannomas presenting with new neurological signs or symptoms can be retreated with radiosurgery. Kano et al.[15] re-irradiated six patients, which resulted in tumor regression in four patients and volume stabilization in two and prevented new neurological symptoms in all.

Selected recurrent salivary tumors involving skull base may also be treated with radiosurgery with good local control and symptomatic relief. All 16 patients treated at University of California San Francisco achieved 1 year freedom from progression and 75% did so at 2 years. Five of seven patients with locoregional failure underwent repeat radiosurgery, successfully achieving control for an additional 4.4–13.4 months in four patients.[16]

Management of Failure after Combined Treatment

These patients are particularly difficult to manage. Principles discussed above—multidisciplinary evaluation of the case, proper imaging studies, etc.—are applicable in this condition. However, in many instances no effective therapy is available. It is important to consider aggressive palliation in selected cases.

Therapy Techniques

Surgical Techniques

It is very important to have access to the detailed record of the previous treatment. In other words, a detailed analysis of the operative report of the previous surgery and/or radiotherapy is essential for adequate planning of the surgical access and the reconstruction.[17] The surgical access usually includes the previous incision, extended to virgin tissues outside of the surgical bed. Conventional bi-coronal craniotomy, combined with some facial approach, such as nasal swing or facial translocation, is the usual way to address these recurrent tumors. However, the head and neck surgeon has to keep in mind that some atypical surgical approaches may be the choice, particularly when dealing with recurrent skin cancers in the skull base. A recent analysis of a series of 484 consecutive patients submitted to major skull base operations in two large Brazilian tertiary centers showed that atypical surgical access procedures were performed in 55.5% of the cases.[18] One of the reasons for this finding was the increased frequency of nonmelanoma skin cancers among those patients. In addition, 58.2% of the patients had already been treated with surgery or radiation therapy.

The goal is to excise the recurrent tumor with free margins, but this can be difficult or at times impossible, especially when there is extensive dural or brain invasion. A very useful technique for evaluating the skin margins of these very extensive recurrent cancers is use of the double-bladed scalpel.[19] In brief, at the beginning of the operation, the surgeon excises the whole perimeter of the lesion with a double-bladed scalpel, carefully mapping—both on the patient and on the excised strip—the corresponding location. The mapped specimen is sent for detailed frozen sectioning, which usually takes several minutes, while the resection of the main body of the tumor goes on. If any positive or suspicious margins are detected, a second strip is excised, until free margins are obtained.

After the tumor is excised, it is imperative to adequately restore the continuity of the craniofacial diaphragm. The best method is the galea-pericranial flap, especially for anterior skull base defects. However, in a reoperative setting, this flap has already been used in many cases and thus has to be excised with the tumor. In these situations, the best and maybe the only option is the microvascular reconstruction.[20] In our experience, the best option to reconstruct the diaphragm along with the large bony and soft tissue craniofacial defect is the rectus abdominis free flap.[21]

Special Considerations[16]

- Try to obtain data from the previous surgical procedure, as well as from the previous adjuvant treatment.
- Imaging studies should include high-resolution CT and MRI for accurate assessment of the bony and soft tissue extent of disease, respectively. The use of PET-CT is helpful in distinguishing post treatment effects from active tumor, and in ruling out systemic disease.
- Interventional radiology is indicated for performing preoperative embolization of highly vascularized tumors, mainly in the lateral skull base. Carotidangiography may also be helpful in mapping out the cerebral circulation, and balloon test occlusion may inform the need for cerebral revascularization in case of injury or sacrifice of the internal carotid artery (ICA).
- Keep in mind that the treatment of skull base tumors requires multidisciplinary input; therefore, surgical strategy must be extensively planned in conjunction with all involved teams. The feasibility of pre- or postoperative adjuvant therapy may be a critical determinant of the decision to pursue surgical resection.
- Frequently, the surgical approach involves atypical incisions, mandated by the extension of the recurrent lesion, especially if there is skin involvement.
- Usually, combined craniofacial resections start with the craniotomy. Do not hesitate to interrupt the procedure when unexpectedly extensive invasion of vital structures is noted (ICA, cavernous sinus (CS), optic chiasm, etc.), especially with very aggressive histological types. Pay special attention to preserving the integrity of the cranial nerves involved within the CS, especially if the ipsilateral eye is still functional. Dural invasion is not a contraindication per se, unless the remaining defect precludes adequate exposure for reconstruction. Similarly, brain invasion may be adequately managed unless vital areas, such as the dominant precentral gyrus, are invaded.
- Always perform a watertight dural closure, using grafts if necessary. In our experience, fascia lata is an excellent alternative.
- Do not hesitate to use microvascular flap reconstruction.

> ! Be very careful when considering a reoperation in the following instances: very aggressive histological types; and extensive involvement of the cavernous sinus, of the intracranial ICA, and of vital parts of the brain or of the optic chiasm.

Complications

The main complications of the craniofacial operations for recurrent tumors, as in every skull base resection, are cerebrospinal fluid fistula, meningitis, flap loss, local wound problems, cranial nerve injuries, hemorrhages, and coma. The frequency of major complications varies from 33%[22] to as high as 95%.[23] The most important measure to avoid complications is a meticulous watertight dural closure, as well as a reliable reconstruction of the craniofacial diaphragm, as cerebrospinal fistula and meningitis are the most common lethal complications.[24]

Case Study

A 42-year-old white salesman had a history of a previous craniofacial oncological resection of an ethmoid adenocarcinoma. Two years later, he developed a local recurrence adherent to

both frontal lobes and underwent a wide excision consisting of orbital exenteration, radical ethmoidectomy, and re-resection of the skull base, with excision of the recurrence adherent to both frontal lobes, using a craniotomy (**Fig. 14.1**).
Reconstruction was performed with a free forearm flap, and the patient received postoperative external beam radiation therapy. The patient had an uneventful posttreatment course, with good quality of life for 4 years. He then had a recurrence in the left orbit, and refused any further treatment.

Radiotherapy Techniques

Typical dose constraints to normal tissues as used for planning IMRT at the Hospital Israelita Albert Einstein and at the Hospital das Clínicas of University of Sao Paulo Medical School are summarized in **Table 14.1**. Deviations from these constraints, often encountered in re-irradiation setting, and potential options are to be discussed among the radiation oncology team and with the patient, including withholding of treatment.

When using single-dose stereotactic radiotherapy, the dose to the optic chiasm and nerves is kept below 8 Gy.

We consider re-irradiation if the interval from the first treatment is at least 1 year. In the setting of single-fraction stereotactic radiosurgery, it is crucial to avoid or minimize overlap. In general, we are less inclined to embark on retreating radioresistant tumors.

In the setting of fractionated radiotherapy, the rule of thumb is to add half of the dose given previously to the actual plan and to respect the cumulative normal tissue dose limits presented above (see following Case Study). The policy is generally to restrict the re-irradiation target to the gross tumor volume (rGTV) only. The use an image-guided system (IGRT) to minimize the day-to-day set-up variation can thereby reduce the margin of target volume expansion on the planning target volume (PTV) to a few millimeters rather than the general accepted ≥5 mm.

Table 14.1 Dose constraints for fractionated[a] radiotherapy of skull base tumors

Structures	Recommendations
Optic Nerves	D_{max}: 50 Gy
Chiasm	D_{max}: 50 Gy
Retina	D_{max}: 54 Gy
Lens	D_{max}: 10 Gy
Cerebral hemisphere without PTV	D_{max}: 60 Gy
Cochlea	D_{max}: 54 Gy; P_{max} 45 Gy: 50%
Brainstem	D_{max}: 54 Gy
Spinal cord C1–C2	D_{max}: 50 Gy
Spinal cord C3 and bellow	D_{max}: 45 Gy
Parotid glands without PTV	P_{max} 24 Gy: 100%; P_{max} 26 Gy: 50%; P_{max} 45 Gy: 25%
Temporomandibular Joint	D_{max}: 70 Gy
Other cranial nerves	D_{max}: 54 Gy

[a] Daily dose between 1.8 Gy and 2.5 Gy. D_{max}: maximum point dose allowed; P_{max}: maximum dose to percentage of the volume.

Case Study

A 49-year-old white man with a diagnosis of stage III—T3N0M0—nasopharyngeal lymphoepithelioma was treated with three cycles of neoadjuvant chemotherapy with docetaxel and cisplatin every 3 weeks followed by 70 Gy IMRT with concomitant cisplatin between July 01, 2008 and August 19, 2008. He achieved complete clinical remission with this treatment, but presented with hypoesthesia and paresthesia of the left face in April 2009. PET-CT and nasofibroscopy with biopsy diagnosed an extensive local tumor recurrence infiltrating the skull base in early July 2009 (**Fig. 14.2a**).
IMRT to the evaluable tumor was delivered between September 09, 2009 and October 22, 2009 to a total dose of 66 Gy in 30 daily fractions. The treatment was planned with fusion of planning CT and MRI, and IGRT with cone beam CT was applied to ensure precision in delivery of radiation. The volume receiving 66 Gy or more is shown in **Fig. 14.2b**, and the volume receiving 25 Gy or more in **Fig. 14.2c**.

Special Considerations

- Make use of CT, MRI, and PET scanning to better delineate the target and normal tissues. Limit the clinical target volume (CTV) to the rGTV.
- Improve dose conformation to target volume and spare normal tissue by using IMRT.
- Follow the normal tissue dose constraints (**Table 14.1**) to minimize morbidity.
- To estimate the normal tissue constraints in case of cancer recurrence 1 year or more after full dose RT, consider 50% recovery of dose tolerance.
- Apply IGRT to improve the accuracy of RT delivery, which allows reduction of the PTV.

!

- Make a complete evaluation of the sequelae of previous RT, including hormonal abnormalities, hearing deficit, visual impairment, and neurological and dental problems before undertaking re-irradiation.
- Discuss the risks and benefits of re-irradiation with the patient and the patient's family. Apply a specific informed consent for each case.

Complications

For re-irradiation, complications include visual impairment, brain necrosis (especially temporal lobe and brainstem), base of skull necrosis, hearing loss, and xerostomia. The precise risk of second treatment–related side effects is difficult to quantify in patients presenting with sequelae caused by the first treatment or recurrent tumor.

From a series of 66 patients with re-irradiated recurrent head and neck tumors reported by Popovtzer et al.,[13] 11 presented base of skull lesions and one developed asymptomatic temporal-lobe necrosis. The risk of this type of complication is probably higher, but if it frequently occurs later in the clinical evolution, the patients may not survive enough time to present it. In a series of 36 patients

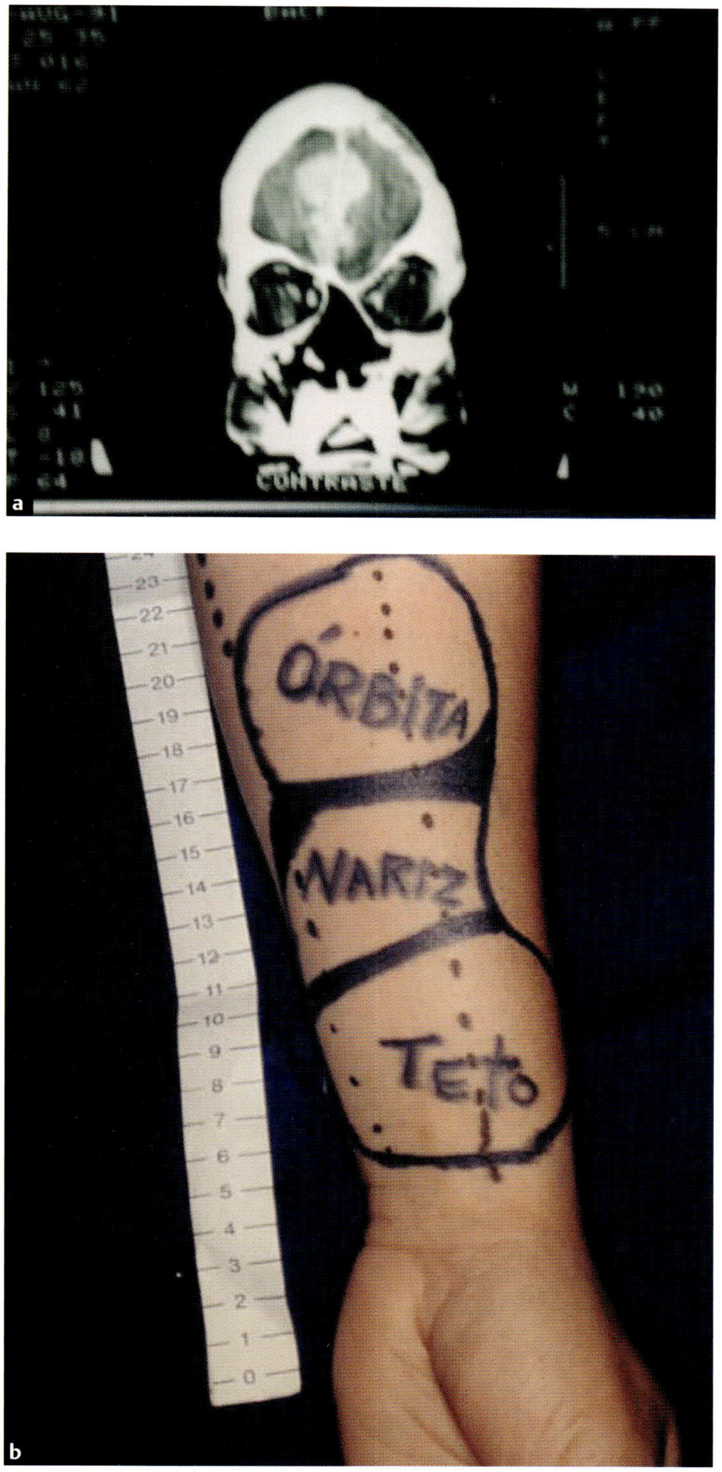

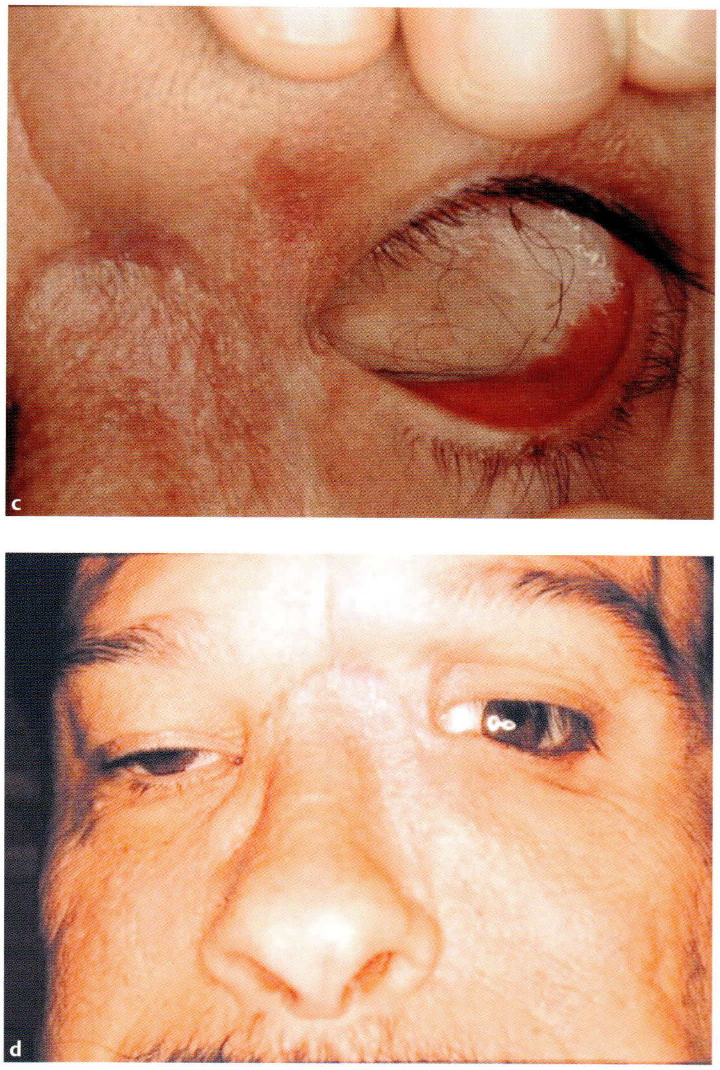

Fig. 14.1a–d Recurrent intracranial adenocarcinoma of the ethmoid, 2 years after craniofacial resection.
a Initial CT scan.
b Forearm flap prepared for harvesting for a multiplanar reconstruction.
c, d Final result of the reconstruction, showing part of the transplanted microvascular bed serving as a crib for a flat ocular prosthesis.

with recurrent head and neck tumors treated with fractionated CyberKnife radiosurgery, 2 of 8 patients with nasopharyngeal carcinoma presented trismus, soft tissue necrosis, and skull base bone necrosis and one of then died from this complication.[7]

Chemotherapy

There are some anecdotal reports of the use of chemotherapy for palliation in otherwise untreatable situations. However, some authors believe that chemotherapy may be a part of multimodality treatment for selected craniofacial cancers, such as olfactory neuroblastomas.[25]

Outcomes

The prognosis of patients with recurrent skull base tumors depends largely on several factors: histology, type of and interval since previous treatment, structures involved, operability, and so on. Moreover, the possibility of actually achieving free margins at the end of the procedure and of delivering adjuvant radiotherapy seems to offer the best survival outcome.

The largest published series of patients with skull base tumors treated at several institutions around the world (including our service at University of Sao Paulo Medical School) comprised 1307 cases.[22] The majority of these patients had recurrent tumors (58.5%). The overall recurrence rate after treatment was 41.7%, and the median time to recurrence was 19 month (1–940 months). The

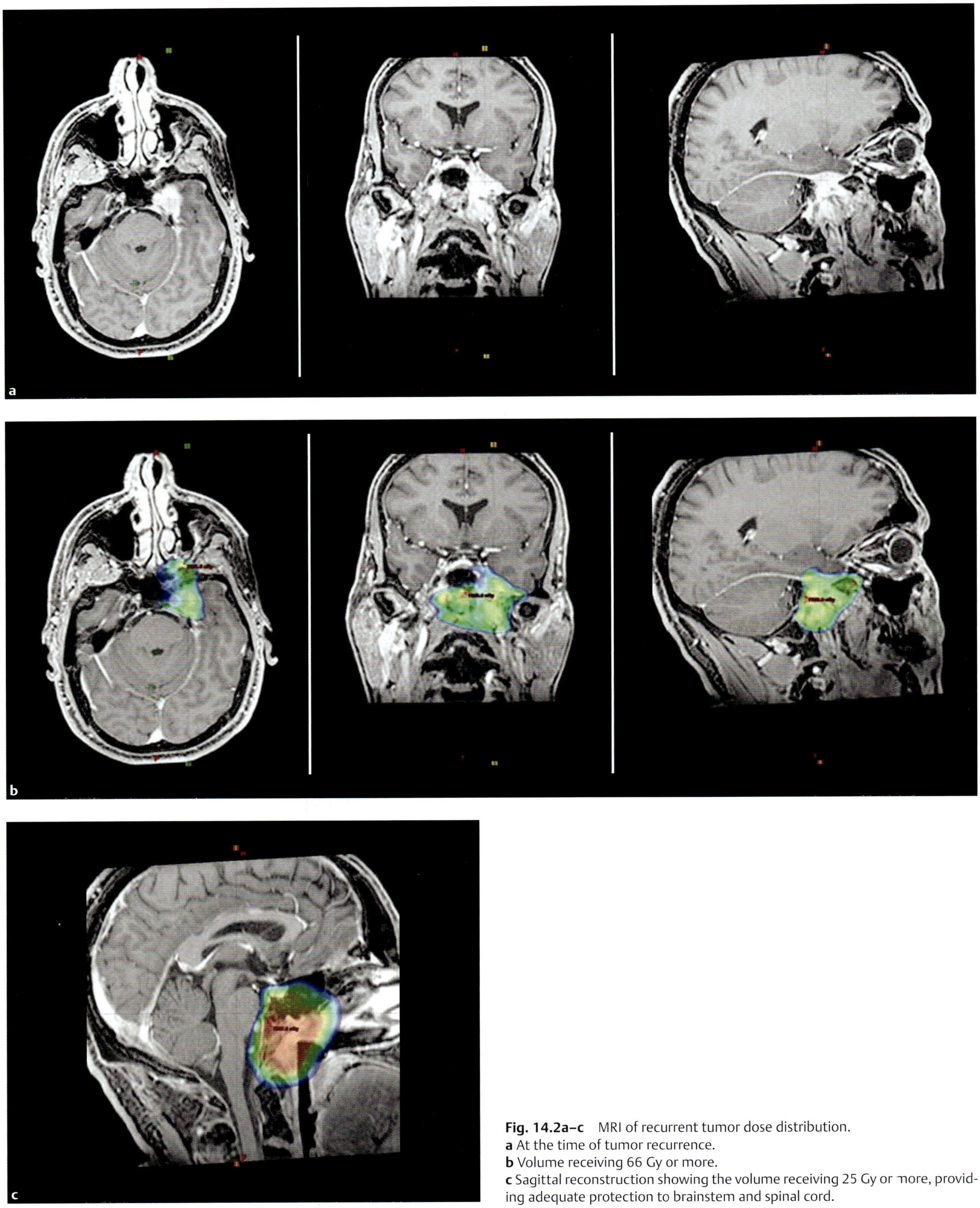

Fig. 14.2a–c MRI of recurrent tumor dose distribution.
a At the time of tumor recurrence.
b Volume receiving 66 Gy or more.
c Sagittal reconstruction showing the volume receiving 25 Gy or more, providing adequate protection to brainstem and spinal cord.

histology of the primary tumor, the extent of intracranial extension, and the status of surgical margins were independently significant predictors of recurrence-free survival. With a median follow-up of 25 months, the 5-year overall, disease-specific, and recurrence-free survival rates for this mixed group of previously untreated and treated patients were 54%, 60%, and 53%, respectively. Again, tumor histology, intracranial extension, and the status of surgical margins were independent predictors of overall, disease-specific, and recurrence-free survival on multivariate analysis.

In our own study, analyses of survival demonstrated a statistically significant negative impact on survival in patients with skull base cancers who underwent previous treatment ($P = 0.0018$).[20]

Undoubtedly, when several cranial nerve deficits occur after the treatment, the quality of life may be severely impaired, despite the length of the survival.[23] This aspect is very well described in a recent publication focusing on survival and quality of life questionnaires in patients with skull base tumors.[26] Woertgen et al. analyzed a limited cohort of 14 cases, using a quality of life questionnaire. At a mean follow-up of 39 months, 36% were alive but only 45% were able to work in their previous occupations 15 months after surgery.

Future Research

- The recent development of oncological endoscopic skull base approaches, with encouraging results, offers a new perspective for the management of recurrent skull base tumors due to a more focused and less invasive approach, with reduced morbidity and mortality.[27,28]
- New advances in targeted therapy directed toward recurrent skull base tumors are eagerly expected to improve local control as well as quality of life[29]. In addition, new surgical tools, such as robotic skull base surgery, are being refined, with an expected increase in surgical accuracy and decrease in operative morbidity.[30,31]

Recommended Reading

- Ganly I, Patel SG, Singh B, et al. Craniofacial resection for malignant paranasal sinus tumors: Report of an International Collaborative Study. Head Neck 2005;27(7):575–584
- Hanna E, DeMonte F, Ibrahim S, Roberts D, Levine N, Kupferman M. Endoscopic resection of sinonasal cancers with and without craniotomy: oncologic results. Arch Otolaryngol Head Neck Surg 2009;135(12):1219–1224
- Nicolai P, Battaglia P, Bignami M, et al. Endoscopic surgery for malignant tumors of the sinonasal tract and adjacent skull base: a 10-year experience. Am J Rhinol 2008;22(3):308–316
- Bristol IJ, Ahamad A, Garden AS, et al. Postoperative radiotherapy for maxillary sinus cancer: long-term outcomes and toxicities of treatment. Int J Radiat Oncol Biol Phys 2007;68(3):719–730
- Hanna EY, Cardenas AD, DeMonte F, et al. Induction chemotherapy for advanced squamous cell carcinoma of the paranasal sinuses. Arch Otolaryngol Head Neck Surg 2011;137(1):78–81

References

1. Ketcham AS, Wilkins RH, Vanburen JM, Smith RR. A combined intracranial facial approach to the paranasal sinuses. Am J Surg 1963;106:698–703
2. Janecka IP, Sen C, Sekhar LN, et al. Cranial base surgery: results in 183 patients. Otolaryngol Head Neck Surg 1994;110(6):539–546
3. Cernea CR, Teixeira GV, Medina dos Santos LR, Vellutini EA, Siqueira MG. Indications for, contraindications to, and interruption of craniofacial procedures. Ann Otol Rhinol Laryngol 1997;106(11):927–933
4. Lee AWM, Foo W, Chappell R, et al. Effect of time, dose, and fractionation on temporal lobe necrosis following radiotherapy for nasopharyngeal carcinoma. Int J Radiat Oncol Biol Phys 1998;40(1):35–42
5. Xia P, Lee N, Liu YM, et al. A study of planning dose constraints for treatment of nasopharyngeal carcinoma using a commercial inverse treatment planning system. Int J Radiat Oncol Biol Phys 2004;59(3):886–896
6. Taylor BW Jr, Marcus RB Jr, Friedman WA, Ballinger WE Jr, Million RR. The meningioma controversy: postoperative radiation therapy. Int J Radiat Oncol Biol Phys 1988;15(2):299–304
7. Kocher M, Voges J, Staar S, Treuer H, Sturm V, Mueller RP. Linear accelerator radiosurgery for recurrent malignant tumors of the skull base. Am J Clin Oncol 1998;21(1):18–22
8. Roh KW, Jang JS, Kim MS, et al. Fractionated stereotactic radiotherapy as reirradiation for locally recurrent head and neck cancer. Int J Radiat Oncol Biol Phys 2009;74(5):1348–1355
9. Sulman EP, Schwartz DL, Le TT, et al. IMRT reirradiation of head and neck cancer-disease control and morbidity outcomes. Int J Radiat Oncol Biol Phys 2009;73(2):399–409
10. Catton C, O'Sullivan B, Bell R, et al. Chordoma: long-term follow-up after radical photon irradiation. Radiother Oncol 1996;41(1):67–72
11. Wang CC. Re-irradiation of recurrent nasopharyngeal carcinoma—treatment techniques and results. Int J Radiat Oncol Biol Phys 1987;13(7):953–956
12. Tanvetyanon T, Padhya T, McCaffrey J, et al. Prognostic factors for survival after salvage reirradiation of head and neck cancer. J Clin Oncol 2009;27(12):1983–1991
13. Popovtzer A, Gluck I, Chepeha DB, et al. The pattern of failure after reirradiation of recurrent squamous cell head and neck cancer: implications for defining the targets. Int J Radiat Oncol Biol Phys 2009;74(5):1342–1347
14. Tokuuye K, Akine Y, Sumi M, et al. Reirradiation of brain and skull base tumors with fractionated stereotactic radiotherapy. Int J Radiat Oncol Biol Phys 1998;40(5):1151–1155
15. Kano H, Kondziolka D, Niranjan A, Flannery TJ, Flickinger JC, Lunsford LD. Repeat stereotactic radiosurgery for acoustic neuromas. Int J Radiat Oncol Biol Phys 2010;76(2):520–527
16. Lee N, Millender LE, Larson DA, et al. Gamma knife radiosurgery for recurrent salivary gland malignancies involving the base of skull. Head Neck 2003;25(3):210–216
17. Cernea CR, Hanna E. Surgical management of recurrent skull base tumors. In: Cernea CR et al., eds. Pearls and Pitfalls in Head and Neck Surgery. Basel: Karger; 2008:146–147
18. Cernea CR, Dias FL, Lima RA, et al. Atypical facial access: an unusually high prevalence of use among patients with skull base tumors treated at 2 centers. Arch Otolaryngol Head Neck Surg 2007;133(8):816–819

19. Cernea CR, Velasco O, Gomes MQ, et al. Double-bladed scalpel: a new option for harvesting margins in head and neck cancers. ORL J Otorhinolaryngol Relat Spec 2006;68(2):83–87
20. Dos Santos LR, Cernea CR, Brandao LG, et al. Results and prognostic factors in skull base surgery. Am J Surg 1994;168(5):481–484
21. Besteiro JM, Aki FE, Ferreira MC, Medina LR, Cernea C. Free flap reconstruction of tumors involving the cranial base. Microsurgery 1994;15(1):9–13
22. Patel SG, Singh B, Polluri A, et al. Craniofacial surgery for malignant skull base tumors: report of an international collaborative study. Cancer 2003;98(6):1179–1187
23. Kaylie DM, Wittkopf JE, Coppit G, Warren FM III, Netterville JL, Jackson CG. Revision lateral skull base surgery. Otol Neurotol 2006;27(2):225–233
24. Dias FL, Sá GM, Kligerman J, et al. Complications of anterior craniofacial resection. Head Neck 1999;21(1):12–20
25. Constantinidis J, Steinhart H, Koch M, et al. Olfactory neuroblastoma: the University of Erlangen-Nuremberg experience 1975–2000. Otolaryngol Head Neck Surg 2004;130(5):567–574
26. Woertgen C, Rothoerl RD, Hosemann W, Strutz J. Quality of Life following Surgery for Malignancies of the Anterior Skull Base. Skull Base 2007;17(2):119–123
27. Nicolai P, Battaglia P, Bignami M, et al. Endoscopic surgery for malignant tumors of the sinonasal tract and adjacent skull base: a 10-year experience. Am J Rhinol 2008;22(3):308–316
28. Hanna E, DeMonte F, Ibrahim S, Roberts D, Levine N, Kupferman M. Endoscopic resection of sinonasal cancers with and without craniotomy: oncologic results. Arch Otolaryngol Head Neck Surg 2009;135(12):1219–1224
29. Johnson MD, Sade B, Milano MT, Lee JH, Toms SA. New prospects for management and treatment of inoperable and recurrent skull base meningiomas. J Neurooncol 2008;86(1):109–122
30. Hanna EY, Holsinger C, DeMonte F, Kupferman M. Robotic endoscopic surgery of the skull base: a novel surgical approach. Arch Otolaryngol Head Neck Surg 2007;133(12):1209–1214
31. O'Malley BW Jr, Weinstein GS. Robotic anterior and midline skull base surgery: preclinical investigations. Int J Radiat Oncol Biol Phys 2007; 69(2, Suppl)S125–S128

15 Recurrent Differentiated Thyroid Cancer

N. Gopalakrishna Iyer, Ashok R. Shaha, R. Michael Tuttle

Summary

- Thyroid cancer predominantly recurs in the lateral cervical compartment, followed by the central compartment and distant metastasis.
- Most patients with differentiated thyroid cancer should be followed up with a combination of serum thyroglobulin and ultrasound scans.
- Prognostication and long-term follow-up strategy is based on risk stratification, which should be modified according to response to initial treatment.
- Watchful waiting is a reasonable option in patients with minimal structural disease and raised thyroglobulin levels.
- Surgery for recurrent disease should aim to remove all gross disease.
- Novel treatment strategies for distant metastases should be used in a clinical trial setting.

Introduction

Thyroid cancer is an umbrella term used to describe a range of different disease processes with a wide range of clinical behavior. At one end of the spectrum lies a group of histological diagnoses classified as differentiated thyroid cancer, with excellent prognosis, good response to therapy, and mortality rates approaching zero. At the other end of the spectrum is undifferentiated or anaplastic thyroid cancer, which has an aggressive course and is nearly always uniformly fatal within months of diagnosis. Several different histological subtypes occupy the middle section, including poorly differentiated cancers (which are thought to be more aggressive variants of differentiated thyroid cancer) and medullary thyroid cancer, both of which can have a variable course.

Despite the large volume of literature available on thyroid cancer, there is limited data that specifically addresses the issue of recurrent thyroid cancer. Since there are no prospective randomized trials in thyroid cancer, most recommendations rely on level 3 and 4 evidence. For recurrent cancers, the level of evidence is more ambiguous, often relying on expert opinion and guidelines from organizations such as the American (ATA), British (BTA) or European (ETA) Thyroid Associations or National Comprehensive Cancer Network (NCCN). This chapter mainly addresses the issue of recurrent differentiated thyroid cancer, which is the commonest type of thyroid cancer encountered in clinical practice. Medullary thyroid cancer is a rare disease, and management of recurrences is far more complex and beyond the scope of this chapter; hence readers are referred to an excellent review article summarizing the ATA's recommendation in managing these patients.[1] As well as clinical evaluation and management principles, this chapter will also highlights the major issues associated with reoperative thyroid surgery.

Differentiated Thyroid Cancer

Differentiated thyroid cancer is a term used to describe tumors arising from thyroid follicular cells. Histological subtypes included in this classification are papillary, follicular and Hurthle cell lesions, and their variants.[2] These tumors represent more than 90% of thyroid cancers. While the different subtypes have traditionally been considered in one category for management decisions, there are some subtle differences in behavior and outcome, which will be highlighted through this section.

Epidemiology

The incidence of differentiated thyroid cancer has undergone a dramatic increase in the last three decades, and the vast majority of newly diagnosed cancers are small, incidentally discovered cancers with questionable clinical relevance.[3,4] Undoubtedly, these cancers are associated with an excellent overall outcome. Disease-specific survival rates for papillary and follicular cancers are 98% and 92% at 10 years and 94% and 84% at 40 years.[5,6] Most patients respond well to initial therapy and are at a low risk for death and recurrence. Despite excellent survival statistics, current data suggest that disease recurrence occurs in 10%–30% of patients depending on the specific series.[5,6] One major caveat to these statistics is that the rates of recurrence depend on the definition, in terms of whether it refers to thyroglobulinemia or structurally identifiable disease. The distinction between persistent disease and recurrent disease is not often made in the older studies. These rates also vary depending on the original histological subtype: patients with papillary thyroid cancer or minimally invasive follicular thyroid cancer have recurrence rates ranging from 5% to 20%, while patients with widely invasive follicular or Hurthle cell carcinomas have recurrence rates ranging from 25% to 73%.[7–10] There is also data from two separate series to suggest that 33%–59% of recurrent cancers tend to have a more aggressive histological subtype than the original tumor.[11,12] Therefore, it is not surprising that disease recurrence is associated with higher mortality rates, with 30-year cancer mortality rates reported as 12% in patients with local recurrence and as high as 43% in patients with distant metastasis.[13]

Classification

Structural disease recurrence can be broadly classified as locoregional or distant metastases. Locoregional recurrence can be further divided into cervical nodal metastasis in the lateral compartment, which represents 85% of cases, or local recurrence in the thyroid bed (including central compartment and superior mediastinal disease), seen in 32% of recurrent thyroid cancer.[14] It may

Table 15.1 Risk stratification for recurrence in differentiated thyroid cancer in patients with complete resection of primary tumor and no evidence of distant metastasis immediately after primary treatment[20]

	Low risk	Intermediate risk	High risk
Primary tumor	Intrathyroidal	Microscopic invasion of perithyroidal tissue	Gross/macroscopic extrathyroidal extension
Primary surgery	Tumor completely resected	Tumor completely resected	Incomplete tumor resection
Histology	Classic PTC	Aggressive histology (tall/columnar cell variant, etc.), vascular invasion	Other than classic PTC
Lymph node involvement or distant metastasis	No regional or distant	Cervical nodal metastasis	Distant metastasis
RAI scan	No uptake outside thyroid bed (if done)	Uptake outside thyroid bed after remnant ablation	Thyroglobulinemia out of proportion to RAI scan

PTC, papillary thyroid carcinoma.

Table 15.2 Variables determined during follow-up that predict response to therapy. (Adapted from Tuttle et al.[19])

	Excellent response	Acceptable response	Incomplete response
Suppressed Tg	Undetectable	Detectable but <1 ng/mL	>1 ng/mL
Stimulated Tg	Undetectable	<10 ng/mL	>10 ng/mL
Trend in suppressed Tg	Undetectable	Declining	Stable or rising
Anti-Tg antibodies	Undetectable	Absent or declining	Persistent or rising
Neck examination	Normal	Normal	Palpable disease
Neck ultrasound	No evidence of disease	Nonspecific changes in thyroid bed Stable millimeter-sized nodes	Significant recurrent/ persistent disease (>1 cm) in thyroid bed Cervical lymph nodes >1 cm
Diagnostic RAI	No evidence of disease	No evidence of disease Faint uptake in thyroid bed only	Persistent/recurrent RAI-avid disease
Sectional imaging (CT, MRI)	No evidence of disease	Nonspecific changes	Structural disease in thyroid bed or lymph nodes
PET scan	No evidence of disease	Nonspecific changes	FDG-avid disease

Tg, thyroglobulin; RAI, radioactive iodine.

often be difficult to distinguish whether local recurrence is due to growth of incompletely excised primary tumor or due to nodal metastasis in the central compartment, especially if there were no preoperative indicators suggesting incomplete excision during the primary surgical procedure. While this may not necessarily impact on management decisions per se, there are important implications with regard to surgical outcome and complications. Distant metastases represent 12% of all recurrences, and tend to be discovered most frequently in the lung (50%), followed by bone (25%), lungs and bone (20%), and other sites (5%).[15–17]

■ Prognostic Factors Based on Risk Groups for Recurrence

Risk stratification is an essential element in the management of differentiated thyroid cancer, and should reflect the clinical balance between the best estimate of the aggressiveness of the disease and the effectiveness (including possible complications) of treatment.[18,19] A critical step in the initial management of patients with differentiated thyroid cancer is to identify patients at high risk for recurrence and disease-specific death and offer them appropriate aggressive therapy and close surveillance.[20] Conversely, identifying low-risk patients is important to spare them from unwanted treatment and unnecessary, expensive, low-yield follow-up studies.[21]

While most prognostic systems have focused on the stratification of mortality rates, these are not always applicable in assessing the risk of disease recurrence. Furthermore, unlike other solid tumors, the risk of death is not always concordant with the risk of death from thyroid cancer. This is a common scenario seen in very young patients with papillary thyroid cancer who have close to 100% survival rates at 40 years, yet have a high incidence of recurrent nodal and distant metastasis. A strategy for initial risk assessment for recurrence in patients with differentiated thyroid cancer is shown in **Table 15.1**, which has been incorporated in the latest ATA guidelines. This system applies to patients with no evidence of distant metastasis and complete primary resection.[20]

In addition, it has been proposed that risk stratification should be a dynamic process, and should take into account the disease evolution with time. Current expert opinion suggests that most patients should be re-assessed after 2–3 years to determine whether they have responded to therapy and the nature of response and so to re-evaluate their risk groups based on treatment response.[19] This approach is important because most patients with thyroid cancer lead long lives and hence have extended periods of follow-up. Given the accuracy and sensitivities of available modalities to detect persistent or recurrent disease and our current understanding of the biological behavior of these events, the physician needs to make a strategic long-term plan for treating these patients. Quick decisions regarding reoperative surgery for

Table 15.3 Follow-up strategy based on risk groups. (Adapted from Tuttle et al.[19])

Initial estimate of risk recurrence during first 2 years of follow-up			
	Low risk	**Intermediate risk**	**High risk**
Suppressed Tg	Q 6 months	Q 6 months	Q 6 months
Stimulated Tg	Not required	1–2 years	1–2 years
Neck ultrasonography	Q 1 year × 2	Q 1 year × 2	Q 1 year × 2
Diagnostic RAI	Not required	1–2 years	1–2 years
Sectional imaging (CT, MRI)	Not required	Not required	If Tg elevated or high clinical suspicion
PET scan	Not required	Not required	If Tg elevated and RAI scan negative
Secondary risk stratification based on response to therapy assessment			
	Excellent	**Acceptable**	**Incomplete**
Ongoing follow-up	Yearly physical examination and yearly suppressed Tg	Yearly physical examination, yearly suppressed Tg and continued assessment of indeterminate structural changes for at least another 2–3 years	Consider additional sectional imaging, possible PET scan and neck for additional therapy

Tg, thyroglobulin; RAI, radioactive iodine; Q, every.

Table 15.4 Shifting paradigms in the detection of recurrent disease

Thyroglobulin/stimulated thyroglobulin
Ultrasound
Ultrasound-guided needle biopsy with cytology or needle-wash for thyroglubulin (nodal disease)
RAI scan
Cross-sectional imaging (CT, MRI scans)
PET scan

low-volume persistent disease, which otherwise has a long natural history, may cause more harm to the patient than a watchful waiting approach.

There are several modalities available to the physician in the long-term follow-up of these patients, and these will be discussed separately below. The predictive values for these modalities are used to modify risk estimates when managing these patients and to divide patients into different treatment response categories: excellent response, acceptable response, and incomplete response (**Table 15.2**).[19] The inclusion of these factors represents a dynamic approach to risk stratification and the need to constantly reevaluate the risk status of any patient over and beyond the initial risk status derived at diagnosis (i.e., based on factors in **Table 15.1**). Thyroglobulin levels shown in **Table 15.2** are most accurate in patients having undergone total thyroidectomy and radioactive iodine ablation (RAI). In patients who undergo lesser procedures, the trend of thyroglobulin levels over time may be more accurate than a single reading of thyroglobulin level. However, the latter group comprise patients who have excellent risk profile and hence have low disease recurrence and long-term mortality rates.

Patients with unmeasurable thyroglobulin levels and no evidence of recurrent disease on imaging are easily managed with routine follow-up.[20] Unfortunately, with increased use and sensitivity of thyroglobulin measurements, we recognize a subset of patients with persistent minimal-volume disease, sometimes even seen on cross-sectional imaging as stable paratracheal nodal disease or nonspecific changes in the thyroid bed. This group of patients falls under the acceptable response category, with disease that is not easily eradicated with additional surgery or RAI. Most of these patients have long progression-free survival and are best managed with observation, reserving additional therapy when evidence of disease progression is documented. Ultimately, the aim is to determine which of these patients develop disease progression that is clinically relevant, and it is hoped that future studies will help to define this subgroup.

The continued use of all detection modalities in all patients is not cost-effective. A risk-stratified follow-up strategy is applied for best utilization of available resources and should be based on initial risk stratification and secondary response to therapy assessment (**Table 15.3**).[19] It is important to note that this approach is mainly directed at patients with complete tumor resection and no evidence of metastatic disease.

■ Investigations and Evaluation

The role of investigative modalities is twofold: first, as a tool for surveillance in patients at risk for recurrence, and second, to confirm the diagnosis of recurrent disease and to aid in planning future therapy (**Table 15.4**).

Surveillance

As stated before, a risk-adapted paradigm should be used for surveillance strategies, given the vast number of modalities available in our armamentarium. The aim of surveillance is to diagnose subclinical disease, at an early point, where therapeutic intervention may be beneficial. There are, however, several caveats to this. First, identification of early disease may not necessarily change treatment or prognosis, such as the detection of miliary lung metastasis, which is not radioiodine avid. Second, in several cases, subclinical disease may not be clinically relevant, such as the aforementioned sub-centimeter thyroid bed nodule or 2–3 mm sized persistent lymph node metastases. The available modalities for surveillance are as follows.

Serum Thyroglobulin

The presence and levels of serum thyroglobulin (Tg) depend on the residual thyroid mass, tumor mass, degree of differentiation, and location of metastasis. After the initial treatment, the presence of thyroglobulin indicates the presence of residual thyroid tissue or recurrence.[22] The former is usually excluded by performing a proper extracapsular total thyroidectomy and sometimes with postoperative radioiodine scan and ablation. A cut-off of 1 ng/mL increases the sensitivity but this is not specific and a time trend may be more useful than a one-time reading. Obviously, higher levels are more specific for recurrent or metastatic disease. For low-risk patients, a single undetectable Tg level post primary treatment confers a 0.5%–1.6% risk of recurrence over a period of 5–12 years.[23–25] Conversely, while surveillance with Tg levels alone may suffice in low-risk patients, for patients with intermediate or high risk, the addition of ultrasound may be important to increase accuracy. There is much interest in the use of stimulated Tg levels as a surveillance tool, using recombinant thyroid-stimulating hormone (TSH), or Thyrogen, to stimulate Tg production. Several studies have shown this to be an excellent marker identifying those patients at lowest risk of recurrence (negative predictive value).[26–28] Once the presence of recurrence is established, it is important to define the location of recurrent disease and in some situations to establish pathological confirmation of recurrence, for treatment planning.

Ultrasound

With improving technology and increasing sensitivity, ultrasound has become one of the most useful tools in evaluating postoperative patients for locoregionally recurrent thyroid cancer. High-resolution imaging of the neck can be achieved with visualization of the thyroid bed and lateral neck compartments.[29] Furthermore, it does not rely on iodine uptake and can identify recurrent disease even when Tg levels are falsely negative. The sensitivity of ultrasound combined with Tg levels exceeds 96%, and has become the primary surveillance tool in all but the very low-risk patient.[22] The main disadvantage of ultrasound is that it relies on imaging criteria, which are not reliable, can be difficult to interpret, and are operator dependent. For nodal disease, these depend on the size, shape (round versus ovoid), and structural details (presence of fatty hilum in benign node; microcalcifications suggest malignant deposits). However, postsurgical changes such as fibrosis, granulation tissue, and parathyroid and thymic tissue may be misinterpreted as recurrent disease. Moreover, ultrasound has limited anatomical coverage and is unable to image paravertebral, retrotracheal, retropharyngeal, and skull base nodal chains (which are all fortunately uncommon sites of metastatic disease). Ultrasound-guided fine-needle aspiration biopsy is a useful adjunct to confirm or refute recurrent disease, and may be used if the diagnosis is in doubt. Its accuracy exceeds 95% when performed by expert radiologists.[30,31]

Radioactive Iodine Whole-body Scan

The radioactive iodine whole-body scan (I-131 WBS) was traditionally the most important modality for surveillance of high-risk patients for recurrent disease. The major advantage was the ability to identify locoregional and distant recurrences, and it had been used as a robust screening tool together with serum Tg levels. However, with a reported sensitivity of only 50%–60%, and the fact that most recurrences occur in the neck, I-131 WBS has been largely superseded by ultrasonography in detecting recurrence.[23,32] As a surveillance tool, it is still useful in patients treated for distant metastasis, to detect new-onset metastatic disease. It is also useful as a diagnostic tool in patients with rising Tg levels, to identify the anatomical location of metastasis.

Diagnosis and Treatment Planning

Fine-needle Aspiration Biopsy

This is a useful adjunct in confirming diagnosis prior to surgery or other treatment modalities, especially with recurrent disease in the neck. It is especially important in patients where the diagnosis is equivocal on imaging, and its accuracy may be increased with ultrasound-guided techniques.[31] The one major disadvantage is that unnecessary needle biopsies in the thyroid bed may be interpreted as atypical, forcing the clinician to plan surgery for clinically irrelevant disease; and with increasing pressure to investigate patients, this may potentially lead to unwanted neck explorations and risk exposing patients unnecessarily to complications of reoperative procedures. Furthermore, the presence of residual thyroid tissue in the thyroid bed is not uncommon, and can be mistakenly read as atypical cells.

Sectional Imaging: CT or MRI

Sectional imaging is important to evaluate either bulky or large volume recurrences or in situations where the anatomy may be altered.[33] It is also important in situations where there is local invasion, and hence there may be a need for more extensive procedures. CT also provides much better visualization of the skull base and retropharyngeal and parapharyngeal nodes, which may rarely be involved by metastatic disease. CT scans should be performed with contrast for maximum image quality and to assess relationship with important vascular anatomy.

Fiberoptic Laryngoscopy

The vocal cords should be evaluated in all patients with recurrent disease where surgical exploration is contemplated.[34,35] Even with a normal voice, a patient could have unsuspected vocal cord paralysis from a previous procedure. Apart from the medicolegal implications arising from this situation, the presence of preexisting vocal cord paralysis may influence the surgeon's decision whether to operate in the contralateral tracheoesophageal groove (especially if there is only low-volume disease) and also to alert the surgeon to take extra precautions with the contralateral recurrent laryngeal nerve, as bilateral cord palsy has a disastrous outcome.

PET Scan

PET scanning has emerged as an important investigational tool for recurrent thyroid cancers, especially in patients with high-grade or aggressive thyroid cancers. While routine use of PET scanning is not indicated in the long-term follow-up of patients, there are two scenarios where it may be invaluable: the first is in patients with rising thyroglobulin levels with no demonstrable disease seen with RAI scans, and the second in patients with metastatic disease. FDG avidity is a direct function of histological aggressiveness, and PET-positive tumors are usually poorly responsive to RAI therapy.[36,37] Hence, patients with recurrent thyroid cancers that are PET-positive have a worse outcome than PET-negative recurrences. Similarly, the extent of FDG avidity and standard uptake values are also important prognostic markers both in patients with locoregional recurrence and in distant metastatic disease.[36]

Principles of Management

Treatment options in managing patients with recurrent thyroid cancer are influenced by several factors, which balance the ability to eradicate disease, establish cure, and prolong life versus the limitations of specific treatment modalities, the complications of treatment, and whether these modalities influence the natural course of the disease process at all.[18] Conventional treatment options include watchful waiting, surgery, radioactive iodine therapy, and external beam radiation. Several novel treatment modalities have also been introduced in the trial setting, but the benefit of these agents remains unproven.

In general, recurrent disease can broadly be grouped into local, regional, and distant recurrences, and treatment options differ between the groups. Generally, all patients with persistent or recurrent disease are on TSH suppressive treatment to reduce the potential risk of TSH-stimulated tumor growth. However, TSH suppression may be of limited value in patients with poorly differentiated tumors. The initial goal of therapy in these high-risk patients is to maintain TSH below 0.1 mIU/mL unless they are at significant risk of or actually develop complications such as thyrotoxic symptoms, osteoporosis, etc.[20,38] If the patient becomes free of disease subsequently, TSH suppression can be moderated to below the lower limit of normal (usually 0.1–0.5 mIU/mL).

Watchful Waiting

With increasing sensitivity of Tg monitoring and ultrasound scans of the thyroid bed, the detection of small, subcentimeter nodules in the thyroid bed and/or small lymph node metastases with borderline Tg levels is coming to pose a common clinical dilemma. Operating in a previously operated thyroid bed is fraught with risks and, given the indolent nature of many of these lesions, the value of surgical resection is questionable. It is also difficult to differentiate the true nature of these thyroid bed abnormalities, as to whether they represent recurrent thyroid cancer, hyperplastic residual thyroid tissue, or nodal disease in the peritracheal region. Some of these abnormalities may even represent granulomas or scar tissue from the initial surgery. Based on the risk-adapted paradigm proposed above, the general philosophy is to appropriately risk stratify these patients and monitor with serial Tg levels and repeat ultrasound at 6–12 month intervals.[19,34] If there is no progression in size or Tg levels, these patients with asymptomatic subcentimeter abnormalities on ultrasound may be safely observed without any intervention. This strategy may even be employed in a situation where a prior needle biopsy shows atypical or malignant thyroid cells, with the caveat that both the clinician and patient accept the advantages and disadvantages of the surveillance scenario. The most recent ATA guidelines recognize these limitations and have endorsed this approach as long as the clinicians managing these patients are clear about their treatment goals and continue to follow up these patients over the long term.[20] In fact, the guidelines specifically recommend not to biopsy lesions less than 5–7 mm by fine-needle aspiration (FNA).

Surgery for Recurrent Disease

Surgery for Lateral Neck Disease

Ultimately, many patients with locoregional recurrence will be treated surgically. The extent of surgery depends on the extent of locally recurrent disease, and every effort should be made to resect all gross tumor thoroughly.[39]

Disease in the lateral neck, which is the most common site of metastatic disease, can easily be managed with an appropriate neck dissection, with minimal morbidity. Most surgeons advocate a selective neck dissection clearing levels II–IV, occasionally including level Vb if there is nodal disease in level IV or V. There is usually no need to dissect level I or level IIb, and thereby place the marginal mandibular or spinal accessory nerves at unnecessary risk, as these nodal stations are rarely involved by metastatic thyroid cancer.

In some cases, patients may develop recurrent neck disease even after a prior lateral neck dissection. In this situation, reoperative neck surgery is always more difficult from a technical point of view, and the surgeon should be familiar with dealing with previously operated necks before embarking on such a procedure (potential complications are listed in **Table 15.5**).[40] Furthermore, there is a real and distinct possibility that the abnormal node may not be found during reoperative surgery, especially if the node is small. Repeat neck dissections may not clear all nodal tissue and patients may develop further lymphadenopathy in the future. Thyroglobulin levels also may not normalize if there is residual microscopic disease. In this situation, the presence of additional positive nodes is reflected by persistent hyperthyroglobulinemia,

Table 15.5 Complications of neck dissection during reoperative surgery[40]

Hypoparathyroidism
Transient
Permanent
Chyle leakage/chyloma
Bleeding and hematoma
Seroma
Wound infection
Nerve injuries
Accessory nerve
Hypoglossal nerve
Ramus mandibularis
Sympathetic chain (Horner syndrome)
Brachial plexus
Phrenic nerve
Cutaneous cervical plexus

and in these circumstances, patients may not be biochemically cured.[34] Patients should be informed of all these issues prior to undertaking the procedure. Most importantly, it is not known whether repeat neck dissections have any effect on prognosis or long-term outcome, especially if disease volume is low and the patient is asymptomatic.

Given the difficulties in performing reoperative neck dissections in patients, several alternate strategies have been developed to eradicate nodal metastases from differentiated thyroid cancer in the hostile neck. These include the use of radiofrequency ablation (RFA), or percutaneous injection of 100% ethanol under ultrasound guidance, directly ablating the abnormal lymph node.[41,42] While the results of these studies appear to be promising for both techniques, patient numbers were small with limited follow-up data available. The authors concluded that these techniques are probably useful for patients not amenable for surgery to attain local control or symptomatic relief.

Surgery for Local/Thyroid Bed Recurrence

Recurrence in the thyroid bed may be more difficult to manage, as there is often scarring from the previous resection.[43] Surgery will be more difficult if the bed has previously been irradiated. If recurrence is due to central compartment nodal disease, care should be taken to preserve the recurrent laryngeal nerve and parathyroid gland. Nerve monitoring may be a useful adjunct in identification and preservation of the recurrent laryngeal nerve.[40,44] If disease is unilateral only, it may be prudent not to dissect the contralateral tracheoesophageal groove unnecessarily. For locally invasive recurrences, it may be necessary to resect adjacent structures with recurrent disease, with extensive procedure.[45,46] These may involve radical resection of the recurrent laryngeal nerve, trachea, cricotracheal complex, esophageal musculature, and the larynx and/or pharynx. The last would involve a formal laryngectomy or pharyngolaryngectomy. The need for a formal laryngectomy is rare, and these should be carefully evaluated in the context of long-term tumor control and quality of life. It should be noted that resection margins for thyroid cancer do not need to be as wide as those for squamous cancer and so a resection margin of 2–3 mm or more is adequate. Occasionally, if there is persistent nodal disease along the trachea into the mediastinum, there may be a role for a median sternotomy and nodal dissection of all mediastinal nodal compartments. This is especially true in situations where there is no evidence of distant metastasis and the disease is PET positive and RAI refractory.

Complications rates are higher during reoperative procedures, with a transient complication rate reported at 8% and permanent morbidity rate of 3.8%.[47] Comparing primary surgery reoperations in the thyroid bed showed higher rates of permanent recurrent laryngeal nerve palsy (3.4% vs. 1.1%) and permanent hypoparathyroidism (3.9% vs. 1.2%).[48] Contraindications to surgical extirpation should always be borne in mind. Apart from patient factors that preclude surgical intervention, extensive tumor invasion involving the prevertebral musculature and carotid encasement are contraindications to surgery. Further, if there is transformation of the original tumor to undifferentiated or anaplastic cancer, the value of surgical resection is limited.

■ Surgery for Distant Metastases

There is a limited role for surgery in the management of distant metastases. Indications are usually palliative to treat symptomatic disease, where serious complications are expected, or to improve quality of life. These situations include metastatic disease to the bone with impending pathological fracture, spinal cord disease with potential cord compression, or brain metastasis with neurological deficits. The role of metastatectomy in a curative setting for disease control has been poorly established. Solitary or limited distant metastasis amenable to curative resection is an uncommon situation. However, there is data from retrospective studies to suggest that, in these situations, complete metastatectomy may be associated with improved survival for localized distant disease, particularly for non–RAI-avid disease.[49–51]

■ Radioactive Iodine

Radioactive iodine (RAI) treatment is used when there is locoregional or metastatic disease that is RAI avid on diagnostic whole-body scans. For locoregional disease, it can be used as adjuvant therapy post surgery for regional nodal metastases or locally invasive disease (involving the upper aerodigestive tract).[20] It can also be used in place of surgery in situations where surgery is considered high-risk or when there is additional metastatic disease; however, its effect on bulky disease may be limited. RAI treatment can be delivered after a period of thyroxine withdrawal (to raise TSH levels to >30 mIU/mL) or using recombinant TSH (rhTSH), hence avoiding the discomfort of thyroxine withdrawal [52–54] However, the use of rhTSH has not been FDA approved as adjunctive therapy for distant metastases (only for whole-body RAI scanning, stimulated thyroglobulin testing, and as adjunct to RAI remnant ablation). There are three dosing methods currently used for RAI treatment and there is no clear evidence that any one method is superior to the others. The NCCN guidelines provide general rules with regard to each of these methods as listed below.[55]

- Empirical fixed dose, which involves administering a fixed dose of 100–200 mCi of I-131 depending on the site of disease.
- Quantitative tumor dosimetry, which estimates the amount of radiation delivered to the lesion per unit of I-131 administered based on the initial dosimetric dose.
- Blood dosimetry, in which a maximum dose of 200 cGy is delivered to the blood while keeping the whole-body retention less than 120 mCi at 48 hours or less than 80 mCi when there is diffuse lung uptake.

In general, posttreatment whole-body scans should be performed to document I-131 uptake by the tumor approximately 2–10 days later. It may also identify additional lesions not seen on diagnostic scans.

External Beam Radiation Therapy

There is limited data on the role of external beam radiation therapy for recurrent thyroid cancer.[56] Indications for use include adjuvant treatment for locally invasive recurrent disease in the thyroid bed, especially when there is suspicion that complete R0 resection was not achieved.[20] Adjuvant radiotherapy (RT) should also be considered for aggressive histological transformation in the recurrent tumor into poorly differentiated or anaplastic variants. In the latter setting, the addition of concurrent chemotherapy (usually doxorubicin) acts as a radiosensitizer, although the evidence for this is limited to small retrospective studies with varying data. Irradiation of the thyroid bed and neck is usually done using intensity-modulated radiation therapy (IMRT), which allows the delivery of high dose to high-risk sites while sparing critical structures.[57] Indeed, there is data showing that external beam RT using IMRT results in better control in patients at higher risk of locoregional recurrence.[58] This approach may be required in patients with persistent or recurrent disease despite multiple attempts at resection. Radiation therapy can also be considered to control tumor growth and symptoms in patients with gross evidence of inoperable disease with local invasion, especially in lesions that are not RAI avid. Finally, RT is an important palliative adjunct in patients with symptomatic metastasis such as painful bony metastasis or metastatic disease to critical structures such as the those that may result in pathological fracture, or spinal metastasis with impending or actual neurological or compressive symptoms that are not amenable to surgery. Brain metastasis may require stereotactic radiosurgery or gamma-knife procedures for symptom control or to prevent complications.

Radiation dosimetry and planning depends on the risk status and nature of disease being treated. For planning of clinical target volumes (CTVs), regions being treated should generally be divided into areas of gross disease, areas with likely microscopic disease (or positive margins), regions at high risk for recurrence, and regions at low risk for recurrence. Suggested radiation doses for these regions include: 66–70 Gy for gross disease, 62–66 Gy for areas with positive margins, 60–64 Gy for high-risk areas, and 54 Gy for areas that are at low risk for microscopic disease or regions being electively irradiated.

■ Systemic Therapy

Conventional chemotherapy plays a limited role in the management of recurrent differentiated thyroid carcinoma. Most agents tested to date have shown minimal to modest response and their use is limited to desperate situations rather than logical, evidence-based use.

The era of targeted therapy underscores a novel paradigm in managing persistent, metastatic, clinically overt disease.[59] These strategies result from our understanding of biological pathways in tumorigenesis and progression of differentiated thyroid cancers, which has paved the way for novel therapeutic options. Recent data have suggested that mutations in one of several genes involved in the receptor tyrosine kinase mitogen-activated protein kinase (MAPK) pathway can be detected in up to 80% of well-differentiated thyroid cancers. Specific mutations include those affecting RET (5%–30% of cases), Ras (10% of cases), and BRAF (40% of cases). Targeting the MAPK pathway has hence been a subject of much investigation in preclinical and early clinical studies (**Table 15.6**). These novel compounds are often used in combination with traditional agents to deliver maximal benefit, although their use is limited to the trial setting. Targeting epigenetic modifiers is an alternative strategy that

Table 15.6 Investigational drugs currently in clinical trial and pathways targeted. (Adapted from Tuttle et al.[59])

Pathways	Specific target	Mechanism	Example (target)
MAPK	TK ligand	Antibody against TK ligand	Bevacizumab (VEGF)
	TK receptor	Antibody against TK receptor	Cetuximab (EGFR) Trastuzumab (EGFR)
		Small molecule inhibitor against TK ligand	Vandetanib (VEGF, EGF,RET) Motesanib (VEGF, PDGF, c-KIT, and RET)
		Small molecule inhibitor against TK receptor	Vatalanib (VEGFR) gefitinib (EGFR) sunitinib (VEGFR and others)
	Downstream targets	Ras inhibition	Ras antisense compounds Phenylacetate (also inhibitor of VEGF) Farnesyl transferase inhibitor (tipifarnib)
		Raf inhibition	Sorafinib
		MEK inhibition	PD 98059 AZD6244
Epigenetic modifiers	DNA methylation	Methylation inhibitor	5-Aza-2-deoxycytidine
	Histone deacetylation	Deacetylase inhibitor	Suberoylanilide hydroxamic acid/SAHA Valproic acid
Nuclear receptors	Retinoic acid receptors and retinoid X receptors	Vitamin A-derived retinoic acids	13-*cis*-Retinoic acid Bexarotene
	Peroxisome proliferators-activated receptors (PPAR)	Thiazolidinediones	Rosiglitazone
Other pathways	Cox-2 pathway	Cox-2 inhibitors	Celecoxib
	Heat-shock protein-90	Hsp inhibitiors	Geldanamycin
	Proteasome	Proteasome inhibitors	Bortezomib
	PI3 kinase pathway	Akt-mTOR inhibitors	Rapamycin analogues

TK, tyrosine kinase.

can be used to re-differentiate thyroid cancer cells and restoring their ability to take up radioactive iodine. Clinical trials are also underway to explore the role of DNA methylation and histone deacetylase inhibitors to this effect. Targeting nuclear receptors such as retinoic acid receptors and peroxisome proliferator-activated receptors can also re-differentiate cells, which in turn increases sodium iodide supporter (NIS) expression and uptake of radioactive iodine. Apart from these agents, there have been scattered reports of promising clinical response to a range of agents used in palliative settings. With increasing number of clinical trials either underway or soon to be opened, the clinician is faced with having to decide which of the available trials would be most beneficial. Unfortunately, currently available data does not allow us to identify the best agent for a particular patient, although the ultimate aim of these strategies is individualized therapy. These questions can only be answered in time and through careful analyses of well-designed, properly controlled prospective clinical trials, to determine which of the many potential novel agents (or combinations) is most effective in treating patients.

Case Studies

Ms. X is a 35-year-old homemaker who presented in July 2007 with a left thyroid nodule. Fine-needle aspiration cytology confirmed this to be consistent with a papillary thyroid carcinoma, and ultrasound scans demonstrated a 2.6 cm left thyroid nodule with microcalcifications and no evidence of nodal disease. She underwent a total thyroidectomy in August 2007. Intraoperatively, there was no evidence of central compartment nodal disease, hence no central compartment dissection was performed. Histopathological evaluation confirmed a 2.5 cm left-sided lower-pole papillary thyroid cancer (well differentiated), with no extrathyroidal extension. She recovered uneventfully with postoperative thyroglobulin was <1 µg/L 3 months after surgery, and hence not deemed to require radioiodine ablation (RAI ablation). She was therefore placed on 125 µg levothyroxine for replacement and TSH suppression, and was followed up with 6-monthly thyroglobulin levels and yearly ultrasound scans. In February 2010, she was found to have elevated thyroglobulin levels of 55 µg/L (**Fig. 15.1**). Ultrasound scans showed small-volume nodal disease in the left tracheoesophageal groove. She subsequently underwent I-131 WBS, which showed RAI-avid disease only in the left tracheoesophageal groove and superior mediastinum. She was therefore treated with an ablative dose of 100 mCi RAI with rTSH. Post ablation, her thyroglobulin levels reduced significantly to 7–10 µg/L but never completely normalized.

Five months after RAI ablation, her thyroglobulin levels were found have risen again to 64.2 µg/L. This time I-131 WBS showed no RAI-avid disease. A PET-CT scan was performed and showed that there was persistent FDG-avid disease in the left tracheoesophageal groove but no further disease in the superior mediastinum (**Fig. 15.2**). She subsequently underwent a reexploration of the left central compartment and a complete dissection of the left tracheoesophageal groove and thymus, taking care to preserve the left recurrent laryngeal nerve and superior parathyroid gland. The contralateral side was not dissected. Histopathological examination of this specimen confirmed residual papillary thyroid cancer in 3 out of 8 nodes dissected from this region. She recovered uneventfully postoperatively with no vocal cord palsy or hypoparathyroidism, and continued on her thyroxine dose of 125 µg daily. Her postdissection thyroglobulin level measured 3 months post surgery was <1 µg/L.

This case illustrates several principles previously mentioned. First, the need for dynamic risk stratification process. Ms. X was initially classified as low risk, but should subsequently be moved to intermediate in her risk for recurrence. Second, detection and management of residual disease requires a multidisciplinary and multimodality approach. Her disease recurrence was identified through rigorous surveillance using thyroglobulin measurements and ultrasound scans. Interestingly, these were shown to be RAI avid, and hence partly responsive to ablation. However, the failure to completely eradicate this disease suggests that there was tumor heterogeneity where non–RAI-avid tumor cells persisted post ablation. This was subsequently identified using FDG-PET, requiring reoperative dissection of the central compartment. Principles of reoperative surgery included careful dissection of the left central compartment with an attempt to identify all critical structures and sparing of the right side, so that both recurrent laryngeal nerves were not placed at risk. Postoperative normalization of thyroglobulin levels justified the surgical procedure, but Ms. X needs to be on close surveillance as she is no longer at low risk for recurrence.

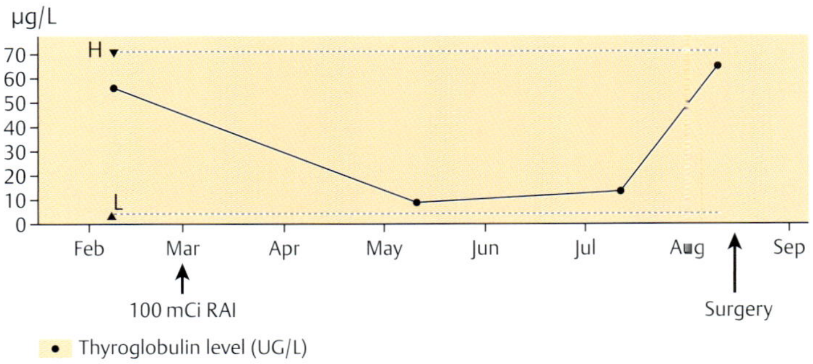

Fig. 15.1 Trend of thyroglobulin with time for Ms. X, with indication of timing for RAI ablation and surgery.

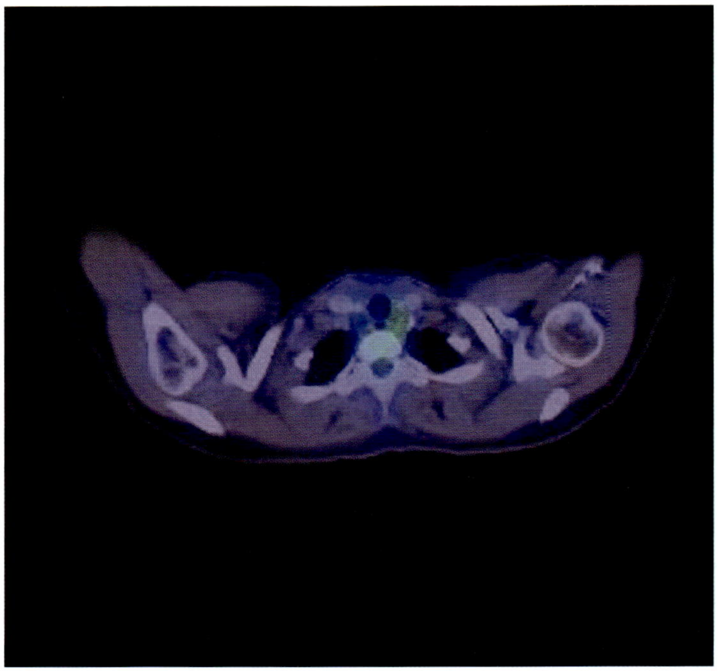

Fig. 15.2 PET-CT scan fused images showing recurrent disease in the left tracheoesophageal groove (paratracheal) nodal chain.

Conclusion

Most patients with differentiated thyroid cancer have excellent prognosis and are cured of disease after initial treatment. Those who develop recurrent disease still have excellent long-term outcome if these are identified early and treated accordingly. Accurate risk stratification, modification of risk profiles, and the institution of effective and appropriate surveillance strategies are paramount to early diagnosis and consequent application of effective treatment options. The few patients who fail these strategies may require a more palliative approach to symptom management or the use of novel target therapeutic agents, although the latter should be used in a trial setting until efficacy can be established. It is hoped that future risk stratification protocols will incorporate all aspects including clinical and molecular profiles to develop a dynamic and more accurate predictive tool when managing these patients, allowing individualized therapeutic options.

Future Research

- Identification of molecular markers that predict early recurrence more accurately than available scoring systems.
- Clinical trials to compare the role of observation versus early surgery for small-volume locoregional recurrent disease.
- Clinical trials to determine the value of novel targeted therapy in patients with metastatic disease, including identification of molecular determinants of response

Recommended Reading

- Kloos RT, Eng C, Evans DB, et al. American Thyroid Association Guidelines Task Force. Medullary thyroid cancer: management guidelines of the American Thyroid Association. Thyroid 2009;19(6):565–612
- Cooper DS, Doherty GM, Haugen BR, et al. American Thyroid Association (ATA) Guidelines Taskforce on Thyroid Nodules and Differentiated Thyroid Cancer. Revised American Thyroid Association management guidelines for patients with thyroid nodules and differentiated thyroid cancer. Thyroid 2009;19(11):1167–1214
- Sherman SI, Angelos P, Ball DW, et al. National Comprehensive Cancer Network Thyroid Carcinoma Panel. Thyroid carcinoma. J Natl Compr Canc Netw 2007;5(6):568–621

References

1. Kloos RT, Eng C, Evans DB, et al. American Thyroid Association Guidelines Task Force. Medullary thyroid cancer: management guidelines of the American Thyroid Association. Thyroid 2009;19(6):565–612
2. Todd WU IV, Wenig BM. Thyroid follicular epithelial cell-derived carcinomas: an overview of the pathology of primary and recurrent disease. Otolaryngol Clin North Am 2008;41(6):1079–1094, vii–viii
3. Davies L, Welch HG. Increasing incidence of thyroid cancer in the United States, 1973–2002. JAMA 2006;295(18):2164–2167
4. Iyer NG, Shaha AR, Silver CE, et al. Thyroid incidentalomas: to treat or not to treat. Eur Arch Otorhinolaryngol 2010;267(7):1019–1026
5. Hay ID, Thompson GB, Grant CS, et al. Papillary thyroid carcinoma managed at the Mayo Clinic during six decades (1940–1999): temporal trends in initial therapy and long-term outcome in 2444 consecutively treated patients. World J Surg 2002;26(8):879–885
6. Shah JP, Loree TR, Dharker D, Strong EW, Begg C, Vlamis V. Prognostic factors in differentiated carcinoma of the thyroid gland. Am J Surg 1992;164(6):658–661
7. Rossi RL, Cady B, Silverman ML, Wool MS, Horner TA. Current results of conservative surgery for differentiated thyroid carcinoma. World J Surg 1986;10(4):612–622
8. Sanders LE, Cady B. Differentiated thyroid cancer: reexamination of risk groups and outcome of treatment. Arch Surg 1998;133(4):419–425
9. Sanders LE, Silverman M. Follicular and Hürthle cell carcinoma: predicting outcome and directing therapy. Surgery 1998;124(6):967–974
10. Stojadinovic A, Ghossein RA, Hoos A, et al. Hürthle cell carcinoma: a critical histopathologic appraisal. J Clin Oncol 2001;19(10):2616–2625
11. Harada T, Ito K, Shimaoka K, Hosoda Y, Yakumaru K. Fatal thyroid carcinoma. Anaplastic transformation of adenocarcinoma. Cancer 1977;39(6):2588–2596
12. Goretzki PE, Simon D, Frilling A, et al. Surgical reintervention for differentiated thyroid cancer. Br J Surg 1993;80(8):1009–1012
13. Mazzaferri EL, Kloos RT. Clinical review 128: Current approaches to primary therapy for papillary and follicular thyroid cancer. J Clin Endocrinol Metab 2001;86(4):1447–1463
14. Schlumberger MJ. Papillary and follicular thyroid carcinoma. N Engl J Med 1998;338(5):297–306
15. Durante C, Haddy N, Baudin E, et al. Long-term outcome of 444 patients with distant metastases from papillary and follicular thyroid carcinoma: benefits and limits of radioiodine therapy. J Clin Endocrinol Metab 2006;91(8):2892–2899
16. Dinneen SF, Valimaki MJ, Bergstralh EJ, Goellner JR, Gorman CA, Hay ID. Distant metastases in papillary thyroid carcinoma: 100 cases observed at one institution during 5 decades. J Clin Endocrinol Metab 1995;80(7):2041–2045
17. Casara D, Rubello D, Saladini G, et al. Different features of pulmonary metastases in differentiated thyroid cancer: natural history and multivariate statistical analysis of prognostic variables. J Nucl Med 1993;34(10):1626–1631
18. Iyer NG, Shaha AR. Management of thyroid nodules and surgery for differentiated thyroid cancer. Clin Oncol (R Coll Radiol) 2010;22(6):405–1412
19. Tuttle RM, Leboeuf R, Shaha AR. Medical management of thyroid cancer: a risk adapted approach. J Surg Oncol 2008;97(8):712–716
20. Cooper DS, Doherty GM, Haugen BR, et al. American Thyroid Association (ATA) Guidelines Taskforce on Thyroid Nodules and Differentiated Thyroid Cancer. Revised American Thyroid Association management guidelines for patients with thyroid nodules and differentiated thyroid cancer. Thyroid 2009;19(11):1167–1214
21. Shaha A. Treatment of thyroid cancer based on risk groups. J Surg Oncol 2006;94(8):683–691

22. Mazzaferri EL, Robbins RJ, Spencer CA, et al. A consensus report of the role of serum thyroglobulin as a monitoring method for low-risk patients with papillary thyroid carcinoma. J Clin Endocrinol Metab 2003;88(4):1433–1441
23. Torlontano M, Attard M, Crocetti U, et al. Follow-up of low risk patients with papillary thyroid cancer: role of neck ultrasonography in detecting lymph node metastases. J Clin Endocrinol Metab 2004;89(7):3402–3407
24. Ashcraft MW, Van Herle AJ. The comparative value of serum thyroglobulin measurements and iodine 131 total body scans in the follow-up study of patients with treated differentiated thyroid cancer. Am J Med 1981;71(5):806–814
25. Frilling A, Görges R, Tecklenborg K, et al. Value of preoperative diagnostic modalities in patients with recurrent thyroid carcinoma. Surgery 2000;128(6):1067–1074
26. Kloos RT, Mazzaferri EL. A single recombinant human thyrotropin-stimulated serum thyroglobulin measurement predicts differentiated thyroid carcinoma metastases three to five years later. J Clin Endocrinol Metab 2005;90(9):5047–5057
27. Baudin E, Do Cao C, Cailleux AF, Leboulleux S, Travagli JP, Schlumberger M. Positive predictive value of serum thyroglobulin levels, measured during the first year of follow-up after thyroid hormone withdrawal, in thyroid cancer patients. J Clin Endocrinol Metab 2003;88(3):1107–1111
28. Dueren C, Dietlein M, Luster M, et al. The use of thyrogen in the treatment of differentiated thyroid carcinoma: An intraindividual comparison of clinical effects and implications of daily life. Exp Clin Endocrinol Diabetes 2010; 118(8):513–519.
29. Frates MC. Ultrasound in recurrent thyroid disease. Otolaryngol Clin North Am 2008;41(6):1107–1116, viii.
30. Sutton RT, Reading CC, Charboneau JW, James EM, Grant CS, Hay ID. US-guided biopsy of neck masses in postoperative management of patients with thyroid cancer. Radiology 1988;168(3):769–772
31. Rodriguez JM, Reus M, Moreno A, et al. High-resolution ultrasound associated with aspiration biopsy in the follow-up of patients with differentiated thyroid cancer. Otolaryngol Head Neck Surg 1997;117(6):694–697
32. Ronga G, Fiorentino A, Paserio E, et al. Can iodine-131 whole-body scan be replaced by thyroglobulin measurement in the post-surgical follow-up of differentiated thyroid carcinoma? J Nucl Med 1990;31(11):1766–1771
33. Aygun N. Imaging of recurrent thyroid cancer. Otolaryngol Clin North Am 2008;41(6):1095–1106, viii viii
34. Shaha AR. Revision thyroid surgery—technical considerations. Otolaryngol Clin North Am 2008;41(6):1169–1183, xx
35. Randolph GW, Kamani D. The importance of preoperative laryngoscopy in patients undergoing thyroidectomy: voice, vocal cord function, and the preoperative detection of invasive thyroid malignancy. Surgery 2006;139(3):357–362
36. Robbins RJ, Wan Q, Grewal RK, et al. Real-time prognosis for metastatic thyroid carcinoma based on 2-[^{18}F]fluoro-2-deoxy-D-glucose-positron emission tomography scanning. J Clin Endocrinol Metab 2006;91(2):498–505
37. Are C, Hsu JF, Ghossein RA, Schoder H, Shah JP, Shaha AR. Histological aggressiveness of fluorodeoxyglucose positron-emission tomogram (FDG-PET)-detected incidental thyroid carcinomas. Ann Surg Oncol 2007;14(11):3210–3215
38. Pacini F, Schlumberger M, Dralle H, Ilisea R, Smith Y, Viersinga V. European consensus on the management of patients with differentiated carcinoma of the thyroid from follicular epithelium. [Article in Russian] Vestn Khir Im I I Grek 2008;167(1):52–56
39. Shaha AR. Management of the neck in thyroid cancer. Otolaryngol Clin North Am 1998;31(5):823–831
40. Gopalakrishna Iyer N, Shaha AR. Complications of thyroid surgery: prevention and management. Minerva Chir 2010;65(1):71–82
41. Dupuy DE, Monchik JM, Decrea C, Pisharodi L. Radiofrequency ablation of regional recurrence from well-differentiated thyroid malignancy. Surgery 2001;130(6):971–977
42. Lewis BD, Hay ID, Charboneau JW, McIver B, Reading CC, Goellner JR. Percutaneous ethanol injection for treatment of cervical lymph node metastases in patients with papillary thyroid carcinoma. AJR Am J Roentgenol 2002;178(3):699–704
43. Richer SL, Wenig BL. Changes in surgical anatomy following thyroidectomy. Otolaryngol Clin North Am 2008;41(6):1069–1078, vii
44. Shindo M, Chheda NN. Incidence of vocal cord paralysis with and without recurrent laryngeal nerve monitoring during thyroidectomy. Arch Otolaryngol Head Neck Surg 2007;133(5):481–485
45. Patel KN, Shaha AR. Locally advanced thyroid cancer. Curr Opin Otolaryngol Head Neck Surg 2005;13(2):112–116
46. Price DL, Wong RJ, Randolph GW. Invasive thyroid cancer: management of the trachea and esophagus. Otolaryngol Clin North Am 2008;41(6):1155–1168, ix–x.
47. Lefevre JH, Tresallet C, Leenhardt L, Jublanc C, Chigot JP, Menegaux F. Reoperative surgery for thyroid disease. Langenbecks Arch Surg 2007;392(6):685–691
48. Menegaux F, Turpin G, Dahman M, et al. Secondary thyroidectomy in patients with prior thyroid surgery for benign disease: a study of 203 cases. Surgery 1999;126(3):479–483
49. Shoup M, Stojadinovic A, Nissan A, et al. Prognostic indicators of outcomes in patients with distant metastases from differentiated thyroid carcinoma. J Am Coll Surg 2003;197(2):191–197
50. Stojadinovic A, Shoup M, Ghossein RA, et al. The role of operations for distantly metastatic well-differentiated thyroid carcinoma. Surgery 2002;131(6):636–643
51. Lee J, Soh EY. Differentiated thyroid carcinoma presenting with distant metastasis at initial diagnosis clinical outcomes and prognostic factors. Ann Surg 2010;251(1):114–119
52. Lippi F, Capezzone M, Angelini F, et al. Radioiodine treatment of metastatic differentiated thyroid cancer in patients on L-thyroxine, using recombinant human TSH. Eur J Endocrinol 2001;144(1):5–11
53. Pacini F, Ladenson PW, Schlumberger M, et al. Radioiodine ablation of thyroid remnants after preparation with recombinant human thyrotropin in differentiated thyroid carcinoma: results of an international, randomized, controlled study. J Clin Endocrinol Metab 2006;91(3):926–932
54. Luster M, Lippi F, Jarzab B, et al. rhTSH-aided radioiodine ablation and treatment of differentiated thyroid carcinoma: a comprehensive review. Endocr Relat Cancer 2005;12(1) 49–64
55. Sherman SI, Angelos P, Ball DW, et al. National Comprehensive Cancer Network Thyroid Carcinoma Panel. Thyroid carcinoma. J Natl Compr Canc Netw 2007;5(6):568–621
56. Cohen EG, Tuttle RM, Kraus DH. Postoperative management of differentiated thyroid cancer. Otolaryngol Clin North Am 2003;36(1):129–157

57. Rosenbluth BD, Serrano V, Happersett L, et al. Intensity-modulated radiation therapy for the treatment of non-anaplastic thyroid cancer. Int J Radiat Oncol Biol Phys 2005;63(5):1419–1426
58. Terezakis SA, Lee KS, Ghossein RA, et al. Role of external beam radiotherapy in patients with advanced or recurrent nonanaplastic thyroid cancer: Memorial Sloan-Kettering Cancer Center experience. Int J Radiat Oncol Biol Phys 2009;73(3):795–801
59. Tuttle RM, Leboeuf R. Investigational therapies for metastatic thyroid carcinoma. J Natl Compr Canc Netw 2007;5(6):641–646

16 Recurrent Salivary Gland Carcinoma and Pleomorphic Adenoma

Alfonsus J.M. Balm, Jan Paul de Boer, Coen R.N. Rasch

Acknowledgment We thank Suzanne Bakker MSc, head of the Central Cancer Library, and coworkers for their support.

Summary

- Salivary gland carcinoma (SGC) is a relatively rare disease and represents a wide spectrum of tumors with different biological behaviors. Approximately 10%–25% of patients recur locally. With the current knowledge it is extremely difficult to determine accurately the prognosis of patients, although prognostic pre- and postoperative scoring models, which incorporate significant prognostic variables, may be helpful in daily clinical decision making for parotid carcinoma management.
- The unpredictable clinical course of locally recurrent SGC makes it of utmost importance to aim at maximizing local control. Combined salvage surgery and radiotherapy are at present the most effective treatment modalities. Treatment-related toxicity and morbidity are related to the extent of surgery and should be minimized and be weighed against the personal requirements and expectations of the individual patient.
- The relatively high chance of occult regional metastases in recurrent SGC is a strong indication for implementing elective treatment of the neck.
- Currently no effective systemic treatment is available for the management of disseminated disease.
- Since there is a high chance of re-recurrent pleomorphic adenoma after surgery, extended parotidectomy is the reoperation of choice. However, it comes at the cost of a high risk of damaging the facial nerve.

Salivary Gland Carcinoma

General Characteristics

Epidemiology

Salivary gland carcinoma (SGC) is a relatively rare disease and accounts for approximately 6% of all head and neck malignancies. It is estimated that in the United States 10 new patients are diagnosed per 1 million inhabitants per year.[1,2] Similar figures are reported for Western European countries.[3] In contrast to head and neck squamous cell carcinomas, there are no specific etiological or genetic factors described that contribute to the origin of SGC. Only the iatrogenic influence of ionizing radiation and radiation from atomic fallout have been reported as etiological factors[4] as well as exposure to several toxic agents (hair dye, rubber industry, nickel, silica dust).[5]

Occurrence

Salivary gland carcinomas can be found in the paired major salivary glands (parotid, submandibular, and sublingual) as well as in the minor salivary glands located in mucosa of the upper aerodigestive tract. This widespread occurrence in the head and neck region implies that for differential diagnostic reasons SGC should always be considered in the differential diagnosis of a suspicious mass. Secondary ulceration may sometimes make it difficult to differentiate SGC macroscopically from even a squamous cell carcinoma.

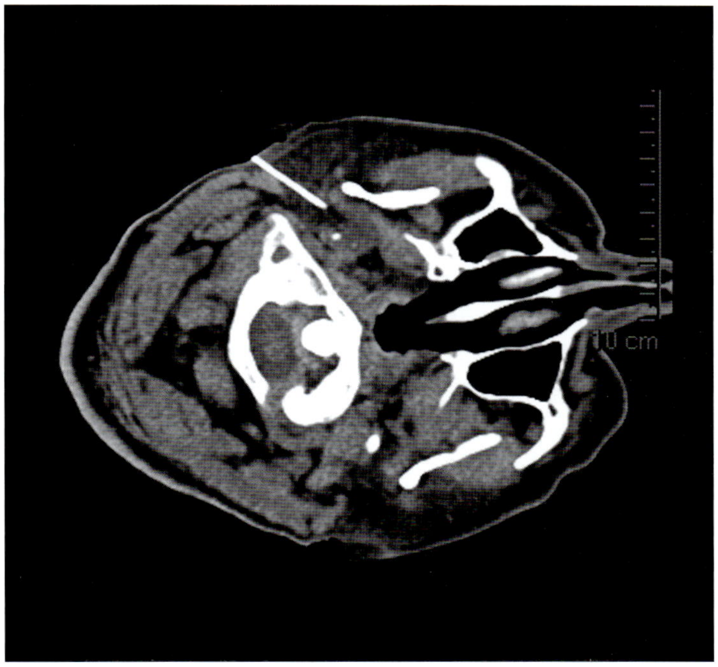

Fig. 16.1 CT scan guided tru cut biopsy of the right parotid gland in a patient with repeated negative aspiration cytologies from a deep lobe tumor, finally diagnosed as an adenocarcinoma.

> **!** The majority of salivary gland tumors, both benign and malignant, occur in the parotid glands (64%–80%), followed by the submandibular glands (7%–11%) and the minor salivary glands (9%–23%), with the last tumors harboring the highest risk of malignancy.[6]

Signs and Symptoms

The clinical presentation depends on the localization of the tumor and there are no specific symptoms related to the disease. However, symptoms like pain, facial nerve palsy, numbness, neck node swelling, and fixation are more related to malignant disease or act as warning signs of occult recurrent SGC. For subcutaneous and submucosal tumors, fine-needle aspiration cytology, guided by ultrasound sonography or CT scan, if indicated, is a very sensitive tool, reaching values of almost 90%, for making the first diagnosis.[7,8] CT-guided tru cut biopsy can serve as a good alternative for open biopsy (**Fig. 16.1**) However. accuracy is strongly dependent on the expertise of the individual pathologist.

Histology

Salivary gland carcinomas display many histological subtypes and several studies have evaluated the relative incidence. Mucoepidermoid carcinoma, adenoid cystic carcinoma, and adenocarcinoma are the most common histological subtypes, accounting for 34%, 22%, and 18%, respectively, of 1278 malignancies.[9] The WHO 2005 histological classification[10] describes a system of 20 different types of carcinomas, which makes it difficult to use in daily clinical practice. To make the system more practicable in the clinical setting, the different tumor types are frequently reclassified according to their clinical behavior. A widely used dichotomy in the WHO classification is the subdivision between low-grade (acinic cell carcinoma, low-grade mucoepidermoid carcinoma) and high-grade malignancies (adenoid cystic carcinoma, adenocarcinoma, carcinoma ex pleomorphic adenoma, high-grade mucoepidermoid carcinoma, squamous cell carcinoma).[11,12] However, the system remains weak for clinical prognostication due to the lack of consensus on histological grading criteria.

Prognosis

Because of the wide spectrum of tumors with different biological behaviors, which are often determined by tumor characteristics such as site, tumor stage, margins, perineural growth, etc. and which often determine prognosis, it is extremely difficult to make an appropriate prediction of the chance of tumor recurrences for the individual patient.

It is estimated that 10%–25% of patients recur locally after surgical resection alone or after combined surgery and radiotherapy.[13–15] In general, the majority of patients with recurrent head and neck cancer, including SGC, will die from a local recurrence[16] and also have a high competing risk of developing distant metastases.[17] The effectiveness of salvage treatment is limited by the site of the primary SGC, by the fact that the majority of patients have undergone postoperative external beam radiotherapy, and by the risk of severe complications after re-irradition.[17] Since it remains impossible with the current knowledge to identify the patients who will have long-term survival after developing local recurrence or development of distant metastases, salvage treatment for local tumor recurrence should only be determined by the use of the various treatment modalities. For reasons of practicality, the most frequently occurring SGCs will be highlighted in the following paragraphs.

Mucoepidermoid Carcinoma

Epidemiology

In many published series on SGC, mucoepidermoid carcinoma (MEC) is considered to be the most common salivary gland carcinoma, comprising 36% of salivary malignancies according to Spiro[9] reporting on 2807 salivary gland tumors. With regard to the minor salivary glands, it competes with adenoid cystic carcinoma as the most frequently occurring SGC in some series.[18]

Occurrence

MECs predominantly arise in the major salivary glands, mainly in the parotid gland.[19]

Grading

There is a known widely diverse biological behavior and an unpredictable outcome among both low-grade and high-grade malignancies. However, the histological grade of mucoepidermoid carcinoma is often reported as having a statistically significant correlation with patients' survival.[20–22]

Different grading schemes and various grading criteria have been proposed over time, indicating the limited utility of grading for predicting prognosis. Traditionally, MECs were histologically classified as low- and high-grade based on the relative proportion of cell types. Others[23] have proposed a grading system based on numerical scores attributed to histological features. This grading system was only applicable for tumors arising in the parotid gland. A three-tiered grading scheme has been developed by Brandwein et al.[24] that includes vascular invasion and type of tumor invasion. Using this classification they reported a more accurate correlation and reported that low-grade tumors showed an excellent prognosis with complete locoregional disease control. The multiple grading schemes and various grading criteria that have been proposed over time are a sign of their limited benefit in predicting prognosis.

Prognosis

Many studies suggest improved locoregional disease control in patients who received adjuvant radiotherapy after surgery, even those with more positive margins.[25,26] Although the efficacy of radiotherapy as sole treatment modality does not exceed 20% in advanced-stage salivary gland carcinoma, Mendenhall et al.[27] state that, despite the lack of randomized studies, adjuvant radiotherapy in salivary malignant tumors improves outcomes of patients with advanced-stage disease, positive margins, and high-grade histology. According to these authors, it is therefore safe to recommend postoperative radiotherapy in bulky tumors with high histological grade regardless of the condition of surgical margins.

Similarly to adenoid cystic carcinoma (ACC), distant metastases of MEC are often of a slowly progressive nature, leading to an average survival of approximately 2.5 years.[28] It has been hypothesized[22] that, irrespective of histological grading, local recurrence is more likely to be the causative factor in the development of distant metastases rather than the original primary tumor. This observation is in direct contrast to the clinical course of disease in patients with ACCs whose distant metastases seem to occur irrespectively of histological grade, margin status, and the presence or absence of locoregional recurrences.[29]

Reported 5-year (disease-specific) survival rates vary widely in the literature from very low percentages (22.5%) to very high (over 90%),[22,30–32] depending on the dichotomous tumor grading. It remains to be elucidated whether the observed high 5-year survival rates are also due to a standardized aggressive surgical treatment and the application of postoperative radiotherapy.

There have been many attempts to predict the risk of recurrence, but the biological behavior of MEC remains to be unraveled. Although histological grade has been suggested to be the most important parameter, with the highest prognostic significance, metastatic disease from low-grade MECs may also occur with lethal consequences. Despite progress in the understanding of the clinical behavior of the various salivary malignancies, the genetic mechanisms of pathogenesis of these tumors are still poorly understood. Gene expression and immunohistochemical profiling are possible promising future tools with which to understand the molecular pathogenesis,[33] but currently no clear genetic differences have emerged between the various histological types. Further studies of MECs at molecular level are needed to define biologically different groups within the same tumor entity and to test the value of various therapeutic modalities, but such challenging goals can only be achieved by an extensive international collaboration to collate a large series of patients.

Adenoid Cystic Carcinoma

Epidemiology

Adenoid cystic carcinoma (ACC) on average accounts for around 20% of all SGC.[9,34] It is a carcinoma of the older age group, commonly presenting during the fifth and sixth decades of life.[35–37]

Occurrence

ACC occurs mainly in the intraoral salivary glands, particularly in the palate, followed in order of frequency by the parotid, submandibular, and sublingual salivary glands. Other sites in the head and neck region can be affected as well, including lacrimal glands, esophagus, and tracheobronchial tree.[38]

Prognosis

Slow and indolent growth seems more or less classical for ACC and the extensive local tissue infiltration and perineural spread results in a high rate of late recurrences,[35,39] even after extensive surgical procedures. Local and distant recurrences are common in ACC, leading to low long-term survival rates.[39] The total failure rate varies from 43% to 70%, with local failures ranging from 31% to 52% and distant metastases from 19% to 52%,[40–42] with lung metastases being the most common.[29,36–38,40,43] Late local recurrence and distant metastasis are frequent in ACC[39] and there are reports describing cases that have recurred even after 9 years of treatment.

Numerous attempts have been undertaken to determine ACC-specific clinicopathological predictors of survival,[37,44] and many prognostic factors have been studied in this respect: Age of the patient, tumor site, histological type and duration of symptoms, clinical stage, modality of treatment, histological subtype, perineural and/or vascular invasion, and presence of positive surgical margins have all been considered.[29,37,38,40,42,44,45]

- Pain and paresthesia are often reported as significant prognostic factors for poor prognosis, but this could not be confirmed by others.[46]
- Advanced clinical stage has been described as a significant predictor of outcome in both univariate and multivariate survival analyses.[37,38,46,47]
- Histological subtype is claimed by some as an important prognostic indicator.[37,40,42,46,47]

Positive surgical margins have emerged as a significant prognostic factor.[29,42,45] Regarding the modalities of treatment, it remains difficult to demonstrate significant differences between groups that received postoperative radiotherapy or surgery alone.[36,40,46] However, some studies showed better local control of the disease with the combined use of surgery and radiotherapy, mainly in cases with surgical positive margins.[27,45,46] Expression of proliferation markers (PCNA, Ki-67) and oncogenes (p53, c-erB-2) has also been correlated with survival,[46,48,49] but so far this has not resulted in independent prognostic factors suitable for clinical practice. Although ACC is one of the most studied SGCs, as in MEC further studies are necessary to better define the relevant prognostic factors and treatment modalities.

Adenocarcinoma

Epidemiology

Adenocarcinomas comprise 16%–20% of the SGCs[5] and include tumors with a wide range of biological behavior. The spectrum extends from the indolent polymorphous low grade adenocarcinoma to the aggressive salivary duct carcinoma. It is postulated that the adenocarcinomas originate from the salivary duct unit of the salivary glands.

Occurrence

The vast majority of the adenocarcinomas are found in the minor salivary glands, followed by the parotid gland and the submandibular gland.[50] The paranasal sinuses are in particular known to be a site of origin. Polymorphous low-grade adenocarcinoma is also mainly found in the minor salivary glands and predominantly involves the oral cavity (usually on the palate, buccal mucosa, and upper lip).[51] Salivary duct carcinoma mainly occurs in the parotid gland.

Prognosis

Adenocarcinomas of the paranasal sinuses have a high chance of recurrence depending on the extent of disease, leading to low 5-year survival rates.[50] For adenocarcinomas in the major salivary glands, survival figures are significantly higher and most probably related to the earlier detection rate for these anatomical sites. Recurrence of polymorphous low-grade adenocarcinoma is rare and occurs late, leading to an excellent 5-year overall survival of exceeding 95%. At the other end of the spectrum is the salivary duct carcinoma, having a very low 5-year survival of 30% with a high chance of local recurrence and distant metastases.[52]

Acinic Cell Carcinoma

Acinic cell carcinoma accounts for approximately 6% of all SGCs[53] and is most frequently found in the parotid gland.[54] It is a low-grade malignancy, with an excellent 5-year survival rate of 80%.[21] Reported local recurrence rates and occurrence of neck node metastases range widely from 0% to 44% and distant metastases are reported to develop in approximately 0%–13%.[54] Like adenoid cystic carcinoma, acinic cell carcinoma has been described to recur many years after the initial treatment.[9]

■ Prediction of Recurrence

In addition to the wide range of reported histological types and grading systems, the many other factors that may influence prognosis, such as increasing age, sex, pain, skin, perineural growth (facial paralysis), skin invasion, and resection margins, not all of which are systematically analyzed in every individual article, make it even more complicated to extrapolate relevant prognostic findings from one setting to the other. Other confounding factors such as the different treatment regimens and differences in the study populations add to the extremely difficult task of finding robust predictive factors for recurrence. In this respect, it may even be questioned whether histology by itself acts as a prognostic feature.

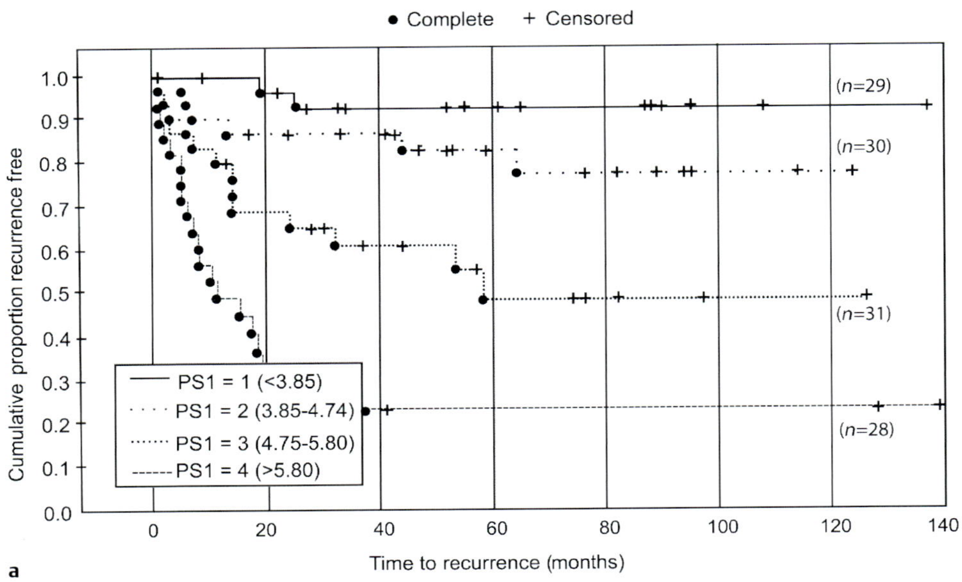

a

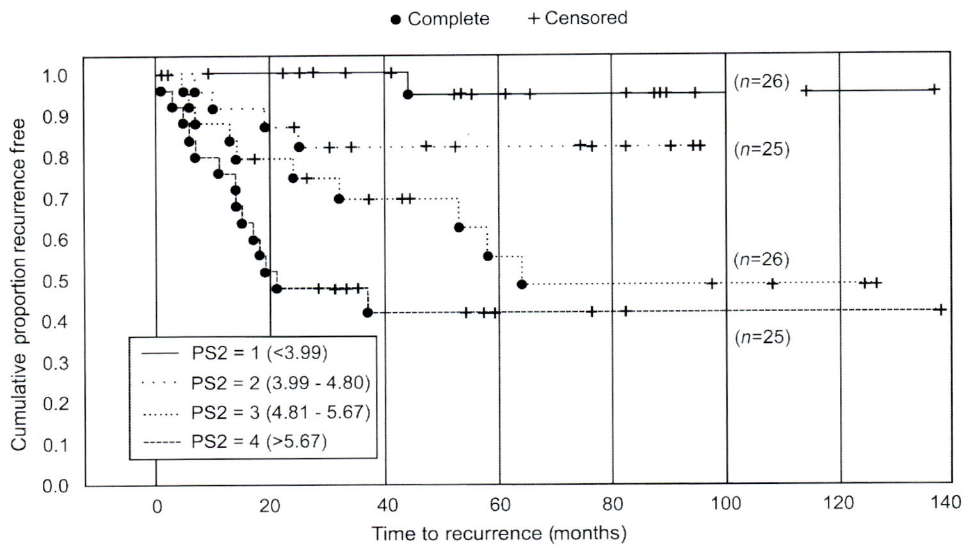

Fig. 16.2a, b Kaplan–Meier recurrence free interval curves by prognostic scores. (Reprinted with permission from V.L.M. Vander Poorten et al. The development of a prognostic score (PS) for patients with parotid carcinoma. Cancer 1999; 85: 2057–67.)

a PS1 based on analysis of pretreatment factors. $PS1 = 0.024A + 0.62P + 0.44T + 0.45N + 0.63S + 0.91F$ where A = age at diagnosis (years), P = pain on presentation (1 = no pain, 2 = pain or numbness), T = clinical T classification (T1 = 0, T2 = 1, T3 = 2, T3 = 2, T4 = 3), N = clinical N classification (N0 = 0, N1 = 1, N2a = 2, N2b = 3, N2c = 4, N3 = 5), S = skin invasion (1 = no invasion, 2 = invasion), F = facial nerve dysfunction (1 = intact function, 2 = (paresis, paralysis).
b PS2 based on the analysis of pretreatment factors together with post-treatment factors. $PS2 = 0.018A + 0.39T + 0.34N + 0.70S + 0.56F + 0.78PG + 0.65PM$ where A = age at diagnosis (years), T = clinical T classification (T1 = 0, T2 = 1, T3 = 2, T3 = 2, T4 = 3), N = clinical N classification (N0 = 0, N1 = 1, N2a = 2, N2b = 3, N2c = 4, N3 = 5), S = skin invasion (1 = no invasion, 2 = invasion). F = facial nerve dysfunction (1 = intact function, 2 = (paresis, paralysis), PG = perineural growth in the resection specimen (1 = no, 2 = yes), PM = positive surgical margins (1 = no; 2 = yes).

Malignant Submandibular Gland Carcinoma and Minor Salivary Gland Carcinomas

Both are rare disease entities and there are few reports available of long-term treatment results and prognostic factors. In a series from our tertiary referral institute with a long-standing stable treatment protocol and long-term follow-up, 5- and 10-year survival rates were found to be 50% and 36%, respectively, for submandibular gland carcinomas and 66% and 57%, respectively, for minor salivary gland carcinomas.[55,56] In both series UICC/AJC TNM classification and stage grouping appeared to be of significance in predicting tumor recurrence, as were perineural growth and skin invasion as recurrence predicting factors in surgical patients. Series of patients with submandibular gland carcinoma and minor salivary gland carcinoma almost never exceed 70 patients in number, thereby making it almost impossible to formulate predictive factors useful for the individual patient.

Parotid Carcinomas

The relatively high incidence of parotid carcinomas makes it possible to identify clinical prognostic factors and combine them in a prognostic model after quantification of their respective weighting in a multivariate analysis. In a cohort of 168 patients, 151 patients were evaluated to assess the prognostic value of clinical and pathological factors in a multivariate proportional hazards analysis. Clinical T(tumor) and N(nodal) classification, pain, age at diagnosis, skin invasion, facial nerve dysfunction, perineural growth, and positive surgical margins acted as major factors predicting recurrence. By a weighted combination of these factors, as present in the individual patient, four subgroups with markedly different prognosis could be identified. Four preoperative (PS1: 1–4) and postoperative (PS2: 1–4) scores were developed, predicting recurrence-free rates ranging from 92%–23% for the preoperative (PS1) scores and from 95% to 42% for the postoperative (PS2) scores, which take into account the histological details of the resection specimen (perineural growth, surgical margin) (**Fig. 16.2**).[57] This prognostic index was externally validated using a nationwide database containing 231 patients from major tertiary referral centers, thereby increasing the statistical and clinical reliability of the prognostic scores.[58] Recently this prognostic index was also validated using a Belgian-German database containing 237 preoperative and postoperative patients. This validation demonstrated that the prognostic indices performed adequately in this international validation sample, warranting prospective generalized use.[59] To make prognostic indices more robust it is important that more external validations are undertaken, with careful attention to the standardized treatment protocols and uniform staging of patients.[60]

■ Diagnostic Work-up

Clinical Investigation

The diagnosis of recurrent salivary gland carcinomas starts with careful registration of complaints, which frequently act as the first sign of a tumor recurrence. In squamous cell carcinoma, pain during follow-up is a sign of tumor recurrence during follow-up, unless proven otherwise.[61] It is reasonable to assume that, *mutatis mutandis*, this statement is applicable to SGC as well. Another important warning sign is referred earache, which is an ominous symptom and should always be carefully investigated, with attention to all the different head and neck subsites.[62] As these tumors, especially adenoid cystic carcinomas, are known for their perineural growth pattern, slowly progressive numbness and/or facial nerve dysfunction may be the first signs of recurrent disease.

Recording of the patient's history should be followed by a thorough ENT examination, including fiberoptic and direct endoscopic examination for the evaluation of the mucosal extension of the recurrent tumor and tumoral tissue sampling. This should be followed by systematic palpation of all levels of the neck in combination with ultrasound-guided aspiration cytology to search for occult neck node recurrences.

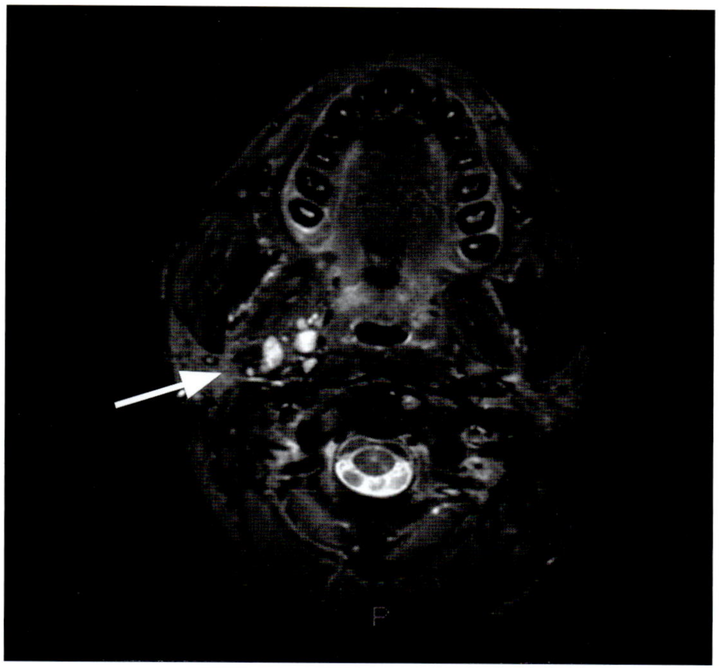

Fig. 16.3 T2-weighted MR image of a patient with multiple recurrent pleomorphic adenoma locations after surgical removal of a right parapharyngeal pleomorphic adenoma. Note the hyperintensity on T2-weighted MR images due to presence of myxoid material in pleomorphic adenoma recurrences (arrow).

Imaging

There is no radiological imaging technique that can accurately diagnose the presence or absence of a recurrent salivary gland carcinoma; they are only helpful in ascertaining the location and the extent of the recurrence.

Computed Tomography and Magnetic Resonance Imaging

Computed tomography (CT) with the administration of intravenous contrast provides an excellent tool for delineation of the tumor mass from the surrounding vascular and bony structures, and identifies cortical bony involvement. Magnetic resonance imaging (MRI) provides superior soft tissue details compared with CT and has the advantage of not requiring ionizing radiation or contrast for visualization of vascular details or ionizing radiation. In general, there is no typical imaging appearance for recurrent salivary gland carcinoma, except for most recurrent pleomorphic adenomas, which are hyperintense on T2-weighted MR images due to presence of myxoid material[63,64] (**Fig. 16.3**). This myxoid subtype has been shown to be the predominant subtype in recurrent pleomorphic adenomas, which makes MRI a valuable tool for radiological follow-up in patients with recurrent pleomorphic adenoma and a high risk of functional deficit after surgery.[65] It is also very suitable for detection of multiple small, recurrent nodules spread over the former operative field in the head and neck. In this respect, it should be emphasized that inadequate surgery for recurrent pleomorphic adenoma implies a high risk for re-recurrence.[66,67]

Positron Emission Tomography with ^{18}F-labeled Fluorodeoxyglucose

There is increasing evidence that PET-FDG is superior to other radiological methods for the initial diagnosis and staging of primary head and neck tumors, and also for detecting recurrent disease and distant metastases during the follow-up period.[68–70] Several studies report on the evaluation of primary salivary gland tumors by PET-FDG,[71–74] with sensitivity rates ranging from 75% to 100%. Positive PET-FDG results are also found in benign salivary gland tumors such as Warthin tumor and pleomorphic adenoma.[71,72,75] However, with knowledge of an already treated malignant salivary gland malignancy in the past, problems of false positivity may not be expected. Otsuka et al.[73] demonstrated that PET-FDG was superior to conventional methods in detecting metastatic disease from SGC during follow-up. In their study, the sensitivity, negative predictive value (NPV), and accuracy of PET-FDG were found to be 93%, 99%, and 94%, respectively, while those of the conventional imaging techniques were 80%, 96%, and 92%. This led to a change in the management of approximately 35% of patients with malignant SGC in their series. In a recently published multicenter, prospective study including 233 patients with newly diagnosed and untreated HNSCC, conventional work-up (CT/MRI head and neck region; thoracic CT) was compared with pretreatment whole-body PET-FDG. The addition of whole-body PET-FDG to the pretherapeutic conventional staging of HNSCC improved the TNM classification of the disease and altered the management of 13.7% of patients.[76]

Several studies have demonstrated that adding PET-FDG (or PET-CT-FDG) to a conventional work-up resulted in a higher staging accuracy: nodal classification is improved, especially in terms of specificity,[77–79] and PET-FDG detects more distant metastases than conventional CT staging.[80–83] However, nodal micrometastases in clinically N0 patients (cN0) remain a source of concern for all imaging techniques, including PET.[77,84] In this respect, in experienced hands ultrasound-guided fine-needle aspiration cytology remains the method of choice for accurate staging of the neck.[85]

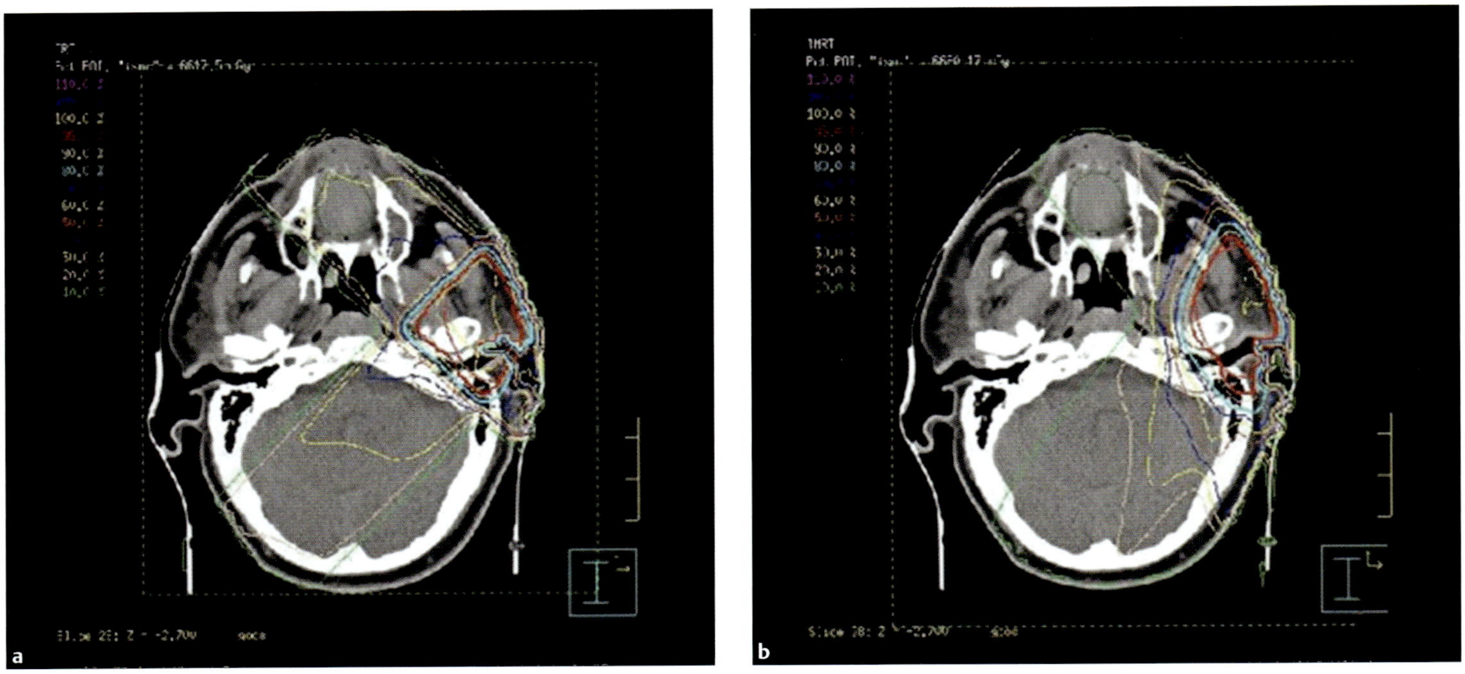

Fig. 16.4a, b Dose distribution for postoperative radiation for parotid gland carcinoma with 3D conformal (**a**) and IMRT (**b**). Note the dose to the internal ear and exiting dose to cerebellum and oral cavity

Principles of Management

Surgery

Surgery is still the mainstay of treatment for salivary gland carcinomas, either primary or recurrent carcinoma. Superficial parotidectomy is the minimum amount of surgery necessary for the parotid gland and can also be performed even after initial enucleation of a primary carcinoma or pleomorphic adenoma. When pretreatment imaging indicates extension of the disease to the deeper lobe of the parotid gland, a total parotidectomy should be performed with preservation of the facial nerve.

The most difficult part in parotid surgery for removal of a (recurrent) parotid carcinoma is sacrificing the facial nerve or nerve branches. By preoperative cytology, with a high rate of sensitivity,[7] most surgeons start parotidectomy with the knowledge of malignant disease. Sacrificing the facial nerve or its branches can therefore be anticipated and the patient should be counseled preoperatively with clear documentation in the medical records. The "rule of thumb" in surgery for parotid carcinoma is that facial nerve preservation is justified if an intact nerve can be dissected from the surrounding tumor tissue leaving behind only microscopic tumor remnants that can be sterilized by postoperative radiotherapy. When the nerve or its branches are running through the tumor mass, transection of the nerve or the branches is unavoidable and the nerve should then be reconstructed by a neural autograft. Nerve grafting with the sural nerve, great auricular nerve, or other sensory nerve is recommended.

Neck Node Recurrence

In a systematic review on treatment outcome of the clinically node-negative neck in primary parotid carcinoma, it was concluded that 83% of parotid carcinomas are clinically N0 but that a substantial proportion of these patients have occult neck node metastases: in 23% of elective neck dissections, neck node metastases were found at a microscopic level. Interestingly, the percentage of neck recurrence in that cohort was approximately 5%, indicating that comprehensive (or selective) elective treatment and/or radiotherapy are indeed effective in reducing the rate of regional recurrences.[86] A well-structured preoperative assessment of the neck by ultrasound-guided aspiration cytology (USFNAC) will certainly also contribute to a higher detection rate of occult neck node metastases. There are no systematic reviews available describing the risk of regional occult metastases in SGCs originating at other subsites, but it may be assumed that similar figures emerge compared with the parotid gland carcinomas. For these nonparotid recurrent carcinomas, maximal effort should be made to optimally stage the neck preoperatively so as to reduce the chance of regional recurrence.

Radiotherapy

Published data on radiotherapy for recurrent SGC is scarce and lacks randomized clinical trials. In general: the indications for radiotherapy are similar to the indications for radiotherapy during the primary treatment.[87,88] Postoperative radiation treatment, (chemo-)radiotherapy, re-irradiation, and radiation for metastatic disease will be discussed.

Postoperative Radiation Treatment

For reasons of involved or close margins and bad prognostic histological signs in the surgical specimen, postoperative radiation treatment is recommended in SGC. Recurrence after SGC surgery is most likely to be the result of incomplete resection and/or tumor spill in the previous resection area. Therefore, radiation portals should include at least the surgical bed of both the first and recurrence surgery.[87,88] Indications for irradiation of the neck should be the same as in the case for a primary treatment, with a recommended elective radiation dose of >46 Gy.

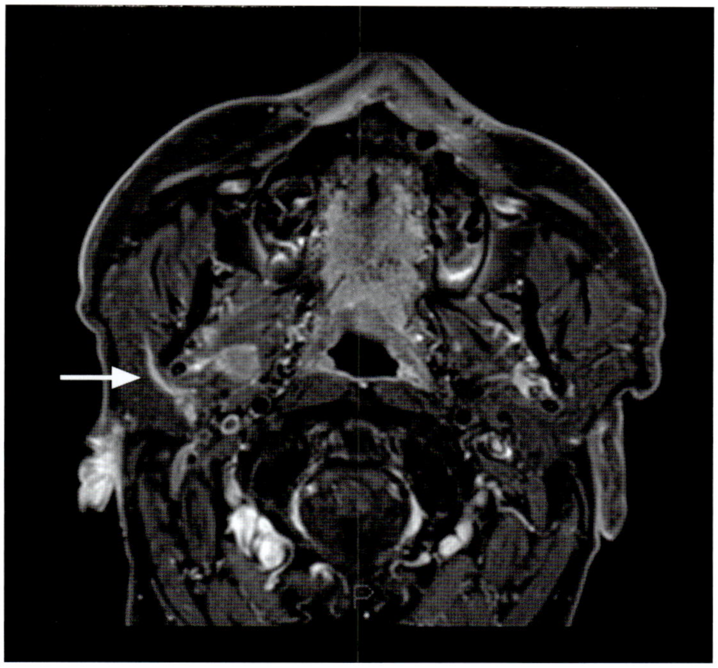

Fig. 16.5 MR imaging of perineural growth of an adenoid cystic carcinoma of the right parotid (arrow).

In case of postoperative irradiation for adenoid cystic carcinoma, better local control (between 85% and 100%) is achieved than in cases that did not receive radiotherapy.[89] In a review of 498 patients, the effective role of postoperative radiation was demonstrated for several clinical conditions: T3–T4 tumors (local control [LC] 84% vs, 18% [no RT]), close resection margins (LC 95% vs. 55%), incomplete resection (LC 82% vs. 44%) bone invasion (LC 86% vs. 54%), and perineural invasion (LC 95% vs. 55%).[88] Radiation portals should cover at least the entire surgical bed of all procedures.[87–89] Since intensity-modulated radiotherapy (IMRT) has been shown to better spare the neighboring organs at risk, this modality is recommended instead of the more conventional radiation techniques[90] (**Fig. 16.4**). Although no clear dose–response data are to be found for postoperative radiation, and possibly since most radiation regimens were in the same range, the recommended dose for postoperative radiation is between 60 and 70 Gy, with a reported median dose of 62 Gy.[88] A special note should be made for adenoid cystic carcinoma (ACC). As mentioned earlier in this chapter, these tumors are often characterized by their perineural growth[89,91] (**Fig. 16.5**). Therefore, in case of recurrent ACC, nerves should be identified and designated as target areas. Given the long doubling time, neutron therapy or charged-particle therapy are theoretically effective.[88] Both techniques have demonstrated their efficacy in the treatment of ACC, with 10-year locoregional control of 81%–65% at 1 and 3 years, respectively, for residual disease for a combination of photon therapy and carbon ions.[92]

Radiation without Surgery

Radiation as primary treatment for recurrent SGC is not the treatment of choice, albeit no comparative trials have been performed. In some cases, however, surgery is not possible or is refused by patients. Radiation should then consist of 66–70 Gy conventional fractionation, for which a 5-year local control of 50% was reported in 38 cases.[88] For mucosal squamous cell carcinomas, concurrent chemotherapy and radiation have shown superiority in advanced cases. Given the poor outcomes in recurrent salivary gland carcinomas, attempts were made for these patients as well.[93–95] A total of 78% local control in unresectable cases has been reported and is indeed promising. However, given the small numbers in the reports so far, the jury is still out and concurrent chemoradiation for recurrent SGC should not be performed outside the scope of a clinical trial.

Re-irradiation

(See also Chapter 4.)

Re-irradiation for salivary gland recurrence in a previously irradiated field carries higher risks of side effects than irradiation in radiation-naive tissues. Late grade III or higher side effects can occur up to 30% of individuals.[96–99] Since these effects are treatment volume–related, it is likely that for the lateralized radiation portals, as used for parotid and submandibular gland cases, a lower incidence of complications may be expected. For those cases where adequate radiation was part of the initial treatment for SGC, consideration should be given to resistance of tumor cells for radiation as well.

Radiation for Metastatic Disease

No trials tailored for metastatic disease of SGC have been published. Accordingly, only general recommendations within the view of the natural course of metastatic salivary gland carcinoma can be made. Since no effective systemic treatment exists, radiation is often remaining the treatment modality available to give relief of symptoms. For bone metastasis, one 8 Gy dose is as good as more prolonged regimens with 70% successful palliation.[100,101] With the advent of more unconventional fractionation regimens, such as three 20 Gy fractions (hypofractionation) for small lung carcinoma and extrathoracic localized diseases, this is increasingly applied for metastatic disease as well.[102] Given the high reported local control of more than 90%, it is a very promising modality, especially in oligometastatic disease. However, there is no scientific proof that it is more effective than palliative hypofractionation of one 8 Gy fraction.

■ Chemotherapy

The heterogeneity of salivary gland carcinoma (SGC) creates a wide difference in response to systemic therapy. Usually, chemotherapy and use of targeted agents are reserved for palliative treatment of disseminated disease or local recurrence with no alternative treatment options. To date a limited number of clinical trials—mainly nonrandomized phase II—have been published containing small numbers of patients with a great variety of tumor histologies and with mixed treatment indications, i.e., locoregional recurrence and disseminated disease. Trials focusing on the three most frequently occurring SGCs will be discussed below.

Mucoepidermoid Carcinoma

In contrast to adenoid cystic carcinoma and adenocarcinoma, some clinical activity has been observed with administration of paclitaxel in mucoepidermoid carcinoma (MEC): Gilbert et al.[103] observed an objective response in 3 out of 14 MEC patients in a phase II study of ECOG. Also some activity has been found using

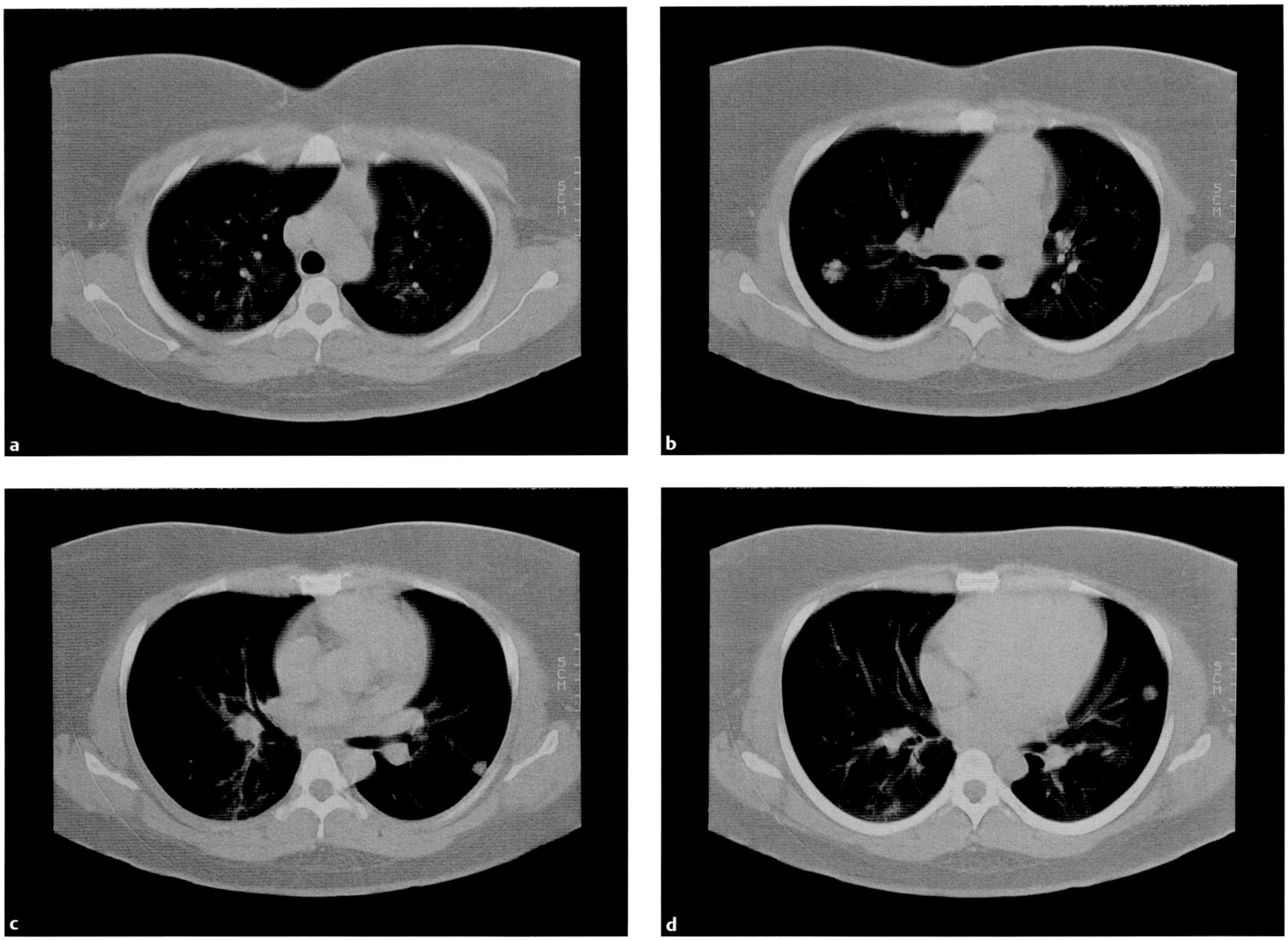

Fig. 16.6a–d CT scan of the thorax, showing multiple lung metastases of an adenoid cystic carcinoma (ACC). This patient has been treated with radiotherapy and adjuvant chemotherapy (cyclophosphamide, Adriamycin, cisplatin) for an ACC of the minor salivary gland in the oral cavity. After an interval of 2 months, demonstrating stable lung disease, major palliative ablative surgery for removal of the intraoral recurrence was undertaken.

cisplatin containing regimens.[104–107] Since in MEC her-2 has shown to be overexpressed in approximately one-third of patients, therapy targeting the her-2 pathway has been studied as well. In a phase II study, Haddad et al.[108] demonstrated a partial response lasting for more than 2 years in 1 out of 3 patients treated with trastuzumab, an anti–human her-2 monoclonal antibody. However, with lapatinib – a dual inhibitor of EGFR and erb-2 tyrosine kinase – no objective response was seen in a phase II study containing 29 non-ACC salivary gland tumors with overexpression of her-2.[109] Thus, single-agent therapy targeting her-2 (based on small numbers of patients) seems so far to be inactive in very limited series of patients. This is surprising, since in head and neck squamous cell carcinoma and breast cancer, the combination of EGFR targeting and other treatment modalities (i.e., radiotherapy of chemotherapy) has been shown to be effective.

Adenoid Cystic Carcinoma

Single-agent or multiagent chemotherapy rarely results in an objective response in adenoid cystic carcinoma (ACC). In prospective trials with single-agent chemotherapy, including vinorelbine, mitoxantrone and epirubicin, response rates ranged from 5% to 12%, although frequently stable disease was observed as well. The latter could also be attributed to the indolent clinical behavior of ACC.[110–113] Cisplatin-based multiagent regimens have been advocated in ACC, i.e., cisplatin–doxorubicin–cyclophosphamide (CAP) and cisplatin–vinorelbine, in which response rates ranging from 27% to 47% were observed, but at the cost of an increased treatment-induced toxicity.[105,114–116] The low number of patients included does not justify the conclusion that multiagent therapy is superior to single-agent therapy.

Since c-Kit and EGFR are overexpressed in 90% and 85% of ACC, studies have been done to explore whether modulation of these targets would be of interest in the treatment of ACC. Hotte et al.[117] treated 17 patients with imatinib, a c-Kit tyrosine kinase inhibitor, and observed no objective response in 15 evaluable patients. In the case of EGFR, Agulnik et al.[109] conducted a phase II study in 29 ACC patients with lapatinib, a dual inhibitor of EGFR and erb2 tyrosine kinase. No objective response was observed in the 19 evaluable patients.

On the basis of the aforementioned experiences, it can be concluded that to date treatment of recurrent and/or metastatic ACC with either chemotherapy or specific targeted agents has shown no or only modest activity. Systemic treatment should therefore be conducted in a patient-tailored manner and, if possible, in a clinical trial setting.

Case Study

A 27-year-old woman was referred to our tertiary referral institute for management of a recurrent adenoid cystic carcinoma of the right oral cavity, with invasion of the mandible and an orocutaneous fistula. Two years before, she had been irradiated for adenoid cystic carcinoma of the floor of mouth (T4N0M1) with a total dose of 4000 Gy in 10 fractions with shrinking fields in a palliative setting. According to the referring specialist, there was a complete macroscopic regression of the tumor process. During treatment, two lung metastases were found in the left lung by chest radiography. After radiotherapy she received six courses of chemotherapy (cyclophosphamide 500 mg/m^2, doxorubicin 50 mg/m^2, cisplatin 50 mg/m^2).

At presentation, she complained of severe pain and leakage of saliva through the orocutaneous fistula. The recurrence was infiltrating the root of the tongue with a massive osteoradionecrosis of the right mandible and tumor invasion of the overlying skin. CT scan of the thorax revealed a progression of distant disease with the presence of six lung metastases in both lungs (**Fig. 16.6**).

The poor quality of life caused by local recurrence, induced pain complaints, and continued dependence on nasogastric tube feeding for food intake, in the presence of distant metastases, made it extremely difficult to create conditions for good palliation. The only viable solution was to perform extensive local surgery with complete removal of the horizontal ramus of the mandible, total glossectomy, and reconstruction of the defects by (free) vascularized flaps. However, the lack of information about the speed of progression of lung metastases made it very difficult to make such a radical decision. In a multidisciplinary tumor board setting, it was decided to postpone surgical palliation and to try to determine the rate of progression of the lung metastases by repeated CT scans of the lungs. Since no growth of lung metastases was observed in a 2-month interval, the planned surgery was performed with reconstruction of the intraoral defect using a free revascularized flap of the fibula and reconstruction of the external skin defect by a pedicled flap of the latissimus dorsi muscle with external split skin coverage. The postoperative course was uneventful with restoration of oral food intake and production of intelligible speech (**Fig. 16.7**). Four weeks postoperatively she was discharged home and was able again to take care of her 3-year-old child. Eight months later there was asymptomatic progression of lung disease. Almost 3 years after completion of the palliative surgery, she died of progressive lung metastases.

The exceptional decision to perform this type of extensive ablative and reconstructive surgery highlights the importance of the incorporation of the individual biological tumor behavior in the clinical decision process in combination with a comprehensive discussion in a multidisciplinary tumor board setting followed by a careful counseling of the patient.

Adenoid cystic carcinoma is often characterized by slow growth but with a high propensity to develop distant metastases. In a series of Spiro et al.[118] the overall incidence of distant metastases was 38%. However, even in the presence of metastatic disease, survival in excess of 10 years has been well established.[118–120] Several studies have examined lung metastasectomy for adenoid cystic carcinoma, but none of them demonstrated a survival-improving effect.[121–123] In a series of the Memorial Sloan-Kettering Institute,[122] no disease-free survivors were encountered in a group of 14 patients undergoing metastasectomy after a follow-up period of 14 years. Longer survival rates were not demonstrated when comparing patients who had undergone histologically complete removal of their lung metastases with those who had had histologically incomplete excision. In a group of 50 patients with radical surgery for an adenoid cystic carcinoma, Bobbio et al.[121] compared 9 patients with lung metastasectomy for a solitary lung lesion—including four re-metastasectomy patients—with 11 patients with distant metastases, who did not undergo surgery. No differences in survival were detected between those two groups. Although the aforementioned studies all concern retrospective analyses, it is reasonable to assume that surgical intervention, even in the presence of a solitary lung lesion, does not contribute to increased survival. Therefore, it is advisable to refrain from surgery in patients with recurrent adenoid cystic carcinoma unless it contributes to the relief of symptoms.

Adenocarcinoma

To date little evidence exists for the effective use of systemic chemotherapy in adenocarcinoma. Administration of vinorelbine resulted in a partial remission in 2 out of 5 patients with adenocarcinoma in a phase II study.[124] In another phase II study with paclitaxel a partial response was observed in 5 out of 17 patients.[103] On the other hand, objective response rates of approximately 60% with cisplatin-containing multiagent chemotherapy have been found.[125,126] As in MEC, some adenocarcinomas do also overexpress EGFR and her-2, but no objective response was detected after administration of trastuzumab.[109] Androgen receptors are also overexpressed in adenocarcinoma, and in one case report partial remission with anti-androgen therapy (goserelin)

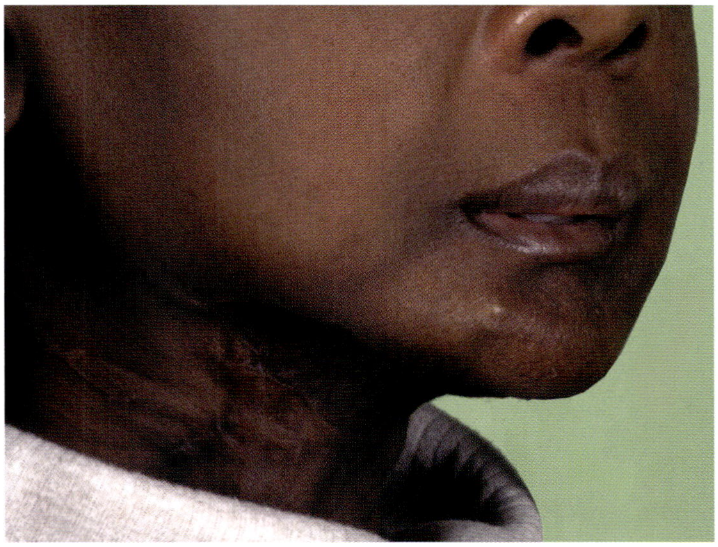

Fig. 16.7 Postoperative appearance of a 27-year-old patient, who had undergone "palliative surgery" consisting of complete horizontal mandibulectomy, total glossectomy and reconstruction of the intraoral defect with a free revascularized fibula flap and extraoral defect closure with a pedicled muscle latissimus dorsi flap. This extensive surgery was performed in the presence of multiple indolent lung metastases (see **Fig. 16.6**). The patient survived 3 years after surgery with comprehensible speech and restored oral intake.

was described.[127,128] In accordance with the successful treatment of paranasal adenocarcinoma with surgical debulking and repeated topical chemotherapy (5-fluorouracil) followed by necrotectomy,[129] this method may also be considered in locally recurrent adenocarcinomas of the paranasal cavity.

Salivary duct carcinoma (SDC) is the most aggressive malignancy among the adenocarcinomas,[52] resulting in an overall survival of 30%. Although no published data are available to support systemic therapy, this low survival warrants consideration of palliative chemotherapy in selected patients. Overexpression of her-2 has been established in this type of carcinoma and durable objective responses have been observed with trastuzumab-containing regimens, i.e., carboplatin, paclitaxel.[130,131] As in adenocarcinoma, androgen receptors are expressed in up to 90% of cases and some cases are also positive for prostate-specific antigen and prostatic acid phosphatase.[132,133] Objective responses have been observed with anti-androgen therapy [134] and anti-androgen therapy might be considered in patients with SDC as well.

Special Considerations: Surgery for SGC of the Parotid

Anterograde Identification of the Facial Nerve

A parotidectomy starts with a Blair's incision with the lower limb extending in a skin crease to minimize visible scar formation postoperatively. An overlying facial skin flap is raised superficially from the musculoaponeurotic sheath and in distal direction superficially from the platysma muscle fibers to prevent damage to the mandibular branches of the facial nerve, which lie deep to the muscle (see **Fig. 16.8**).

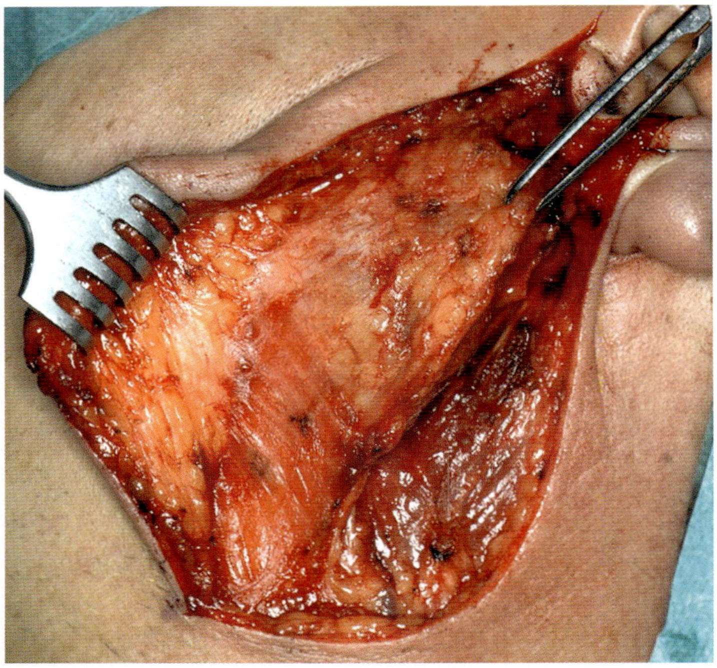

Fig. 16.8 Raised skin flap in parotidectomy lateral to the musculoaponeurotic sheath and superficial from the platysma muscle fibers, preventing damaging of mandibular branches of the facial nerve.

After visualization of the anterior border of the sternocleidomastoid (SCM) muscle, dissection is continued upward to the tendinous attachment of the muscle to the mastoid. Complete exposure of the sternocleidomastoid muscle tendon is important because it ensures that one stays behind the capsule of the parotid gland, thereby minimizing the chance of unintended diffuse bleeding. After identification of the mastoid tip, the posterior belly of the digastric muscle is dissected from the surrounding tissues. Then the cartilaginous tragal pointer of the external auditory canal is identified as being the third important landmark (posterior belly of the digastric, mastoid, tragal pointer). Thereafter, identification of the main stem of the facial nerves starts by careful dissection of the collagenous fibers lying laterally to the facial nerve. Although many geometrical descriptions exist in the literature that presume a more helpful mathematical method for identification of the nerve, these appear of less value during a stressful surgical procedure, especially for recurrent disease. Even for experienced head and neck surgeons, final visualization of the nerve may remain difficult until the very last moment, when the nerve is covered by a thin layer of less than 1 mm of collagen fibers. After identification of the main trunk of the facial nerve, the branches are dissected through the parotid tissue.

Retrograde Identification of the Facial Nerve

Reoperation for recurrent parotid tumors is hampered by scar tissue formation, which makes it almost impossible to discriminate nerve fibers from the surrounding fibrous tissue. The solution is to start a retrograde identification of the facial nerve branches outside the former operation field, thus minimizing the risk of damaging the nerve. The retromandibular vein is used to identify the marginal branch, but surgery can also start with identification of the zygomatic branches, which are located inferior to the lower border of the zygomatic arch. This all depends on the position of the recurrent tumor. The centripetal dissection of the nerve is continued to identify the bifurcation and trunk of the facial nerve, but is preferably done under combined visualization of buccal, mandibular, cervical, zygomatic, and temporal branches to stay in the right surgical plane and to prevent accidental transection of connecting nerve fibers. Intraoperative monitoring is advised in recurrent tumor surgery, but there is no absolute guarantee of preservation of neural structures since nerve branches remain at risk of surgical damage after identification. Under certain circumstances, the use of electromyographic monitoring can make the identification of branches of the facial nerve easier.[135] O'Regan et al.[136] investigated facial nerve morbidity after retrograde nerve dissection in a group of 136 patients who had surgery for benign disease and found 99% normal nerve function 6 months postoperatively, with only one patient showing a persistent marginal mandibular nerve paresis. In general, soft tissue landmarks (retromandibular vein, parotid duct) are much easier to identify than is commonly thought, and in recurrent parotid tumor surgery unnecessary exposure of the main trunk of the facial nerve can be avoided, thereby lowering the risk of more damage to the facial nerve.[137]

Occasionally, tumors have to be removed by extended parotidectomy including resection of the ascending branch of the mandible or in combination with a transoral approach, particularly in case of parapharyngeal tumors.

Surgery for SGC of the Submandibular Gland and Minor Salivary Gland

Primary or recurrent SGCs of the submandibular gland are approached by a transcervical incision, running from the submental area to the anterior border of the sternocelidomastoid muscle. After a subplatysmal flap is raised, the marginal branch of the facial nerve is identified and mobilized cranially. But when the nerve branches are running too close to the (recurrent) carcinoma, the surgical plane should be planned lateral to the platysma mucle with the calculated risk of sacrificing the marginal facial nerve branch. The facial vessels are clamped and ligated at the inferior border of the mandible. After exposure of the posterior border of the mylohyoid muscle, lingual and hypoglossal nerves are identified. The submandibular ganglion (parasympathetic ganglion) originating from the lingual nerve is sacrificed. The gland is then retracted posteriorly and, after ligation of the facial artery over the posterior belly of the digastric muscle, the tumor can be removed. Sometimes tumor extension requires en bloc resection of levels II/III, to achieve free tumor margins (formerly termed "supraomohyoidal dissection").

The majority of minor salivary gland carcinomas arise in the hard and soft palate and can be removed by local transoral excision, sometimes extended to partial or total maxillectomy. The remainder of the minor salivary gland tumors can arise in the mucosa of the upper areodigestive tract and types of surgical removal are indicated by a specific location. For lesions from the oral cavity this may sometimes lead to a commando procedure depending on the local extension of the disease with surgical defect reconstruction using free revascularized flaps (free radial forearm, rectus abdominis, lateral thigh, etc.) or pedicled flaps (pectoralis major muscle, latissimus dorsi muscle, etc.).

Recurrent Pleomorphic Adenoma

Epidemiology

Pleomorphic adenomas make up almost 50% of all salivary gland tumors and are mainly found in the parotid gland.[9] Malignant transformation of pleomorphic adenoma can occur in 3%–15% of patients.[138] The parotid gland is most frequently involved. It is an aggressive type of SGC, with a high local recurrence rate of 42% mainly in patients with submaxillary and minor salivary gland tumors.[5] It is suggested that the risk of malignant degeneration increases with the duration of the presence of a pleomorphic adenoma ranging from 1.5% in the first 5 years to almost 10% after 15 years.

Chance of Recurrence

After simple enucleation there is a high chance of recurrence.[66,139] The lobulated growth pattern and surgical dissection close to the pseudocapsule increase the risk of incomplete resection or of capsular rupture.[139,140] The pseudocapsule contains often no more than a couple of cell layers, which makes it almost impossible, even for experienced head and neck pathologists, to confirm histologically the completeness of resection. The preoperative judgment of the individual surgeon is therefore decisive in histologically doubtful cases. Recurrence rates drop to 5% in patients treated by (superficial) parotidectomy.[141–144]

Presumably because surgeons tend to make small skin incisions to improve cosmesis, recurrent pleomorphic adenomas are frequently found in young and female patients.[66,145] A large number of recurrent nodules are located far beyond the incisions from prior surgery and microscopically more than 100 nodules can be found.[66]

Surgical Treatment

Revision surgery in the parotid area is extremely difficult and has a higher risk of damaging the facial nerve, because the course of the nerve is distorted after previous surgery. Discrimination of the nerve from surrounding fibrous scar tissue remains always very difficult.[146] Since there is a high chance of re-recurrence in 10%–63% of cases after revision surgery,[66,147–149] different types of treatment are recommended, ranging from local excision to radical resection sacrificing the facial nerve, and even to no treatment or radiotherapy.[150–154] Since the number of nodules is probably much higher than is clinically evident or even detectable by T2-weighted MRI,[63,64] a surgical technique should aim at complete removal of all tumor nodules with as much normal surrounding gland tissue as possible, significantly reducing the probability of rerecurrence.[66] Revision surgery contributes to a higher risk of permanent facial nerve dysfunction than primary surgery,[150,152] except for enucleation without exposure of the facial nerve.

Adjuvant Radiotherapy

It remains controversial whether adjuvant radiotherapy has a role in recurrent pleomorphic adenoma. In their review on salivary gland pleomorphic adenoma, Mendenhall et al.[155] state that local control is improved in a subgroup of patients demonstrating inadequate margins and/or multinodular recurrence. This statement is based on retrospective series and there is no study available comparing surgery versus surgery combined with radiotherapy or radiotherapy alone. Nevertheless, adjuvant radiotherapy might be indicated when a residual tumor or massive spillage at revision surgery is reported.[148,152] The postoperative tumor dose for recurrent pleomorphic adenoma is 50 Gy for radical treatment and more than 60 Gy in the case of residual disease,[87–89] all given as 1.8–2 Gy per fraction, five times a week (conventional fractionation). If surgery is not possible or is refused, radiation can be applied but data on its efficacy in recurrent adenoma are lacking.

Metastatic Pleomorphic Adenoma

Metastatic pleomorphic adenoma is a very rare disease, with around 50 cases reported in the international literature.[156] It is a clinical paradox, since both primary and metastatic pleomorphic adenoma have the same benign histological appearance. No histological criteria, clinical characteristics, or even genetic factors have been identified that might explain the exceptional metastatic nature of the disease. In most cases, tumor recurrence precedes the metastasis.[156–158] If metastatic, pleomorphic adenoma usually gives rise to hematogenous metastases to the lungs, bone, and other organs, but lymphatic metastases have been described as well.[157] Metastatic pleomorphic adenoma is in principle a lethal disease and is sometimes classified as low-grade malignant salivary gland carcinoma.[150]

Some hypothesize that previous radiation of the primary tumor or previous surgical intervention may play a role in increasing the metastatic potential of the primary tumor by favoring permeation of vessels by tumor cells, followed by metastatic spread. However, there is no scientific data to support this.[156] It may be postulated that accumulation of chromosomal losses, as observed in metastasizing carcinoma ex-pleomorphic adenoma, may be of greater importance for the metastatic potential of pleomorphic adenoma.[159] From the foregoing it can be concluded that presumably local recurrence may be the first step in the metastatic process of pleomorphic adenoma, which highlights the essential role of radical primary surgery and postoperative radiotherapy if indicated.

Case Study

A 35-year-old woman presented with a pleomorphic adenoma of the right submandibular gland, which was resected by a general ENT surgeon with limited experience in head and neck surgery. The referring specialist reported that the tumor had been histologically completely removed at the time. Six years later, the woman developed a painless subcutaneous 2 cm bilobular nodule located just below the right mandibular angle. Fine-needle aspiration cytology (FNAC) from the lesion revealed a recurrent pleomorphic adenoma, which was removed by a selective neck dissection (level I–III) and en bloc resection of the lower pole of the parotid gland, after excision of the incisional scar. Although the marginal branch of the facial nerve was visualized during surgery, it remained paralyzed postoperatively. Histological examination of the resection specimen showed a solitary, completely removed pleomorphic adenoma, with no signs of microscopic recurrent disease in the scar tissue at the former incision site. The multidisciplinary tumor board decided not to irradiate her postoperatively and recommended regular outpatient follow-up.

Three years later she developed low back pain radiating to the left leg. After 2 years of increasing doses of pain medication, she came back to the hospital. CT scan and bone scan demonstrated a suspicious mass in the left sacroiliac joint and a metastatic pleomorphic adenoma was confirmed by FNAC (**Fig. 16.9**). After preoperative radiotherapy (60 Gy in 30 fractions) she underwent a subtotal sacral bone resection. The postoperative course was complicated by an *E. coli* infection of the urinary tract and bladder incontinence, successfully treated by intravenous administration of antibiotics (ciprofloxacin). As a late sequela of this last surgical procedure, the patient suffered a persistent bilateral peroneus paralysis with dystrophic problems of both legs and an instability of the iliac crest, for which she needed long-term orthopedic rehabilitation.

A couple of months later she developed a third cytologically proven submucosal recurrence at the medial side of the mandible with infiltration into the mandible. A segmental mandibular resection was done with AO-plate reconstruction of the mandibular defect. At histological examination, the recurrent tumor showed extensive bone destruction and appeared to be completely removed. The patient received postoperative radiotherapy to a total dose of 58 Gy in 28 fractions.

Two years postoperatively the AO plate fractured, resulting in a more or less stable position of both parts of the metal fragments with preservation of the overlying atrophic skin. Her history of surgery and radiotherapy implied a high risk of osteomyelitis and skin necrosis, so no attempts were made to remove the AO plate material. The fourth recurrence occurred in the right lung almost 9 years after the commando procedure and was removed by a wedge excision. She is now 6 years recurrence free and remains under follow-up with regular PET scans.

This case demonstrates the tragic course of a recurrent pleomorphic adenoma with multiple invalidating surgical procedures and permanent uncertainty about development of future manifestations of this seemingly benign disease.

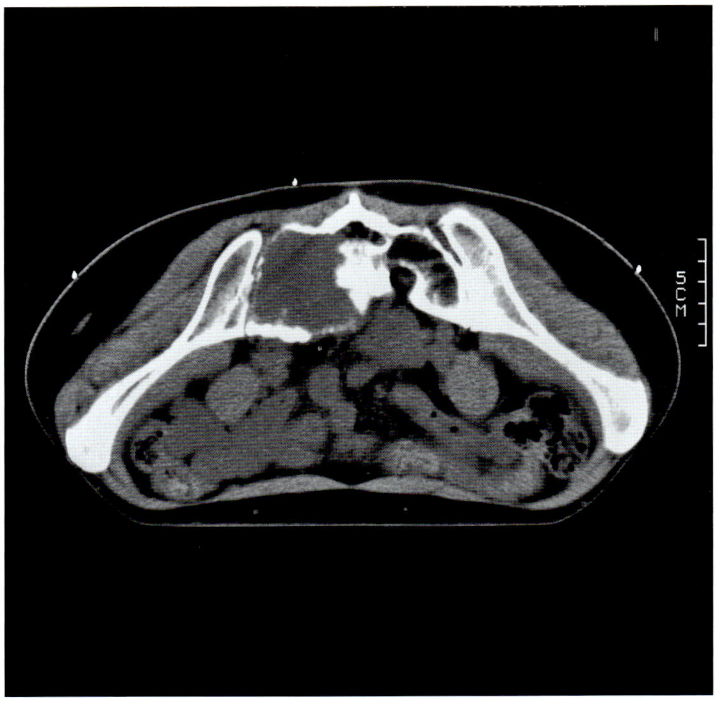

Fig. 16.9 Large metastatic pleomorphic adenoma in the left sacroiliac joint with bone destruction in a 38-year-old woman who had undergone surgical removal of the primary tumor in the submaxillary gland 3 years before.

Future Research

- The rare incidence of salivary gland carcinomas is a limiting factor by itself to setting up well-organized prospective analyses of treatment results and prognostic factors for each individual histological subtype. It is of utmost importance that efforts are undertaken by the international Head and Neck Oncology community to set up an international database of SGC and to agree upon internationally accepted histological entities as well as diagnostic and treatment protocols.
- Further research should concentrate on the prediction of indolent growth of recurrent SGC, as is often encountered in adenoid cystic carcinoma, to avoid palliative treatment modalities leading to high comorbidity.
- To improve the implementation of novel drugs and small molecules, multicenter clinical trials should be conducted with special emphasis on cell receptor expression and intracellular regulatory pathways. A good example of this strategy is a multicenter phase II trial of the University of Chicago Cancer Center (i.e., UCCRC-16691B) for patients with recurrent or metastatic salivary gland tumors, in which patients are divided ino ACC and non-ACC tumors and several biomarkers will be assessed, for example, c-Kit, c-scr, scr signal transduction, PDGFR.
- With the absence of high-level evidence for or against radiation in recurrent salivary gland carcinoma, the case for randomized clinical trials is clear. For recurrent SGC this seems not to be feasible, however. Future efforts should therefore should be aiming at better selection of patients by microarray or biological markers for prognostic and treatment-related facts.

Recommended Reading

- Chen AM, Garcia J, Bucci MK, et al. Recurrent salivary gland carcinomas treated by surgery with or without intraoperative radiation therapy. Head Neck 2008; 30(1):2–9. (One of the few articles on the treatment options for recurrent salivary gland carcinoma that report a significantly improved disease control after intraoperative radiation therapy (IORT) in a series of 99 patients.)
- Lonneux M, Hamoir M, Reychler H, et al. Positron emission tomography with [18F]fluorodeoxygucose improves staging and patient management in patients with head and neck squamous cell carcinoma: a multicenter prospective study. J Clin Oncol 2010;28(7):1190–1195. (This article, describing a large multicentre prospective study, nicely demonstrates that adding PET-FDG imaging significantly improved detection of metastatic or additional disease in 233 HNSCC patients. Provided that similar PET FDG activity may be expected in recurrent SGC, this imaging modality has significant impact on treatment planning and should be implemented in the routine work-up.)
- Spiro RH. Salivary neoplasms: overview of a 35-year experience with 2807 patients. Head Neck Surg 1986;8(3):177–184. (The largest series of salivary gland tumors in the international literature, containing representative epidemiological information on salivary gland carcinomas.)
- Poorten VV, Hart A, Vauterin T, et al. Prognostic index for patients with parotid carcinoma: international external validation in a Belgian-German database. Cancer 2009;115(3):540–550. (This is a unique international validation of prognostic indices for recurrence-free intervals in patients with parotid carcinoma after a successful national validation process. The value of prospective generalized use seems to be demonstrated.)
- Wittekindt C, Streubel K, Arnold G, Stennert E, Guntinas-Lichius O. Recurrent pleomorphic adenoma of the parotid gland: analysis of 108 consecutive patients. Head Neck 2007;29(9):822–828. (A report on 108 patients with recurrent pleomorphic adenoma demonstrating the high risk of re-recurrence after inadequate surgery for recurrent pleomorphic adenoma and emphasizing the importance of extended parotid surgery for this recurrent disease.)

References

1. Spiro JD, Spiro RH. Salivary Tumors. Hamilton, ON: BC Decker; 2001
2. Pinkston JA, Cole P. Incidence rates of salivary gland tumors: results from a population-based study. Otolaryngol Head Neck Surg 1999;120(6):834–840
3. Vander Poorten VLM. Salivary Gland Carcinoma [Thesis]. Leuven: Acco; 2002
4. Land CE, Saku T, Hayashi Y, et al. Incidence of salivary gland tumors among atomic bomb survivors, 1950–1987. Evaluation of radiation-related risk. Radiat Res 1996;146(1):28–36
5. Simental A, Carrau RL. Malignant neoplasms of the salivary gland. In: Cummings Otolaryngology Head and Neck Surgery. 4th ed. Philadelphia: Elsevier Mosby; 2005:1378–1405
6. Laurie SA, Licitra L. Systemic therapy in the palliative management of advanced salivary gland cancers. J Clin Oncol 2006;24(17):2673–2678
7. Postema RJ, van Velthuysen ML, van den Brekel MW, Balm AJ, Peterse JL. Accuracy of fine-needle aspiration cytology of salivary gland lesions in the netherlands cancer institute. Head Neck 2004;26(5):418–424
8. Zhang S, Bao R, Bagby J, Abreo F. Fine needle aspiration of salivary glands: 5-year experience from a single academic center. Acta Cytol 2009;53(4):375–382
9. Spiro RH. Salivary neoplasms: overview of a 35-year experience with 2807 patients. Head Neck Surg 1986;8(3):177–184
10. Barnes LB, Eveson JW, Sidransky D. Pathology and Genetics of Head and Neck Tumors. Lyon: IARC Press; 2005
11. Ward MJ, Levine PA. Salivary gland tumors. In: Close LG, Larson DL, Shah JP, eds. Essentials of Head and Neck Oncology. New York: Thieme; 1998
12. Million RR, Cassisi NJ, Mancuso AA. Major salivary gland tumors. In: Million PR, Cassisi NJ, eds. Managmenet of Head and Neck Cancer: A Multidisciplinary Approach. 2nd ed. Philadelphia: JB Lippincott; 1994: 711–735
13. Mendenhall WM, Morris CG, Amdur RJ, Werning JW, Villaret DB. Radiotherapy alone or combined with surgery for salivary gland carcinoma. Cancer 2005;103(12):2544–2550
14. Le QT, Birdwell S, Terris DJ, et al. Postoperative irradiation of minor salivary gland malignancies of the head and neck. Radiother Oncol 1999;52(2):165–171
15. Garden AS, el-Naggar AK, Morrison WH, Callender DL, Ang KK, Peters LJ. Postoperative radiotherapy for malignant tumors of the parotid gland. Int J Radiat Oncol Biol Phys 1997;37(1):79–85
16. Hong WK, Bromer RH, Amato DA, et al. Patterns of relapse in locally advanced head and neck cancer patients who achieved complete remission after combined modality therapy. Cancer 1985;56(6):1242–1245
17. Chen AM, Garcia J, Bucci MK, et al. Recurrent salivary gland carcinomas treated by surgery with or without intraoperative radiation therapy. Head Neck 2008;30(1):2–9
18. Sadeghi A, Tran LM, Mark R, Sidrys J, Parker RG. Minor salivary gland tumors of the head and neck: treatment strategies and prognosis. Am J Clin Oncol 1993;16(1):3–8
19. Ellis GL, Auclair PL. The normal salivary glands. In: Ellis GL, Auclair PL, eds. Tumors of the Salivary Glands. Washington DC: Armed Forces Institute of Pathology; 1996: 1–23
20. Ellis GL, Auclair PL. Atlas of tumor pathology. In: Ellis GL, Auclair PL, eds. Tumors of the Salivary Glands. Washington, DC: Armed Forces Institue of Pathology; 1996: 155–373
21. Bhattacharyya N, Fried MP. Determinants of survival in parotid gland carcinoma: a population-based study. Am J Otolaryngol 2005;26(1):39–44
22. Rapidis AD, Givalos N, Gakiopoulou H, et al. Mucoepidermoid carcinoma of the salivary glands. Review of the literature and clinicopathological analysis of 18 patients. Oral Oncol 2007;43(2):130–136
23. Goode RK, Auclair PL, Ellis GL. Mucoepidermoid carcinoma of the major salivary glands: clinical and histopathologic analysis of 234 cases with evaluation of grading criteria. Cancer 1998;82(7):1217–1224
24. Brandwein MS, Ivanov K, Wallace DI, et al. Mucoepidermoid carcinoma: a clinicopathologic study of 80 patients with special reference to histological grading. Am J Surg Pathol 2001;25(7):835–845

25. Chung CT, Sagerman RH, Ryoo MC, King GA, Yu WS, Dalal PS. The changing role of external-beam irradiation in the management of malignant tumors of the major salivary glands. Radiology 1982;145(1):175–177
26. Hosokawa Y, Shirato H, Kagei K, et al. Role of radiotherapy for mucoepidermoid carcinoma of salivary gland. Oral Oncol 1999;35(1):105–111
27. Mendenhall WM, Morris CG, Amdur RJ, Werning JW, Hinerman RW, Villaret DB. Radiotherapy alone or combined with surgery for adenoid cystic carcinoma of the head and neck. Head Neck 2004;26(2):154–162
28. Auclair PL, Goode RK, Ellis GL. Mucoepidermoid carcinoma of intraoral salivary glands. Evaluation and application of grading criteria in 143 cases. Cancer 1992;69(8):2021–2030
29. Rapidis AD, Givalos N, Gakiopoulou H, et al. Adenoid cystic carcinoma of the head and neck. Clinicopathological analysis of 23 patients and review of the literature. Oral Oncol 2005;41(3):328–335
30. Guzzo M, Andreola S, Sirizzotti G, Cantu G. Mucoepidermoid carcinoma of the salivary glands: clinicopathologic review of 108 patients treated at the National Cancer Institute of Milan. Ann Surg Oncol 2002;9(7):688–695
31. Clode AL, Fonseca I, Santos JR, Soares J. Mucoepidermoid carcinoma of the salivary glands: a reappraisal of the influence of tumor differentiation on prognosis. J Surg Oncol 1991;46(2):100–106
32. Plambeck K, Friedrich RE, Schmelzle R. Mucoepidermoid carcinoma of salivary gland origin: classification, clinical–pathological correlation, treatment results and long-term follow-up in 55 patients. J Craniomaxillofac Surg 1996;24(3):133–139
33. Leivo I, Jee KJ, Heikinheimo K, et al. Characterization of gene expression in major types of salivary gland carcinomas with epithelial differentiation. Cancer Genet Cytogenet 2005;156(2):104–113
34. Oplatek A, Ozer E, Agrawal A, Bapna S, Schuller DE. Patterns of recurrence and survival of head and neck adenoid cystic carcinoma after definitive resection. Laryngoscope 2010;120(1):65–70
35. Kim KH, Sung MW, Chung PS, Rhee CS, Park CI, Kim WH. Adenoid cystic carcinoma of the head and neck. Arch Otolaryngol Head Neck Surg 1994;120(7):721–726
36. Kokemueller H, Eckardt A, Brachvogel P, Hausamen JE. Adenoid cystic carcinoma of the head and neck—a 20 years experience. Int J Oral Maxillofac Surg 2004;33(1):25–31
37. Nascimento AG, Amaral AL, Prado LA, Kligerman J, Silveira TR. Adenoid cystic carcinoma of salivary glands. A study of 61 cases with clinicopathologic correlation. Cancer 1986;57(2):312–319
38. Spiro RH, Huvos AG. Stage means more than grade in adenoid cystic carcinoma. Am J Surg 1992;164(6):623–628
39. van der Wal JE, Becking AG, Snow GB, van der Waal I. Distant metastases of adenoid cystic carcinoma of the salivary glands and the value of diagnostic examinations during follow-up. Head Neck 2002;24(8):779–783
40. Khan AJ, DiGiovanna MP, Ross DA, et al. Adenoid cystic carcinoma: a retrospective clinical review. Int J Cancer 2001;96(3):149–158
41. Matsuba HM, Spector GJ, Thawley SE, Simpson JR, Mauney M, Pikul FJ. Adenoid cystic salivary gland carcinoma. A histopathologic review of treatment failure patterns. Cancer 1986;57(3):519–524
42. Prokopakis EP, Snyderman CH, Hanna EY, Carrau RL, Johnson JT, D'Amico F. Risk factors for local recurrence of adenoid cystic carcinoma: the role of postoperative radiation therapy. Am J Otolaryngol 1999;20(5):281–286
43. Sung MW, Kim KH, Kim JW, et al. Clinicopathologic predictors and impact of distant metastasis from adenoid cystic carcinoma of the head and neck. Arch Otolaryngol Head Neck Surg 2003;129(11):1193–1197
44. Eby LS, Johnson DS, Baker HW. Adenoid cystic carcinoma of the head and neck. Cancer 1972;29(5):1160–1168
45. Avery CME, Moody AB, McKinna FE, Taylor J, Henk JM, Langdon JD. Combined treatment of adenoid cystic carcinoma of the salivary glands. Int J Oral Maxillofac Surg 2000;29(4):277–279
46. da Cruz Perez DE, de Abreu Alves F, Nobuko Nishimoto I, de Almeida OP, Kowalski LP. Prognostic factors in head and neck adenoid cystic carcinoma. Oral Oncol 2006;42(2):139–146
47. Friedrich RE, Bleckmann V. Adenoid cystic carcinoma of salivary and lacrimal gland origin: localization, classification, clinical pathological correlation, treatment results and long-term follow-up control in 84 patients. Anticancer Res 2003;23(2A):931–940
48. Zhu QR, White FH, Tipoe GL. p53 oncoprotein accumulation in adenoid cystic carcinoma of parotid and palatine salivary glands. Pathology 1997;29(2):154–158
49. Kiyoshima T, Shima K, Kobayashi I, et al. Expression of p53 tumor suppressor gene in adenoid cystic and mucoepidermoid carcinomas of the salivary glands. Oral Oncol 2001;37(3):315–322
50. Spiro RH, Huvos AG, Strong EW. Adenocarcinoma of salivary origin. Clinicopathologic study of 204 patients. Am J Surg 1982;144(4):423–431
51. Paleri V, Robinson M, Bradley P. Polymorphous low-grade adenocarcinoma of the head and neck. Curr Opin Otolaryngol Head Neck Surg 2008;16(2):163–169
52. Batsakis JG, Luna MA. Low-grade and high-grade adenocarcinomas of the salivary duct system. Ann Otol Rhinol Laryngol 1989;98(2):162–163
53. O'Brien CJ, Soong SJ, Herrera GA, Urist MM, Maddox WA. Malignant salivary tumors—analysis of prognostic factors and survival. Head Neck Surg 1986;9(2):82–92
54. Greig SR, Chaplin JM, McIvor NP, Izzard ME, Taylor G, Wee D. Acinic cell carcinoma of the parotid gland: Auckland experience and literature review. ANZ J Surg 2008;78(9):754–758
55. Vander Poorten VL, Balm AJ, Hilgers FJ, et al. Prognostic factors for long term results of the treatment of patients with malignant submandibular gland tumors. Cancer 1999;85(10):2255–2264
56. Vander Poorten VL, Balm AJ, Hilgers FJ, Tan IB, Keus RB, Hart AA. Stage as major long term outcome predictor in minor salivary gland carcinoma. Cancer 2000;89(6):1195–1204
57. Vander Poorten VL, Balm AJ, Hilgers FJ, et al. The development of a prognostic score for patients with parotid carcinoma. Cancer 1999;85(9):2057–2067
58. Vander Poorten VL, Hart AA, van der Laan BF, et al. Prognostic index for patients with parotid carcinoma: external validation using the nationwide 1985–1994 Dutch Head and Neck Oncology Cooperative Group database. Cancer 2003;97(6):1453–1463
59. Poorten VV, Hart A, Vauterin T, et al. Prognostic index for patients with parotid carcinoma: international external validation in a Belgian-German database. Cancer 2009;115(3):540–550
60. Vander Poorten VL, Balm A, Hart A. Reflections on Takahama Jr. et al's "Comparison of two prognostic scores for patients with parotid carcinoma". Head Neck 2010;32(2):274–275, author reply 275–277
61. Smit M, Balm AJ, Hilgers FJ, Tan IB. Pain as sign of recurrent disease in head and neck squamous cell carcinoma. Head Neck 2001;23(5):372–375

62. de Bondt RB, Balm AJ, Hilgers FJ, Tan IB. [Referred earache; an important symptom of head-and-neck cancers]. Ned Tijdschr Geneeskd 1998;142(31):1753–1756
63. Moonis G, Patel P, Koshkareva Y, Newman J, Loevner LA. Imaging characteristics of recurrent pleomorphic adenoma of the parotid gland. AJNR Am J Neuroradiol 2007;28(8):1532–1536
64. Tsushima Y, Matsumoto M, Endo K, Aihara T, Nakajima T. Characteristic bright signal of parotid pleomorphic adenomas on T2-weighted MR images with pathological correlation. Clin Radiol 1994;49(7):485–489
65. Stennert E, Wittekindt C, Klussmann JP, Arnold G, Guntinas-Lichius O. Recurrent pleomorphic adenoma of the parotid gland: a prospective histopathological and immunohistochemical study. Laryngoscope 2004;114(1):158–163
66. Wittekindt C, Streubel K, Arnold G, Stennert E, Guntinas-Lichius O. Recurrent pleomorphic adenoma of the parotid gland: analysis of 108 consecutive patients. Head Neck 2007;29(9):822–828
67. Myssiorek D, Ruah CB, Hybels RL. Recurrent pleomorphic adenomas of the parotid gland. Head Neck 1990;12(4):332–336
68. Stokkel MP, ten Broek FW, van Rijk PP. The role of FDG PET in the clinical management of head and neck cancer. Oral Oncol 1998;34(6):466–471
69. Braams JW, Pruim J, Freling NJ, et al. Detection of lymph node metastases of squamous-cell cancer of the head and neck with FDG-PET and MRI. J Nucl Med 1995;36(2):211–216
70. Laubenbacher C, Saumweber D, Wagner-Manslau C, et al. Comparison of fluorine-18-fluorodeoxyglucose PET, MRI and endoscopy for staging head and neck squamous-cell carcinomas. J Nucl Med 1995;36(10):1747–1757
71. Keyes JW Jr, Harkness BA, Greven KM, Williams DW III, Watson NE Jr, McGuirt WF. Salivary gland tumors: pretherapy evaluation with PET. Radiology 1994;192(1):99–102
72. Okamura T, Kawabe J, Koyama K, et al. Fluorine-18 fluorodeoxyglucose positron emission tomography imaging of parotid mass lesions. Acta Otolaryngol Suppl 1998;538:209–213
73. Otsuka H, Graham MM, Kogame M, Nishitani H. The impact of FDG-PET in the management of patients with salivary gland malignancy. Ann Nucl Med 2005;19(8):691–694
74. McGuirt WF, Keyes JW Jr, Greven KM, Williams DW III, Watson NE Jr, Cappellari JO. Preoperative identification of benign versus malignant parotid masses: a comparative study including positron emission tomography. Laryngoscope 1995;105(6):579–584
75. Matsuda M, Sakamoto H, Okamura T, et al. Positron emission tomographic imaging of pleomorphic adenoma in the parotid gland. Acta Otolaryngol Suppl 1998;538:214–220
76. Lonneux M, Hamoir M, Reychler H, et al. Positron emission tomography with [18F]fluorodeoxyglucose improves staging and patient management in patients with head and neck squamous cell carcinoma: a multicenter prospective study. J Clin Oncol 2010;28(7):1190–1195
77. Kyzas PA, Evangelou E, Denaxa-Kyza D, Ioannidis JP. ^{18}F-fluorodeoxyglucose positron emission tomography to evaluate cervical node metastases in patients with head and neck squamous cell carcinoma: a meta-analysis. J Natl Cancer Inst 2008;100(10):712–720
78. Yamazaki Y, Saitoh M, Notani K, et al. Assessment of cervical lymph node metastases using FDG-PET in patients with head and neck cancer. Ann Nucl Med 2008;22(3):177–184
79. Roh JL, Yeo NK, Kim JS, et al. Utility of 2-[^{18}F] fluoro-2-deoxy-d-glucose positron emission tomography and positron emission tomography/computed tomography imaging in the preoperative staging of head and neck squamous cell carcinoma. Oral Oncol 2007;43(9):887–893
80. Basu D, Siegel BA, McDonald DJ, Nussenbaum B. Detection of occult bone metastases from head and neck squamous cell carcinoma: impact of positron emission tomography computed tomography with fluorodeoxyglucose F 18. Arch Otolaryngol Head Neck Surg 2007;133(8):801–805
81. Kim SY, Roh JL, Yeo NK, et al. Combined ^{18}F-fluorodeoxyglucose-positron emission tomography and computed tomography as a primary screening method for detecting second primary cancers and distant metastases in patients with head and neck cancer. Ann Oncol 2007;18(10):1698–1703
82. Krabbe CA, Pruim J, van der Laan BF, Rödiger LA, Roodenburg JL. FDG-PET and detection of distant metastases and simultaneous tumors in head and neck squamous cell carcinoma: a comparison with chest radiography and chest CT. Oral Oncol 2009;45(3):234–240
83. Gourin CG, Watts TL, Williams HT, Patel VS, Bilodeau PA, Coleman TA. Identification of distant metastases with positron-emission tomography-computed tomography in patients with previously untreated head and neck cancer. Laryngoscope 2008;118(4):671–675
84. Nahmias C, Carlson ER, Duncan LD, et al. Positron emission tomography/computerized tomography (PET/CT) scanning for preoperative staging of patients with oral/head and neck cancer. J Oral Maxillofac Surg 2007;65(12):2524–2535
85. van den Brekel MW, Castelijns JA. Imaging of lymph nodes in the neck. Semin Roentgenol 2000;35(1):42–53
86 Valstar MH, van den Brekel MW, Smeele LE. Interpretation of treatment outcome in the clinically node-negative neck in primary parotid carcinoma: a systematic review of the literature. Head Neck 2010;32(10):1402–1411
87. Terhaard CH. Postoperative and primary radiotherapy for salivary gland carcinomas: indications, techniques, and results. Int J Radiat Oncol Biol Phys 2007; 69(2, Suppl):S52–S55
88. Terhaard CH, Lubsen H, Rasch CR, et al. Dutch Head and Neck Oncology Cooperative Group. The role of radiotherapy in the treatment of malignant salivary gland tumors. Int J Radiat Oncol Biol Phys 2005;61(1):103–111
89. Iseli TA, Karnell LH, Preston TW, et al. Facial nerve sacrifice and radiotherapy in parotid adenoid cystic carcinoma. Laryngoscope 2008;118(10):1781–1786
90. Nutting CM, Rowbottom CG, Cosgrove VP, et al. Optimisation of radiotherapy for carcinoma of the parotid gland: a comparison of conventional, three-dimensional conformal, and intensity-modulated techniques. Radiother Oncol 2001;60(2):163–172
91. Iseli TA, Harris G, Dean NR, Iseli CE, Rosenthal EL. Outcomes of static and dynamic facial nerve repair in head and neck cancer. Laryngoscope 2010;120(3):478–483
92. Schulz-Ertner D, Nikoghosyan A, Jäkel O, et al. Feasibility and toxicity of combined photon and carbon ion radiotherapy for locally advanced adenoid cystic carcinomas. Int J Radiat Oncol Biol Phys 2003;56(2):391–398
93. Sasiaja M, Funa N, Kamata M, Furutani K, Matsumoto A, Kodaira T. Unresectable adenoid cystic carcinoma of the trachea treated with chemoradiotherapy. Clin Oncol (R Coll Radiol) 2000;12(4):272

94. Haddad RI, Posner MR, Busse PM, et al. Chemoradiotherapy for adenoid cystic carcinoma: preliminary results of an organ sparing approach. Am J Clin Oncol 2006;29(2):153–157
95. Maruya S, Namba A, Matsubara A, et al. Salivary gland carcinoma treated with concomitant chemoradiation with intraarterial cisplatin and docetaxel. Int J Clin Oncol 2006;11(5):403–406
96. De Crevoisier R, Bourhis J, Domenge C, et al. Full-dose reirradiation for unresectable head and neck carcinoma: experience at the Gustave-Roussy Institute in a series of 169 patients. J Clin Oncol 1998;16(11):3556–3562
97. De Crevoisier R, Domenge C, Wibault P, et al. Full dose reirradiation combined with chemotherapy after salvage surgery in head and neck carcinoma. Cancer 2001;91(11):2071–2076
98. Langendijk JA, Kasperts N, Leemans CR, Doornaert P, Slotman BJ. A phase II study of primary reirradiation in squamous cell carcinoma of head and neck. Radiother Oncol 2006;78(3):306–312
99. Langendijk JA, Bourhis J. Reirradiation in squamous cell head and neck cancer: recent developments and future directions. Curr Opin Oncol 2007;19(3):202–209
100. Steenland E, Leer JW, van Houwelingen H, et al. The effect of a single fraction compared to multiple fractions on painful bone metastases: a global analysis of the Dutch Bone Metastasis Study. Radiother Oncol 1999;52(2):101–109
101. Nielsen OS, Bentzen SM, Sandberg E, Gadeberg CC, Timothy AR. Randomized trial of single dose versus fractionated palliative radiotherapy of bone metastases. Radiother Oncol 1998;47(3):233–240
102. Kavanagh BD, McGarry RC, Timmerman RD. Extracranial radiosurgery (stereotactic body radiation therapy) for oligometastases. Semin Radiat Oncol 2006;16(2):77–84
103. Gilbert J, Li Y, Pinto HA, et al. Phase II trial of taxol in salivary gland malignancies (E1394): a trial of the Eastern Cooperative Oncology Group. Head Neck 2006;28(3):197–204
104. Airoldi M, Fornari G, Pedani F, et al. Paclitaxel and carboplatin for recurrent salivary gland malignancies. Anticancer Res 2000;20(5C):3781–3783
105. Dimery IW, Legha SS, Shirinian M, Hong WK. Fluorouracil, doxorubicin, cyclophosphamide, and cisplatin combination chemotherapy in advanced or recurrent salivary gland carcinoma. J Clin Oncol 1990;8(6):1056–1062
106. Kaplan MJ, Johns ME, Cantrell RW. Chemotherapy for salivary gland cancer. Otolaryngol Head Neck Surg 1986;95(2):165–170
107. Posner MR, Ervin TJ, Weichselbaum RR, Fabian RL, Miller D. Chemotherapy of advanced salivary gland neoplasms. Cancer 1982;50(11):2261–2264
108. Haddad R, Colevas AD, Krane JF, et al. Herceptin in patients with advanced or metastatic salivary gland carcinomas. A phase II study. Oral Oncol 2003;39(7):724–727
109. Agulnik M, Cohen EW, Cohen RB, et al. Phase II study of lapatinib in recurrent or metastatic epidermal growth factor receptor and/or erbB2 expressing adenoid cystic carcinoma and non adenoid cystic carcinoma malignant tumors of the salivary glands. J Clin Oncol 2007;25(25):3978–3984
110. Airoldi M, Bumma C, Bertetto O, Gabriele P, Succo G, Pedani F. Vinorelbine treatment of recurrent salivary gland carcinomas. Bull Cancer 1998;85(10):892–894
111. Mattox DE, Von Hoff DD, Balcerzak SP. Southwest Oncology Group study of mitoxantrone for treatment of patients with advanced adenoid cystic carcinoma of the head and neck. Invest New Drugs 1990;8(1):105–107
112. Verweij J, de Mulder PH, de Graeff A, et al.; EORTC Head and Neck Cancer Cooperative Group. Phase II study on mitoxantrone in adenoid cystic carcinomas of the head and neck. Ann Oncol 1996;7(8):867–869
113. Vermorken JB, Verweij J, de Mulder PH, et al. Epirubicin in patients with advanced or recurrent adenoid cystic carcinoma of the head and neck: a phase II study of the EORTC Head and Neck Cancer Cooperative Group. Ann Oncol 1993;4(9):785–788
114. Airoldi M, Gabriele AM, Gabriele P, et al. Concomitant chemoradiotherapy followed by adjuvant chemotherapy in parotid gland undifferentiated carcinoma. Tumori 2001;87(1):14–17
115. Licitra L, Cavina R, Grandi C, et al. Cisplatin, doxorubicin and cyclophosphamide in advanced salivary gland carcinoma. A phase II trial of 22 patients. Ann Oncol 1996;7(6):640–642
116. Dreyfuss AI, Clark JR, Fallon BG, Posner MR, Norris CM Jr, Miller D. Cyclophosphamide, doxorubicin, and cisplatin combination chemotherapy for advanced carcinomas of salivary gland origin. Cancer 1987;60(12):2869–2872
117. Hotte SJ, Winquist EW, Lamont E, et al. Imatinib mesylate in patients with adenoid cystic cancers of the salivary glands expressing c-kit: a Princess Margaret Hospital phase II consortium study. J Clin Oncol 2005;23(3):585–590
118. Spiro RH. Distant metastasis in adenoid cystic carcinoma of salivary origin. Am J Surg 1997;174(5):495–498
119. Renehan A, Gleave EN, McGurk M. An analysis of the treatment of 114 patients with recurrent pleomorphic adenomas of the parotid gland. Am J Surg 1996;172(6):710–714
120. Harbo G, Bundgaard T, Pedersen D, Søgaard H, Overgaard J. Prognostic indicators for malignant tumours of the parotid gland. Clin Otolaryngol Allied Sci 2002;27(6):512–516
121. Bobbio A, Copelli C, Ampollini L, et al. Lung metastasis resection of adenoid cystic carcinoma of salivary glands. Eur J Cardiothorac Surg 2008;33(5):790–793
122. Liu D, Labow DM, Dang N, et al. Pulmonary metastasectomy for head and neck cancers. Ann Surg Oncol 1999;6(6):572–578
123. Locati LD, Guzzo M, Bossi P, et al. Lung metastasectomy in adenoid cystic carcinoma (ACC) of salivary gland. Oral Oncol 2005;41(9):890–894
124. Jennings T, Li Y, Pinto H. Phase II trial of paclitaxel in advanced or metastatic salivary gland malignancies: An Eastern Cooperative Oncology Group Oncology study. Proc Am Soc Clin Oncol 2001;20:236a
125. Belani CP, Eisenberger MA, Gray WC. Preliminary experience with chemotherapy in advanced salivary gland neoplasms. Med Pediatr Oncol 1988;16(3):197–202
126. Creagan ET, Woods JE, Rubin J, Schaid DJ. Cisplatin-based chemotherapy for neoplasms arising from salivary glands and contiguous structures in the head and neck. Cancer 1988;62(11):2313–2319
127. Locati LD, Perrone F, Losa M, et al. Treatment relevant target immunophenotyping of 139 salivary gland carcinomas (SGCs). Oral Oncol 2009;45(11):986–990
128. van der Hulst RW, van Krieken JH, van der Kwast TH, et al. Partial remission of parotid gland carcinoma after goserelin. Lancet 1994;344(8925):817
129. Knegt PP, Ah-See KW, vd Velden LA, Kerrebijn J. Adenocarcinoma of the ethmoidal sinus complex: surgical debulking and topical fluorouracil may be the optimal treatment. Arch Otolaryngol Head Neck Surg 2001;127(2):141–146

130. Nabili V, Tan JW, Bhuta S, Sercarz JA, Head CS. Salivary duct carcinoma: a clinical and histologic review with implications for trastuzumab therapy. Head Neck 2007;29(10):907–912
131. Prat A, Parera M, Reyes V, et al. Successful treatment of pulmonary metastatic salivary ductal carcinoma with trastuzumab-based therapy. Head Neck 2008;30(5):680–683
132. Nasser SM, Faquin WC, Dayal Y. Expression of androgen, estrogen, and progesterone receptors in salivary gland tumors. Frequent expression of androgen receptor in a subset of malignant salivary gland tumors. Am J Clin Pathol 2003;119(6):801–806
133. Fan CY, Wang J, Barnes EL. Expression of androgen receptor and prostatic specific markers in salivary duct carcinoma: an immunohistochemical analysis of 13 cases and review of the literature. Am J Surg Pathol 2000;24(4):579–586
134. Locati LD, Quattrone P, Bossi P, Marchianò AV, Cantù G, Licitra L. A complete remission with androgen-deprivation therapy in a recurrent androgen receptor-expressing adenocarcinoma of the parotid gland. Ann Oncol 2003;14(8):1327–1328
135. Harner SG, Daube JR, Beatty CW, Ebersold MJ. Intraoperative monitoring of the facial nerve. Laryngoscope 1988;98(2):209–212
136. O'Regan B, Bharadwaj G, Bhopal S, Cook V. Facial nerve morbidity after retrograde nerve dissection in parotid surgery for benign disease: a 10-year prospective observational study of 136 cases. Br J Oral Maxillofac Surg 2007;45(2):101–107
137. Zhao K, Qi DY, Wang LM. Functional superficial parotidectomy. J Oral Maxillofac Surg 1994;52(10):1038–1041
138. Lüers JC, Wittekindt C, Streppel M, Guntinas-Lichius O. Carcinoma ex pleomorphic adenoma of the parotid gland. Study and implications for diagnostics and therapy. Acta Oncol 2009;48(1):132–136
139. Buchman C, Stringer SP, Mendenhall WM, Parsons JT, Jordan JR, Cassisi NJ. Pleomorphic adenoma: effect of tumor spill and inadequate resection on tumor recurrence. Laryngoscope 1994;104(10):1231–1234
140. Natvig K, Søberg R. Relationship of intraoperative rupture of pleomorphic adenomas to recurrence: an 11–25 year follow-up study. Head Neck 1994;16(3):213–217
141. Laccourreye H, Laccourreye O, Cauchois R, Jouffre V, Ménard M, Brasnu D. Total conservative parotidectomy for primary benign pleomorphic adenoma of the parotid gland: a 25-year experience with 229 patients. Laryngoscope 1994;104(12):1487–1494
142. Leverstein H, van der Wal JE, Tiwari RM, van der Waal I, Snow GB. Surgical management of 246 previously untreated pleomorphic adenomas of the parotid gland. Br J Surg 1997;84(3):399–403
143. Guntinas-Lichius O, Kick C, Klussmann JP, Jungehuelsing M, Stennert E. Pleomorphic adenoma of the parotid gland: a 13-year experience of consequent management by lateral or total parotidectomy. Eur Arch Otorhinolaryngol 2004;261(3):143–146
144. Maynard JD. Management of pleomorphic adenoma of the parotid. Br J Surg 1988;75(4):305–308
145. McGregor AD, Burgoyne M, Tan KC. Recurrent pleomorphic salivary adenoma—the relevance of age at first presentation. Br J Plast Surg 1988;41(2):177–181
146. Jackson SR, Roland NJ, Clarke RW, Jones AS. Recurrent pleomorphic adenoma. J Laryngol Otol 1993;107(6):546–549
147. Laskawi R, Schott T, Schröder M. Recurrent pleomorphic adenomas of the parotid gland: clinical evaluation and long-term follow-up. Br J Oral Maxillofac Surg 1998;36(1):48–51
148. Carew JF, Spiro RH, Singh B, Shah JP. Treatment of recurrent pleomorphic adenomas of the parotid gland. Otolaryngol Head Neck Surg 1999;121(5):539–542
149. Glas AS, Vermey A, Hollema H, et al. Surgical treatment of recurrent pleomorphic adenoma of the parotid gland: a clinical analysis of 52 patients. Head Neck 2001;23(4):311–316
150. Bradley PJ. Recurrent salivary gland pleomorphic adenoma: etiology, management and results. Curr Opin Otolaryngol Head Neck Surg 2001;9:100–108
151. Barton J, Slevin NJ, Gleave EN. Radiotherapy for pleomorphic adenoma of the parotid gland. Int J Radiat Oncol Biol Phys 1992;22(5):925–928
152. Renehan A, Gleave EN, Hancock BD, Smith P, McGurk M. Long-term follow-up of over 1000 patients with salivary gland tumours treated in a single centre. Br J Surg 1996;83(12):1750–1754
153. Maimaris CV, Ball MJ. Treatment of parotid gland tumours by conservative parotidectomy. Br J Surg 1986;73(11):897
154. Dallera P, Marchetti C, Campobassi A. Local capsular dissection of parotid pleomorphic adenomas. Int J Oral Maxillofac Surg 1993;22(3):154–157
155. Mendenhall WM, Mendenhall CM, Werning JW, Malyapa RS, Mendenhall NP. Salivary gland pleomorphic adenoma. Am J Clin Oncol 2008;31(1):95–99
156. Rodríguez-Fernández J, Mateos-Micas M, Martínez-Tello FJ, et al. Metastatic benign pleomorphic adenoma. Report of a case and review of the literature. Med Oral Patol Oral Cir Bucal 2008;13(3):E193–E196
157. Wenig BM, Hitchcock CL, Ellis GL, Gnepp DR. Metastasizing mixed tumor of salivary glands. A clinicopathologic and flow cytometric analysis. Am J Surg Pathol 1992;16(9):845–858
158. Yoshizaki T, Kinsen H, Minato H, Kita T, Furukawa M. Metastasizing mixed tumour of the parotid gland presenting as multiple lung metastases. J Laryngol Otol 2004;118(9):724–726
159. Johns MM III, Westra WH, Califano JA, Eisele D, Koch WM, Sidransky D. Allelotype of salivary gland tumors. Cancer Res 1996;56(5):1151–1154

17 Recurrent Melanotic and Nonmelanotic Skin Cancer

Michael Veness, Gary Morgan, Julie Howle

Summary

- Skin cancer is diagnosed more frequently than any other malignancy and optimal treatment will reduce the risk of recurrence.
- Initial treatment dictates the subsequent management of patients with recurrence.
- Patients may be candidates for multimodality salvage treatment.
- Locoregional recurrence of nonmelanoma skin cancer is the dominant clinical scenario.
- Salvage treatment has potential cosmetic and functional consequences.
- Salvage surgery often requires excising and repairing previously irradiated tissue.
- The evidence to support definitive re-irradiation in patients with recurrent skin cancer is limited.
- Patients with recurrent head and neck skin cancer are frequently encountered and should be managed in a multidisciplinary setting. The evidence to support many of the recommendations in managing these patients is limited and of low level (level 4 evidence) or often only the expert opinion (level 5 evidence) of experienced clinicians.

Epidemiology

Nonmelanoma Skin Cancer

Nonmelanoma skin cancer (NMSC) is the commonest malignancy worldwide. It is a consequence of chronic mutagenic ultraviolet (UV) exposure in fair-skinned caucasians, especially males.[1] Most patients are older (60–70 years) and 75%–80% will have a basal cell carcinoma (BCC) with the remainder (20%–25%) having a squamous cell carcinoma (SCC). The sun-exposed head and neck is the most frequently involved site (70%–80%) followed by the extremities. Collectively, BCC and SCC comprise 95% of all NMSC.

Merkel cell carcinoma (MCC) is an uncommon small cell (neuroendocrine) cutaneous malignancy typically arising in elderly white patients and characterized by high rates of relapse. The head and neck is involved in 50%–60% of cases. The incidence is markedly increased in immunocompromised individuals and the presence of nodal metastases is a powerful predictor of outcome. In some series 30%–40% of patients die from recurrent MCC.[2]

The worldwide incidence of NMSC has increased since the 1960s. In Australia between 1985 and 2002 the annual incidence of BCC increased from 657/100 000 to 884/100 000 and that of SCC more than doubled.[3] Australia has the highest incidence of NMSC. In regions of Northern Australia the annual incidence of SCC in males exceeds 1300/100 000 population.[4] In 2002 the incidence of NMSC in Australia was more than 5 times that of all other cancers combined with an annual rate of 1170/100 000.[3] In the United States over 1 million new cases of NMSC are diagnosed annually.

Malignant Melanoma

Malignant melanoma accounts for approximately 5% of skin malignancies but accounts for 75% of all skin cancer deaths. Melanoma is the third commonest cancer in Australia with over 10 000 cases diagnosed annually and is increasing in incidence worldwide.[5] In the United States, the incidence has tripled between 1975 and 2005.[6] In contrast to NMSC, melanoma is less related to chronic sun exposure, with only 20% occurring on the head and neck, and is common in younger patients. Intermittent sun exposure and a history of sunburn are risk factors.[7] Desmoplastic melanoma is a variant that commonly occurs in the head and neck with a propensity for perineural invasion and local recurrence rates ranging from 6% to 50%.[8]

Prognostic Factors

Nonmelanoma Skin Cancer

Despite being locally invasive, death from a BCC is rare in contrast to patients diagnosed with SCC, MCC, or melanoma. Despite this, patients with incompletely excised mid-face BCC (especially nasolabial fold), or with invasive/infiltrative or sclerosing histology, are at risk of local recurrence and associated morbidity, and are often referred to as having a "high-risk" BCC.[9]

In patients with SCC, tumor thickness (>5–6 mm), location near the parotid gland, recurrent primary lesions, and immunosuppression (organ transplant recipient/hematological malignancy) are risk factors for poor outcome and recurrence (usually nodal)[10] (level 2 evidence). Factors such as tumor grade, lymphovascular invasion, and perineural invasion also contribute to this risk and are often present in association with other factors. Clinicians should be aware that immunosuppressed patients are at exceptionally high risk of developing skin cancer, mainly immunogenic SCC and MCC, which is often aggressive with an increased risk of recurrence and death[11] (**Fig. 17.1**). Death may occur as a consequence, with an Australian tumor registry study documenting 120 skin cancer deaths over a 5-year period accounting for approximately 1% of all cancer related deaths.[12] In a US study of patients with SCC, local recurrence at presentation was significantly associated with worse disease-specific survival, with 10% of patients dying from their disease.[13]

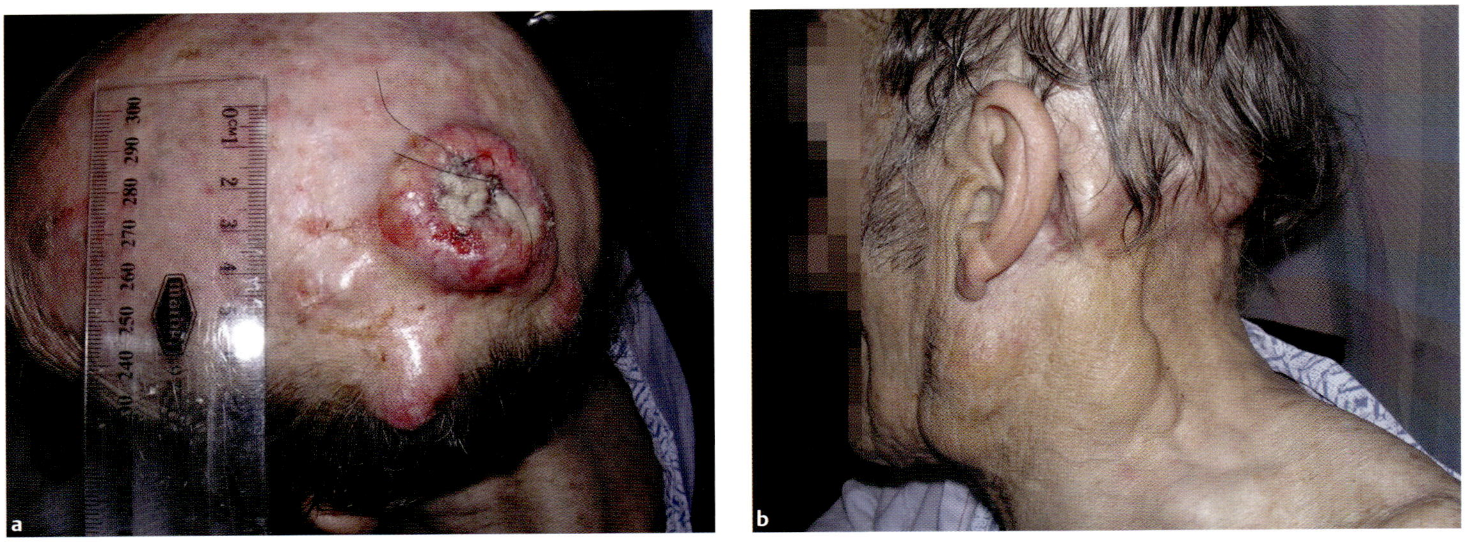

Fig. 17.1a, b Squamous cell carcinoma.
a A 76-year-old man with a rapidly growing posterior scalp squamous cell carcinoma in the setting of chronic lymphocytic leukemia (CLL). Note the nearby in-transit metastases.
b Multiple enlarged lymph nodes were present in the posterior neck, with biopsies confirming some nodes containing metastatic squamous cell carcinoma and others enlarged due to CLL. The patient was treated with palliative intent with radiotherapy (25 Gy in 5 fractions) alone.

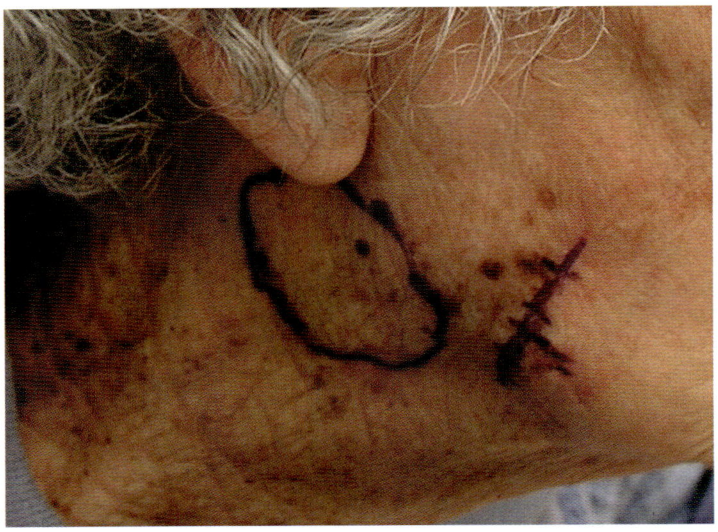

Fig. 17.2 An 82-year-old woman with a previously excised 8 mm right-sided lower-face MCC (as marked) presenting now with a 3 cm right-sided upper neck metastatic lymph node. Investigations did not identify any distant disease. The patient was recommended right hemi-neck radiotherapy and received a dose of 55 Gy in 25 fractions using megavoltage photons.

Malignant Melanoma

Tumor thickness (Breslow thickness), the presence of ulceration, and mitoses >1/mm² are important prognostic factors in primary melanoma. A patient with a 1 mm thick lesion and no ulceration has a 10-year survival of just under 90%, whereas a patient with a lesion >4 mm thick with ulceration has a 10-year survival of only 30%.[14] The poor outcome is dictated by the increased risk of recurrence and disease-specific mortality. The pathological status of the sentinel lymph node is the most important prognostic factor for predicting recurrence and survival in malignant melanoma.[15]

Patterns of Recurrence

Nonmelanoma Skin Cancer

In patients with SCC, MCC, or malignant melanoma, the risk of recurrence extends beyond the primary site to also include in-transit (or satellite), regional, and distant recurrence (including perineural invasion). In patients with NMSC, locoregional recurrence predominates.

The site of first recurrence is influenced by the initial treatment. In patients with SCC and MCC, regional recurrence in untreated first-echelon lymph nodes is frequently the first site of failure (**Fig. 17.2**). In contrast, patients who have undergone nodal treatment may first recur in a distant site, although regional recurrence can still occur as a first site of relapse in treated nodal basins, especially in patients with SCC. In most cases a patient with NMSC developing distant recurrence should be considered incurable and treated palliatively. However, selected patients with a solitary site of recurrence may be candidates for metastasectomy.[16]

Malignant Melanoma

Patients with malignant melanoma are more likely than patients with NMSC to experience relapse, with 20%–25% of patients recurring. A patient recurring with melanoma has a worse prognosis than a patient recurring with SCC or BCC. Recurrences can be categorized as local, in-transit, regional, and distant. An Australian study of 873 patients who relapsed reported distant recurrence as the commonest site (45%), followed by regional (34%), local (11%), and in-transit metastases (10%).[17]

Primary Lesion Treatment

Initial treatment impacts on the subsequent management of recurrence. Patients treated surgically may be offered further sur-

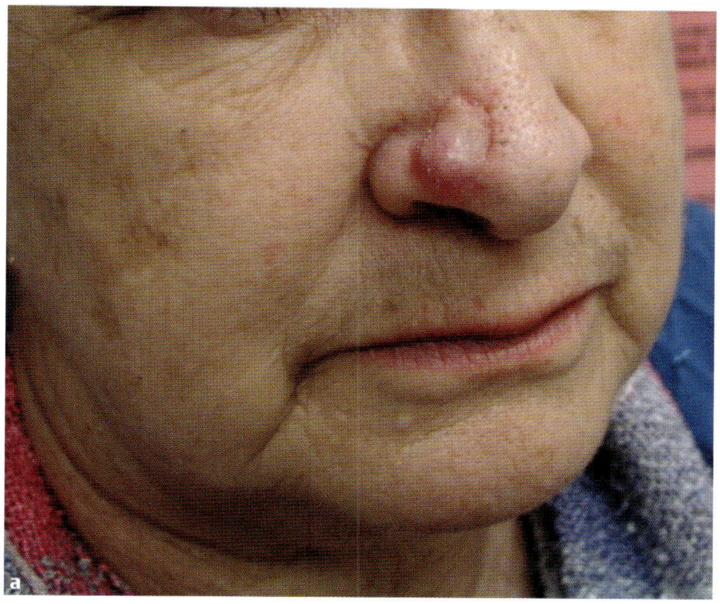

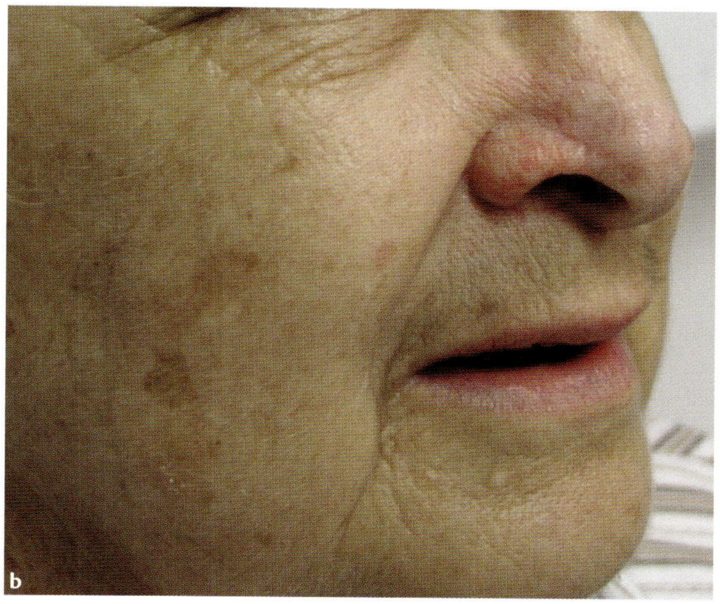

Fig. 17.3a, b Recurrence of lower-nose SCC.
a Recurrence of a poorly differentiated right lower-nose SCC in a previously grafted site 3 months after surgery. Excision pathology confirmed a positive deep margin with no further treatment recommended.
b The patient proceeded to a course of local radiotherapy receiving 55 Gy in 25 fractions using orthovoltage energy photons. At 3 months follow-up she had experienced complete regression of the SCC. The regional lymph nodes were not electively treated and the patient was placed on close observation.

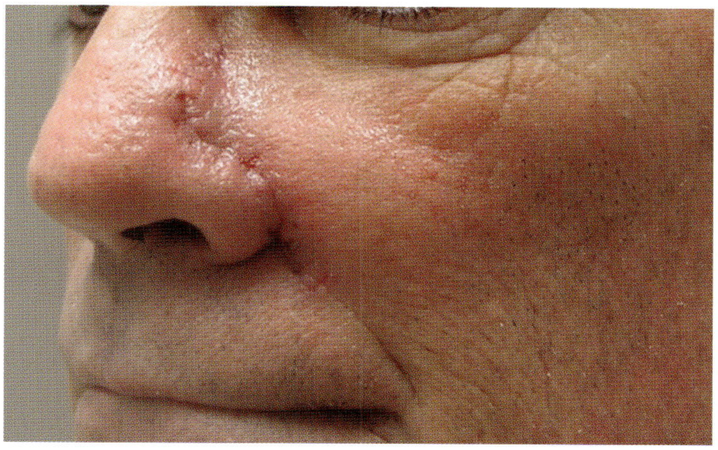

Fig. 17.4 A 55-year-old man following recent excision of a 10 mm infiltrative BCC from his left-side nasolabial fold. Surgical pathology confirmed a close deep excision margin at 0.5 mm. A recommendation was made for further treatment and he received a course of adjuvant radiotherapy (50 Gy in 20 fractions) to reduce his risk of undetected deep recurrence.

gery, whereas patients treated with radiotherapy (RT) may not necessarily be considered candidates for further RT. In this section, we review the principles of treatment of primary cancers, since suboptimal initial management has a significant factor in the development and subsequent management of recurrence.

Squamous and Primary Basal Cell Carcinoma

Surgery for Primary Squamous Cell Carcinoma

The importance of adequate excision is relevant when determining risk of local relapse. Up to 50% of patients with an incompletely excised SCC may recur locally and these patients have an increased risk of developing nodal metastases[18] (**Fig. 17.3**). A patient with an incompletely (positive or close margin) excised SCC remains at risk of locoregional recurrence and should undergo re-excision or adjuvant RT (level C recommendation). Observation alone is not recommended, as many patients will not return for regular clinic follow-up.

Surgery for Primary Basal Cell Carcinoma

Following excision, 10%–15% of specimens will be reported as incompletely excised.[19] Lesions located on the head and neck region or recurrent or morpheic (sclerosing) subtypes have higher rates of incomplete excision (40%–50%). Without further treatment up to 20%–30% of incompletely excised BCC recur locally and those with both deep and peripherally involved margins are at the highest risk (**Fig. 17.4**).

Definitive Radiotherapy for Squamous Cell and Basal Cell Carcinoma

Definitive RT is an option where the outcome—cosmetic (e.g., nasal BCC) and/or functional—is considered better with RT than with surgery. The cosmetic result for well-fractionated RT (2–3 Gy fraction sizes) is excellent and this is an option for patients where other modalities may have failed or are considered less optimal.[20] As an example, in a case series of patients from MD Anderson Cancer Center with SCC of the eyelid treated with definitive RT, the authors documented an excellent 5-year local control of 89%.[21]

Adjuvant Radiotherapy for Squamous Cell and Basal Cell Carcinoma

Adjuvant local RT is an effective option when excision is incomplete and re-excision is not possible. A retrospective institutional study of patients with lower lip SCC documented a 37% local recurrence rate in excised patients not receiving adjuvant RT (27% close/positive margins) compared with 6% local recurrence rate in patients treated with surgery and adjuvant RT (94% close/positive

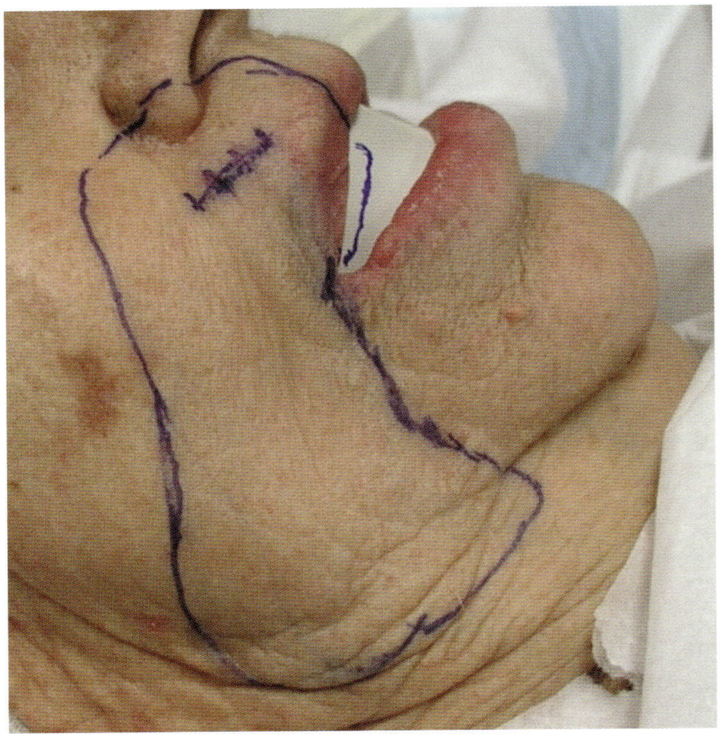

Fig. 17.5 An 85-year-old woman following recent excision of a 9 mm MCC from her right-side upper lip. Closest excision margin was 2 mm and lymphovascular invasion was present. The patient proceeded to wide-field adjuvant radiotherapy to widely encompass the excision site, in-transit tissues, and first-echelon lymph nodes (as marked). A dose of 50 Gy in 20 fractions was prescribed using 9 MeV electrons and 1 cm tissue equivalent bolus. At 13 months follow-up she remains relapse free.

margins).[22] In a retrospective study of 187 Canadian patients, all with incompletely excised BCC (93% located on HN), 119 underwent adjuvant RT (median dose 35 Gy in 5 fractions) versus expectant treatment (salvage surgery or RT) in 67. Recurrence free rates were markedly lower in the adjuvant group (91 vs. 61% at 5 years; $P = 0.00001$); however, following salvage treatment most patients were cured and the 10-year actuarial control rates were equivalent (92 vs. 90%; $P = 0.05$).[23]

Merkel Cell Carcinoma

Excision is the initial treatment in patients with operable MCC and will establish a diagnosis. However, achieving wide excision margins (2–3 cm), noting also that intradermal spread is well documented in MCC, is difficult in the head and neck. More than any other skin cancer, local (including satellite) recurrence is well documented even in the setting of a negative excision margin. Surgical margins (4–5 mm) recommended for SCC/BCC patients are inadequate in MCC patients. But with the addition of wide-field adjuvant RT the need for wide excision margins is not necessary.[24] In a review of 1024 cases of MCC, the mean relapse rate with the addition of adjuvant RT was 10% compared with 53% not receiving RT ($P = 0.00001$).[25] Most studies support a benefit in locoregional control and survival with the addition of adjuvant RT. A meta-analysis of 1254 patients reported a significant reduction in local (HR, 0.27; $P < 0001$) and regional recurrence (HR, 0.34; $P < 0.001$) and a benefit in overall survival (HR, 0.63; $P = 0.04$) in patients treated with surgery and adjuvant RT compared with surgery alone[26] (**Fig. 17.5**).

Table 17.1 Excision margins for primary melanoma

Breslow thickness	Margin of excision
Melanoma in situ	5 mm
<1 mm	1 cm
1–2 mm	1–2 cm
2–4 mm	1–2 cm
>4 mm	2 cm

Malignant Melanoma

Primary melanoma should be treated with wide local excision ± sentinel lymph node biopsy (SLNB). The recommendations for the clinical margin of excision are based on the Breslow thickness of the primary tumor (**Table 17.1**).[27] Lesions located on the head and neck often require appropriate reconstruction to achieve a balance between adequate excision and maintaining form and function. The National Comprehensive Cancer Network (NCCN) and Australian and New Zealand guidelines recommend that sentinel lymph node biopsy be offered to patients with primary melanoma >1 mm thick and should be considered in patients who have a primary melanoma 0.75–1 mm thick with adverse features (ulceration, mitoses >1/mm^3, lymphovascular invasion, or young patient age).[27,28]

Regional Treatment

Regional Treatment of Malignant Melanoma

Therapeutic nodal dissection is recommended in patients with biopsy-proven clinical nodal metastases. After surgery, the risk of regional (and systemic) recurrence may justify adjuvant RT (48 Gy in 20 fractions), with a recent multicenter randomized study ($n = 250$) from Australia showing a significant reduction in regional recurrence from 31% to 19% (HR 1.77; 1.02–3.08, $P = 0.041$) (level 1b evidence) in patients randomized to surgery and adjuvant RT.[29] With a median survival of only 27 months, a significant difference in median survival was not shown ($P = 0.14$). Therefore, most patients relapsing in a nodal basin (or presenting with nodal metastases) should be recommended to have adjuvant nodal RT (grade A recommendation).

Regional Treatment of Squamous Cell Carcinoma

Patients with SCC can recur in nodal metastases, although only a minority (2%–3%) do so. High-risk patients have an incidence of 10%–20% of developing nodal metastases[30] (**Fig. 17.6**). Only 20%–30% of nodal metastases are concomitant with the primary lesion, with most recurring within 12–18 months of treatment to the primary. Twenty to thirty percent may not have an identifiable index lesion. In a large prospective cohort study ($n = 653$), patients with SCC >6 mm thick were at significantly higher risk of developing nodal metastasis and local recurrence. Sixteen percent of patients with a thick SCC (>6 mm) developed metastases[10] (level

1b evidence) and no patient with a tumor <2 mm thick developed metastases. Similarly, immunosuppressed patients had a higher rate of developing metastases (16 vs. 4%; $P = 0.002$). Patients with high-risk SCC should have regular 3- to 4-monthly follow-up for 3–4 years.

Patients with regional metastases are at risk of morbidity and death. The addition of adjuvant regional RT significantly improves freedom from relapse and survival.[31] Patients should be recommended surgery and adjuvant RT (60 Gy in 30 fractions) as best practice with single-modality treatment associated with a worse outcome (grade C recommendation).

Regional Treatment of Merkel Cell Carcinoma

Patients with MCC are at high risk (30%–40%) of harboring occult regional metastases.[32] Sentinel lymph node biopsy may improve the ability to detect subclinical nodal metastases. Despite the results from small studies, the role for sentinel lymph node biopsy in patients with MCC is unclear, with most patients receiving elective nodal RT in any case. We do not recommend sentinel lymph node biopsy as a routine procedure, although identification of the sentinel node may be advantageous in planning RT fields (grade D recommendation).

Patients with regional relapse (or nodal metastases at diagnosis) in previously untreated nodal basins often die from distant metastases. There is recent evidence that patients with relatively small-volume (2–3 cm) nodal metastases may be adequately treated with RT alone (level 4 evidence). In a large US study that included patients treated with RT alone for palpable metastatic lymph nodes, the 2-year regional relapse-free survival was 78%.[33] In an Australian series, the authors documented a 5-year overall survival of 37% in 43 patients treated with RT alone. Most patients had nodal relapse, with the majority dying from distant relapse while maintaining an in-field control rate of 75%.[34]

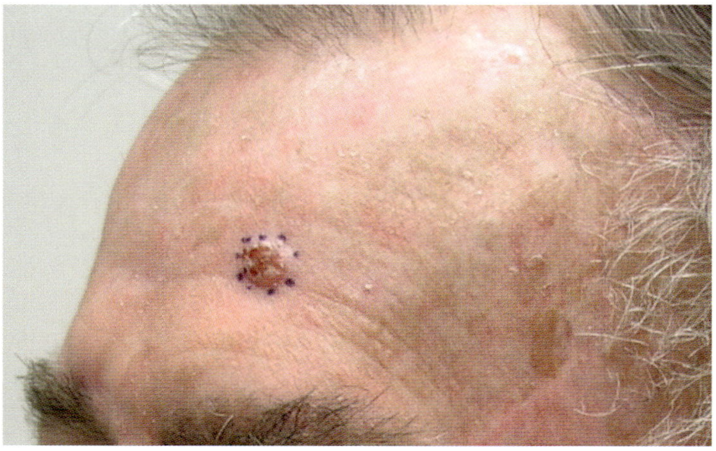

Fig. 17.6 A 70-year-old man with a recurrent left forehead SCC presenting with a concomitant 2 cm metastatic left preauricular node. The patient proceeded to excision of the recurrent primary, superficial parotidectomy, and upper neck dissection. Both surgical sites received adjuvant radiotherapy.

Recurrence

Prognostic Factors

Recurrent Nonmelanoma Skin Cancer

Patients developing recurrence have a worse outcome, with various factors predictive for outcome.

Site

Patients developing local recurrence are in a favorable group compared with patients with nodal relapse. Patients with distant relapse are essentially incurable. In the rare cases of isolated distant metastases, surgery may be considered.

Extent of Recurrence

Patients must be carefully evaluated to establish operability. Some consideration must be given to the functional and cosmetic morbidity of salvage locoregional surgery. Patients presenting with multiple fixed metastatic lymph nodes, with skull base invasion (in the case of parotid recurrence) or involving neurovascular structures are usually inoperable. Similarly, recurrent perineural invasion from a previously treated periorbital SCC that extends beyond the skull base or orbital apex should also be considered inoperable—patients should be offered RT (**Fig. 17.7**). Previously unirradiated patients have the option of RT as a salvage treatment, which may be of radical intent, or in some cases palliative (5–10 fractions) to improve quality of life in an incurable patient.

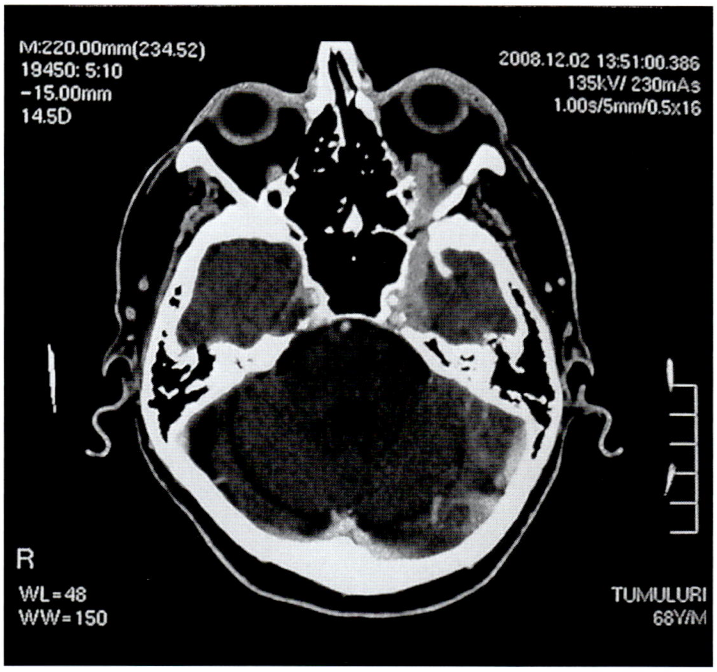

Fig. 17.7 Axial CT scan slice highlighting advanced perineural extension beyond the left orbital apex into the intracranial cavity from a previously excised left supraorbital SCC. Because of disease extension beyond the orbital apex, he received a course of CT-planned multifield multiphase radiotherapy to a total dose of 55 Gy in 30 fractions.

Time to Recurrence

Most recurrences will occur within 12–18 months of initial treatment. Late recurrences raise the possibility of a second primary, although the management is often similar. Early relapse within 2–3 months usually implies aggressive disease and portends a worse outcome. Of note, recurrent BCC can occur late, even 4–5 years after treatment.

Previous Radiotherapy

Previous RT may preclude this as an option for re-treatment, although cases need to be considered individually. Ideally, RT relapses should be excised, although re-irradiation may also be considered. However, outcome is probably better if an operation is feasible. Important factors that need to be considered in re-irradiating include the previous RT field and dose fractionation schedule. An estimation of the dose received at the skin surface and at depth, and of the structures previously irradiated, is also important. Converting total doses to a 2 Gy biological equivalent dose (BED) using equivalence tables allows[35] some estimation of the risk of re-irradiating, although the data to support this option is very limited (level 4 evidence). In cases of patients undergoing extensive salvage surgery with removal of previously irradiated tissues, further RT may also be considered.

Patient Factors

Consideration must be given to the impact that salvage treatment will have on a patient. Elderly patients with significant medical comorbidity may be better treated with palliative intent. RT is effective in palliating advanced recurrent disease associated with pain and bleeding.

Recurrent Malignant Melanoma

Site of recurrence is the most important prognostic factor, with survival following local recurrence better than in-transit, followed by regional and lastly distant relapse.[36] Increasing tumor thickness and location (head and neck or trunk) are associated with a worse survival in patients developing local recurrence. Similarly, in patients with regional recurrence, the presence of concurrent local and regional disease is associated with a worse prognosis.[37] The extent of locoregional recurrence is also prognostic.

Prognosis is poor in patients with distant metastases and is dependent on the number of distant sites and the presence of visceral involvement. Patients with local or regional recurrences have a 5-year survival rate of 30%–40% and patients with distant metastases have a survival rate of less than 10% at 5 years. Most recurrent events occur within 5 years of diagnosis and the majority of late recurrences after 5 years are to distant sites.

■ Investigations

Recurrent Nonmelanoma Skin Cancer

Biopsy Confirmation

Biopsy confirmation is required in clinically suspected recurrence. Complete clinical regression of primary cutaneous lesions or metastatic nodes after RT may take weeks to months and therefore a biopsy performed in this early setting may be difficult to interpret. It is important to note that RT-induced cellular changes (i.e., atypia) could be incorrectly reported as residual malignancy.[38] Pathologists receiving biopsy material in this setting must be aware of the history of previous RT.

Anatomical Imaging

Contrast-enhanced computed tomography (CT) scans of the involved site allow accurate determination of the underlying extent of recurrence. In cases of well-defined early local recurrence (e.g., BCC), the additional information may not add more to clinical examination. Periorbital recurrences often require imaging to exclude subclinical orbital involvement. Regional scanning frequently identifies abnormal nodes in the clinically negative setting that require further investigation (i.e., ultrasound-guided biopsy). Patients at risk of developing distant metastases should be considered for CT scanning of the chest and abdomen/pelvis. In the setting of presumed perineural invasion, a magnetic resonance imaging (MRI) scan with contrast is the investigation of choice because of the ability to identify enlarged and enhancing nerves, skull base involvement, and intracranial extension.[39] CT and MRI scans often provide complimentary information around the skull base.

Functional Imaging

Patients at risk of developing distant metastases may benefit from functional investigations such as a bone scan or positron emission tomography–CT (PET-CT) scan. Recent onset of bone pain is often a symptom suggesting skeletal metastases and warranting a bone scan. Patients with relapsed MCC should always be considered for a PET-CT scan because of the high propensity for distant disease, which may not be identified on anatomical imaging alone.[40] PET-CT scans have the sensitivity to detect FDG-avid disease as small as 5 mm.

Recurrent Malignant Melanoma

Recurrent malignant melanoma must be confirmed with either a fine-needle aspiration biopsy for nodal or large soft tissue recurrences or an excision biopsy for dermal metastases. Although there are no randomized trials, we recommend that all patients with recurrent malignant melanoma be re-staged to determine the extent of metastatic disease. The results may influence management since if there is widespread metastatic disease it may be more appropriate for the patient to undergo systemic treatment. For re-staging the patient, we also recommend CT scans of the head and neck, chest, and abdomen/pelvis and MRI of the brain, ± PET-CT (level D recommendation).

A recent prospective study comparing CT to PET scans found no difference in the upstaging of patients. However, PET scanning was able to detect more metastatic sites.[41] PET-CT scanning has been found to be more accurate than PET or CT scanning alone for the detection of metastatic disease, with sensitivity and specificity reported as 98% and 94%, respectively.[42] Given the high FDG avidity and unpredictable metastatic spread of malignant melanoma, a PET-CT scan is an appropriate investigation in most patients with recurrence. Sentinel lymph node biopsy has been performed in patients with isolated local or in-transit recurrence; however, there is currently no evidence to suggest that this improves survival.[43]

Principles of Management

Indications in Nonmelanoma Skin Cancer

Local Recurrence after Surgery

Local BCC recurrence after excision will necessitate further surgery, if possible, with a strong recommendation for the addition of adjuvant local RT to reduce the risk of further recurrence, particularly if excision margins are inadequate. Patients may be considered for Moh's surgery. Recent level 1 evidence supports Moh's surgery as the optimal surgery for recurrent BCC of the face with better control rates than with non-Moh's excision. In a large study of primary ($n = 488$) and recurrent BCC ($n = 202$) (not necessarily after RT), patients with recurrent BCC treated with Moh's surgery had significantly fewer further recurrences (2.4 vs. 12.1%; $P = 0.015$) when compared with those undergoing wide excision with 3 mm clinical margins.[44] Following excision clinicians may elect to observe, even with close/positive margins. However, patients with mid-face lesions should receive adjuvant RT as further recurrences may be inoperable or require morbid surgery.

In the case of recurrent primary SCC, excision with clear margins and adjuvant RT is recommended, and as with BCC Moh's surgery is an option. The risk of developing subclinical metastatic nodal metastases may warrant consideration of electively treating regional nodes (surgery or RT), although there is no high-level evidence to support this approach and each case should be considered on its own merits. The parotid gland nodes are the most frequently involved nodes for metastatic skin cancer of the head and neck. Therefore, patients who do proceed to adjuvant RT for a recurrent SCC in proximity to the parotid gland could be treated with an en bloc RT field that electively treats the parotid gland (grade D recommendation).

Regional Recurrence after Surgery

Regional SCC recurrence after a previous neck dissection should be reoperated on, if possible. The extent of recurrence will dictate the type and extent of surgery, and may require the excision of overlying involved skin and require flap reconstruction. All patients should be offered adjuvant RT and patients with small-volume limited-level nodal recurrence may be treated with selective neck dissection followed by adjuvant RT, which should encompass the surgical bed and the uninvolved next echelon nodes. Elective treatment to the parotid following neck relapse may be warranted, especially for upper neck relapse. Both elective parotid RT or superficial parotidectomy are options, although with most patients receiving adjuvant neck RT adding a parotid RT field is an option. Recurrent SCC in the parotid bed following nerve-sparing parotidectomy may require salvage radical parotidectomy with sacrifice of the facial nerve with patients also receiving regional adjuvant RT.

Recurrent locoregional MCC is potentially treated nonsurgically with RT alone, especially noting the competing risks of distant relapse and the elderly population that develop MCC.[33,34] Five-year survival was significantly worse in patients with MCC treated in the setting of locoregional recurrence compared than in those without recurrence (22 vs. 52%; $P = <0.001$).[45] However, if surgery is contemplated, all patients should receive adjuvant RT, and it is therefore not necessary to achieve wide excision margins at the expense of form or function. RT should follow without undue delay within 2–4 weeks of surgery to decrease the risk of further recurrence.[46]

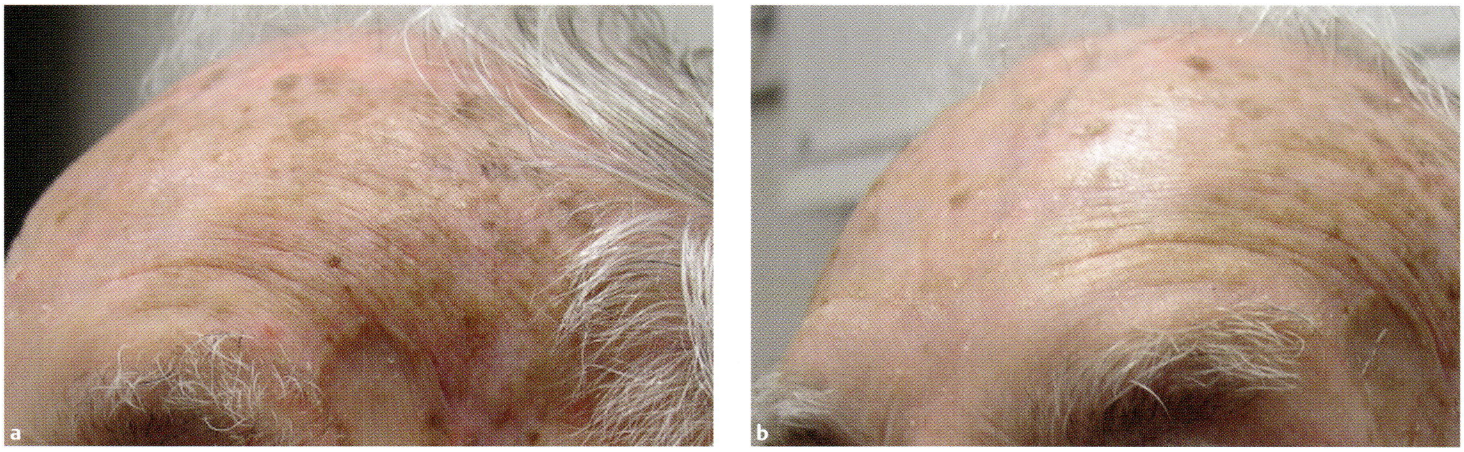

Fig. 17.8a, b Recurrence of SCC.
a A 90-year-old man who developed a 2 cm dermal based recurrence 9 months after excision and grafting of a nearby SCC. It was felt, based on the location and dermal-based nature of the recurrence, that radiotherapy offered the best chance of achieving local control and maintaining function.
b The patient received 55 Gy in 25 fractions using orthovoltage energy photons following the insertion of an internal eye shield. At 6 months post treatment the patient had obtained an excellent cosmetic and functional outcome but subsequently recurred in his ipsilateral parotid gland, requiring parotidectomy and adjuvant radiotherapy.

Other Recurrence after Surgery

Dermal-based (or in-transit) SCC or MCC recurrences are relatively uncommon (compared with malignant melanoma) and because of the multicentric nature are usually treated with wide-field RT. Patients with limited dermal lesions may undergo excision but all should also proceed to wide-field adjuvant RT, or alternatively receive RT alone. The primary site is often in close proximity and therefore may also be included in the treatment field (**Fig. 17.8**). At least one small study documented an excellent outcome (80% disease free) following treatment.[47] Dermal metastases well away from the primary site are possibly hematogenous metastases and usually a surrogate marker for the development of further distant metastases.

Patients can present with cranial nerve palsies and neuropathic symptoms secondary to recurrent perineural invasion from a previously excised lesion, typically in the trigeminal nerve distribution, from a forehead or periorbital SCC. Recurrent disease that has spread beyond the skull base or orbit is inoperable and patients should undergo RT using CT-planned conformal treatment (including intensity-modulated radiotherapy [IMRT]) to doses of approximately 60 Gy[48] (grade C recommendation). Despite the poor prognosis, patients can still be cured with high-dose RT. However, late orbital and central nervous system side effects need to be considered. Hyperfractionated RT and the addition of concomitant chemotherapy have been used in this setting.[49] The natural history of perineural invasion, unlike other recurrent sites, may extend over many years as disease progression is usually slow.

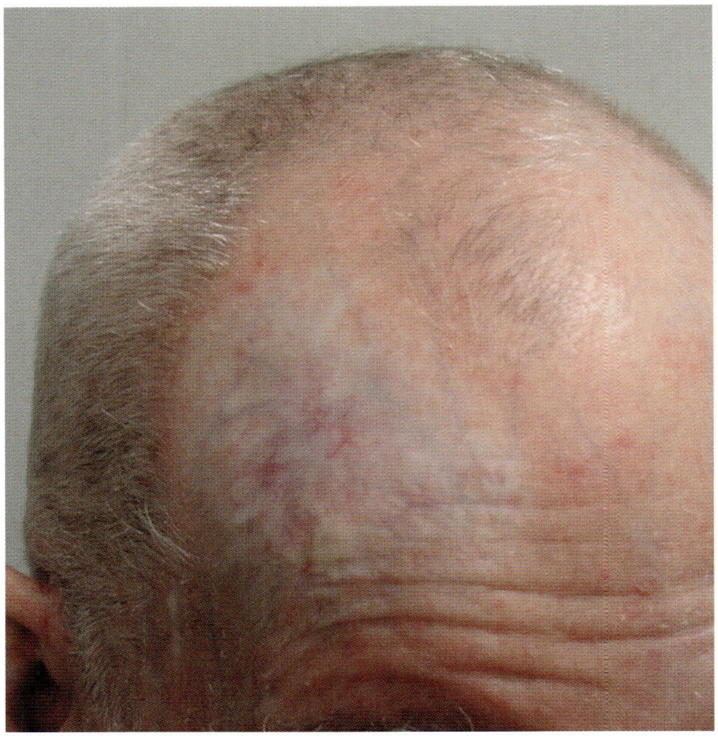

Fig. 17.9 A 70-year-old man 4 years post adjuvant radiotherapy to his right-side upper forehead in the setting of a high-risk cutaneous SCC. The patient received a total of 50 Gy in 20 fractions using superficial energy photons. Note the presence of in-field hypopigmentation, scattered telangiectasia, and epidermal atrophy. He has also previously received treatment to his lower nose. This patient would not be a candidate for re-irradiation if he were to develop in-field recurrence or a nearby second cutaneous primary.

In-field Recurrence after Radiotherapy for Non-melanoma Skin Cancer

Patients recurring after RT may be candidates for further RT. The details of previous treatment, including the prescribed dose/fractionation schedule, must be reviewed, but these are not always available. Clinical assessment is very important and patients exhibiting late RT changes such as in-field cutaneous hypo- (or hyper-) pigmentation, telangiectasia, epidermal atrophy, or fibrosis should not be re-irradiated (**Fig. 17.9**).

The most common scenario for in-field recurrence is local recurrence of a mid-face BCC after definitive RT. Recurrent BCC, especially after RT, can be a difficult management problem.[50] Deep invasion, especially of the mid-face, may be present and patients are best approached with salvage surgery rather than further RT.

Local Re-irradiation

There is very little evidence documenting re-irradiation as an option in the setting of in-field (or marginal) recurrence. In a small series of 17 irradiated patients with recurrent head and neck NMSC (8 BCC, 9 SCC), all were re-irradiated to a cumulative median biological equivalent dose (BED) of 103 Gy.[51] This achieved local control in 10/17 patients (59%), with two developing subsequent skin defects. The authors concluded that patients receiving an initial BED of <55 Gy at 5 mm depth and a cumulative BED of no more than 110 Gy at the skin surface had the best outcome, with re-treatment fraction sizes limited to 2 Gy to further reduce late tissue reactions. Interestingly, on review of the initial RT details, the authors documented suboptimal initial treatment in 10 of the 17 patients, further reinforcing the need for optimal initial treatment as a means to reduce the risk of recurrence. In contrast to the aforementioned series, 5 lesions were re-irradiated by a Spanish group. No details of the RT doses were available and 3 patients recurred, with the authors suggesting a benefit in only selected patients.[52] There is preclinical animal data to suggest, at least for pig dermal tissue, a re-treatment tolerance of more than 90% for late dermal necrosis after an 18 Gy single dose and further RT.[53] However, extrapolating this data to the human subject following fractionated cutaneous RT needs to be done with caution. We therefore do not recommend local re-irradiation as a first option, but it may be considered in select patients (grade D recommendation).

Perhaps not as well appreciated is that patients who have already been diagnosed with NMSC are at risk of developing metachronous lesions. This risk has been estimated at 10 times that of the general population.[54] New primary lesions may be close enough (5–10 mm) to a previous RT field to limit further RT as a first option in the new untreated lesion.

Regional Re-irradiation

Regional recurrence after RT, usually adjuvant, (i.e., parotid and/or neck metastatic SCC, MCC, or MM) poses a more difficult problem as patients will usually have had a large volume (e.g., ipsilateral parotid ± hemi-neck) of normal tissue (e.g., mandible, soft tissue, brainstem/spinal cord, nerves, carotid artery) irradiated to 50–60 Gy. Following appropriate re-staging, operable patients should proceed to surgery. For inoperable patients, the evidence available for re-irradiation relates predominantly to treating mucosal head and neck SCC patients. In this analogous setting, recent evidence has emerged supporting the use of highly conformal

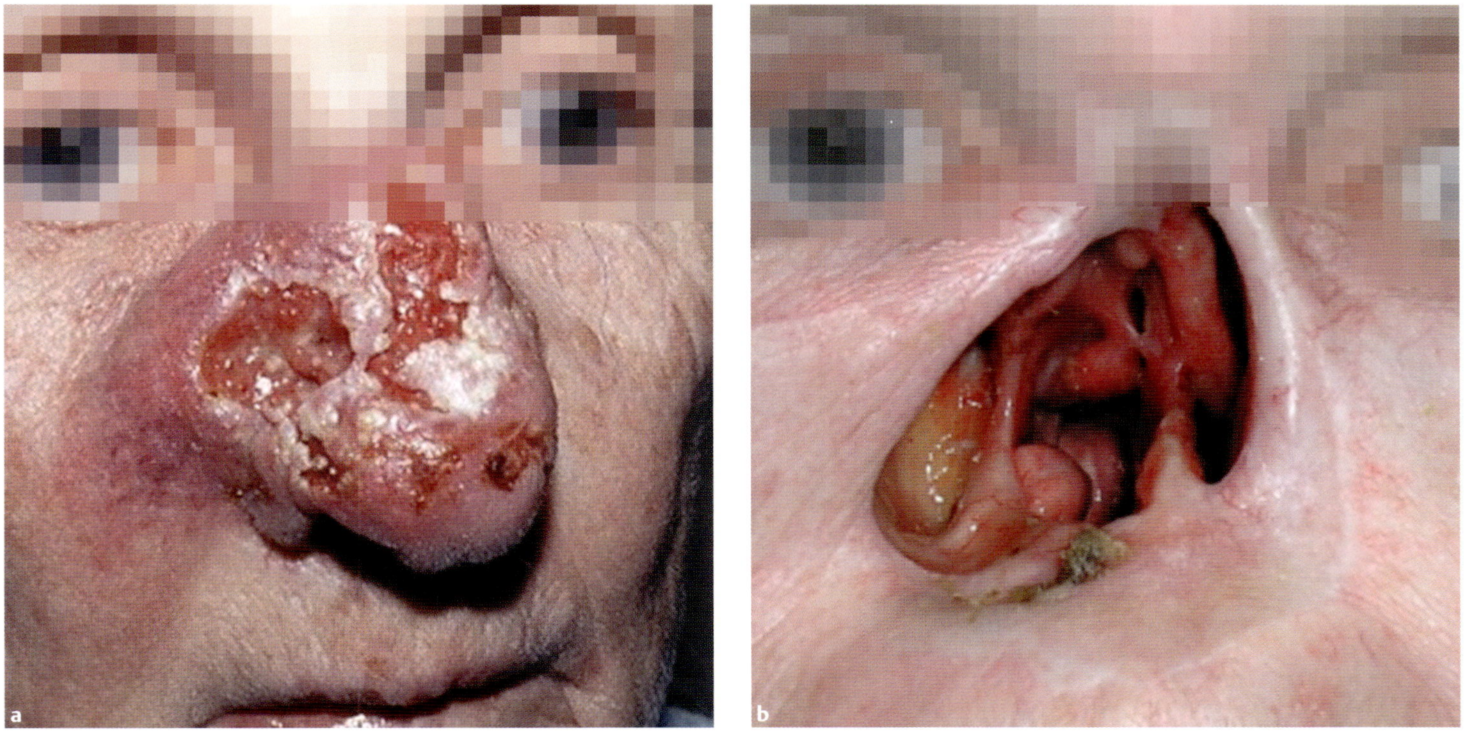

Fig. 17.10a, b A 72-year-old woman after rhinectomy for a recurrent locally advanced nasal squamous cell carcinoma previously treated with local radiotherapy. Pathology indicated close margins and the presence of perineural invasion and she proceeded to further radiotherapy. Essentially all of the previously irradiated tissue has been removed. The decision not to reconstruct using tissue transfer means easy visual access for monitoring for evidence of recurrence.

IMRT.[55,56] Patients retreated with IMRT are likely to have a better outcome (improved locoregional control and decreased severe late effects) compared with conventional 3D conformal re-irradiation. The best results are achieved with radical re-irradiation doses of approximately 60–70 Gy in 2 Gy daily fractions and re-treatment volumes limited to approximately 2 cm around gross disease or the resection bed. The spine, brainstem, and optic chiasm should receive a limited re-treatment dose (15–25 Gy) if previously irradiated to tolerance. Of note, even when utilizing IMRT, serious late toxicity and treatment-related deaths are reported in around 20% of patients. The addition of concurrent chemotherapy to re-irradiation has also been recommended in selected patients with mucosal SCC. The role of re-irradiation after salvage nodal surgery is less well defined, but in patients with unfavorable pathology (i.e., close/positive excision margins, extranodal spread) it should be considered, along with concurrent chemotherapy.

Case Study

A 72-year-old woman presented with a 2-month history of a rapidly growing ulcerative lesion occupying most of her nose. Biopsy confirmed a poorly differentiated SCC. Of note she had previously received definitive RT for a right-sided nasal SCC treated to 50 Gy in 20 fractions using orthovoltage energy photons. Examination revealed involvement of the entire nose, with extension onto the right medial face. CT confirmed gross destruction of underlying cartilage and nasal bones. There was no evidence of regional or distant recurrence and she was therefore staged as having a recurrent T4N0M0 nasal SCC.

The patient proceeded to total rhinectomy with the intention of fitting a nasal prosthesis. Pathology confirmed a deeply invasive recurrent SCC that involved multiple margins. Because all previously irradiated tissue had been excised and also because of her unfavorable pathology, she proceeded to adjuvant RT, receiving 60 Gy in 30 fractions to the mid-face and nasal cavity using an appositional 9 MeV electron field with nasal packing. At review 4 months after RT she remained disease free (**Fig. 17.10**).

Indications in Malignant Melanoma

Recurrence after Surgery

Local recurrence with malignant melanoma is often ill defined in the literature. True local recurrence develops from residual melanoma following excision and often arises within the surgical scar. Local recurrence rates are generally of the order of 3%–5%. There is no consensus as to what constitutes an appropriate margin of excision in locally recurrent malignant melanoma, and we recommend margins used to excise primary melanoma (see **Table 17.1**). Local recurrences that are not contiguous with the scar and have no epidermal involvement should be considered metastatic disease and investigated appropriately for evidence of nodal or distant disease.

In-transit recurrences are cutaneous or subcutaneous deposits that occur between the primary site and the regional lymph nodes, and represent intralymphatic spread. They arise in approximately 10% of patients with reported 5-year survival rates of approximately 50%.[27] In-transit recurrence may present in a variety of

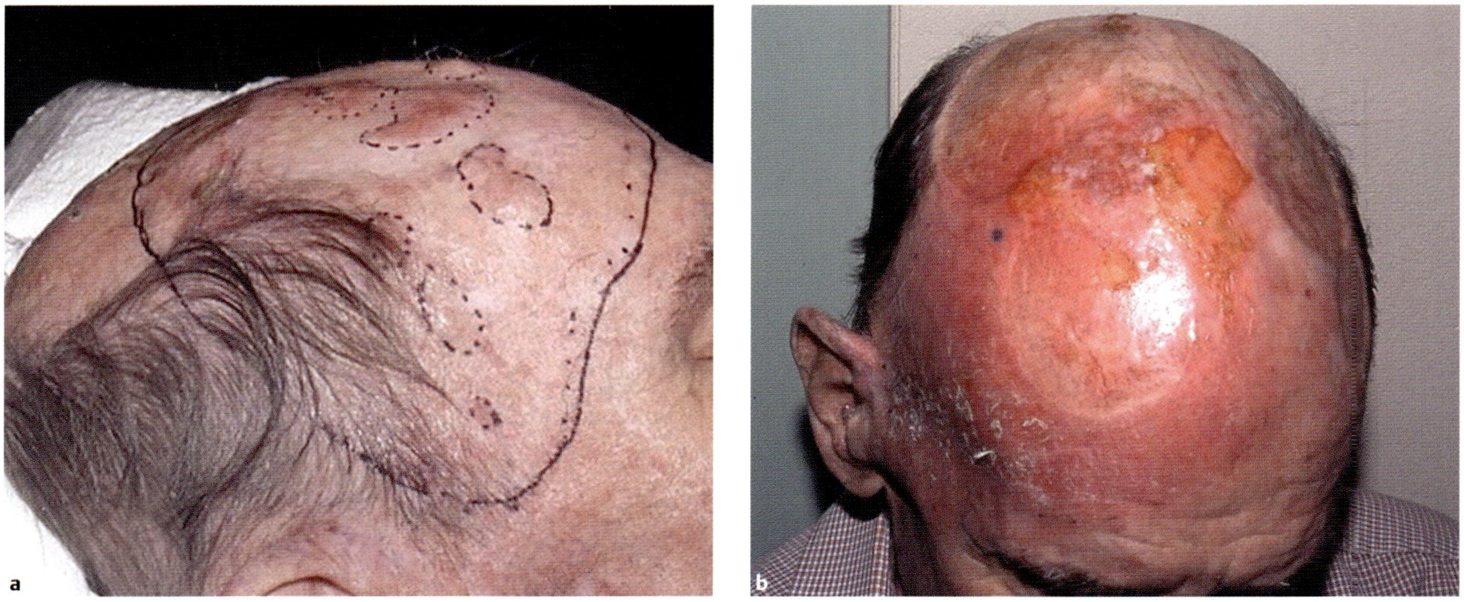

Fig. 17.11a, b Recurrence of malignant melanoma.
a A 62-year-old man presented with a rapidly growing 3.5 cm × 2.5 cm dermal-based recurrence 9 months following excision of a 15 mm maximum dimension, 2.5 mm thick, malignant melanoma from his right-side scalp.
b He underwent wide excision and rotation flap reconstruction. Excision pathology confirmed a close (0.5 mm) deep margin and he was recommended for adjuvant local RT (50 Gy in 20 fractions).

ways and there is often variation in the number and distribution of deposits. The condition can be uncomfortable and disabling, and if left untreated may ulcerate. As in-transit disease is considered to be of advanced stage, the choice of local treatment is unlikely impact on survival, which is often dictated by the development of distant metastases. Local treatment should therefore be viewed as palliative, even if staging investigations provide no evidence of distant disease. The type and extent of surgery should be tailored to the type and extent of disease. Resectable disease should be treated surgically with narrow but clear margins. With multiple dermal deposits, carbon dioxide laser ablation can be used, but the recurrence rate is high and this technique is limited to lesions less than 1 cm in diameter.[57] Other modalities include RT, cryotherapy, and electrochemotherapy. Intralesional injections of bleomycin and various other agents, including Rose Bengal, have provided documented responses.[58] Topical immunotherapy agents such as diphencyprone may also be considered in patients when surgery is inappropriate.[59]

Up to 9% of patients have been reported to develop regional recurrence following a negative sentinel lymph node biopsy and rates of up to 12.5% have been reported following a positive one.[60] The rate of regional recurrence following a therapeutic lymph node dissection ranges from 14% to 34%.[61] Risk factors for recurrence in this setting include the presence of extranodal spread, more than three involved nodes, and involved nodes more than 3 cm in size.[62] The prognosis of these patients is poor, with 10-year overall survival rates ranging from 25% to 40%.[63] Patients who are considered operable should proceed to surgery and most should also receive adjuvant nodal RT. Previously operated and irradiated nodal basins are often difficult to reoperate on because of tissue fibrosis, and subsequently surgical wounds may be slow to heal postoperatively.

Stage IV melanoma is often viewed with pessimism as the 5 year survival is less than 10%. However, selected patients with limited sites and numbers of metastases should be considered for resection. A randomized trial examining the effect of Canvaxin, a melanoma vaccine, in patients who had undergone complete resection of stage IV disease reported that patients with resectable disease had a 5-year survival exceeding 45% associated with aggressive resection.[64] Patients with distant skin/subcutaneous or lymph node disease have a better survival after resection than those with distant disease at other sites.[65]

Case Study

A 62-year-old man presented with a rapidly growing 3.5 cm × 2.5 cm dermal-based recurrence 9 months following excision of a 15 mm maximum dimension, 2.5 mm thick, malignant melanoma from his right-side scalp (**Fig. 17.11a**). Investigations prior to surgery identified multiple small pulmonary nodules suspicious for metastases. Despite the presence of distant metastases it was felt that he should undergo surgery and the patient subsequently proceeded to wide excision and rotation flap reconstruction (**Fig. 17.11b**). Excision pathology confirmed a close (0.5 mm) deep margin and he was recommended for adjuvant local RT (50 Gy in 20 fractions).

■ Systemic Treatment

Recurrent Malignant Melanoma

Systemic treatment is reserved for those with widespread and/or unresectable disease. However, results from the use of conventional chemotherapy are poor. Dacarbazine and its active metabolite temozolomide remain the most active single agents, with clinical response rates in approximately 15% of patients and complete response in approximately 5% of patients with a median duration of response of 4–6 months.[66] Interleukin-2 (immunotherapy) is similarly effective, with response rates of around 20% and complete response in 6%, but can be associated with significant toxicity. Interleukin-2 used in combination with conventional chemotherapeutic agents has not been shown to improve overall survival.[67] There has been extensive research into the use of targeted molecular therapy, for example BRAF inhibitors. BRAF is mutated in 70% of malignant melanoma arising in skin that is not sun-damaged, in 15% of chronically sun-damaged skin, and in acral and mucosal malignant melanoma. Early clinical trials have shown excellent initial response rates in patients treated with a BRAF inhibitor.[68]

Recurrent Non-melanoma Skin Cancer

Patients with recurrent SCC are rarely candidates for systemic treatment. There is currently a randomized trial going on under the auspices of the Australian and New Zealand Trans Tasman Radiation Oncology Group (TROG) investigating the addition of weekly carboplatin chemotherapy to adjuvant RT following surgery for patients with metastatic nodal SCC (Post Operative Skin Trial [POST] 05.01, www.trog.com.au). Pending the results from this trial, adjuvant chemo/RT may become best practice in the future management of these patients. Selected good-performance patients may also be recommended for palliative chemotherapy, often platinum-based, although response rates and duration of responses are low. Palliative local RT (20–30 Gy in 5–10 fractions) to symptomatic sites (e.g., painful bone metastasis, bleeding site) is usually beneficial. Recent novel treatments include epidermal growth factor receptor (EGFR) inhibitors[69] and intralesional interferons (IFNs).[70]

Merkel cell carcinoma (MCC) is a chemoresponsive disease with response rates of 60%–70% to platinum-based regimes.[71] The role of chemotherapy in the adjuvant setting is unclear and is not recommended.[72] However, patients with recurrent metastatic MCC may be recommended for chemotherapy, although median survival is measured in months and toxicity (bone marrow suppression) is a concern in this mainly elderly population.

■ Techniques

Surgical Techniques for Treating Local Relapse

Moh's versus non-Moh's Excision

The benefits of Moh's surgery in malignant melanoma, and to a lesser extent in NMSC, remain controversial, as it is a technique that is highly operator dependent. However, proponents suggest that the outcome for patients with malignant melanoma may be better than with non-Moh's excision.[73] There is little evidence for undertaking Moh's surgery in locally recurrent malignant melanoma, with a small study of 50 patients demonstrating a 5-year disease free survival of 66%. The authors recommended 2 cm excision margins (including the scar) to adequately treat patients with true local recurrence.[74] Moh's surgery may offer the benefit of a narrower excision margin, if this is desirable. However, there is insufficient evidence currently to routinely recommend Moh's surgery over conventional wide excision.

Primary Closure versus Flap/Graft Reconstruction

The method of closure following excision of local or in-transit recurrence depends on the site and size of the defect, and functional and cosmetic considerations. It has been shown not to affect survival in head and neck melanoma patients.[75] Where possible, an elliptical excision with primary closure should be employed, with the excision oriented appropriately with respect to relaxed skin tension lines.

For small to moderately sized defects where primary closure is not possible, local flaps or full/split thickness skin grafts may be used, with consideration given to cosmesis and functional outcome. A variety of different local flaps may be used in the head and neck, including transposition, rotational, and advancement flaps, with the choice of flap dictated mainly by the site and size of the defect[76] (**Fig. 17.12**). In terms of cosmesis, local flaps are often preferable to skin grafts, as there is better matching of skin color and texture, and less contour deformity. When planning to close

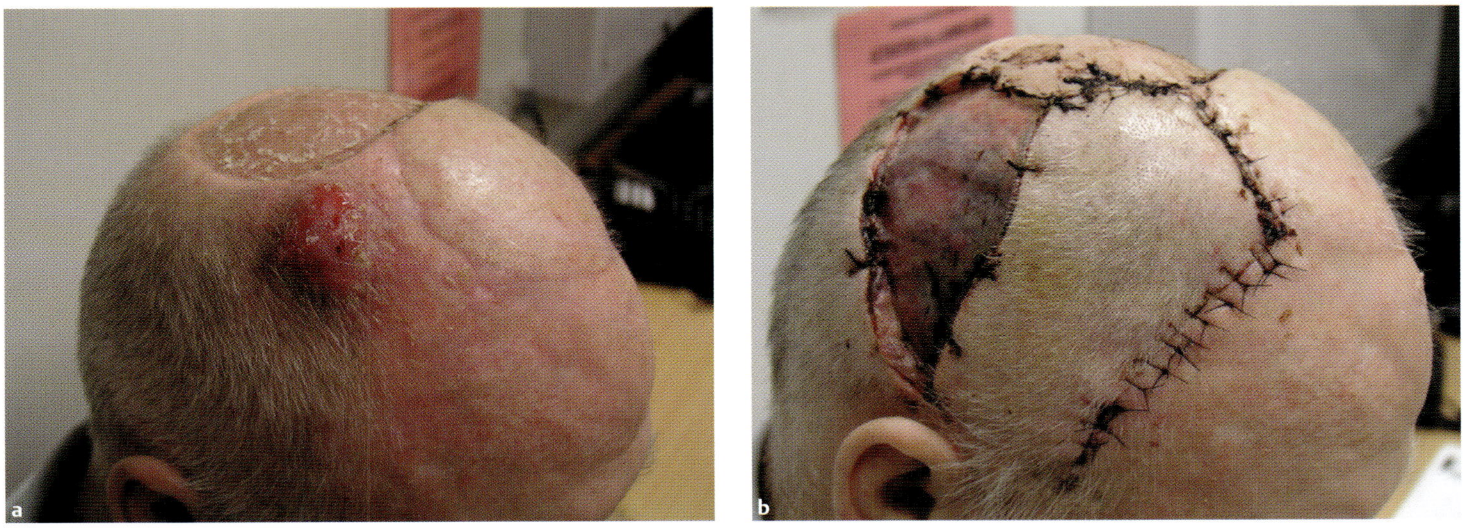

Fig. 17.12a, b Scalp squamous cell carcinoma.
a A 58-year-old man with a 4 cm × 3 cm dermal-based right-sided scalp squamous cell carcinoma in close proximity to a previously excised scalp lesion.
b The patient underwent wide local excision and reconstruction with a local rotation scalp flap. Pathology supported a positive deep excision margin and the patient therefore proceeded to adjuvant scalp radiotherapy.

a defect with a local flap, the flap should originate from the same aesthetic unit of the face as the defect, if possible.

Another important consideration is previous RT or surgery, which may reduce tissue vascularity due to microvascular occlusion and decrease distensibility due to fibrosis. Previous RT generally precludes the use of local flaps to the site. Conversely, if adjuvant RT is given, the reconstructed area needs to be well vascularized and sufficiently robust to withstand RT.

Split skin grafts, including the epidermis with variable thicknesses of dermis, generally have better survival rates than full-thickness skin grafts but may have inferior cosmetic results. In a small study of 30 split-skin grafts (in nonirradiated tissue) followed by adjuvant RT, there were only two cases of partial skin graft loss and one total loss. The authors suggest that RT should start no sooner than 6 weeks and that grafts be placed on healthy vascularized tissue.[77] We recommend that, where skin grafts are placed over irradiated tissue, RT should not start until complete graft healing is achieved.

In the setting of locoregional relapse, regional/pedicled flaps or distant/free flaps are frequently required for reconstruction, particularly for large or complex defects and sites where a local flap would not be viable due to previous RT. Pedicle flaps used in the head and neck include the pectoralis major, deltopectoral, latissimus dorsi, and trapezius flaps. Their use, however, is limited by a relative lack of mobility and bulkiness, and is more useful in the reconstruction of defects in the neck rather than on the face.

Free flaps are often utilized in reconstruction of large or complex defects in the head and neck. Two of the most frequently used free flaps in head and neck reconstruction are the radial forearm and anterolateral thigh free flaps. When planning the reconstruction of a defect, previous neck dissection needs to be taken into account, as there may be a resultant lack of suitable recipient vessels.

> **!**
> - Remember that the first priority is adequate treatment of the tumor.
> - Where possible close defects primarily.
> - Local flaps generally have a more aesthetically pleasing outcome than skin grafting.
> - Take into account previous surgery and RT when planning reconstruction.
> - Be aware that the histological extent of any tumor recurrence is often much greater than indicated by clinical examination and imaging, especially in irradiated tissue.
> - Ensure the local flap is designed to minimize downward tension on the lower eyelid so as to avoid ectropion.

Surgical Techniques for Treating Regional Relapse

Relapse in a Previously Dissected Neck

There is sparse evidence regarding the treatment of recurrent melanoma or NMSC in a previously dissected nodal basin. However, patients should be considered for surgery as it may offer a survival benefit provided there are no other metastases. In the setting of malignant melanoma some authors recommend, if there is concern that the previous dissection was inadequate, that the entire nodal basin be re-dissected.[78] However, in the neck the benefits of this approach may be outweighed by the risk of injury to neurovascular structures and this risk is dependent on the extent of prior surgery. Previous RT further complicates surgery because of fibrosis and the increased risk of delayed wound healing. We recommend that patients undergoing salvage surgery should have a completion or extended neck dissection, except where reoperation would entail carotid artery resection. In that circumstance, balloon occlusion may be used as a predictor of neurological outcome, noting that long-term survival is uncommon when carotid artery resection is undertaken.

Relapse in an Untreated Neck

There is no consensus regarding the extent of lymphadenectomy. Traditionally, radical neck dissection was considered the most appropriate treatment for melanoma and NMSC metastatic to the neck. More recently, modified radical neck dissection (in which levels I–V are resected but which preserves one or more of the accessory nerve, the internal jugular vein, and the sternomastoid muscle) and selective lymphadenectomy (where there is preservation of one or more lymph node groups) have been proposed as effective approaches.[79–81] For most patients with palpable metastatic disease in the neck, we recommend that a modified radical, or selective, neck dissection be performed followed by adjuvant RT.

Patients who relapse in the parotid and have a clinically node-negative neck should undergo parotidectomy and selective neck dissection of levels I–III, as it has been shown that there is a high incidence (30%–40%) of cervical node involvement in these patients.[82] Selective or modified radical neck dissection may be considered in the palliative setting in selected patients who have distant disease to minimize the morbidity of uncontrolled metastatic disease in the neck.

Radiotherapy Techniques

Patients considered candidates for local re-irradiation should have treatment limited to the site of recurrence with appropriate field margins to encompass subclinical extension. The selection of the energy of the orthovoltage photon beam should aim to ensure adequate coverage of deep tumor involvement, which can usually be assessed clinically. Electron beam RT is an alternative technique. However, use of small-field low-energy (5–6 MeV) electron beams raises issues of skin sparing and the need to add tissue-equivalent bolus as well as issues of wide treatment field penumbra, dose constriction, and rapid dropoff at depth.[83]

RT fraction sizes should be limited to around 1.8–2 Gy to further reduce the risk of late tissue changes. With limited evidence to guide clinicians, it is recommended that re-treatment total doses be limited to 50–55 Gy at 5 mm depth and that the cumulative skin dose not exceed 110 Gy. The role of hyperfractionation using 1.1–1.3 Gy fractions twice daily in this setting as a means to reduce the risk of late effects is unsupported by clinical data but is potentially another option.

Re-irradiating nodal basins carries a greater risk of late complications because of the increased volume of tissue and the number of structures re-irradiated. In keeping with data from the head and neck mucosal SCC literature, re-treatment volumes should be limited to the operative bed or to gross disease with 2–3 cm margins using IMRT or CT-planned conformal treatment. Elective nodal treatment should be avoided and neural tissue should receive no greater than a 50 Gy cumulative dose. The treatment toxicity will be greater than with local site re-irradiation and patients should therefore be of good performance status.

Brachytherapy

Brachytherapy uses radioactive emitting sources to treat skin cancers by direct contact, using either surface molds or interstitial needles. Its role is well established in the primary treatment of NMSC, with excellent cure rates of 90%–95% and minimal complications.[84] The concept of brachytherapy lends itself to the re-treatment of suitable RT recurrences because of the limited re-treatment of surrounding tissue. Despite this, data to support this approach as a re-treatment are lacking and brachytherapy remains an option only in centers with the expertise to deliver it.

Future Research

- Further studies to investigate the role of systemic therapy, in conjunction with radiotherapy, to enhance locoregional control in patients with MCC and SCC are required.
- Research leading to a better understanding of the clinical and radiobiological consequences of tissue re-irradiation could assist clinicians in better deciding on re-irradiation schedules.
- Future improvements in investigations, especially functional imaging, may offer the benefits of early detection of recurrent disease

Recommended Reading

- Mendenhall WM, Amdur RJ, Hinerman RW, Cognetta AB, Mendenhall NP. Radiotherapy for cutaneous squamous cell and basal cell carcinomas of the head and neck. Laryngoscope 2009;119(10):1994–1999
- Veness MJ. The important role of radiotherapy in patients with non-melanoma skin cancer and other cutaneous entities. J Med Imaging Radiat Oncol 2008;52(3):278–286. (Both articles are a useful resource for non–radiation oncologists who wish to understand further the role of radiotherapy in patients with skin cancer.)
- Moncrieff MD, Thompson JF, Quinn MJ, Stretch JR. Reconstruction after wide excision of primary cutaneous melanomas: part I-the head and neck. Lancet Oncol 2009;10(7):700–708. (This review article provides an excellent overview on methods of reconstruction in patients with melanoma and is written by recognized world experts in this field.)
- Baker SR. Local Flaps in Facial Reconstruction. 2nd ed. Philadelphia: Mosby Elsevier; 2007. (A well-written reference textbook on reconstructive surgery in facial skin cancers.)
- Merkel Cell Carcinoma. Seattle, WA: Seattle Cancer Care Alliance; 2011. Available at: www.merkelcell.org (accessed November 22, 2011). (Clinicians wanting relevant information on the management of patients with Merkel cell carcinoma can access current and updated information at this site.)
- Stasko T, Brown MD, Carucci JA, et al. International Transplant-Skin Cancer Collaborative; European Skin Care in Organ Transplant Patients Network. Guidelines for the management of squamous cell carcinoma in organ transplant recipients. Dermatol Surg 2004;30(4 Pt 2):642–650. (Immunosuppressed patients make up a disproportionate number of patients with recurrent skin cancer and clinicians should have a clear understanding of current management.)

References

1. de Vries E, van de Poll-Franse LV, Louwman WJ, de Gruijl FR, Coebergh JWW. Predictions of skin cancer incidence in the Netherlands up to 2015. Br J Dermatol 2005;152(3):481–488
2. Veness MJ, Palme CE, Morgan GJ. Merkel cell carcinoma: a review of management. Curr Opin Otolaryngol Head Neck Surg 2008;16(2):170–174
3. Staples MP, Elwood M, Burton RC, Williams JL, Marks R, Giles GG. Non-melanoma skin cancer in Australia: the 2002 national survey and trends since 1985. Med J Aust 2006;184(1):6–10
4. Buettner PG, Raasch BA. Incidence rates of skin cancer in Townsville, Australia. Int J Cancer 1998;78(5):587–593
5. Tracey EA, Chen S, Baker D, Bishop J, Jelfs P. Cancer in New South Wales: Incidence and Mortality 2004. Sydney: Cancer Institute NSW; 2006
6. Surveillance Epidemiology and End Results (SEER) Bethesda MD: National Cancer Institute, Surveillance Research Program; 2011. Available at: http://www.seer.cancer.gov (accessed 22 November, 2011)
7. Garbe C, Leiter U. Melanoma epidemiology and trends. Clin Dermatol 2009;27(1):3–9
8. Chen JY, Hruby G, Scolyer RA, et al. Desmoplastic neurotropic melanoma: a clinicopathologic analysis of 128 cases. Cancer 2008;113(10):2770–2778
9. Garcia L, Nagore E, Llombart B, et al. Basal cell carcinoma of the nasolabial fold: an apparently 'benign' tumour that often needs complex surgery. J Eur Acad Dermatol Venereol 2006;20(8):926–930
10. Brantsch KD, Meisner C, Schonfisch B, et al. Analysis of risk factors determining prognosis of cutaneous squamous-cell carcinoma: a prospective study.. Lancet Oncol 2008;9(8):713–720
11. Neubauer KE, Goldstein GD, Plumb SJ. Squamous cell carcinoma of the scalp in organ transplant recipients: exploring mechanisms for recurrence and treatment guidelines. Dermatol Surg 2010;36(2):185–193
12. Nolan RC, Chan MT, Heenan PJ. A clinicopathologic review of lethal nonmelanoma skin cancers in Western Australia. J Am Acad Dermatol 2005;52(1):101–108
13. Clayman GL, Lee JJ, Holsinger FC, et al. Mortality risk from squamous cell skin cancer. J Clin Oncol 2005;23(4):759–765
14. Balch CM, Soong SJ, Gershenwald JE, et al. Prognostic factors analysis of 17600 melanoma patients: validation of the American Joint Committee on Cancer melanoma staging system. J Clin Oncol 2001;19(16):3622–3634
15. Leong SP, Accortt NA, Essner R, et al. Sentinel Lymph Node Working Group. Impact of sentinel node status and other risk factors on the clinical outcome of head and neck melanoma patients. Arch Otolaryngol Head Neck Surg 2006;132(4):370–373

16. Shiono S, Kawamura M, Sato T, et al. Metastatic Lung Tumor Study Group of Japan. Pulmonary metastasectomy for pulmonary metastases of head and neck squamous cell carcinomas. Ann Thorac Surg 2009;88(3):856–860
17. Francken AB, Accortt NA, Shaw HM, et al. Prognosis and determinants of outcome following locoregional or distant recurrence in patients with cutaneous melanoma. Ann Surg Oncol 2008;15(5):1476–1484
18. Huang CC, Boyce SM. Surgical margins of excision for basal cell carcinoma and squamous cell carcinoma. Semin Cutan Med Surg 2004;23(3):167–173
19. Su SY, Giorlando F, Ek EW, Dieu T. Incomplete excision of basal cell carcinoma: a prospective trial. Plast Reconstr Surg 2007;120(5):1240–1248
20. Swanson EL, Amdur RJ, Mendenhall WM, Morris CG, Kirwan JM, Flowers F. Radiotherapy for basal cell carcinoma of the medial canthus region. Laryngoscope 2009;119(12):2366–2368
21. Petsuksiri J, Frank SJ, Garden AS, et al. Outcomes after radiotherapy for squamous cell carcinoma of the eyelid. Cancer 2008;112(1):111–118
22. Babington S, Veness MJ, Cakir B, Gebski VJ, Morgan GJ. Squamous cell carcinoma of the lip: is there a role for adjuvant radiotherapy in improving local control following incomplete or inadequate excision? ANZ J Surg 2003;73(8):621–625
23. Liu FF, Maki E, Warde P, Payne D, Fitzpatrick P. A management approach to incompletely excised basal cell carcinomas of skin. Int J Radiat Oncol Biol Phys 1991;20(3):423–428
24. Poulsen M, Harvey J. Is there a diminishing role for surgery for Merkel cell carcinoma of the skin? A review of current management. ANZ J Surg 2002;72(2):142–146
25. Medina-Franco H, Urist MM, Fiveash J, Heslin MJ, Bland KI, Beenken SW. Multimodality treatment of Merkel cell carcinoma: case series and literature review of 1024 cases. Ann Surg Oncol 2001;8(3):204–208
26. Lewis KG, Weinstock MA, Weaver AL, Otley CC. Adjuvant local irradiation for Merkel cell carcinoma. Arch Dermatol 2006;142(6):693–700
27. Australian Cancer Network Melanoma Guidelines Revision Working Party. Clinical practice guidelines for the management of melanoma in Australia and New Zealand. Wellington, NZ: Cancer Council Australia and Australian Cancer Network, Sydney and New Zealand Guidelines Group, Wellington; 2008
28. NCCN Clinical Practice Guidelines in Oncology v.2. Fort Washington, PA: National Comprehensive Cancer Network; 2010. Available at: http://www.nccn.org/professionals/physician_gls/f_guidelines.asp (accessed November 22, 2011)
29. Henderson MA, Burmeister B, Thompson JF, et al. Adjuvant radiotherapy and regional lymph node control in melanoma patients after lymphadenectomy: Results of an intergroup randomiszed trial (ANZMTG 01.02/TROG 02.01). J Clin Oncol 2009;27:18s Abstract No. LBA 9084
30. Veness MJ, Palme CE, Morgan GJ. High-risk cutaneous squamous cell carcinoma of the head and neck: results from 266 treated patients with metastatic lymph node disease. Cancer 2006;106(11):2389–2396
31. Veness MJ, Morgan GJ, Palme CE, Gebski V. Surgery and adjuvant radiotherapy in patients with cutaneous head and neck squamous cell carcinoma metastatic to lymph nodes: combined treatment should be considered best practice. Laryngoscope 2005;115(5):870–875
32. Gupta SG, Wang LC, Peñas PF, Gellenthin M, Lee SJ, Nghiem P. Sentinel lymph node biopsy for evaluation and treatment of patients with Merkel cell carcinoma: The Dana-Farber experience and meta-analysis of the literature. Arch Dermatol 2006;142(6):685–690
33. Fang LC, Lemos B, Douglas J, Iyer J, Nghiem P. Radiation monotherapy as regional treatment for lymph node-positive Merkel cell carcinoma. Cancer 2010;116(7):1783–1790
34. Veness M, Foote M, Gebski V, Poulsen M. The role of radiotherapy alone in patients with Merkel cell carcinoma: Reporting the Australian experience of 43 patients. Int J Radiat Oncol Biol Phys 2010;78(3):703–709
35. Barton M. Tables of equivalent dose in 2 Gy fractions: a simple application of the linear quadratic formula. Int J Radiat Oncol Biol Phys 1995;31(2):371–378
36. Francken AB, Accortt NA, Shaw HM, et al. Prognosis and determinants of outcome following locoregional or distant recurrence in patients with cutaneous melanoma. Ann Surg Oncol 2008;15(5):1476–1484
37. Leong SP, Accortt NA, Essner R, et al. Sentinel Lymph Node Working Group. Impact of sentinel node status and other risk factors on the clinical outcome of head and neck melanoma patients. Arch Otolaryngol Head Neck Surg 2006;132(4):370–373
38. Magi-Galluzzi C, Sanderson H, Epstein JI. Atypia in nonneoplastic prostate glands after radiotherapy for prostate cancer: duration of atypia and relation to type of radiotherapy. Am J Surg Pathol 2003;27(2):206–212
39. Williams LS, Mancuso AA, Mendenhall WM. Perineural spread of cutaneous squamous and basal cell carcinoma: CT and MR detection and its impact on patient management and prognosis. Int J Radiat Oncol Biol Phys 2001;49(4):1061–1069
40. Concannon R, Larcos GS, Veness M. The impact of ^{18}F-FDG PET-CT scanning for staging and management of Merkel cell carcinoma: results from Westmead Hospital, Sydney, Australia. J Am Acad Dermatol 2010;62(1):76–84
41. Bastiaannet E, Wobbes T, Hoekstra OS, et al. Prospective comparison of [^{18}F]fluorodeoxyglucose positron emission tomography and computed tomography in patients with melanoma with palpable lymph node metastases: diagnostic accuracy and impact on treatment. J Clin Oncol 2009;27(28):4774–4780
42. Strobel K, Dummer R, Husarik DB, Pérez Lago M, Hany TF, Steinert HC. High-risk melanoma: accuracy of FDG PET/CT with added CT morphologic information for detection of metastases. Radiology 2007;244(2):566–574
43. Yao KA, Hsueh EC, Essner R, Foshag LJ, Wanek LA, Morton DL. Is sentinel lymph node mapping indicated for isolated local and in-transit recurrent melanoma? Ann Surg 2003;238(5):743–747
44. Mosterd K, Krekels GAM, Nieman FHM, et al. Surgical excision versus Mohs' micrographic surgery for primary and recurrent basal-cell carcinoma of the face: a prospective randomised controlled trial with 5-years' follow-up. Lancet Oncol 2008;9(12):1149–1156
45. Poulsen MG, Rischin D, Porter I, et al. Does chemotherapy improve survival in high-risk stage I and II Merkel cell carcinoma of the skin? Int J Radiat Oncol Biol Phys 2006;64(1):114–119
46. Tsang G, O'Brien P, Robertson R, Hamilton C, Wratten C, Denham J. All delays before radiotherapy risk progression of Merkel cell carcinoma. Australas Radiol 2004;48(3):371–375

47. Carucci JA, Martinez JC, Zeitouni NC, et al. In-transit metastasis from primary cutaneous squamous cell carcinoma in organ transplant recipients and nonimmunosuppressed patients: clinical characteristics, management, and outcome in a series of 21 patients. Dermatol Surg 2004;30(4 Pt 2):651–655
48. Gluck I, Ibrahim M, Popovtzer A, et al. Skin cancer of the head and neck with perineural invasion: defining the clinical target volumes based on the pattern of failure. Int J Radiat Oncol Biol Phys 2009;74(1):38–46
49. Galloway TJ, Morris CG, Mancuso AA, Amdur RJ, Mendenhall WM. Impact of radiographic findings on prognosis for skin carcinoma with clinical perineural invasion. Cancer 2005;103(6):1254–1257
50. Smith SP, Grande DJ. Basal cell carcinoma recurring after radiotherapy: a unique, difficult treatment subclass of recurrent basal cell carcinoma. J Dermatol Surg Oncol 1991;17(1):26–30
51. Chao CKS, Gerber RM, Perez CA. Reirradiation of recurrent skin cancer of the face. A successful salvage modality. Cancer 1995;75(9):2351–2355
52. Hernández-Machin B, Borrego L, Gil-García M, Hernández BH. Office-based radiation therapy for cutaneous carcinoma: evaluation of 710 treatments. Int J Dermatol 2007;46(5):453–459
53. Simmonds RH, Hopewell JW, Robbins ME. Residual radiation-induced injury in dermal tissue: implications for retreatment. Br J Radiol 1989;62(742):915–920
54. Marcil I, Stern RS. Risk of developing a subsequent nonmelanoma skin cancer in patients with a history of nonmelanoma skin cancer: a critical review of the literature and meta-analysis. Arch Dermatol 2000;136(12):1524–1530
55. Duprez F, Madani I, Bonte K, et al. Intensity-modulated radiotherapy for recurrent and second primary head and neck cancer in previously irradiated territory. Radiother Oncol 2009;93(3):563–569
56. Sulman EP, Schwartz DL, Le TT, et al. IMRT reirradiation of head and neck cancer-disease control and morbidity outcomes. Int J Radiat Oncol Biol Phys 2009;73(2):399–409
57. Kandamany N, Mahaffey P. Carbon dioxide laser ablation as first-line management of in-transit cutaneous malignant melanoma metastases. Lasers Med Sci 2009;24(3):411–414
58. Good LM, Miller MD, High WA. Intralesional agents in the management of cutaneous malignancy: a review. J Am Acad Dermatol 2011;64(2):413–422
59. Damian DL, Shannon KF, Saw RP, Thompson JF. Topical diphencyprone immunotherapy for cutaneous metastatic melanoma. Australas J Dermatol 2009;50(4):266–271
60. Clary BM, Brady MS, Lewis JJ, Coit DG. Sentinel lymph node biopsy in the management of patients with primary cutaneous melanoma: review of a large single-institutional experience with an emphasis on recurrence. Ann Surg 2001;233(2):250–258
61. Mack LA, McKinnon JG. Controversies in the management of metastatic melanoma to regional lymphatic basins. J Surg Oncol 2004;86(4):189–199
62. Lee RJ, Gibbs JF, Proulx GM, Kollmorgen DR, Jia C, Kraybill WG. Nodal basin recurrence following lymph node dissection for melanoma: implications for adjuvant radiotherapy. Int J Radiat Oncol Biol Phys 2000;46(2):467–474
63. Warso MA, Das Gupta TK. Melanoma recurrence in a previously dissected lymph node basin. Arch Surg 1994;129(3):252–255
64. Morton DL, Thompson JF, Kelly M, et al. MMAIT-IV Clinical Trial Group. Multicenter double-blind phase 3 trial of Canvaxin vs. placebo as post surgical adjuvant in metastatic melanoma. Presented at the Society of Surgical Oncology's 59th Annual Cancer Symposium, San Diego, California, 2006
65. Essner R, Lee JH, Wanek LA, Itakura H, Morton DL. Contemporary surgical treatment of advanced-stage melanoma. Arch Surg 2004;139(9):961–966, discussion 966–967
66. Hill GJ II, Krementz ET, Hill HZ. Dimethyl triazeno imidazole carboxamide and combination therapy for melanoma. IV. Late results after complete response to chemotherapy (Central Oncology Group protocols 7130, 7131, and 7131A). Cancer 1984;53(6):1299–1305
67. Atkins M, Lee S, Flaherty L, et al. A prospective randomized phase III trial of concurrent biochemotherapy (BCT) with cisplatin, vinblastine, dacarbazine (CVD), IL-2 and interferon-alpha-2b (IFN) versus CVD alone in patients with metastatic melanoma (E3695): an ECOG-coordinated intergroup trial. Proc Am Soc Clin Oncol 2003;22:708 Abstract 2847
68. Flaherty K, Pusanov I, Sosman J, et al. Phase I study of PLX4032: proof of concept for V600E BRAF mutation as a therapeutic target in human cancer. J Clin Oncol 2009;27(Suppl):9000 Abstract
69. Bauman JE, Eaton KD, Martins RG. Treatment of recurrent squamous cell carcinoma of the skin with cetuximab. Arch Dermatol 2007;143(7):889–892
70. Anasagasti-Angulo L, Garcia-Vega Y, Barcelona-Perez S, Lopez-Saura P, Bello-Rivero I. Treatment of advanced, recurrent, resistant to previous treatments basal and squamous cell skin carcinomas with a synergistic formulation of interferons. Open, prospective study. BMC Cancer 2009;9:262–274
71. Voog E, Biron P, Martin JP, Blay JY. Chemotherapy for patients with locally advanced or metastatic Merkel cell carcinoma. Cancer 1999;85(12):2589–2595
72. Garneski KM, Nghiem P. Merkel cell carcinoma adjuvant therapy: current data support radiation but not chemotherapy. J Am Acad Dermatol 2007;57(1):166–169
73. Bricca GM, Brodland DG, Ren D, Zitelli JA. Cutaneous head and neck melanoma treated with Mohs micrographic surgery. J Am Acad Dermatol 2005;52(1):92–100
74. Brown CD, Zitelli JA. The prognosis and treatment of true local cutaneous recurrent malignant melanoma. Dermatol Surg 1995;21(4):285–290
75. Lent WM, Ariyan S. Flap reconstruction following wide local excision for primary malignant melanoma of the head and neck region. Ann Plast Surg 1994;33(1):23–27
76. Moncrieff MD, Thompson JF, Quinn MJ, Stretch JR. Reconstruction after wide excision of primary cutaneous melanomas: part I-the head and neck. Lancet Oncol 2009;10(7):700–708
77. Bui DT, Chunilal A, Mehrara BJ, Disa JJ, Alektiar KM, Cordeiro PG. Outcome of split-thickness skin grafts after external beam radiotherapy. Ann Plast Surg 2004;52(6):551–556, discussion 557
78. Coit D, Ferrone C. Recurrent regional metastases of melanoma. In: Balch C, Houghton A, Soong S-J, Atkins M, Thompson J, eds. Cutaneous Melanoma. 5th ed. St Louis, MO: Quality Medical Publishing; 2009:487–498
79. O'Brien CJ, Petersen-Schaefer K, Ruark D, Coates AS, Menzie SJ, Harrison RI. Radical, modified, and selective neck dissection for cutaneous malignant melanoma. Head Neck 1995;17(3):232–241
80. Byers RM. Treatment of the neck in melanoma. Otolaryngol Clin North Am 1998;31(5):833–839
81. Gooris PJJ, Vermey A, de Visscher JGAM, Burlage FR, Roodenburg JLN. Supraomohyoid neck dissection in the management of cer-

vical lymph node metastases of squamous cell carcinoma of the lower lip. Head Neck 2002;24(7):678–683

82. O'Brien CJ, McNeil EB, McMahon JD, Pathak I, Lauer CS. Incidence of cervical node involvement in metastatic cutaneous malignancy involving the parotid gland. Head Neck 2001;23(9):744–748

83. Zablow AI, Eanelli TR, Sanfilippo LJ. Electron beam therapy for skin cancer of the head and neck. Head Neck 1992;14(3):188–195

84. Guix B, Finestres F, Tello JI, et al. Treatment of skin carcinomas of the face by high-dose-rate brachytherapy and custom-made surface molds. Int J Radiat Oncol Biol Phys 2000;47(1):95–102

18 Prognosis of Recurrent Head and Neck Cancer

R.J. Baatenburg de Jong, M.P. van der Schroeff

Summary

- Recurrence rates depend on initial tumor stage, localization, histological markers, treatment, and biomarkers and genomic markers.
- The occurrence and timing of recurrences influence prognosis heavily.
- Patients with recurrent head and neck cancer need updated prognostic information to balance the burden of the new treatment against the possible gain in life expectancy and quality of life.
- Dynamic, multivariate prognostic models could offer accurate and individualized estimates of prognosis in recurrent disease.

Introduction

Optimal counseling and treatment of patients with recurrent head and neck cancer require an accurate estimate of their prognosis. Patients need updated prognostic information to balance the burden of the new treatment against the possible gain in life expectancy and quality of life. In addition, they need to reorganize their lives and to adapt to the new situation. As clinicians we need prognostic information to assist our patients in these important decisions. In primary head and neck cancer, a lot of research is devoted to the identification of prognostic factors, and numerous papers on this subject are published every month. Unfortunately, information on determinants of prognosis in recurrent cancer is scarce. In this chapter we aim to present an overview of available information on this topic. In addition, we will present an instrument to integrate available information and the corresponding hazard ratios into an individualized prognosis for the patient with recurrent cancer.

Head and neck squamous cell carcinoma (HNSCC) invades locally and tends to metastasize to regional lymph nodes. Locoregional control is paramount in the optimization of disease-free and overall survival. To improve local and regional control in early-stage and locally advanced HNSCC, new treatment modalities have been developed and implemented. In recent years, for example, laser surgery, intensity-modulated radiation therapy (IMRT), chemoradiation, and biologics have been introduced. These changes in treatment modalities make recurrence rates over longer periods of time difficult to interpret. However, in general 15%–50% of all HNSCC patients will recur.[1–6] Recurrence rates depend on initial tumor stage, localization, histological markers, and treatment. In addition, tumor volume, biomarkers and genomic markers (such as DNA copy number variation and loss of heterozygosity) have been shown to be associated with recurrence of HNSCC.[7–9] Up to 50% of the patients who die from HNSCC have locoregionally recurrent disease as the sole site of failure.[10] Treatment options for locally recurrent disease are of course dependent on the extent of disease and previous treatment.

Prognostic Factors

Prognosis in head and neck cancer, but also in cancer generally, is based on characteristics known at the time of diagnosis. However, the prognosis is not static. During follow-up there are various factors that might change from the situation at diagnosis, such as age (obviously patients get older during follow-up), developing comorbidity (especially in comorbidity-prone patients such as head and neck cancer patients) and the occurrence of recurrences. Dynamic predictions of head and neck cancer survival can be done using conditional relative prognosis. We published the results of such an approach, which showed that the overall conditional relative prognosis of 7255 patients with primary HNSCC reached a plateau after approximately 4 years: long term HNSCC survivors exhibited a permanent 20%–25% excess mortality (compared with age- and sex-matched counterparts in the general population).[11]

The single most important event during follow-up is the occurrence and timing of local, regional, or distant recurrence. It is common knowledge that these adverse events greatly influence prognosis.[12] Little is published about the effect on actual survival and the natural course of recurrent head and neck cancer. Obviously, a study on the natural course of recurrent disease is unethical if treatment is considered beneficial. Most studies examine the effect of (novel) cytotoxic agents or salvage surgery. Effectiveness differs with patient selection (e.g., previous treatment, tumor localization). In 2000, Goodwin published a meta-analysis on salvage surgery in recurrent HNSCC.[13] It contained 32 published reports with 1080 patients from 28 different institutions. The weighted average of 5-year survival was 39%. No comparison can be made with a group of patients who refused treatment and therefore serve as a reflection of natural history. Goodwin also reported on a prospective review of 109 consecutive patients undergoing salvage surgery for the treatment of recurrent squamous cell carcinoma of the upper aerodigestive tract.[14] Survival time was strongly dependent on the TNM stage of recurrent disease at the time of surgical salvage and weakly dependent on the site of disease.

An (as yet unpublished) analysis of our own patients data is in line with the data published by Goodwin (**Table 18.1**). Our database consists of 2927 consecutive patients with a primary HNSCC, diagnosed between January 1980 and November 2006. Follow-up ranged from 0 to 319 months, with a median of 34 months. Overall 5-year survival was 50.2%. The number of recurrences and metastases during follow-up was 1087 (37.1%), occurring in 838 patients (**Table 18.1**). Glottic and oral cancer were associated with

Table 18.1 Cohort characteristics

	Cohort (n = 2927 patients)	Recurrence (n = 838 patients)	KM-estimatea 5-years	No recurrence (n = 2089 patients)	KM-estimatea 5-years
Sex (n,%)					
Female	707 (24)	199 (24)	30.0%	508 (24)	57.8%
Male	2220 (76)	639 (76)	30.2%	1581 (76)	60.0%
Age (mean, in years)	63	61		64	
Localization (n,%)					
Larynx, glottic	769 (26)	182 (22)	48.6%	587 (28)	74.1%
Larynx, supraglottic	351 (12)	110 (13)	34.2%	241 (11)	52.2%
Hypopharynx	269 (9.2)	99 (12)	9.80%	170 (8.1)	38.5%
Oropharynx	501 (17)	146 (17)	16.0%	355 (17)	48.3%
Nasopharynx	73 (2.5)	21 (2.5)	21.5%	52 (2.5)	67.0%
Oral cavity	557 (19)	190 (23)	25.3%	367 (18)	52.0%
Lip	224 (7.7)	31 (3.7)	62.8%	193 (9.2)	72.4%
Other	183 (6.3)	59 (7.0)	24.7%	124 (5.9)	50.5%
Initial treatment					
Surgery	550 (19)	127 (15)	41.3%	423 (20)	66.4%
Radiotherapy	1362 (46)	398 (47)	37.6%	964 (46)	61.3%
Surgery with radiotherapy	636 (22)	219 (26)	14.6%	417 (20)	67.2%
Radiotherapy with chemotherapy	186 (6.4)	65 (7.8)	21.4%	121 (5.8)	46.5%
Chemotherapy	19 (0.6)	9 (1.1)	–	10 (0.5)	–
Other treatments	174 (5.9)	13 (1.6)	–	154 (7.4)	70.6%
Time to local recurrence (mean, in months)	–	29	–	–	–
Time to regional recurrence (mean, in months)	–	47	–	–	–
Time to distant recurrence (mean, in months)	–	57	–	–	–

[a] Kaplan–Meier estimate: cumulative proportion surviving 5 years.

Table 18.2 Salvage rates

	1-year survival	2-year survival	5-year survival
Local recurrence	54%	41%	29%
Regional recurrence	38%	27%	14%
Locoregional recurrence	41%	25%	12%
Distant metastasis	13%	4.3%	1.8%

the highest incidences of recurrence, 22% and 23%, respectively. Interestingly, chance of surviving a recurrence of glottic cancer was nearly 50%, which is favorable compared with all other subsites, except recurrence of lip cancer. Five-year survival rate for a recurrence of lip cancer was as high as 62.8%.

These results are probably biased by treatment of the primary tumor: both early glottic and lip cancer may be treated by irradiation or limited surgery, providing the possibility of salvage treatment. Other subsites are more likely to have received multimodality treatment with limited possibilities for salvage treatment. Indeed, in our series of patients, 5-year survival rates of patients treated with single modality compared favorably with patients treated with a combination of radiation and surgery or radiation and chemotherapy (**Fig. 18.1**). In local recurrence, other predictors of survival, for example, tumor size and age, may play a role too (**Figs. 18.2 and 18.3**). Treatment of the index tumor, not the recurrence, influences treatment options when diagnosed with a recurrence.

These univariate survival analyses after the diagnosis of recurrence produce probable, but not definite, predictors of length of survival. Multivariate analysis would account for confounders but requires larger numbers of patients. Salvage rates are shown in **Table 18.2**.

■ Timing and Time-dependent Effects

In addition to the occurrence of recurrent cancer, its timing is of prognostic importance. Approximately 80%–90% of all recurrences will occur within the first 2–4 years after treatment with curative intent.[15,16] In general the prognosis for a group of HNSCC patients

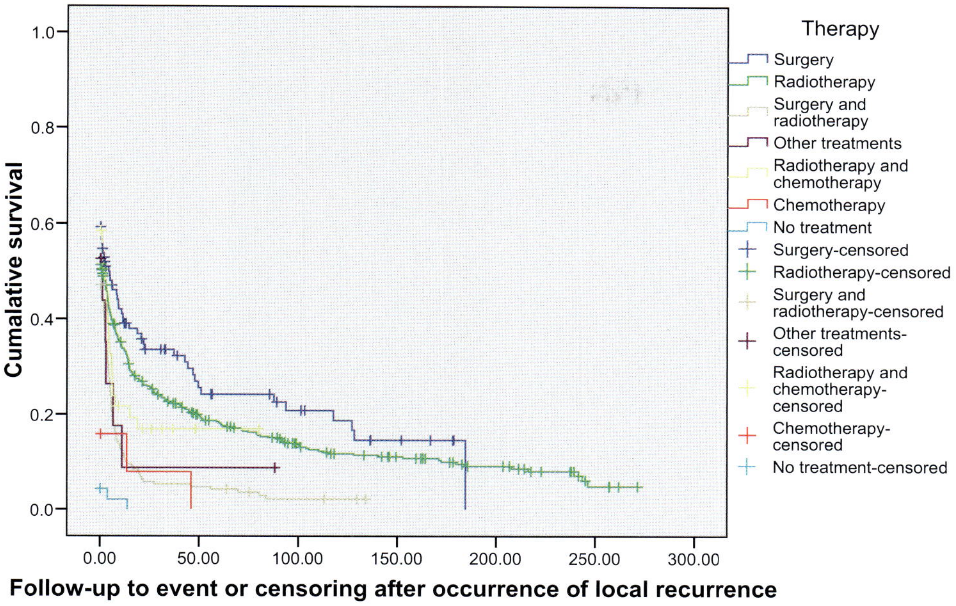

Fig. 18.1 Univariate survival analysis (Kaplan–Meier) on therapy, after occurrence of local recurrence.

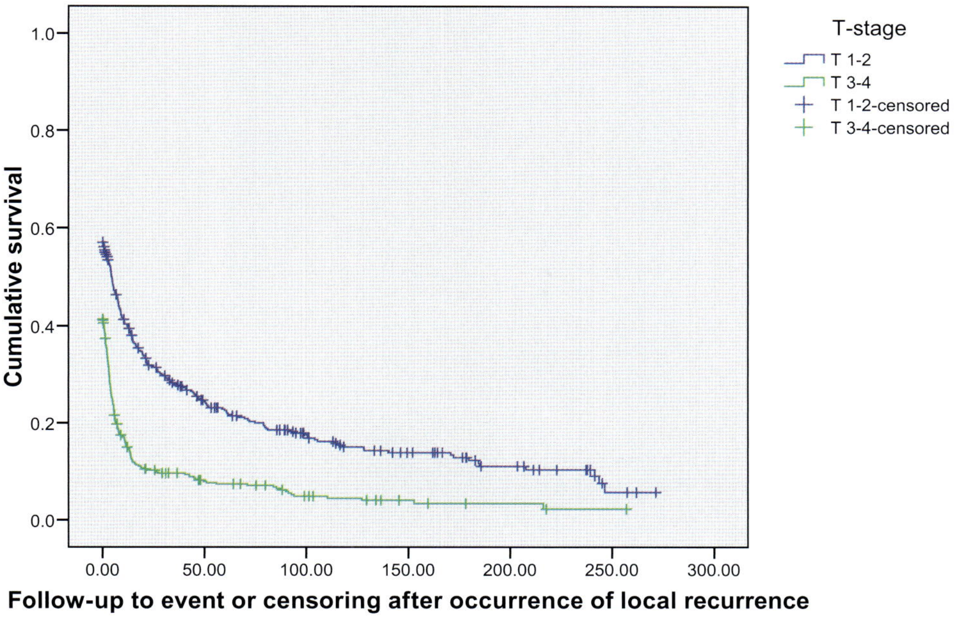

Fig. 18.2 Univariate survival analysis (Kaplan–Meier) on T-stage, after occurrence of local recurrence.

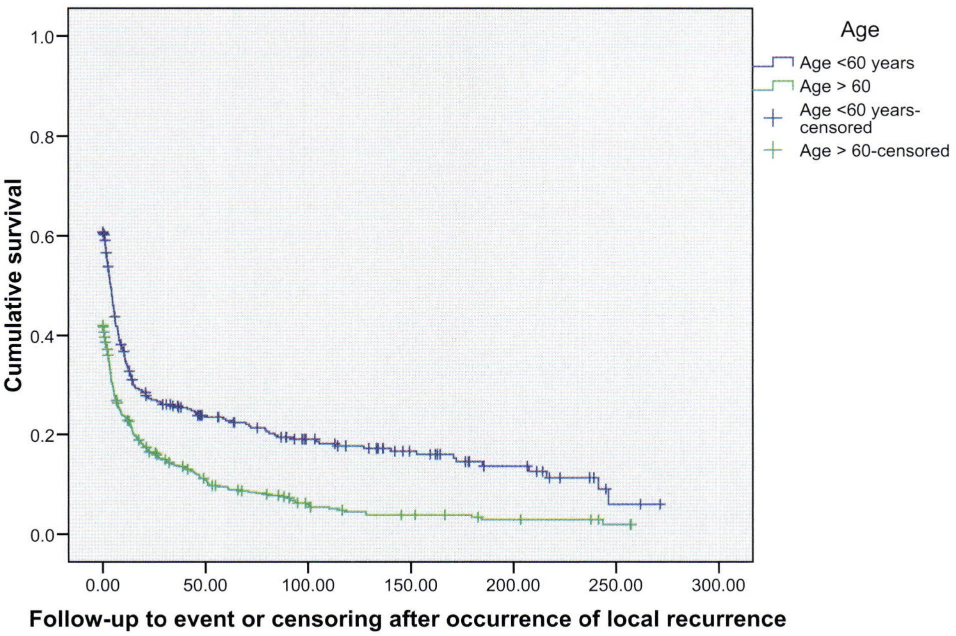

Fig. 18.3 Univariate survival analysis (Kaplan–Meier) on age, after occurrence of local recurrence.

improves after they survive the first few critical years after treatment of the index tumor. This is because patients with a very poor prognosis, possibly in the more advanced stages of the disease, die early, leaving those with relatively favorable prognosis.[11] At an individual level, early failures of control might reflect a more aggressive index tumor. In **Table 18.1**, the mean time to recurrence is shown for our cohort: 29 months for a local, 47 months for a regional, and 57 months for a recurrence at a distant site.

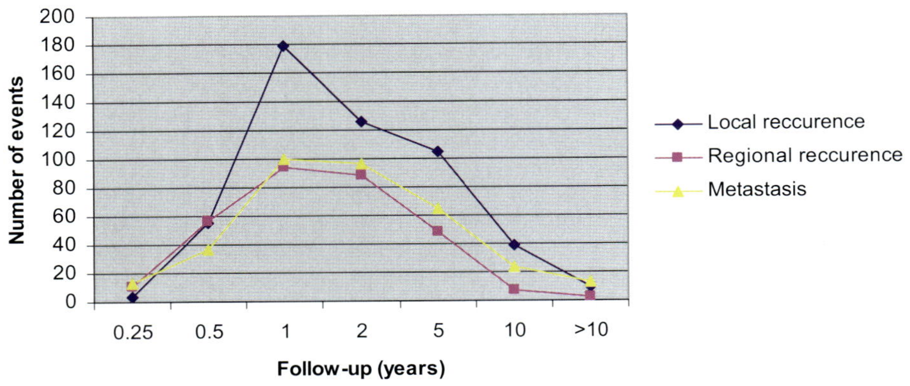

Fig. 18.4 Recurrence and metastasis during follow up.

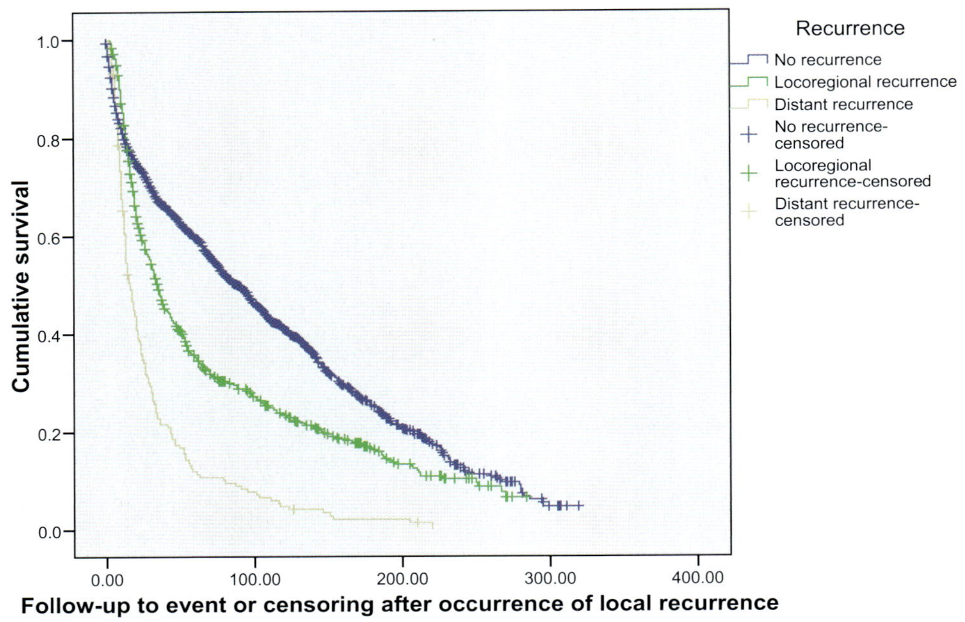

Fig. 18.5 Univariate survival analysis (Kaplan–Meier) on type of recurrence.

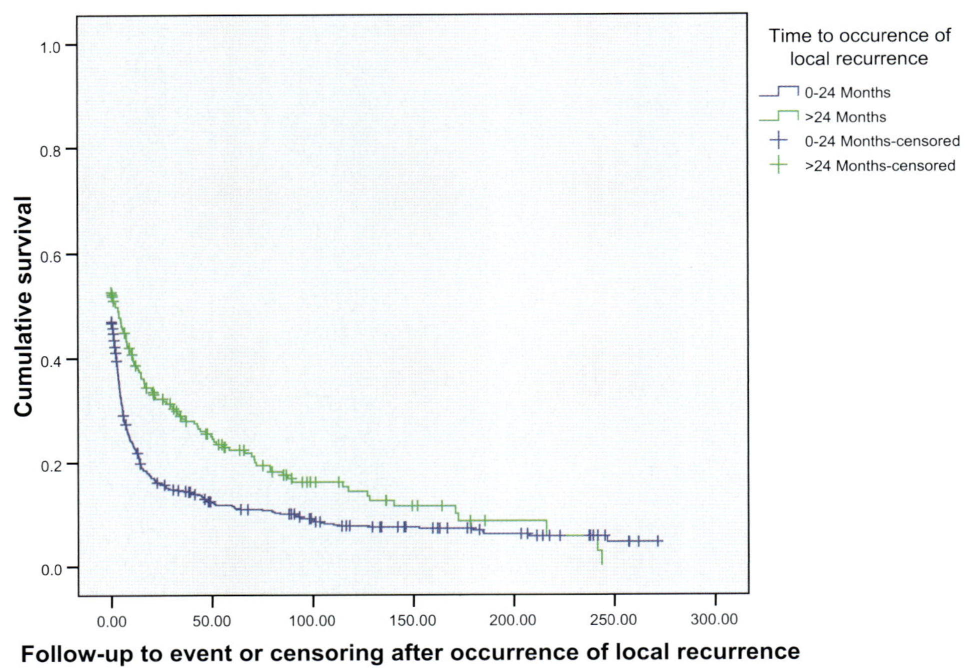

Fig. 18.6 Univariate survival analysis (Kaplan–Meier) on timing of recurrence.

Figure 18.4 shows the distribution of occurrences during follow-up. A steep curve is seen up to 1 year after treatment of the index tumor, which is followed by a gradual decline.

We performed a period analysis in which we studied those patients who had a recurrence and the predictors of length of survival after this diagnosis. **Figure 18.5** displays the effect on predicted survival of a locoregional or distant recurrence, the first showing a better prognosis. In **Fig. 18.6**, the difference in effect on survival between an early versus late local recurrence is illustrated, the latter showing better prognosis.

Individualized Prognosis in Recurrent HNSCC

A predictive model based on a multivariate analysis using the Cox proportional hazards model was built. To investigate follow-up time-dependent effects and to incorporate local and regional recurrences as well as delayed distant metastases, we produced further follow-up models at different time points after initial diagnosis and treatment.[17] This stepwise approach allows for dynamic predictions taking into account only those patients still alive at

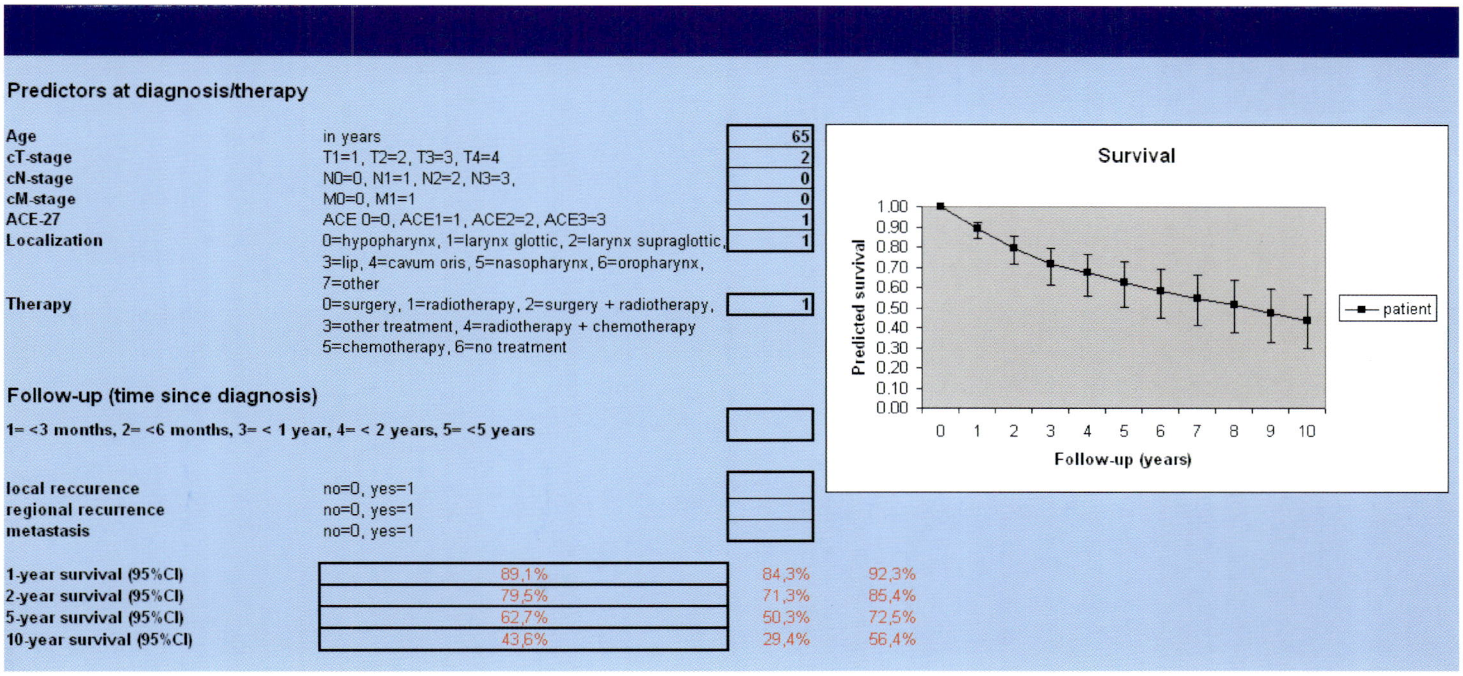

Fig. 18.7 Desktop interface showing survival estimates for a 65-year-old patient with mild comorbidity and a T2N0M0 glottic carcinoma, treated with radiotherapy. No follow-up data at this point in time.

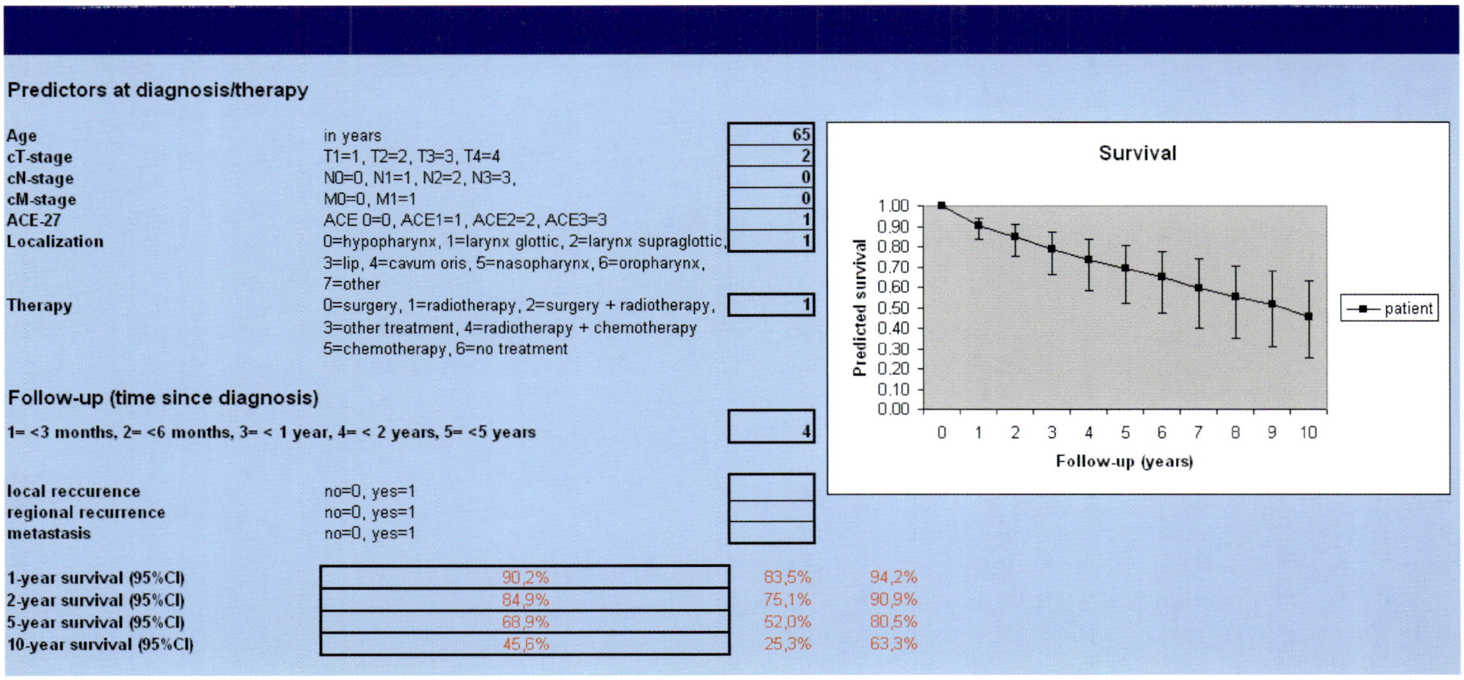

Fig. 18.8 Desktop interface showing survival estimates for a 65-year-old patient with mild comorbidity and a T2N0M0 glottic carcinoma, treated with radiotherapy. No recurrence up to 2 years of follow-up.

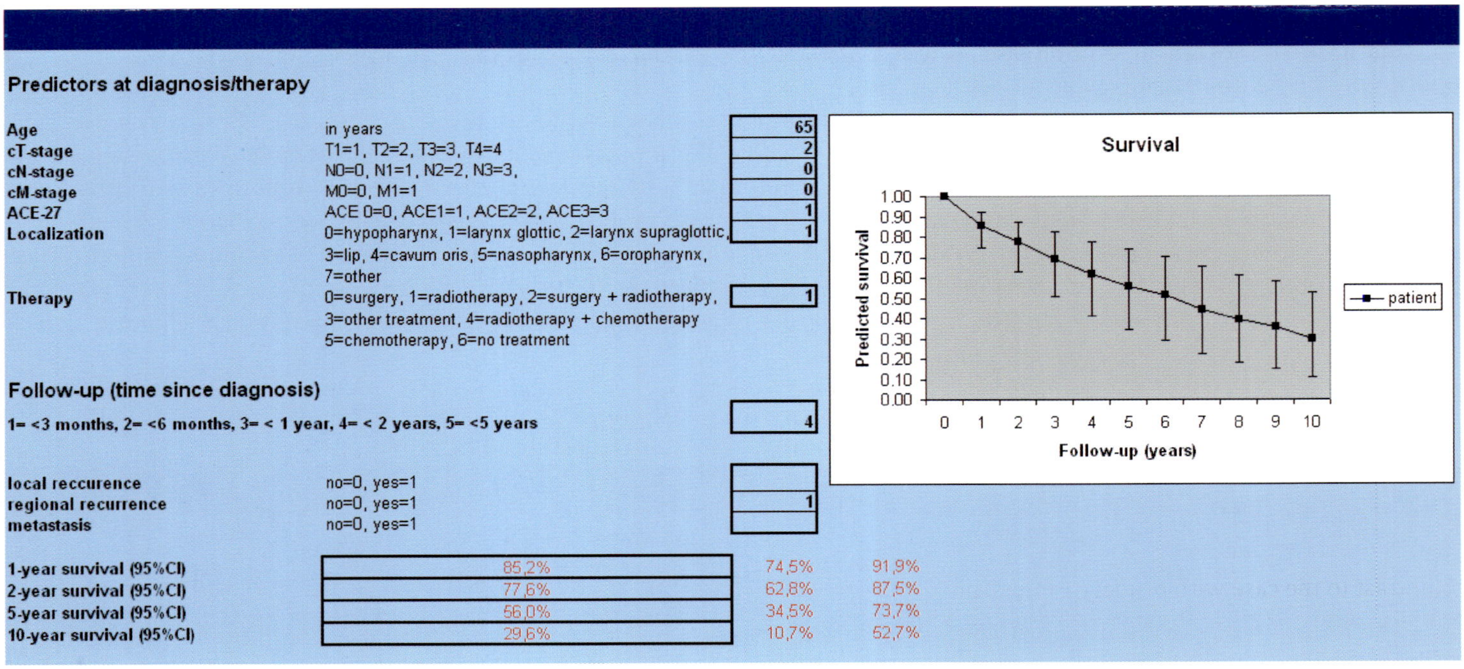

Fig. 18.9 Desktop interface showing survival estimates for a 65-year-old patient with mild comorbidity, a T2N0M0 glottic carcinoma, treated with radiotherapy, and a regional recurrence within 2 years of follow-up.

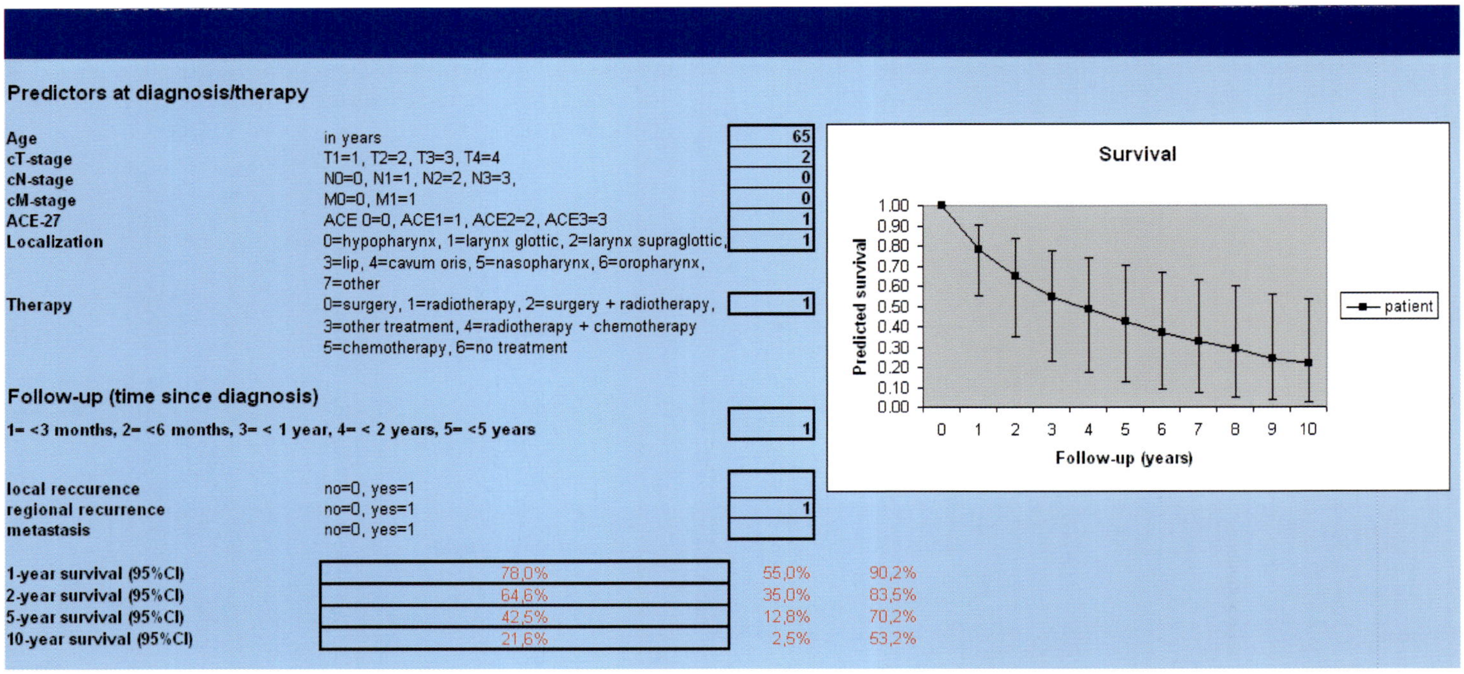

Fig. 18.10 Desktop interface showing survival estimates for a 65-year-old patient with mild comorbidity, a T2N0M0 glottic carcinoma, treated with radiotherapy, and a regional recurrence within 3 months of follow-up.

certain time points, the progression of age, and the occurrence of locoregional and distant recurrences. The final models were incorporated into a desktop interface (**Figs. 18.7–18.10**) For example: a 65-year-old patient with a T2N0M0 glottic laryngeal carcinoma treated with radiotherapy and known to have mild comorbidity (ACE-27[18] score 1) has an estimated 5-year overall survival of 62.7% (95% CI, 50.3%–72.5%). When still alive after 2 years of follow-up, the predicted 5-year overall survival increases to 68.9% (95% CI, 52.0%–80.5%). This improved predicted prognosis is caused by the survival of the first two critical years. On the other hand, the effect is muted by advancing age. If a regional recurrence has occurred after 2 years of follow-up, the estimated 5-year overall survival drops to 56.0% (95% CI, 34.5%–73.7%). If this particular patient had experienced an early recurrence (for example, within 3 months), the predicted 5-year overall survival would have been even worse (42.5%). The broad 95% confidence intervals indicate uncertainty of estimation, a question of power.

Routine Follow-up and Recurrent Disease

A Norwegian study on recurrence rates during follow-up showed the overall recurrence "pick-up rate" of 1 recurrence in 36 consultations.[15] This concerned 661 consecutive and previously untreated patients with confirmed squamous cell carcinoma of the head and neck, considered "free of disease" 6 weeks after the completion of the therapy. Ritoe et al. studied the effect of routine follow-up after treatment of laryngeal cancer on life expectancy and mortality.[19] Their simulation model showed only slight gains in life expectancy when discovering recurrences at an asymptomatic stage during routine follow-up compared with no follow-up. The lead time, estimated to be less than 2 months,[19,20] produced a gain in life expectancy in the range of 0.3 years to 1.5 years that decreased with advancing age. Routine follow-up therefore seems not very effective in the detection of recurrences. However, a very modest improvement of life expectancy may be expected.

Conclusion

In contrast to the case with primary tumors, prognostic research into recurrences is scarce. Commonly used adages on the detrimental effect of recurrences would benefit from more statistical foundation. In general, recurrences worsen prognosis; the earlier the recurrence, the worse the prognosis. Dynamic, multivariate prognostic models could offer accurate and individualized estimates of prognosis in recurrent disease.

Future Research

- External validation of prognostic models.
- Prospective research into the applicability and desirability of usage of prognostic models in daily practice.

Recommended Reading

- van der Schroeff MP, van de Schans SA, Piccirillo JF, Langeveld TP, Baatenburg de Jong RJ, Janssen-Heijnen ML. Conditional relative survival in head and neck squamous cell carcinoma: Permanent excess mortality risk for long-term survivors. Head Neck 2010;32(12):1613–1618. (Conditional relative survival estimates are dynamic by nature and show us the long-lasting effects of hazardous behavior such as smoking and alcohol abuse.)
- Goodwin WJ Jr. Salvage surgery for patients with recurrent squamous cell carcinoma of the upper aerodigestive tract: when do the ends justify the means? Laryngoscope 2000; 110(3 Pt 2, Suppl 93)1–18. (A well conducted meta-analysis of salvage surgery for recurrent head and neck cancer.)

References

1. Bourhis J, Le Maître A, Baujat B, Audry H, Pignon JP; Meta-Analysis of Chemotherapy in Head, Neck Cancer Collaborative Group; Meta-Analysis of Radiotherapy in Carcinoma of Head, Neck Collaborative Group; Meta-Analysis of Chemotherapy in Nasopharynx Carcinoma Collaborative Group. Individual patients' data meta-analyses in head and neck cancer. Curr Opin Oncol 2007;19(3):188–194
2. Brockstein B, Haraf DJ, Rademaker AW, et al. Patterns of failure, prognostic factors and survival in locoregionally advanced head and neck cancer treated with concomitant chemoradiotherapy: a 9-year, 337-patient, multi-institutional experience. Ann Oncol 2004;15(8):1179–1186
3. Bernier J, Domenge C, Ozsahin M, et al. European Organization for Research and Treatment of Cancer Trial 22931. Postoperative irradiation with or without concomitant chemotherapy for locally advanced head and neck cancer. N Engl J Med 2004;350(19):1945–1952
4. Cooper JS, Pajak TF, Forastiere AA, et al. Radiation Therapy Oncology Group 9501/Intergroup. Postoperative concurrent radiotherapy and chemotherapy for high-risk squamous-cell carcinoma of the head and neck. N Engl J Med 2004;350(19):1937–1944
5. Forastiere AA, Goepfert H, Maor M, et al. Concurrent chemotherapy and radiotherapy for organ preservation in advanced laryngeal cancer. N Engl J Med 2003;349(22):2091–2098
6. Hall SF, Groome PA, Irish J, O'Sullivan B. The natural history of patients with squamous cell carcinoma of the hypopharynx. Laryngoscope 2008;118(8):1362–1371
7. van den Broek GB, Rasch CR, Pameijer FA, et al. Pretreatment probability model for predicting outcome after intraarterial chemoradiation for advanced head and neck carcinoma. Cancer 2004;101(8):1809–1817
8. Chen Y, Chen C. DNA copy number variation and loss of heterozygosity in relation to recurrence of and survival from head and neck squamous cell carcinoma: a review. Head Neck 2008;30(10):1361–1383
9. Duffy SA, Taylor JM, Terrell JE, et al. Interleukin-6 predicts recurrence and survival among head and neck cancer patients. Cancer 2008;113(4):750–757
10. Hong WK, Bromer RH, Amato DA, et al. Patterns of relapse in locally advanced head and neck cancer patients who achieved complete remission after combined modality therapy. Cancer 1985;56(6):1242–1245
11. van der Schroeff MP, van de Schans SA, Piccirillo JF, Langeveld TP, Baatenburg de Jong RJ, Janssen-Heijnen ML. Conditional relative survival in head and neck squamous cell carcinoma: permanent excess mortality risk for long-term survivors. Head Neck 2010;32(12):1613–1618
12. Colevas AD. Chemotherapy options for patients with metastatic or recurrent squamous cell carcinoma of the head and neck. J Clin Oncol 2006;24(17):2644–2652
13. Goodwin WJ Jr. Salvage surgery for patients with recurrent squamous cell carcinoma of the upper aerodigestive tract: when do the ends justify the means? Laryngoscope 2000; 110(3 Pt 2, Suppl 93)1–18
14. Arnold DJ, Goodwin WJ, Weed DT, Civantos FJ. Treatment of recurrent and advanced stage squamous cell carcinoma of the head and neck. Semin Radiat Oncol 2004;14(2):190–195
15. Boysen M, Lövdal O, Tausjö J, Winther F. The value of follow-up in patients treated for squamous cell carcinoma of the head and neck. Eur J Cancer 1992;28(2–3):426–430
16. Ritoe SC, Krabbe PF, Kaanders JH, van den Hoogen FJ, Verbeek AL, Marres HA. Value of routine follow-up for patients cured of laryngeal carcinoma. Cancer 2004;101(6):1382–1389
17. van der Schroeff MP, Steyerberg EW, Wieringa MH, Langeveld TP, Molenaar J, Baatenburg de Jong RJ. Prognosis: a variable parameter. Dynamic prognostic modeling in head and neck squamous cell carcinoma. Head Neck 2011. Epub ahead of print. doi: 101002/hed.2169

18. Piccirillo JF, Tierney RM, Costas I, Grove L, Spitznagel EL Jr. Prognostic importance of comorbidity in a hospital-based cancer registry. JAMA 2004;291(20):2441–2447
19. Ritoe SC, de Vegt F, Scheike IM, et al. Effect of routine follow-up after treatment for laryngeal cancer on life expectancy and mortality: results of a Markov model analysis. Cancer 2007;109(2):239–247
20. Ritoe SC, Verbeek AL, Krabbe PF, Kaanders JH, van den Hoogen FJ, Marres HA. Screening for local and regional cancer recurrence in patients curatively treated for laryngeal cancer: definition of a high-risk group and estimation of the lead time. Head Neck 2007;29(5):431–438

19 Rehabilitation after Treatment for Recurrent Head and Neck Cancer

Alison Perry, Julia Maclean

Summary

- Rehabilitation is integral to each head and neck (H&N) cancer patient's care; it is not an "add on" once treatment is completed.
- Refer early, and refer well, to key members of the supportive care team.
- Establish clear, comfortable communication with a patient/family members and the key staff in a supportive care team.
- Many unpleasant sequelae of H&N cancer treatments can be well managed (**Table 19.1**).
- Identify the needs of significant others, as well as the patient, and ensure these are addressed.
- Supportive care needs to be provided across the care pathway, from a patient's initial presentation to cancer services, through treatment, to survivorship/palliation.

Introduction

Effective management of people with H&N cancer(s) involves a skilled multidisciplinary team of professional staff who can offer supportive care to the cancer patient and their family. Although most cancer supportive care teams are based at a cancer unit, staff members may undertake home visits and/or see patients outside that unit where necessary.

It is important for successful continuity of care that people who develop a recurrent cancer feel confident and comfortable with the members of the supportive care team, which usually comes after some months—or even years—of regular contact. It may seem clichéd to state this but, for successful supportive care, patients and their families need to feel that they are *known* and *understood*, not just seen as a series of symptoms and/or walking tumor stages.

In a busy outpatient cancer clinic it is sometimes difficult to engender a supportive atmosphere, which is when a H&N cancer-specific, experienced member of a supportive care team may make a positive difference.

A Supportive Care Team

Head and neck cancer is a complex disease with physical, psychological, economic, legal, vocational, social, ethical, and spiritual implications for the individual, the health-care system, and society as a whole.

It must be managed by a highly skilled team that will include medical oncologists, surgeons, radiation oncologists, diagnostic radiologists, neurologists, palliative care physicians, dentists, pharmacists, speech pathologists, dietitians, psychologists, psychiatrists, social workers, nurses, physiotherapists and occupational therapists, as well as, sometimes, clergy and cancer survivor volunteers.[1]

A team-based approach provides continuity through the cancer patient's care, which includes screening and prevention, diagnosis, staging, treatment, supportive care, rehabilitation, palliative care, home care, and (possibly) hospice care.[1]

A recent UK audit of H&N cancer patients[2] showed that 93% of people were reviewed by a multidisciplinary team (MDT), which was an improvement on previous data, but the National Institute of Clinical Excellence (NICE) guidelines state that 100% of cases should be thus reviewed, so some work in this area remains to be done.

Rehabilitation Needs of Patients with Recurrent Cancer

Approaches to Assess Unmet Needs

The World Health Organization recognizes "health" as a multidimensional concept and includes in its classification (The International Classification of Functioning, Disability, and Health, or ICF), the components of body structures and functions (Impairment Level), and functioning in daily life from both individual (Activity Limitation), and societal (Participation Restriction) perspectives.[3]

The ICF may be used to classify the key presenting problems that patients are concerned about across Impairment, Activity and/or Participation health domains. It is desirable to add to these a fourth domain—Well-being/Distress, assessed from a patient and family perspective.

However, applying this ICF classification to patients may present a challenge. In their recent paper, Sanson-Fisher et al.[4] describe the difficulty in eliciting cancer patients' perceptions of their need for help, and this may especially be the case with H&N cancer patients. H&N cancer is predominantly a disease of males, who typically have lower medical consultation rates than females for all symptoms and so may present late to treatment; many find it difficult to express their psychosocial needs, especially when confronted with a tumor recurrence and the implications of further treatment (or not).

Most attempts to ascertain cancer patients' needs has come from what Samson-Fisher et al.[4] term a "top down" approach, whereby the health professionals take responsibility for determining patients' needs. This usually demands the use of psychological tests to determine whether a patient is depressed, anxious, or has other psychological concerns that need attention. Some of the standardized tests commonly used for assessment include the Hospital Anxiety and Depression Scale,[5] the Depression, Anxiety and Stress Scale,[6] the Brief Symptom Inventory,[7] and the Beck Depression Inventory.[8] Such standardized tests do not, however,

Table 19.1 Impairments and their management (with their evidence base)

Disorder	Notes/management advice	Level of evidence[a] (reference)
Dysphagia	Undertake a *pretreatment* VFSS for formal diagnostic assessment. Prior swallowing function has been shown to be the best predictor of subsequent posttreatment swallowing outcomes	Level 2b[18]
Odynophagia	Diet modification (use of soft, "slidy" foods)	Level 5[19]
	Adherence to scrupulous oral hygiene	Level 2b[27]
Mucositis	Use of benzydamine mouth rinse reduces mucositis in H&N patients having radiotherapy	Level 2a[26]
	Chamomile tea reportedly has anti-inflammatory effects and promotes mucosal healing so may be used for prevention of mucositis	Level 2c[22]
	Benzydamine (Difflam C) has been shown to reduce mucositis pain in patients undergoing radiotherapy	Level 5[23]
Xerostomia	Regular sipping of tap water Use of lanolin-based lip balm	Level 2b[27]
	Sugar-free gels or lozenges may help stimulate saliva in people with suppressed production	Level V5[28]
	Sialogogues are effective in the presence of functional residual salivary gland tissue	Level 2a[27]
Thick, sticky saliva	Patients use steam inhalations to hydrate the oropharynx and/or gargle with mild effervescent antacids or water with salt and soda	Level 5[23,28]
Dysgeusia	High-dose zinc supplementation may be useful in treating dysgeusia. (A recent double-blind placebo trial has refuted this, however)	Level 2B[29]
	Meticulous mouth care, treatment of xerostomia. and dietary modification have been shown to improve disturbances of taste	Level 5 (http://www.cancersupportivecare.com/oral.html)
Trismus	TheraBite mobilization device to increase jaw mobility	Level 5[31]
Communication	Teach the use artificial larynges or other augmentative communication aids for assisting communication	Level 5[35]

[a] Ranked using the NHS R&D Centre for Evidence Based Medicine's Levels of Evidence classification.

take into account a patient's views about their well-being or their willingness to accept treatment.[4]

An alternative, "bottom up," approach[4] acknowledges the need to involve patients in decision making about their own care and well-being. In this model, the cancer patient has equal "expert" status, alongside the health-care professionals, and therefore has a choice about whether or not to seek assistance. This is in line with the concept of patient-centered care, but it has disadvantages—for example, some patients may not be aware of being depressed, so may not seek help; and/or they may not be aware of the availability of effective interventions.[4]

In most H&N cancer units, a hybrid approach is increasingly accepted whereby a screening tool is used to first ascertain those deemed at risk, and then a clinical assessment follows in which the cancer patient is encouraged to decide which problems they want to have specifically addressed. This is important, both for clearly determining the needs of the patient and for involving them in their own symptom management. The best outcome occurs when each patient is treated as an autonomous person—not managed as a walking tumor with a person attached!

Scales and Questionnaires

Only limited work has been undertaken to develop questionnaires that document the unmet needs of people with advanced cancer and of those who are terminally ill (and they were not specifically developed with H&N cancer patients). Among these is a scale devised by Rainbird et al.,[9,10] *The Needs Assessment for Advanced Cancer Patients* that was developed after a literature review and professional consensus. Seven domains are covered—psychological/emotional; medical information/communication; social; symptom; daily living; spiritual needs; and financial needs.

Similarly, only recently has there been an attempt to identify the unmet needs of significant others, such as partners, relatives, or friends. *The Support Persons' Unmet Needs Survey*[11] has 76 items on a self-report scale. It is used to measure the unmet needs of the primary support person of a cancer survivor. Six factors are identified: informational needs; personal and family concerns; emotional and mental health issues; medical care needs; concerns about the future; and emotional support.[11]

An alternative, *The Cancer Survivors' Partners' Unmet Needs* measure, is a 35-item scale covering five factors: relationships; information; partner issues; comprehensive care; and emotional support.[12] This scale has been shown to have high internal consistency and good convergent validity but only moderate test–retest reliability. Many scales in current clinical use have not been subjected to rigorous psychometric testing and/or have been developed either for one cancer population, or in one country, so caution is needed when considering their use/validity in a different setting.

Influence of Unmet Needs on Outcomes

There is ongoing work by researchers to examine whether high unmet needs scores predict future outcomes.[3] For example, do high scores on unmet needs measures predict that patients will have depression, or that they will use more emergency medicine or supportive care services?

When cancer recurs, it is often experienced as more traumatic than at the first diagnosis, which reinforces the importance of periodic screening of patients for distress throughout the cancer journey, including the survivorship phase.[13]

It is common for people with H&N cancer to adopt a "positive attitude" in the belief that this may contribute to longer survival. For some patients, this strategy may confer a sense of control and optimism, but for others it represents a burden, especially if there is pressure (which may be subtle) to avoid discussing and confronting issues. "The belief that one's force of will and attitude can influence the course of cancer poses a burden if the cancer recurs, with an implication that the person has not tried hard enough."[2,13]

Researchers in Australia have found several issues that are specific to people from culturally and linguistically diverse (CALD) backgrounds, which may be a source of additional distress.[13]

For example, in some Chinese, Greek, and Arabic communities, cancer is perceived as incurable, with the connotation of "certain" and "imminent" death, so that it is a source of stigma that should be kept private in families. In some parts of the Greek and Chinese communities, cancer is believed to be contagious.[14–16]

Many people from CALD communities, especially if they have difficulty in both written and oral language, have difficulty in navigating a Western health-care system, and in understanding the (sometimes subtle) nuances of, for example, "treatment with a palliative intent." This may result in patients having difficulty when making informed decisions about treatments and/or using supportive care services.

There may be occasions where a surrogate decision-maker will need to be consulted, if a patient is deemed not to be competent in decision making or does not have the requisite cognitive or language skills to fully consent to proposed treatment/intervention.

Understanding the context in which a patient is operating and living is critical to establishing clear, comfortable communication between the patient and key members of the care team. This, in turn, is likely to result in a more successful engagement of the patient with decisions about their treatment—which is not approached as "one size fits all." Rather, a tailored approach should be taken with each patient, understanding their reality, their fears and concerns, and trying to address these with empathy and respect. We need a strong evidence base upon which to develop culturally appropriate policies and practices, to improve the well-being of people with recurrent cancer.

Symptoms and Their Management

There are many unpleasant and uncomfortable symptoms that occur as sequelae of H&N cancer treatment, regardless of whether surgery, radiation, chemotherapy or multimodal approaches are used as the primary treatment. Treatment of a recurrent tumor may be associated with more severe acute symptoms and, for those salvaged successfully, with long-term side effects.

Impairments may include, but are not limited to, *dysphagia* either resulting from mechanical problems (due to limited/no movements of oral structures) or due to *odynophagia*. Dysphagia often coexists with *mucositis* or *xerostomia*. Other swallowing-related problems include *cachexia*, *dysgeusia*, *trismus*, and *osteoradionecrosis*.

Communication (speech or voice) problems may include:

- Dysarthria (reduced control of motor function resulting in slurred speech that may, at times, be unintelligible)
- Dysphonia (hoarse, husky voice)

For postlaryngectomy patients, a recurrent tumor may mean an inability to use their previously satisfactory communication aid or their tracheoesophageal voice prosthesis (see Exemplary Case Studies). Such reduced communication may mean isolation and frustration for a patient and/or for their close others, so this is an urgent symptom to address.

Some of the above impairments can, fortunately, be well managed. However, many interventions have little or no evidence base to support their effectiveness. This situation has arisen because of the proliferation of small studies that lack the power to adequately evaluate interventions. Few studies have been replicated, and successive studies often have different interventions, populations or outcomes, making aggregation of data and/or assessment of quality very difficult. The recommendations for best practice are therefore mainly level C and D recommendations, unless stated otherwise (**Table 19.1**).

The impact of the above impairments (**Table 19.1**) on other health domains—activity, participation, and well-being (ICF-WHO)[3]—can be profound. Often, when swallowing becomes difficult and meals take much longer to eat, food becomes a trial instead of a pleasure. In countries such as Australia and the UK, where so much socialization revolves around food, this can negatively impact on the social dynamics of patients and their families. Patients with dysphagia may feel embarrassed when eating in public, so they will withdraw and become reclusive. This results in isolation and a diminishing of psychological well-being/quality of life—not only for patients, but also for their partners and families.

Australian Therapy Outcome Measures

The Australian Therapy Outcome Measures (AusTOMs)[17] are valid and reliable sets of scales for assessing the health domains (ICF-WHO) of individual patients.[3] The various scales are designed for use in physiotherapy, occupational therapy, and speech pathology practices. All three sets were designed and validated in the context of Australian health care.[3]

The AusTOMs are not measures of QoL, nor of general health; rather, they are tools for assessing change over time, usually in patients who are undergoing an episode of therapy.

The Speech Pathology set of the AusTOMs has a Swallowing Scale that includes three of the ICF domains—Impairment; Activity Limitation; and Participation Restriction—with a fourth domain added: Distress/Well-being. Rating of a patient is made by a clinician across each of the speech pathology's four health domains, matching the patient to written descriptions. Each domain is rated independently, from 0, representing "complete" difficulty to 5 representing "no" difficulty. The AusTOMs are quick and easy to use and have demonstrated good psychometric properties.[17] The Swallowing Scale of the AusTOMs is for the assessment of any person with dysphagia—it was not specifically designed for H&N cancer patients—but it is widely used in Australia with this population.[18]

Dysphagia

Signs and Symptoms

Marked dysphagia may mean that a patient cannot eat in public, or needs to use alternative feeding via a gastrostomy or a nasogastric (n-g) tube that will limit their eating in cafes or restaurants. This, in turn, reduces their activity and social participation and may result in changes to family meals and to social dynamics.

Diagnostic

Dysphagia should be examined using a videofluoroscopic swallowing study (VFSS), which is the clinical standard for assessment of swallowing. The standard VFSS protocol has been well described[19,20] and is now in use in many centers worldwide.

Regardless of etiology (whether from original surgery, radiotherapy, combined treatment, or a tumor recurrence), a patient with a recurrent cancer and dysphagia needs to have a thorough diagnostic examination, not just a screening test of aspiration/penetration of a liquid or semisolid bolus. The cause of a patient's dysphagia should be ascertained using a diagnostic evaluation. For example, if aspiration occurs, the exact point in the swallow sequence when this happens (before, during, or after the triggering of the swallow reflex) should be noted, and then a hypothesis generated about *why* aspiration is occurring at that time. A VFSS is the only instrumental assessment that enables such a precise diagnosis to occur.

Risk Factors

Of concern, in the recent audit of H&N cancer patients,[2] pretreatment dietetic and speech pathology assessments were reportedly higher than in earlier reports, but still "represented a small number of cases."[2] This is despite a recent publication in which, using multiple regression analysis, previous swallowing function was shown to be the best predictor of subsequent posttreatment swallowing outcomes in a prospective cohort of 81 patients.[18]

It is important to establish baseline functional status (speech, swallowing, pain, etc.) when patients present with recurrence, so that any changes may be attributed to treatment and morbidity from such therapies can be properly documented and audited. It is only in this way that informed consent to treatment can be provided, once patients know what are the expected treatment outcomes and side effects.

Management

Management of dysphagia should include trials of any/all direct or indirect therapies that are deemed to be suitable during the VFSS. This may include altering the consistency of food and/or liquids to reduce aspiration, changing head/neck posture, or teaching "safer swallowing" maneuvers. Any positive change to swallowing safety can be documented, then used in therapy while the VFSS is kept for future comparison. The baseline study provides an objective record of the patient's swallowing at that point in their cancer treatment, against which any future changes can be compared. The involvement of a dietitian is important at this stage, to ensure that nutritional needs are being met while a patient combats their recurrent cancer.

■ Odynophagia

Odynophagia is caused by irritation of the mucosa and usually occurs during, or immediately after, radiotherapy treatment. It can result in a lack of appetite and marked weight loss, as swallowing becomes very painful.

Management

Management of odynophagia may involve using an oral lubricant, such as a salad oil or grape seed oil, rinsed around the patient's mouth before eating. This can enable them to swallow more easily, so that swallowing small amounts of viscous ("slidy") foods, such as small pieces of tinned fruit, spoons of yoghurt or of ice cream, can be commenced. In cases with marked weight loss because of painful swallowing, nonoral feeding (via the use of a gastrostomy or nasogastric tube) should be instigated for the patient's hydration and nutritional needs to be met. The involvement of a dietitian is essential at this stage for advice about initiating and maintaining nonoral feeding. It is important that oral hygiene is always scrupulously followed, to clean and buffer the oral cavity, avoiding any infection from accumulated food debris.

■ Mucositis

Mucositis is a painful condition in which the lining of the mucous membrane of the mouth and throat is inflamed. In 1998, the Joanna Briggs Institute for Evidence Based Nursing and Midwifery in South Australia published an evidence-based information sheet for health professionals, "Prevention and treatment of oral mucositis in cancer patients."[21] Updated evidence-based guidelines for the prevention and treatment of mucositis were also published by the American Cancer Society in 2007.[22]

Management

Management of mucositis presents a significant problem for many H&N cancer patients treated with (chemo)radiotherapy. The emphasis should be on pain relief, so that swallowing and oral comfort can be promptly reestablished.

Chamomile tea reportedly has anti-inflammatory effects and promotes mucosal healing[23] so this may be legitimately suggested for the prevention and treatment of early mucositis.

Usually, during and after (chemo)radiotherapy treatment, a staged approach to managing a patient's mucositis is used. First a mouthwash mixed with water may be gargled throughout the day. Clinically, benzydamine (Difflam C) has been noted to reduce mucositis pain in patients undergoing radiotherapy.[24] Second, viscous xylocaine (5 mL four times a day), can be swallowed (it may be mixed with 5 mL mucaine). Third, 0.5% cocaine mouthwash (5–10 mL rinsed around the mouth and gargled four times a day). Last, 1 mL Nilstat can be swilled and swallowed four times a day. Alongside this regimen, systemic analgesia is essential for effective pain relief.[24]

Analgesia is also applied in a stepwise fashion. First, soluble acetaminophen (1 g four times a day) is used; then panadine forte (acetaminophen and codeine phosphate) ; then morphine elixir (2 mg/mL, starting 4 mL × 4 hourly, then 2 mL as required and titrate). Last, MS contin (controlled-release morphine sulfate) suspension (30 mg is the lowest available dose) is given, and then the morphine elixir may be increased by 30%–50% every 24 hours as required.[25]

Cryotherapy, using ice chips for 5 minutes prior to using fluorouracil (5-FU) and for a further 25 minutes following administration, can reduce mucositis in patients receiving chemoradiotherapy,[26] except in those who have a continuous infusion of 5-FU or with serums that have a long half-life.[22] Frequent sipping of salt and baking soda (½ teaspoon each in a cup of water) cleans and soothes sore mucosa.[25]

■ Xerostomia

Xerostomia and its treatment have been well reviewed by Guijarro Guijarro et al.[27] Ionizing radiation can cause irreversible damage to the salivary glands, and the severity of hypofunction is directly related to the radiation dose involved. These authors state that if salivary secretion has ceased 5 weeks after radiotherapy, it rarely recovers, so the importance of using parotid-sparing radiotherapy techniques needs to be emphasized.[27]

Signs and Symptoms

Despite a lack of salivary secretions, a patient's sense of profound oral dryness can diminish over a period of 1–12 months, partly as a result of compensatory hypertrophy of nonirradiated gland tissue and, in part, due to their tolerating, and adjusting to, the continued sensation of oral dryness.[27]

In addition to oral dryness, xerostomia can manifest itself as an alteration to speech, or as a swallowing difficulty (especially of dry foods), or a taste alteration (dysgeusia) with a reportedly metallic taste, or itching/burning when eating spicy foods.

Oral infections, such as candidacies, can occur from xerostomia, with fissures or ulceration of the corners of the mouth and a sensation of burning or itching of the tongue. Halitosis (due to food stagnation), dental caries (due to promotion of plaque formation), and salivary gland swelling and/or pain may also occur.[27]

Management

Management of xerostomia includes regular sipping of tap water, using a lanolin based balm or lubricant to moisten the lips, and the "swishing and rinsing" of grape seed oil (or a flavorless salad oil) around the oral cavity to alleviate a dry mouth.[28]

Where a degree of salivary gland function remains, then stimulation by chewing of gustative (taste-intensive) substances should be encouraged.[26] Sugar-free chewing gums, gels, or lozenges can be recommended,[26] or, if there is no mucositis or other confounding factors, foods that require severe mastication (such as carrots and celery) may be used several times a day.

Acidic beverages and lemonades should be avoided, as they stimulate dental demineralization. A salt and baking soda mouthwash (½ teaspoon each, dissolved in a cup of water) neutralizes acidity. This can be gargled and dissolves thick, sticky oral secretions,[26] giving relief to patients with xerostomia.

Sialogogues are systemically administered drugs that stimulate saliva secretion, but they are only effective in the presence of functional residual salivary gland tissue.[27]

Saliva substitutes—"artificial saliva," such as the proprietary formulations Mouth Kote, Biotene or Aquaea—provide palliative therapy, with varying degree of success, for patients whose salivary gland function is lost. These substitutes are available as liquid solutions, aerosol sprays, gels, or tablets and can be used as often as needed throughout the day, being retained in the mouth for a period of time. An artificial saliva solution can, in fact, easily be made, consisting of 20 mL of a 4% methylcellulose solution, 10 mL of glycerin, a drop of lemon oil, and sufficient saline solution to prepare a final volume of 90 mL.[27]

Milk has been proposed as a saliva substitute[27] as it lubricates dehydrated mucosa and it neutralizes oral acids, reduces enamel solubility, and can contribute calcium and phosphorus to a patient's diet. New methods and devices continue to be trialed and developed in an attempt to secure a more effective management of xerostomia, and the interested reader is directed to the review by Guijarro Guijarro et al.[27]

Thick, Sticky Saliva

Signs and Symptoms

The presence of *thick, sticky saliva* may give a feeling of a persistent "frog in the throat" or result in constant throat-clearing or debilitating bouts of coughing. Patients may also have poor saliva control (due to reduced lip closure or poor oral control) and so may prandially aspirate saliva.

Management

The management can be assisted by the patient using regular daily steam inhalations (thus "artificially" hydrating the oropharynx and larynx) and/or by them gargling with mild effervescent antacids or water with salt and baking soda.[26]

Hydrating dry atmospheres (such as occurs when air conditioning or central heating is being used) by use of a humidifier or regular nebulized saline, or by simply placing saucers of water around a room, can be helpful in reducing atmospheric dryness. Keeping well hydrated (directly, by daily drinking plenty of water and indirectly, by adding moisture to the surrounding home or work atmosphere) helps to reduce a patient's production of thick, sticky saliva.

Dysgeusia

Dysgeusia is a sensory disturbance of taste, which may occur following chemotherapy and/or radiotherapy. The mechanisms of this dysfunction are complex and may result from the direct effects on acinar cell function and/or conditioned food aversions. Changes in salivary function are thought to contribute further to this condition. Hypogeusia (partial loss of taste) or ageusia (complete loss of taste) may occur secondarily to direct injury to taste buds from radiation and/or chemotherapy agents. Usually, recovery of taste occurs 4–6 months following completion of treatment as taste buds regenerate; however, complete recovery may not occur.

Management

Management of dysgeusia has included high-dose zinc supplementation. It has been suggested that this aids in the recovery of taste, although a recent phase III trial has not supported this proposition.[29] Treatment of xerostomia and meticulous oral hygiene may decrease dysgeusia during treatment and in the recovery phase.

Trismus

Signs and Symptoms

Trismus ("lockjaw") is a prolonged tonic spasm of the muscles of the jaw and, in extreme cases, this may mean a patient is unable to open their mouth wide enough to be able to insert a spoon or fork of food. Jaw excursion is very painful, making mastication difficult or impossible.

Management

Management of trismus includes the instigation of jaw exercises from the beginning of cancer treatment. This can help to keep the range of jaw movement usable for speech and swallowing.[30] If trismus has become established, one of the simplest interventions is to use a stack of tongue depressors, placed one on top of another, and begin by sliding two along the patient's molar ridge or gum line (if edentulous), between the mandible and maxilla, and then insert a third between the two. Hold these for as long as the patient finds comfortable, and then gradually increase the number of tongue depressors that can be tolerated in the stack. In this way, a greater degree of jaw opening is encouraged and the jaw is gradually pushed open until a suitable stage is reached for mastication and swallowing to occur.

There are commercial devices such as TheraBite, which is a stretching device that act is a similar way to improve mandibular mobility after composite surgery or after radiotherapy treatments. In one small study, using six repetitions of holding the mouth open with TheraBite for six seconds, six times daily, the mean change in maximal inter-incisor opening in five patients who had undergone midline mandibulotomy improved, from a mean of 30 mm to 40 mm, over 12 weeks post surgery.[31]

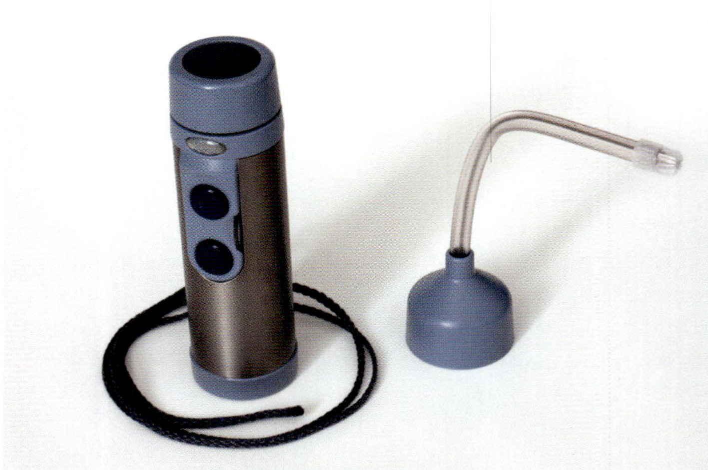

Fig. 19.1 A Servox communication aid. (Image courtesy of St. George Hospital, Helen Phelan, Kogarah [Sydney], NSW, Australia 2010.)

Osteoradionecrosis

Osteoradionecrosis is a particularly difficult problem that results in pain and can give difficulty in both speech and swallowing.

Data from one paper have shown an overall incidence of 8.2% and a 3-fold higher incidence for men than for women.[32] Osteoradionecrosis was most commonly located in the body of the mandible. Concerning the risk factors, a negative influence was shown for advanced tumors, segmental resections of the mandible, radiation dose, and pre/postradiation tooth extractions. Tooth extractions were found to be responsible for 50% of all cases.[32]

Management

Treatment includes hyperbaric oxygen and aggressive surgery, used in a progressively staged manner for "complete resolution of osteoradionecrosis,"[33] but the use of hyberbaric oxygen treatment (HBO) remains controversial, with some clinicians fearing it could exacerbate tumor growth.

In one recently reported study, mice underwent a fractionated course of radiotherapy that simulated the dose used to treat cancer in the mandible and, one week following the completion of radiotherapy, one half of the total animals underwent a 4-week course of HBO. Two animals were sacrificed from each group at 4 week intervals until 36 weeks.

Histological sections of their tissue clearly showed continued growth of teeth and maintenance of specialized tissues, such as salivary glands and bone, in the treated group compared with the nontreated group. Thus, HBO did not revive dead or dying tissue that lay within the field of radiation; rather, it simply revascularized the hypoxic tissue. This experimental model, the authors state, provides preliminary evidence of "HBO being effective in reducing the long-term side effects of radiation to normal tissue."[34]

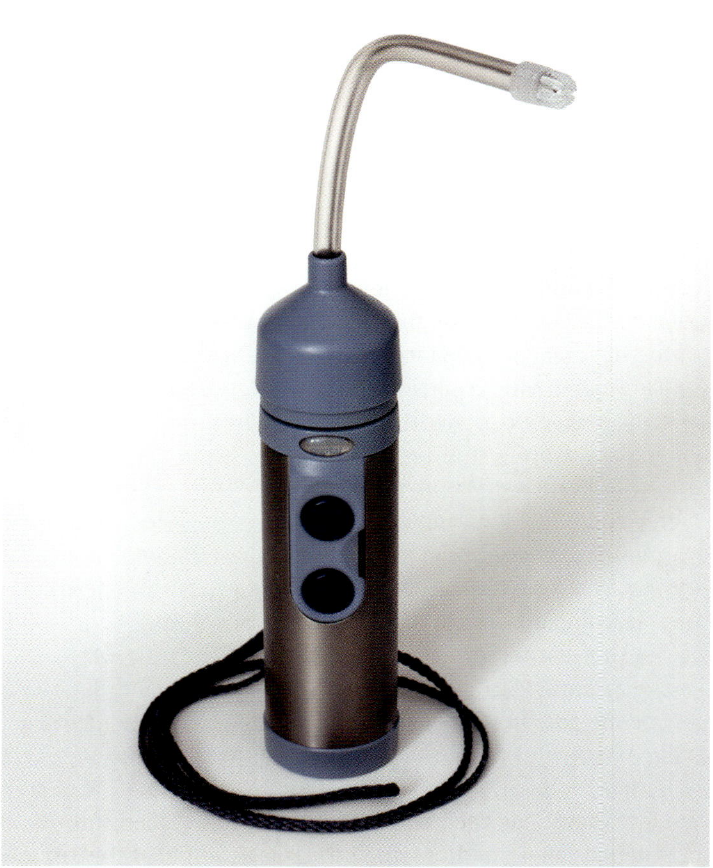

Fig. 19.2 A Servox aid with intraoral adaptor fitted (Image courtesy of St. George Hospital, Helen Phelan, Kogarah [Sydney], NSW, Australia 2010.)

Communication Difficulties

Communication can be a major problem for patients who have a recurrent cancer. This may be directly due to a motor speech problem, for example, if the nerve supply to any of the articulators is affected by the recurrent tumor, or if a recurrent tumor impacts on a laryngectomy patient's stoma, thereby eliminating their ongoing use of a voice prosthesis (see Exemplary Case Studies).

However, reduced communication may also be due to comorbid depression or anxiety. This needs to be established and, if present, treated with psychological support (counseling), medication, or both. Counseling may involve assistance for the family, as well as for the patient.

There are many alternative and augmentative communication systems available, and a speech pathologist will be able to assist with assessment of a patient's needs and then recommend/provide the most suitable communication aid. Artificial larynges, commonly used by laryngectomy patients, consist of either a pneumatic (lung-powered) system, such as the Tokyo pneumolarynx,[35] or an electronic (battery-driven) type of aid. The latter may be either an intraoral device, such as the Cooper-Rand[35] or a transcervical (neck type) communication aid, such as the Servox (**Fig. 19.1**).

Many neck-type artificial larynges, such as the Servox, have an intraoral adaptor, which is useful if a patient reaches a stage where they cannot place an aid against their neck tissues, due to soreness and/or discomfort. In this way, they continue to use a "familiar"

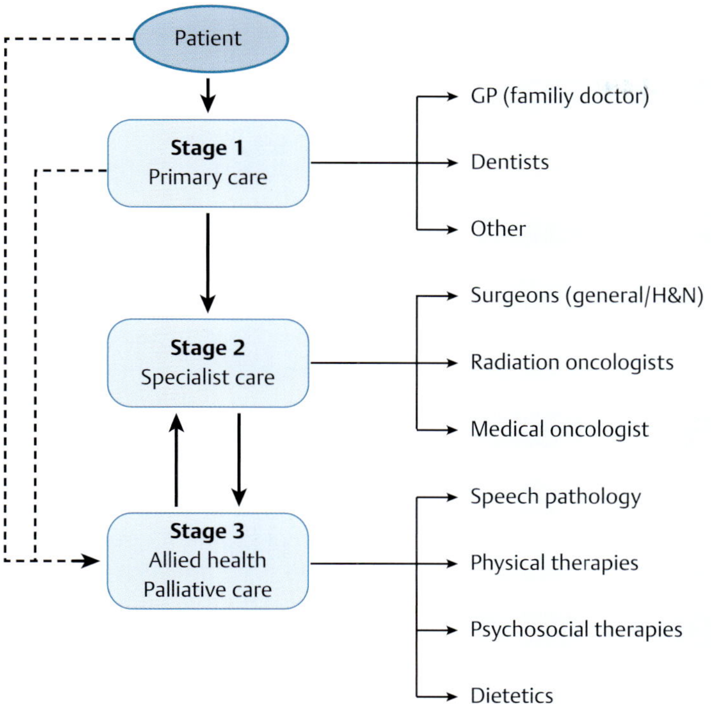

Fig. 19.3 A model of supportive care pathways for people with head and neck cancer.

communication aid, simply moving the placement of the vibratory source from transmission through the neck tissues to transmission inside the oral cavity, via its tube adaptor[35] (**Figs. 19.1 and 19.2**).

There are many sophisticated communication aids available, offering computerized written systems or synthesized speech that is "spoken" from written text input. However, the reality is that most H&N cancer patients are older men, most of whom are not highly computer-literate. At a time when they need to communicate, while facing very confronting issues of morbidity and mortality, it may not be desirable for them to be spending their precious time learning how to use a complex communication system.

For this reason, writing (where the patient is literate) may well be the communication mode of choice. In this case, it is important to *give the patient time* to get their message across, to *be patient* while waiting for them to complete the writing of messages, and then to read the message back and *discuss its contents*, reinforcing the fact that it has been read and understood. A plentiful supply of notepads, pens, and/or wipe boards is essential at this time.

This may be a very frustrating and distressing time for families, patient, and staff but it is essential to keep the lines of communication open, so that patients feel supported, "heard," and understood by staff and families.

Supportive Care Services; "Surviving Survivorship"

Facing issues of morbidity and mortality is confronting for all concerned, but distress may be eased when staff ensure that the surrounding atmosphere is supportive and comforting for both the patient and the family. There is an increasing recognition that cancer survivors require continued care, beyond diagnosis and treatment.[36]

We do not currently have good data about how and when best to support patients and families who are undergoing H&N cancer treatments or who are living with the aftermath and symptom burden of their treatment. It is, however, likely that many people are unaware of services on offer and therefore may not receive timely help in such a way that they might benefit.

Much work remains to be done to examine survivorship and the common concerns of head and neck cancer patients and families. A more developed model of supportive care needs to be developed along the care continuum as, currently, once patients complete their cancer treatment it is often difficult for them to access ongoing care, especially when living in very rural or remote areas of Australia or the UK.

Figure 19.3 profiles a "typical" model of supportive care pathways for people who are undergoing head and neck cancer treatment; allied health assistance is sometimes not offered until stage 3 (post treatment).

It has been suggested that a full review of psychological and adjustment issues should be incorporated into an optimal model of survivorship care.[4] Psychological interventions and allied health assistance may improve symptoms as they arise or recur, and these should be discussed as part of tailored care. Unfortunately, all too often, the delivery of survivorship care is fragmented and inconsistent, which adds to the survivorship burden for patients and families.

Greater development of new initiatives, such as clear care plans, screening tools, education and training programs, and the development of evidence-based guidelines, is crucial to improving the care provided to this population.[36]

The Cancer and Rehabilitation Workforce Project in the UK went online in 2010.[37] The website (www.cancer.nhs.uk/rehabilitation) links the reader to a series of rehabilitation intervention care pathways that are evidence based, one of which is for patients with H&N cancer. This is the culmination of over 3 years of work by the NHS National Cancer Action Team, examining evidence for intervention from dietetics, occupational therapy, physiotherapy, speech pathology, and lymphodema practitioners.

In addition to the clear review of evidence for rehabilitation, several barriers were identified that inhibit the delivery of good-quality rehabilitation services. One of the more salutary barriers is a "misconception of rehabilitation as something additional, but not integral, to the patient's" care, making rehabilitation not valued by patient's or professional groups."

The overview report on the website indicates the extent of this project as, for example, 1405 references were initially sourced, using strict criteria of including only prospective intervention studies (one-group studies, trials, or randomized controlled trials), or systematic reviews including such studies. Of these, 174 were relevant and only 80 pieces of evidence were used for the final report.

Further work is underway to incorporate the specification and metrics into the UK's cancer commissioning toolkit and guidance for commissioners. Rollout of the H&N care pathway continues across the NHS Cancer Networks in England and Wales into 2012 and beyond.

Exemplary Case Studies

Rehabilitation after Surgical Therapy

Patient History and Examination

Charlie, at 67 years old, presented to his ENT surgeon following a 4-week history of hemoptysis and increased shortness of breath on exertion. He had undergone radiotherapy 2 years previously for a T2N0M0 SCC of the right (R) vocal fold. Charlie is married, lives with his wife, and has three adult children. He is a retired builder with a 50-year history of smoking a pack of 20 cigarettes a day, and drinking 60–70 g ethanol daily. His mother died of lung cancer at 55 years of age, and his father died of a brain tumor at 60 years of age.

Investigations

The ENT clinical evaluation revealed a recurrent tumor on the (R) vocal cord extending to the subglottis. The (R) vocal fold was noted to be fixed and there was some decreased movement of the (L) vocal fold. Staging procedures, including a CT scan, chest radiograph, and biopsy, were performed. Charlie proceeded to surgery.

Management Plan

Charlie had a total laryngectomy and primary voice restoration. He recovered well following surgery and a Blom-Singer low-pressure voice prosthesis was inserted on the tenth postoperative day. He obtained excellent voice with his prosthesis, and quickly became independent in managing it. Charlie was reviewed following his surgery by the multidisciplinary H&N team.

Twelve months after surgery, he presented to the speech pathologist for routine follow-up. During this visit, he reported that his voice prosthesis had become more difficult to insert and, when changing it, he had noticed some bleeding.

On assessment, his voice via the prosthesis was noted to have decreased slightly in loudness and bleeding was observed when the prosthesis was changed in the clinic. There appeared to be some mucosal changes adjacent to the voice prosthesis at the tracheoesophageal puncture (TEP) site.

The ENT surgeon reviewed him and undertook a biopsy, which revealed a stomal recurrence.

Following discussions with Charlie and his wife, palliative chemotherapy was commenced. At this time, the speech pathologist inserted a Blom-Singer indwelling voice prosthesis to decrease any trauma that might occur from regular changing of the original voice prosthesis. As the loudness of his voice fluctuated, Charlie was also given a Servox artificial larynx to use (see **Fig. 19.1**). He was taught how to place the Servox against the skin of his neck, but he did not like the mechanical sound of this battery-operated device. Charlie was reviewed regularly by the speech pathologist during his chemotherapy treatment. His voice prosthesis worked intermittently, but this remained his preferred method of communication. He was encouraged to practice and become proficient with the Servox, in case his voice prosthesis failed and he needed to use the telephone in an emergency.

Three months following the completion of his chemotherapy, he returned to the speech pathologist to report that he had noticed intermittent leaking from the voice prosthesis when he drank fluids (**Fig. 19.4**). An ENT evaluation confirmed that the tumor had increased in size, and there was destruction of the stomal tissue around the voice prosthesis. Charlie was adamant that he still wanted to use his voice prosthesis as his primary method of communication.

An indwelling voice prosthesis was modified, using increased diameters of the tracheal and esophageal flanges, to provide larger, more tightly adherent surfaces, to prevent the likelihood of leakage of fluids around the prosthesis (**Fig. 19.5**). This modified prosthesis was hand-folded into the Blom-Singer gel-cap insertion system to prevent any trauma on insertion.

This modification worked well and Charlie continued to use his prosthesis to speak. At this time, Charlie was finding it increasingly difficult to swallow soft foods, secondary to compression of the pharynx and esophagus from the recurrent tumor. Following a review by the dietitian, he was commenced on high-protein oral fluid supplements. Charlie was never able to speak well using his prosthesis after drinking, as a result of marked pharyngeal pooling. During these times, he used his Servox to communicate with his wife. With encouragement from his wife and the speech pathologist, Charlie slowly became more accepting of his "mechanical voice" as it gave him an efficient method of communicating. In the subsequent 4 months Charlie continued to deteriorate physically until he was admitted to a hospice for palliative care. At this time, he was more reliant on his Servox (see **Figs. 19.1 and 19.2**) for communication, as his stoma had become very tender as a result of extensive tumor growth.

Charlie said he often felt hungry, but he was experiencing worsening dysphagia, which he found distressing. Following discussions with Charlie, his wife, and the ENT surgeon, the speech pathologist recommended removing the indwelling voice prosthesis to insert a

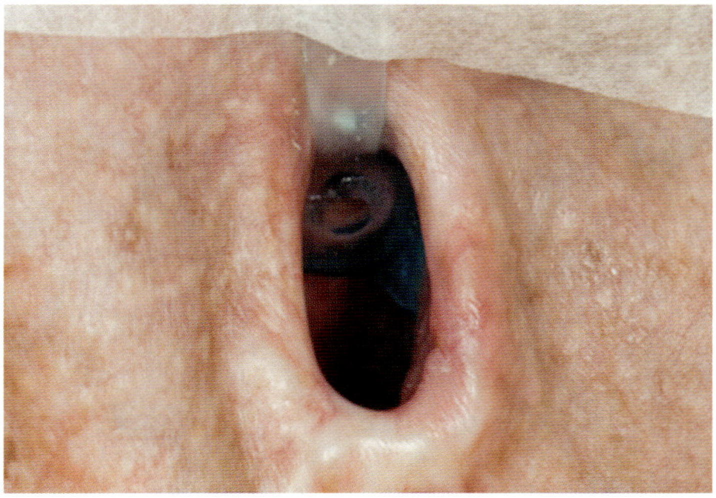

Fig. 19.4 Leakage of liquids from around a voice prosthesis, visualized by adding blue food coloring to a liquid bolus.(Image courtesy of Royal Darwin Hospital, Kara Burns, Royal Darwin Hospital, Darwin NT, Australia 2010.)

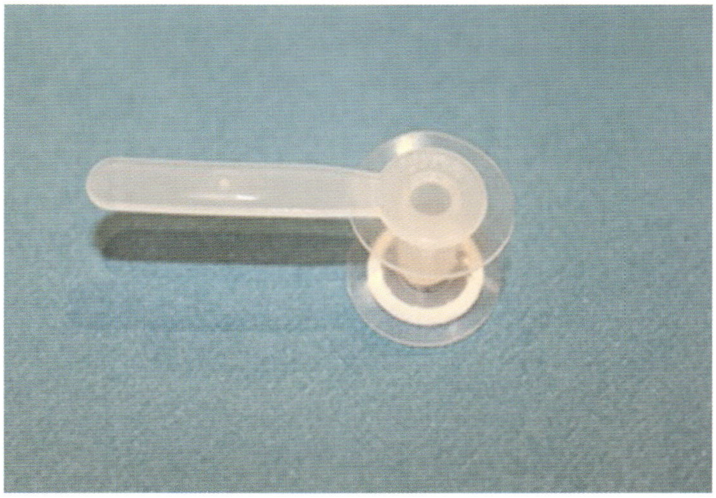

Fig. 19.5 Indwelling Blom–Singer prosthesis modified with increased tracheal and esophageal flange diameters. (Image courtesy of Main Medical Pty Ltd, Church Point, NSW, Australia 2010)

tracheogastric feeding tube through the TEP site, allowing feeding to bypass the tumor site and thus alleviate Charlie's hunger.

The feeding tube was inserted and Charlie continued to receive medications and liquid food supplements through this tube as he desired/needed.

During this time, Charlie continued to use his Servox to communicate. However, as he became progressively weaker, he tended just to mime words to his wife, who endeavored to lip-read and interpret his utterances. As a result of further tumor extension, Charlie's breathing became more difficult and the palliative care consultants reviewed his medications. He slowly became less alert and died peacefully at the hospice two days later, with his wife present.

■ Rehabilitation after Radiotherapy

Patient History and Examination

Max, aged 54 years, presented to the head and neck multidisciplinary team (H&N MDT) with an 8-week history of discomfort in the region of his right tonsillar fossa. He was married and lived with his wife; they had a married daughter who was supportive and lived nearby. Max currently worked at manufacturing sheepskin bedding underlays, and had been in the textile industry for the past 30 years. He had a 30-year history of smoking 10 cigarettes a day and consuming 40–50 g ethanol daily. He ceased smoking at the time of his cancer diagnosis. His mother was alive and well, his father died of a myocardial infarction at 62 years. There was no reported family history of malignancy.

His general practitioner (GP) had recently assessed him and prescribed 7 days of antibiotics and throat lozenges. When reviewed by his GP, there had been no improvement to his symptoms and he reported some right-sided otalgia. At that time he was referred to an ENT surgeon, after which an examination under anesthesia and biopsy of the right tonsil were undertaken.

Investigations

CT of his head and neck region and a chest radiograph were also performed. The CT revealed some fullness of the right side of the hypopharynx, extending to the margin of the epiglottis, but his chest radiograph was clear. The biopsy confirmed a squamous cell carcinoma, which was staged as T2N0M0 SCC (R) tonsil.

Management Plan

Max underwent definitive radiotherapy receiving a cumulative dose of 70 Gy in 35 fractions to the primary site and 50 Gy in 25 fractions to his ipsilateral neck. He tolerated his treatment well, suffering only from mild odynophagia, which was relieved with soluble acetaminophen (paracetamol) and a topical anesthetic agent. His weight remained stable throughout his treatment and he did not require any enteral nutrition to supplement his oral intake.

Max was seen, following radiotherapy, by the ENT surgeon and a radiation oncologist. He remained disease-free, with a stable weight. At the fifth anniversary of his initial treatment, the ENT surgeon noticed some mucosal changes on Max's soft palate.

A biopsy revealed carcinoma in situ and this was treated definitively with carbon dioxide laser ablation. The following year, during routine follow-up, a biopsy of the (L) retromolar trigone revealed carcinoma in situ. Max underwent repeat biopsies and, 12 months later, an invasive SCC was identified in this area.

At the second visit to the H&N MDT, it was recommended that he should undergo surgical excision involving a (L) paramedian mandibulotomy, excision of the tumor, and reconstruction using a radial forearm free flap. This was conducted the following month, and he then underwent radiotherapy to the operative bed, receiving 60 Gy in 30 fractions. During his treatment, he tolerated a soft moist diet and normal fluids with a minimal odynophagia, requiring soluble acetaminophen only. He remained well, and attended his follow-up appointments diligently.

At his 12-month follow-up, Max was noted to have marked xerostomia and trismus, so the speech pathologist recommended he use a TheraBite to improve his jaw opening.[31] It was further observed that his weight had decreased by 2 kg from his last clinic appointment, 3 months previously. He stated that he was still able to manage his normal diet at this time.

At his next clinic appointment, some 3 months later, his jaw opening was a little improved but his weight had decreased by a further 6 kg to 52 kg. He reported a gradual increase in symptoms of dysphagia, and having difficulty initiating a swallow. He reportedly required foods to be cut into very fine pieces; he was not experiencing any difficulty with swallowing fluids, and had no signs of aspiration. At this time a videofluoroscopy swallowing study (VFSS) was performed to assess Max's oropharyngeal swallowing function and to ascertain whether any therapeutic maneuvers might improve his swallowing efficiency.

VFSS Findings

A speech pathologist and radiologist together undertook a VFSS. Max was seated throughout the procedure; and swallowed 3 mL each of undiluted liquid barium, puree, soft fruit pieces, and bread. Lateral and anteroposterior (A-P) views were recorded.

- **Oral phase:** There was adequate lip seal, mastication of solid food, and good oral bolus manipulation. Max held the bolus anteriorly in his oral cavity, after which a delay in the initiation of the swallow and piecemeal deglutition was observed. There was no post-swallow residue seen in the lateral sulci or on the tongue surface.
- **Pharyngeal phase:** The swallow was effortful in nature and there was significant pharyngeal residue noted following all swallows. Max required 3–4 swallows to clear a small bolus. Decreased hyolaryngeal excursion was observed and there was one episode of silent penetration of a liquid bolus during the swallow (**Fig. 19.6**). An instructed cough was effective in clearing the penetrated material from the laryngeal vestibule. The pharynx appeared to be "crowded" with extensive edema. The appearance of a long hypopharyngeal stricture and poor relaxation of cricopharyngeus muscle was noted, resulting in significant pharyngeal residue and slow transit of all boluses into the esophagus (**Fig. 19.6**). Bread remained in the left vallecula despite multiple swallows (**Fig. 19.7**) and Max required water to clear the bolus. The residual material was noted to be symmetrical in A-P view.
- **Therapeutic maneuvers:** There is (level 3) evidence to support the use of certain therapeutic maneuvers to improve swallowing following treatment for head and neck cancer.[38] It is recommended that all such maneuvers be assessed during a VFSS to assure their clinical effectiveness.[38]

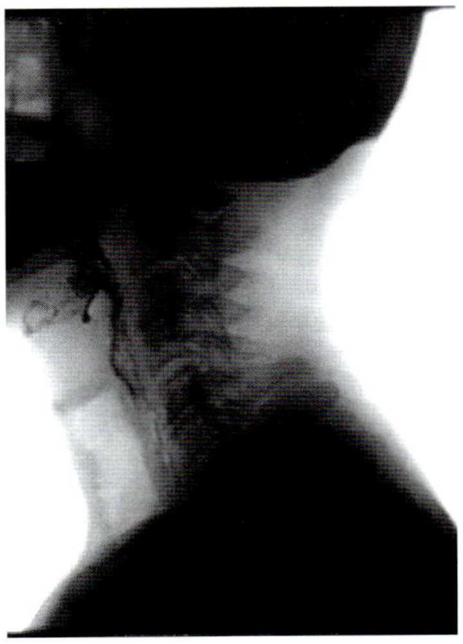

Fig. 19.6 Lateral radiograph, showing laryngeal penetration with liquids, diffuse pooling in the pharynx, and generalized pharyngeal edema.

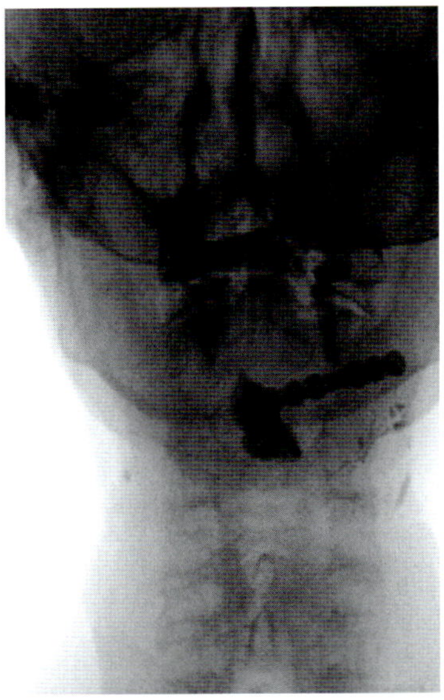

Fig. 19.7 A-P radiograph, displaying bread bolus remaining in vallecula following a swallow and (L) mandibular fixation plate.

During Max's VFSS, his three most significant impairments were:

- Poor clearance of a bolus through the pharynx
- Decreased hyolaryngeal excursion
- Laryngeal penetration of liquids

An effortful swallow and a Mendelsohn maneuver were applied[20] to assist bolus clearance and to improve Max's hyolaryngeal excursion. A Mendelsohn maneuver requires a patient to voluntarily "hold" their larynx for several seconds at its maximum height of excision, thereby prolonging the duration of cricopharyngeal opening.

A super-supraglottic swallow (designed to close the airway entrance before and during the swallow) was used to improve Max's airway protection. A Mendelsohn maneuver has been shown to be an effective therapeutic maneuver for people who demonstrate poor laryngeal elevation (and consequent risk of aspiration) after H&N cancer treatment.[38] This maneuver was, indeed, effective in reducing the amount of residual bolus material in the pharynx following Max's swallows. He practiced this strategy in the clinic with the speech pathologist.

Dilation of the cricopharyngeus and pharyngeal strictures/webs is widely used, with clinical evidence (level 5) of improvement. However, the true effectiveness of dilation has not been scientifically examined, as all available data are from uncontrolled studies.[39]

The results of the VFSSs were explained to Max. A modified soft diet and use of nutritional supplements were recommended in addition to using the effortful swallow and the Mendelsohn maneuver. Regular assessments with a dietitian were arranged, as it was likely that Max would require a gastrostomy tube for long-term enteral nutrition if his weight continued to decrease.

Max was instructed to present to his GP should he suspect he was aspirating, especially if he became febrile and/or had an increase in productive sputum.

A review by a gastroenterologist, to seek an opinion about the benefit of empirical dilation of the hypopharynx and cricopharyngeus, was also suggested.

Max underwent endoscopic dilation the following month. Two weeks following the procedure he was contacted by the speech pathologist and asked whether he felt there had been any improvement in swallowing. He reported that he was just sitting down to his lunch, of steak and fries, and was delighted that he was able to swallow foods of a normal consistency.

Future Research

- Design of evidence-based therapy before and during H&N cancer treatment for better functional outcomes (speech, swallowing) post treatment.
- Development of an evidence-based model of supportive care: how/when to support patients and family members who are living with the aftermath and symptom burden of these H&N cancer treatments.
- Better management of people with H&N cancers from culturally and linguistically diverse (CALD) backgrounds.

Recommended Reading

- National Cancer and Palliative Care Rehabilitation Workforce Project. NHS, UK. www.cancer.nhs.uk/rehabilitation/workforce_project (accessed January 14, 2010). (The culmination of three years of work by the National Cancer Action Team in the UK to design/provide evidence-based care pathways, one of which is for patients with H&N cancer.)
- Sullivan PA, Guilford AM. Swallowing Intervention in Oncology. San Diego, London: Singular Publishing Group; 1999. (An excellent text book examining dysphagia in H&N cancer patients and the management thereof.)
- New Voice. Laryngectomy speech rehabilitation. 2006. CD-ROM demonstrating all forms of alaryngeal speech and voice restoration. School of Human Communication Sciences, La Trobe University, Melbourne, Australia. http://www.latrobe.edu.au/communication-clinic/resources.html. (Postlaryngectomy communication, illustrated with diagrams and videos, is presented. Content includes esophageal speech, artificial larynges, and TEP speech.)

References[1]

1. Sullivan PA, Guilford AM. Swallowing Intervention in Oncology. San Diego, London: Singular Publishing Group; 1999 **

1 References with asterisks indicate the most important reference articles on the topic.

2. National Head and Neck Cancer Audit published: http://www.ic.nhs.uk/news-and-events/news/national-head-and-neck-cancer-audit-published (accessed 19th April, 2012)
3. International Classification of Functioning. Disability and Health: ICF. Geneva: World Health Organization; 2001*
4. Sanson-Fisher R, Carey M, Paul C. Measuring the unmet needs of those with cancer; a critical overview. Cancer Forum 2009;33(3):198–201*
5. Bjelland I, Dahl AA, Haug TT, Neckelmann D. The validity of the Hospital Anxiety and Depression Scale. An updated literature review. J Psychosom Res 2002;52(2):69–77
6. Ng F, Trauer T, Dodd S, Calley T, Campbell S, Beck AT. Use of the Beck depression inventory for primary care to screen for major depression disorders. Gen Hosp Psychiatry 1999;21(2):106–111
7. Zabora J, BrintzenhofeSzoc K, Jacobsen P, et al. A new psychosocial screening instrument for use with cancer patients. Psychosomatics 2001;42(3):241–246
8. Furlanetto LM, Mendlowicz MV, Romildo Bueno J. The validity of the Beck Depression Inventory-Short Form as a screening and diagnostic instrument for moderate and severe depression in medical inpatients. J Affect Disord 2005;86(1):87–91
9. Rainbird KJ, Perkins JJ, Sanson-Fisher RW. The Needs Assessment for Advanced Cancer Patients (NA-ACP): a measure of the perceived needs of patients with advanced, incurable cancer. A study of validity, reliability and acceptability. Psychooncology 2005;14(4):297–306
10. Rainbird KJ, Perkins JJ, Sanson-Fisher R, Rolfe I, Anseline P. The needs of patients with advanced, incurable cancer. Br J Cancer 2009;101(5):759–764
11. Campbell HS, Sanson-Fisher R, Taylor-Brown J, Hayward L, Wang XS, Turner D. The cancer support person's unmet needs survey: psychometric properties. Cancer 2009;115(14):3351–3359
12. Hodgkinson K, Butow P, Hobbs KM, Hunt GE, Lo SK, Wain G. Assessing unmet supportive care needs in partners of cancer survivors: the development and evaluation of the Cancer Survivors' Partners Unmet Needs measure (CaSPUN). Psychooncology 2007;16(9):805–813
13. Boyes A, Hodgkinson K, Aldridge L, Turner J. Issues for cancer survivors in Australia. Cancer Forum 2009;33(3):164–167*
14. Goldstein D, Thewes B, Butow P. Communicating in a multicultural society. II: Greek community attitudes towards cancer in Australia. Intern Med J 2002;32(7):289–296
15. Sze M, Duggal-Beri P, Bulow P, et al. Low psychological service utilisation in cancer—does it mean CALD patients cope better? Asia Pac J Clin Oncol 2007;3:A96
16. Lui CW, Ip D, Chui WH. Ethnic experience of cancer: a qualitative study of Chinese-Australians in Brisbane, Queensland. Soc Work Health Care 2009;48(1):14–37
17. Perry A, Skeat J. AusTOMs for speech pathology. Melbourne: La Trobe University; 2004
18. Frowen J, Cotton SM, Corry J, Perry A. Impact of demographics, tumor characteristics, and treatment factors on swallowing after (chemo)radiotherapy for head and neck cancer. Head Neck 2010; 32(4)513–528
19. Logemann JA. Manual for the Videofluorographic Study of Swallowing. 2nd ed. Austin, TX: Pro-Ed; 1986*
20. Logemann JA. Evaluation and Treatment of Swallowing Disorders. 2nd ed. Austin, TX: Pro-Ed; 1998**
21. Levels of Evidence from Joanna Briggs Institute, Australia. In: Reilly S, et al. Evidence Based Practice in Speech Pathology. London: Whurr publishers; 1994
22. Keefe DM, Schubert MM, Elting LS, et al. Updated clinical practice guidelines for the prevention and treatment of mucositis. 2007. American Cancer Society. Online 5th Feb 2007. www.interscience.wiley.com (accessed December 2009)*
23. Clarkson JE, Worthington HV, Furness S, McCabe M, Khalid T, Meyer S. Interventions for treating oral mucositis for patients with cancer receiving treatment (Cochrane Review) http://onlinelibrary.wiley.com/doi/10.1002/14651858.CD001973.pub4/pdf/standard (accessed 17 April, 2012)
24. Head & Neck Clinic Staff Handout. Mucositis Management. Melbourne, Australia: Peter MacCallum Cancer Centre; 2009
25. Rubenstein EB, Peterson DE, Schubert M. Clinical practice guidelines for the prevention and treatment of cancer therapy-induced oral and gastrointestinal mucositis. Cancer 2004;100(9 Suppl):2026–2046
26. Oral Complications of Cancer Treatment: What the Dental Team Can Do. National Institute of Dental and Craniofacial Research, NIH, USA. http://www.nidcr.nih.gov/OralHealth/Topics/Cancer-Treatment/OralComplicationsCancerOral.htm (accessed 17 April, 2012)
27. Guijarro Guijarro B, López Sánchez AF, Hernández Vallejo G. Treatment of xerostomia. A review. Med Oral 2001;6(1):7–18
28. Clinical Guidelines—The Oral Management of Oncology Patients Requiring Radiotherapy: Chemotherapy: Bone Marrow Transplants. http://www.bsdh.org.uk/guidelines/oncolradio.pdf (accessed 19 April, 2012)
29. Halyard MY, Jatoi A, Sloan JA, et al. Does zinc sulfate prevent therapy-induced taste alterations in head and neck cancer patients? Results of phase III double-blind, placebo-controlled trial from the North Central Cancer Treatment Group (N01C4). Int J Radiat Oncol Biol Phys 2007;67(5):1318–1322
30. Appleton J, Machin J. Working with Oral Cancer. Oxford, UK: Winslow Press; 1995
31. Cohen EG, Deschler DG, Walsh K, Hayden RE. Early use of a mechanical stretching device to improve mandibular mobility after composite resection: a pilot study. Arch Phys Med Rehabil 2005;86(7):1416–1419
32. Reuther T, Schuster T, Mende U, Kübler A. Osteoradionecrosis of the jaws as a side effect of radiotherapy of head and neck tumour patients—a report of a thirty year retrospective review. Int J Oral Maxillofac Surg 2003;32(3):289–295
33. Marx RE. A new concept in the treatment of osteoradionecrosis. J Oral Maxillofac Surg 1983;41(6):351–357
34. Williamson R. The role of hyperbaric oxygen in osteoradionecrosis; the present and the future. Conference Abstract. August 8, 2009. Australia & New Zealand Head and Neck Society (ANZHNS) conference, Perth, Australia
35. New Voice. Laryngectomy speech rehabilitation. 2006. CD-ROM demonstrating all forms of alaryngeal speech and voice restoration. School of Human Communication Sciences, La Trobe University, Melbourne, Australia. http://www.latrobe.edu.au/communication-clinic/resources.html (accessed 19 April, 2012)*
36. Lotfi-Jam K, Schofield P, Jefford M. What constitutes ideal survivorship care? Cancer Forum 2009; 33(3)
37. National Cancer and Palliative Care Rehabilitation Workforce Project. NHS, UK. http://www.ncat.nhs.uk/our-work/ensuring-better-treatment/multi-disciplinary-team-development (accessed 19 April, 2012)**

38. McCabe D, Ashford J, Wheeler-Hegland K, et al. Evidence-based systematic review: Oropharyngeal dysphagia behavioral treatments. Part IV—impact of dysphagia treatment on individuals' postcancer treatments. J Rehabil Res Dev 2009;46(2):205–214

39. Cook IJ. Oropharyngeal dysphagia. Gastroenterol Clin North Am 2009;38(3):411–431

20 Psychosocial Aspects of Recurrent Head and Neck Cancer

Marinella P.J. Offerman, Maarten F. de Boer, R.J. Baatenburg de Jong, Jean F.A. Pruyn

Introduction

The Psychosocial Impact of Recurrent Cancer in General

Despite the prevalence of recurrent cancer, psychosocial research on the experience of cancer recurrence and quality of life outcomes after recurrence has been limited.[1–3] Burnet and Robinson indicated in their paper that research on the psychosocial adjustment of cancer has been mainly focused on *newly* diagnosed cancer patients and not on cancer recurrence experiences.[1] It was more than three decades ago that Weisman suggested that "strangely enough" little investigation into cancer recurrence has been done, whereas this phase may be the most discouraging that a patient has to face.[4]

Earlier research has found that recurrence of cancer can be equally as stressful as or more stressful than the original diagnosis of cancer.[2] Complex treatment regimes, unclear explanations, and exhaustion caused by the accumulation of earlier experiences with cancer may leave families overwhelmed and confused. The relapse of cancer can bring back negative emotions and different psychosocial concerns that could be more intense than and different from those after first diagnosis. There is often more uncertainty about the patient's future than at the time of the initial diagnosis and treatment. Vivar et al.[3] suggested that recurrence is a distressing experience for survivors and families because they have to face again psychosocial effects of cancer. The authors identified in their review three main categories that explained survivors' and families' experiences of recurrent cancer:

- Fear of recurrence during survivorship, which is one of the most frequently mentioned components of distress among cancer survivors and is often triggered by medical follow-up
- Facing new challenges as a family when cancer recurs, like dealing with the diagnosis of recurrent cancer, living with uncertainty, and facing treatment again
- Distress caused by recurrence

In earlier research it is suggested that knowing the cancer had returned was devastating because, although patients knew the chances of recurrence, they were not prepared for this shock.[2] Individuals are faced with adapting to changing circumstances, living with uncertainty, letting go of some relationships and reinforcing others, including those with spouses and family.[1] In contrast, other research suggested that levels of distress in patients with recurrence were statistically not significantly different from those of patients newly diagnosed with cancer.[3] Yang et al.[5] concluded in a mixed cancer population that patients with disease recurrence report gains in their psychological functioning and quality of life. Their hypothesis was that patients' familiarity with the cancer experience would ease the psychological impact at the time of the recurrence diagnosis.

The findings in the literature concerning whether the recurrence experience is more or less distressing than that of the primary cancer are contradictory and debatable. Burnet and Robinson mentioned that the question that is more relevant in this context is: "What is distressing and upsetting about the recurrence experience and what can healthcare professionals do to help?"[1] More research is needed to better understand the psychosocial impact of recurrence. The goal of this chapter is to shed some more light on the psychosocial aspects of recurrence in head and neck cancer patients, as well as in relation to the first diagnosis. By providing more information about this underreported subject in the literature on head and neck cancer, we hope that health-care professionals can better fine-tune their services for this specific group of cancer patients.

A Context of the Impact of Recurrence in Head and Neck Cancer

Head and neck (H&N) cancer can be described as a psychologically highly traumatic cancer type. Many vital functions, such as mastication, swallowing, speech, taste, smell, and appearance can be affected. Even minor disturbances of anatomy by surgery may lead to significant dysfunction and disfigurement, and hence to psychosocial complaints.[6] The survival of head and neck cancer is approximately 50%,[7] with average survival rates at 5 years ranging from zero to 40%.[8] In a retrospective review over a period of 5 years, 19% of the head and neck cancer patients developed a recurrence.[9] The recurrence risk in orofacial cancer patients is relatively high in comparison to other cancers.[10] One-third of all head and neck cancer patients are confronted with a recurrence at some time in their lives.[11] Patients who develop a recurrent head and neck cancer have a poor prognosis; to a large extent because the initial course of treatment substantially reduces the flexibility and intensity of re-treatment.[12] The main cause of death in patients with advanced head and neck cancer is locoregional recurrence, occurring in approximately 40%–60% of patients.[13,14]

Studies on Psychosocial Response after Head and Neck Cancer Recurrence

A literature search was performed to identify the maximum possible number of papers on our topic of psychosocial aspects of head and neck cancer recurrence. With our research team, in cooperation with a professional research librarian, we have undertaken a search with specific search terms using the databases PubMed, EMbase, Web of Science, and PsycInfo (see the box). In total we found 254 articles, of which 106 were duplicates, leaving a total of $N = 148$ articles. Of this total number of 148 papers, the great majority (133) were not related to quality of life in head and neck cancer recurrence in terms of psychosocial aspects. In most cases these papers deal either with the meaning of different surgery types or therapy options in the management of recurrent head and neck cancer, or with quality of life of patients with recurrent head and neck cancer treated with treatment X or Y.

! Search Terms of the Literature Research

- With these search terms: (head and neck neoplas*[tw] OR neck cancer*[tw] OR mouth neoplasms[mesh] OR otorhinolaryngologic neoplasms[mesh]) AND (recurr*[ti] OR relap*[ti]) AND (psychology, social[mesh] OR psychosocial[tw] OR life style*[tw] OR lifestyle*[tw] OR life change event*[tw] OR stressful event*[tw] OR life experien*[tw] OR psychol*[tw] OR quality of life[tw] OR life qualit*[tw] OR qol[tw]) → we found in *PubMed 76 articles*.
- With these search terms: ('head and neck cancer'/syn OR 'mouth cancer'/syn OR ((neck OR mouth OR otorhinolaryngol* OR head OR tongue OR pharyn* OR hypophar* OR nasopharyn* OR oropharyn* OR laryn* OR otolaryn*) NEAR/3 (neoplasm* OR cancer* OR tumo* OR carcinom*)):ti,ab,de) AND (recurr*:ti OR relap*:ti) AND ('social psychology'/syn OR psychosocial:ti,ab,de OR life style*:ti,ab,de OR lifestyle*:ti,ab,de OR ((life OR stressful) NEAR/3 (event* OR experien*)):ti,ab,de OR psychol*:ti,ab,de OR (quality NEAR/3 life):ti,ab,de OR qol:ti,ab,de) → we found in EMbase: 95 articles, of which after removing all duplicates from PubMed there remained in *EMbase 36 articles*.
- With these search terms: (neck OR mouth OR otorhinolaryngol* OR head OR tongue OR pharyn* OR hypophar* OR nasopharyn* OR oropharyn* OR laryn* OR otolaryn*) AND (neoplasm* OR cancer* OR tumo* OR carcinom*) AND (ti=recurr* OR ti=relap*) AND (social AND psychol* OR psychosocial OR life style OR lifestyle* OR ((life OR stressful) AND (event* OR experien*)) OR psychol* OR (quality AND life) OR qol) → we found in Web of Science: 78 articles, of which after removing all duplicates from PubMed there remained in *Web of Science 36 articles*.
- With these search terms: (neck OR mouth OR otorhinolaryngol* OR head OR tongue OR pharyn* OR hypophar* OR nasopharyn* OR oropharyn* OR laryn* OR otolaryn*) AND (neoplasm* OR cancer* OR tumo* OR carcinom*) AND (recurr*.ti. OR relap*.ti.) AND (social AND psychol* OR psychosocial OR life style OR lifestyle* OR ((life OR stressful) AND (event* OR experien*)) OR psychol* OR (quality AND life) OR qol) → we found in PsycInfo: 5 articles, of which after removing all duplicates from PubMed there remained in *PsycInfo 0 articles*.

Of the remaining 15 papers, we found only one paper that examined psychological response in patients with head and neck cancer recurrence.[15] The key outcomes of this study will be discussed in the next section.

Nine papers dealt with fear of head and neck cancer recurrence, of which the key conclusions will be discussed later in this chapter.

One paper specifically discussed the need for close follow-up in patients previously treated for oral/oropharyngeal squamous cell carcinoma because the majority of the patient population were unaware of the recurrence of their disease.[9] The authors conclude that a close follow-up in the first 2 years is essential.

Additionally, there is a study in which recurrence is also discussed as an outcome measure for head and neck cancer patients.[16] With respect to psychosocial predictors, they found that patients who perceived themselves as more physically self-efficacious were more likely to survive and less likely to have a recurrence. And patients who expressed a higher intensity of negative feelings in regard to their illness were less likely to develop a recurrence than those patients who were unable to express such feelings.

In one study the association between depression and disease recurrence in patients with head and neck cancer is examined.[18] The authors concluded that depressed patients with head and neck cancer may have a higher mortality and recurrence rate. Therefore, diagnosis, prevention, and treatment of depression in head and neck cancer may provide an avenue to improve survival.

Furthermore, we found one recent review discussing the relevant literature concerning quality of life considerations in treatment of recurrent unresectable head and neck cancer.[8] According to these authors, the management of locoregional recurrence is a complex problem. The best choice for treatment is related to interplay of patient and tumor variables. This paper discusses the background to the question why it is not straightforward to assess and interpret quality of life scores in recurrent head and neck cancer patients. The authors suggest that this group is difficult to assess because many patients are too unwell to comply, which leads to high attrition rates and less possibility for long-term follow-up. Sample sizes are often small and all existing validated quality of life instruments are only suitable for comparing populations of patients and not individual scores. No instrument has been correlated with clinical anchor states in recurrent head and neck cancer so as to direct decisions on the best form of management. The paper concluded that this population has the most to lose if treatment processes cause deterioration in quality of life, owing to their limited lifespan. It is, therefore, of the utmost importance to ensure that they have the highest attainable quality of life even if survival might not be prolonged. All in all, results of treatment are poor; thus quality of life outcome should play a major role in the choice of treatment.

To focus on our chapter topic, we share the main thoughts of the one study that examined the psychosocial experience of head and neck cancer recurrence.[15] The authors used a qualitative method and did research with 9 head and neck cancer patients of whom three had two or more recurrences. They collected their data by making use of a semistructured interview schedule in a flexible and adaptive approach. The authors identified five core themes. The first three themes were (a) emotional reactions, such as shock, fear, or denial; (b) reevaluation; such as reappraisal of life; and (c) active coping strategies, such as striving for hope and normality, fighting spirit, or thinking positively. The authors called these themes "internal or psychological" effects of cancer recurrence. The other two themes were (d) life changes, such as limitations or physical problems; and (e) support, such as the positive impact on relations. These two themes were considered as "external" effects of cancer recurrence. An additional theme was found concerning improvement in relationships, such as more closeness within familial relationships due to the recurrence of the cancer. One of the main conclusions shared in this paper was that even though there was a wide variation of individual differences reported, a common experience of heightened emotional vulnerability was seen across participants with recurrent illness. The level of consequential emotional burden expressed was strongly determined by how patients were able to comprehend, reappraise, and adjust to the circumstances they found themselves in. Furthermore, they said that the patient's journey through specialist services was not always smooth and sometimes added to their burden. Therefore, increased provision of support for both patients who experience recurrence and their caregivers seems to be a vital addition to head and neck oncology services that wish to meet the emotional and psychological needs of their patients. These needs are likely to be complex and significant after a diagnosis of oral cancer recurrence.

Studies on Fear of Recurrence

Earlier studies in different types of cancer patients indicated fear of recurrence as one of the major concerns that cancer survivors report. Distress because of the fear of recurrence in cancer is clearly established in the literature.[3] When we look specifically at the subject of fear of recurrence in the population of head and neck cancer patients, there is some relatively recent literature available.[10,19–25] The key conclusions of these papers dealing with fear of head and neck cancer recurrence are:

- A majority (80%) of patients expressed their concern about the possibility of recurrence at 3 months post treatment and 72% of the patients at 7 months post treatment.[10]
- Many head and neck cancer patients have a wish to discuss their fear of recurrence concerns during the outpatient review.[19]
- A third of HNC patients at diagnosis reported relatively high levels of fears of recurrence, with 12% still reporting similar levels of fear 6–8 months after treatment.[25]
- Patients aged 65 or above were significantly less concerned about recurrence.[10]
- Carers recorded higher recurrence concerns on average than patients.[21]
- A low level of cancer concern persisted in about half of the long-term head and neck cancer survivors.[20]
- Cancer concern is associated with continued pain, disfigurement, and limitations on eating in public.[20]
- Patients who have more severe long-term effects will be more likely to be concerned about the recurrence of their cancer.[20]
- Fear of cancer recurrence after treatment was directly predicted by pretreatment fears and optimism.[25]
- Future research is required into the triggers of fear of recurrence and to identify the aspects of fear of recurrence and concerns and how best to give information to patients about the likelihood of further disease.[19]

Current Research

To further build on the findings of the sparse literature on psychosocial experiences of head and neck cancer recurrence with the one and only paper,[15] we have set up some further research as follows:

- **Research question:** How can we fine-tune our health-care services for the specific group of head and neck cancer patients experiencing recurrence of the disease?
- **Research goal:** Obtain knowledge to describe the psychosocial responses after the recurrence message and the impact of the illness experience on the life of the patient.

Methods

Sample

Purposeful criterion-based sampling was performed. This meant that patients were selected in a purposeful way so that it was not a coincidence to be included in the research. We used an up-to-date database with our H&N oncology patients treated in the Erasmus Medical Center Rotterdam, the Netherlands, and followed the trend of our data, i.e., the division in our total database of first recurrence tumors belonging to a first primary tumor and to second primary tumors. We decided to include 10 patients who had recurrence of the illness; 8 of them received curative treatment and 2 patients received palliative treatment (**Table 20.1**). Medically speaking, a recurrence means that *the same cancer* (related to the first cancer) comes back after some time. However, we defined recurrence from the perspective of the patient, i.e., the patient has been treated successfully for the first cancer experience and, after a period, they experience cancer in the same area for a second time. We therefore included locoregional second primary head and neck cancer, as from the patient perspective, this is recurrence

Table 20.1 Demographic and medical data participants $N = 10$

	Sex	Age (years)	Nature of tumor	Tumor belongs to	Treatment recurrence
P1	Male	63	2nd primary	–	Curative surgery Jan. 2010
P2	Male	83	1st recurrence	1st primary tumor	Curative surgery and RT Oct. 2009
P3	Male	72	1st recurrence	1st primary tumor	None, palliative control visits As of Feb. 2010
P4	Male	46	1st recurrence	1st primary tumor	Curative surgery Sep. 2009
P5	Female	62	1st recurrence	1st primary tumor	Curative surgery Dec. 2009
P6	Female	39	1st recurrence	1st primary tumor	None, palliative control visits As of summer 2009
P7	Male	49	1st recurrence	1st primary tumor	Curative surgery and CRT Jan. 2010
P8	Male	64	2nd primary	–	Curative RT Nov. 2009
P9	Female	74	2nd primary	–	Curative surgery and RT Aug. 2009
P10	Male	59	2nd primary	–	Curative RT Nov. 2009

RT= radiotherapy; CRT= chemoradiation therapy.

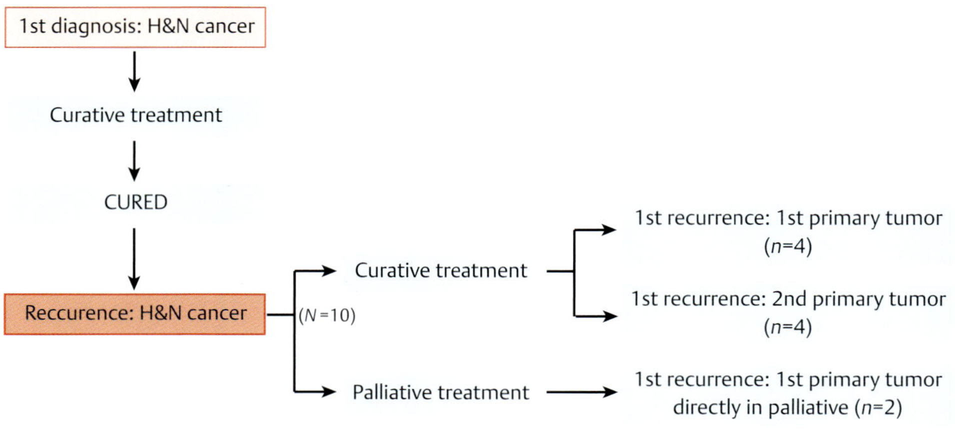

Fig. 20.1 Progression of patients

as well, since the disease came back, despite the fact that with a second primary tumor, it is not a recurrence in the pure sense of the word. For further information, see **Fig. 20.1**. Additional inclusion criteria were adequate knowledge of the Dutch language and no significant cognitive deficits of the patient.

Patients were selected from our database and their status of locoregional recurrence was checked by a head and neck surgeon. After this first selection, the candidates were handed over to the specialized head and neck nurses who have regular contact with the patients. They know best whether the patient is in a good condition to be interviewed or whether he or she can speak the Dutch language. The nurses made the first contact with the candidates and they asked permission of the patients for a research psychologist to contact them. This psychologist made the second call to the patient and gave further background and an introduction of the interview. And the end of the telephone call an appointment was made for a home visit.

Set-up Interview

In-depth qualitative interviews were set up with a well-structured questionnaire containing five main blocks of questions. Each block had a primary question to start the interview with. First there was time for open reactions. Each primary question was then followed by a series of questions to follow through on the subject.

The five **main blocks** were:

- Primary reactions (thoughts, emotions, and behavior) of the patient directly after the recurrence message (second diagnosis) given by the surgeon.
- The differences in primary reactions of the message between the second and first diagnoses.
- Psychosocial responses in the period from receiving the news of recurrence until now (when the first "shock" is over).
- The differences between the second and first diagnoses in terms of psychosocial responses in the period after the first "shock."
- Wants and needs for health care in H&N cancer patients experiencing recurrence.

Examples of questions per main block were:

- What were your first thoughts after the receiving the news of the recurrence? How did you behave? How did the surgeon behave? Can you describe your emotions? With what expectations did you enter the doctor's room? Did you have any idea of why the recurrence took place?
- Did you enter the doctor's room with another expectation than the first time? Were your feelings or was your behavior different compared with the first diagnosis?
- How do you try and cope with your situation of recurrence? Did you think about how you want to spend/change your life from then on? Do you have fear for a second recurrence and possible death?
- Do you have other thoughts on your mind compared with the first diagnosis? Are the consequences of the disease on your social life and partner different from those from the first diagnosis?
- What questions did you have when you received the news about the recurrence? What kind of support did you need? Was there room for your emotions? How was the support afterwards? Current needs?

The results and conclusion of the research will be described in the following sections. We will go step by step through the process that the patient follows more or less chronologically from the receipt of the recurrence message. The psychosocial consequences after recurrence are described starting right after the news and in the period following the recurrence message when the first "shock" has "sunk in." Furthermore, we describe the differences in experience between the first and the second diagnosis of head and neck cancer.

The Doctor's Message: "The Cancer is Back"

The main question in this chapter is: Is it even worse for patients getting this message for the second time? Awaiting a possible diagnosis of cancer, expected or not, can be an important stress factor in itself for both patient and partner. Imagine that you had received the message of a "diagnosis head and neck cancer" two years ago. After a successful treatment, the doctor said: "We have removed the cancer." You are getting better and better with time and you are returning more or less to your normal lifestyle. This morning you had your control visit. And then the doctor said: "I don't have good news for you. The cancer is back" (**Fig. 20.2**). For some patients this message will come completely out of the blue and for others it is a confirmation of already anxious foreboding.

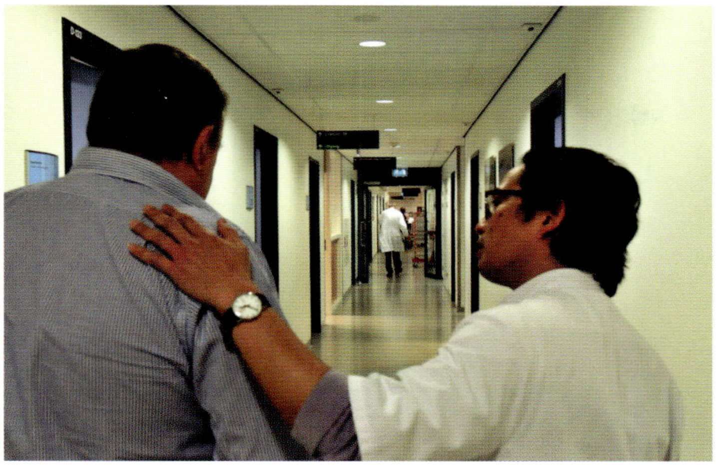

Fig. 20.2 The doctor's message: "The cancer is back."

For health-care professionals, it would be interesting to know whether people experience this second message differently than the first. More knowledge about the psychosocial impact of the recurrence message can better prepare professionals in their work with patients and their partners. This part of the chapter goes deeper into the inner thoughts and feelings of patients who experience head and neck cancer recurrence. It describes the first thoughts, emotions after the message is received, and also the patients' own ideas of why the cancer came back. This part of the chapter ends with a description of the difference experienced between the news of the second and of the first head and neck cancer.

■ First Thoughts after the Recurrence Message

We asked the participants to describe their very first thoughts when they were in the doctor's room receiving the recurrence message. Four out of 10 patients had a resigned attitude, letting things take their course: "I'll wait and see what happens. I have to follow this treatment, otherwise I will die, the doctor says."

Three out of 10 patients had angry reactions; anger against the professional, such as "The doctors did not react adequately earlier on." Also anger against the situation—"Damn, again an operation, I thought everything was OK and now I have to follow the same process again..."—or anger in the sense of rebellion, as one patient says after receiving a palliative diagnosis as a recurrence message: "One way or the other, I am going to make it. This does not fit with the idea I had for myself and the future."

Additionally, there were two reactions of disbelief, including the question "Why is this happening to me again" and one reaction of "shock."

■ First Emotions after the Recurrence Message

The participants described their very first emotions after the recurrence message of the doctor. Four out of 10 patients had a down-to-earth attitude with feelings of acceptance of the situation. One example is "I looked at it soberly. I knew from the first time how things were going and I completely entrusted my situation to the doctors again."

Three out of 10 patients were distressed and felt sad: "I roared with sadness and I cried. The doctor tried to calm me down." Other reactions were anger, anxiety, and powerlessness.

■ Expectations and Explanations of the Patient

We asked all participants about what expectations they had when they entered the doctor's room. Four out of 10 had a premonition about the cancer coming back. One example is: "I already had an idea that it was not good as the doctor mentioned before the tests that he saw an abnormality. I have known my doctor for more than one year and he does not say something like that when it is not true."

The complete opposite was reported by the same number of participants; 4 out of 10 persons were completely shocked as they did not expect the recurrence: "I thought I was 100% OK, as I had not noticed anything and I did not feel ill. I entered the doctor's room with fresh courage; however, I was thrown off my balance right after the recurrence message."

The other two reactions were open-minded and patients did not have any specific foreboding.

When we asked the participants whether they thought they were completely cured after the first head and neck cancer experience, 7 out of 10 said that they had had the feeling that they were completely cured after the first time. For example: "After the first treatment, the doctor said that it was gone." The three others were neutral in their reaction: "I did not know if I was cured. They never told me that I got rid of it or that (some of) it was still there." Two of the neutral reactions also mentioned the critical period of 5 years had not passed; only then you can say you are cured or not, participants said.

We also asked the participants if they had an idea of why the cancer came back. It seems that everyone had his or her own *ideas* of explanations of the cancer recurrence. One person said that his work in the petrochemical industry might have had negative influence on his health and could have caused the first and second cancers. Another said that cancer runs in the family. The other eight persons did not such fixed ideas of the origin of the recurrence as the previous two patients, but they either had no idea or had speculative ideas such as "Maybe some cells were left behind and could have caused the recurrence" or "Probably it was not gone in the first place."

■ Reaction of the Doctor

We can conclude from all the interviews that the doctors informed the patient of the news of recurrence in a direct manner. All patients' experience was that, in terms of communicating the message, the doctor immediately came to the point. A majority of the patients (8 out of 10) found that in essence a good approach. People in general want the doctor to be honest with them. An example of that approach is: "I do not have good news for you. If we don't do anything, you have no longer than four months to live." One person says that it is good that the doctor was straightforward. However, the patient would have liked the doctor to have built up the message a bit more toward the bad news—it was too harsh.

Table 20.2 Verbatim reactions after news of recurrence

Shock recurrence message	Example verbatim
Recurrence was bigger shock than the first experience (50%)	"The second time is a bigger shock because you theoretically know that it can come back but now I really experienced that it did." "The second time is a bigger shock because you think why isn't the cancer gone after the first time? I have always lived a healthy life and still I am confronted with cancer twice!"
Recurrence was less of a shock than the first experience (30%)	"The first time was a bigger shock because I did not know what cancer was and I thought I was going to die. Now that I have not, I think that the second time I will survive as well." "The first time was a bigger shock because that message came totally unexpected whereas the second time was something I always thought of as a possibility."
Recurrence was equal to first experience (20%)	"Both experiences were the same in terms of impact, but they are separate from each other. Both times bad luck." "Both experiences were equal to each other in terms of shock as both times I already expected it."

Table 20.3 Type of reaction after news of recurrence

Type 1 "move on"	*N* = 8, of whom one patient was in the palliative phase	"Actually there hasn't been that much change since the recurrence. The only thing is that I have physical implications which I have to accept. My goal is to come back on track into my old life pattern as much as possible." "I don't want to do new things in life, and I don't see life differently. I just want to move back into my old lifestyle." "I just want to live my life as I normally do."
Type 2 "depressed"	*N* =1 This patient was in the palliative phase	"I have nothing to look forward to now I know that I don't have a future anymore. The joy of living disappears bit by bit and I am more withdrawn from others. I feel defeated."
Type 3 "life change"	*N* = 1	"I don't want to completely get back to my "old self'. I used to work more than 60 hours per week. Now I know that I can be replaced at work, I want to enjoy other aspects of life more. I enjoy the moment in itself because you never know how long it takes. I try to do that more consciously than before."

One of the patients receiving the message of palliative treatment had the feeling that the doctor, in a figurative sense, had stepped aside. The message was more or less "This is it." The doctor could not offer a curative treatment. In addition, the patient had the feeling that the doctor was letting her down in a way by sending her home with this bad message to deal with by herself.

Reaction of the Partner

Four out of 10 partners had the same down-to-earth attitude as the patient, with feelings of acceptance of the situation. One patient said: "My partner accepted the situation just as much as I did. That gives me calm and peaceful feeling." The rest had a variety of reactions such as: anger, sadness, anxiety, loss of control, and feeling numb. An example of the latter is "When we entered the doctor's room my partner had good faith in a positive message and she cheered me up all the time. When she heard that the cancer was back, she was really stunned."

Difference: Recurrence Message versus the First Message

We asked the participants to describe the differences, if any, between the news of recurrence compared with the news of the first diagnosis of head and neck cancer (**Table 20.2**). We asked this question in terms of possible differences in "shock" between the two. Half of the respondents found the news of recurrence a bigger "slap in the face" than the first experience; 3 out of 10 found the opposite and said that the first message was a bigger shock for them. Two out of 10 found both messages equally shocking.

After the News of Recurrence ... How to Go On?

Type of Patients' Reactions to Recurrence

Along with the doctor's news that the cancer is back, the uncertainties come back too. At the top of one's mind, the question often is: "Can I be cured for the second time?" What are the psychosocial experiences of patients when cancer recurs? How do they deal with this second experience? We asked patients whether anything radically changed in their lives after the news of the recurrence. We clustered the reactions in a characterization of three different types (**Table 20.3**):

- The type of person who wants to move on with life as normally as possible and try to get back to the same level
- The type of person who becomes depressed and cannot get back into the old situation
- The type of person who sees the recurrence experience as an event to change one's life perspective

Eight out of 10 patients said that after the first shock of the recurrence they wanted to move on as before (type 1), even though for many of these patients their lives have been changed in many aspects. Some of them can only eat via tube feeding for the rest of their lives, feel extremely tired, or experience psychological distress. However, they try to do their utmost to move on with their lives and find more or less their old lifestyle. One patient was depressed (type 2) and was not able to go on as before; and another patient saw the disease as a turning point to see their life differently (type 3).

Table 20.4 Coping styles of patients

Coping style	Patients (N = 10)									
	P1	P2	P3	P4	P5	P6	P7	P8	P9	P10
Put in perspective	×									
Acceptance [a]	×	×			×			×	×	×
Positive attitude	×	×								
Active coping [b]			×			×	×	×		
Step by step coping			×			×				
Turn off feelings							×			
Humor					×		×			
Express feelings			×	×						
Find distraction [c]			×	×	×					
Give up						×				
Hope						×				

[a] The coping style that is most frequently used is "acceptance." This strategy is used by 6 out of 10 patients. Patients said: "Even if the message was bad after my treatment of the recurrent cancer, I accept that. Who am I to say that I will become 90 years old when so many people around me died earlier than me?" Or another reaction: "I have just accepted the whole situation and had the feeling to bravely go on."
[b] "Active coping" was used by 4 out of 10 patients. Examples of active coping are: "I try to go on life live normally and be with other people as much as possible. I don't want to sit in a corner doing nothing."
[c] The coping strategy "find distraction" has been used by nearly one-third of the patients. Examples of distraction are closely related to active coping: "I want to find distraction so I returned to my work very quickly as I can't stay at home."

Coping with Recurrent Head and Neck Cancer

Table 20.4 gives an overview of the coping styles that patients said they mostly used after the first shock of the news of recurrence in trying to deal with the (consequences of) the situation. The results show that there are several strategies used by patients. The style of coping is not limited to one specific strategy. Only two patients showed a single strategy (acceptance); all the rest used two or more strategies to cope with the situation. Furthermore, the results show that the patients in the palliative phase (patient 3 and patient 6) used the most coping strategies (four).

Current Fears

We asked all participants whether they have current fears as an open question. When patients asked "fear of what?" we explained that this could be different aspects of fear such as fear of death, of recurrence, of pain, of follow-up visits, an so on. One patient in the palliative phase and 5 patients in the curative phase did not experience fears. Reactions from this group were: "I don't have fears, not even of pain or death. I would say that it would be a pity when I die." "I don't make myself anxious about fear of second recurrence. I cannot control it so it does not make any sense." "I do not fear death. I will see when it is my time to go."

Four out of 10 patients, including one in the palliative phase, reported having fears of different backgrounds. One patient described a strong sense of fear of a second recurrence. "My biggest fear is related to the follow-up visit as my biggest concern is that the cancer has spread. In five months I have my follow-up visit with a lung scan again and I worry about this already."

Table 20.5 Difficulties in coping with recurrence compared with the initial cancer

Equal	Recurrence is less difficult	Recurrence is more difficult
N = 2	*N* = 3	*N* = 5
Two patients had equal feelings of coping	Three patients found coping with recurrence less difficult than the first cancer	Five patients found coping with recurrence more difficult than with the first cancer

Another patient described his fear of another recurrence. Since the first recurrence, there have been stronger thoughts and fears that the cancer can come back for a third time: "The follow-up visits with the scans, these are very scary." Another patient, in a palliative phase, described fear of agony and fear for her young son that she cannot raise and help grow up. A further patient had fear of pain that would not go away.

Difference in Coping with Cancer Recurrence Compared with the first Cancer Experience

Half of the patients found coping with recurrent head and neck cancer more difficult than the first head and neck cancer experience. Patients felt they had more to cope with because of experiencing several different feelings, such as feeling more defeated (in case the recurrence meant a palliative diagnosis), feeling that the recurrence was not expected, feeling that the recurrence treatment was harder (for example, in the case of patients who the first time only had surgery and now face surgery including radiation therapy with a lot of negative consequences), or because they had more questions, mainly driven by the need for more information on the cause of the disease recurrence (**Table 20.5**).

For three patients, the coping with recurrence was less difficult than the first experience as there were more feelings of acceptance and there were fewer emotions. For two patients it was equally difficult both times.

Patients' Suggestions for the Professional

We asked all patients an open question to give us suggestions regarding the best way of informing patients of the news of recurrence. Seven out of 10 patients spontaneously said that doctors in general should come directly to the point. Doctors must be open and honest when answering the patients' questions because they want to know exactly what is going on and what their options are when it comes to treatment. Patients certainly do not want doctors to raise false hope or to disguise any information.

Other preferred doctors' skills during the phase of bringing the recurrence message mentioned were:

- The ability to listen well to the patient in the case of questions or expressing their wishes
- The ability to let the patient finish talking
- The ability to take time for the patient, or at least give the patient *the feeling* that the doctor has time for the patient even if that is not the case

- The ability to set the right expectations in terms of treatment; for example, when the operation is serious or when the radiation treatment will be difficult, especially later in the trajectory

Additionally, one patient who received a recurrence message, which in this case also mentioned a palliative diagnosis, mentioned that it is very important that doctors tell the patients in such a situation to bring someone with them, so that they are not alone when they receive such a message.

When it comes to support right after the message, most patients mentioned that it is of key importance to get a telephone number of a direct contact person who can be called for support or with questions when the news has "sunk in."

Summary

- The psychosocial aspects of head and neck cancer recurrence are under-reported in the literature.
- One of the main conclusions of the only paper dealing with the psychosocial impact of head and neck cancer recurrence was that a common experience of heightened emotional vulnerability was seen across patients with recurrent illness. Increased provision and attention to both patients and partners seems to be a vital addition to head and neck oncology services.
- Our study aimed to describe the psychosocial responses of patients after receiving the news of the recurrence of head and neck cancer, and the impact of the illness experience as compared with the impact of the initial diagnosis. An in-depth qualitative interview with 10 patients was held covering five main aspects:
  1. Primary reactions of the patients directly after receiving the news that the cancer had recurred
  2. The difference between initial reactions to the news after the second and after the first diagnosis
  3. The psychosocial response in the period after receiving the news of recurrence
  4. The difference in psychosocial responses in the period following the first emotional shock after the second and the after first diagnosis
  5. Suggestions for health-care professionals in communicating the news of a recurrence
- The key results of the current study were:
  – Half of the respondents found that the news of recurrence caused them a bigger shock than the first diagnosis. Three out of 10 patients found the news of recurrence less of a shock and 2 out of 10 were equally shocked after receiving the news on both occasions.
  – After the recurrence experience, the great majority of patients want to move on with life as normally as possible.
  – Half of the patients found coping with the cancer recurrence more difficult than coping with the first diagnosis.
  – Four out of 10 patients experience fears, especially for a second recurrence. These fears can be triggered by the follow-up visits.
  – Patients have the need for an explanatory model of the cause of their recurrent disease.

Concluding Thoughts

In the literature, little attention has been paid to the psychosocial impact of head and neck cancer recurrence. Only one earlier paper investigated this subject within this specific patient group.[15] The current research reported on in this chapter has added to this by comparing the recurrence situation with the experience of the initial diagnosis to better understand the experiences and their contexts.

We point out that the study results are based on a small sample size. Furthermore, the retrospective method of the research could have caused errors in the recall of information given the timing of the interview after the treatment of the cancer recurrence. To minimize recall bias, we have designed a well-structured questionnaire that we followed for our qualitative interviews. These findings provide useful insights into the under-reported subject of the psychosocial experience of head and neck cancer recurrence. This subject deserves more attention because one-third of all head and neck cancer patients whom we treat will be confronted with a recurrence sometime in their lives. On the basis of the findings of this study, future quantitative research with a larger sample size should be carried out.

Recurrence experiences can be broadly divided into two types. One group of patients manage and cope with the consequences of the disease quite well, while another, more vulnerable, group of patients will need more attention. In the current study half of the patients experienced a bigger shock on receiving the news of the cancer recurrence than on receiving the news of the initial diagnosis. Also, half of the patients found it more difficult to cope with the recurrent cancer than with the initial cancer experience. Both findings strongly suggest that this substantial patient group should get extra attention from health-care professionals.

Explanations for the larger difficulties experienced in coping with recurrent cancer could be that the recurrence was not expected, or that patients with recurrence were struggling with questions about how the recurrence could have happened. It seemed that everyone had his or her own ideas and explanations about the possible causes of the cancer recurrence. This cognitive process can be explained by the attribution theory within the field of social psychology, introduced by Heider.[26] Attribution means that someone ascribes (attributes) causes to certain events or behavior. People make attributions all the time. We all try to determine what caused a certain event. There is a general tendency in people to see reality in their own way and to give meaning to it in their own way. When people enter into an insecure situation like a cancer recurrence, there can be a great need for some kind of explanation to provide more control of the insecure situation. The cognitive process of attribution will be followed by a response of coping. Coping refers to both cognitive and behavioral efforts to manage situations that are perceived as stressful.[27] The majority of the patients were not limited to one coping style, and they used a variety of strategies. The most frequently used coping styles were "acceptance" and "active coping." This is in line with earlier research among advanced head and neck cancer patients.[28] These patients used a broad array of coping strategies of which the most prominent were "religion, acceptance, and active coping." Another finding of this study is that patients who respond to the disease with denial or avoidance may be at heightened risk of psychosocial morbidity. More recently, this finding has been confirmed in a paper indicating that the use of avoidance coping was associated with more depressive symptoms and a worse quality of life.[29]

There is more to be said about how people live on after the treatment of head and neck cancer recurrence. The majority of patients did not radically change their life and/or lifestyle after the recurrence experience. Eighty percent said that after the first shock of the recurrence, they wanted to move on with their lives. They wanted to find their old lifestyle level again as much as possible. This is in line with earlier research on goal importance among head and neck cancer patients. The short-term goals were mainly focused on building up physical condition and living life as normally as possible.[30] It is also in concordance with earlier research in head and neck cancer patients in the palliative phase in which patients also strived to return to a normal lifestyle.[31] Furthermore this kind of attitude fits with the logic of the most frequently used coping styles of "acceptance" and "active coping."

What do these results mean for health-care professionals in hospitals? As we concluded, our findings justify extra attention for this vulnerable group of patients who experience the recurrence as a bigger shock and find it more difficult to cope with. This means that professionals should systematically screen which of their patients belong to the "vulnerable group." This systematic screening should be part of a fixed procedure or protocol. Earlier research confirmed the efficacy of a specific head and neck cancer screening and referral instrument for patients with psychosocial problems. This screening method was developed at the Erasmus Medical Center, Rotterdam.[32] General suggestions from patients were that doctors should be open and honest and should have good listening skills. Furthermore, they suggested that doctors should carefully observe whether their patients experienced strong emotions or clammed up after receiving the message that the cancer had recurred. Physicians should pay attention to these more vulnerable patients and offer them and their partners for the option of another visit in the coming days so that the patient and partner can ask questions that may come up later. Alternatively, additional time with a specialized nurse could be offered in case patients experience the recurrence as a bigger shock, accompanied by strong emotions (**Fig. 20.3**).

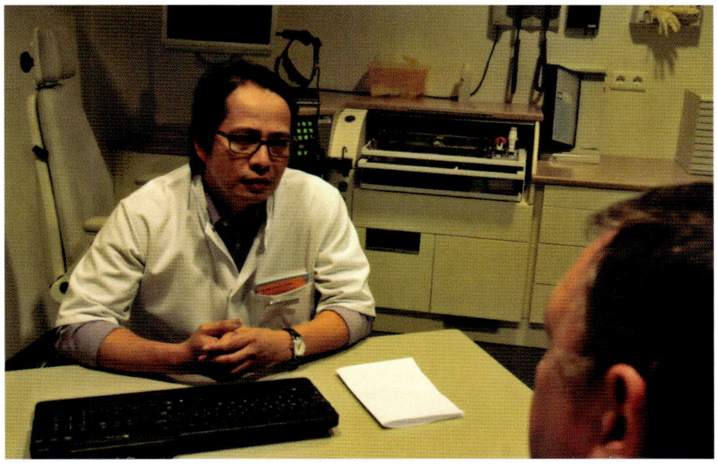

Fig. 20.3 Physicians should pay attention to more vulnerable patients and offer them the option of another visit in the coming days so that the patient can ask questions that may come up later.

And what do the psychological processes of coping and attribution mean for the patient–doctor communication? First, we stress that although there is often no single straightforward explanation for the cancer recurrence, doctors should realize that patients may need to make sense out of the situation. Patients have the need for an explanatory model of the cause of their recurrent disease. Doctors therefore should, wherever they can, help patients in looking for possible explanations. Patients may want to receive information to decrease their feeling of insecurity, to get more control over the situation. Second, during the course of the disease, physicians should ask the patients how they are coping with the situation. Patients who rigidly deny the reality of the disease or refuse to allow themselves to think about it should elicit the physician's concern.[28] We add that denial in itself is not necessarily wrong and could be an adaptive coping response in a given situation, like any other coping style for that matter. Coping is not a static process and how patients react during their disease trajectory can change, also because of changing circumstances. Therefore there is no wrong coping style in itself, as each coping style is a means for the patient to deal with her or his distress. It is important to stay in open communication with patients about their coping. One specific question that a doctor can ask is: "Do you think you are capable of dealing with this situation of cancer recurrence, or do you think you will need additional support from us?" In this way, physicians can understand what the cancer recurrence means to their patients and find out whether patients might get stuck somewhere in the process of dealing with the consequences of the recurrent disease.

Future Research

More research is needed in the following areas:

- Identifying the psychosocial needs of patients after recurrence with different types of cancer and covering both female and male patient groups. Specifically, the literature lacks data on the psychosocial response and the psychosocial needs of head and neck cancer patients experiencing recurrence.
- How to best screen head and neck cancer patients on the fear of recurrence.
- Understanding how best to set up supportive care both for the head and neck cancer patient and the spouse, and for the family dealing with such a traumatic experience as a recurrence.
- How the doctor can help the patients to understand the cause of their recurrent head and neck cancer (need for an explanatory model).

Recommended Reading

- Griffiths MJ, Humphris GM, Skirrow PM, Rogers SN. A qualitative evaluation of patient experiences when diagnosed with oral cancer recurrence. Cancer Nurs 2008;31(4):E11–E17. (This is one of the scarce articles in the literature giving more in-depth insight into patients' psychosocial response to head and neck cancer recurrence.)
- Rogers SN, Scott B, Lowe D, Ozakinci G, Humphris GM. Fear of recurrence following head and neck cancer in the outpatient clinic. Eur Arch Otorhinolaryngol. 2010;267(12):1943–1949. (This paper makes a direct link with clinical practice and

stresses the importance of good screening for fear of recurrence as patients with high fear of recurrence tend to have significant problems associated with their fear.)

- McLarnon C, Kulloo P, Mehanna H, Kelly C, Paleri V. Quality-of-life considerations in treatment of unresectable, recurrent head and neck cancer. Expert Rev Anticancer Ther 2010;10(3):345–352. (These authors suggest that there are insufficient data on the effects of different treatment modalities on the quality of life of recurrent head and neck cancer patients. This vulnerable group of patients have the most to lose if treatment processes cause deterioration in quality of life because of their limited lifespan.)
- Vivar CG, Canga N, Canga AD, Arantzamendi M. The psychosocial impact of recurrence on cancer survivors and family members: a narrative review. J Adv Nurs. 2009;65(4):724–736. (These authors state that the impact of cancer recurrence is as bad or even more devastating for family members. This review analyses both the psychosocial experience of cancer recurrence for survivors and for their family members.

References

1. Burnet K, Robinson L. Psychosocial impact of recurrent cancer. Eur J Oncol Nurs 2000;4(1):29–38
2. Mahon SM, Casperson DM. Exploring the psychosocial meaning of recurrent cancer: a descriptive study. Cancer Nurs 1997;20(3):178–186
3. Vivar CG, Canga N, Canga AD, Arantzamendi M. The psychosocial impact of recurrence on cancer survivors and family members: a narrative review. J Adv Nurs 2009;65(4):724–736
4. Weisman AD. A model for psychosocial phasing in cancer. Gen Hosp Psychiatry 1979;1(3):187–195
5. Yang HC, Thornton LM, Shapiro CL, Andersen BL. Surviving recurrence: psychological and quality-of-life recovery. Cancer 2008;112(5):1178–1187
6. De Boer MF, McCormick LK, Pruyn JF, Ryckman RM, van den Borne BW. Physical and psychosocial correlates of head and neck cancer: a review of the literature. Otolaryngol Head Neck Surg 1999;120(3):427–436
7. Ledeboer QC, Velden LA, Boer MF, Feenstra L, Pruyn JF. Physical and psychosocial correlates of head and neck cancer: an update of the literature and challenges for the future (1996–2003). Clin Otolaryngol 2005;30(4):303–319
8. McLarnon C, Kulloo P, Mehanna H, Kelly C, Paleri V. Quality-of-life considerations in treatment of unresectable, recurrent head and neck cancer. Expert Rev Anticancer Ther 2010;10(3):345–352
9. Kissun D, Magennis P, Lowe D, Brown JS, Vaughan ED, Rogers SN. Timing and presentation of recurrent oral and oropharyngeal squamous cell carcinoma and awareness in the outpatient clinic. Br J Oral Maxillofac Surg 2006;44(5):371–376
10. Humphris GM, Rogers S, McNally D, Lee-Jones C, Brown J, Vaughan D. Fear of recurrence and possible cases of anxiety and depression in orofacial cancer patients. Int J Oral Maxillofac Surg 2003;32(5):486–491
11. van der Schroeff MP, Steyerberg E, Wieringa MH, Langeveld TPM, Molenaar J, Baatenburg de Jong RJ. Prognosis: a variable parameter. Dynamic prognostic modeling in head and neck squamous cell carcinoma. Head Neck. 2011 Feb 14. doi: 101 002/hed.21 693. [Epub ahead of print]
12. Sher DJ, Haddad RI, Norris CM Jr, et al. Efficacy and toxicity of reirradiation using intensity-modulated radiotherapy for recurrent or second primary head and neck cancer. Cancer 2010;116(20):4761–4768
13. Coatesworth AP, Tsikoudas A, MacLennan K. The cause of death in patients with head and neck squamous cell carcinoma. J Laryngol Otol 2002;116(4):269–271
14. Woolgar JA, Rogers S, West CR, Errington RD, Brown JS, Vaughan ED. Survival and patterns of recurrence in 200 oral cancer patients treated by radical surgery and neck dissection. Oral Oncol 1999;35(3):257–265
15. Griffiths MJ, Humphris GM, Skirrow PM, Rogers SN. A qualitative evaluation of patient experiences when diagnosed with oral cancer recurrence. Cancer Nurs 2008;31(4):E11–E17
16. De Boer MF, Van den Borne B, Pruyn JF, et al. Psychosocial and physical correlates of survival and recurrence in patients with head and neck carcinoma: results of a 6-year longitudinal study. Cancer 1998;83(12):2567–2579
17. Lazure KE, Lydiatt WM, Denman D, Burke WJ. Association between depression and survival or disease recurrence in patients with head and neck cancer enrolled in a depression prevention trial. Head Neck 2009;31(7):888–892
18. Rogers SN, Scott B, Lowe D, Ozakinci G, Humphris GM. Fear of recurrence following head and neck cancer in the outpatient clinic. Eur Arch Otorhinolaryngol 2010;267(12):1943–1949
19. Campbell BH, Marbella A, Layde PM. Quality of life and recurrence concern in survivors of head and neck cancer. Laryngoscope 2000;110(6):895–906
20. Hodges LJ, Humphris GM. Fear of recurrence and psychological distress in head and neck cancer patients and their carers. Psychooncology 2009;18(8):841–848
21. Humphris G, Ozakinci G. The AFTER intervention: a structured psychological approach to reduce fears of recurrence in patients with head and neck cancer. Br J Health Psychol 2008;13(Pt 2):223–230
22. Humphris GM, Rogers SN. The association of cigarette smoking and anxiety, depression and fears of recurrence in patients following treatment of oral and oropharyngeal malignancy. Eur J Cancer Care (Engl) 2004;13(4):328–335
23. Llewellyn CD, Weinman J, McGurk M, Humphris G. Can we predict which head and neck cancer survivors develop fears of recurrence? J Psychosom Res 2008;65(6):525–532
24. Heider F. Social perception and phenomenal causality. Psychol Rev 1944; 51:358–374
25. Lazarus R, Folkman P. Stress, Appraisal, and Coping. New York: Springer; 1984
26. Sherman AC, Simonton S, Adams DC, Vural E, Hanna E. Coping with head and neck cancer during different phases of treatment. Head Neck 2000;22(8):787–793
27. Derks W, Leeuw JR, Hordijk GJ, Winnubst JA. Differences in coping style and locus of control between older and younger patients with head and neck cancer. Clin Otolaryngol 2005;30(2):186–192
28. Offerman MP, Schroevers MJ, van der Velden LA, de Boer MF, Pruyn JF. Goal processes & self-efficacy related to psychological distress in head & neck cancer patients and their partners. Eur J Oncol Nurs 2010;14(3):231–237

29. Goldstein NE, Genden E, Morrison RS. Palliative care for patients with head and neck cancer: "I would like a quick return to a normal lifestyle." JAMA 2008;299(15):1818–1825

30. Pruyn JF, Heule-Dieleman HA, Knegt PP, et al. On the enhancement of efficiency in care for cancer patients in outpatient clinics: an instrument to accelerate psychosocial screening and referral. Patient Educ Couns 2004;53(2):135–140

21 Palliative and Psychosocial Issues in Advanced Head and Neck Cancer

Dan Munday, Cherith J. Semple

Summary

- Effective management of advanced head and neck cancer demands an integrated multidisciplinary approach.
- Pain in head and neck cancer is common and often complex and can be difficult to manage effectively.
- Surgery and treatment with chemoradiotherapy can lead to significant morbidity and impact on quality of life.
- Malnutrition resulting from dysphagia has a major impact on outcome and quality of life. Use of enteral feeding tubes should be carefully planned in advance.
- Head and neck cancer sufferers share all common psychosocial issues with other cancer patients, compounded by disfigurement and dysfunction.
- Most deaths in head and neck cancer are not dramatic, the mode of death being similar to that of other malignant diseases. However, a significant minority die from bleeding and respiratory obstruction, which can be extremely distressing to the patient, to carers, and to attendant health-care staff.

Introduction

Effective management of patients with advanced cancer requires a multidisciplinary approach, since cancer has a major impact on the whole of a patient's life. As the illness progresses, patients frequently suffer a marked reduction in quality of life through the development of unpleasant symptoms related to their disease and treatment, anxiety about the future and depression resulting from multiple losses through increasing functional impairment and the inability to maintain social roles. Patients with advanced head and neck cancer have to contend with a particularly high symptom burden related both to the disease and to treatment, which can in itself lead to high levels of morbidity. They have a particularly high incidence of neuropathic pain, which is frequently difficult to control. Neuropathic pain can also be associated with impaired swallowing, communication problems, disfiguring facial changes, and fungating lesions which can be particularly distressing and lead to social isolation. Not surprisingly psychosocial morbidity is particularly high for these patients.

Most head and neck tumors are etiologically linked to a history of smoking and alcohol use, which has historically led to a higher incidence in men than women and continues to disproportionately affect people from lower socioeconomic groups. A significant number of these patients have poor access to health care and lack social support structures.[1]

Through its common etiology with respiratory and cardiovascular diseases, patients with head and neck cancer also have a higher incidence of serious medical comorbidities, raising further complications for their effective management.

Despite the importance of providing effective palliative and supportive care for patients with head and neck cancer, little attention in the past had been devoted to this area.[2] However, in 2004, the UK's National Institute for Health and Clinical Excellence (NICE) Service Guidance on Improving Outcomes in Head and Neck Cancer included a section on palliative intervention and care, highlighting the importance of a multidisciplinary approach.[3] More recently, the British Association of Head and Neck Oncologists published standards for head and neck cancer care.[4] These emphasize the importance of developing policies for the provision of palliative care within individual centers in partnership with local palliative care consultants and the need for all health-care professionals to be familiar with the route of referral for palliative care.

While palliative and supportive care management for patients suffering from head and neck cancer holds much in common with that of other cancers, there are important areas that merit special consideration. In this chapter, we explore some of the common but challenging palliative and supportive care issues central to the effective management of advanced head and neck cancer. We will specifically concentrate on: management of oral problems, swallowing and nutrition; management of complex wounds; and management of psychosocial problems resulting from disfigurement and dysfunction. We will also consider the management of the last few days of life and advance care planning, which focuses on exploring a patient's priorities for end-of-life care. For other symptoms, readers are encouraged to also access general palliative care texts and we give some suggestions in the Recommended Reading section at the end of the chapter.

First we will consider pain control and its particular challenges in advanced head and neck cancer.

Pain Control in Advanced Head and Neck Cancer

Pain is a common symptom in patients with advanced head and neck cancers, with case series reporting incidence of between 62% and 84%.[5–7] Pain is also a frequent occurrence at diagnosis, with one study reporting that 48% of patients had pain on presentation.[8] For this reason, clinicians who care for these patients need to have the knowledge and skills to assess and treat pain effectively.

Etiological Aspects

Pain in advanced head and neck cancer can also be difficult to treat because of its complex etiology.[9] This complexity is a feature of the anatomy of the head and neck, with a multiplicity of nerves, bone, highly innervated soft tissue, and restricted spaces where tumor expansion is likely to cause pain through pressure effects. It is not only the underlying disease process that leads to pain; post-treatment effects may also be the underlying cause. Long-term postsurgical pain sequelae are not infrequent with, most notably, shoulder or arm pain occurring after neck dissection.[10] Mucositis commonly causes distressing mouth pain following chemoradiotherapy[11] and osteoradionecrosis of the jaw is a relatively uncommon but devastating complication.[12] As a result, the pain encountered in patients with advanced head and neck cancer frequently has a mixed etiology, with often two or more pains occurring simultaneously, each one requiring careful assessment to enable effective management.

Achieving good control of pain is also likely to be challenging because of psychological and emotional factors. Exploring such issues through a meticulous holistic approach has been recognized as a central task in providing effective palliative care from the earliest days of the specialty[13]; failing to do so is likely to affect not just the patient's mood and psychological state but also the likelihood of controlling their physical pain effectively.

Management of Different Types of Pain

The importance of establishing the cause of pain lies in the fact that different types of pain will respond to different therapeutic approaches and will be resistant to others. It is therefore helpful to have a framework for assessing pain (**Table 21.1**).

Nociceptive Pain

Nociceptive pain caused by stimulation of nociceptors in pain-transmitting neurons may be subdivided into somatic or visceral. Visceral pain, such as from enlarging cervical nodes typically produces pain with a deep, aching quality, which is poorly localized and is normally responsive to opioids.

Somatic Pain

Somatic pain, caused by infiltration of bone, joint, or muscle might be more easily localized, may present as aching or sharp in quality, and typically worsens with movement. While it is partially responsive to opioids, pain control in somatic pain can be improved by adding nonsteroidal anti-inflammatory drugs as an adjuvant analgesic. For all patients with pain of whatever etiology, it is helpful for them to take acetaminophen even if they are taking opioids, as this does give additional analgesic benefit through a synergistic effect.[14]

Table 21.1 Pain classification according to etiology

Type of pain	Therapeutic approach
Nociceptive pain: results from tissue damage and caused by stimulation of nociceptors in pain transmitting neurons	
Visceral pain	Opioid sensitive
Somatic pain	Partially opioid sensitive. Responds to NSAIDs
Neuropathic pain: caused by disruption of sensory neurons through compression, tumor infiltration, surgical section, or other pathological process (e.g., chemotherapy induced)	Opioids are frequently ineffective or insufficient to control the pain Management relies on co-analgesics particularly tricyclic antidepressants and anticonvulsants

Neuropathic Pain

Neuropathic pain in head and neck cancer will typically be caused by nerve damage as a result of compression from an expanding tumor, malignant infiltration, surgical section, or toxic damage following chemotherapy. Neuropathic pain has traditionally been considered as opioid resistant and coanalgesic agents such as tricyclic antidepressants and anticonvulsants either individually or in combination are typically used for pain control in this situation. The tricyclic antidepressant most commonly prescribed and with which many clinicians have the most experience is amitriptyline (10–75 mg daily). Randomized controlled trials have, however, demonstrated that amitriptyline is in fact no more effective than other tricyclic antidepressants such as nortryptyline and desipramine, which have considerably fewer side effects.[15]

In the United Kingdom the most popular anticonvulsants used in neuropathic pain are gabapentin (100–3600 mg in divided doses) and pregabalin (75–600 mg in divided doses). These drugs are similar in action and efficacy and are the only drugs licensed specifically for the treatment of neuropathic pain[14]). Most RCTs suggest that the number needed to treat (NNT) for anticonvulsants and antidepressants is around 3.[15] Frequently, the dose of drug that may be given is limited by side effects, leading to further challenges in achieving a therapeutic dose. Amitriptyline causes somnolescence even if taken in a single night-time dose and it frequently leads to a dry mouth, which might be particularly problematic in patients with salivary gland dysfunction, which is common in head and neck cancer. Pregabalin and gabapentin seem to be better tolerated, but need to be given in divided doses (two to three times daily), which can be more problematic for patients already on a plethora of medication.

While neuropathic pain has been commonly considered as opioid resistant, this has not been confirmed by randomized controlled trials. These have demonstrated effectiveness for the common opioids used in clinical practice that is similar to the other drugs frequently used in neuropathic pain[16] with the NNT for opioids being around 3, similar to anticonvulsants and antidepressants.[15] Caution needs to be taken in interpreting these results, because as with all randomized controlled trials for neuropathic pain, they have largely been undertaken in patients with noncancer causes of pain, typically diabetes or postherpetic neuropathy. However, it is probably reasonable to assume that patients with head and neck cancer who have neuropathic pain should be managed with adequate levels of opioid analgesics in addition to coanalgesics.

Route of Administration

In head and neck cancer patients who have difficulty swallowing, delivering analgesics by the parenteral route is a useful alternative. The practical alternatives for long-term analgesia when a patient is unable to manage oral medications, particularly in the community setting, are transdermal patches or, alternatively, subcutaneous opioids delivered by a syringe driver.

Transdermal Route

Transdermal patches enable the patient to remain in control of their analgesia by changing the patch every 3 days or weekly, depending on the type of patch used. They are designed to deliver a standard dose of drug over a unit time across the skin and the "size" of patch denotes this dose (e.g., a fentanyl "25" patch delivers 25 µg of the drug per hour).

The two drugs available in patch form are fentanyl and buprenorphine. Fentanyl is similar to morphine, being a pure opioid agonist at the mu receptor, and has no theoretical ceiling dose. Buprenorphine is a partial agonist at the mu receptor and antagonist at kappa and sigma receptors but has a similar clinical spectrum of action to morphine. Recent case reports have indicated that buprenorphine may have a particular use in neuropathic pain, although this effect has not been tested in randomized controlled trials.[17] Effectiveness in neuropathic pain may make buprenorphine a particularly suitable analgesic in head and neck cancer, and certainly the author of this chapter has found it to be frequently effective in these patients.

Fentanyl and buprenorphine are highly lipophilic agents, a necessary property to allow transdermal absorption. Once absorbed, the drugs form a subcutaneous deposit from which they are slowly absorbed into the circulation. For this reason it can take 12–24 hours for the patch to exert an appreciable analgesic effect and up to 72 hours for it to reach steady state. In addition, once the patch is discontinued the drug will continue to be absorbed from the subcutaneous deposit with appreciable levels of drug remaining in circulation for up to 24 hours. Care therefore needs to be taken when starting a patch, to ensure the patient has sufficient alternative analgesia for the first 24 hours. Similarly, when discontinuing the patch and rotating onto another opioid, a lower dose of the new analgesic needs to be given for the first 24 hours after the patch is removed.

There is wide variability among individuals in the rate of absorption of transdermal opioids. Absorption is affected by the thickness of the stratum corneum layer of skin and cutaneous blood flow, with higher rates of absorption through warm, vasodilated skin. As a consequence there is a wide range of dose equivalence with morphine. Fentanyl is 100 times more potent than morphine, with a "25 micrograms patch" equivalent to a 24-hourly dose of morphine of around 90 mg, with a range of 60–120 mg. There has been recent debate about the dose equivalence for buprenorphine, with previous advice being that it was about half as potent as fentanyl when given transdermally (such that buprenorphine 50 µg per hour was equivalent to 25 µg per hour of fentanyl). Current advice from recent comparative studies suggests that the two drugs should be seen as equipotent.[17]

Syringe Drivers

Syringe drivers provide an important route for delivery of drugs in head and neck cancer patients who have difficulty swallowing oral medication. Their introduction into practice some 25 years ago had a major impact on the practice of palliative care as it enabled patients needing parenteral medication for symptom control to be effectively managed in the community.[18] Analgesics, antiemetics, sedatives and anticholinergics are the commonest drugs administered via this route either individually or in combination. If used in combination, it is vital that compatible drugs are mixed together. Compatibility data are available from www.palliativedrugs.com, a free to use web site available for all health-care professionals.

Enteral Route

Drugs, including many analgesics, can be delivered through enteral feeding tubes, but care needs to be taken to ensure that the tube does not become blocked, that there is no interaction with the feed, or that the drug's bioavailability is not altered by administration via this route. Information about individual drugs can be obtained from the British Pharmaceutical Nutrition Group (www.bapen.org.uk) and from www.palliativedrugs.com.

Transmucosal Route

Recent years have seen the development of novel drug delivery systems for fentanyl using the oral and intranasal transmucosal route, with the drug being absorbed through the mucosa to produce rapid-onset analgesia. As fentanyl also has a high volume of distribution, it will be redistributed rapidly, leading to a fall in blood levels over a few minutes. This makes fentanyl given by this route "rapid onset" and "rapid offset." It is therefore particularly useful for pain of short duration, such as with a dressing change or with "incident pain," i.e., pain brought on by movement.[19] Patients can take the preparation before the activity, with the drug starting to become effective after around 5 minutes and lasting for around 40 minutes to 1 hour. Several fentanyl preparations are now available including sublingual tablets, lozenges for buccal absorption, and intranasal sprays. It is too early to tell whether one preparation is preferable to another and decisions will be based on patient characteristics and personal preference of the prescribing clinician.

Oral Problems in Head and Neck Cancer

Oral problems are common in head and neck cancer and may arise as a result of the disease, treatment, or concomitant problems. Some problems are generic and common to any patient with an advanced malignancy and others are specific to head and neck cancer. As with pain, it is important that a thorough assessment is made so that the cause of the problem may be ascertained, since it may be possible to address or remove the underlying cause (particularly where it is the side effect of a drug), provide appropriate treatment, and consider or exclude any other problems causing oral symptoms.

Xerostomia/Dry Mouth

Etiology

Xerostomia is certainly not confined to patients with head and neck cancer and is present in around 80% of patients with advanced neoplasia.[20] However, while it is one of the most common symptoms found in patients with advanced disease, it often remains undiagnosed and poorly managed.[21] This may be a result of patients frequently viewing it as inevitable and trivial in the

Table 21.2 Causes of xerostomia

General causes (shared with other sites)	Specific causes in head and neck cancer
Cancer	**Cancer**
Hypercalcemia with dehydration	Replacement of salivary gland with tumor Erosion of buccal mucosa
Treatment related	**Treatment related**
Drugs: particularly opioids, antimuscarinics (hyoscine, tricyclics, antihistamines), cyclizine, diuretics, NSAIDs Oxygen therapy (unhumidified) Proprietary mouthwashes	Local surgery Local radiotherapy Chemoradiotherapy
Other causes	**Other causes**
Debility, dehydration, mouth breathing, diabetes, oral candidiasis, smoking, alcohol, caffeine	As for general causes, but patients are much more likely to develop secondary infections/dry mouth through loss of normal mouth-cleaning processes

(Adapted from reference [20].)

context of more serious problems, and clinicians may not ask patients directly about it.

Multiple causes are responsible for xerostomia and frequently a patient will have more than one concomitant cause; for example, the patient has previously had radiotherapy leading to posttreatment salivary gland dysfunction and is now taking opioids (**Table 21.2**).

Signs and Symptoms

Xerostomia is not only unpleasant for the patient but may have other adverse effects. Oral discomfort and difficulty chewing and swallowing may increase feelings of anorexia and lead to poor oral intake and weight loss and contribute to general deterioration. Saliva has an antimicrobial protective effect, so that xerostomia may lead to candidiasis or bacterial oral infections and also acceleration of dental caries. Halitosis and discomfort when speaking and eating can lead to isolation, with patients avoiding social contact.

Prevention

Patients who have had radiotherapy to the head and neck will frequently develop salivary gland dysfunction. This reduction in salivary flow is often evident soon after the radiotherapy starts and worsens throughout its course. Partial recovery may occur following its completion, but some residual dysfunction is likely to be permanent.[11] Attempts may be made to reduce the likelihood of radiation damage to the salivary glands by a variety of techniques, including conformal radiotherapy, in which the salivary glands are spared through altering the shape of the field by using lead tissues shields; and intensity-modulated radiotherapy (IMRT), where the dose of radiation delivered to salivary glands is reduced using complex radiotherapy planning techniques and the use of amifostine, a cytoprotective agent that reduces the likelihood of radionecrosis in normal tissue.[11] The main side-effect of amifostine is nausea, and this, in association with the need for a daily intravenous infusion, makes it unpopular with patients with advanced head and neck cancer.

Management

Management of xerostomia includes the removal of the cause, if at all possible. Drugs with anticholinergic side effects, such as amitriptyline, should be stopped if appropriate and substituted with drugs less likely to dry the mouth, for example, gabapentin/pregabalin. Diuretics should be reviewed and discontinued if this is feasible, since these are frequently prescribed for hypoalbuminemic peripheral edema in advanced cancer, with limited effectiveness. Oxygen should always be humidified when delivered to the patient. Patients with dry mouth may be helped by regular sips of water, crushed ice, and salivary stimulation by chewing gum or sucking boiled sweets such as acid drops.[14] Artificial saliva sprays and saliva replacement gels are available, but these may need to be used every 30–60 minutes to achieve the desired effect. pH-neutral agents should be used preferentially as prolonged use of acidic artificial salivas causes demineralization of the teeth.[20] If simple local measures are not effective, salivary flow can be stimulated using the parasympathomimetic agents pilocarpine or bethanacol. These agents are only effective in patients with some residual salivary gland function and their use is restricted because of side effects including sweating, flushing, nausea, intestinal colic, and urinary frequency.[17]

■ Drooling

Signs and Symptoms

Drooling is not uncommon in patients with head and neck cancer. In most instances when drooling is apparent the patient's saliva production is normal, but there is failure to handle saliva effectively. This may be due to anatomical distortion of the mouth or lips as a result of the disease or following surgery, or to inability to swallow saliva due to pharyngeal obstruction.

Management

Referral to speech and language therapy is helpful for assessment and management, which will include training in head positioning or exercises to improve swallowing.[21] Drug therapy utilizing the antisecretory effects of anticholinergic drugs such as hyoscine hydrobromide (Scopoderm) patches, or alternatively oral glycopyronium or propanthaline can be effective in reducing saliva flow.[17] Use of amitriptyline is an alternative and can be particularly appropriate if required for pain control, for sedation, or as an antidepressant. Rarely if drooling cannot be effectively controlled with drug measures, radiotherapy to salivary glands will reduce salivary flow and provide effective palliation.

■ Stomatitis and Mucositis

Etiology

Stomatitis is a diffuse inflammation of the oral mucous membranes, often with erosions or ulceration, which commonly occurs in patients who are debilitated from any cause including those with advanced cancer. Colonization of the mouth with organisms such as *Candida albicans* or Gram-negative bacteria often underlies the condition. This is more prevalent in patients in whom there has been a loss of the cytoprotective effect of saliva either from salivary gland dysfunction or through drying of the mouth with prolonged mouth breathing or use of unhumidified oxygen.[20]

Severe stomatitis found in head and neck cancer patients following local radiotherapy or in any patient receiving chemotherapy is termed **mucositis.**[1] Mucositis arises as a result of damage to basal keratinocytes of the oral mucosa and is characterized by marked ulceration in the mouth as the normal mucosal repair mechanisms are rendered ineffective. As a result of this process, there is colonization of the mouth by Gram-negative coliform organisms, which accelerate the inflammation and ulceration. When head and neck radiotherapy and chemotherapy are combined, they will have a synergistic effect, frequently causing severe mucositis.[11]

Prevention

Since mucositis is very common in patients with head and neck cancer receiving chemoradiotherapy, preventative measures form a very important aspect of its overall management. These should include pretreatment dental consultation and therapy, regular mouth washes with hypotonic saline or sodium bicarbonate, and the avoidance of irritants such as spicy food or alcohol during and for 6 weeks after treatment.

Management

A detailed discussion of the management of established mucositis is beyond the scope of this chapter; however, in summary, management usually involves the use of locally active mucosal coating agents (e.g., sucralfate, gelclair), anti-inflammatories (benzydamine, corticosteroid mouthwash), antiseptic mouthwashes, antimicrobials (antibiotic lozenges, antifungal agents), immunomodulators (granulocyte colony-stimulating factor: G-CSF), anesthetic agents (lignocaine, benzocaine), and analgesics (e.g., topical morphine).[10] There is little robust evidence for the use of any particular topical therapy for mucositis[22] and most services will have their own protocols based on evidence, local preference, and cost. Systemic antifungals or antibiotics might also be used in the treatment of severe mucositis and many patients will also require systemic analgesics such as opioids and NSAIDs.[10]

Swallowing and Nutrition

Dysphagia

Dysphagia, defined as difficulty swallowing or inability to swallow safely, is present in over 50% of patients with head and neck cancer and is significantly associated with decreased survival. Dysphagia has been reported as the second most prevalent symptom in the last 6 months of life for patients with advanced head and neck cancer.[6]

Etiology

Patients with advanced head and neck cancer are at risk of developing dysphagia for several reasons. These include the physical presence of the tumor obstructing swallow, cranial nerve deficiencies, trismus (inability to open the mouth normally), surgical resection, radiotherapy and chemotherapy, and cancer-related fatigue.

Signs and Symptoms

Research suggests that health-care professionals are generally poor at recognizing signs and symptoms of dysphagia. Furthermore, patients can see the condition as an inevitable part of aging or the disease process. Commonly, individuals experiencing dysphagia will exhibit effortful swallows or a delay in initiating a swallow. Drooling or the accumulation of food in the mouth can be noted in patients with poor lingual movement. Difficulties with swallowing often elicit a cough reflex, nasal or oral regurgitation, or the presence of a "wet" voice quality. It is important to recognize these overt signs of dysphagia, as individuals with advanced head and neck cancer are at high risk of aspiration. Aspiration is most commonly attributed to decreased laryngeal elevation and a delay in triggering the pharyngeal swallow.

In addition to the risk of aspiration, weight loss and malnutrition may be a consequence of dysphagia. Approximately one-third of patients with advanced head and neck cancer are severely malnourished and another third are mildly malnourished.[23] Malnutrition can also be related to alcohol abuse, odynophagia (pain on swallowing), and side effects related to treatment such as xerostomia (dry mouth), dysgeusia (altered taste), and dysosmia (altered smell). Some patients develop food aversions, while others experience thick, ropy saliva that interferes with adequate oral intake. Weight loss in patients with advanced head and neck cancer can also be attributed to fatigue, depression, and cancer cachexia.

It is important to understand the difference between cachexia and starvation, because they are distinctly different entities:

- In starvation, lean body mass is conserved, and there is a preferential increase in fat metabolism to supply energy. These patients have lower resting energy expenditure, which matches their reduced energy intake.
- Cancer cachexia appears to be a different process with preferential loss of skeletal muscle over adipose tissue and involves inappropriate elevation of resting energy expenditure. Patients with cachexia have marked unintentional weight loss, anemia, anorexia, and emotional and mental fatigue.

Dysphagia has a profound and multidimensional impact on the lives of patients with advanced head and neck cancer and their families. Normal routines are altered, which can change the meaning that patients with head and neck cancer attribute to food. Patients may require extra time to eat, or may avoid eating with others due to embarrassment resulting from oral incontinence, thus affecting interactions with family members. Reduced enjoyment from food is often reported, as many patients require a modified diet or have altered taste. Not surprisingly, dysphagia impacts considerably on quality of life. Patients with dysphagia have described feelings such as anger, frustration, lack of confidence, and poor self-esteem.[24]

Management

Having established that dysphagia is a common problem for patients with advanced head and neck cancer and can lead to aspiration, malnourishment, and reduced quality of life, it should there-

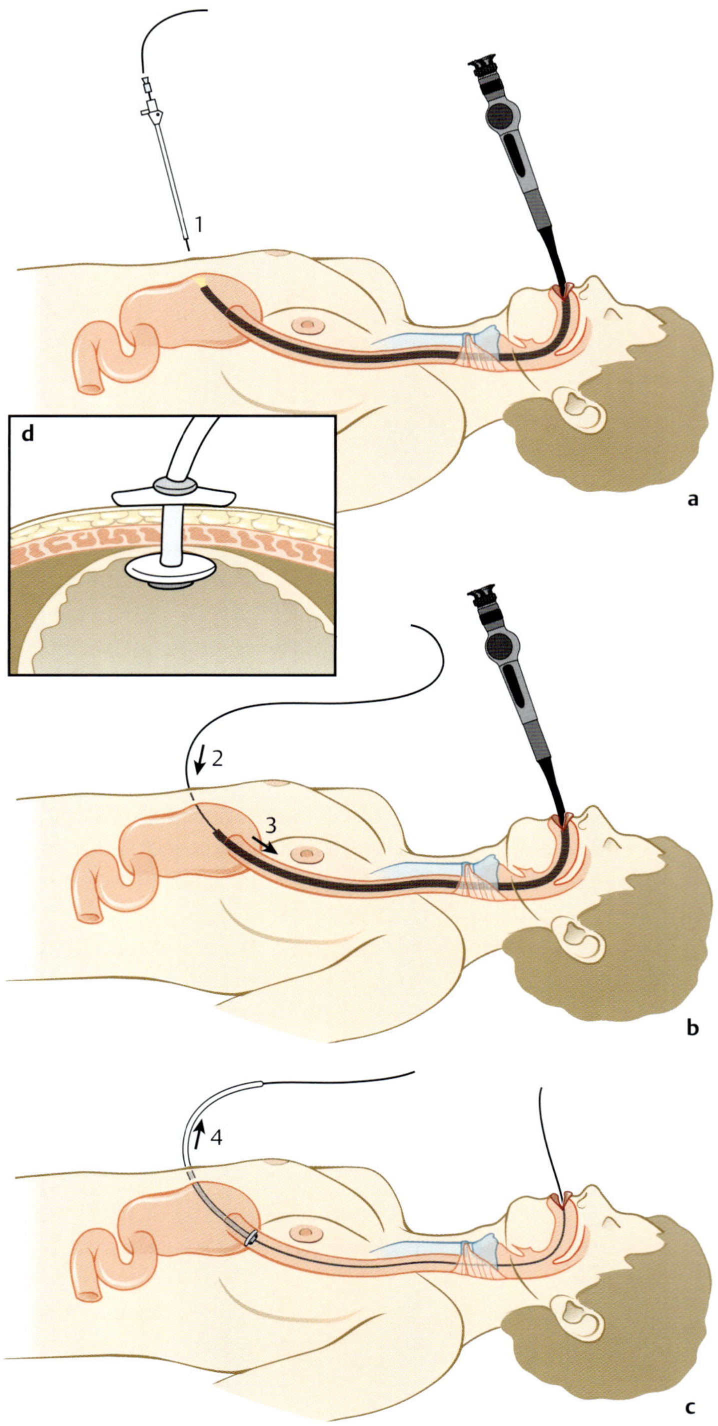

Fig. 21.1a–d Percutaneous endoscopic gastrostomy (PEG).
a A flexible endoscope is used to transilluminate the gastric wall. A sharp needle (1) is used to perforate the gastric wall at the illuminated point.
b A guide wire is introduced (2) and is retracted with the esophagoscope (3) and led out of the mouth.
c The gastrostomy tube is connected to the guide wire. The wire is retracted through the gastric wall together with the tube (4).
d A double-layered plate is used to seal the gastric wall.

fore be assessed in a multidisciplinary manner. Patients should be referred to a speech and language therapist (SLT). Assessment of the patient's current swallow status will involve a clinical bedside observation, but may also include a FEES (fiberoptic endoscopic evaluation of swallowing) and/or videofluoroscopy (modified barium swallow) if insufficient information is gained from the bedside assessment.

Following assessment, dysphagia may be managed by:
- Simple measures such as recommendations by the SLT on diet modification
- Enteral feeding
- Surgical management

Recommendations from the SLT to minimize swallowing deficits and compensate for problems may include a variety of intervention strategies such as:
- Manipulating the progress of the food bolus by modifying the consistency and viscosity of the food. This may include advice such as alternating liquid and solid foods, use of puréed foods, or use of thicker liquids.
- Altering the head and neck posture to slow or direct the passage of the food bolus.
- Specific therapy techniques such as chin-down posture for patients with reduced laryngeal closure as this will put the epiglottis in a more protective position and narrow the laryngeal entrance.

Where the implementation of the above simple interventions may be impractical due to fatigue or is inadequate to sustain nutritional needs, or if the patient is aspirating, then enteral nutrition (tube feeding) may be appropriate. The timing for tube placement is often a reflection of clinical judgment and patient preference. Generally, enteral feeding should not be instituted in the last week of life; such intervention would usually be seen as inappropriate, but prognostication is not always straightforward.

■ Enteral Tube Feeding

It is imperative that the use of enteral tube feeding is considered carefully by the multidisciplinary team and fully discussed with the patient and their carers. The ability for the individual patient and/or carer to manage will vary as some patients and carers may be taught to manage the feeding themselves, while others may require substantial support in the home setting. The advantages and disadvantages of the different types of enteral tube feeds should also be considered by the multidisciplinary team and fully discussed with the patient/carer. The two most common types of enteral feeding tubes are a nasogastric tube or a gastrostomy tube.

Nasogastric (NG) tube feeding may be the route of choice for patients requiring relatively short-term feeding (less than 4–6 weeks); for example, for a patient with oral mucositis, where it is anticipated that patient will resume oral nutrition when mucositis has resolved. An NG tube may also be used as an interim measure, while a gastrostomy is being scheduled. On occasions, an NG tube may be the preferred mode of enteral feeding if an individual is clinically fragile. Fine-bore tubes made from soft polyurethane or silicone are the NG tubes of choice as they are more comfortable. Placement of NG tubes may be difficult in some patients with advanced head and neck cancer who have altered anatomy as a result of tumor, surgery, and/or treatment. NG feeding can be associated with complications such as patient discomfort, laryngeal irritation, and persistent gastroesophageal reflux. NG feeding tubes are at risk of tube displacement and blockage and are often socially unacceptable.

Gastrostomy tube insertions may be considered for patients who are likely to require longer-term feeding (i.e., for periods of greater than 4 weeks). The gastrostomy tube can be placed endo-

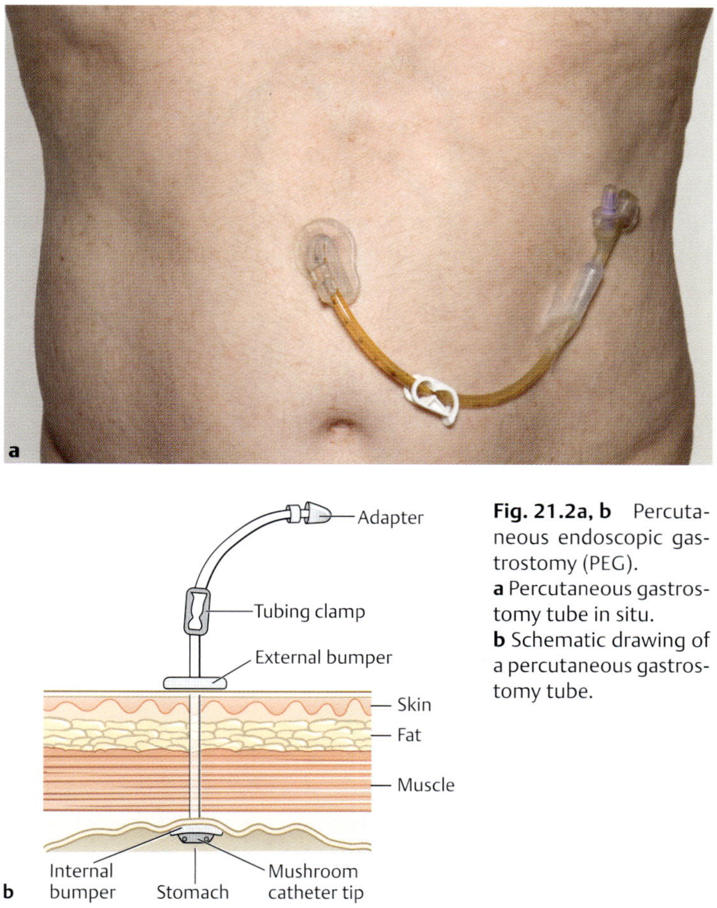

Fig. 21.2a, b Percutaneous endoscopic gastrostomy (PEG).
a Percutaneous gastrostomy tube in situ.
b Schematic drawing of a percutaneous gastrostomy tube.

scopically in a procedure known as a percutaneous endoscopic gastrostomy (PEG, **Fig. 21.1**), or radiologically in a procedure known as a radiologically inserted gastrostomy (RIG). A PEG (**Fig. 21.2**) is the most common type of gastrostomy tube placement, but passage of an endoscope may be difficult in patients with extensive disease and/or trismus. If this is the case, then a RIG should be considered.

Evidence from both prospective and retrospective studies indicated that PEGs may have potential advantages over NG tubes during radiotherapy, through enhanced mobility and improved quality of life. Comparison between the two mechanisms of enteral feeding has not been conducted in patients who have advanced cancer and are receiving supportive care. Nevertheless, gastrostomy placement is not without complications and patients who are being consented should be counseled about the risk of local site infection, leakage around the gastrostomy site, local pain, granulation tissue around the site, migration of the tube, gastric erosion, intraperitioneal leakage, and death from peritonitis. A Swedish study showed that fatal or severe complications of PEG placement occurred in 26% of cases over 2 years,[25] whereas other studies have demonstrated complications rates ranging from 4% to 70%. However, serious complications from placement of a PEG would appear to be low in departments with greater levels of expertise. Once the feeding regimen is established and patients/carers are educated in managing the PEG, community nurses and dietitians should be involved to provide support at home.

Role of Surgery

When swallow is impaired due to strictures, dilation may be performed under local (using flexible endoscopes) or general anesthetic. If the problem is considered to be a result of muscle spasm involving the cricopharyngeus, this may be addressed by injection of botulinum toxin. Extensive unresectable tumor recurrences within the pharynx may cause dysphagia. Sometimes, it is possible to perform transoral laser or diathermy resection of tumor masses to improve swallow. Nonetheless, patients need to be selected carefully and managed appropriately by an experienced surgeon.

> **!**
> - Dysphagia is commonly experienced by patients with advanced head and neck cancer and can have adverse sequelae including aspiration, malnourishment, tube dependency and reduced quality of life.
> - Dysphagia should be managed within the context of a specialist multidisciplinary team, with STLs and dietitians playing a vital role in helping patients and families cope and adapt to changes in their swallowing function.
> - Optimal management of dysphagia is important as it not only minimizes distressing symptoms such as choking but also reduces the risk of medical complications (dehydration, respiratory infection) and hospitalization.

Management of Complex Wounds

Complex wounds in head and neck cancer are predominantly related to disease progression. There are no exact statistics on the occurrence of malignant wounds in head and neck cancer, but estimates vary from 5% to 10%. Despite their infrequent occurrence, they are always distressing and pose a considerable challenge to the patient, carers, the individual's social network, and health-care professionals.

Pathophysiology

A cancerous wound that erupts through the surface of the skin is known as a "fungating wound" (**Fig. 21.3**). Fungating wounds are the visible markers of underlying malignant disease. In most cases, the wounds are a direct invasion from the primary site into the cutaneous facial structures, or a consequence of local or distant metastases from the primary tumor. The malignant wound usually presents as either raised nodules similar in appearance to cauliflower (proliferating) or a craterlike ulcer (destructive process), extending into the epithelium and its supporting lymph and blood vessels. As the mass increases and loses its vascularity, capillaries rupture and necrosis occurs and subsequent infection often develops. This produces a malodorous purulent wound.

Unless amenable to anticancer treatments, the infiltration extends and the wound progresses, with disruption of the blood and lymphatic systems. Without efficient circulation of blood and lymph, skin function is severely impaired, resulting in congestion and build up of waste materials in the tissues, ultimately causing tissue death. Anaerobic and aerobic bacteria proliferate in these conditions and are sources of malodor and exudate. The disease burden increases further if an orocutaneous fistula or lymphedema develops.

Signs and Symptoms

The most common physical symptoms of a fungating wound are malodor, exudate, pain, and bleeding. The assault to the individual,

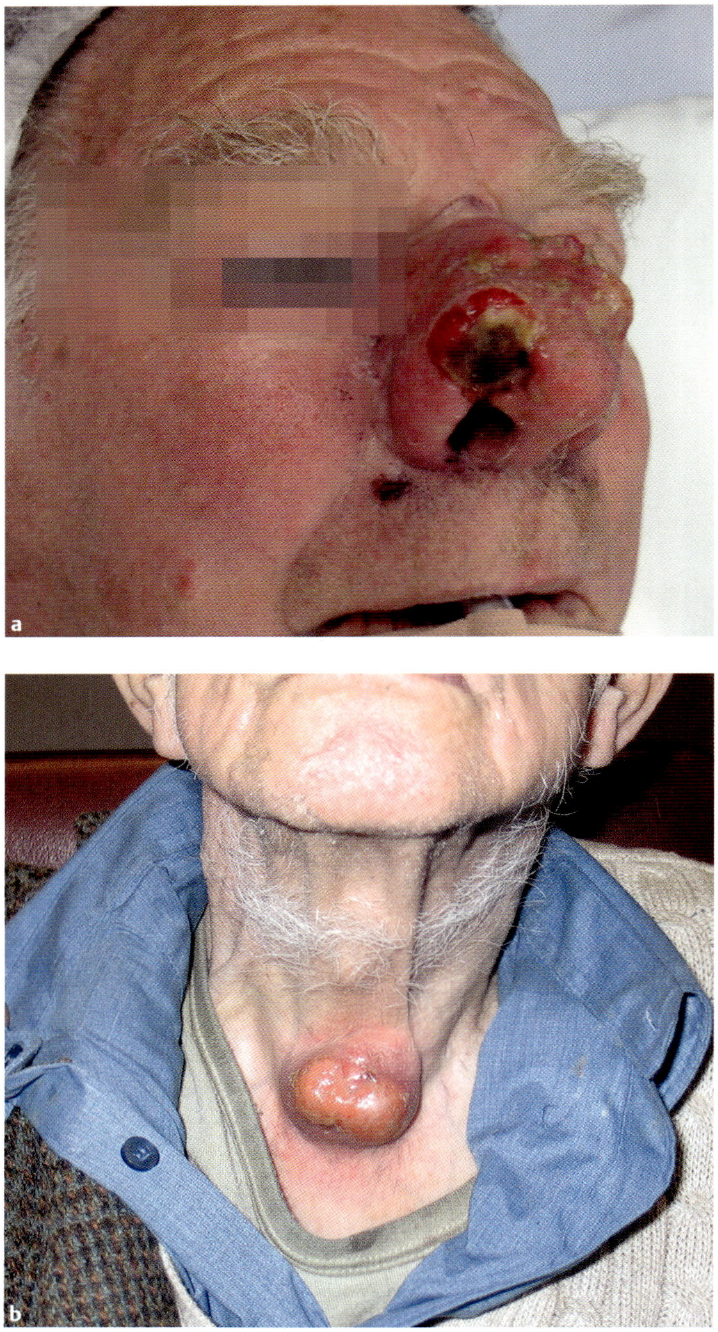

Fig. 21.3a, b Fungating lesions.
a Fungating recurrent tumor of the nose.
b Fungating skin metastasis from a recurrent hypopharyngeal cancer.

both physically and psychosocially, of uncontrolled tumor infiltration is immense. According to Grocott, skin is not only the largest and an important body organ with numerous physical functions, it plays a pivotal role in individuals' socialization, including how they perceive themselves and their acceptance in the social world.[26] The full impact may amount to a loss of self on behalf of the individual but also a separation from family and friends attributable to revulsion from loss of control over bodily fluids (exudate) and malodor. Unless fungating wounds are contained under wound dressings, the patient's life can center on leakage of exudate, soiling, changing of dressings, and laundry. Fungating wounds have far-reaching consequences, which may include anxiety, diminished self-esteem, social isolation, stigma, altered relationships, and loss of personhood and independence.

Management

The management of fungating wounds requires commitment from the multidisciplinary team. Consideration should be given to the use of oncological treatment to reduce the tumor size or promote healing of the wound. Radiotherapy can be a useful measure to reduce exudate, control bleeding, and alleviate pain. If fungation has not yet occurred, it may also delay this happening. It is important to note that any radiation therapy has the potential to cause skin reactions such as dry desquamation and erthyema. These should be managed according to local guidelines, but treatment side effects should never cause additional distress to the patient. Surgery is rarely used in the management of fungating wounds due to the local extension of the wound to underlying structures. In certain circumstances, it may be possible to remove a lesion to prevent progression of tumor infiltration. Despite the use of oncological treatment options for management of fungation, it is not uncommon to see tumor recurrence within a short time and the patient, family, and clinicians have to face the problems of living with a fungating tumor all over again. Individualized symptom control measures (local and systemic) alongside wound dressings are the mainstay of management once oncological treatments have been exhausted.

A comprehensive, individualized assessment is imperative and should not only focus on the wound history and properties but also address nutritional status, ability to self-care, psychosocial issues (mood, body image, sexuality), social support, current morbidities, and spiritual and cultural needs. Constant reassessment and tailoring of management to meet the changing needs is particularly important. When possible, a consultation with tissue viability/wound care teams should be sought.

> **!** Only wounds that are producing exudate, purulence, or serous fluids require wound cleansing. This can be achieved by gentle irrigation with normal saline 0.9% at room temperature to avoid further trauma, pain, or bleeding. It is also accepted that this cleansing can be done adequately with showering.

■ Exudate

Signs and Symptoms

Fungating wounds can produce large amounts of exudate, sometimes over a liter per day. This is due to the increased permeability to fibrinogen and plasma colloid of the tumor microvasculature, secretion of vascular permeability factor (VPF) by tumor cells, and inflammatory processes associated with infection.

Management

It is important to use an absorbent dressing with a good seal to minimize the risk of leakage. It is also important to choose a dressing that maintains a moist wound bed. *Alginates* (Kaltostat, Sorbsan) and *hydrofiber* dressings (Aquacel) may be used as a primary dressing and are useful in absorbing medium to high amounts of exudate. Caution should be exercised on removal if they are adherent. *Foams* (Allevyn, Tielle Plus) can be used as primary or secondary dressings (in combination with other dressings). Protection of the surrounding skin should also be considered to prevent further breakdown of the wound. A protective *non-alcohol skin barrier film* such as Cavilon is recommended. The use of a *stoma bag appliance* may be helpful for discrete fungating wounds with intact surrounding skin. In the authors' clinical area, more extensive wounds with orocutaneous fistulas are referred to the maxillofacial technician; an individualized wound management appliance made from silicone has been found to be of some benefit.

Malodor

Signs and Symptoms

This is often described as one of the most distressing symptoms for the patient and family and can have an overwhelming effect on quality of life. The characteristic smell that is associated with a fungating wound is due to anaerobic bacteria, such as those found in the genera *Bacteroides* and *Clostridium*. The bacteria flourish in the accessible necrotic tissue, where their metabolic processes produce particularly pungent volatile short-chain fatty acids as an end product.

Management

According to Grocott,[26] the three main approaches to be adopted for the management of odor are systemic antibiotics, topical metronidazole, and charcoal dressings.

Systemic metronidazole is used as a presumptive measure to reduce bacterial colonization and control the offensive odor from volatile metabolic end-products. One of the limitations of its use is poor acceptability to the patients, due to gastric side effects. Some suggest that metronidazole could be used in a lower dose of 200 mg three times a day, with fewer side effects without losing the therapeutic effect on the odour.[14]

Topical metronidazole gel (0.8%–0.9%) may overcome the limitations of the systemic route, however, in extensive necrotic wounds sufficient inhibitory concentration of metronidazole to deodorize may not be reached. Metronidazole gel can be mixed with other hydrogels to facilitate debridement. Use is recommended for 5–7 days, but may be repeated to manage odor.

Clearance of dead tissue by **surgical debridement** is generally not an option for fungating wounds because of the bleeding potential. Autolytic debridement with topical hydrating materials may be appropriate, but the clinical gains need to be assessed critically. Honey and enzymatic debriding agents are forms of autolytic debridement and reduce odor significantly. Nonetheless, these agents inevitably increase exudate as the devitalized tissue is liquefied and separated from the wound bed. This exudate has to be contained with wound dressings otherwise the patients experience a further unpleasant problem or the aggravation of an existing problem.[26]

Activated charcoal dressings (Clinisorb, Carboflex) act as filters to absorb the volatile malodorous chemicals from the wound, before they pass into the air. Charcoal dressings become ineffective if they become wet, or if they cannot be fitted as a sealed unit. Some charcoal dressings are impregnated with silver and claims are made that the dressing has bacteriostatic properties in addition to adsorbing odor-forming molecules (Actisorb Silver).

Bleeding

Signs and Symptoms

In patients with advanced head and neck cancer, bleeding from a wound can be a common reason for an emergency admission. Ethunandan et al. reported that 29% of emergency admissions were as a result of bleeding.[5]

Malignant wounds often have bleeding and clotting irregularities due to abnormal vasculature in the advancing tumor. Bleeding can also be related to the application of an inappropriate dressing; hence careful selection of dressings is imperative. Although certain fibrous alginates are promoted as hemostatic dressings, fibers can become intertwined in the tumor, causing mechanical damage and bleeding on removal. Alternative nonadherent systems include Mepitel with a simple pad or Mesorb.

Management

The following treatments should also be considered for the management of bleeding from eroding blood vessels in a wound:

- **Epinephrine 1:1000** soaked in gauze can be applied with pressure. However, the vasoconstrictive effects of epinephrine are associated with ischemic necrosis if it is used liberally.
- **Oral antifibrinolytics,** such as tranexamic acid given orally or via a feeding tube can be given for the prevention of bleeding.
- **Surgical hemostatic sponges** (e.g., Spongostan) are very useful in fast capillary bleeding. Unfortunately, they are very difficult for community staff to access; they are expensive and are not available on the Drug Tariff in many countries. **Sucralfate** suspension applied directly to the wound has been advocated as a cost-effective alternative, but robust evidence for its use is lacking and its performance should be evaluated in clinical trials

Pain

The physical sensation of pain in malignant wounds may be caused by:

- Pressure from the tumor on nerves and blood vessels
- Exposure of dermal nerve endings
- Recurrent infection
- Surrounding edema and/or excoriated skin
- Dressing changes

Accurate assessment of pain is vital. Pain as a complex phenomenon has been dealt with earlier in this chapter.

Pruritus

The causes of pruritus in advanced cancer are diverse, but commonly include dehydrated skin, uremia, thrombocytosis, and an over-abundance of histamine, serotonin, or opioids. If it occurs around the margin of the wound, a gentle moisturizing cream can be applied.

> !
> - Fungating wounds are a challenge to the patient and family, requiring a multidisciplinary approach to a complex man-

agement issue. They are a distressing additional burden to an individual with advanced head and neck cancer.
- Comprehensive and ongoing assessment of the evolving situation is paramount. Assessment of malodor and exudate is particularly important.

Psychosocial Issues

A diagnosis of head and neck cancer, as of any other cancer, brings with it significant psychosocial problems including uncertainty, fear, and loss. Individuals with cancer in the head and neck region have very specific and vast needs because of the location of their disease. Many patients face the reality of an altered appearance that is highly visible, and changes to their speech, swallowing, and breathing. The burden of head and neck cancer may be even more traumatic than that of other cancers and can manifest in psychosocial distress, which can have a negative impact on quality of life.[28]

Anxiety and Depression

Social Anxiety and Posttraumatic Stress Disorder

Prevalence

Studies have found that patients with head and neck cancer have some of the highest documented rates of anxiety and depression when compared with other tumor groups.[29] For instance, rates of clinically significant depression range from 19% to 40% in patients with head and neck cancer, with similar rates for clinically significant anxiety. Furthermore, research would suggest that social anxiety and posttraumatic stress disorder (PTSD) might be more frequent in head and neck cancer patients than in people with other cancers. Psychological distress has been correlated with patient characteristics, disease-related factors, and treatment-related factors.

- **Patient characteristics:** A recent review by Haisfield-Wolfe et al.[30] identified that within the head and neck cancer population the following patient characteristics are associated with depression: male, unmarried, less educated, younger (<40 years), smoking history, and those with lower physical functioning. On the other hand, individuals with higher levels of social support have reported fewer depressive symptoms.
- **Disease-related factors**: Some studies appear to suggest an interrelationship between psychological and physical symptoms. For example, if a patient has a feeding tube, with speech or swallowing difficulties they are more likely to experience depression.[31] Other studies have consistently indicated that anxiety and depression are more common in patients with advanced cancer.
- **Treatment related factors:** Patients receiving combined treatment modalities and more aggressive treatment are most at risk of psychological distress. Although psychological problems cannot be attributed to a single physical, disease, or treatment characteristic, knowledge of the multiple factors that contribute to distress may help clinicians to identify patients at greater risk.

In clinical practice there would appear to be a tendency for healthcare professionals to accept anxiety and low mood as "understandable" symptoms given the patient's current situation, which leads to a delay in diagnosis or to psychological problems not being detected. Anxiety is particularly prevalent at certain junctures of the cancer trajectory—for example, waiting on test results about recurrence. Anxiety is also common among patients with advanced disease, especially if death is impending but it may also result from an underlying anxiety disorder, pain, or other poorly managed symptoms.

Management

Optimal management of anxiety in patients with advanced head and neck cancer, without obvious organic contributions, often incorporates both anxiolytic pharmacotherapy and relaxation exercises or other behavioral interventions. Most experts consider short-acting benzodiazepines the drugs of choice for anxiety in patients with advanced cancer. To date, no agent has been studied in prospective clinical trials for patients with advanced cancer.

Depression and Adjustment Disorder

Signs and Symptoms

Many patients experience a low mood in response to a stressor such as receiving bad news but do not develop a depressive illness. This type of emotional reaction is called an **adjustment disorder** as there is a clear relationship to a stressor, and the reaction is limited in its duration. Furthermore, symptoms related to an adjustment disorder often fluctuate and patients can be distracted from their distress. However, **depression** is a major mood disorder consisting of a cluster of symptoms, representing a marked departure from an individual's habitual lifestyle. The DSM-IV criteria define a major depressive episode as the presence of five or more symptoms that include either depressed mood or loss of interest/pleasure for at least two consecutive weeks. Other symptoms may include significant weight loss or gain (change of >5% of body weight in 1 month), insomnia or hypersomnia, fatigue or loss of energy, feelings of worthlessness, or excessive or inappropriate guilt, diminished ability to concentrate or make decisions, and recurrent thoughts of death or suicidal ideation, planned or attempted.

Diagnostic

The assessment of distress can be facilitated by the use of a validated self-report screening instrument, such as the Hospital Anxiety and Depression Scale (HADS), General Health Questionnaire 28 (GHQ 28), Beck Depression Inventory (BDI) or distress thermometer. These questionnaires are brief, convenient and easily completed even by patients with advanced disease. Although these screening instruments possess a high degree of sensitivity in detecting clinical levels of anxiety and depression, no self-report measure is sufficient by itself. Follow-up with a clinician is required as specific forms of distress can have an organic cause, such as brain metastases or being medication-induced.

Management

Despite depression being a common condition for individuals with advanced cancer, evidence for effective treatment is sparse. There are too few adequate studies to draw clear conclusions about management of depression in the palliative setting. The treatment of depression in patients with advanced disease must, for now, be informed by the larger body of evidence on effective treatments for depression in patients with either no physical illness or less severe medical conditions.

To optimally manage depression, treatment of pain and other reversible physical symptoms should be instituted before or with initiation of specific antidepressant treatment. Antidepressant medications should be considered for the treatment of moderate-to-severe major depression in patients with advanced cancer. Current evidence does not support the relative superiority of one pharmacological treatment over another. The choice of an antidepressant should be informed by individual medication and patient factors: the side effect profiles of the medication, tolerability of treatment (including the potential for interaction with other current medications), response to prior treatment, and patient preference.

Based on evidence from the general population and other medically ill populations, combined approaches of pharmacological and psychosocial interventions may be the most effective way of managing depression for patients with advanced cancer. Recent research efforts have paid particular attention to psychological interventions, with cognitive behavioral therapy (CBT) approaches being most evaluated and showing some encouraging results. However, when treating a patient with a major depressive disorder, it may be more appropriate to delay formal psychotherapy until improvement has been noted from antidepressant therapy. Consideration should be given to prescribing antidepressants in elixir form for patients with advanced head and neck cancer with dysphagia.

Suicidal Ideation

Risk Factors

The risk of suicide is thought to be higher in patients' with cancer than in the general population. This risk increases with advanced stages of the disease as individuals' experience physical impairment and loss of autonomy, preceding an inexorable death. Expression of the following factors has been strongly correlated with suicidal ideation: poorly controlled physical symptoms, poor prognosis, depression, exhibiting hopelessness and helplessness, loss of control of the situation, preexhibiting psychopathology, and inadequate social support. This suicidal crisis can be considered as a way for the patient to escape an intolerable situation (uncontrolled pain or other symptoms) and maintain self-control and decisional autonomy.

Management

Management of suicidal crisis in patients with advanced cancer includes careful attention to the patient's distress without inducing any guilt. The primary goal is to identify issues that are contributing to the suicidal ideation. Appropriate control of physical symptoms is warranted, including screening and treating any mood disorder, associated anxiety, or organic mental disorder. However, if the patient is actively suicidal, then the expertise of Liaison Psychiatry and specialist mental health professionals may be necessary. Nevertheless, those engaged in the care of the patient with advanced disease should continue to provide input and offer ongoing psychological support.

Disfigurement

The face plays an extremely important role in an individual's sense of who they are and is focal when communicating with others. Individuals with head and neck cancer often experience an altered appearance as a result of the treatment or disease progression. Facial disfigurement profoundly affects self-concept, social interaction, and emotional well-being. Those at greatest risk of psychosocial difficulties would appear to be female patients and those with limited social support. A central finding has been that the degree of distress experienced by an individual is poorly related to objective disfigurement, indicating that disfigurement is subjectively experienced.

Although, degree of objective disfigurement may not be associated with quality of life, altered facial appearance often results in people feeling isolated and restricting their social activities. Social support is seen as an important factor in alleviating emotional distress experienced by patients with facial disfigurement. There is also evidence to suggest that patients with posttreatment difficulties that include disfigurement can benefit from intervention based on CBT, utilizing social skills training.

Family Issues

Supporting key family members is an important part of holistic care for the patient with advanced head and neck cancer. Existing literature suggests that partners of patients with advanced head and neck cancer have levels of anxiety equal to or higher than those of patients themselves.[31] Family members are often dealing with their own emotional response to their loved one's illness but often take on the role as caregiver, laden with multiple responsibilities. The factors that contribute to spouses' or family members' emotional distress are often the presence of a feeding tube, a fungating wound, not being able to take action to improve the difficult situation, and disruption in their daily schedule as a result of caring responsibilities, especially if the patient has eating or drinking difficulties. Mealtimes are dramatically changed and caregivers frequently choose not to attend social functions. Ross et al.[32] have suggested that caregivers' experience of psychological distress is associated with the greater time spent in caregiving. Informal caregivers of patients with advanced head and neck cancer require psychological support to cope with the stressors and demands of the situation. It is important for health-care professionals to recognize that family members are in a unique position of both giving and requiring support.

As a direct consequence of the increased incidence rates of head and neck cancer in the younger population (<40 years), more parents of young children are being diagnosed with this illness. Parents with cancer are confronted with the fears of missing milestones in the life of their children and are uncertain about how best to deal with their children's needs, along with balancing the physical effects of the illness. There is an overwhelming consensus that parents feel unsupported by professionals and require support on how to discuss their illness with the children, the transition of role change within the family, and how to prepare their children for the death of a parent.[33] Parents should be encouraged to provide honest, clear information in an age-appropriate language, with time to ask and process questions. Children also need structure and a sense of normality and continuity, and require extra security at this time. They need a trusted adult: one they know will offer support and counsel in the future. Children may also need help making sense of death and time to talk about challenging existential issues and a safe space in which to be listened to and heard and to share lonely feelings, possibly with a professional. It is important that professionals provide realistic information about a patient's prognosis as this helps parents prepare the children for their death. This may also encompass memory-making activates, to include fun times with the children.

■ Communication

Communication is imperative in developing and maintaining relationships, with verbal communication having a vital role in one's lifestyle and self-concept. Patients with advanced head and neck cancer can experience communication difficulties as a result of the physical presence of their tumor or treatment; for example, speech may be impaired due to the presence of a tracheostomy. Patients' satisfaction with their communication would appear to be directly related to perception of voice quality in terms of telephone intelligibility, volume, pitch, and natural abilities to communicate vocally.[34] If communication attempts are unsuccessful, patients can experience frustration, fear, and high levels of anxiety. As communication is a necessary part of socializing, it is not uncommon for patients with head and neck cancer to experience changes to their social patterns such as possible rejection of friends, distancing of children, and being misunderstood or having difficulty in conveying messages to the public. Loss of voice or unintelligible speech can lead to emotional and social changes that may result in withdrawal and depression.

Management

Patients who are voiceless or have unintelligible speech generally require augmentative and alternative communication (AAC) tools and strategies to facilitate communication.[35] To increase effective communication, the following AAC tools and strategies should be considered: unaided AAC such as gestures, facial expression, or sign language, and/or aided AAC. This may include pictures, alphabet boards for direct selection of messages, and pencil and paper. Nonetheless, patients who are frail and weak may find it difficult to write or point to pictures or words or may lack the concentration to spell out and/or read. The utility of such aids can be also be compromised if patients have impaired vision or are illiterate. As technology advances, there may be greater availability of electronic voice-output communication aids to enhance communication for patients with head and neck cancer.

The ultimate goal is to enable the patient to engage and communicate with family, friends, and health-care professionals. Engaging with a patient who has complex communication needs is generally slower, and even slower as the patient becomes medically fragile. Other important strategies include establishing a quiet and conducive communication environment and pausing to give the patient extra time and maintaining eye contact with the patient. This clearly reinforces the communication opportunity for the patient and indicates that their interaction and input are wanted. It may also be necessary to repeat back and confirm that the message is interpreted correctly before acting on it. Professionals should capitalize on the patient's nonverbal cues (eye gaze, body language, facial expressions). Input should also be sought from speech and language therapists.

> **!**
> - Patients with head and neck cancer may be more prone to experiencing distress than patients from other tumor groups.
> - Health-care professionals must be alert to manifestations of distress and these should not simply be regarded as an "understandable" symptom of having cancer.
> - If distress is left untreated, it can produce serious and negative consequences for the patient and their family.
> - Combined approaches of pharmacological and psychosocial interventions may be the most effective way of managing psychological distress for patients with advanced head and neck cancer.

■ Management of the Last Days of Life

The problems faced by patients with head and neck cancer in the last days of life are much the same as for those with other forms of terminal cancer. In the terminal phase patients tend to become weaker, spend longer periods of time asleep, take little orally, and frequently have signs of delirium. A minority of patients with head and neck cancer die suddenly from a catastrophic complication of their disease—either massive hemorrhage or upper airways obstruction.[7] (For details about the general management of the terminal phase, readers are referred to a general text on symptom control in palliative care; see Recommended Reading at the end of the chapter.)

> **!** Sudden death through hemorrhage or airways obstruction occurs in between 5% and 8% of patients with head and neck cancer.[6,7] These should be seen as palliative care emergencies and are very distressing for all those present.

■ Massive Hemorrhage

Massive bleeds are often heralded by minor warning bleeds. It is, however, difficult to predict which patients with minor bleeds will progress to catastrophic bleeding, making it good practice to be prepared for heavy bleeding in all patients where there is a warning bleed. As mentioned earlier, measures such as use of epinephrine 1:1000-soaked gauze, alginate dressing, or tranexamic acid, either orally or topically, can help to reduce minor bleeding if it is arising from a superficial site that is accessible and suitable to be treated locally. Heavier bleeds may stop spontaneously and there is often prognostic uncertainty about whether a heavy bleed will be a terminal event. In all situations, it is important that a health-care professional who is able to manage the situation with confidence stays with the patient through the period of a heavy bleed. If the bleeding settles and the patient survives for 24 hours, then transfusion may be indicated.

Catastrophic bleeding normally occurs as a result of the erosion of a major vessel. Little can be done to prevent such bleeds although there are case reports of successful stenting in patients at risk of "carotid blowout"[36]. In the event of a massive bleed, the patient and their carers are likely to become very distressed. In these situations, it is the role of the most senior health-care professional present to take charge of the situation and provide direction for the management and support for all involved. The standard management of such an event is to use sedative drugs (buccal, IV, or IM midazolam 10 mg),[17] unless there has already been loss of consciousness, and to try to mask the extent of the bleeding by the use of green or red towels to soak up blood. Clearly the management of such an event will be easier in an in-patient unit than at home, and it may be appropriate to offer hospice admission to a patient who is at high risk of a catastrophic bleed and for whom such an event occurring in the community might be a particular concern—for example, with the presence of children in the home.

Witnessing such an event can be an extremely distressing experience for anyone present, particularly family members and others close to the patient. Family members are likely to suffer complicated grief following such an event and it is important that they are followed up and offered bereavement counseling at the appropriate time. Health-care professionals may also be adversely affected and should be provided with support and offered counseling. Whether to warn family members and those caring for the patient before such an event occurs can be a difficult judgment, particularly as only the minority of patients who have warning bleeds will progress to massive hemorrhage.[37]

■ Airway Obstruction

Although airway obstruction is a common complication in head and neck cancer, particularly of the larynx, base of tongue, and thyroid, and metastatic disease in the neck, it is a cause of death in only a minority of patients. Many patients will have undergone a tracheostomy earlier in their disease. For patients who are at risk of developing an obstruction during the palliative phase of their illness, it is important to have developed a management plan and for this to be reviewed regularly. As the disease progresses and life expectancy and quality of life decrease, it may become less appropriate for a patient to be subjected to a tracheostomy even if this might be technically feasible. Patients who have disease recurrence at their tracheostomy site are particularly at risk of developing airway obstruction, either from the tumor mass or from bleeding from the tumor into the airway. Any airway obstruction is a medical emergency whether the aim of management is symptom control and supportive care or surgical intervention to relieve the obstruction.

Patients with acute dyspnea as a result of airway obstruction will be highly anxious and as the work of breathing increases they will become fatigued. All patients should have constant support from a member of the health-care staff, who should maintain an air of calm and give support to both the patient and their family. Patients should be given supplementary oxygen at a high dose (at least 40%) and oxygen saturations should be monitored. If an emergency tracheotomy is planned and the patient is becoming fatigued with the increased work of breathing, the risk of cardiopulmonary arrest becomes high. In this situation, Heliox (a helium–oxygen mixture) can temporarily improve breathing. Helium has a lower density than nitrogen, making it easier than oxygen-enriched air to draw through a narrowed airway in which there is turbulent flow.[38]

If the patient is not to receive surgical intervention, the situation should still be considered as a palliative care emergency, but the focus of treatment should be on managing the patient's anxiety and attempting to allow a peaceful death through sedation. Frequently only small doses of sedative, such as midazolam 2.5–5 mg subcutaneously, will be sufficient to sedate the patient in extremis, but occasionally higher doses will be needed. Doses should be repeated every 10–15 minutes until the patient is comfortable. Intravenous midazolam in this situation may be easier to titrate in doses of 1 mg injected slowly over 2 minutes and repeated according to response.[37] For either of these routes, the placement of an indwelling cannula will facilitate titration of several doses. Sedation is likely to worsen airways obstruction, particularly if the obstruction is supraglottic, when the risk is that the patent airway may be lost through muscle relaxation in the pharynx. However, if a patient is dying through obstruction and no active treatment is planned, it is important to provide adequate palliation and the fear of precipitating total obstruction should not prevent adequate doses of sedative being administered.

■ Advance Care Planning

Clinical management for all patients with advanced cancer should be patient-centered. The patient should be able to make decisions about their treatment having been given all the information they need in a way they can understand and having been supported in making the decision by the health-care professionals who are managing their care. This process can take considerable time, it requires good communication skills and must enable the patient to ask questions for which they receive a clear and honest answer. This can be extremely challenging, particularly when there is a high level of uncertainty about prognosis, outcome of treatment, or development of complications. A recent Dutch study highlighted that information needs of head and neck cancer patients at the end of life were often poorly met.[39]

Advance care planning is the process by which patients can discuss their illness, the likely prognosis, and their priorities and preferences for future care. They may want to make specific decisions about treatments they would not wish to have if they lacked the capacity to be involved in decision-making at a later date.[40] This situation could arise particularly in patients with advanced head and neck cancer who develop respiratory obstruction and have to make a decision about emergency tracheotomy.

Advance care planning should be voluntary and the subject should be sensitively broached with patients, as some do not wish to address issues concerning their prognosis or future decisions.[41] It should also be regularly reviewed since the patient's wishes are likely to change over time. As well as expressing their preferences and priorities, the patient may also want to appoint someone to make decisions on their behalf should they lack capacity. Many countries have systems for allowing a proxy to be nominated and it is important that the correct procedure is followed. In the United Kingdom, for example, such a nominated person will only be able to legally act on the patient's behalf if they are registered as having Lasting Power of Attorney (LPA) with the Office of the Public Guardian.[42] LPA may cover financial and "health and welfare" decisions. The scope of the powers must be explicitly stated and a patient may register more than one LPA. If someone has LPA for health and welfare on behalf of a patient, they will be able to make health-related decisions as if they were the patient themselves, but only when the patient lacks capacity, and these will always be expected to be consistent with the patient's best interest.

Advance care plans can take two forms in the United Kingdom:

- Advance statements of wishes for future care
- Advance decisions to refuse treatment (ADRTs), previously called living wills

Advance Statements

Advance statements cover patient preferences and priorities in general and may include indications about how active the patient would wish future disease management to be, who the important people to be involved in making decisions for them are, and whether the patient would want to be cared for at home in their final days. These statements are not legally binding because some of the preferences may be dependent on the situation at the time and possibly difficult to achieve—such as dying at home. However, when a patient has expressed their preferences for future care, these should be respected as far as possible and taken into account when making a clinical decision on behalf of the patient.

The process of preparing an advance statement encourages open communication and also enables clinicians to have a clearer idea of what treatments the patient may wish to consider even if they do not lose capacity. Any expressed wishes should be clearly written in the patient's clinical record by the professional having the discussion with the patient so that other team members are aware of the patient's preferences.

However, patients will often be under more than one clinical team and it is likely that not all clinicians will have access to the records in which the patient's wishes are recorded. Patient-held documents can help resolve this issue and a number have been designed in recent years and are available for use (further information available at www.endoflifecare.nhs.uk). Patient-held advance statements enable the patient to be in control of the process, so they can elect whether or not to have one, they can record anything they feel is relevant within it, they can make alterations as their preferences change, and they can use it to open up discussions with family and friends.[40]

Advance Decisions to Refuse Treatment

Advance decisions to refuse treatment (ADRTs) are legally binding documents and must be respected by clinicians. A valid ADRT which states, for example, that the patient would not want a tracheotomy if they developed acute respiratory obstruction as a result of head and neck cancer must be accepted as their decision. For an ADRT to be valid when the treatment being refused is potentially life-saving, it must be written and signed, it must refer to a specific situation, and it must indicate that the person knows that they are likely to die if they do not receive the treatment. A clinician may decide an ADRT is not valid if the patient's choices or behavior since the document was written indicate that the patient might have changed their mind.[42]

Lack of Capacity and Best-interest Decisions

The Mental Capacity Act[43] for England and Wales sets out how a diagnosis of lack of capacity should be made. These criteria, of course, may differ in other countries according to national and professional statutes. First and importantly, all patients are presumed to have capacity unless there is reason to suspect that there is a problem leading to potential lack of capacity. Capacity to make a decision should be assessed for each decision individually as patients might have capacity to make some decisions and not others. The Act describes the process of deciding on capacity, which involves a two-stage test:

- First, the patients must have an impairment of the brain or mind which lead to them losing capacity.
- Second, a functional test with several elements needs to be performed. This should indicate that the patient either:
  - cannot understand the issue in question
  - cannot retain the information long enough to process it
  - cannot perform the necessary mental processing to come to a decision, or
  - cannot communicate their decision

Clinicians must make every reasonable effort to improve the patient's capacity; for example, by communicating the information in ways that the patient can understand or by making sure that the patient has communication aids available to be able to make their decision known.[44]

If when following this process it is decided that a patient does lack capacity, the management decision needs to be taken on the basis of the patient's best interest. Best-interest decisions should take into account the clinical situation and the likely outcome of different options. They should take into account what is known about the patient's wishes and preferences and the opinions of those close to the patient in shedding light on what the patient's preferences might be. The decision taken should be that which is the least burdensome to the patient if several decisions are otherwise equally justified. All decisions need to be taken carefully, weighing up all of the relevant factors, which in complex cases will frequently require a high level of clinical knowledge and experience. Clinicians should be aware of their particular perspective on the issue and the possibility of different views being held by other clinical team members. Such decisions should therefore involve multidisciplinary discussion as far as is practical. The patient also should be involved in the process as much as possible, because even if they are unable to reach a decision independently, they may well have the capacity to understand some of the issues and express an opinion. Finally, the factors taken into account in making the decision should be clearly recorded including, importantly, the reason why the clinicians considered the patient to lack capacity to make a decision.

Conclusion

In providing effective management for patients with advanced head and neck cancer it is essential that their palliative and supportive care needs are not overlooked. Since they experience high levels of physical, psychological, social, and spiritual distress, their management requires a well coordinated multidisciplinary approach from a wide range of health-care professionals.[1] It is vital that all members of the multidisciplinary team are aware of the role of professionals from other disciplines, of which patients to refer for specific services, and of local referral pathways to secure these services. Only in this way will patients receive the care they need at the time they need it. Effective management will require forward planning and anticipation of problems as well as prompt reaction as they emerge. It is vital that a patient-centered approach is taken at all times. Finally, further research is needed to explore the experience of patients and their families when they have reached the final stages of their illness so that management can be based on clearer and more robust evidence.[45]

Case Study

A.A. was a 38-year-old woman who presented in August 2002 with a biopsy-proven squamous cell carcinoma (SCC) to her right retromolar trigone. Her past medical history included breast abscess and chronic back pain. A.A. was on Step 2 of the WHO Analgesic Ladder, as she regularly took weak opioids and nonsteroidal anti-inflammatory medication. She was prescribed an SSRI antidepressant by her family doctor for low mood resultant from martial difficulties, including separation from her husband 6 months prior to cancer diagnosis. At diagnosis, she lived with her 6- and 15-year-old daughters and had a very good social network which included her parents, siblings, extended family, and a few close friends. A.A. had stopped smoking 3 years prior to her cancer diagnosis and took occasional alcohol when socializing with friends. Examination under anesthetic (EUA) of oral cavity revealed a T2 SCC of the retromolar pad, encroaching onto the buccal mucosa and anterior pillar. Following staging investigations and discussion with A.A. and her parents, she underwent a modified radical neck dissection, mandibulectomy, and in-continuity tumor resection with the rim of mandible, followed by 6 weeks of radiotherapy. She tolerated the treatment well, maintaining her nutrition in spite of trismus and mucositis.

At first treatment review her oral cavity was difficult to visualize but there was an impression of altered mucosa in the right retromolar region. It was agreed that she should have a further EUA of this area and biopsy, and the results demonstrated that no tumor cells were evident. Within 9 months this patient discovered a lump on the left side of her neck, which proved on fine-needle aspiration (FNA) to be metastatic SCC. A modified radical neck dissection was performed on the contralateral neck with adjuvant radiotherapy. At posttreatment review following symptoms that were evident were trismus, dysphagia, pain, and psychosocial distress that centered on fear of recurrence and altered appearance. She received regular input from the SLT and Head and Neck Clinical Nurse Specialist (CNS) to facilitate management of these side-effects and concerns. In April 2007 A.A. was disease-free and discharged to the care of her GP.

Eighteen months after discharge from the head and neck team (November 2008), she experienced marked increase in pain with additional trismus, leading to an assessment with her family doctor, who noticed an ulcer in her right upper alveolus. An urgent referral was made to the head and neck team, who scheduled investigations to include EUA, CT, and biopsy. Histology confirmed a new primary SCC in the right upper alveolus with extensive bone involvement. This proved to be difficult news for this parent as she contemplated having to tell her children about this new cancer diagnosis. The conclusion from the Multidisciplinary Team Meeting in December 2008 indicated that further radiotherapy was not a suitable option and the only potential curative option was further radical surgery in the form of a partial maxillectomy with obturator. A PET scan was performed to ascertain whether she had any distant disease. The PET scan confirmed the primary disease, but also indicated a small right submental node (9 mm in diameter) with low-grade uptake (maximum SUV 2.3) and abnormal uptake of SUV in relation to the left external auditory meatus. Direct visualization of this area confirmed infection. An ultrasound-guided FNA of the right submental node proved to be reactive, with no evidence of malignancy. This information was discussed with the patient and her parents, and after carefully weighing up the relevant factors the consensus was to pursue this surgical option. After one further lengthy preoperative consultation surrounding the functional implications of this surgery, the maxillectomy was scheduled for late December 2008. Pathology report indicated T4 moderately differentiated SCC, as tumor was invading into the bone of the alveolar crest with low-grade dysplasia at the margins. Despite an uneventful postoperative recovery the consequences of this surgery led to additional symptoms including drooling, occasional nasal regurgitation of liquids, and further deterioration of speech quality. Nevertheless, she remained stoical and felt the need to be strong for her two daughters, often placing priority on her parental role to minimize disruption to family life. A.A. reported that the most apparent change to family life was at mealtimes, as she required puréed food and supplements. At first review appointment, which was 1 month after surgery, she had the additional sequelae of denture stomatitis and right otalgia. Fluconazole proved very effective for the stomatitis and a modest dose of pregabalin was added as a coanalgesic to oxycodene, acetaminophen, and the NSAID she was currently prescribed. Nine months after her maxillectomy, ulceration was noted to the right posterior tongue, as well as increased pain, swallowing difficulties, and fatigue. Given the symptomatology, concerns were expressed about recurrence and a further EUA and biopsy was organized. The pathology report confirmed the clinical suspicion of recurrent disease. Sharing these results, of what was now a progressive and an incurable illness, proved challenging. There was an initial sense of disbelief on the patient's behalf, as this was the first time in her seven-year cancer journey that no active treatment option was available. Following the consultation with the clinician, time was spent with the CNS discussing this difficult news, and how best to share this diagnosis with her daughters and appropriateness of referral to a local palliative care team. During this consultation she expressed concerns about the evident behavioral changes in her youngest daughter and it was agreed that a referral would also be made to a family support worker for children who have an adult with cancer, which proved an invaluable support to the family.

As her swallowing difficulties increased, she struggled more and more to maintain her weight but refused a gastrostomy. The rationale for her decision was complex but included issues around promoting normality for her daughters. She had frequent input from the community dietitian and SLT, trialing and rotating several nutritional supplements to prevent taste fatigue. One of the main reasons for declining enteral feeding at this juncture of her illness was the imminent desire to go on a holiday with her two daughters. This proved to be one of the most enjoyable times in the last 3 months of her life, as many positive memories were created, such as engaging in water sports with her two daughters. On her return from this holiday, attention was given to creating memory books and a family portrait and organizing the home.

A.A. was well supported socially by her family and also had regular input from the local palliative care team, dietitian, and SLT, and invaluable support from her family doctor. She remained at home for several weeks with one short in-patient stay for symptom management at the hospice due to the complexity of her disease burden. As her disease progressed and her symptoms increased to include pain with a neuropathic element, repeated episodes of candida, xerostomia, trismus, poor sleep pattern with irritating cough, aspiration on thin fluids, nausea, constipation, fatigue (low hemoglobin), episodes of intraoral bleeding, and low mood, she agreed to a further admission to the hospice, where every endeavor was made to promote a "good death."

In Reflection on this Case Study, the Key Aspects of Care Should Be Highlighted:

- The necessity for a multidisciplinary approach to care.
- Liaison between primary care and the Head and Neck Team in the acute setting.
- A holistic approach to care, with the patient identifying priorities for care.
- Patient involvement in decision making.
- The need for honesty, which facilitates family planning and creating memories for the children.
- This is an arduous pathway for some patients.

Recommended Reading

- Booth S, Davies P. Palliative Care Consultations: Head and Neck Cancer. Oxford: University Press; 2006
- Davies A, Epstein J. Oral Complications of Cancer and Its Management. Oxford: University Press; 2010
- Twycross R, Wilcock A, Stark-Toller C. Symptom Management in Advanced Cancer. Nottingham: Palliativedrugs.com Ltd; 2009
- www.Palliativedrugs.com (accessed November 242 011) (A free to use website with a comprehensive palliative care formulary, discussion forum and many other resources)

References[1]

1. Specht L. Oral complications in the head and neck radiation patient. Introduction and scope of the problem. Support Care Cancer 2002;10(1):36–39
2. Lovel T. Palliative care and head and neck cancer. Br J Oral Maxillofac Surg 2000;38(4):253–254
3. Improving Outcomes for Patients with Head and Neck Cancer. The Manual. London: National Institute for Health and Clinical Excellence (NICE): 2004**
4. British Association of Head & Neck Oncologists. Standards for the Process of Head and Neck Cancer Care. BAHNO; 2009. Available from www.bahno.org.uk (accessed November 24, 2011)
5. Ethunandan M, Rennie A, Hoffman G, Morey PJ, Brennan PA. Quality of dying in head and neck cancer patients: a retrospective analysis of potential indicators of care. Oral Surg Oral Med Oral Pathol Oral Radiol Endod 2005;100(2):147–152
6. Price KA, Moore EJ, Moynihan T, Price DL. Symptoms and terminal course of patients who died of head and neck cancer. J Palliat Med 2009;12(2):117–118
7. Forbes K. Palliative care in patients with cancer of the head and neck. Clin Otolaryngol Allied Sci 1997;22(2):117–122
8. Chaplin JM, Morton RP. A prospective, longitudinal study of pain in head and neck cancer patients. Head Neck 1999;21(6):531–537
9. Mercadante S. Opioid responsiveness in patients with advanced head and neck cancer. Support Care Cancer 1998;6(5):482–485
10. Webster M, Hagen N. Pain management in advanced and recurrent disease. In: Booth S, Davies P, eds. Palliative Care Consultations in Head and Neck Cancer. Oxford: Oxford University Press; 2006: 139
11. Calman F. The non-surgical management of advanced head and neck cancer. In: Booth S, Davies P, eds Palliative Care Consultations in Head and Neck Cancer. Oxford: Oxford University Press; 2006: 9–32**
12. Jereczek-Fossa BA, Orecchia R. Radiotherapy-induced mandibular bone complications. Cancer Treat Rev 2002;28(1):65–74
13. Saunders C. A personal therapeutic journey. BMJ 1996;313(7072):1599–1601
14. Twycross R, Wilcock A, Stark-Toller C. Symptom Management in Advanced Cancer. Nottingham: Palliativedrugs.com Ltd.; 2009**
15. Freynhagen R, Bennett MI. Diagnosis and management of neuropathic pain. BMJ 2009;339:b3002
16. Davis MP. What is new in neuropathic pain? Support Care Cancer 2007;15(4):363–372
17. Twycross R, Wilcock A. Palliative Care Formulary, Nottingham: Palliativedrugs.com Ltd.; 2007.*
18. Graham F, Clark D. The syringe driver and the subcutaneous route in palliative care: the inventor, the history and the implications. J Pain Symptom Manage 2005;29(1):32–40
19. Davies AN, Dickman A, Reid C, Stevens AM, Zeppetella G; Science Committee of the Association for Palliative Medicine of Great Britain and Ireland. The management of cancer-related breakthrough pain: recommendations of a task group of the Science Committee of the Association for Palliative Medicine of Great Britain and Ireland. Eur J Pain 2009;13(4):331–338
20. Davies A. Oral problems. In: Booth S, Davies P, eds. Palliative Care Consultations in Head and Neck Cancer. Oxford: Oxford University Press; 2006: 77–90 **
21. Machin J. Improving swallowing and communication. In: Booth S, Davies P, eds. Palliative Care Consultations in Head and Neck Cancer. Oxford: Oxford University Press; 2006: 91–106 *
22. Clarkson J, Worthington H, Eden TO. Interventions for treating oral mucositis for patients with cancer receiving treatment. Oxford: Cochrane Collaboration; 2007
23. Goodwin WJ Jr, Byers PM. Nutritional management of the head and neck cancer patient. Med Clin North Am 1993;77(3):597–610

1 References with asterisks indicate the most important reference articles on the topic.

24. Chasen MR, Bhargava R. A descriptive review of the factors contributing to nutritional compromise in patients with head and neck cancer. Support Care Cancer 2009;17(11):1345–1351
25. Ehrsson YT, Langius-Eklöf A, Bark T, Laurell G. Percutaneous endoscopic gastrostomy (PEG) - a long-term follow-up study in head and neck cancer patients. Clin Otolaryngol Allied Sci 2004;29(6):740–746
26. Grocott P. Care of patients with fungating malignant wounds. Nurs Stand 2007;21(24):57–58, 60, 62 passim
27. Grocott P, Browne N, Cowley S. Quality of life: assessing the impact and benefits of care to patients with fungating wounds. Wounds 2005;17(1):8–15
28. Semple CJ, Dunwoody L, George Kernohan W, McCaughan E, Sullivan K. Changes and challenges to patients' lifestyle patterns following treatment for head and neck cancer. J Adv Nurs 2008;63(1):85–93
29. Zabora J, BrintzenhofeSzoc K, Curbow B, Hooker C, Piantadosi S. The prevalence of psychological distress by cancer site. Psychooncology 2001;10(1):19–28
30. Haisfield-Wolfe ME, McGuire DB, Soeken K, Geiger-Brown J, De Forge BR. Prevalence and correlates of depression among patients with head and neck cancer: a systematic review of implications for research. Oncol Nurs Forum 2009;36(3):E107–125.**
31. Verdonck-de Leeuw IM, Eerenstein SE, Van der Linden MH, Kuik DJ, de Bree R, Leemans CR. Distress in spouses and patients after treatment for head and neck cancer. Laryngoscope 2007;117(2):238–241
32. Ross S, Mosher CE, Ronis-Tobin V, Hermele S, Ostroff JS. Psychosocial adjustment of family caregivers of head and neck cancer survivors. Support Care Cancer 2010;18(2):171–178
33. Semple CJ, McCance T. Experience of parents with head and neck cancer who are caring for young children. J Adv Nurs 2010;66(6):1280–1290
34. Happ MB, Roesch T & Kagav SH. Communication needs, methods, and perceived voice quality following head and neck cancer surgery: a literature review. Cancer Nurs 2004;27(1):1–9
35. Beukelman DR, Mirenda P. Augmentative Alternative Communication. Supporting adults and children with complex communication needs. Baltimore: Paul H. Brooks Publishing Co; 2005
36. Desuter G, Hammer F, Gardiner Q, et al. Carotid stenting for impending carotid blowout: suitable supportive care for head and neck cancer patients? Palliat Med 2005;19(5):427–429
37. Thompson E, Davies A. The last few days of life. In: Booth S, Davies P, eds. Palliative Care Consultations in Head and Neck Cancer. Oxford: Oxford University Press; 2006:175
38. Gibbins N, Jani P. Management of airway problems in advanced or recurrent disease. In: Booth S, Davies P, eds. Palliative Care Consultations in Head and Neck Cancer. Oxford: Oxford University Press; 2006:55–76
39. Ledeboer QC, Offerman MP, van der Velden LA, de Boer MF, Pruyn JF. Experience of palliative care for patients with head and neck cancer through the eyes of next of kin. Head Neck 2008;30(4):479–484
40. Advance Care Planning. A Guide for Health and Social Care Staff. Leicester: End of Life Care Programme; EOLCP 2007
41. Randall F, Downie RS. End of Life Choices: Consensus and Controversy. Oxford, New York: Oxford University Press; 2010
42. Mental Capacity Act: Code of Practice. London: Department of Constitutional Affairs: DCA 2007*
43. Department of Constitutional Affairs. Mental Capacity Act (2005) Code of Practice. London. TSO 2007
44. Nicholson TR, Cutter W, Hotopf M. Assessing mental capacity: the Mental Capacity Act. BMJ 2008;336(7639):322–325
45. Ledeboer QC, Velden LA, Boer MF, Feenstra L, Pruyn JF. Physical and psychosocial correlates of head and neck cancer: an update of the literature and challenges for the future (1996–2003). Clin Otolaryngol 2005;30(4):303–319

Subject Index

Page numbers in *italics* refer to illustrations or tables

D

Programming in Visual Basic

Version 5.0

Statement	Effect	Text Page
`Load` *FormName*	Loads a form into memory.	198
`LOF(`*FileNumber*`)`	Function; returns the length of a data file in bytes.	333
`Mid(`*String*, *StartPosition* `[,`*NumberOfCharacters*`])`	Function; returns a string from StartPosition to end of string or the specified number of characters.	247
`[`*Object*`.]Move` *Left* `[,` *Top*`[,` *Width*`[,` *Height*`]]]`	Move the specified object.	483
`MsgBox "`*Message String*`" [,` *Buttons/Icon*`] [, "`*Caption*`"]`	Displays a dialog box with a message, buttons, and an optional icon.	134
`MsgBox ("`*Message String*`" [,` *Buttons/Icon*`] [, "`*Caption*`"])`	Function; returns a value indicating the button pressed by the user.	245
`Next [{`*LoopIndex*`|`*ElementName*`}]`	Terminates a `For/Next` or a `For Each` loop.	242
`On Error GoTo` *LineLabel*	Enables error trapping and specifies the line label of the error-handling routine.	319
`On Error Go To 0`	Turns off error trapping.	320
`Open "`*FileName*`" For {Input|Output|Append|Random} As #`*FileNumber* `[Len =` *RecordLength*`]`	Opens a data file.	313
`Pmt (`*InterestRate*, *Periods*, *Principal*`)`	Function; returns the payment amount.	547
`[`*Object*`.]Print` *ItemsToPrint*	Sends output to named object; may be Printer, Debug, a form, or a picture box control.	250
`[`*Object*`.]PSet (`*x*, *y*`) [,` *Color*`]`	Draws a dot on the named object.	474
`Public` *Identifier* `[As` *DataType*`]` `Public Const` *Identifier* `[As` *DataType*`] =` *Value*	Declares a variable or constant as public.	201
`Put #`*FileNumber*, `[`*RecordNumber*`],` *RecordName*	Writes data from a record variable into a random file in RecordNumber position. If the record number is omitted, the record is written in the next position.	332

`Resume`
`Resume Next`
`Resume` *LineLabel*
	Resumes execution after error trapping with `On Error GoTo`.	323

`Right(`*String*, *NumberOfCharacters*`)`	Function; returns a string of the specified number of characters from the right end of the string.	247
`Rnd`	Function; returns a random number between 0 and 1.	474
`RGB(`*RedValue*, *GreenValue*, *BlueValue*`)`	Function; returns a color.	472
`[`*Object*`.]Scale` $(x_1, y_1) - (x_2, y_2)$	Changes the coordinates for the object.	488
`Seek(`*FileNumber*`)`	Function; returns the current record number.	334
`Select Case` *Expression*	Begins a Case structure. (Ends with `End Select`.)	273
`[`*FormName*`.]Show [0|1]`	Shows a form.	196
`Static` *Identifier* `[As` *DataType*`]`	Declares a variable as static.	201
`[{Private|Public}] Sub` *ProcedureName* `[{`*Parameters*`}]`	Begins a sub procedure. (Ends with `End Sub`.)	174
`Type` *VariableType*	Defines a data structure with one or more elements. (Ends with `End Type`.)	281
`Ucase(`*String*`)`	Function; returns the uppercase representation of the string.	126
`Unload FormName`	Unloads a form from memory.	198
`Val(`*String*`)`	Function; returns the numeric value of the string.	89
`With` *ObjectName*	Begins a block of code relating to a single object. (Ends with `End With`.)	61
`Write #`*FileNumber*, *ListOfFields*	Writes data in a sequential file.	316

Programming in Visual Basic

Version 5.0

Julia Case Bradley
Mt. San Antonio College

Anita C. Millspaugh
Mt. San Antonio College

Irwin McGraw-Hill

Boston, Massachusetts Burr Ridge, Illinois Dubuque, Iowa
Madison, Wisconsin New York, New York San Francisco, California St. Louis, Missouri

Irwin/McGraw-Hill

A Division of The ***McGraw-Hill*** *Companies*

PROGRAMMING IN VISUAL BASIC, VERSION 5.0

This book is printed on acid-free paper.

4 5 6 7 8 9 0 VNH/VNH 9 0 9 8 (U.S. Edition)
4 5 6 7 8 9 0 VNH/VNH 9 0 9 8 (International Edition)

ISBN 0-256-25941-0

Vice president and editorial director: *Michael W. Junior*
Sponsoring editor: *Rhonda Sands*
Editorial coordinator: *Carrie Berkshire*
Marketing manager: *James Rogers*
Project manager: *Robert A. Preskill/Margaret Rathke*
Production supervisor: *Scott Hamilton*
Senior designer: *Crispin Prebys*
Designer: *Becky Lemma*
Cover illustration: *Peter Siv*
Compositor: *GTS Graphics, Inc.*
Typeface: *11/13 Bodoni Book*
Printers: *Von Hoffmann Press, Inc.*

Library of Congress Cataloging-in-Publication Data

Bradley, Julia Case.
Programming in Visual Basic, version 5.0 / Julia Case Bradley, Anita C. Millspaugh.
p. cm.
Includes index.
ISBN 0-256-25941-0
1. BASIC (Computer program language) 2. Microsoft Visual BASIC.
I. Millspaugh, A. C. (Anita C.) II. Title.
QA76.73.B3B724 1998
005.26'8—dc21 97-21935

INTERNATIONAL EDITION

When ordering this title, use ISBN 0-07-115432-9.

http://www.mhcollege.com

Preface

As the world turns to graphical user interfaces, computer programming languages are changing to accommodate the shift. Visual Basic 5 is designed to allow the programmer to develop applications that run under Windows without the complexity generally associated with Windows programming. With very little effort, the programmer can design a screen that holds standard Windows elements such as command buttons, check boxes, option buttons, text boxes, and list boxes. Each of these Windows objects operates as expected, producing a "standard" Windows user interface.

Visual Basic is easy to learn, which makes it an excellent tool for understanding elementary programming concepts. In addition, it has evolved into such a powerful and popular product that skilled Visual Basic programmers are in demand in the job market.

About This Text

This textbook is intended for use in an introductory programming course, which assumes no prior knowledge of computer programming. However, many of the later chapters are appropriate for an advanced-level course. The later chapters are also appropriate for professional programmers who are learning a new language to upgrade their skills.

This text assumes that the student is familiar with the Windows operating environment.

Approach

The authors have successfully taught Visual Basic to beginning and advanced programming students for several years. This text incorporates the basic concepts of programming, problem solving, programming logic, as well as the design techniques of an event-driven language.

Chapter topics are presented in a sequence that allows the programmer to learn how to deal with a visual interface while acquiring important programming skills such as creating projects with loops, decisions, and data management.

The later chapters may be used in various sequences to accommodate the needs of beginning and advanced-level courses, as well as a shorter quarter system or a semester-long course. For a shorter course, the professor may choose to skip the chapter on data files and cover only the first of the two database chapters.

New in Visual Basic 5

This latest version of Visual Basic is bound to be a success with students as well as professional application developers.

Visual Basic 5:

- Runs much faster than previous versions and incorporates more features required for professional application development. VB5 will be competitive with C++ for object-oriented program development.
- Incorporates many helpful new features in the editor, making it easier for beginners as well as advanced programmers to enter and edit code. For example:
  - Drag-and-drop editing for moving and copying lines.
  - Pop-up lists of available datatypes when declaring variables.
  - Pop-up lists of allowable properties and methods for controls.
  - Tips showing formats and arguments for functions and statements that appear automatically as you enter program code.
- Is easier to debug than previous versions. For example:
  - Data tips, similar to tool tips, display the current contents of variables, properties, and expressions, and pop up when you point to the expression during break time.
  - You can easily set breakpoints in code by clicking in the margin of a statement.
  - During break time, you can drag the highlighted line to set the next statement to execute.
- Includes many new controls. For example:
  - Many ActiveX controls for programming on the Web.
  - A new Web browser control that allows you to retrieve and display Web pages in an application.

New in This Edition of the Text

This edition is a major revision of the text. In addition to the update to Windows 95 and Visual Basic 5, many sections have been reorganized and expanded. This edition places more emphasis on the planning steps of project design to encourage students to develop good programming habits from the start.

In response to many helpful suggestions from students and reviewers, several topics have been rearranged. Control arrays now appear in the same chapter as variable arrays. The grid control is presented along with database handling. Do/Loops and For/Next loops now appear together in one chapter. The numeric functions have been moved to an appendix. Also, topics are now organized so that those teaching a short course can use only a few chapters.

Numerous new examples and tutorials are included in this revision. A new step-by-step tutorial demonstrates debugging techniques. Another tutorial illustrates how to create a new folder in Windows 95 and save projects into the new folder. Many new examples now appear in the chapters on calculations and decisions, and a new section covers string functions. The advanced techniques chapter (Chapter 14) now includes sections on creating a new class and Crystal Reports.

The screens for all projects have been modified to reflect the look and feel of Windows 95. New controls include the tabbed dialog control, the Web browser control, and ActiveX controls, including instructions on creating your own ActiveX controls.

Students and instructors will appreciate the new appendix, "Tips and Shortcuts for Mastering the VB Environment." This reference brings together many helpful tips that can save a programmer a significant amount of time.

The instructor materials are also updated and expanded. New materials include suggested coding standards and masters of forms for project planning that can be reproduced and distributed to students. The solutions to all exercises are available for download on the Web.

Chapter Organization

Each chapter begins with identifiable objectives and a brief overview. Numerous coding examples as well as hands-on projects with guidance for the coding appear throughout. Thought-provoking feedback questions give students time to reflect on the current topic and to evaluate their understanding of the details. The end-of-chapter items include a chapter review, questions, programming exercises, and two case studies. The case studies provide a continuing-theme exercise that may be used throughout the course.

Chapter 1 walks the student through the creation of a first Visual Basic project, incorporating command buttons and labels. The programming environment is introduced along with the concepts of objects and their related properties, methods, and events.

Chapter 2 continues coverage of controls, including text boxes, option buttons, check boxes, frames, images, lines, and shapes. It also covers some of the finer points of using the environment and working with keyboard access keys, multiple controls, and alignment. The color constants are used at this point to lead the novice programmer into Chapter 3, which introduces variables and constants. The text includes a naming convention to make the scope and data type of a variable or constant easier to determine from the coding syntax. Standards also provide for the use of Option Explicit to force the declaration of all variables and constants.

Chapter 4 introduces the relational and logical operators and their use with the If statement. Input validation and message boxes are also covered. In Chapter 5 students learn to set up custom menus and to write their own sub functions and sub procedures. Multiple forms, global variables, and standard code modules are presented in Chapter 6.

Chapter 7 incorporates list boxes and combo boxes into the projects, providing the opportunity to discuss looping procedures and printing lists of information. The list concept leads logically into the use of variable arrays and control arrays in Chapter 8 and to writing the information to disk in Chapter 9. Chapter 9 covers both sequential and random files, but the material may be covered in sections.

Chapters 10 and 11 deal with the use of Visual Basic as a front end for database programming. The projects display and update tables created by a database application such as Microsoft Access. Chapter 11 includes using a data-bound grid, error trapping, and writing queries in SQL.

The drag-and-drop feature of Windows programming is introduced in Chapter 12. This chapter normally brings great enthusiasm from students as they learn to deal with the source and target objects. The examples and assignments provide a blend of practical and just-for-fun applications. This approach is also true of Chapter 13, which introduces the graphics methods and graphics controls.

Chapter 14, the final chapter, covers various topics that build a bridge from Visual Basic to other applications. These include using and creating ActiveX controls, creating a new object class, the Windows API, DLLs, OLE, and Visual Basic for Applications.

Acknowledgments

We would like to express our appreciation to the many people who have contributed to the successful completion of this text. Most especially, we thank our students at Mt. San Antonio College who helped class-test the material and who greatly influenced the manuscript.

Many people have worked very hard to design and produce this text, including Carrie Berkshire, Robert A. Preskill, Crispin Prebys, Garrett Glanz, and June Waldman. A special thank you goes to Rhonda Sands, our editor, whose help has been invaluable.

We greatly appreciate Diane Murphey, Theresa Berry, and Dennis Fraser for their thorough technical reviews, constructive criticism, and many valuable suggestions. Thanks also to Theresa for writing the Instructors Manual and to Dennis for preparing the exercise solutions. And most importantly, we are grateful to Dennis, Andy, Eric, and Tricia for their support and understanding through the long days and busy phone lines.

We want to thank our reviewers, who have made many helpful suggestions:

Gary R. Armstrong
Shippensburg University

Ronald L. Burgher
Metropolitan Community College

Diane Murphey
Oklahoma Panhandle State University

Sheila J. Pearson
Southern Arkansas University

Thomas S. Pennington
Maple Woods Community College

Hwang Santai
Purdue University–Fort Wayne

Judy Yaeger
Western Michigan University

The Authors

We have had fun teaching and writing about Visual Basic. We hope that this feeling is evident as you read this book and that you will enjoy learning or teaching this outstanding programming language.

Julia Case Bradley
Anita C. Millspaugh

To the Student

The best way to learn to program in Visual Basic is to do it. If you enter and run the sample projects, you will be on your way to writing Windows applications. Reading the examples without trying to run them is like trying to learn a foreign language or mathematics just by reading about it. Enter the projects, look up your questions in Visual Basic's excellent Help files, and make those projects *run*.

Format Used for Visual Basic Statements

Visual Basic statements and functions are shown in `this font`. Any values you must supply are in *`italics`*. Optional items are in [square brackets]. Braces and a vertical bar indicate that you must choose one or the other value {one | other}.

Example:

```
Open "FileName" For {Input|Output|Append|Random} As #FileNumber [Len=RecLength]
```

As you work your way through this textbook, note that you may see a subset of the available options for a Visual Basic statement. Generally, the options that are included will reflect those covered in the chapter. If you want to see the complete format for any statement, refer to online Help.

J.C.B.
A.C.M.

Contents

3 Variables, Constants, and Calculations 77

4 Decisions and Conditions 115

5 Menus, Sub Procedures, and Sub Functions 159

C H A P T E R

1

Introduction to Visual Basic

At the completion of this chapter, you will be able to . . .

1. Describe the process of visual program design and development.
2. Explain the term *event-driven programming.*
3. Explain the concepts of objects, properties, and methods.
4. List and describe the three steps for writing a Visual Basic project.
5. Describe the various files that make up a Visual Basic project.
6. Identify the elements in the Visual Basic environment.
7. Explain the differences among design time, run time, and break time.
8. Write, run, save, print, and modify your first Visual Basic project.
9. Identify compile errors, run-time errors, and logic errors.
10. Look up Visual Basic topics in Help.

Writing Windows Applications with Visual Basic

Using this text, you will learn to write computer programs that run in the Microsoft Windows environment. Your projects will look and act like standard Windows programs. Visual Basic (VB) provides the tools you need to create windows with familiar elements like menus, text boxes, command buttons, option buttons, check boxes, list boxes, and scroll bars. Figure 1.1 shows some sample Windows user interfaces.

Figure 1.1

Graphical user interfaces for application programs designed with Visual Basic.

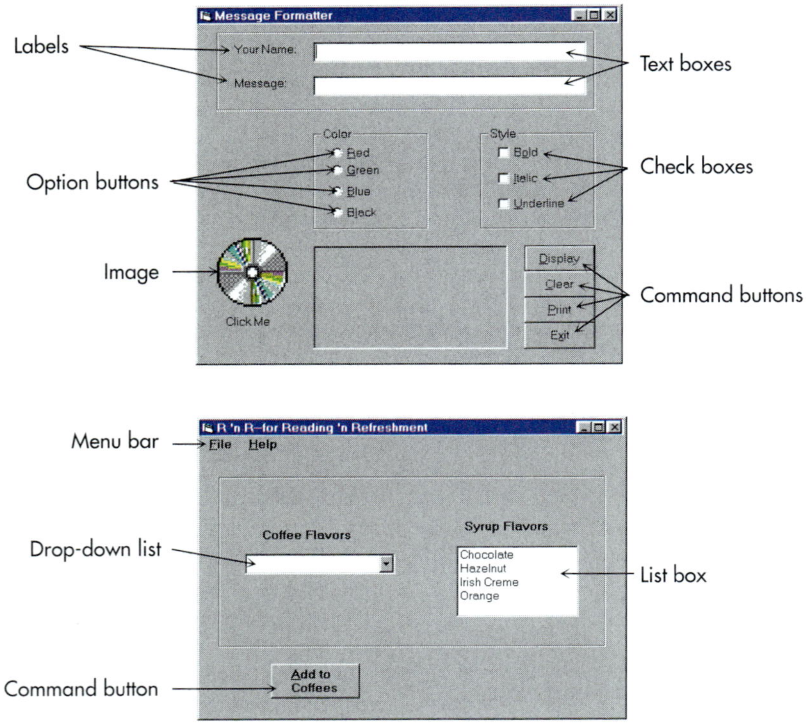

The Windows Graphical User Interface

Microsoft Windows uses a **graphical user interface**, or **GUI** (pronounced "gooey"). The Windows GUI defines how the various elements look and function. As a Visual Basic programmer, you have available a toolbox of these elements. You will create new windows, called **forms**. Then you will use the toolbox to add the various elements, called **controls**. The projects that you will write follow a relatively new type of programming, called ***event-driven programming***.

Programming Languages—Procedural, Object Oriented, and Event Driven

There are literally hundreds of programming languages. Each was developed to solve a particular type of problem. Most traditional languages, such as

BASIC, C, COBOL, FORTRAN, PL/I, and Pascal are considered *procedural* languages. That is, the program specifies the sequence of all operations step-by-step. Program logic determines the next instruction to execute in response to conditions and user requests.

The newer programming languages, such as C++ and Visual Basic, use a different approach: **object-oriented programming** (OOP) and event-driven programming. Microsoft refers to Visual Basic as an event-driven programming language, which has many (but not all) elements of an object-oriented language such as C++. Each release of Visual Basic moves it a little closer to a true object-oriented language.

In the event-driven model, programs are no longer procedural; they do not follow a sequential logic. You, as the programmer, do not take control and determine the sequence of execution. Instead, the user can press keys and click on various buttons and boxes in a window. Each user action can cause an *event* to occur, which triggers a Basic procedure that you have written. For example, the user clicks on a command button labeled Calculate. The clicking causes the button's Click event to occur, and the program automatically jumps to a procedure you have written to do the calculation.

The Object Model

In Visual Basic you will work with **objects**, which have **properties** and **methods**.

Objects

Think of an object as a thing, or a noun. Examples of objects are forms and controls. *Forms* are the windows and dialog boxes you place on the screen; *controls* are the elements you place inside a form, such as text boxes, command buttons, and list boxes.

Properties

Properties tell something about an object, such as its name, color, size, location, or how it will behave. You can think of properties as adjectives that describe objects.

When you refer to a property, you first name the object, add a period, and then name the property. For example, refer to the Caption property of a form called Form1 as Form1.Caption (say "form1 dot caption").

Methods

Actions associated with objects are called methods. Methods are the verbs of object-oriented programming. Some typical methods are Move, Print, Resize, and Clear.

You refer to methods as Object.Method ("object dot method"). For example, a Print method can apply to different objects. Printer.Print sends the output to the printer object; Form1.Print sends output to the form called Form1.

Versions of Visual Basic

Microsoft Visual Basic for Windows comes in a **Learning Edition**, a **Professional Edition**, and an **Enterprise Edition**. Anyone planning to do professional application development that includes the advanced features of database management should use the Professional Edition or Enterprise Edition. Another version runs under DOS, but it is considerably different from the Windows version and is not covered here.

In addition to the various editions of Visual Basic, you must also be aware of the release number. This text is based on release 5.0, the current release. Release 5.0 is significantly different from earlier releases. Although most of the projects in this text can be written with release 4.0, the menus and screens will not look the same as the text screen shots. Also, several new elements and statements were added in release 5.0. In short, you should use release 5.0 with this text.

Next to each new or changed feature you will see an icon (see margin).

New to VB 5!

Writing Visual Basic Projects

When you write a Visual Basic project, you follow a three-step process for planning the project and then repeat the process for creating the project. The three steps involve setting up the user interface, defining the properties, and then creating the code.

The Three-Step Process

Planning

1. *Design the user interface.* When you plan the **user interface**, you draw a sketch of the screens the user will see when running your project. On your sketch, show the forms and all the controls that you plan to use. Indicate the names that you plan to give the form and each of the objects on the form. Refer to Figure 1.1 for examples of user interfaces.

   Before you proceed with any more steps, consult with your user and make sure that you both agree on the look and feel of the project.
2. *Plan the properties.* For each object, write down the properties that you plan to set or change during the design of the form.
3. *Plan the Basic code.* This step is where you plan the procedures that will execute when your project runs. You will determine which events require action to be taken and then make a step-by-step plan for those actions.

   Later, when you actually write the Visual Basic **code**, you must follow the language syntax rules. But during the planning stage, you will write out the actions using **pseudocode**, which is an English expression or comment that describes the action. For example, you must plan for the event that occurs when the user clicks on the Exit command button. The pseudocode for the event could be *Terminate the project.*

Programming

After you have completed the planning steps and have agreement from your user, you are ready to begin the actual construction of the project. You will use the same three step process that you used for planning.

1. *Define the user interface.* When you define the user interface, you create the forms and controls that you designed in the planning stage.

Think of this step as *defining* all of the objects you will use in your project.

2. *Set the properties.* When you set the properties of the objects, you give each object a name and define such attributes as the contents of a label, the size of the text, and the words that appear on top of a command button and in the form's title bar.

   You might think of this step as *describing* each object.
3. *Write the Basic code.* You will use Basic programming statements (called Basic code) to carry out the actions needed by your program. You will be surprised and pleased by how few statements you need to create a powerful Windows program.

   You can think of this third step as defining the *actions* of your program.

Visual Basic Projects

Each Visual Basic project consists of at least two, and usually more, files.

1. The .VBP file, called the ***project file***, is a small text file that holds the names of the other files in the project, as well as some information about the VB environment. *Note:* If you are using release 2.0 or 3.0 of Visual Basic, project files have a .MAK extension.
2. Each form in your project is saved in a file with a .FRM extension. To begin, your projects will have only one form (and therefore one **form file**). Later, you can expect your projects to have several forms, with one .FRM file for each form.

   A form file holds a description of all objects and their properties for the form, as well as the Basic code you have written to respond to the events.

   In Visual Basic each of these form files is referred to as a ***form module***.
3. Optionally, your project can have .BAS extension files. These files hold Basic statements that can be accessed from any form. As soon as you begin writing multiform projects, you will need .BAS files.

   .BAS files are called ***standard code modules***.
4. Additional controls, called *custom controls*, are stored in files with an .OCX extension. If you include controls in your project that are not part of the standard control set, the .OCX file names will be included in the project.
5. After you save a project, Visual Basic automatically adds one more file to your project with an extension of .VBW. This file holds information about each of your project's forms.

Tip

Before creating any files for your project, first create a new folder on disk. Save your .VBP file, .FRM files, and .BAS files into the new folder. Then if you want to copy or move the project to another disk, you will get all the pieces. It is easy to miss parts of a project unless all files are together in one folder.

New to VB 5!

The Visual Basic Environment

The **Visual Basic environment** is where you create and test your projects. Figure 1.2 shows the various windows in the Visual Basic environment. Note that each window can be moved, resized, opened, and closed. Your screen may not look exactly like Figure 1.2; in all likelihood you will want to customize the placement of the various windows.

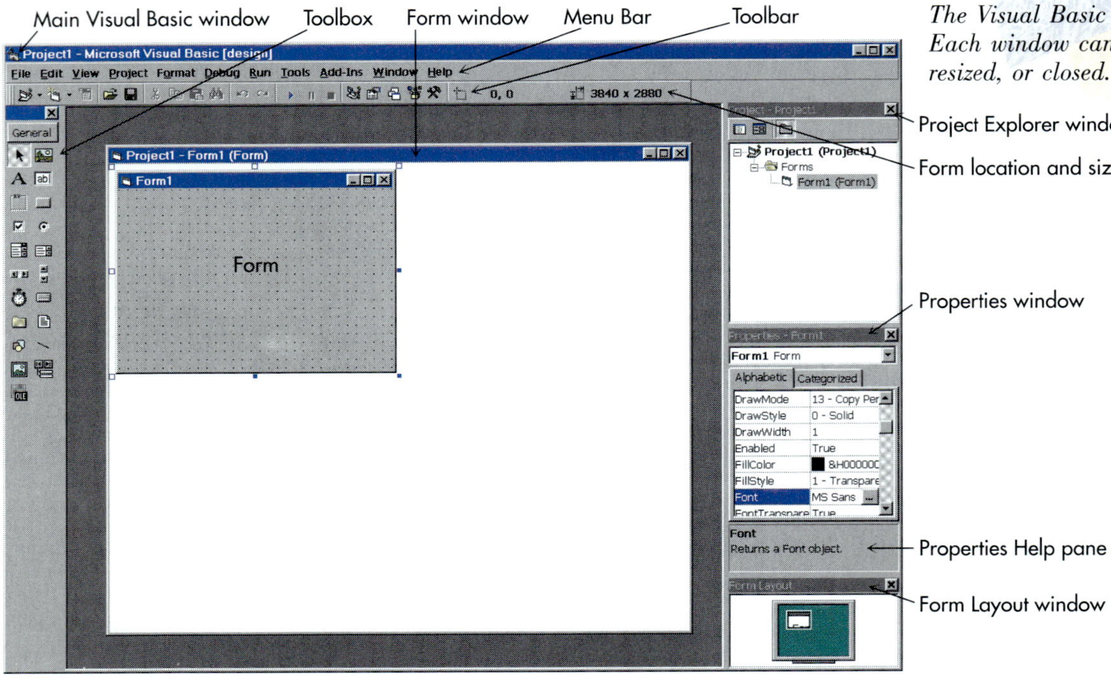

Figure 1.2

The Visual Basic environment. Each window can be moved, resized, or closed.

The Form Window

The **Form window** is where you design the forms that make up your user interface. You can use standard Windows techniques to change the size and location of the form.

When you begin a new project, Visual Basic gives your new form the default name *Form1*. As soon as you save the file, you will give it a new (more meaningful) name.

The Project Explorer Window

The **Project Explorer window** holds the filenames for the files included in your project. The window's title bar holds the name of your project (.VBP) file, which is *Project1* by default until you save it with a new name.

The Properties Window

You use the **Properties window** to set the properties for the objects in your project. See "Set Properties" later in this chapter for instructions on changing properties.

The Form Layout Window

The position of the form in the form layout window determines the position of the form on the desktop when execution of the project begins.

The Toolbox

The **toolbox** holds the tools you use to place controls on a form. You may have more or different tools in your toolbox, depending on the edition and release of Visual Basic you are using. See Figure 1.3 for a labeled version of the toolbox.

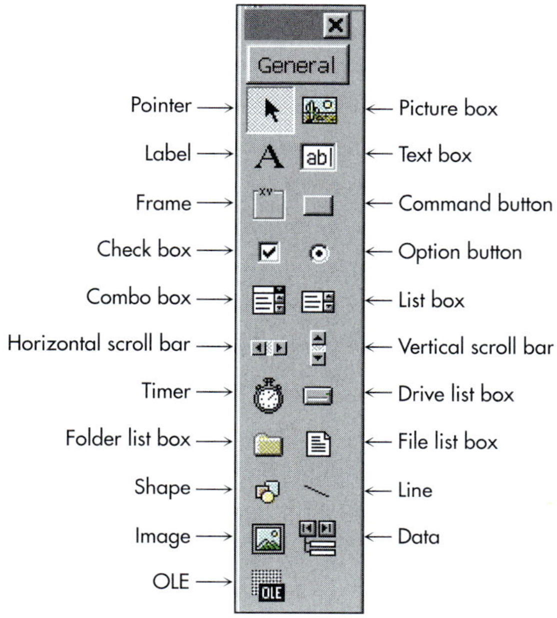

Figure 1.3

The toolbox for the Visual Basic Professional Edition. Your toolbox may have more or fewer tools, depending on the edition and release you are using.

The Main Visual Basic Window

The Main Visual Basic window holds the VB menu bar, the toolbar, and the form location and size information.

The Toolbar

You can use the buttons on the **toolbar** as shortcuts for frequently used operations. Each button represents a command that can also be selected from a menu. Figure 1.4 shows the toolbar buttons.

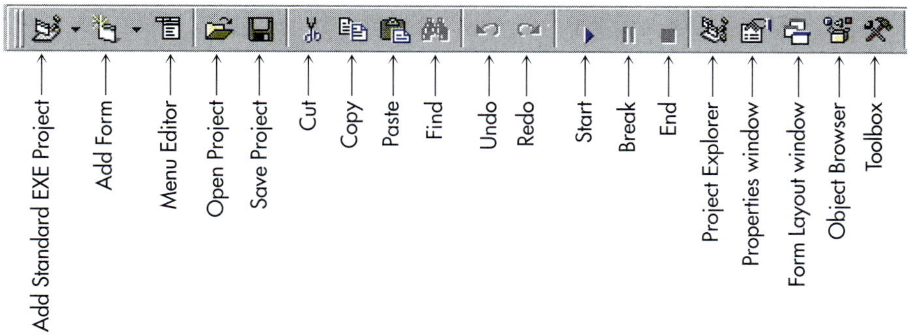

Figure 1.4

The Visual Basic toolbar. Each button represents a command that you can execute by clicking the button or by choosing a command from a menu.

The Form Location and Size Information

The two small diagrams at the right end of the Visual Basic toolbar (refer to Figure 1.2) show the position of the form on the screen along with the size of the form.

Help

Visual Basic has an extensive Help facility. It includes most of the reference manual, as well as many coding examples. In addition to the Help Index and Books Online, you will find Microsoft on the Web with a submenu containing various resources. Take some time to investigate the options on the Help menu.

Design Time, Run Time, and Break Time

Visual Basic has three distinct modes. While you are designing the user interface and writing code, you are in **design time**. When you are testing and running your project, you are in **run time**. If you get a run-time error or pause project execution, you are in **break time**. Notice the title bar notation in Figure 1.2, indicating that the project is currently in design time.

Writing Your First Visual Basic Project

For your first event-driven project, you will create a form with three controls (see Figure 1.5). This simple project will display the message "Hello World" when the user clicks the Push Me command button and will terminate when the user clicks the Exit button.

Figure 1.5

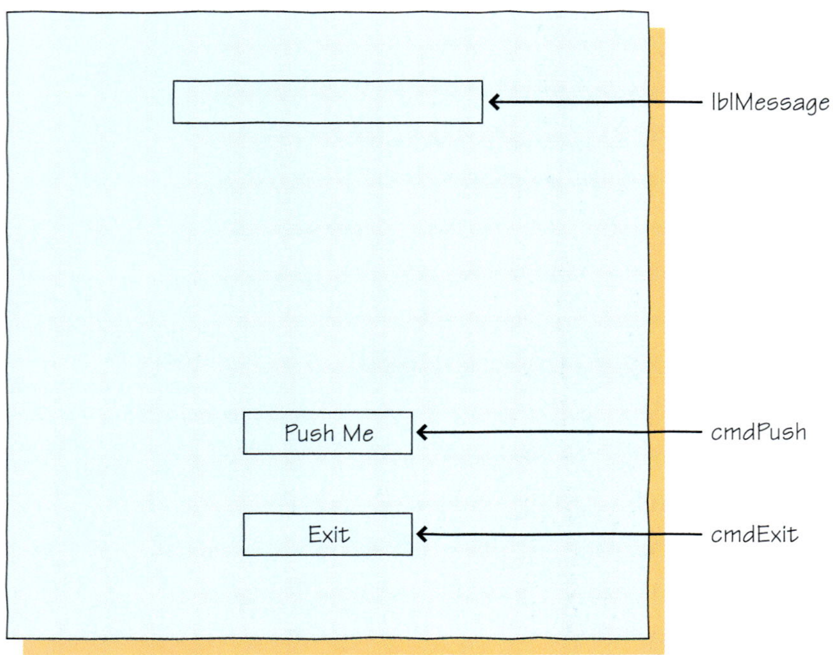

The Hello World form. The "Hello World" message will appear in the label when the user clicks on the Push Me command button.

Set Up Your Visual Basic Workspace

Before you can begin a project, you must run Visual Basic and set up your workspace the way you want it.

Run Visual Basic

STEP 1: Click on the Start button and move the mouse pointer to *Programs*.
STEP 2: Locate *Microsoft Visual Basic 5.0*.
STEP 3: Click on *Visual Basic 5.0* (Figure 1.6) in the submenu.

Note: If you see the dialog box pictured in Figure 1.7, check the box that says *Don't show this dialog in the future*. If you are using a shared computer lab, check with your instructor before checking this box.

The Visual Basic project will begin and display the VB environment on the screen (refer to Figure 1.2).

Figure 1.6

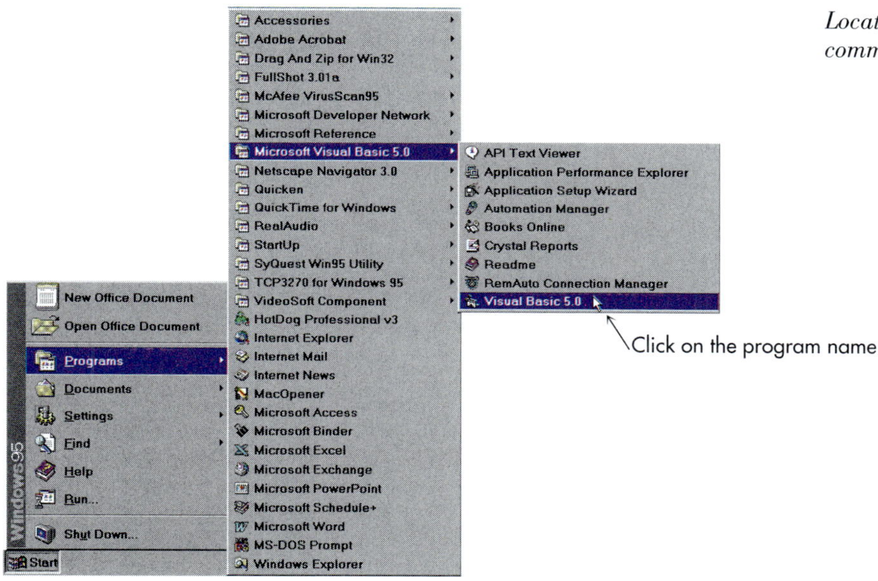

Locate the Visual Basic 5.0 command and click on it.

Figure 1.7

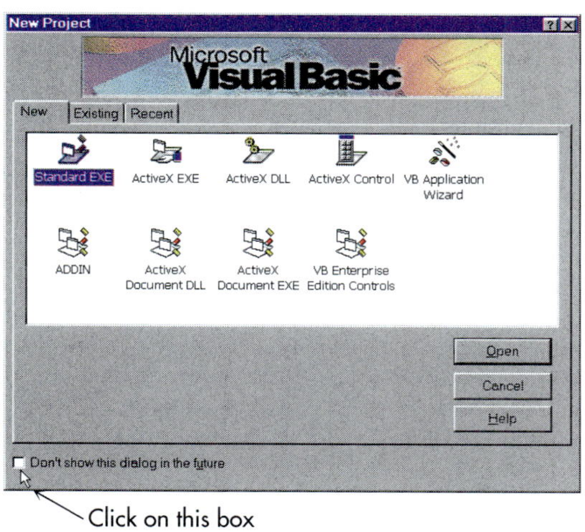

The New Project *dialog box may appear when you start Visual Basic. Click on the check box to prevent the box from appearing for each project.*

Set Up Your Workspace

STEP 1: Open the Visual Basic *Tools* menu and choose *Options*. Select the *Editor* tab if necessary. Then check each of these options, changing any that do not match (Figure 1.8).

New to VB 5!

Figure 1.8

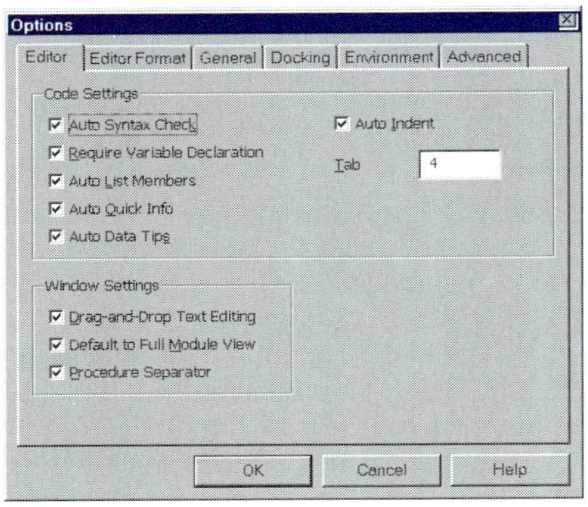

Choose Options from the Tools menu and select the Editor tab; make sure the options are properly set.

Code Settings:	
Auto Syntax Check	Selected
Require Variable Declaration	Selected
Window Settings:	
Drag-and-Drop Text Editing	Selected
Default to Full Module View	Selected
Procedure Separator	Selected

STEP 2: Click on the *General* tab of the Options window and make sure the following options are selected (Figure 1.9). When you are finished, click OK.

New to VB 5!

Form Grid Settings:	
Show Grid	Selected
Align Controls to Grid	Selected
Show ToolTips	Selected

Figure 1.9

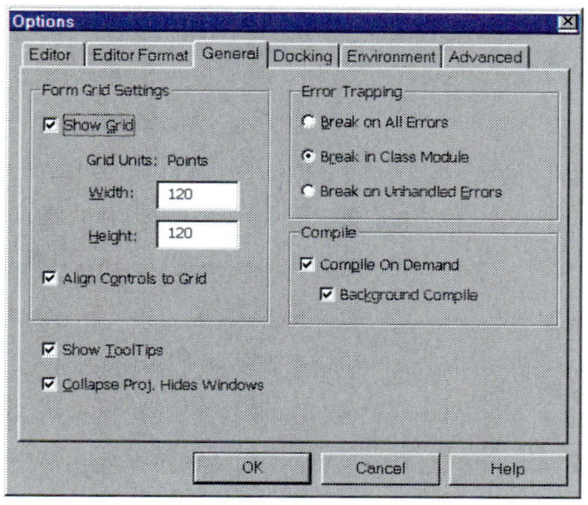

Set these options on the General tab of the Options window.

STEP 3: If the Project Explorer window is not displaying, open the *View* menu and select *Project Explorer.*

STEP 4: If the Properties window is not displaying, open the *View* menu and select *Properties Window.* (You may move or resize the Form window by dragging its title bar.)

STEP 5: If the toolbox is not displaying, open the *View* menu and select *Toolbox.*

STEP 6: Maximize the Form window by clicking on its Maximize button.

STEP 7: Adjust the size and location of the various windows if necessary. You can point to the divider between the Project Explorer window and the Properties window and drag to resize. Each window may be floating or docked, so your screen may not look like the examples. Try to make your screen layout similar to Figure 1.10.

Figure 1.10

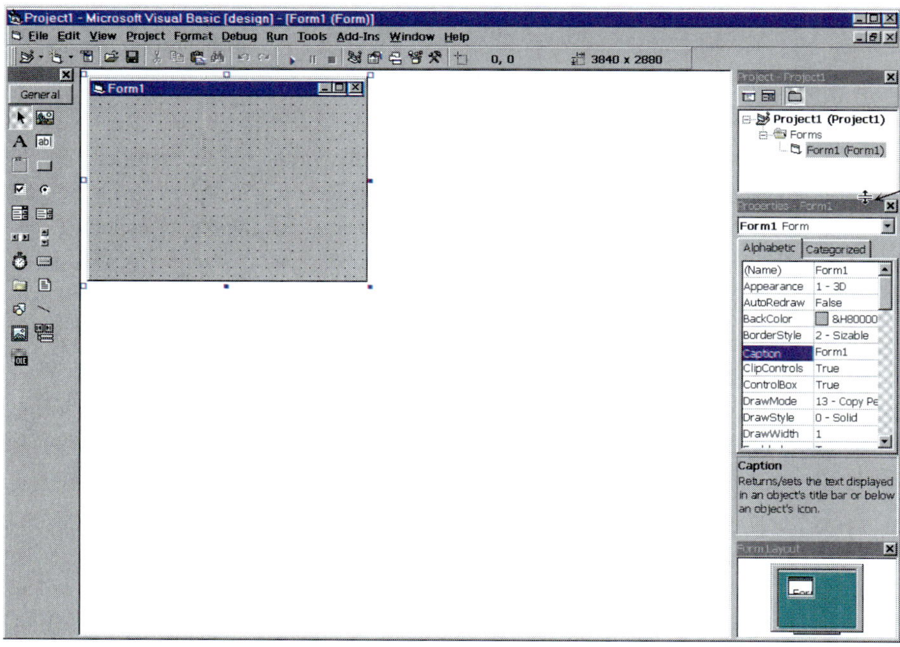

Resize windows with resizing pointer

Move and resize the windows so that all are visible.

Plan the Project

The first step in planning is to design the user interface. Figure 1.11 shows a sketch of the form that includes a label and two command buttons. You will refer to the sketch as you create the project.

Figure 1.11

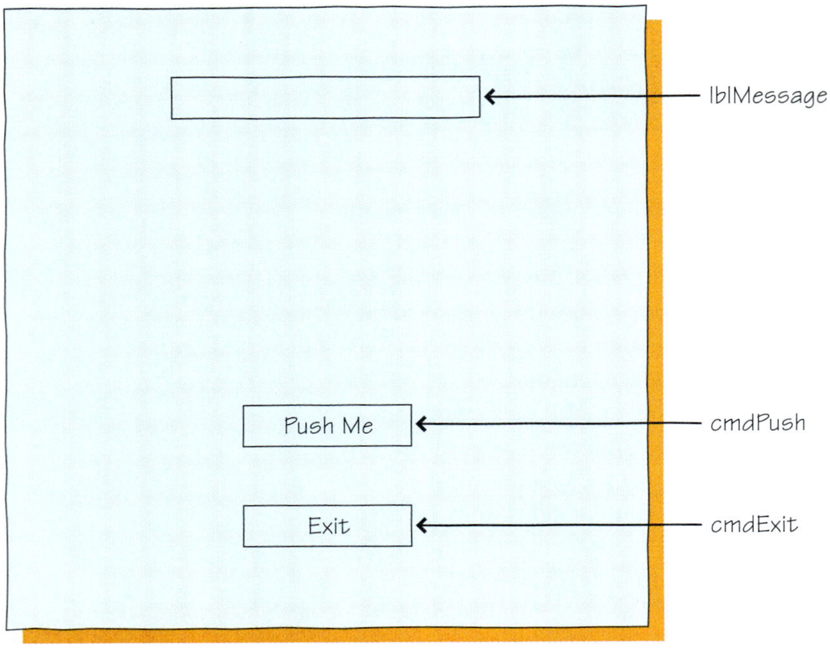

A sketch of the Hello World form for planning.

The next two steps, planning the properties and the code, have already been done for this first sample project. You will be given the values in the steps that follow.

Define the User Interface

Set Up the Form

Notice that the new form in the Form window has all the standard Windows features, such as a title bar, maximize and minimize buttons, and a close button.

STEP 1: Resize the form in the Form window: Drag the handle in the lower-right corner down and to the right (see Figure 1.12 on page 13).

STEP 2: Look at the Form Layout window in the lower-right corner of the screen (refer to Figure 1.12). The small picture of a form on the monitor shows the location where your form will appear when the project runs. You may drag the picture to a different location. (*Note:* Monitors have differing resolutions, and the location you choose when designing your project may not appear the same on a different monitor.)

Figure 1.12

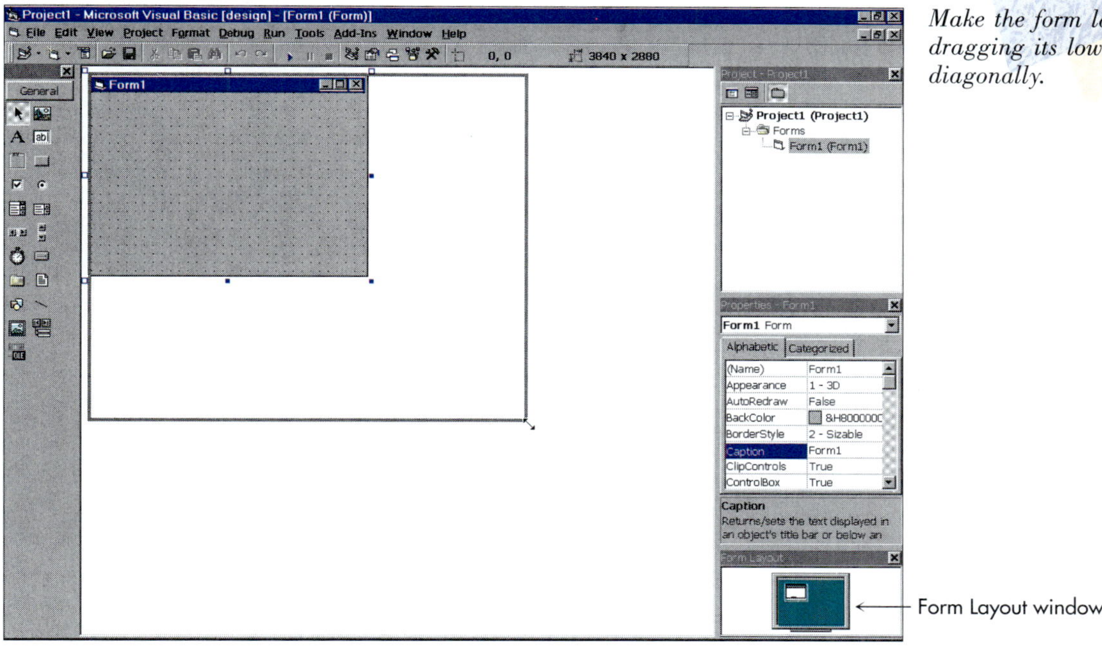

Make the form larger by dragging its lower-right handle diagonally.

Place Controls on the Form

You are going to place three controls on the form: a **label** and two **command buttons**.

STEP 1: Point to the label tool in the toolbox and click. Then move the pointer over the form. Notice that the pointer becomes a crosshair, and the label tool looks like it has been pressed, indicating it is the active tool (Figure 1.13).

Figure 1.13

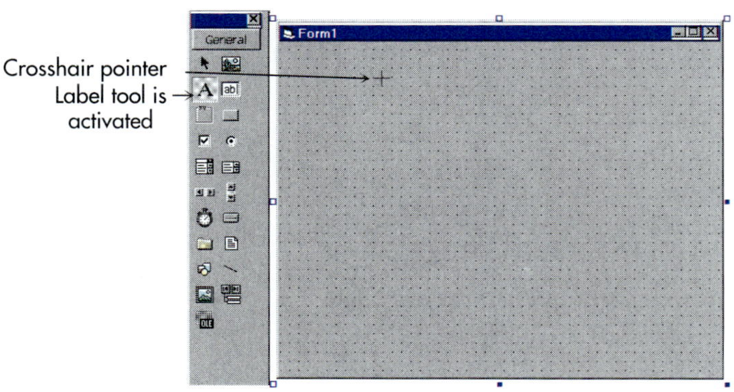

When you click on the label tool in the toolbox, the tool's button is activated and the mouse pointer becomes a crosshair.

STEP 2: Point to the upper-left corner where you want the label to begin, press the mouse button, and drag the pointer to the opposite corner (Figure 1.14). When you release the mouse button, the label and its default contents (Label1) will appear (Figure 1.15).

Figure 1.14

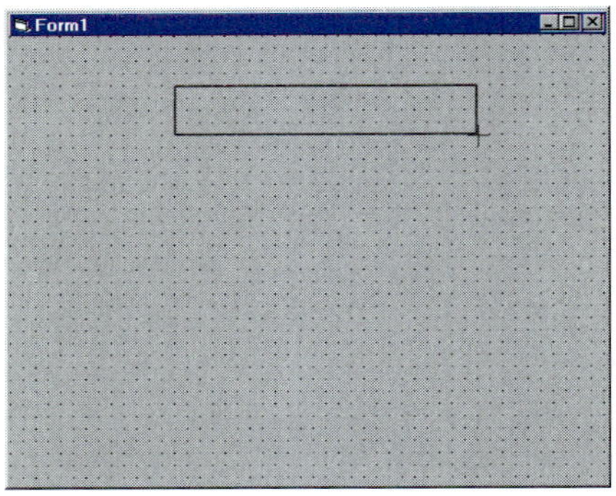

Drag the mouse pointer diagonally to draw the label on the form.

Figure 1.15

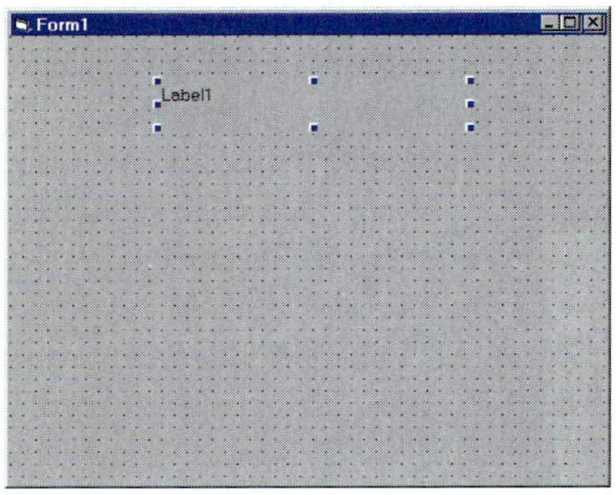

The newly created label has eight small handles, indicating that it is selected. Notice that the contents of the label are set to Label1 by default.

When you pause, Visual Basic's ToolTip pops up, indicating the size of the control in *twips,* which is a printer's measurement system. 1 twip = 1/1440 inch.

The label has eight small square **handles**, indicating that the control is currently selected. While a control is selected, you can delete it, resize it, or move it. Refer to Table 1.1 for instructions for selecting, deleting, resizing, and moving controls. Click outside of a control to deselect it.

Table 1.1

Selecting, deleting, resizing, and moving controls on a form.

Select a control	Click on the control.
Delete a control	Select the control and then press the Delete key on the keyboard.
Move a control	Select the control, point inside the control (not on a handle), press the mouse button, and drag it to a new location.
Resize a control	Make sure the control is selected; then point to one of the handles, press the mouse button, and drag the handle. Drag a side handle to change the width, a bottom or top handle to change the height, or a corner handle to resize in two directions.

STEP 3: Draw a command button on the form: Click on the Command button tool in the toolbox, position the crosshair pointer for one corner of the button, and drag to the diagonally opposite corner (Figure 1.16).

The new command button should have selection handles.

Figure 1.16

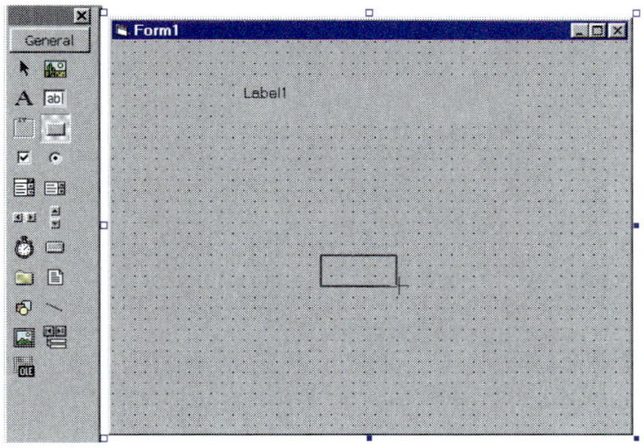

Select the Command button tool and drag diagonally to create a new command button control.

STEP 4: Create another command button using this alternative method: Point to the Command button tool in the toolbox and double-click. A new command button of the default size will appear in the center of the form (Figure 1.17).

Figure 1.17

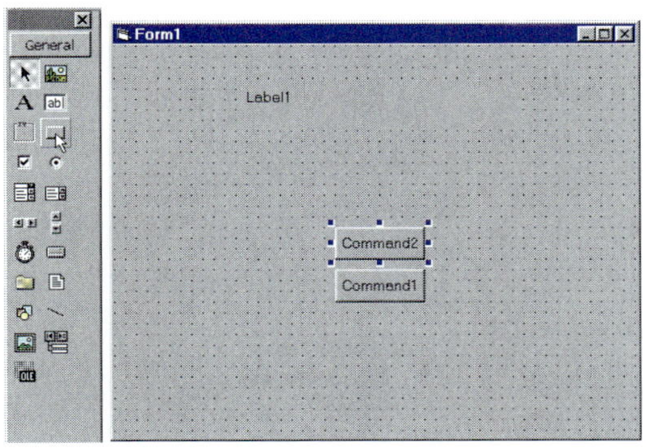

Place a new command button on the form by double-clicking the Command button tool in the toolbox. The new button appears in the center of the form.

STEP 5: Keep the new command button selected, point anywhere inside the button (not on a handle), and drag the button below your first button (Figure 1.18). As you drag the control, you see only its outline; when you release the mouse button, the control is actually moved to its new location.

Figure 1.18

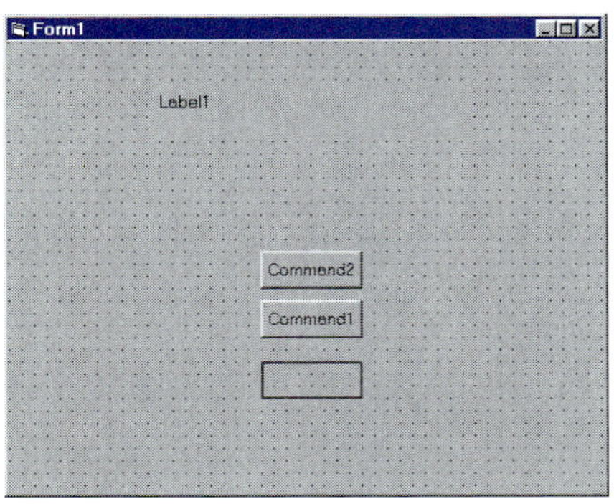

Drag the new command button (Command2) below Command1. An outline of the control shows the new location for the control.

STEP 6: Select each control and move and resize the controls as necessary. Make the two buttons the same size and line them up.

STEP 7: Point anywhere on the form except on a control and click the right mouse button. On the Shortcut menu, select *Lock Controls* (Figure 1.19). Locking prevents you from accidentally moving the controls. When your controls are locked, you see white handles, rather than the dark handles, around a selected control.

Note: You can unlock the controls at any time if you wish to redesign the form. Just click on *Lock Controls* on the Shortcut menu again to deselect it.

Figure 1.19

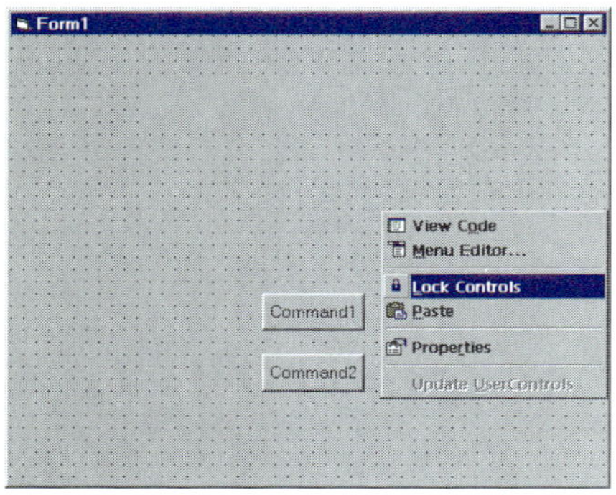

After the controls are placed into the desired location, lock them in place by selecting Lock Controls *from the shortcut menu.*

At this point you have designed the user interface and are ready to set the properties.

Set Properties

Set the Name and Caption Properties for the Label

Tip

If the Properties window is not visible, you can press the F4 key to show it.

STEP 1: Click on the label you placed on the form; selection handles will appear. Next click on the title bar of the Properties window to make it the active window (Figure 1.20).

Figure 1.20

The currently selected control is shown in the Properties window.

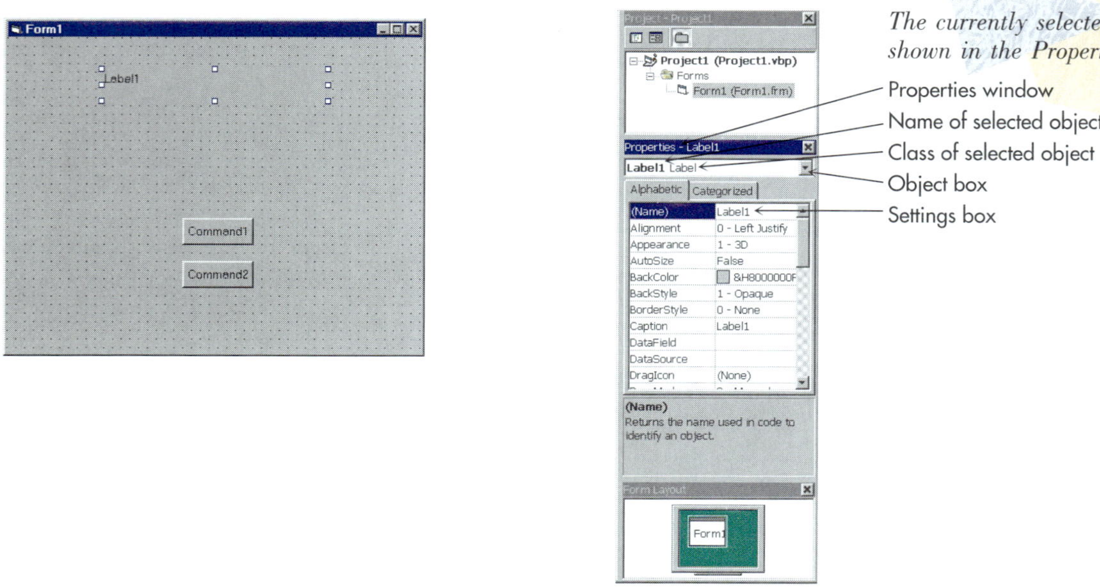

Notice that the Object box at the top of the Properties window is showing *Label1* (the name of the object) and *Label* (called the ***class*** of the object).

STEP 2: Select the Name property. Click on *(Name)* and notice that the Settings box shows *Label1,* the default name of the label (Figure 1.21).

Figure 1.21

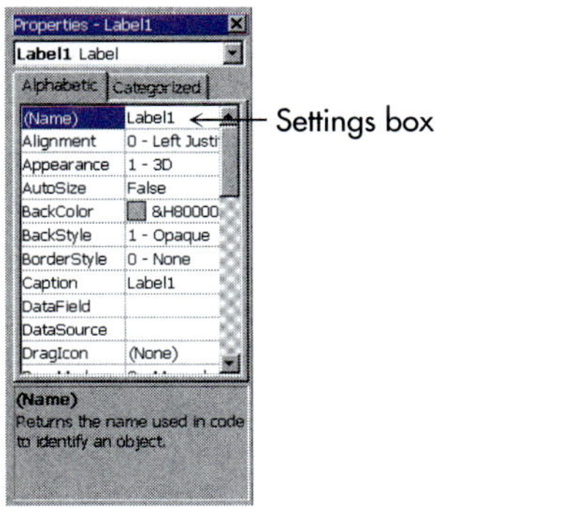

The Properties window. Click on the Name property to change the value in the Settings box.

STEP 3: Type "lblMessage" (without the quotation marks). See Figure 1.22.

Figure 1.22

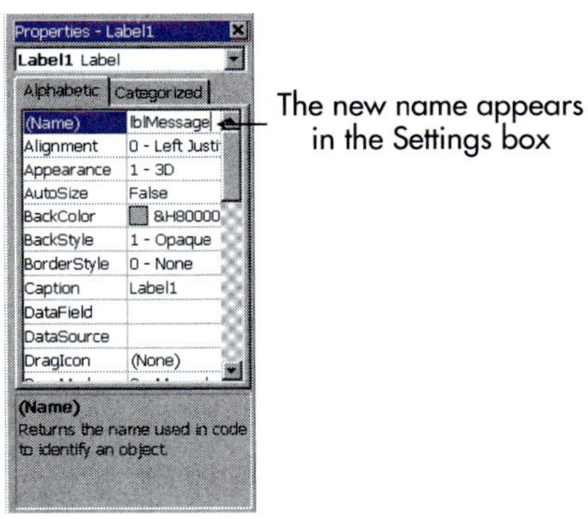

Type "lblMessage" into the Settings box for the Name property.

STEP 4: Click on the Caption property to select it. Scroll the list if necessary.

The **Caption** property of a label determines what will be displayed on the form. Since nothing should display when the project begins, you must delete the value of the Caption property (as described in the next two steps).

STEP 5: Double-click on *Label1* in the Settings box; the entry should appear selected (highlighted). See Figure 1.23.

Figure 1.23

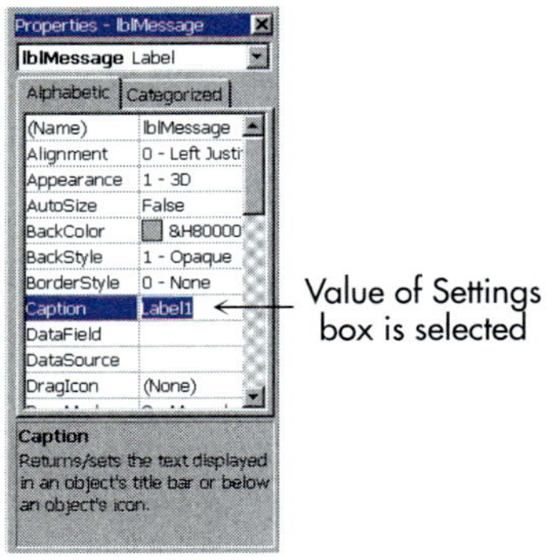

Double-click in the Settings box to select the entry.

STEP 6: Press the Delete key to delete the value of the Caption property. Notice that the label on the form now appears empty (Figure 1.24).

Figure 1.24

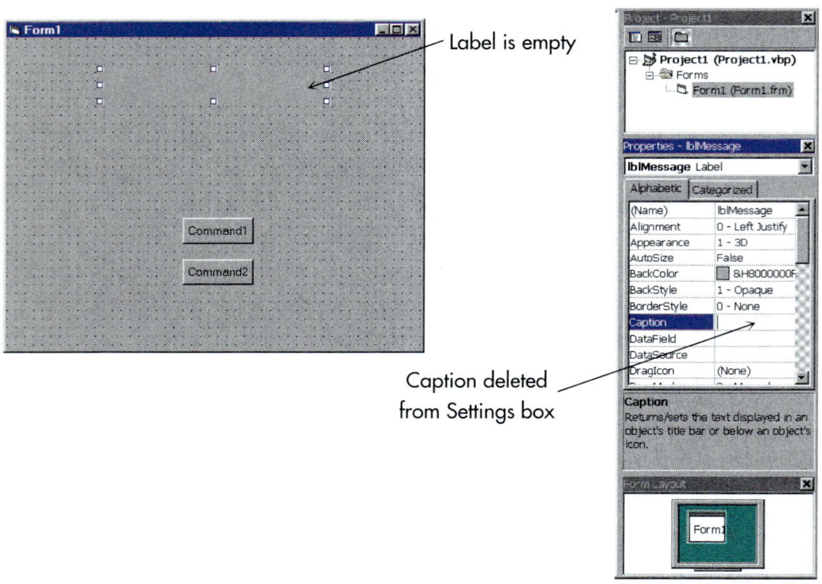

Delete the value for the Caption property from the Settings box; the label on the form also appears empty.

Set the Name and Caption Properties for the First Command Button

STEP 1: Click on the first command button (Command1) to select it and then look at the Properties window. The Object box should show the name *(Command1)* and class *(CommandButton)* of the command button. See Figure 1.25.

Problem? If you should double-click and another window appears, simply close the window by clicking on the new window's close button.

STEP 2: Change the Name property of the command button to "cmdPush" (without the quotation marks).

Tip

Don't confuse the Name property with the Caption property. You will use the Name property to refer to the control in your Basic code. The Caption property tells what the user will see on the form. Visual Basic sets both of these properties to the same value by default, and it is easy to confuse them.

Figure 1.25

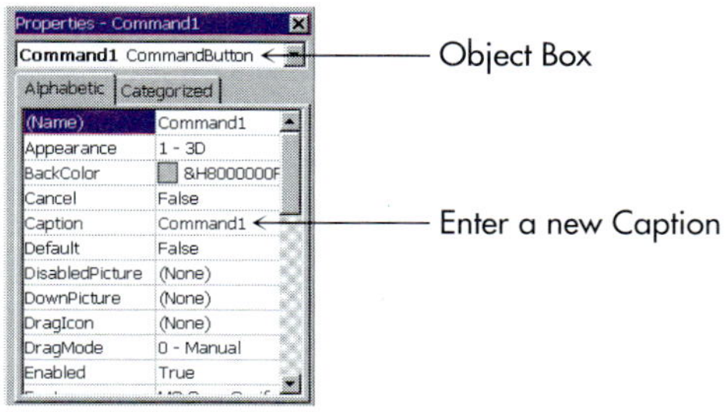

Change the Caption property for the first command button.

Although the project would work fine without this step, we prefer to give this button a meaningful name, rather than use Command1, its default name.

STEP 3: Change the Caption property to "Push Me" (without the quotation marks). This changes the words that appear on top of the button.

Tip

Always set the Name property of controls before writing code. If you change the name of an object after the code is typed, the code becomes separated from its object and the program does not run properly.

Set the Name and Caption Properties for the Second Command Button

STEP 1: Select Command2 and change its Name property to "cmdExit".

STEP 2: Change the Caption property to "Exit".

Change the Caption Property for the Form

STEP 1: Click anywhere on the form, except on a control. The Properties window Object box should now show the form as the selected object (*Form1* as the object's name and *Form* as its class).

STEP 2: Change the Caption property to "Hello World by *Your Name*" (again, no quotation marks).

The Caption property of a form determines the text to appear in the title bar. Your screen should now look like Figure 1.26.

Figure 1.26

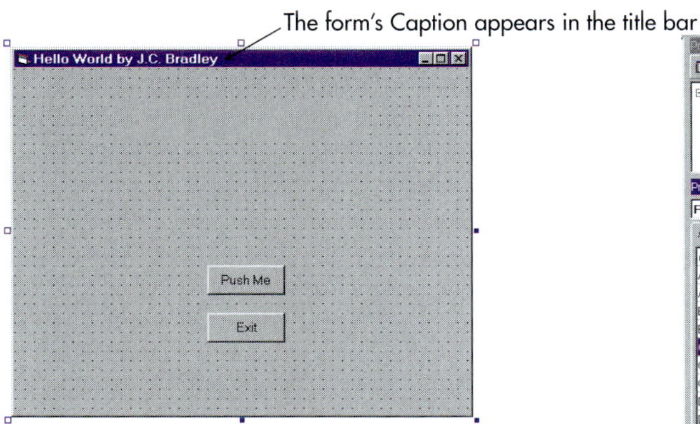

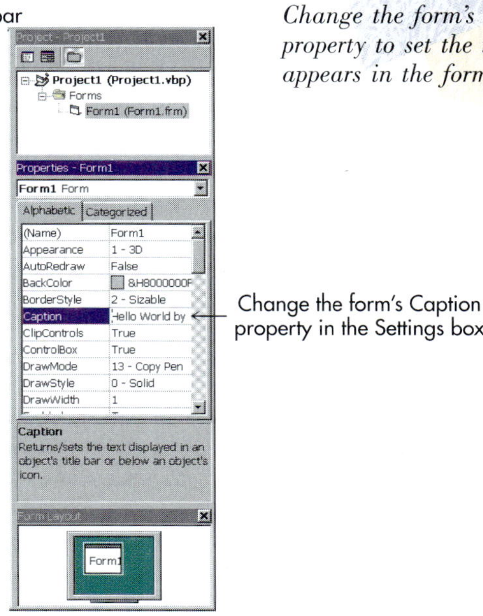

Change the form's Caption property to set the text that appears in the form's title bar.

Write Code

Visual Basic Events

While your project is running, the user can do many things, such as move the mouse around; click on either button; move, resize, or close your form's window; or jump to another application. Each action by the user causes an **event** to occur in your Visual Basic project. Some of the events you care about (like clicking on a command button), and some events you do not care about (like moving the mouse and resizing the window). If you write Basic code for a particular event, then Visual Basic will respond to the event and automatically execute your procedure. *VB ignores events for which no procedures are written.*

Visual Basic Event Procedures

You write code in Visual Basic in **procedures**. For now, each of your procedures will be a **sub procedure**, which begins with the words *Private Sub* and ends with *End Sub*. (Later you will also learn about function procedures.) *Note:* Many programmers refer to sub procedures as *subprograms* or *subroutines*. *Subprogram* is OK; *subroutine* is not, because Basic actually has a different statement for a subroutine, which is not the same as a sub procedure.

Visual Basic automatically names your **event procedures**. The name consists of the object name, an underscore (_), and the name of the event. For example, the Click event for your command button called cmdPush will be *cmdPush_Click*. For the sample project you are writing, you will need a cmdPush_Click procedure and a cmdExit_Click procedure.

Visual Basic Code Statements

This first project requires three Visual Basic statements: the **remark**, the **assignment statement**, and the **End statement**.

The Remark Statement

Remark statements, sometimes called *comments*, are used for project documentation only. They are not considered "executable" and have no effect when the project runs. The purpose of remarks is to make the project more readable and understandable by the people who read it.

Good programming practices dictate that programmers include remarks to clarify their projects. Every sub procedure should begin with a remark that describes the purpose of the sub. Every project module should have remarks that tell the purpose of the module, as well as provide identifying information such as the name of the programmer and the date the module was written and/or modified. In addition, it is a good idea to place remarks within the logic of a project, especially if the purpose of any statements might be unclear.

When you try to read someone else's project, or your own after a period of time, you will appreciate the generous use of remarks.

Visual Basic remarks begin with an apostrophe. Most of the time your remarks will be on a separate line that starts with an apostrophe. You can also add an apostrophe and a remark to the right end of a line of code.

The Remark Statement—Examples

```
'This project was written by Jonathon Edwards
'Exit the project
lblMessage.Caption = "Hello World" 'Assign the message to the Caption property
```

The Assignment Statement

The assignment statement assigns a value to a property or variable (you'll learn about variables in Chapter 3). Assignment statements operate from right to left; that is, the value appearing on the right side of the equal sign is assigned to the property named on the left of the equal sign. It is often helpful to read the equal sign as "is replaced by." For example, the assignment statement in the previous example box would read "lblMessage.Caption is replaced by Hello World."

The Assignment Statement—General Form

```
[Let] Object.Property = value
```

The value named on the right side of the equal sign is assigned to (or placed into) the property named on the left. The `Let` is optional and may be included if you wish. You may find that using `Let` improves the readability of your projects.

The Assignment Statement—Examples

```
lblTitle.Caption = "A Snazzy Program"
lblAddress.Caption = "1234 South North Street"
lblTitle.FontSize = 12
Let lblTitle.FontBold = True
```

Notice that when the value to assign is some actual text (called a *literal*), it is enclosed in quotation marks. This allows you to type any combination of alpha and numeric characters. If the value is numeric, do not enclose it in quotation marks. And do not place quotation marks around the terms *True* and *False*, which Visual Basic recognizes as special key terms.

The End Statement

The `End` statement stops execution of a project. In most cases, you will include an `End` statement in the sub procedure for an Exit button or an *Exit* menu choice.

The End Statement—Example

```
End
```

Code the Event Procedures for Hello World

Code the Click Event for the Push Me Button

STEP 1: Double-click on the Push Me command button. The Visual Basic **Code window** will open with the first and last lines of your sub procedure already in place (Figure 1.27).

Figure 1.27

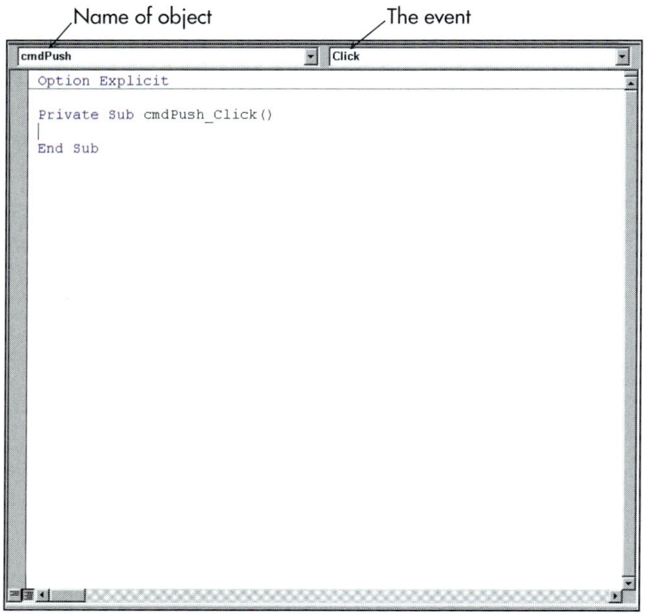

The Code window, showing the first and last lines of the sub procedure.

STEP 2: Press the Tab key once to indent and then type this remark statement:

```
'Display the Hello World message
```

STEP 3: Press Enter and notice that Visual Basic automatically changes remarks to green (unless you or someone else has changed the color with the Environment option).

Follow good coding conventions and indent all lines between Private Sub and End Sub. Also, always leave a blank line after the remarks at the top of a sub procedure.

STEP 4: Press Enter again and then type this assignment statement:

```
lblMessage.Caption = "Hello World"
```

Note: When you type the period after lblMessage, a list box appears showing the properties and methods available for a label control. Although you can type the entire word *Caption*, you can allow the Visual Basic editor to help you. As soon as you type the *C*, the list automatically scrolls to the word *Caption*. You can press the space bar to select the word and continue typing the rest of the statement.

This assignment statement assigns the literal "Hello World" to the Caption property of the control called lblMessage. Compare your screen to Figure 1.28.

Figure 1.28

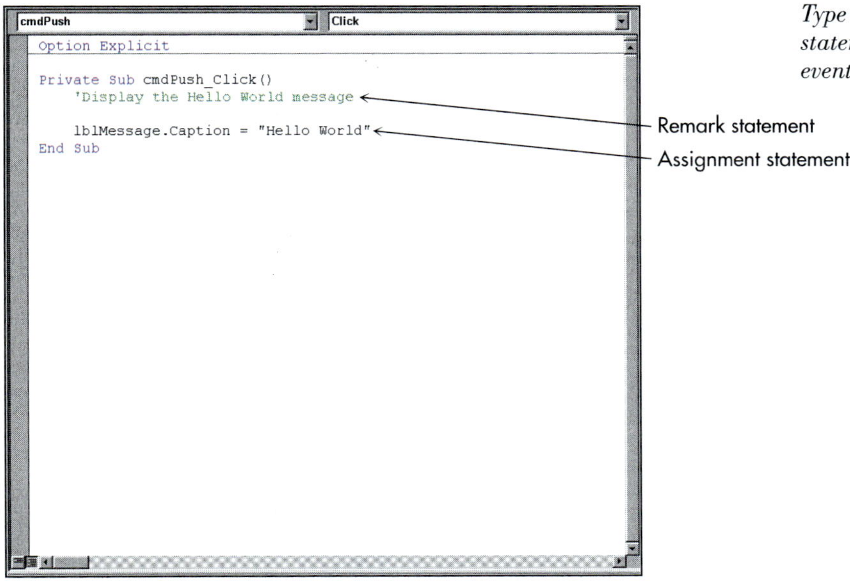

Type the remark and assignment statement for the cmdPush_Click event.

STEP 5: Return to the form by clicking on the View Object button on the Project Explorer window (Figure 1.29).

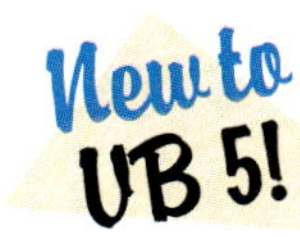

Figure 1.29

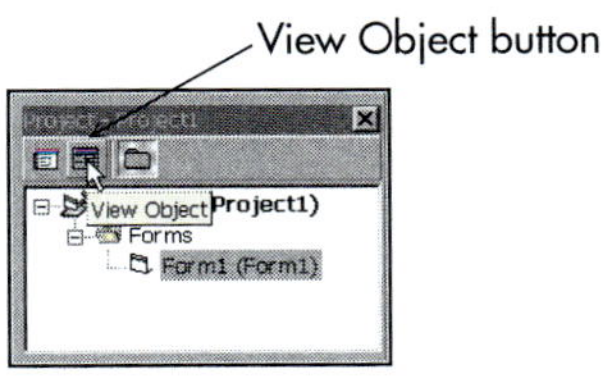

Click on the View Object button to return to the form.

Code the Click Event for the Exit Button

STEP 1: Double-click on the Exit command button to open the Code window for the cmdExit_Click event.

STEP 2: Press Tab once and type this remark:

```
'Exit the project
```

STEP 3: Press Enter twice and type this Basic statement:

```
End
```

STEP 4: Make sure your code looks like Figure 1.30 and then click on the Code window's Close button.

Figure 1.30

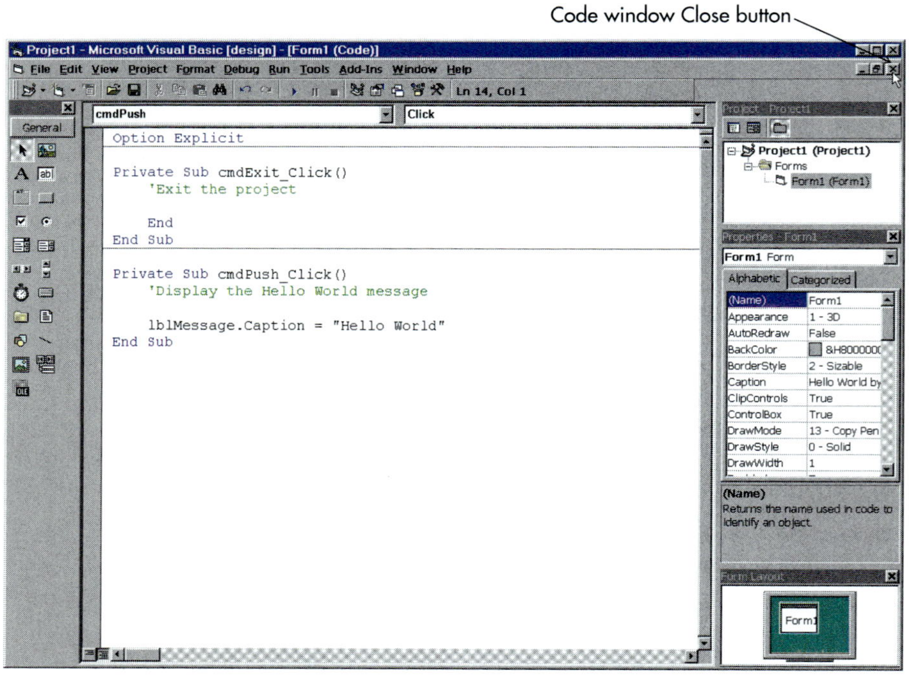

Type the remark and End statement for the cmdExit_Click event and close the Code window.

Run the Project

After you have finished writing the code, you are ready to run the project. Use one of these three methods:

1. Open the *Run* menu and choose *Start*.
2. Press the Start button on the toolbar.
3. Press F5, the shortcut key for the *Start* command.

Start the Project Running

STEP 1: Choose one of the three methods shown above to start your project running.

Notice that the Visual Basic title bar now indicates that you are in run time and that the grid dots have disappeared from your form (Figure 1.31). (The grid dots help you align the controls; you may turn them off if you prefer.)

Figure 1.31

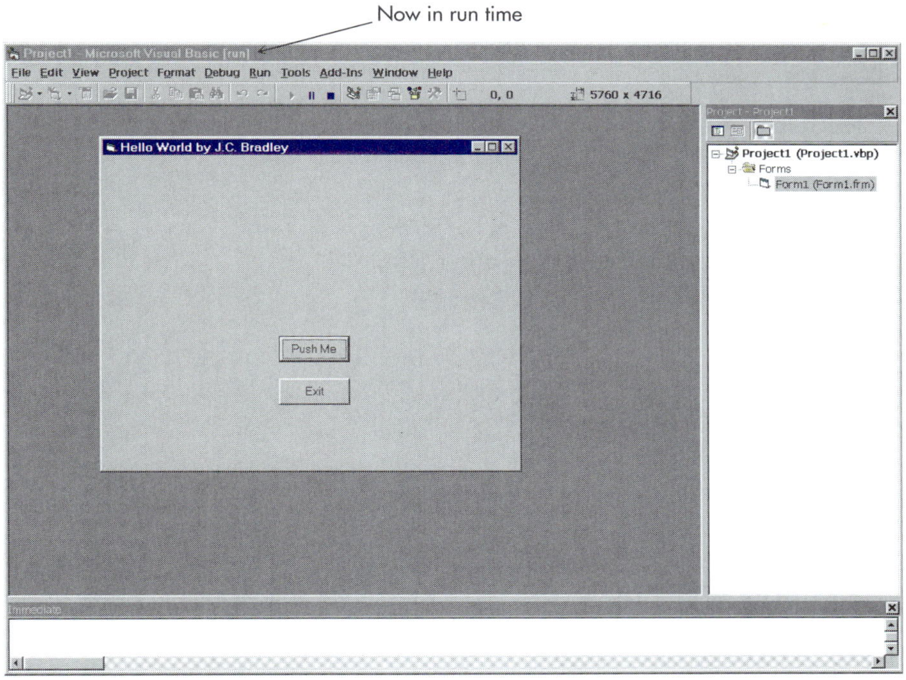

When you run the project, the Visual Basic title bar indicates run time and the form's grid dots disappear.

Click the Push Me Button

STEP 1: Click the Push Me button. Your "Hello World" message appears in the label (Figure 1.32).

Figure 1.32

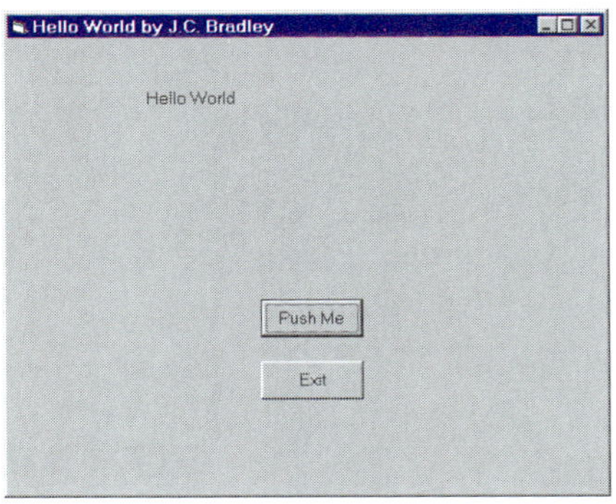

Click on the Push Me button and "Hello World" appears in the label.

Click the Exit Button

STEP 1: Click the Exit button. Your project terminates, and you return to Visual Basic design time.

(Problems? See "Finding and Fixing Errors" later in this chapter.)

Save the Project

Of course, you must always save your work often. Except for a very small project like this one, you will usually save your work as you go along.

Create a Folder

It is very easy to lose parts of a Visual Basic project and neglect to include all of the files when you copy a project from disk to disk. Therefore, you should always create a new folder on disk before saving your first file.

Note: Because of the way Visual Basic stores its project files, it is sometimes difficult to make it recognize that you have changed the location of a file. Always create your folder *first* and save into the folder—do not save somewhere else first and plan to organize later.

Save the Form File

STEP 1: Open the Visual Basic *File* menu and choose *Save Form1 As*. This option allows you to save the current form.

STEP 2: Check the *Save in* box and change to the correct drive.

STEP 3: Click on the *Create New Folder* button (Figure 1.33).

Figure 1.33

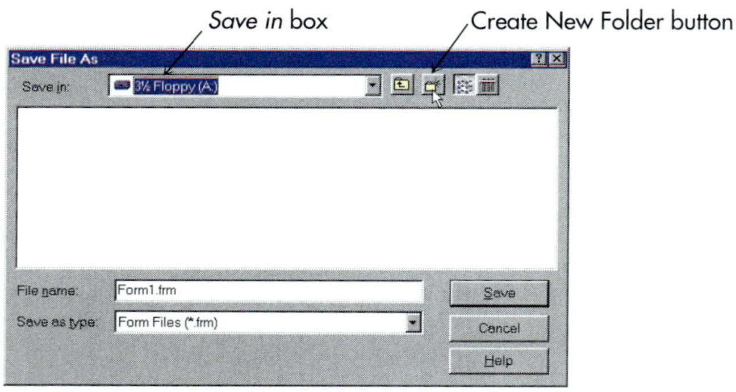

The Save Form As dialog box. Click on the Create New Folder button and name the new folder.

STEP 4: Type the name of your new folder as "Hello" (without the quotation marks) and press Enter.

STEP 5: Open the new folder by double-clicking on it.

STEP 6: In the *File name* box, type "Hello" (without the quotation marks; see Figure 1.34). Visual Basic will add the correct .FRM extension to the filename.

Figure 1.34

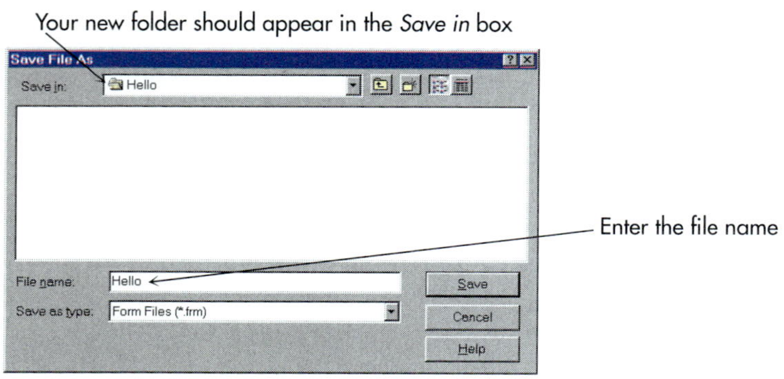

Double-click on your new folder so that it appears in the Save in box. Then enter the new file name.

STEP 7: Check the *Save in* list again to make sure the file will be saved in your new folder. Then press Enter or click *Save* to save the form file.

Save the Project File

STEP 1: Open the *File* menu and select *Save Project As.* This will allow you to save the project (.VBP) file.

STEP 2: Check the *Save in* box; your new folder should still be showing.

STEP 3: In the *File name* box, type "Hello" (without the quotation marks; see Figure 1.35). This file will be saved as *Hello.vbp*, since Visual Basic adds the correct file extension.

Figure 1.35

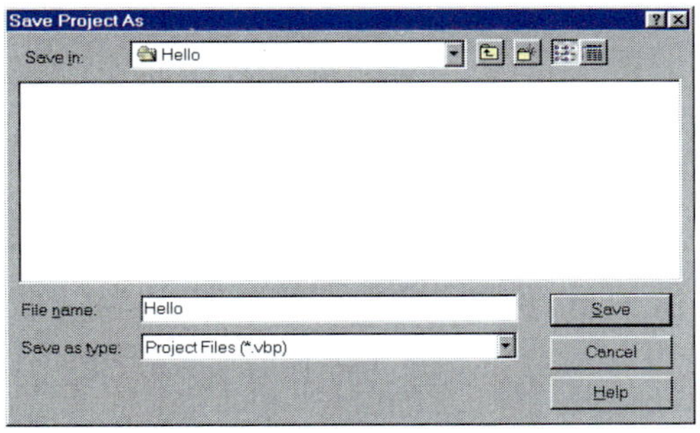

The Save Project As dialog box. Make sure the correct folder is selected and type the name of the project file in the File name box.

STEP 4: Press Enter or click *Save* to save the project file.

Open the Project

Now is the time to test your save operation by opening the project from disk.

Open the Project File

STEP 1: Either click on the Open Project button on the toolbar or choose *Open Project* from the *File* menu.

STEP 2: In the *Open Project* dialog box, check the *Look in* box. Your Hello folder should still be set correctly.

When you begin a new session, you will need to change to your drive and directory before you can open a project.

STEP 3: You should see your project name, Hello.vbp, in the file list box (Figure 1.36). Click on the filename and then click on the *Open* button (or double-click on the filename).

Figure 1.36

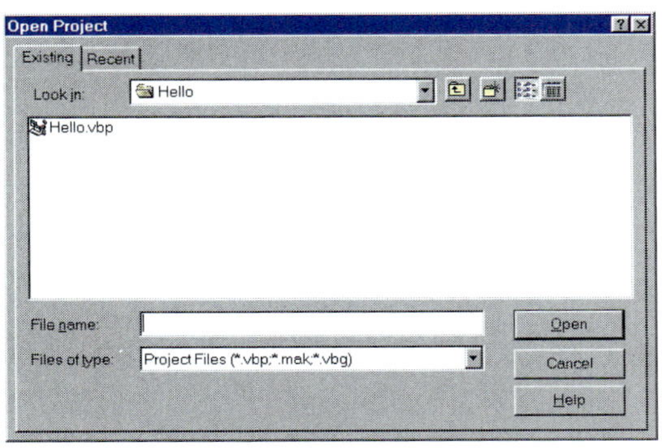

The Open Project dialog box. Select the correct folder and find your project name in the file list.

STEP 4: If you do not see your form on the screen, check the Project Explorer window—it should say *Hello.vbp* for the project. Click on the View Object button, and your form will appear.

Modify the Project

Now it's time to make some changes to the project. We'll change the size of the "Hello World" message, display the message in two different languages, and display the programmer name (that's you) on the form. We'll also provide a button that will print the form.

Change the Size and Alignment of the Message

STEP 1: Right-click somewhere on the form to display the *Shortcut* menu and select *Lock Controls* to unlock the controls so that you can make changes.

STEP 2: Click on the label on your form, which will make dark selection handles appear. (If your selection handles are white, you must unlock the controls, as described in Step 1.)

STEP 3: Widen the label on both ends by dragging the handles wider. (Drag the right end farther right and the left end farther left.)

STEP 4: With the label still selected, scroll to the Font property, and click to select it. The Settings box shows the currently selected font.

Notice the new button with an ellipses on top, which appears in the Settings box (Figure 1.37). The button is called the *Properties* button; the ellipses indicates that clicking on the button will display a dialog box with choices.

Figure 1.37

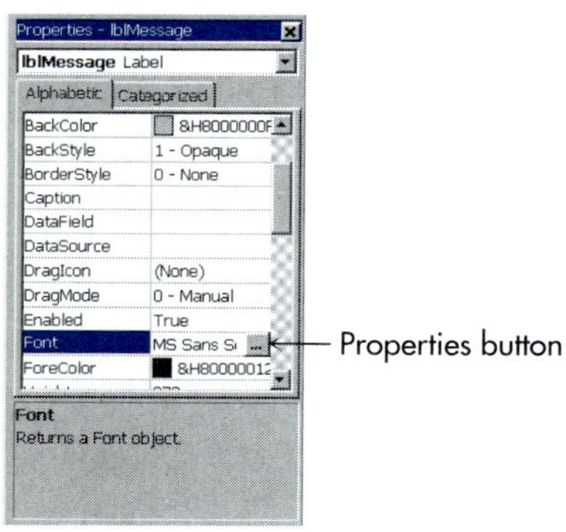

Click on the Properties button to see the choices for the Font property.

STEP 5: Click on the Properties button to display the *Font* dialog box (Figure 1.38). Select 12 point if it is available. (If it isn't available, choose another number larger than the current setting.) Close the *Font* dialog box.

Figure 1.38

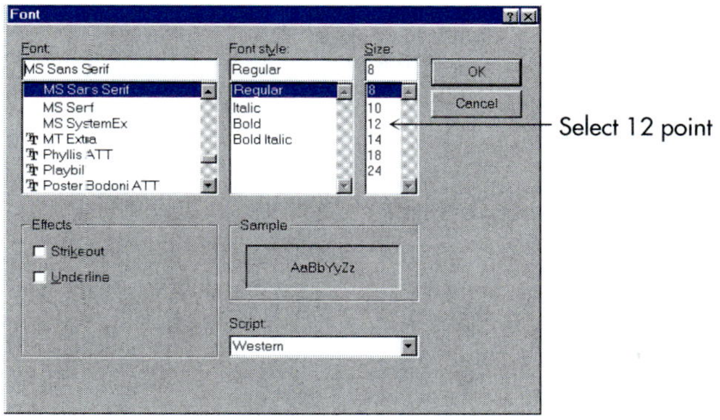

Choose 12 point from the Font dialog box.

STEP 6: Select the Alignment property. The Properties button that appears with the down-pointing arrow indicates a drop-down list of choices. Drop down the list and choose *2—Center.*

Add a New Label for Your Name

STEP 1: Click on the Label tool in the toolbox and create a new label along the bottom edge of your form (Figure 1.39). (You can resize the form if necessary.)

Figure 1.39

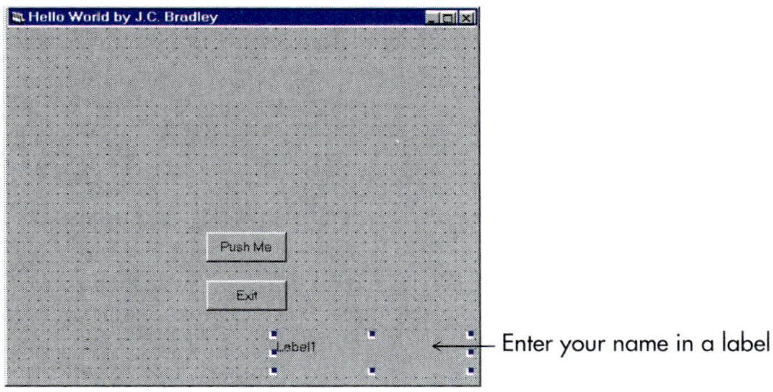

Add a new label for your name at the bottom of the form.

STEP 2: Change the label's Caption property to "by Your Name". (Use your name and omit the quotation marks.)

Change the Location and Caption of the Push Me Button

Since we plan to display the message in one of two languages, we'll change the caption on the Push Me button to English and move the button to allow for a second command button.

STEP 1: Select the Push Me button and change its Caption property to English.

STEP 2: Move the English button to the left to make room for a Spanish button (see Figure 1.40).

Figure 1.40

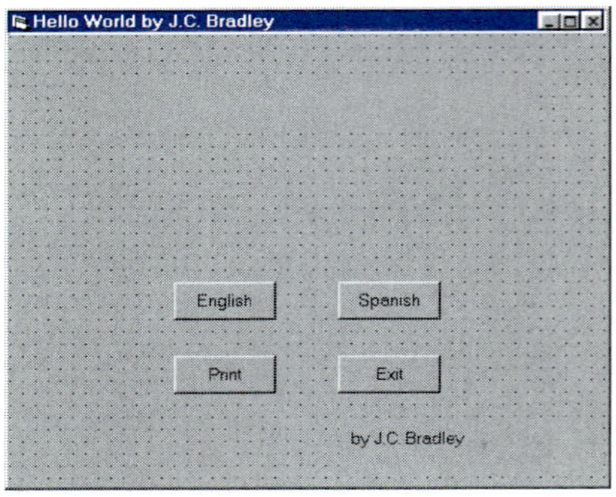

Move the English button to the left and add a Spanish button and a Print button.

Add a Spanish Button

STEP 1: Add a new command button. Move and resize it as necessary, referring to Figure 1.40.
STEP 2: Change the Name property of the new button to cmdSpanish.
STEP 3: Change the Caption property of the new button to Spanish.

Add an Event Procedure for the Spanish Button

STEP 1: Double-click on the Spanish button to open the Code window for cmdSpanish_Click.
STEP 2: Press the Tab key once and add a remark:

```
'Display the Hello World message in Spanish
```

STEP 3: Press Enter twice and type the following Basic code line:

```
lblMessage.Caption = "Hola Mundo"
```

STEP 4: Close the Code window.

Add a Print Button

STEP 1: Move the Exit button to the right to make room for the Print button.
STEP 2: Add a new command button; move and resize it to match Figure 1.40.
STEP 3: Change the Name property of the new button to cmdPrint.
STEP 4: Change the Caption property of the new button to Print.

Lock the Controls

STEP 1: When you are satisfied with the placement of the controls on the form, display the Shortcut menu and select *Lock Controls* again.

Add an Event Procedure for the Print Button

To print the form, we will use the PrintForm method, which prints the current form without its title bar or borders.

STEP 1: Double-click on the Print button to open the Code window for the cmdPrint_Click event.
STEP 2: Indent and add a remark that tells what you plan to do in the subprogram.

STEP 3: Leave a blank line and indent the following code statement:

```
PrintForm
```

That's all there is to it. The actual format for a method is Object.Method (object dot method). However, we can leave off the object in this case, since it defaults to the current form.

Save and Run the Project

STEP 1: Save your project again. You can use the *Save File* and *Save Project* menu options or click on the Save button on the toolbar, which saves both.

STEP 2: Close the Code window and run your project again. Try clicking on the English button and the Spanish button. You can click on the Print button any time you wish. (Problems? See "Finding and Fixing Errors" later in this chapter.)

Add General Remarks

Good documentation guidelines require some more remarks in the project. Always begin each procedure with remarks that tell the purpose of the procedure. In addition, each project file needs identifying remarks at the top.

The **General Declarations section** is a good location for these remarks.

STEP 1: Click on the View Code button in the Project Explorer window; the Code window appears.

Your Code window may appear with or without an `Option Explicit` statement at the top. If you *do* see the `Option Explicit` statement, click at the left end of the line and press Enter; then skip to Step 3. (You will learn about the `Option Explicit` statement in Chapter 3. If it doesn't appear for this project, that's OK.)

STEP 2: Using the Code window's scroll bar, scroll to the top of the Code window. Then click in front of the first line and press Enter, creating a blank line.

STEP 3: Move the insertion point up to the blank line and type the following remarks, one per line (Figure 1.41):

```
'Hello World project
' by Your Name (use your own name here)
'Today's date (fill in today's date)
'This project will display a "Hello World" message in two different
' languages, and print the form on the printer.
```

Figure 1.41

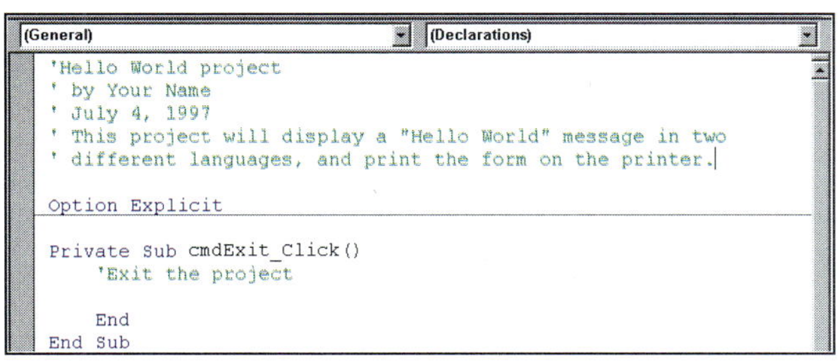

Enter remarks in the General Declarations section of the form module.

Explore the Code Window

STEP 1: Notice the two drop-down lists at the top of the Code window.

You can use these lists to move to any procedure in the Code window.

STEP 2: Click on the left down-pointing arrow to view the list of objects. Notice that every object in your form is listed there (Figure 1.42). At the top of the list, you see *(General)*.

Figure 1.42

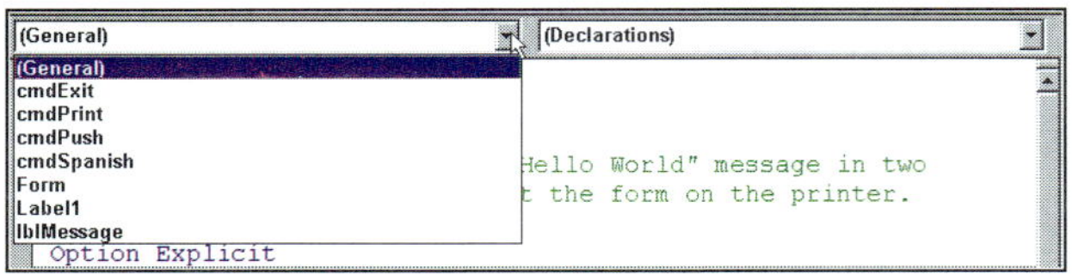

View the list of objects in this form module by dropping down the object list. Select an object from the list to display the sub procedures for that object.

STEP 3: Click on *(General)* to select it. Then notice the Procedure list, on the right, which says *(Declarations)*. This is the quick way to jump to the General Declarations section of a module.

STEP 4: Drop down the Object list, (the left list) and select *cmdSpanish*. The insertion point jumps to the event procedure for cmdSpanish.

STEP 5: Look at the Procedure list box, (the right list box); it says *Click*. You are currently viewing the cmdSpanish_Click event procedure.

To write code for more than one event for an object, use the Procedure drop-down list.

STEP 6: Drop down the Procedure list and view the list of events available for the selected object. You can jump to another procedure by selecting its name from the list.

Finish Up

STEP 1: Close the Code window.

STEP 2: Save the project again.

Print the Project Documentation

Select the Printing Options

STEP 1: Open the *File* menu and choose *Print*. The *Print* dialog box appears (Figure 1.43).

Figure 1.43

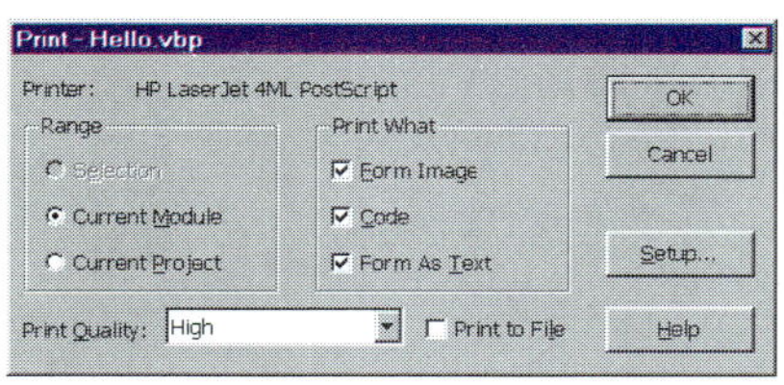

Select the options you want in the Print dialog box.

STEP 2: Click on the check boxes to select the printing options you want.

Range	
Selection	This option is available only when you have selected (highlighted) text in the Code window.
Current Module	This option will print all of the current module (form file).
Current Project	This option will print all modules in the project. Since this project has only one module, the two options give the same result.
Print What	
Form Image	Print a picture of the form as it appears at design time.
Code	Print all procedures and the General Declarations section.
Form as Text	Print a description of every object and its properties.

STEP 3: Select all three check boxes for *Print What* and click OK.

Sample Printout

This is the output produced when you choose to print the form image, the code, and the form as text.

The Form Image

When you select *Form Image*, the form prints without its title bar or borders. See Figure 1.44.

Figure 1.44

The form prints without its title bar or border.

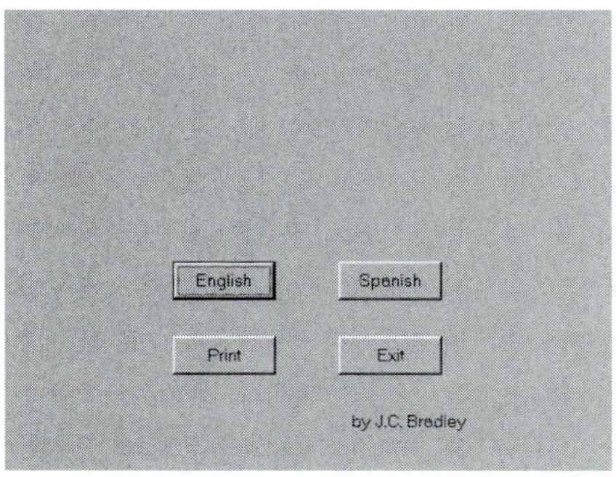

The Code

The *Code* selection prints all module procedures, as well as the General Declarations section.

```
'Hello World project
' by Your Name
' July 4, 1997
' This project will display a "Hello World" message in two
' different languages, and print the form on the printer.
Option Explicit
```

```
Private Sub cmdExit_Click()
    'Exit the project

    End
End Sub
```

```
Private Sub cmdPrint_Click()
    'Print the form

    PrintForm
End Sub
```

```
Private Sub cmdPush_Click()
    'Display the Hello World message

    lblMessage.Caption = "Hello World"
End Sub
```

```
Private Sub cmdSpanish_Click()
    'Display the Hello World message in Spanish

    lblMessage.Caption = "Hola Mundo"
End Sub
```

The Form as Text

The output produced when you select *Form as Text* lists the objects and properties in the module.

```
VERSION 5.00
Begin VB.Form Form1
   Caption              =  "Hello World by J.C. Bradley"
   ClientHeight         =  4392
   ClientLeft           =  48
   ClientTop            =  276
   ClientWidth          =  5664
   LinkTopic            =  "Form1"
   LockControls         =  -1 'True
   ScaleHeight          =  4392
   ScaleWidth           =  5664
   StartUpPosition      =  3 'Windows Default
   Begin VB.CommandButton cmdPrint
      Caption           =  "Print"
      Height            =  372
      Left              =  1560
      TabIndex          =  5
      Top               =  3120
      Width             =  972
   End

   Begin VB.CommandButton cmdSpanish
      Caption           =  "Spanish"
      Height            =  372
      Left              =  3120
      TabIndex          =  4
      Top               =  2400
      Width             =  972
   End

   Begin VB.CommandButton cmdExit
      Caption           =  "Exit"
      Height            =  372
      Left              =  3120
      TabIndex          =  2
      Top               =  3120
      Width             =  972
   End

   Begin VB.CommandButton cmdPush
      Caption           =  "English"
      Height            =  372
      Left              =  1560
      TabIndex          =  1
      Top               =  2400
      Width             =  972
   End
```

```
   Begin VB.Label Label1
      Caption         =  "by J.C. Bradley"
      Height          =  372
      Left            =  3240
      TabIndex        =  3
      Top             =  3840
      Width           =  2292
   End
   Begin VB.Label lblMessage
      BeginProperty Font
         Name           =  "MS Sans Serif"
         Size           =  12
         Charset        =  0
         Weight         =  400
         Underline      =  0  'False
         Italic         =  0  'False
         Strikethrough  =  0  'False
      EndProperty
      Height          =  372
      Left            =  840
      TabIndex        =  0
      Top             =  480
      Width           =  4092
   End
End
Attribute VB_Name = "Form1"
Attribute VB_GlobalNameSpace = False
Attribute VB_Creatable = False
Attribute VB_PredeclaredId = True
Attribute VB_Exposed = False
```

Finding and Fixing Errors

You may have already seen some errors as you entered the first sample project. Programming errors come in three varieties: **compile errors**, **run-time errors**, and **logic errors**.

Compile Errors

As Visual Basic attempts to convert your project code to machine language (called *compiling the code*), it finds any compile errors. You get compile errors when you break the syntax rules of Basic and sometimes when you use an illegal object or property.

For example, try spelling *End* as *ennd* or using the word *Quit* instead of *End*. The compiler can only translate the exact spelling of a word and cannot recognize either of these words; they would both cause a Compile Error message box.

You also receive a compile error if you accidentally use the wrong punctuation or place the punctuation in the wrong place. The compiler cannot understand `lblMessage,Caption` or `lblMessage.Caption;`.

Compile errors may be found by the editor as you move off the offending line. Or the compile error may not be found until you try to run the project. Before Visual Basic can actually run your code, it attempts to compile the code into machine language. If VB finds compile errors, it displays the Code window, highlights the offending line, and enters break time.

After you have corrected your compile errors, you can click the Run button to continue the compile and run, or click the Stop button to end.

One type of compile error that is all too common for beginning programmers is the inconsistent spelling of object names. For example, if you set a label control's Name property to `lblMessage`, you must always refer to it with that exact spelling. The following line of code will generate a compile error. Can you spot the problem?

```
lblMessages.Caption = "Hello World"
```

Run-Time Errors

If your project halts during execution, that's a run-time error. Visual Basic displays a dialog box, goes into break time, and highlights the statement causing the problem. Statements that cannot execute correctly cause run-time errors. The statements are correctly formed Basic statements that pass the syntax checking of the compiler; however, the statements fail to execute. Run-time errors can be caused by attempting to do impossible arithmetic operations such as calculate with nonnumeric data, divide by zero, or find the square root of a negative number.

Logic Errors

With logic errors, your project runs but produces incorrect results. Perhaps the results of a calculation are incorrect or the wrong text appears or the text is OK but appears in the wrong location.

Beginning programmers often overlook their logic errors. If the project runs, it must be right—right? All too often, that statement is not correct. You may need to use a calculator to check the output. Check all aspects of the project output: computations, text, and spacing.

For example, the Hello World project in this chapter has event procedures for printing "Hello World" in English and in Spanish. If the contents of the two procedures were switched, the program would work but the results would be incorrect.

The following code does not give the proper instructions to display the message in Spanish:

```
Private Sub cmdSpanish_Click
   'Display the Hello World Message in Spanish

   lblMessage.Caption = "Hello World"
End Sub
```

Project Debugging

If you talk to any computer programmer, you will learn that programs don't have errors, but that programs get "bugs" in them. Finding and fixing these bugs is called **debugging**.

For compile errors and run-time errors, your job is easier. Visual Basic displays the Code window with the offending line highlighted. However, you must identify and locate logic errors yourself.

If you are able to see the problem and fix it, you can continue project execution from that location by clicking on the Run button, pressing F5, or choosing *Start* from the *Run* menu. You can restart execution from the beginning by selecting *Restart* from the *Run* menu or by pressing Shift + F5.

Visual Basic has some very helpful tools to aid in debugging your projects. The debugging tools are covered in Chapter 4.

Naming Rules and Conventions for Objects

Using good, consistent, names for objects can help make a project easier to read and understand, as well as easier to debug. You *must* follow the Visual Basic rules for naming objects, procedures, and variables. In addition, conscientious programmers will also follow certain naming conventions.

The Naming Rules

When you select a name for an object, Visual Basic requires the name to begin with a letter. The name can be up to 40 characters in length and can contain letters, digits, and underscores. An object name cannot include a space or punctuation mark.

The Naming Conventions

This text follows the industrywide naming conventions, which help make projects more understandable: Always begin a name with a lowercase three-letter prefix, which identifies the object type (such as label, command button, or form) and capitalize the first character after the prefix (the "real" name of the object). For names with multiple words, capitalize each word in the name. All names must be meaningful and indicate the purpose of the object.

Examples

lblMessage
cmdExit
frmDataEntry
lblDiscountRate

Do not keep the default names assigned by Visual Basic, such as Command1 and Label3. Also, do not name your objects with numbers. The exception to this rule is for labels that never change during project execution. These labels usually hold items such as titles, instructions, and labels for other controls. Leaving these labels with their default names is perfectly acceptable and is practiced in this text.

Refer to Table 1.2 for the list of object prefixes.

Table 1.2

Recommended naming conventions for Visual Basic objects.

Object Class	Prefix	Example
Form	frm	frmDataEntry
Command button	cmd	cmdExit
Text box	txt	txtPaymentAmount
Label	lbl	lblTotal
Option button	opt	optBold
Check box	chk	chkPrintSummary
Frame	fra	fraSelection
Horizontal scroll bar	hsb	hsbRate
Vertical scroll bar	vsb	vsbTemperature
Image	img	imgLogo
Picture box	pic	picLandscape
Combo box	cbo	cboBookList
List box	lst	lstIngredients
Shape	shp	shpBox

Visual Basic Help

The Visual Basic **Help** facility is great! With Help, you really don't need a printed manual. You can look up any Basic statement, object, property, method, or programming concept. Many coding examples are available, and you can copy and paste the examples into your own project, modifying them if you wish.

The *Search Master Index* option helps you access the online manuals. There is also an option to get additional information from the Internet, including a Web tutorial.

New to VB 5!

You can look up topics in Help by using the Help Contents list (like a table of contents) or Search (which resembles an index). Also, you can use **context-sensitive Help**, which automatically jumps to the Help topic relating to what you are working on at the moment. For context-sensitive Help, select any object on the screen and press F1; VB automatically displays the relevant Help page.

Feedback 1.1

Note: Answers for all Feedback questions are shown in Appendix A.

1. Use the *Help* menu's *Microsoft Visual Basic Help Topics.* Select the *Index* tab and type "label". Display and print the information for the Label control. Click on Properties and view the list of available properties for a

Label control. Repeat the procedure for the Command Button control—display the options for command button and then display the information for the Command Button control. Print out the information page; then view the list of properties for a Command Button control.

2. If you are connected to the Internet, check out the Help option *Microsoft on the Web.*
3. Display the code window of your Hello World project. Place the mouse pointer on the keyword `End` in your Exit procedure. Press the F1 key to view context-sensitive help.

New to VB 5!

Summary

1. Visual Basic is an event-driven language used to write application programs that run in the Windows operating environment.
2. The object model of programming has objects that have properties and methods.
3. The current release of Visual Basic is 5.0. There is a Learning Edition, a Professional Edition, and an Enterprise Edition.
4. To plan a project, first sketch the user interface and then list the objects and properties needed. Then plan the necessary event procedures.
5. The three steps to creating a Visual Basic project are (1) define the user interface, (2) set the properties, and (3) write the Basic code.
6. A Visual Basic project consists of at least a .VBP file and an .FRM file and may have multiple .FRM files, .BAS files, .OCX files, and a .VBW file.
7. The VB environment consists of the Form window, the Project Explorer window, the Properties window, the Form Layout window, the toolbox, the menu bar, and the toolbar.
8. VB has three modes: design time, run time, and break time.
9. Visual Basic code is written in procedures. Sub procedures begin with the words *Private Sub* and end with *End Sub*.
10. Project remarks are used for documentation. Good programming practices require remarks in every procedure and in the General Declarations section of a module.
11. Assignment statements assign a value to a property or a variable. Assignment statements work from right to left, assigning the value on the right side of the equal sign to the property named on the left side of the equal sign.
12. The `End` statement terminates project execution.
13. Each event to which you want to respond requires an event procedure.
14. You must save both the form file and the project file to properly save a Visual Basic project. The recommended practice is to first create a folder to hold the files.
15. The PrintForm method prints the current form on the printer.
16. You can print out an image of the form; the code, which is a listing of the Basic statements in the project; and the form text, which is a listing of all objects and their properties.
17. Three types of errors can occur in a Visual Basic project: compile errors (which violate the syntax rules of Basic statements), run-time errors

(which contain a statement that cannot execute properly), and logic errors (which produce erroneous results).
18. Finding and fixing programming errors is called *debugging*.
19. Following good naming conventions can help make a project easier to debug.
20. Visual Basic Help has very complete descriptions of all project elements and their uses. You can use the Contents list, Index, or context-sensitive Help. Additional help is available on the Web.

Key Terms

assignment statement *20*
break time *8*
Caption *17*
class *17*
code *4*
Code window *22*
command button *13*
compile error *36*
context-sensitive Help *39*
control *2*
debugging *38*
design time *8*
End statement *20*
Enterprise Edition *3*
event *20*
event-driven programming *2*
event procedure *20*
form *2*
form file *5*
form module *5*
Form window *6*
General Declarations section *31*
graphical user interface (GUI) *2*
handle *14*
Help *39*
label *13*
Learning Edition *3*
logic error *36*
method *3*
object *3*
object-oriented programming *3*
procedure *20*
Professional Edition *3*
project file *5*
Project Explorer window *6*
Properties window *6*
property *3*
pseudocode *4*
remark *20*
run time *8*
run-time error *36*
standard code module *5*
sub procedure *20*
toolbar *7*
toolbox *7*
user interface *4*
Visual Basic environment *5*

Review Questions

1. What are objects and properties? How are they related to each other?
2. What are the three steps for planning and creating Visual Basic projects? Describe what happens in each step.
3. What is the purpose of these Visual Basic file types: .VBP, .FRM, .BAS, and .OCX?
4. When is Visual Basic in design time? run time? break time?
5. What is the purpose of the Name property of a control?
6. What property determines what appears on the form for a label control?

7. What is the purpose of the Caption property of a command button? the Caption property of a form?
8. What does *cmdPush_Click* mean? To what does cmdPush refer? To what does Click refer?
9. What is a Visual Basic event? Give some examples of events.
10. What property must be set to center text in a label? What should be the value of the property?
11. What is the General Declarations section of a form module? What belongs there?
12. What is a compile error, when does it occur, and what might cause it?
13. What is a run-time error, when does it occur, and what might cause it?
14. What is a logic error, when does it occur, and what might cause it?
15. Tell the class of control and the likely purpose of each of these object names:

    lblAddress
    cmdExit
    txtName
    optTextBlue

16. What does *context-sensitive Help* mean? How can you use it to see the Help page for a command button?

Programming Exercises

1.1 For your first Visual Basic exercise, you must first complete the Hello World project. Then add command buttons and event procedures to display the "Hello World" message in two more languages. You may substitute any other languages for those shown. Use Figure 1.44 as a guideline but feel free to modify the user interface to suit yourself (or your instructor).

Make sure to use meaningful names for your new command buttons, following the naming conventions in Table 1.2. (Begin the name with lowercase "cmd".) Include remarks at the top of every procedure and in the General Declarations section of the module.

"Hello World" in French: *Bonjour tout le monde*
"Hello World" in Italian: *Ciao Mondo*

1.2 Write a new Visual Basic project, which displays a different greeting, or make it display the name of your school or your company. Include at least three command buttons to display the greeting, print the form, and exit the project.

Include a label that holds your name at the bottom of the form and change the Caption property of the form to something meaningful.

Follow good naming conventions for object names; include remarks at the top of every procedure and in the General Declarations section of the module.

Select a different font name and font size for the greeting label. If you wish, you can also select a different color for the font. Select each font attribute from the *Font* dialog box, from the Properties window.

1.3 Write a project that displays four sayings, such as "The early bird gets the worm" or "A penny saved is a penny earned." (You will want to keep the sayings short, as each must be entered on one code statement. However, when the saying displays on your form, long lines will wrap within the label if the label is large enough.)

Make a command button for each saying with a descriptive Caption for each, as well as command buttons to print the form and to exit the project.

Include a label that holds your name at the bottom of the form. Also, make sure to change the Caption property of the form to something meaningful.

You may change the Font properties of the large label to the font and size of your choice.

Make sure the label is large enough to display your longest saying and that the command buttons are large enough to hold their entire Captions.

Follow good naming conventions for object names; include remarks at the top of every procedure and in the General Declarations section of the module.

1.4 Write a project to display company contact information. Include command buttons and labels for contact person, department, and phone. When the user clicks on one of the command buttons, display the contact information in the corresponding label. Include command buttons to print the form and to exit.

Include a label that holds your name at the bottom of the form and change the Caption property of the form to something meaningful.

You may change the Font properties of the labels to the font and size of your choice.

Follow good naming conventions for object names; include remarks at the top of every procedure and in the General Declarations section of the module.

CASE STUDIES

Very Busy (VB) Mail Order

If you don't have the time to look for all those hard-to-find items, tell us what you're looking for. We'll send you a catalog from the appropriate company or order for you.

We can place an order and ship it to you. We also help with shopping for gifts; your order can be gift wrapped and sent anywhere you wish.

The company title will be shortened to VB Mail Order. This name should appear as the Caption on the first form of every project that you create throughout the text for this case study.

Your first job is to create a project that will display the name and telephone number for the contact person for the customer relations, marketing, order processing, and shipping departments.

Include a command button for each department. When the user clicks on the button for a department, display the name and telephone number for the contact person in two labels. Also include identifying labels with Captions "Department Contact" and "Telephone Number".

Be sure to include a command button for Exit and another for Print Form.

Include a label at the bottom of the form that holds your name and give the form a meaningful Caption.

Test Data

Department	Department Contact	Telephone Number
Customer Relations	Tricia Mills	500-1111
Marketing	Michelle Rigner	500-2222
Order Processing	Kenna DeVoss	500-3333
Shipping	Eric Andrews	500-4444

Valley Boulevard (VB) Auto Center

Valley Boulevard Auto Center will meet all of your automobile needs. The center has facilities with everything for your vehicles including sales and leasing for new and used cars and RVs, auto service and repair, detail shop, car wash, and auto parts.

The company title will be shortened to VB Auto Center. This name should appear as the Caption on the first form of every project that you create throughout the text for this case study.

Your first job is to create a project that will display current notices.

Include four command buttons with the Captions: "Auto Sales", "Service Center", "Detail Shop", and "Employment Opportunities". One label will be used to display the information when the command buttons are clicked. Be sure to include command buttons for Exit and Print Form.

Include your name in a label at the bottom of the form.

Test Data

Command Button	Label Caption
Auto Sales	Family wagon, immaculate condition $12,995
Service Center	Lube, oil, filter $25.99
Detail Shop	Complete detail $79.95 for most cars
Employment Opportunities	Sales position contact Mr. Mann 551-2134 x475

CHAPTER

2

More Controls

At the completion of this chapter, you will be able to . . .

1. Use text boxes, frames, check boxes, option buttons, images, shapes, and lines effectively.
2. Set the Appearance property to make controls appear flat or three-dimensional.
3. Select multiple controls and move them, align them, and set common properties.
4. Make your projects easy for the user to understand and operate by defining access keys, setting a default and a cancel button, controlling the tab sequence, and resetting the focus during program execution.
5. Clear the contents of text boxes and labels.
6. Change font attributes, such as bold, italic, underline, size, and color, during program execution.
7. Code multiple statements for one control using the `With` and `End With` statements.
8. Concatenate (join) strings of text.
9. Make a control visible or invisible by setting its Visible property.

Introducing More Controls

In Chapter 1 you learned to use labels and command buttons. In this chapter you will learn to use several more control types: text boxes, frames, check boxes, option buttons, image controls, shapes, and lines. Figure 2.1 shows the toolbox with the tools for these controls labeled. Figure 2.2 shows some of these controls on a form.

Each class of controls has its own set of properties. If you want to see a complete list of the properties for any class of control, you can (1) place a control on a form and examine the properties list or (2) click on a tool or a control and press F1 for context-sensitive Help. VB will display the Help page for that control, and you can view a list of the properties and an explanation of their use.

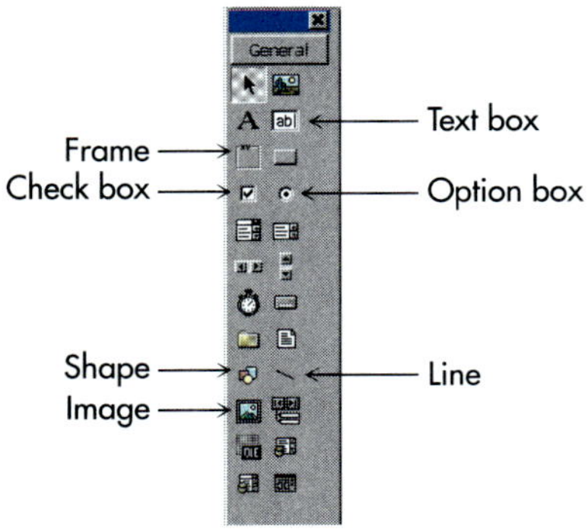

Figure 2.1

The toolbox showing the controls that will be covered in this chapter.

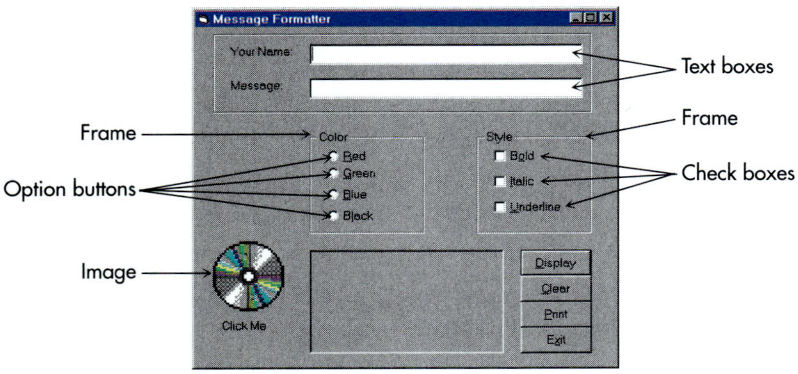

Figure 2.2

A form designed using text boxes, frames, check boxes, option buttons, and an image.

Text Boxes

Use a **text box** control when you want the user to type some input. The form in Figure 2.2 has two text boxes. The user can move from one box to the next, make corrections, cut and paste if desired, and click the Display button when finished. In your program code you can use the **Text property** of each text box.

Example

```
lblName.Caption = txtName.Text
```

In this example whatever the user enters into the text box is assigned to the Caption property of lblName. If you want to display some text in a text box during program execution, assign a literal to the Text property:

```
txtMessage.Text = "Watson, come here."
```

You can set the **Alignment property** of text boxes to change the alignment of text within the box. However, you must also set the **Multiline property** to True, or Visual Basic ignores the Alignment.

The values for the Alignment property, which can be set only at design time (not at run time), are

0 – Left Justify
1 – Right Justify
2 – Center

The three-letter prefix for naming a text box is "txt".

Examples

txtTitle
txtCompany

Frames

Frames are used as containers for other controls. Usually, groups of option buttons or check boxes are placed in frames. Using frames to group controls makes your forms easier to understand.

Set a frame's Caption property to the words you want to appear on the top edge of the frame. The three-letter prefix for naming a frame is "fra".

Examples

fraColor
fraStyle

Check Boxes

Check boxes allow the user to select (or deselect) an option. In any group of check boxes, any number may be selected. The **Value property** of a check box is set to 0 if unchecked, 1 if checked, or 2 if grayed (disabled). You can write an event procedure to execute when the user clicks in the box. In Chapter 4, when you learn about `If` statements, you can take one action when the box is checked and another action when it is unchecked.

Use the Caption property of a check box for the text you want to appear next to the box. The three-letter prefix for naming a check box is "chk".

Examples

chkBold
chkItalic

Option Buttons

Use **option buttons** when only one button of a group may be selected. Any option buttons placed directly on the form (not in a frame) function as a group. A group of option buttons inside a frame function together. The best method is to first create a frame and then to create each option button inside the frame. You must be careful to create the button inside the frame; don't create it on the form and drag it inside the frame—it still belongs to the form's group, not the frame's group. Therefore, you should not create an option button by double-clicking on its toolbox tool; instead, click to select the tool and use the crosshair pointer to draw the option button control.

The Value property of an option button is set to True if selected or to False if unselected.

You can write an event procedure to execute when the user selects an option button. In Chapter 4 you will learn to determine in your code whether or not a button is selected.

Set an option button's Caption property to the text you want to appear next to the button. The three-letter prefix for naming an option button is "opt".

Examples

optRed
optBlue

Images

An **image** control holds a picture. You can set an image's **Picture property** to a file with an extension of .BMP, .WMF, .ICO, .DIB, .GIF, .JPG, .EMF, or .CUR. First place the image control on a form and then select its Picture property in the Properties window. Click on the Properties button (Figure 2.3) to display the `Load Picture` dialog box where you can select a filename (Figure 2.4).

You can use any picture file (with the proper format) that you have available. You will find many icon files included with Visual Basic. Look in the Icons folder, under the Graphics folder, beneath the VB folder (Figure 2.5).

Default path for icon files:

```
Program Files
    DevStudio
       VB
          Graphics
             Icons
```

Figure 2.3

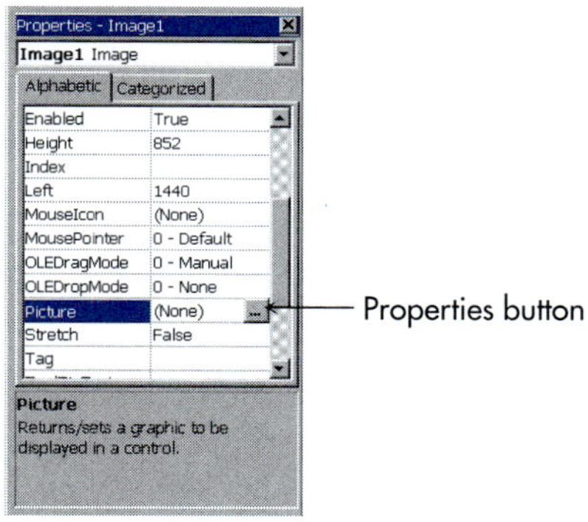

Click on the Picture property for an image control, and a Properties button appears. Click on the Properties button to view the Load Picture *dialog box.*

Figure 2.4

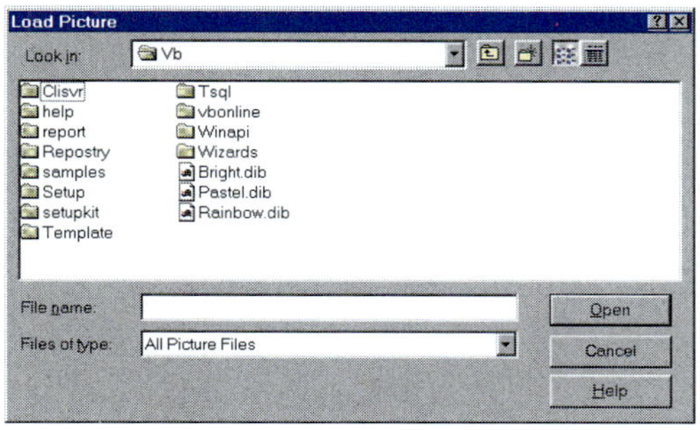

The Load Picture *dialog box. Make your selection here for the picture file you want to appear in the image control.*

Figure 2.5

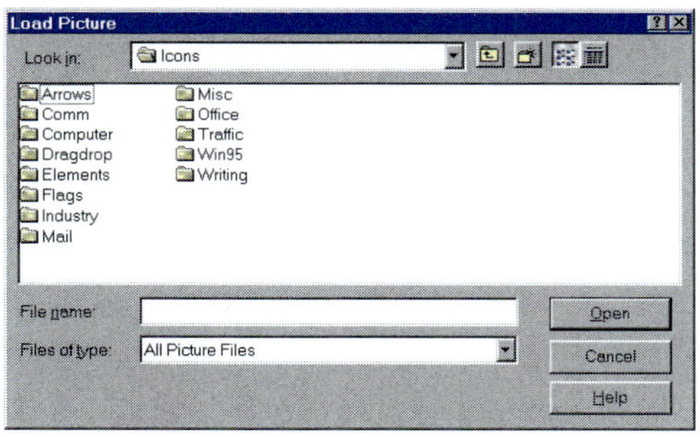

Find the Visual Basic icon files in several folders beneath the VB\Graphics\Icons folder.

Image controls have several useful properties that you can set at design time or run time. For example, set the **Stretch property** to True to make the picture enlarge to fill the control. You can set the **Visible property** to False to make the image disappear.

For example, to make an image invisible at run time, use this code statement.

```
imgLogo.Visible = False
```

The three-letter prefix for naming an image is “img”.

Setting a Border and Style

Most controls can appear to be three-dimensional (refer to Figure 2.2) or flat. Labels, text boxes, check boxes, option buttons, and images all have an **Appearance property**, with choices of 0 – Flat, or 1 – 3D. In order to make a label or an image appear three-dimensional, you must first give it a border. Set the BorderStyle to 1 – Fixed Single. The Appearance property defaults to 1 – 3D.

Tip

To remove a picture from a form or image, select the Picture property value in the Properties window and press the Delete key.

Feedback 2.1

Create an image control that displays an enlarged icon and appears in a "sunken" box. (Make up a name that conforms to this textbook's naming convention.)

Property	Setting
Name	
Stretch	
Appearance	
BorderStyle	
Visible	

The Shape Control

You can place rectangles, squares, ovals, and circles on a form using the **shape control** (Figure 2.6). Shapes can enhance the readability of a screen or add some fun. You may wish to use shapes to create a company logo or to separate a form into sections.

Figure 2.6

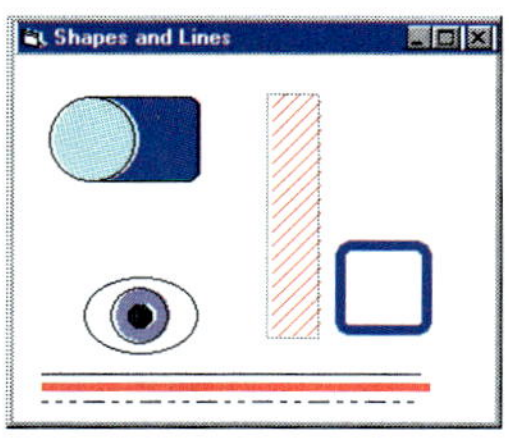

Shapes and lines created with the shape control and the line control.

Use the shape tool in the toolbox (refer to Figure 2.1) to draw a shape on the form. Then you can determine its shape by setting its Shape property. The property values are

0 – Rectangle
1 – Square
2 – Oval
3 – Circle
4 – Rounded Rectangle
5 – Rounded Square

You can draw, move, and resize shape controls in the same manner as the other controls. By changing properties, you can select the style and color of the shape's outline, the color of its fill, and whether it is transparent or solid.

The naming prefix for shape controls is "shp", such as *shpRectangle*.

The Line Control

You can draw a line on a form by using the **line control**. You may want to include lines when creating a logo, or you may simply want to divide the screen by drawing a line. Click on the line tool (refer to Figure 2.1) and use the crosshair pointer to drag a line; you may rotate the line in any direction and stretch it until releasing the mouse button.

Change other properties of line controls to set the color and style of the line. You can determine the thickness of a line by changing its Borderwidth property.

The naming prefix for a line control is "lin", for example, *linLogo*.

Working With Multiple Controls

You can select more than one control at a time, which means that you can move the controls as a group, set similar properties for the group, and align the controls.

Selecting Multiple Controls

There are two methods of selecting multiple controls. If the controls are near each other, the easiest method is to use the mouse to drag a selection box around the controls. Point to one corner of a box surrounding the controls, press the mouse button, and drag to the opposite corner (Figure 2.7). When you release the mouse button, each control will have light gray selection handles (Figure 2.8).

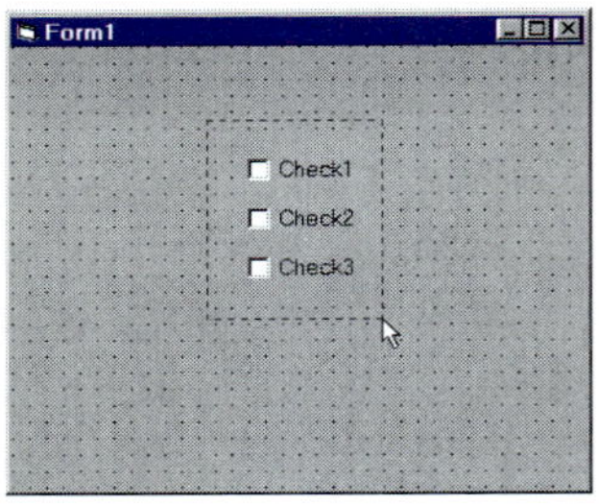

Figure 2.7

Using the pointer, drag a selection box around the controls you wish to select.

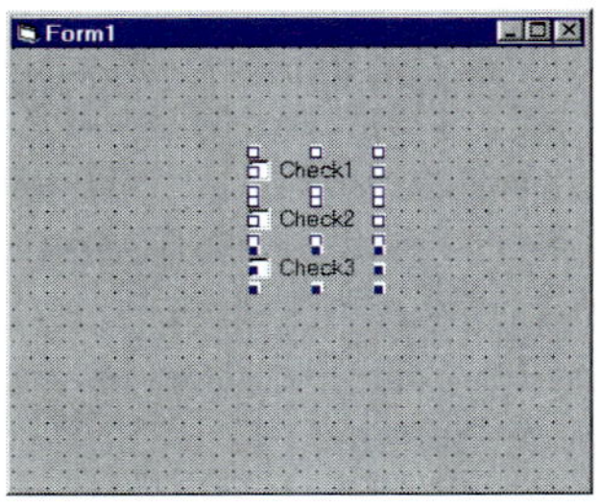

Figure 2.8

When multiple controls are selected, each has selection handles.

You can also select multiple controls, one at a time. Click on one control to select it, hold down the Ctrl key or the Shift key, and click on the next control. You can keep the Ctrl or Shift key down and continue clicking on controls you wish to select. Ctrl–click (or Shift–click) on a control a second time to deselect it without changing the rest of the group.

When you want to select most of the controls on the form, use a combination of the two methods. Drag a selection box around all of the controls to select them all and then Ctrl–click on the ones you want to deselect.

Deselecting a Group of Controls

When you are finished working with a group of controls, it's easy to deselect them. Just click anywhere on the form (not on a control) or select another (single) control.

Moving Controls as a Group

After selecting multiple controls, you can move them as a group. Point inside one of the selected controls, press the mouse button, and drag the entire group to a new location (Figure 2.9). As you drag the mouse pointer, an outline of the controls moves. When you release the mouse button, the controls move to their new location.

Figure 2.9

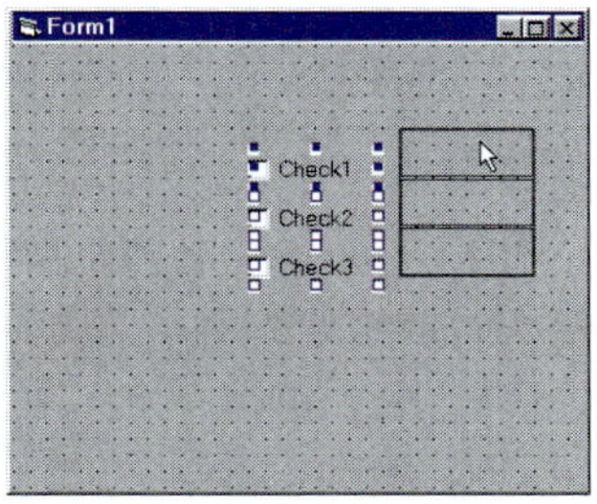

Drag a group of selected controls. An outline of the controls moves as you drag, and then the group moves when you release the mouse button.

Setting Properties for Multiple Controls

You can set some common properties for groups of controls. After selecting the group, check the Properties window. Any properties shown in the window are shared by all of the controls and can be changed all at once. For example, you may want to set the appearance for all your controls to three-dimensional or change the font used for a group of labels.

Aligning Controls

After you select a group of controls it is easy to resize and align them using the options on the *Format* menu. Figure 2.10 shows the *Align* submenu, and Figure 2.11 shows the *Make Same Size* submenu. Select your group of controls and first choose *Make Same Size*, then use the *Align* option. You may also find it necessary to move the entire group to a new location.

New to VB 5!

Figure 2.10

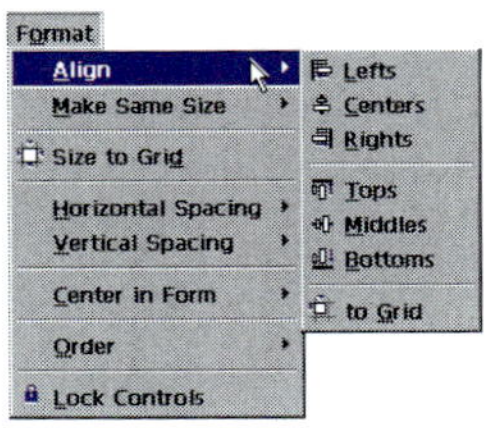

Choose the alignment for multiple selected controls from the Align submenu.

Figure 2.11

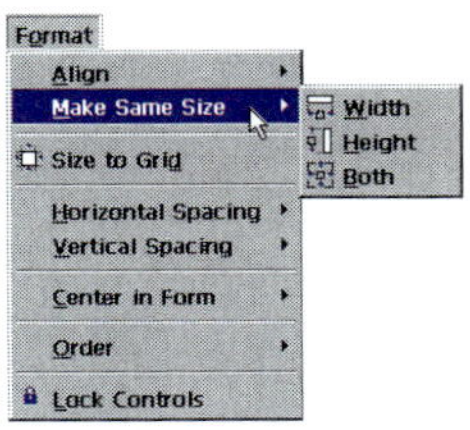

Resize multiple selected controls to make them all the same size using the Make Same Size submenu.

You can also set the spacing between controls using the *Horizontal Spacing* (Figure 2.12) and/or *Vertical Spacing* (Figure 2.13) options on the *Format* menu. Using these options you can create equal spacing between controls, or you can increase or decrease the space between controls.

Figure 2.12

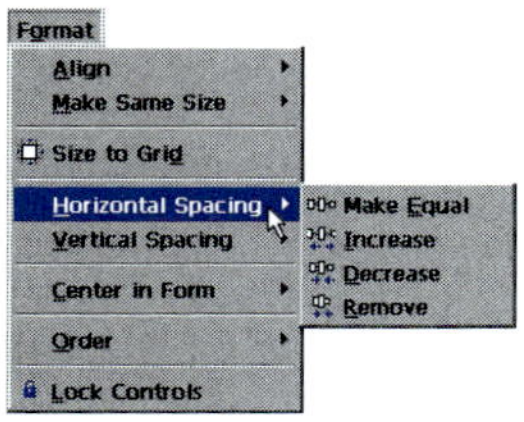

Change the horizontal alignment of multiple selected controls using the Horizontal Spacing submenu.

Figure 2.13

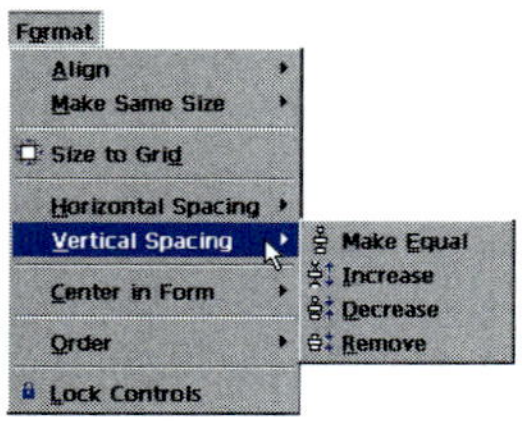

Change the vertical alignment of multiple selected controls using the Vertical Spacing submenu.

Another way to align controls on a form is to select them and set their location using properties. For example, if you have a group of controls to align vertically, select them all and set their Left property to the same value. You can also set the Width property so the controls are all the same size. If you want to set the controls to align horizontally, set them to the same Top property. See Figure 2.14.

Figure 2.14

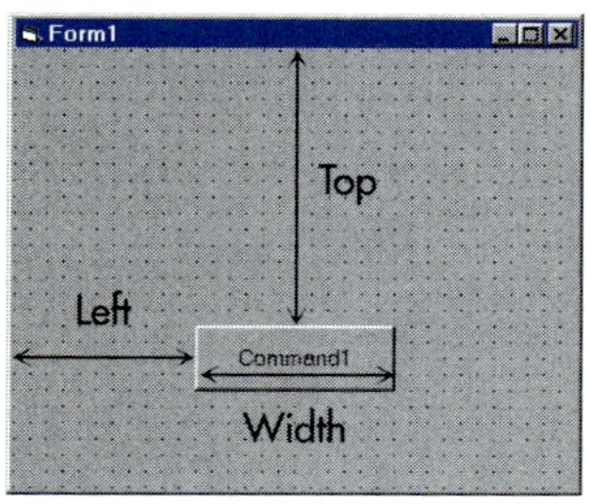

A control's Top property is its distance in twips from the top of the form; the Left property is its distance from left edge of the form, and the Width property is the width of the control.

The numbers you see in the Settings box for Left, Top, and Width may look strange. The measurements are shown in twips, which is a measuring system from the printing industry. One **twip** is 1/20 of a printer's point or 1/1440 of an inch. If you define a control to be 1440 twips wide, theoretically it is 1 inch wide. Actually, when it prints on the printer, it is 1 inch. However, on the screen it may be smaller or larger, depending on the resolution of monitors.

Designing Your Applications for User Convenience

One of the goals of good programming is to create programs that are easy to use. Your user interface should be clear and consistent. One school of thought says that if users misuse a program, it's the fault of the programmer, not the users. Since most of your users will already know how to operate Windows programs, you should strive to make your programs look and behave like other Windows programs. Some of the ways to accomplish this goal are to use controls in the standard way, define keyboard access keys, set a default command button, and make the Tab key work correctly.

Designing the User Interface

The design of the screen should be easy to understand and "comfortable" for the user. The best way that we can accomplish these goals is to follow industry standards in relation to color, size, and placement of controls. Once users become accustomed to a screen design, they will expect (and feel more familiar with) applications that follow the same design criteria. Design your applications to match other Windows applications. Take some time to examine the screens and dialog boxes in Microsoft Office as well as those in Visual Basic.

Microsoft has done extensive program testing with users of different ages, genders, nationalities, and disabilities. We should take advantage of this research and follow the guidelines.

One recommendation about interface design concerns color. You have probably noticed that Windows applications are predominantly gray. A reason is that many people are color blind. Also, gray is easiest and best for the majority of users. Although you may personally prefer brighter colors, if you want your applications to look professional, you will stick with gray.

Colors can indicate to the user what is expected. Use a white background for text boxes to indicate that the user is to input information. Use a gray background for labels, which the user cannot change. Labels that will display a message or result of a calculation should have a border around them; labels that provide a caption on the screen should have no border (the default).

Group your controls on the form to aid the user. A good practice is to create frames to hold related items, especially those controls that require user input. This visual aid helps the user understand the information that is being presented or requested.

Use a sans serif font on your forms, such as the default MS Sans Serif, and do not make them boldface. Limit large font sizes to a few items, such as the company name.

Defining Keyboard Access Keys

Many people prefer to use the keyboard, rather than use a mouse, for most operations. Windows is set up so that most everything can be done with either the keyboard or a mouse. You can make your projects respond to the keyboard by defining **access keys**. For example, in Figure 2.15 you can select the OK button with Alt + o and the Exit button with Alt + x.

Figure 2.15

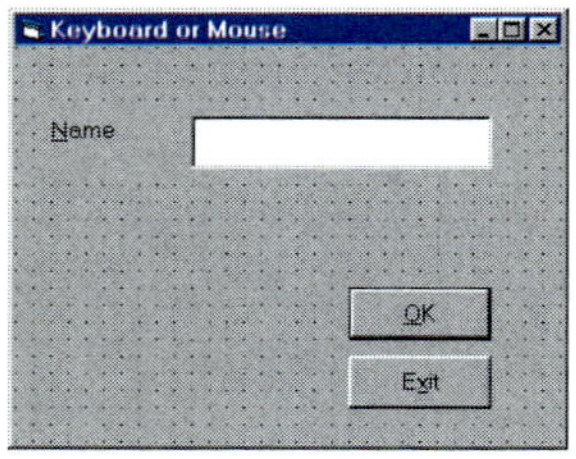

The underlined character in a Caption defines an access key. The user can select the OK button by pressing Alt + o and the Exit button with Alt + x.

You can set access keys for command buttons, option buttons, and check boxes when you define their Caption properties. Type an ampersand (&) in front of the character you want for the access key; Visual Basic underlines the character.

For example, type the following Captions:

&OK	for OK
E&xit	for Exit

When you define access keys, you need to watch for several pitfalls. First, try to use the Windows-standard keys whenever possible. For example, use the x of Exit and the S of Save. Second, make sure you don't give two controls the same access key—it confuses the user. The first time he presses the access key, it selects the first button; the next time he presses the same key, it selects a different button.

Setting the Default and Cancel Properties of Command Buttons

Are you a keyboard user? If so, do you mind having to pick up the mouse and click a button after typing text into a text box? Once a person's fingers are on the keyboard, most people prefer to press the Enter key, rather than to click the mouse. If one of the command buttons on the form is the *default button,* pressing Enter is the same as clicking the button. You can always identify the default button on a form by its darker outline. Referring to Figure 2.15, the OK button is the default.

You can make one of your command buttons the default button by setting its **Default property** to True. When the user presses Enter, that button is automatically selected.

You can also select a *cancel button*. The cancel button is the button that is selected when the user presses the Esc key. You can make a command button the cancel button by setting its **Cancel property** to True. An example of a good time to set the Cancel property is on a form with OK and Cancel buttons. You may want to set the Default property to True for the OK button and the Cancel property to True for the Cancel button.

Setting the Tab Order for Controls

In Windows programs, one control on the form always has the **focus**. You can see the focus change as you Tab from control to control. For controls such as command buttons and option buttons, the focus appears as a light dotted line. For text boxes, the insertion point (also called the cursor) appears inside the box.

Some controls can receive the focus; others cannot. For example, text boxes and command buttons can receive the focus, but labels and images cannot.

The Tab Order

Two properties determine whether the focus stops on a control and the order in which the focus moves. Controls that are capable of receiving focus have a **TabStop property**, which you can set to True or False. If you do not want the focus to stop on a control when the user presses the Tab key, set the TabStop property to False.

The **TabIndex property** determines the order the focus moves as the Tab key is pressed. As you create controls on your form, Visual Basic assigns the TabIndex property in sequence. Most of the time that order is correct, but if you want to Tab in some other sequence or if you add controls later, you will need to modify the TabIndex properties of your controls.

When your program begins running, the focus is on the control with the lowest TabIndex (usually 0). Since you want the insertion point to appear in the first text box on the form, its TabIndex should be set to 0. The next text box should be set to 1; the next to 2; and so forth.

You may be puzzled by the properties of labels, which have a TabIndex property, but not a TabStop. A label cannot receive focus, but it has a location in the tab sequence. This fact allows you to create keyboard access keys for text boxes. When the user types an access key, such as Alt + N, the focus jumps to the first TabIndex following the label. See Figure 2.16.

Figure 2.16

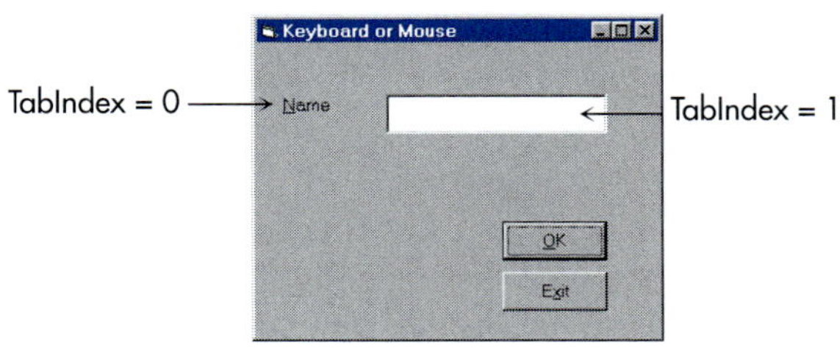

To use keyboard access keys for a text box, the TabIndex of the label must precede the TabIndex of the text box.

Setting the Form's Location on the Screen

New to VB 5!

When your project runs, the form will appear in the upper-left corner of the screen by default. The easiest way to choose a location for your form is to use the (new to VB 5) Form Layout window (Figure 2.17). Drag the image of the form to the screen location where you want the form to appear. Figure 2.18 shows the setting to make your form appear centered on the screen.

Figure 2.17

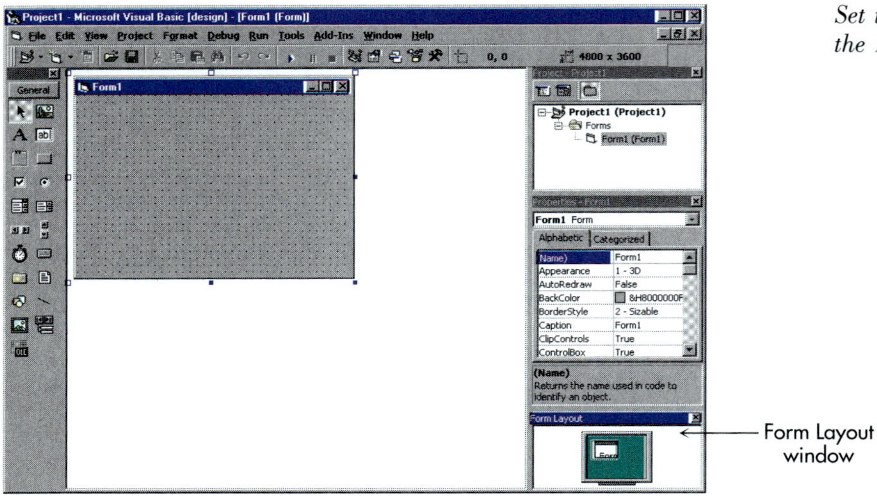

Set the position of the form in the Form Layout window.

Figure 2.18

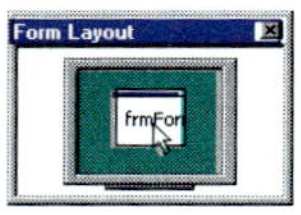

Drag the form to the center of the screen.

You can also set the form's screen position by setting the StartupPosition property of the form. Figure 2.19 shows your choices for the property setting. To center your form on the user's screen, set the StartupPosition property to *2-Center Screen.*

Figure 2.19

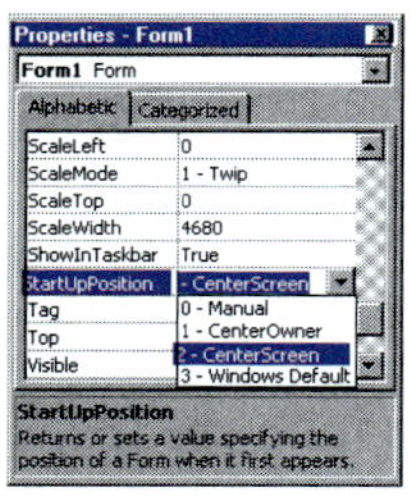

Set the StartupPosition property of the form to 2-Center Screen to make the form appear in the center of the screen.

Coding for the Controls

You already know how to set initial properties for controls at design time. You may also want to set some properties in code, as your project executes. You can clear out the contents of text boxes and labels; reset the focus; and change font attributes, such as bold, underline, italic, and the color of text.

Clearing Text Boxes and Labels

You can clear out the contents of a text box or label by setting the property to an **empty string**. Use "" (no space between the two quotation marks). This empty string is also called a *null string.*

Examples

```
txtName.Text = ""           'Clear the contents
lblMessage.Caption = ""     'Clear the contents
```

Resetting the Focus

As your program runs, you want the insertion point to appear in the text box where the user is expected to type. The focus should begin in the first text box. But what about later? If you clear the form's text boxes, you should reset the focus to the first text box. The **SetFocus method** handles this situation. Remember, the convention is Object.Method, so the statement to set the insertion point in the text box called txtName is

```
txtName.SetFocus   'Make the insertion point appear here
```

Setting the Value Property of Option Buttons and Check Boxes

Of course, the purpose of option buttons and check boxes is to allow the user to make selections. However, often you need to select or deselect an option in code. You can select or deselect option buttons and check boxes at design time (to set initial status) or at run time (to respond to an event).

To make an option button appear selected initially, set its Value property to True in the Properties window. In code, assign True to its Value property:

```
optRed.Value = True   'Make button selected
```

For check boxes, the procedure is slightly different, since the Value property has three settings: 0 – unchecked, 1 – checked, and 2 – grayed. You can set the initial state by making a selection in the Properties window. At run time, use these code statements:

```
chkBold.Value = 1     'Make box checked
chkItalic.Value = 0   'Make box unchecked
```

You can also use the Basic keywords `Checked` and `Unchecked` to set the Value property in code:

```
chkBold.Value = Checked       'Make box checked
chkItalic.Value = Unchecked   'Make box unchecked
```

Although a check box's Value property is set to 0, 1, or 2, sometimes you can treat its Value as True or False. For example, you can assign the Value of a check box to another property that must be True or False:

```
optDisplay.Value = chkScreen.Value    'Set option button Value _
                                         to check box Value
```

In the previous example, the Value of the option button will be set to True if the check box is checked and to False if the check box is unchecked.

Feedback 2.2

1. Write the Basic statements to clear the text box called txtCompany and reset the insertion point into the box.
2. Write the Basic statements to clear the label called lblCustomer and place the insertion point into a text box called txtOrder.
3. What will be the effect of each of these Basic statements?
   (a) `chkPrint.Value = 1`
   (b) `optColor.Value = False`
   (c) `imgDrawing.Visible = False`
   (d) `lblLocation.BorderStyle = 1`
       `lblLocation.Appearance = 1`
   (e) `lblCity.Caption = txtCity.Text`

Changing the Font Properties of Controls

It is easy to define initial properties of a text box or a label. You just select *Font* in the Properties window and display the *Font* dialog box. There you can change the name of the font, the size, the style (bold, italic, underline), and the color. But what if you want to change Font properties while the program is running? For that, you need to set Font properties in code.

Visual Basic has a special object called a **Font object**. A Font object has several properties, including Name, Size, Bold, Italic, Underline, and StrikeThrough. You can set each of the properties for the Font object and access it through the Font property of a control.

Examples

```
txtName.Font.Bold = True        'Set the font to bold
lblMessage.Font.Size = 12       'Change to 12-point font
lblTitle.Font.Italic = True     'Set the font to italic
```

Changing the Color of Text

You can change the color of text by changing the **ForeColor property** of a control. Actually, most controls have a ForeColor and a BackColor property. The ForeColor property changes the color of the text; the BackColor property controls the color around the text.

The Color Constants

Visual Basic provides an easy way to specify some of the most-used colors. These eight names are called **color constants**.

```
vbBlack
vbRed
vbGreen
vbYellow
vbBlue
vbMagenta
vbCyan
vbWhite
```

Examples

```
txtName.ForeColor = vbRed
lblMessage.ForeColor = vbWhite
```

Changing Multiple Properties of a Control

By now you can see that there are times when you want to change several properties of a single control. In versions of Visual Basic previous to version 4, you had to write out the entire name (Object.Property) for each statement.

Examples

```
txtTitle.Visible = True
txtTitle.ForeColor = vbWhite
txtTitle.Font.Bold = True
txtTitle.Font.Italic = True
txtTitle.SetFocus
```

Of course, you can still specify the statements this way, but now Visual Basic provides a statement to make this task easier—the `With` and `End With`.

The With and End With Statements—General Form

```
With ObjectName
       Statement(s)
End With
```

You specify an object name in the **`With`** statement. All subsequent statements until the **`End With`** relate to that object.

The With and End With Statements—Examples

```
With txtTitle
       .Visible = True
       .ForeColor = vbWhite
       .Font.Bold = True
       .Font.Italic = True
       .SetFocus
End With
```

The statements beginning with `With` and ending with `End With` are called a *With block*. The statements inside the block are indented for readability. Although indentation is not required by VB, it is required by good programming practices.

The real advantage of using the `With` statement, rather than spelling out the object for each statement, is that `With` is more efficient. Your Visual Basic projects will run a little faster if you use `With`. On a large, complicated project, the savings can be significant.

Concatenating Text

At times you need to join strings of text. For example, you may want to join a literal and a property. You can "tack" one string of characters to the end of another, in the process called **concatenation**. Use an ampersand (&), preceded and followed by a space, between the two strings.

Examples

```
lblMessage.Caption = "Your name is: " & txtName.Text
txtNameAndAddress.Text = txtName.Text & txtAddress.Text
lblFontSize.Caption = "The current fontsize is " & txtMessage.Font.Size & " points."
```

Continuing Long Program Lines

Basic interprets the code on one line as one statement. You can type *very* long lines in the Basic Code window; the window scrolls sideways and allows you to keep typing. However, this method is inconvenient. It isn't easy to see your program code, and printers can't handle the extra width. (Some printers wrap long lines to the next line; others just drop the extra characters.)

When a Basic statement becomes too long for one line, use a **line-continuation character**. You can type a space and an underscore, press Enter, and continue the statement on the next line. It is OK to indent the continued lines. The only restriction is that the line-continuation character must appear between elements; you cannot place a continuation in the middle of a literal or split the name of an object or property.

Tip

Although Basic allows concatenation with the + operator, the practice is not advised. Depending on the contents of the text box, the compiler may interpret the + operator as an addition operator rather than a concatenation operator, giving unpredictable results.

Examples

```
lblGreetings.Caption = "Greetings " & txtName.Text & ": " & _
     "You have been selected to win a free prize. " & _
     "Just send us $100 for postage and handling."
```

Using the Default Property of a Control

Each class of control has one property that is the default property. When you use the default property of a control, you do not have name the property. For example, the Text property is the default property for a text box. Therefore, these two statements are equivalent:

```
txtCompany.Text = "R 'n R — for Reading 'n Refreshment"
txtCompany = "R 'n R — for Reading 'n Refreshment"
```

This text uses the complete form for consistency, readability, and understandability. You may choose to refer to the default property of controls in your projects, however. Table 2.1 shows controls and their default properties.

Table 2.1

Controls and their default properties.

Control	Default Property
Check box	Value
Combo box	Text
Command button	Value
Frame	Caption
Horizontal scroll bar	Value
Image	Picture
Label	Caption
Line	Visible
List box	Text
Menu	Enabled
Option button	Value
Picture box	Picture
Shape	Shape
Text box	Text
Timer	Enabled
Vertical scroll bar	Value

Your Hands-On Programming Example

For this example you will write a program that uses many of the new controls and topics introduced in this chapter. The program will input the user's name and a message, display the two items concatenated in a label, and change the format of the label. Using option buttons and check boxes for selection, the user can make the label bold, underlined, or italic, and change its color.

You will include command buttons to display the message in the label, clear the text boxes and label, print the form, and exit. Include keyboard access keys for the command buttons; make the Display button the default button and make the Clear button the cancel button.

Place a logo on the form. Actually, you will place two images with different sizes for the logo on the form. Each time the user clicks on the logo, it will toggle the large and small versions of the logo.

Planning the Project

Sketch a form (Figure 2.20), which your users sign off as meeting their needs. *Note:* Although this may seem unnecessary, it is standard programming practice and documents that your users have been involved and approve the design.

Figure 2.20

A planning sketch of the form for the hands-on programming example.

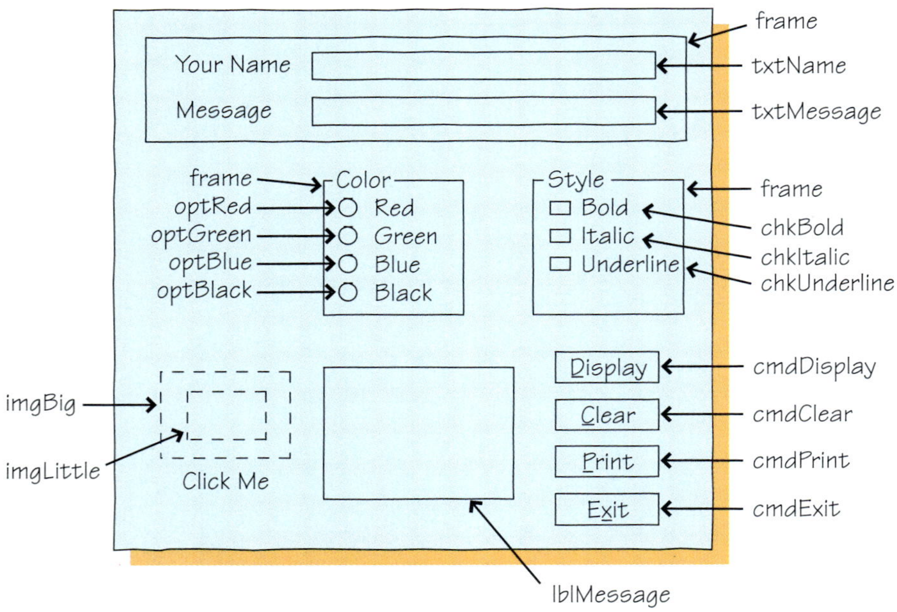

Plan the Objects and Properties

Plan the property settings for the form and for each control.

Object	Property	Setting	
Label1	Caption	Your Name:	
txtName	Name	txtName	
	Text	(blank)	
Label2	Caption	Message:	*Hint:* Do not change the name of this label.
txtMessage	Name	txtMessage	
	Text	(blank)	

(continued)

Object	Property	Setting	
fraColor	Name	fraColor	
	Caption	Color	
optRed	Name	optRed	*Hint:* Don't forget to draw the option buttons *inside* the frame.
	Caption	&Red	
optGreen	Name	optGreen	
	Caption	&Green	
optBlue	Name	optBlue	
	Caption	&Blue	
optBlack	Name	optBlack	
	Caption	B&lack	
fraStyle	Name	fraStyle	
	Caption	Style	
chkBold	Name	chkBold	
	Caption	B&old	
chkItalic	Name	chkItalic	
	Caption	&Italic	
chkUnderline	Name	chkUnderline	*Hint:* If you can't see option button or checkbox captions, make your objects wider.
	Caption	&Underline	
imgBig	Name	imgBig	
	Stretch	True	
	Picture	VB\ICONS\COMPUTER\CDROM01.ICO	
	Visible	True	
imgLittle	Name	imgLittle (Note that the two images are in the same location, one on top of the other.)	
	Stretch	True	
	Picture	VB\ICONS\COMPUTER\CDROM02.ICO	
	Visible	False	
Label3 (or some other number)	Caption	Click Me	
lblMessage	Name	lblMessage	
	Caption	(blank)	
	Alignment	2 - Center	
	Appearance	1 - 3D	

(continued)

Object	Property	Setting
lblMessage	Name	lblMessage
	BorderStyle	1 - Fixed Single
cmdDisplay	Name	cmdDisplay
	Caption	&Display
	Default	True
cmdClear	Name	cmdClear
	Caption	&Clear
	Cancel	True
cmdPrint	Name	cmdPrint
	Caption	&Print
cmdExit	Name	cmdExit
	Caption	E&xit

Plan the Event Procedures

You will need event procedures for each command button, option button, check box, and image.

Procedure	Actions—Pseudocode
cmdDisplay_Click	Set lblMessage to both the name and message from the text boxes (concatenate them).
cmdClear_Click	Clear the two text boxes and label. Reset the focus in the first text box.
cmdPrint_Click	Print the form.
cmdExit_Click	End the project.
optRed_Click	Make the ForeColor of lblMessage red.
optGreen_Click	Make the ForeColor of lblMessage green.
optBlue_Click	Make the ForeColor of lblMessage blue.
optBlack_Click	Make the ForeColor of lblMessage black.
chkBold_Click	Set lblMessage's Font.Bold property to match the check box (selected or deselected).
chkItalic_Click	Set lblMessage's Font.Italic property to match the check box (selected or deselected).
chkUnderline_Click	Set lblMessage's Font.Underline property to match the check box (selected or deselected).
imgBig_Click	Make imgBig invisible (Visible = False). Make imgLittle visible (Visible = True).
imgLittle_Click	Make imgLittle invisible. Make imgBig visible.

Write the Project

Follow the sketch in Figure 2.20 to create the form. Figure 2.21 shows the completed form.

- Set the properties of each of the objects, as you have planned.
- Working from the pseudocode, write each event procedure.
- When you complete the code, thoroughly test the project.

Figure 2.21

The form for the hands-on programming example.

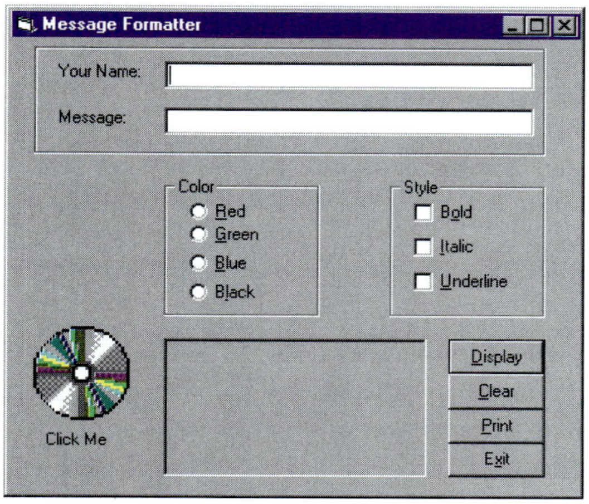

The Project Coding Solution

```
'Project:       Chapter Example 2.1
'Date:          July 1997
'Programmer:    J.C. Bradley
'Description:   This project uses labels, text boxes, option buttons,
'               check boxes, images, and command buttons to change
'               the properties of text.
'Folder:        Ch0201
Option Explicit
```

```
Private Sub chkBold_Click()
    'Change the message text to/from bold

    lblMessage.Font.Bold = chkBold.Value
End Sub
```

```
Private Sub chkItalic_Click()
    'Change the message text to/from italic

    lblMessage.Font.Italic = chkItalic.Value
End Sub
```

```
Private Sub chkUnderline_Click()
    'Change the message text to/from underline

    lblMessage.Font.Underline = chkUnderline.Value
End Sub
```

```
Private Sub cmdClear_Click()
    'Clear the text controls

    With txtName
        .Text = ""    'Clear the text box
        .SetFocus     'Reset the insertion point
    End With
    lblMessage.Caption = ""
    txtMessage.Text = ""
End Sub
```

```
Private Sub cmdDisplay_Click()
    'Display the text in the message area

    lblMessage.Caption = txtName.Text & ": " & txtMessage.Text
End Sub
```

```
Private Sub cmdExit_Click()
    'Exit the project

    End
End Sub
```

```
Private Sub cmdPrint_Click()
    'Print the form

    PrintForm
End Sub
```

```
Private Sub imgBig_Click()
    'Switch the icon

    imgBig.Visible = False
    imgLittle.Visible = True
End Sub
```

```
Private Sub imgLittle_Click()
    'Switch the icon

    imgLittle.Visible = False
    imgBig.Visible = True
End Sub
```

```
Private Sub optBlack_Click()
    'Make label black

    lblMessage.ForeColor = vbBlack
End Sub
```

```
Private Sub optBlue_Click()
    'Make label blue

    lblMessage.ForeColor = vbBlue
End Sub
```

```
Private Sub optGreen_Click()
    'Make label green

    lblMessage.ForeColor = vbGreen
End Sub
```

```
Private Sub optRed_Click()
    'Make label red

    lblMessage.ForeColor = vbRed
End Sub
```

Programming Hints

1. To make the text in a text box right justified or centered, you must set the Multiline property to True, in addition to setting the Alignment property.
2. You can use the Value property of a check box to set other properties that must be True or False. For example:

```
txtMessage.Font.Bold = chkBold.Value   'Sets Bold property to True or _
                                         False to match check box
```

3. Always test the tab order on your forms. Fix it if necessary by changing the TabIndex properties.
4. You can create multiple controls of the same type without clicking on the tool in the toolbox every time. To create the first of a series, Ctrl–click on the tool; the tool will remain active and allow you to keep drawing more controls. Click on the pointer tool (the arrow) when you are finished.
5. Always remember to create an option button inside its frame. If you double-click to create an option button, it does not belong to the frame. You can make an option button belong to a frame by cutting and pasting it inside the frame.
6. Use text boxes when you want the user to enter or change the text. Use label controls when you do not want the user to change the data. You can set the BorderStyle and BackColor properties of a label so that it looks just like a text box, but cannot be changed.

Summary

1. Text boxes are used primarily for user input. The Text property holds the value input by the user. You can also assign a literal to the text property during run time.
2. Frames are used as containers for other controls and to group like items on a form.
3. Check boxes and option buttons allow the user to make choices. In a group of option buttons, only one can be selected; but in a group of check boxes, any number of the boxes may be selected.
4. Image controls hold a graphic, which is assigned to the Picture property.
5. The Appearance property of many controls can be set to 0 – Flat or 1 – 3D, which determines whether the control appears flat or three-dimensional.
6. You can select multiple controls and treat them as a group, including setting common properties at once, moving them, or aligning them.
7. Make your programs easier to use by following Windows standard guidelines for colors, control size and placement, access keys, default and cancel buttons, and tab order.
8. Define keyboard access keys by including an ampersand in the caption of command buttons, option buttons, and check boxes.
9. Set the Default property of one command button to True so that the user can press Enter to select the button. If you set the Cancel property to True, the button will be selected when the user presses the Esc key.
10. The focus moves from control to control as the user presses the Tab key. The sequence for tabbing is determined by the TabIndex properties of the controls.
11. Clear the Text property of a text box or the Caption property of a label by setting it to an empty string.
12. To place the insertion point into a text box as the program is running, use the SetFocus method.
13. To change font attributes of a text box or a label, use the Font property of the control. The Font property refers to a Font object with properties for bold, italic, underline, size, etc.
14. Change the color of text in a control by changing the ForeColor property.
15. You can use the Visual Basic color constants to change colors during run time.
16. The `With` and `End With` statements provide an easy way to refer to an object multiple times without repeating the object's name.
17. Joining two strings of text is called *concatenation* and is accomplished by placing an ampersand between the two elements. (A space must precede and follow the ampersand.)
18. Use a space and an underscore to continue a long statement on another line.
19. Using the default property of a control allows you to refer to an object without naming the property.

Key Terms

access key 55
Alignment property 47
Appearance property 50
Cancel property 56
Check box 47
color constant 60
concatenation 62
Default property 56
empty string 59
focus 57
Font object 60
ForeColor property 60
Frame 47
image 48
Line control 51
line-continuation character 62
Multiline property 47
option button 48
Picture property 48
SetFocus method 59
Shape control 50
Stretch property 49
TabIndex property 57
TabStop property 57
text box 46
Text property 46
twip 54
Value property 47
Visible property 49
`With` and `End With` statements 61

Review Questions

1. You can display program output in a text box or a label. When should you use a text box? When is a label appropriate?
2. How does the behavior of option buttons differ from the behavior of check boxes?
3. If you want two groups of option buttons on a form, how can you make the groups operate independently?
4. Explain how to make a graphic appear in an image control.
5. Describe how to select several labels and set them all to 12-point font size with one command.
6. What is the purpose of keyboard access keys? How can you define them in your project? How do they operate at run time?
7. Explain the purpose of the Default and Cancel properties of command buttons. Give an example of a good use for each.
8. What is the focus? How can you control which object has the focus?
9. Assume you are testing your project and don't like the initial position of the insertion point. Explain how to make the insertion point appear in a different text box when the program begins.
10. During program execution you want to return the insertion point to a text box called txtAddress. What Basic statement will make that happen?
11. What Basic statements will clear the current contents of a text box and a label?
12. Explain how to change a label's Caption to italic at design time and at run time.
13. How are the `With` and `End With` statements used? Give an example.
14. What is concatenation and when would it be useful?
15. Explain how to continue a very long Basic statement onto another line.
16. What is the default property of a control? Give an example.

Programming Exercises

2.1 Create a project that will switch a light bulb on and off, using the user interface shown below as a guide.

Form: Include a text box for the user to enter his/her name. Create two images, one on top of the other. Only one will be visible at a time. Use option buttons to select the color of the text in the label beneath the light bulb image.

Include keyboard access keys for the option buttons and the command buttons. Make the Print button the default button and the Exit button the cancel button.

Project operation: The user will enter a name and click an option button for the color (not necessarily in that order). When the light bulb is clicked, display the other image and change the message below it. Concatenate the user name to the end of the message.

The two icon files are

VB\ICONS\MISC\LIGHTOFF.ICO
VB\ICONS\MISC\LIGHTON.ICO

(You will need to find the location of the VB directory in order to find the icons.)

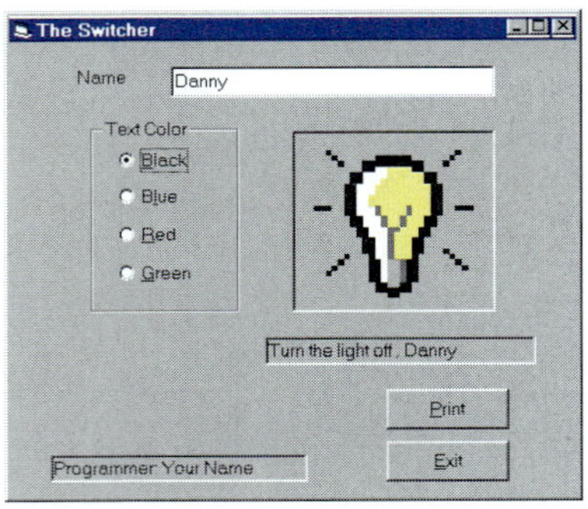

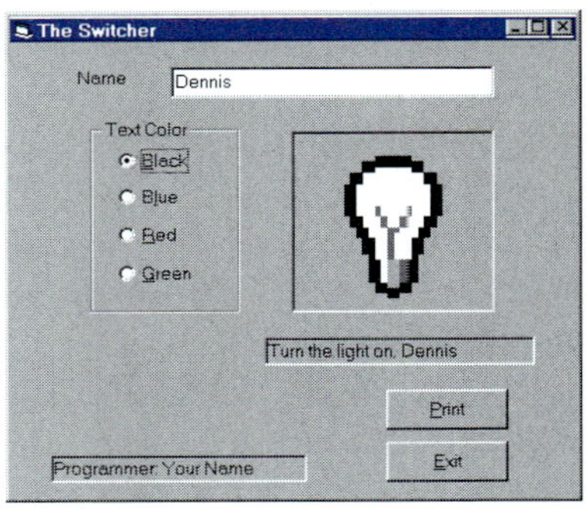

Coding: In the click event for each Color option button, change the color of the message below the light bulb. In the click event for the Print command button, print the form.

2.2 Write a project that will display the flags of four different countries, depending on the setting of the option buttons. In addition, display the name of the country in the large label under the flag image. The user can also choose to display or hide the form's title, the country name, and the name of the programmer. Use check boxes for the display/hide choices.

Include keyboard access keys for all option buttons, check boxes, and command buttons. Make the Print button the default button and the Exit button the cancel button.

You can choose the countries and flags. You will find more than 20 flag icons in VB\ICONS\FLAGS.

Hints: When a project begins running, the focus goes to the control with the lowest TabIndex. Since that is likely an option button, one button will appear selected. You must either display the first flag to match the option button or make the focus begin in a different control. You might consider beginning the focus on one of the command buttons.

Set the Visible property of a control to the Value property of the corresponding check box. That way when the check box is selected, the control becomes visible.

Since all three selectable controls will be visible when the project begins, set the Value property of the three check boxes to *1 - Selected* at design time. Set the images to *Visible = False* so they won't appear at startup. (If you plan to display one image at startup, its Visible property must be set to True.)

Rather than stack the images as was done in the chapter example, you might consider another method of setting up the four flag images. Try placing four small invisible flag icons near the bottom of the form. When the user selects a different country's flag, set the Picture property of the large flag image to the Picture property of one of the small, invisible images.

Example:

```
imgFlag.Picture = imgMexico.Picture
```

Make sure to set the Stretch property of the large image control to True.

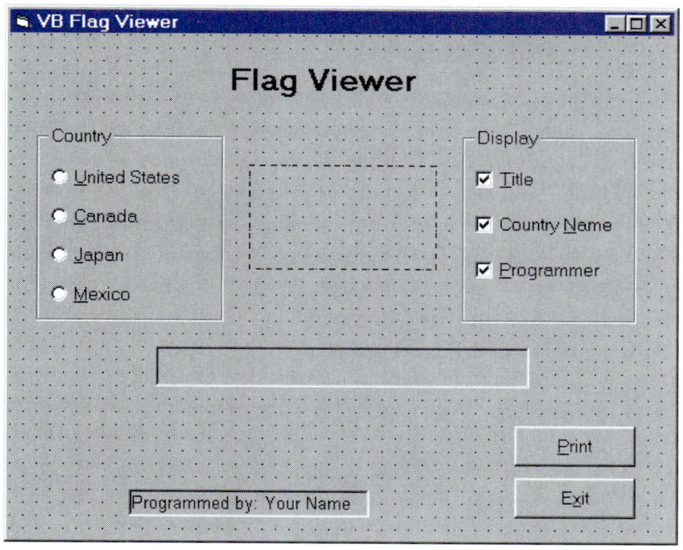

2.3 Write a project that will display a weather report. The user can choose one of the option buttons and display an icon and a message. The message should give the weather report in words and include the person's name (taken from the text box at the top of the form). For example, if the user chooses the Sunny button, you might display "It looks like sunny weather today, John" (assuming that the user entered "John" in the text box).

Include keyboard access keys for the option buttons and command buttons. Make the Exit button the cancel button.

You might consider the method of hiding and displaying images described in the hints for exercise 2. The four icons displayed are in the VB\ICONS\ELEMENTS subdirectory and are called CLOUD.ICO, RAIN.ICO, SNOW.ICO, and SUN.ICO.

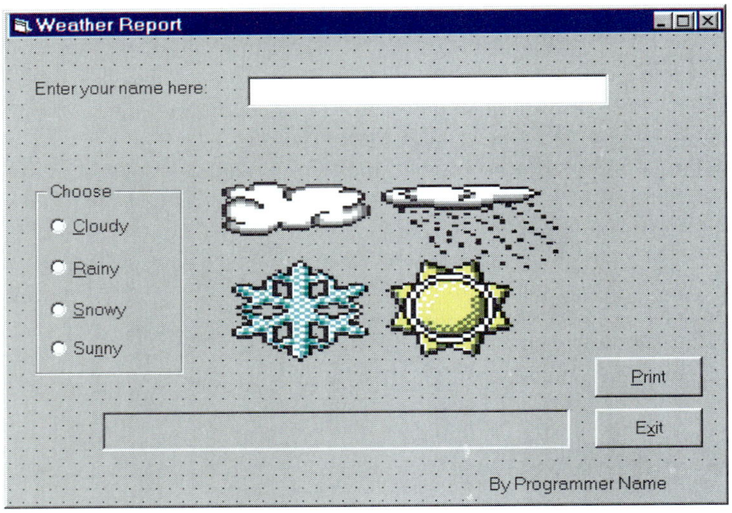

2.4 Write a project that will input the user name and display a message of the day in a label, along with the user's name. Include command buttons (with keyboard access keys) for Display, Clear, Print, and Exit. Make the Display button the default button and the Clear button the cancel button.

Include a group of option buttons for users to select the font size of the message. Give them a choice of three different sizes. *Hint:* Display the *Font* dialog box from the Properties window to determine the available sizes. Make sure your message label is large enough to display the longest message in the largest font size.

Make your form display a changeable image. You can use the happy face icon files or any other images you have available (VB\ICONS\MISC\FACE01.ICO, FACE02.ICO, and FACE03.ICO).

You may choose to have only one message of the day, or you can have several that the user can select from option buttons. You might want to choose messages that go with the different face icons.

Optional extra: Include check boxes to change the font attributes of the message. Include Bold, Underline, Italic, and StrikeThru. Make sure to include keyboard access keys.

2.5 Create a project that will allow the user to input information and then display the lines of output for a mailing label.

Remember that fields to be input by the user require text boxes while information to be displayed belongs in labels. Use text boxes for first name, last name, street address, city, state, and ZIP code; give meaningful names to the text boxes and set the Captions to blank. Add appropriate labels to each text box to indicate to the user what data will be entered into each box.

Use command buttons for Display Label Info, Clear, Print Form, and Exit. Make the Display button the default button and the Clear button the cancel button.

Use three labels for displaying the information for Line 1, Line 2, and Line 3.

A click event on the Display Label Info command button will display the following:

Line 1—The first name and last name concatenated together.
Line 2—The street address.
Line 3—The city, state, and ZIP code concatenated together. (Make sure to concatenate a comma and a space between the city and state using ", ", and 2 spaces between the state and ZIP code).

CASE STUDIES

VB Mail Order

Design and code a project that has shipping information.

Use an appropriate image in the upper-left corner of the form.

Use text boxes with labels attached for Catalog Code, Page Number, and Part Number.

Use two groups of option buttons on the form; enclose each group in a frame. The first frame should have a Caption of Shipping and contain buttons for Express and Ground. Use a Caption of Payment Type on the second frame and include buttons for Charge, COD, and Money Order.

Use a check box for New Customer.

Add command buttons for Print Form, Clear, and Exit. Make the Clear button the cancel button.

VB Auto Center

Modify the project from the Chapter 1 VB Auto Center case study, replacing the command buttons with images. Place a label above each image that indicates which department or command the image represents. A click on an image will produce the appropriate information in the special notices label.

Add an image that allows the form to be printed as well as an image that will clear the special notices label.

Add two option buttons that will allow the user to view the special notices label in 10-point font or 14-point font. Make sure that the label is large enough to hold the 14-point message.

Include a check box labeled Hours. When the check box is selected, a new label will display the message "Open 24 Hours--7 days a week".

Department/Command	Image
Auto Sales	vb\graphics\icons\industry\cars
Service Center	vb\graphics\icons\industry\wrench
Detail Shop	vb\graphics\icons\elements\water
Employment Opportunities	vb\graphics\icons\mail\mail12
Exit	vb\graphics\icons\computer\msgbox1
Print Form	vb\graphics\icons\dragdrop\drag1pg

CHAPTER

3

Variables, Constants, and Calculations

At the completion of this chapter, you will be able to . . .

1. Distinguish between variables, constants, and controls.
2. Differentiate among the various data types.
3. Apply naming conventions incorporating standards and indicating scope and data type.
4. Declare variables using the `Dim` statement.
5. Select the appropriate scope for a variable.
6. Convert text input to numeric values using the `Val` function.
7. Perform calculations using variables and constants.
8. Accumulate sums and generate counts.
9. Format data for output.
10. Modify the environment to require `Option Explicit`.

In this chapter you will learn to do calculations in Visual Basic. You will start with text values input by the user, convert them to numeric values, and perform calculations on them. You will also learn to format the results of your calculations and display them for the user.

Although the calculations themselves are quite simple (adding, subtracting, multiplying, and dividing), there are some important issues to discuss first. You must learn about variables and constants, the various types of data used by Visual Basic, and how and where to declare variables and constants. Variables are declared differently, depending on where you want to use them and how long you need to retain their values.

The code below is a small preview that shows calculating the product of two text boxes. The first group of statements (the `Dims`) declares the variables and their data types. The second group of statements converts the text box contents to numeric and places the values into the variables. The last line performs the multiplication and places the result into a variable. The following sections of this chapter describe how to set up your code for calculations.

```
'Dimension the variables
Dim iQuantity             As Integer
Dim cPrice                As Currency

'Convert input text to numeric and assign values to variables
iQuantity = Val(txtQuantity.Text)
cPrice = Val(txtPrice.Text)

'Calculate the product
cExtendedPrice = iQuantity * cPrice
```

Data—Variables and Constants

So far, all data you have used in your projects have been properties of objects. You have worked with the Text property of Text Boxes and the Caption property of Labels. Now it is time to consider working with values that are not properties. Basic allows you to set up locations in memory and give each location a name. You can visualize each memory location as a scratch pad; the contents of the scratch pad can change as the need arises. In this example, the memory location is called *iMaximum.*

```
iMaximum = 100
```

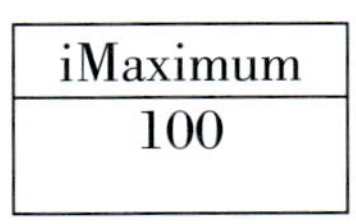

After executing this statement, the value of iMaximum is 100. You can change the value of iMaximum, use it in calculations, or display it in a control.

In the preceding example, the memory location called iMaximum is a **variable**. Memory locations that hold data that can be changed during project execution are called *variables;* locations that hold data that cannot change during execution are called ***constants***. For example, a customer's name will vary as the information for each individual is being processed. However, the name of the company and the sales tax rate will remain the same (at least for that day).

When you declare a variable or a named constant, Visual Basic reserves an area of memory and assigns it a name, called an ***identifier***. You specify identifier names according to the rules of Basic as well as some recommended naming conventions.

The **declaration** statements establish your project's variables and constants, give them names, and specify the type of data they will hold. The statements are not considered executable; that is, they are not executed in the flow of instructions during program execution.

Here are some sample declaration statements:

```
Dim stName As String                       'Declare a string variable
Dim iCounter As Integer                    'Declare an integer variable
Const cDISCOUNT_RATE As Currency = .15 'Declare a named constant
```

The next few paragraphs describe the data types, the rules for naming variables and constants, and the format of the declarations.

Data Types

The **data type** of a variable or constant indicates what type of information will be stored in the allocated memory space: perhaps a name, a dollar amount, a date, or a total. Note that the default data type is **variant**. If you do not specify a data type, your variables and constants will be variants. The advantage of using variant data type is that it's easy, and the variables and constants change their appearance as needed for each situation. The disadvantage is that variants are less efficient than the other data types; they require more memory and operate less quickly. The best practice is to always specify the data type.

Data Type	Use For
Boolean	True or False values.
Byte	A single ASCII character (code 0 to 255).
Currency	Decimal fractions, such as dollars and cents.
Date	An eight-character date.
Double	Double-precision floating-point numbers with 14 digits of accuracy.
Integer	Whole numbers in the range −32,768 to 32,767.
Long	Larger whole numbers.
Single	Single-precision floating point numbers with six digits of accuracy.
String	Alphanumeric data: letters, digits, and other characters.
Variant	Converts from one type to another, as needed.

The most common types of variables and constants we will use are string, integer, and currency. When deciding which data type to use, follow this guideline: If the data will be used in a calculation, then it must be numeric (usually integer or currency); if it is not used in a calculation, it will be string. Use currency as the data type for any decimal fractions in business applications; single and double data types are generally used in scientific applications.

Consider the following examples:

Contents	**Data Type**	**Reason**
Social Security number	String	Not used in a calculation.
Pay rate	Currency	Used in a calculation, contains a decimal point.
Hours worked	Currency	Used in a calculation, may contain a decimal point. (Currency can be used for any decimal fraction, not just dollars.)
Phone number	String	Not used in a calculation.
Quantity	Integer	Used in calculations, contains a whole number.

Naming Rules

Each programmer has to name (identify) the variables and named constants that will be used in a project. Basic requires identifiers for variables and named constants to follow these rules: names must be 1 to 255 characters in length; they may consist of letters, digits, and underscores; they cannot contain any spaces or periods; and they may not be reserved words. (Reserved words, also called *keywords,* are words to which Basic has assigned some meaning, such as *print, name,* and *value.*)

Naming Conventions

When naming variables and constants, you *must* follow the rules of Basic. In addition, you *should* follow some naming conventions. Conventions are the guidelines that separate good names from bad (or not so good) names. The meaning and use of all identifiers should always be clear.

Just as we established conventions for naming objects in Chapter 1, in this chapter we will adopt conventions for naming variables and constants. The following conventions are widely used in the programming industry:

1. Identifiers must be meaningful. Choose a name that clearly indicates its purpose. Do not abbreviate unless the meaning is obvious, and do not use very short identifiers, such as *X* or *Y.*
2. Precede each identifier with a lowercase prefix that specifies the data type. This convention is similar to the convention we already adopted for naming objects.
3. For variable names, capitalize each word of the name (following the prefix). Use mixed case for variable names, never all uppercase.

4. For named constants, use all uppercase following the prefix. Use underscore characters between the words to make names easier to read.

This text uses the following prefixes to specify data types:

b	Boolean
c	Currency
d	Double-precision floating point
i	Integer
l	Long integer
s	Single-precision floating point
st	string
v	Variant

Sample identifiers

Field of Data	Possible Identifier
Social Security number	`stSocialSecurityNumber`
Pay rate	`cPayRate`
Hours worked	`cHoursWorked`
Phone number	`stPhoneNumber`
Quantity	`iQuantity`
Tax rate (constant)	`cTAX_RATE`
Quota (constant)	`iQUOTA`
Population	`lPopulation`

Feedback 3.1

Indicate whether each of the following identifiers conforms to the rules of Basic and to the naming conventions. If invalid, give the reason. Remember, the answers to all Feedback questions are found in Appendix A.

1. `omitted`
2. `i#Sold`
3. `i Number Sold`
4. `i.Number.Sold`
5. `s$Amount`
6. `Sub`
7. `stSub`
8. `Caption`
9. `conMaximum`
10. `MINIMUM_RATE`
11. `cMAXIMUM_CHECK`
12. `stCOMPANY_NAME`

Constants—Named and Intrinsic

Constants provide a way to use words to describe a value that doesn't change. In Chapter 2 you used the Visual Basic constants vbBlue, vbRed, vbYellow, and so on. Those constants are built into Visual Basic—you don't need to define them anywhere. The constants that you define for yourself are called *named constants;* those that are built into VB are called *intrinsic constants.*

Named Constants

You declare named constants using the keyword `Const`. You give the constant a name, a data type, and a value. Once a value is declared as a constant, its value cannot be changed during the execution of the project. The data type that you declare and the data type of the value must match. For example, if you declare an integer constant, you must give it an integer value.

You will find two important advantages to using named constants rather than the actual values in code. The code is easier to read; for example, seeing the identifier cMAXIMUM_PAY is more meaningful than seeing a number, such as 1000. In addition, if you need to change the value at a later time, you need to change the constant declaration only once and not change every reference to it throughout the code.

Const Statement—General Form

```
Const Identifier [As Datatype] = Value
```

Naming conventions for constants require a prefix that identifies the data type and puts the name portion entirely in uppercase. The purpose of the uppercase is to make it obvious in other parts of the code that the identifer is a constant and therefore cannot have a new value assigned to it.

Although the data type is optional, the best practice is to always declare the data type. When you don't declare the data type, Visual Basic looks at the value given and chooses an appropriate data type.

This example sets the company name, address, and the sales tax rate as constants:

Const Statement—Examples

```
Const stCOMPANY_NAME As String = "R 'n R for Reading 'n Refreshment"
Const stCOMPANY_ADDRESS As String = "101 S. Main Street"
Const cSALES_TAX_RATE As Currency = .08
```

Assigning Values to Constants

The values you assign to constants must follow certain rules. You have already seen that a text (string) value must be enclosed in quotation marks; numeric values are not so enclosed. However, you must be aware of some additional rules.

Numeric constants may contain only the digits (0–9), a decimal point, and a sign (+ or −) at the left side. You cannot include a comma, dollar sign, any other special characters, or a sign at the right side.

String literals (also called *string constants*) may contain letters, digits, and special characters, such as $ # @ % & *. The only problem comes when you want to include quotation marks inside a string literal, since quotation marks enclose the literal. The solution is to use two quotation marks together inside the literal; Visual Basic will interpret the pair as one symbol.

Example

`"He said, ""I like it."""` produces this string: `He said, "I like it."`

Although you can use numeric digits inside a string literal, remember that these numbers are text and cannot be used for calculations.

The string values are referred to as **string literals** because they contain exactly (literally) whatever is inside the quotation marks.

Example constants

Data Type	Constant Value Example

Integer	`5`
	`+25`
	`-170`
	`2000`

Single or currency	`101.25` `-5.0`

String literals	`"Visual Basic"`
	`"ABC Incorporated"`
	`"1415 J Street"`
	`"102"`
	`"She said ""Hello."""`

Intrinsic Constants

Intrinsic constants are system-defined constants. Several sets of intrinsic constants are stored in library files and available for use in your Visual Basic programs. For example, the color constants you used in Chapter 2 are intrinsic constants.

Intrinsic constants use a two character prefix to indicate the source, such as *vb* for Visual Basic, *db* for Data Access Objects, and *xl* for Excel. In the next chapter we will use intrinsic constants for creating message boxes.

Declaring Variables

Although there are several ways to declare a variable, the most commonly used statement is the `Dim` statement.

Dim Statement—General Form

```
Dim Identifier [As Datatype]
```

If you omit the optional data type, the variable's type defaults to variant. It is best to always declare the type, even when you intend to use variants.

Dim Statement—Examples

```
Dim stCustomerName    As String
Dim iTotalSold        As Integer
Dim sTemperature      As Single
Dim cPrice            As Currency
Dim vChanging                        'Defaults to Variant type
```

The reserved word `Dim` is really short for *dimension,* which means "size." When you declare a variable, the amount of memory reserved depends on its data type. Table 3.1 shows the amount of memory allocated for each data type.

Table 3.1

The amount of memory allocated for each data type.

Data Type	Number of Bytes of Memory Allocated
Boolean	2
Byte	1
Currency	8
Date	8
Double	8
Integer	2
Long	4
Single	4
String (variable length)	10 bytes plus 1 byte for each character in the string.
Variant	Holding numbers—16 bytes. Holding characters—22 bytes plus 1 byte for each character in the string.

Note: Visual Basic does not require you to declare a variable before using it—see "Programming Hints" at the end of this chapter for details.

Entering Dim Statements

New to VB 5!

Visual Basic's Auto Fill In feature helps you enter `Dim` statements. After you type the space that follows `Dim VariableName As`, a shortcut menu pops up (Figure 3.1). This list shows the possible entries for data type to complete the statement. The easiest way to complete the statement is to begin typing the correct entry; the list automatically scrolls to the correct section (Figure 3.2). When the correct entry is highlighted, press Enter, Tab, or the space bar to select the entry, or double-click if you prefer using the mouse.

Figure 3.1

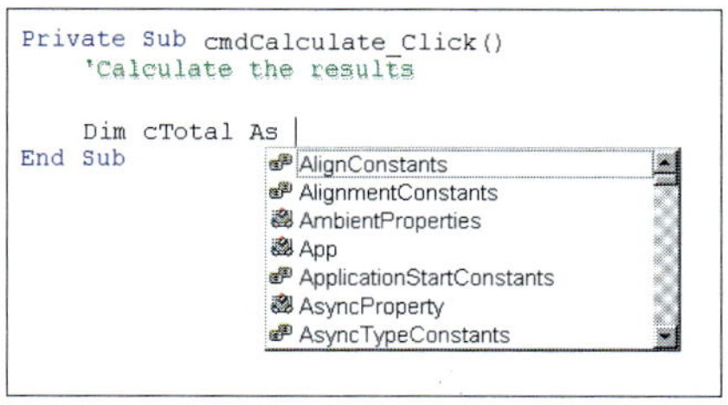

As soon as you type the space after `As`*, the Auto Fill In menu pops up. You can make a selection from the list with your mouse or the keyboard.*

Figure 3.2

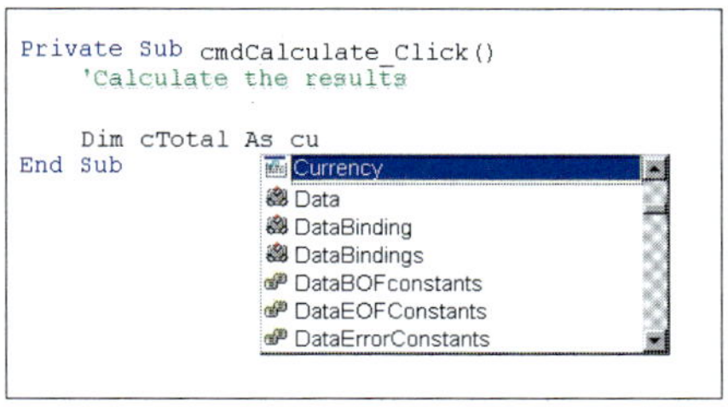

Type the first few characters of the data type and the Auto Fill In list will quickly scroll to the correct section. When the correct word is highlighted, press Enter, Tab, or the space bar to select the entry.

Note: Some people find the Auto Fill In feature annoying rather than helpful. You can turn off the feature by selecting *Tools/Options/Editor tab* and deselecting *Auto List Members.*

Feedback 3.2

Write a declaration for the following situations; make up an appropriate variable identifier.

1. You need variables for payroll processing to store the following:
   (a) Single-precision number of hours.
   (b) String employee's name.
   (c) Department number (not used in calculations).
2. You need variables for inventory control to store the following:
   (a) Integer quantity.
   (b) Description of the item.
   (c) Part number.
   (d) Cost.
   (e) Selling price.

Scope of Variables

A variable may exist and be visible for an entire project, for only one form, or for only one procedure. The visibility of a variable is referred to as its **scope**. *Visibility* really means "can this variable be used or 'seen' in this location." The scope is said to be global, module level, or local. A **global** variable may be used in all procedures of a project and will be discussed in

Chapter 6. **Module-level** variables are accessible from all procedures of a form. A **local** variable may be used only within the procedure in which it is declared.

The scope of a variable declared with a `Dim` statement is determined by where the declaration statement is made.

Variable Lifetime

When you create a variable, you must be aware of its **lifetime**. The *lifetime* of a variable is the period of time that the variable exists. The lifetime of a local variable is normally one execution of a procedure. For example, each time you execute a sub procedure, the local `Dim` statements are executed. Each variable is created as a "fresh" new one, with an initial value of 0 for numeric variables and an empty string for string variables. When the procedure finishes, its variables disappear; that is, their memory locations are released.

The lifetime of a module-level variable is the entire time the form is loaded, generally the lifetime of the entire project. If you want to maintain the value of a variable for multiple executions of a procedure, for example to calculate a running total, you must use a module-level variable (or a variable specified as Static, which is discussed in Chapter 6).

Local Declarations

Any variable that is declared inside a procedure is local in scope; it is known only to that procedure. A `Dim` statement may appear anywhere inside the procedure, as long as it appears prior to the first use of the variable in a statement. However, good programming practices dictate that all `Dim`s appear at the top of the procedure, prior to all other code statements (after the remarks).

```
Private Sub cmdCalculate_Click()
    'Calculate the price and discount

    Dim iQuantity           As Integer
    Dim cPrice              As Currency
    Dim cExtendedPrice      As Currency
    Dim cDiscount           As Currency
    Dim cDiscountedPrice    As Currency
    Const cDISCOUNT_RATE    As Currency = 0.15

    'Convert input values to numeric variables
    iQuantity = Val(txtQuantity.Text)
    cPrice = Val(txtPrice.Text)

    'Calculate values
    cExtendedPrice = iQuantity * cPrice
    cDiscount = cExtendedPrice * cDISCOUNT_RATE
    cDiscountedPrice = cExtendedPrice - cDiscount
```

Notice the `Const` statement in the preceding example. You can declare named constants to be local, module-level, or global in scope, just as you can variables.

Module-Level Declarations

At times you need to be able to use a variable or constant in more than one procedure of a form. When you declare a variable or constant as module-level, it may be used anywhere in that form. Place the declarations (`Dim` or `Const`) for module-level variables and constants in the general declarations section of the form. (Recall that you have been using the general declarations section for remarks since Chapter 1.) If you wish to accumulate a sum or count items for multiple executions of a procedure, you should declare the variable at the module level.

Figure 3.3 illustrates the locations for coding local variables and module-level variables.

Figure 3.3

The variables you dimension inside a procedure are local. Variables that you dimension in the General Declarations section of a form are module level.

```
(General Declarations section)

Option Explicit
Dim ModuleLevelVariables
Const ModuleLevelConstants
________________________________
Private Sub cmdCalculate_Click
   Dim LocalVariables
   Const LocalConstants

   ...
End Sub
________________________________
Private Sub cmdSummarize_Click
   Dim LocalVariables
   Const LocalConstants

   ...
End Sub
________________________________
Private Sub cmdInitialize_Click
   Dim LocalVariables
   Const LocalConstants
   ...
End Sub
________________________________
```

```
'General Declarations section of a form

Option Explicit

'Dimension module-level variables
Dim miQuantitySum          As Integer
Dim mcDiscountSum          As Currency
Dim miSaleCount            As Integer
```

Including the Scope in Identifiers

When you use variables and constants, it is important to know their scope. For that reason you should include scope information in your naming conventions. To indicate a module-level variable or constant, place a prefix of `m` before the identifier. Local variables and constants do not have an additional prefix, so any variable without an initial `m` can be assumed to be local.

Examples

```
Dim mcTotalPay As Currency
```

Note that the `m` stands for module level, and the `c` stands for currency data type.

```
Const miNUMBER_QUESTIONS As Integer = 50
```

The `m` stands for module level, and the `i` stands for integer data type.

Coding Module-Level Declarations

To enter module-level declarations, you must be in the Code window, in the General Declarations section (Figure 3.4). Recall how to display the General Declarations section:

Figure 3.4

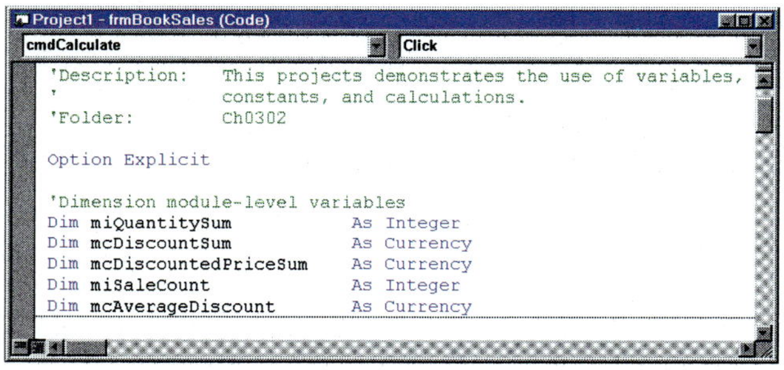

Code module-level declarations in the General Declaration section of a form module.

1. Select *Code* from the *View* menu or click on the *View Code* button in the *Project Explorer* window.
2. In the Object list, select *(General)*.
3. In the Procedure list, select *(Declarations)*.
4. Place the `Dim` (or `Const`) statements in this section of code, after the `Option Explicit` statement.

Feedback 3.3

Write the declarations (`Dim` or `Const` statements) for each of the following situations and indicate where each statement will appear.

1. The total of the payroll that will be needed in a Calculate event procedure and in a Summary event procedure.
2. The sales tax rate that cannot be changed during execution of the program but will be used by multiple procedures.
3. The number of participants that are being counted in the Calculate event procedure but not displayed until the Summary event procedure.

Calculations

In programming you can perform calculations with variables and with the properties of certain objects.

The properties you will use, such as the Text property of a text box and the Caption property of a label, are actually strings of text characters. These character strings, such as "Howdy" or "12345" should not be used directly in calculations. Visual Basic tries to make assumptions about the property values you use in calculations. Those assumptions are correct most of the time, but are incorrect often enough that we must take steps to convert all property values to numeric before using them in calculations.

Use the `Val` function to convert the property of a control to its numeric form before you use the value in a calculation:

```
'Convert input values to numeric variables
iQuantity = Val(txtQuantity.Text)
cPrice = Val(txtPrice.Text)

'Calculate the extended price
cExtendedPrice = iQuantity * cPrice
```

Val Function

Visual Basic supplies many functions that you can use in your programs. A **function** performs an action and returns a value. The expression to operate upon, called the ***argument***, (or multiple arguments, in some cases), must be enclosed in parentheses.

The first Basic function we will use is `Val`. (Think of *val* as an abbreviation for *value*.) The `Val` function converts text data into a numeric value.

The Val Function—General Form

```
Val(ExpressionToConvert)
```

The expression you wish to convert can be the property of a control, a variable, or a constant.

A function cannot stand by itself. It returns (produces) a value that can be used as a part of a statement, such as the assignment statements in the following examples.

The Val Function—Examples

```
iQuantity = Val(txtQuantity.Text)
cPrice = Val(txtPrice.Text)
lCustomerNumber = Val(mstCUSTOMER_NUMBER)
```

When the `Val` function converts an argument to numeric, it begins at the argument's left-most character. If that character is a numeric digit, decimal point, or sign, `Val` converts the character to numeric and moves to the next character. As soon as a nonnumeric character is found, the operation stops. Here are some examples of the values returned by the `Val` function:

Contents of Argument	Numeric Value Returned by the Val function
(blank)	0
123.45	123.45
$100	0
1,000	1
A123	0
123A	123
4B5	4
−123	−123
+123	123
12.34.8	12.34

Arithmetic Operations

The arithmetic operations you can perform in Visual Basic include addition, subtraction, multiplication, division, and exponentiation.

Operator	Operation
+	Addition
−	Subtraction
*	Multiplication
/	Division
^	Exponentiation

Order of Operations

The order in which operations are performed determines the result. Consider the expression 3 + 4 * 2. What is the result? If the addition is done first, the result is 14. However, if the multiplication is done first, the result is 11.

The hierarchy of operations or **order of precedence** in arithmetic expressions from highest to lowest is

1. Exponentiation
2. Multiplication and division
3. Addition and subtraction

In the previous example, the multiplication is done before addition, and the result is 11. To change the order of evaluation, use parentheses: (3 + 4) * 2 will yield 14 as the result. One set of parentheses may be used inside another set. In that case, the parentheses are said to be nested.

Example

```
((iScore1 + iScore2 + iScore3)/3) * 1.2
```

Extra parentheses can always be used for clarity. The expressions

`2 * cCost * cRate` and `(2 * cCost) * cRate`

are equivalent, but the second is easier to understand.

Multiple operations at the same level (such as multiplication and division) are performed from left to right. The example 8 / 4 * 2 yields 4 as its result, not 1. The first operation is 8 / 4, and 2 * 2 is the second.

Evaluation of an expression occurs in this order:

1. All operations within parentheses. Multiple operations within the parentheses are performed according to the rules of precedence.
2. All exponentiation. Multiple exponentiation operations are performed from left to right.
3. All multiplication and division. Multiple operations are performed from left to right.
4. All addition and subtraction are performed from left to right.

Although the precedence of operations in Basic is the same as in algebra, take note of one important difference: There are no implied operations in Basic. The following expressions would be valid in mathematics, but they are not valid in Basic:

Mathematical Notation	Equivalent Basic Function
2A	2 * A
3(X +Y)	3 * (X + Y)
(X + Y)(X − Y)	(X + Y) * (X − Y)

Feedback 3.4

What will be the result of the following calculations using the order of precedence?

Assume that: X = 2, Y = 4, Z = 3

1. X + Y ^ 2
2. 8 / Y / X
3. X * (X + 1)

4. X * X + 1
5. Y ^ X + Z * 2
6. Y ^ (X + Z) * 2
7. (Y ^ X) + Z * 2
8. ((Y ^ X) + Z) * 2

Using Calculations in Code

Calculations are performed in assignment statements. Recall that whatever appears on the right side of an = (assignment operator) is assigned to the item on the left. The left side may be the property of a control or a variable. It cannot be a constant.

Examples

```
cAverage = cSum / iCount
lblAmountDue.Caption = cPrice - (cPrice * cDiscountRate)
txtCommission.Text = cSalesTotal * cCOMMISION_RATE
```

In the preceding examples, the results of the calculations were assigned to a variable, the Caption property of a label, and the Text property of a text box. In most cases you will assign calculation results to variables or to the Caption properties of labels. Text boxes are usually used for input from the user, not for program output.

Formatting Data

When you want to **format** data for display, either on the printer or on the screen, use the `Format` function. To *format* means to control the way the output will look. For example, 12 is just a number, but $12.00 conveys more meaning for dollar amounts. The *currency* format is used to display dollar amounts.

The Format Function—General Form

```
Format[$](ExpressionToFormat [, "FormatDescription"])
```

The optional dollar sign in the function name specifies that the formatted value be a string. Without the dollar sign, the value returned is a variant data type. In most situations the results are the same, but using the dollar sign is more efficient.

The expression to be formatted may be numeric or string, a variable, a literal, or a property. In most cases you will use formats for numeric data to control the number of decimal positions. Formats are not generally needed for integer values.

The format description can take one of several forms. Visual Basic provides several predefined formats for the most common types of output. To select one of these formats, include the format name in quotation marks. You may also design your own format for the output, which will be covered shortly.

Predefined Format Names	Description
Currency	A dollar sign; two digits to the right of the decimal; a comma for thousands, if needed; negative numbers in parentheses.
Fixed	Two digits to the right of the decimal point; displays 0 to left of decimal if the value is less than one; no comma for thousands.
General Number	Displays the number as it appears.
Medium Time*	A 12-hour time format; uses hours and minutes and AM or PM.
On/Off	Displays the word Off if the value is 0; all other values will display as On.
Percent	Number multiplied by 100 with percent sign on right; two digits to the right of the decimal point.
Scientific	Standard scientific notation (E notation).
Short Date	Uses the system date format.
Short Time	A 24-hour time format, with hours and minutes, such as 15:30.
Standard	Two digits to the right of the decimal point and a comma for thousands if necessary.
True/False	Displays False if the value is 0; all other values display as True.
Yes/No	Displays No if the value is 0; all other values display as Yes.

*Time and Date may be Medium, Short, or Long.

The Format Function—Examples

```
lblTotal.Caption = Format$(cTotalAmount, "Currency")
lblDate.Caption = Format$(iBirthdate, "Short Date")
```

One extremely nice feature of the `Format` function is that it rounds fractional values to the requested number of decimal places. Note that the value is rounded for output; the stored value does not change. Any future calculations will be done with the nonrounded value.

These statements produce the following values displayed in the labels:

Statements	Displayed Output
`sNumber = 1234.2766`	
`lblFormattedCurrency.Caption = Format$(sNumber, "Currency")`	$1,234.28
`lblFormattedStandard.Caption = Format$(sNumber, "Standard")`	1,234.28
`lblFormattedFixed.Caption = Format$(sNumber, "Fixed")`	1234.28
`lblFormattedScientific.Caption = Format$(sNumber, "Scientific")`	123E+03
`bFirstTime = True`	
`lblDisplay1.Caption = Format$(bFirstTime, "Yes/No")`	Yes
`lblDisplay2.Caption = Format$(bFirstTime, "True/False")`	True
`lblDisplay3.Caption = Format$(bFirstTime, "On/Off")`	On
`iScore = 45`	
`iPossible = 50`	
`sPercentCorrect = iScore / iPossible`	
`lblDisplay4.Caption = sPercentCorrect`	0.9
`lblDisplay1.Caption = Format$(sPercentCorrect, "Percent")`	90.00%
`dToday = Now 'Function to retrieve system clock`	
`Print Format$(dToday, "Short Date")`	6/15/97
`Print Format$(dToday, "Short Time")`	21:12
`Print Format$(dToday, "Medium Time")`	09:12 PM

Feedback 3.5

Give the line of code that assigns the formatted output and tell how the output would be displayed for the specified value.

1. A calculated variable called mcAveragePay has a value of 123.456 and will be displayed in a label called lblAveragePay.
2. The variable sCorrect, which contains .76, must be displayed as a percentage in the label called lblPercentCorrect.
3. The total amount collected in a fund drive is being accumulated in a variable called mcTotalCollected. What statement will display the variable in a label called lblTotal with commas and two decimal positions but no dollar signs?

Creating Custom Numeric Formats

If the predefined numeric formats don't give the results you want, you can create your own formats. For example, you might want to display whole-dollar amounts without the pennies or to show leading zeros.

The following sections describe how to create custom numeric formats. You can also create custom formats for strings and date/time values; see the Help topics *User-Defined Date/Time Formats* and *User-Defined String Formats* for help creating these formats.

Symbol	Description	Purpose
0	Zero placeholder	Displays a digit in the position; if there is no digit, a zero will display.
#	Null placeholder	Displays a digit in the position; if there is no digit, nothing will display.
.	Decimal point	Displays the decimal point in the position.
,	Thousand separator	Inserts appropriate commas when the number is greater than or equal to 1,000.
%	Percentage	Multiplies the value by 100 and adds the percentage symbol.

Custom Numeric Format—Examples

Statements	Output
`sAmount = 1542.788`	
`lblAmount1.Caption = Format$(sAmount, "####.#")`	1542.8
`lblAmount2.Caption = Format$(sAmount, "#,###")`	1,543
`lblAmount3.Caption = Format$(sAmount, "$##,###")`	$1,543
`sAmount = 542`	
`lblAmount4.Caption = Format$(sAmount, "###")`	542
`lblAmount5.Caption = Format$(sAmount, "###.##")`	542.
`lblAmount6.Caption = Format$(sAmount, "###.00")`	542.00
`lblAmount7.Caption = Format$(sAmount, "00000.00")`	000542.00
`sAmount = 0.5462`	
`lblAmount8.Caption = Format$(sAmount, "##.#%")`	54.6%
`lblAmount9.Caption = Format$(sAmount, "00.00%")`	54.62%
`lblAmount10.Caption = Format$(sAmount, "#%")`	55%

Feedback 3.6

What will be displayed for each of the following?

```
Dim cAmount as Currency
cAmount = 1.345
```

1. `lblAmount1.Caption = Format$(cAmount, "##.##")`
2. `lblAmount2.Caption = Format$(cAmount, "00.00")`
3. `lblAmount3.Caption = Format$(cAmount, "##.#")`
4. `lblAmount4.Caption = Format$(cAmount, "$#,###")`
5. `lblAmount5.Caption = Format$(cAmount, "$##.#")`

A Calculation Programming Example

R 'n R—For Reading 'n Refreshment—needs to calculate prices and discounts for books sold. The company is currently having a big sale, offering a 15 percent discount on all books. In this project you will calculate the amount due for a quantity of books, determine the 15 percent discount, and deduct the discount, giving the new amount due—the discounted amount.

Planning the Project

Sketch a form (Figure 3.5) that meets the needs of your users.

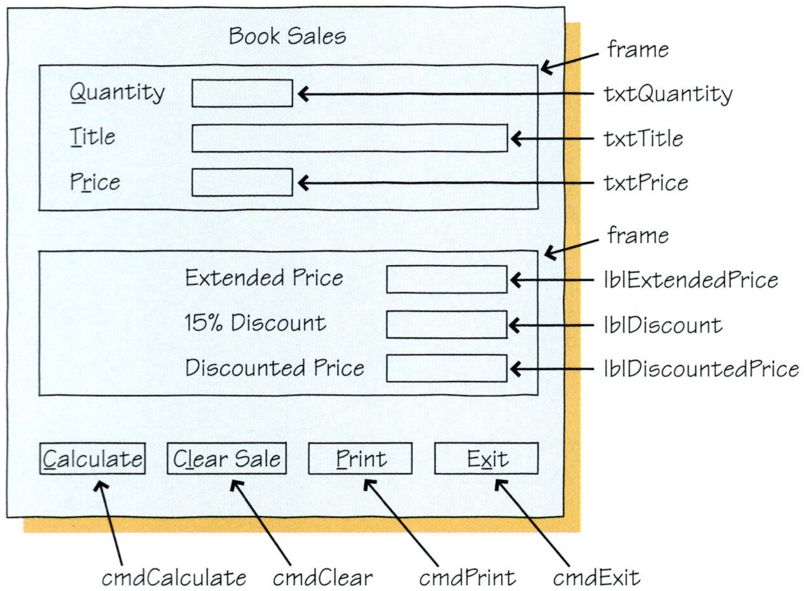

Figure 3.5

A planning sketch of the form for the calculation programming example.

Plan the Objects and Properties

Plan the property settings for the form and each of the controls.

Object	Property	Setting
Form	Name	frmBookSales
	Caption	R 'n R for Reading 'n Refreshment
Label1	Name	Label1
	Caption	Book Sales
	Font	Bold, 12 point
fraInput	Name	fraInput
	Caption	(blank)

(continued)

Object	Property	Setting
Label2	Name	Label2
	Caption	&Quantity
txtQuantity	Name	txtQuantity
	Text	(blank)
Label3	Name	Label3
	Caption	&Title
txtTitle	Name	txtTitle
	Text	(blank)
Label4	Name	Label4
	Caption	P&rice
txtPrice	Name	txtPrice
	Text	(blank)
fraOutput	Name	fraOutput
	Caption	(blank)
Label5	Name	Label5
	Caption	Extended Price
lblExtendedPrice	Name	lblExtendedPrice
	Caption	(blank)
	Alignment	Right Justify
	BorderStyle	Fixed Single
Label6	Name	Label6
	Caption	15% Discount
lblDiscount	Name	lblDiscount
	Caption	(blank)
	Alignment	Right Justify
	BorderStyle	Fixed Single
Label7	Name	Label7
	Caption	Discounted Price
lblDiscountedPrice	Name	lblDiscountedPrice
	Caption	(blank)
	Alignment	Right Justify
	BorderStyle	Fixed Single
cmdCalculate	Name	cmdCalculate
	Caption	&Calculate

(continued)

Object	Property	Setting
cmdClear	Name	cmdClear
	Caption	C&lear Sale
cmdPrint	Name	cmdPrint
	Caption	&Print
cmdExit	Name	cmdExit
	Caption	E&xit

Plan the Event Procedures

Since you have four command buttons, you need to plan the actions for four event procedures.

Event Procedure	Actions—Pseudocode
cmdCalculate_Click	Dimension the variables and constants. Convert the input Quantity and Price to numeric. Calculate Extended Price = Quantity * Price. Calculate Discount = Extended Price * Discount Rate. Calculate Discounted Price = Extended Price − Discount. Format and display output in labels.
cmdClear_Click	Set each text box and label to blanks. SetFocus in the first text box.
cmdPrint_Click	Print the form.
cmdExit_Click	Exit the project.

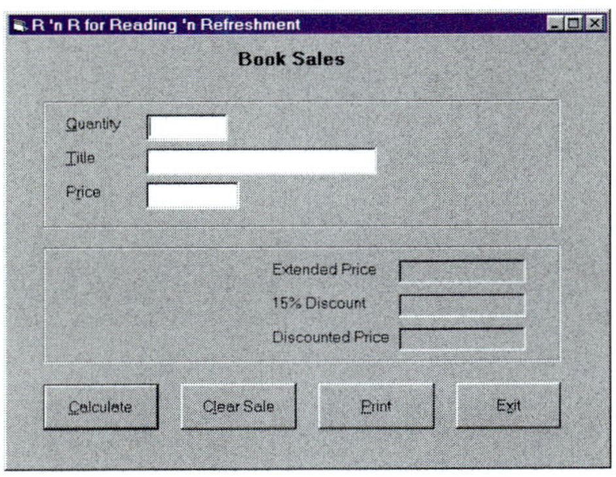

Figure 3.6

The form for the calculation programming example.

Write the Project

Follow the sketch in Figure 3.5 to create the form. Figure 3.6 shows the completed form.

- Set the properties of each object, as you have planned.
- Write the code. Working from the pseudocode, write each event procedure.
- When you complete the code, use a variety of test data to thoroughly test the project.

The Project Coding Solution

```
'Project:        Chapter Example 3.1
'Date:           February 1997
'Programmer:     J.C. Bradley
'Description:    This project demonstrates the use of variables,
'                constants, and calculations.
'Folder:         Ch0301

Option Explicit
```

```
Private Sub cmdCalculate_Click()
    'Calculate the price and discount

    Const cDISCOUNT_RATE      As Currency = 0.15
    Dim iQuantity             As Integer
    Dim cPrice                As Currency
    Dim cExtendedPrice        As Currency
    Dim cDiscount             As Currency
    Dim cDiscountedPrice      As Currency

    'Convert input values to numeric variables
    iQuantity = Val(txtQuantity.Text)
    cPrice = Val(txtPrice.Text)

    'Calculate values
    cExtendedPrice = iQuantity * cPrice
    cDiscount = cExtendedPrice * cDISCOUNT_RATE
    cDiscountedPrice = cExtendedPrice - cDiscount

    'Format and display answers
    lblExtendedPrice.Caption = Format$(cExtendedPrice, "currency")
    lblDiscount.Caption = Format$(cDiscount, "currency")
    lblDiscountedPrice.Caption = Format$(cDiscountedPrice, "currency")
End Sub
```

```
Private Sub cmdClear_Click()
    'Clear previous amounts from the form

    txtQuantity.Text = ""
    txtTitle.Text = ""
    txtPrice.Text = ""
    lblExtendedPrice.Caption = ""
    lblDiscount.Caption = ""
    lblDiscountedPrice.Caption = ""
    txtQuantity.SetFocus
End Sub
```

```
Private Sub cmdExit_Click()
    'Exit the project

    End
End Sub
```

```
Private Sub cmdPrint_Click()
    'Print the form

    PrintForm
End Sub
```

Counting and Accumulating Sums

Programs often need to sum numbers. For example, in the previous programming exercise each sale is displayed individually. If you want to accumulate a total of the sales amounts, of the discounts, or of the number of books sold, you need some new variables and new techniques.

As you know, the variables you declare inside a procedure are local to that procedure. They are re-created each time the procedure is called; that is, their lifetime is one time through the procedure. Each time the procedure is entered, you have a new fresh variable with an initial value of 0. If you want a variable to retain its value for multiple calls, in order to accumulate totals, you must declare the variable as module level. (Another approach, using Static variables, is discussed in Chapter 6.)

Summing Numbers

The technique for summing the sales amounts for multiple sales is to dimension a module-level variable for the total. Then, in the cmdCalculate_Click event for each sale, add the current amount to the total:

```
mcDiscountedPriceSum = mcDiscountedPriceSum + cDiscountedPrice
```

Reading this assignment statement from right to left, it says to add the cDiscountedPrice and the current contents of mcDiscountedPriceSum and place the result into mcDiscountedPriceSum. The effect of the statement is to add the current value for cDiscountedPrice into the sum held in mcDiscountedPriceSum.

Counting

If you want to count something, such as the number of sales in the previous example, you need another module-level variable. Dimension a counter variable as integer:

```
Dim miSaleCount as Integer
```

Then in the cmdCalculate_Click event procedure, add one to the counter variable:

```
miSaleCount = miSaleCount + 1
```

This statement, reading from right to left, adds one and the current contents of miSaleCount, placing the result in miSaleCount.

Calculating an Average

To calculate an average, divide the sum of the items by the count of the items. In the R 'n R book example, we can calculate the average sale by dividing the sum of the discounted prices by the count of the sales.

```
mcAverageDiscountedSale = mcDiscountedPriceSum / miSaleCount
```

Note: Error checking for division by zero is covered in Chapter 4.

Your Hands-On Programming Example

In this project, R 'n R—For Reading 'n Refreshment—needs to expand its book sale project done previously in this chapter. In addition to calculating individual sales and discounts, management wants to know the total number of books sold, the total number of discounts given, the total discounted amount, and the average discount per sale.

Planning the Project

Sketch a form (Figure 3.7) that your users sign off as meeting their needs.

Figure 3.7

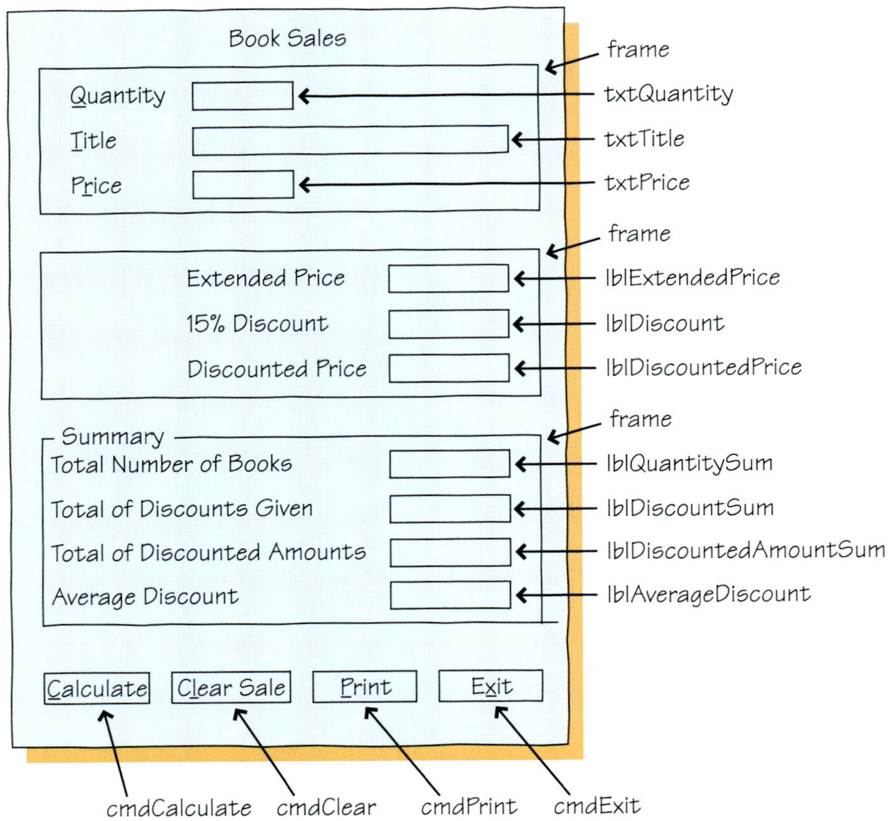

A planning sketch of the form for the hands-on programming example.

Plan the Objects and Properties

Plan the property settings for the form and each control. These objects and properties are the same as the previous example, with the addition of the summary information beginning with fraSummary.

Object	Property	Setting
Form	Name	frmBookSales
	Caption	R 'n R for Reading 'n Refreshment
Label1	Name	Label1
	Caption	Book Sales
	Font	Bold, 12 point
fraInput	Name	fraInput
	Caption	(blank)
Label2	Name	Label2
	Caption	&Quantity

(continued)

Object	Property	Setting
txtQuantity	Name	txtQuantity
	Text	(blank)
Label3	Name	Label3
	Caption	&Title
txtTitle	Name	txtTitle
	Text	(blank)
Label4	Name	Label4
	Caption	P&rice
txtPrice	Name	txtPrice
	Text	(blank)
fraOutput	Name	fraOutput
	Caption	(blank)
Label5	Name	Label5
	Caption	Extended Price
lblExtendedPrice	Name	lblExtendedPrice
	Caption	(blank)
	Alignment	Right Justify
	BorderStyle	Fixed Single
Label6	Name	Label6
	Caption	15% Discount
lblDiscount	Name	lblDiscount
	Caption	(blank)
	Alignment	Right Justify
	BorderStyle	Fixed Single
Label7	Name	Label7
	Caption	Discounted Price
lblDiscountedPrice	Name	lblDiscountedPrice
	Caption	(blank)
	Alignment	Right Justify
	BorderStyle	Fixed Single
cmdCalculate	Name	cmdCalculate
	Caption	&Calculate
cmdClear	Name	cmdClear
	Caption	C&lear Sale

(continued)

Object	Property	Setting
cmdPrint	Name	cmdPrint
	Caption	&Print
cmdExit	Name	cmdExit
	Caption	E&xit
fraSummary	Name	fraSummary
	Caption	Summary
Label8	Name	Label8
	Caption	Total Number of Books
lblQuantitySum	Name	lblQuantitySum
	Caption	(blank)
	Alignment	Right Justify
	BorderStyle	Fixed Single
Label9	Name	Label9
	Caption	Total Discounts Given
lblDiscountSum	Name	lblDiscountSum
	Caption	(blank)
	Alignment	Right Justify
	BorderStyle	Fixed Single
Label10	Name	Label10
	Caption	Total of Discounted Amounts
lblDiscountedAmountSum	Name	lblDiscountedAmountSum
	Caption	(blank)
	Alignment	Right Justify
	BorderStyle	Fixed Single
Label11	Name	Label11
	Caption	Average Discount
lblAverageDiscount	Name	lblAverageDiscount
	Caption	(blank)
	Alignment	Right Justify
	BorderStyle	Fixed Single

Plan the Event Procedures

The planning that you did for the previous example will save you time now. The only procedure that requires more steps is the cmdCalculate_Click event.

Event Procedure	Actions—Pseudocode

cmdCalculate_Click	Dimension the variables and constants.
	Convert the input Quantity and Price to numeric.
	Calculate Extended Price = Quantity * Price.
	Calculate Discount = Extended Price * Discount Rate.
	Calculate Discounted Price = Extended Price – Discount.
	Calculate the summary values:
	  Add Quantity to Quantity Sum.
	  Add Discount to Discount Sum.
	  Add Discounted Price to Discounted Price Sum.
	  Add 1 to Sale Count.
	  Calculate Average Discount = Discount Sum / Sale Count.
	Format and display sale output in labels.
	Format and display summary values in labels.

cmdClear_Click	Set each text box and label to blanks. SetFocus in the first text box.
cmdPrint_Click	Print the form.
cmdExit_Click	Exit the project.

Write the Project

Following the sketch in Figure 3.7 create the form. Figure 3.8 shows the completed form.

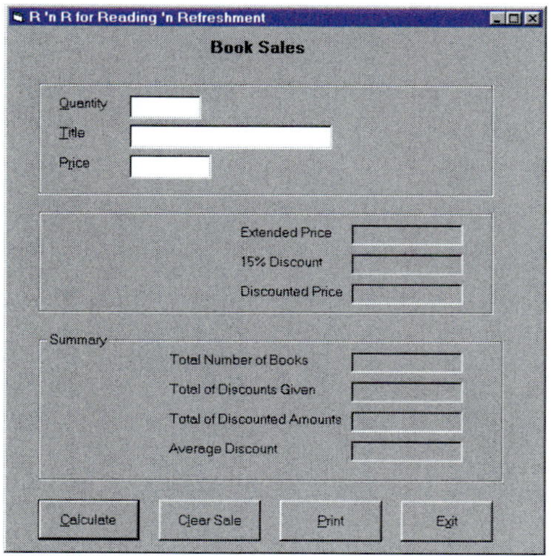

Figure 3.8

The form for the hands-on programming example.

- Set the properties of each of the objects, as you have planned.
- Write the code. Working from the pseudocode, write each event procedure.
- When you complete the code, use a variety of test data to thoroughly test the project.

The Project Coding Solution

```
'Project:         Chapter Example 3.2
'Date:            February 1997
'Programmer:      J.C. Bradley
'Description:     This project demonstrates the use of variables,
                  constants, and calculations.
'Folder:          Ch0302

Option Explicit

'Dimension module-level variables
Dim miQuantitySum          As Integer
Dim mcDiscountSum          As Currency
Dim mcDiscountedPriceSum   As Currency
Dim miSaleCount            As Integer
Dim mcAverageDiscount      As Currency
```

```
Private Sub cmdCalculate_Click()
    'Calculate the price and discount
    Const cDISCOUNT_RATE    As Currency = 0.15
    Dim iQuantity           As Integer
    Dim cPrice              As Currency
    Dim cExtendedPrice      As Currency
    Dim cDiscount           As Currency
    Dim cDiscountedPrice    As Currency
    Dim cAverageDiscount    As Currency

    'Convert input values to numeric variables
    iQuantity = Val(txtQuantity.Text)
    cPrice = Val(txtPrice.Text)

    'Calculate values for sale
    cExtendedPrice = iQuantity * cPrice
    cDiscount = cExtendedPrice * cDISCOUNT_RATE
    cDiscountedPrice = cExtendedPrice - cDiscount

    'Calculate summary values
    miQuantitySum = miQuantitySum + iQuantity
    mcDiscountSum = mcDiscountSum + cDiscount
    mcDiscountedPriceSum = mcDiscountedPriceSum + cDiscountedPrice
    miSaleCount = miSaleCount + 1
    mcAverageDiscount = mcDiscountSum / miSaleCount

    'Format and display answers for sale
    lblExtendedPrice.Caption = Format$(cExtendedPrice, "currency")
    lblDiscount.Caption = Format$(cDiscount, "currency")
    lblDiscountedPrice.Caption = Format$(cDiscountedPrice, "currency")
```

```
    'Format and display summary values
    lblQuantitySum.Caption = miQuantitySum
    lblDiscountSum.Caption = Format$(mcDiscountSum, "currency")
    lblDiscountedAmountSum.Caption = Format$(mcDiscountedPriceSum, "currency")
    lblAverageDiscount.Caption = Format$(mcAverageDiscount, "currency")
End Sub
```

```
Private Sub cmdClear_Click()
    'Clear previous amounts from the form

    txtQuantity.Text = ""
    txtTitle.Text = ""
    txtPrice.Text = ""
    lblExtendedPrice.Caption = ""
    lblDiscount.Caption = ""
    lblDiscountedPrice.Caption = ""
    txtQuantity.SetFocus
End Sub
```

```
Private Sub cmdExit_Click()
    'Exit the project

    End
End Sub
```

```
Private Sub cmdPrint_Click()
    'Print the form

    PrintForm
End Sub
```

Programming Hints

Use the `Option Explicit` statement to help avoid common coding errors.

Visual Basic does not require you to declare a variable before using it. When the variable is first used in the code, it will automatically become type Variant. However, good programming style suggests the declaration of all variables. The specification of a data type will save memory space. It is also to the programmer's advantage to declare all variables.

As an example of what might occur if the `Option Explicit` is not used, look at the following code:

```
Sub cmdCalcPay_Click()
    'Calculate Pay

    cHours = Val(txtHours.Text)
    cPayRate = Val(txtPayRate.Text)
    cPay = Hours * PayRate
    mcTotalPay = mcTotlPay + cPay
End Sub
```

Look carefully at this code, which does not generate any Visual Basic errors. What will be the values in cPay and mcTotalPay? This type of error is difficult to spot visually and, unfortunately, very easy to make. *Hint:* The code has three errors.

Are you ready for the answers? cPay and mcTotalPay will both be 0. Notice the different spellings of the variable names cHours/Hours, cPayRate/PayRate, and mcTotalPay/mcTotlPay.

You can avoid this type of error completely by setting the option that requires all variables to be declared prior to use. This technique will help in debugging projects because the compiler will detect misspelled variable names when the project is run.

The steps to setting `Option Explicit` are

1. From the *Tools* menu select *Options.*
2. On the *Editor* tab, make sure that *Require Variable Declaration* is selected.
3. Click the OK button.

When you turn on the *Require Variable Declaration* option, Visual Basic automatically adds the `Option Explicit` statements to all new forms you create after that point. VB does not add an `Option Explicit` statement to a form that has already been created. You can add an `Option Explicit` statement yourself to any existing form.

Summary

1. Variables and constants are temporary memory locations that have a name (called an *identifier*), a data type, and a scope. The value stored in a variable can be changed during the execution of the project; the values stored in constants cannot change.
2. The data type determines what values may be stored in a variable or constant. The most common data types are string, integer, currency, single precision, and Boolean. Any variable not explicitly given a data type defaults to variant.
3. Identifiers for variables and constants must follow the Visual Basic naming rules and should follow good naming standards, called *conventions.* An identifier should be meaningful and have a lowercase prefix that indicates the data type and the scope. Variable names should be mixed upper- and lowercase. The name for a constant should be uppercase, following the lowercase prefix.
4. Instrinsic constants, such as vbRed and vbBlue, are predefined and built into Visual Basic. Named constants are programmer-defined constants and are declared using the `Const` statement. The location of the `Const` statement determines the scope of the constant.
5. Variables are declared using the `Dim` statement; the location of the statement determines the scope of the variable.

6. The scope of a variable may be global, module level, or local. Local variables are available only within the procedure in which they are declared; module-level variables are accessible in all procedures within a form; global variables are available in all procedures of all modules in a project with multiple modules.
7. A Visual Basic function performs an action and returns a value. The expressions named in parentheses are called *arguments*.
8. Use the `Val` function to convert text values to numeric before performing any calculations.
9. Calculations may be performed using the values of numeric variables, constants, and the properties of controls. The result of a calculation may be assigned to a numeric variable or to the property of a control.
10. A calculation operation with more than one operator follows the order of precedence in determining the result of the calculation. Parentheses alter the order of operations.
11. The `Format` and `Format$` functions indicate how information should appear when it is displayed or printed out. Formatting can be used to specify the number of decimal positions and request commas, dollar signs, and percent signs. There are predefined numeric formats for standard, fixed, or currency. You can also create custom formats.
12. You can calculate a sum by adding each transaction to a module-level variable. In a similar fashion, you can calculate a count by adding to a module-level variable.
13. A frequent cause of errors in Basic programming is the misspelling of variable names. You can avoid this error by including the `Option Explicit` statement in the General Declarations section of each module. VB will automatically add the `Option Explicit` statement to all new modules if you set the option to *Require Variable Declaration.*

Key Terms

argument *89*
constant *79*
data type *79*
declaration *79*
format *92*
function *89*
global *85*
identifier *79*
intrinsic constant *83*
lifetime *86*
local *86*
module-level *86*
order of precedence *90*
scope *85*
string literal *83*
variable *78*
variant *79*

Review Questions

1. Name and give the purpose of five types of data available in Visual Basic.
2. What does *declaring a variable* mean?
3. What effect does the location of a `Dim` statement have upon the variable it declares?
4. Explain the difference between a constant and a variable.
5. What is the purpose of the `Val` function?
6. Explain the order of precedence of operators for calculations.
7. What statement(s) can be used to declare a variable?
8. When would it be necessary to define a format string for numeric data?
9. Should the `Format` function be included for all captions and text display in a program? Justify your answer.

Programming Exercises

3.1 Create a project that calculates the total of fat, carbohydrate, and protein calories. Allow the user to enter (in text boxes) the grams of fat, the grams of carbohydrate, and the grams of protein. Each gram of fat is nine calories, while a gram of protein or carbohydrate is four calories.

Display the total calories for the current food item in a label. Use two other labels to display an accumulated sum of the calories and a count of the items entered.

Form: The form should have three text boxes for the user to enter the grams for each category. Include labels next to each text box indicating what the user is to enter.

Include command buttons to Calculate, to Clear the text boxes, to Print, and to Exit.

Make the form's caption "Calorie Counter".

Code: Write the code for each of the command buttons.

3.2 Lennie McPherson, proprietor of Lennie's Bail Bonds, needs to calculate the amount due for setting the bail. Lennie requires something of value as collateral, and his fee is 10 percent of the bail amount. He wants the screen to provide boxes to enter the bail amount and the item being used for collateral. The program must calculate the fee. He needs to print the screen form so that he can attach it to the legal documents.

Form: Include text boxes for entering in the amount of bail and the description of the collateral. Label each text box.

Include command buttons for Calculate, Clear, Print Form, and Exit.

The caption for the form should be "Lennie's Bail Bonds".

Code: Include event procedures for the click event of each command button. Calculate the amount due as 10 percent of the bail amount and display it in a label, formatted as Currency.

3.3 In retail sales, management needs to know the average inventory figure and the turnover of merchandise. Create a project that allows the user to enter the beginning inventory, the ending inventory, and the cost of goods sold.

Form: Include labeled text boxes for the beginning inventory, the ending inventory, and the cost of goods sold. After calculating the answers, display the average inventory and the turnover formatted in labels.

Include command buttons for Calculate, Clear, Print Form, and Exit. The formulas for the calculations are

$$\text{Average inventory} = \frac{\textit{Beginning inventory} + \textit{Ending inventory}}{2}$$

$$\text{Turnover} = \frac{\textit{Cost of goods sold}}{\textit{Average inventory}}$$

Note: The average inventory is expressed in dollars; the turnover is the number of times the inventory turns over.
Code: Include procedures for the click event of each of the command buttons. Display the results in labels. Format the average inventory as Currency and the turnover as Standard.

Test Data

Beginning	Ending	Cost of Goods Sold
58500	47000	400000
75300	13600	515400
3000	19600	48000

Check Figures

Average Inventory	Turnover
$52,750.00	7.58
$44,450.00	11.60
$11,300.00	4.25

3.4 A local recording studio rents its facilities for $200 per hour. Management charges only for the number of minutes used. Create a project in which the input is the name of the group and the number of minutes it used the studio. Your program calculates the appropriate charges, accumulates the total charges for all groups, and computes the average charge and the number of groups that used the studio.
Form: Use labeled text boxes for the name of the group and the number of minutes used. The charges for the current group should be displayed formatted in a label. Create a frame for the summary information. Inside the frame, display the total charges for all groups, the number of groups, and the average charge per group.
Code: Use a constant for the rental rate per minute.

Test Data

Group	Minutes
Pooches	95
Hounds	5
Mutts	480

Check Figures

Total Charges for Group	Total Number of Groups	Average Charge	Total Charges for All Groups
$317.00	1	$317	$317.00
$17.00	2	$167	$334.00
$1,600.00	3	$645	$1,934.00

3.5 Create a project that determines the future value of an investment at a given interest rate for a given number of years. The formula for the calculation is

Future value = Investment amount * (1 + Interest rate) ^ Years

Form: Use labeled text boxes for the amount of investment, the interest rate (as a decimal fraction), and the number of years the investment will be held. Display the future value in a label.

Include command buttons for Calculate, Clear, Print Form, and Exit. Format all dollar amounts.

Test Data

Amount	Rate	Years
2000.00	.15	5
1234.56	.075	3

Check Figures

Future Value
$4,022.71
$1,533.69

3.6 Write a project that calculates the shipping charge for a package if the shipping rate is $0.12 per ounce.
Form: Use labeled text boxes for the package-identification code (a six-digit code) and the weight of the package—one box for pounds and another one for ounces. Use a label to display the shipping charge.

Include command buttons for Calculate, Clear, Print Form, and Exit.
Code: Include event procedures for each of the command buttons. Use a constant for the shipping rate, calculate the shipping charge, and display it formatted in a label.
Calculation hint: There are 16 ounces in a pound.

Test Data

ID	Weight
L5496P	0 lb. 5 oz.
J1955K	2 lb. 0 oz.
Z0000Z	1 lb. 1 oz.

Check Figures

Shipping Charge
$0.60
$3.84
$2.04

3.7 Create a project for the local car rental agency that calculates the rental charges. The agency charges $15 per day plus $0.12 per mile.
Form: Use text boxes for the customer name, address, city, state, ZIP code, beginning odometer reading, ending odometer reading, and the number of days the car was used. Use labels to display the miles driven and the total charge.

Include command buttons for Calculate, Clear, Print Form, and Exit.
Code: Include an event procedure for each command button. For the calculation, subtract the beginning odometer reading from the ending odometer reading to get the number of miles traveled. Use a constant for the $15 per day charge and the $0.12 mileage rate.

3.8 Create a project that will input an employee's sales and calculate the gross pay, deductions, and net pay. Each employee will receive a base pay of $900 plus a sales commission of 6 percent of sales.

After calculating the net pay, calculate the budget amount for each category based on the percentages given.

Pay

Base pay	$900; use a named constant
Commission	6% of sales
Gross pay	Sum of base pay and commission
Deductions	18% of gross pay
Net pay	Gross pay minus deductions

Budget

Housing	30% of net pay
Food and clothing	15% of net pay
Entertainment	50% of net pay
Miscellaneous	5% of net pay

Form: Use text boxes to input the employee's name and the dollar amount of the sales. Use labels to display the results of the calculations.

Provide command buttons for Calculate, Clear, Print Form, and Exit.

CASE STUDIES

VB Mail Order

The company has instituted a bonus program to give its employees an incentive to sell more. For every dollar the store makes in a four-week period, the employees receive 2 percent of sales. The amount of bonus each employee receives is based upon the percentage of hours he or she worked during the bonus period (a total of 160 hours).

The screen will allow the user to enter the employee's name, the total hours worked, and the amount of store's total sales. The amount of sales needs to be entered only for the first employee. (*Hint:* Don't clear it.)

The Calculate command button will determine the bonus earned by this employee, and the Clear button will clear only the name and hours worked fields. A Print Form button will be available only after the calculation has been made—it will be disabled until the Calculate button is pressed the first time. When the Clear button is pressed, the Print Form button will become disabled (Enabled = False).

VB Auto Center

Salespeople for used cars are compensated using a commission system. The commission is calculated based on the costs incurred for the vehicle.

Commission =
 Commission rate × (Sales price − Cost value)

The screen will allow for the user to enter the salesperson's name, the selling price of the vehicle, and the cost value of the vehicle. Use a constant of 20 percent for the commission rate.

The Calculate command button will determine the commission earned by the salesperson; the Clear button will clear the text boxes. A Print Form button will be available only after the calculation has been made—it will be disabled until the Calculate button is pressed the first time. When the Clear button is pressed, the Print Form button will become disabled (Enabled = False).

C H A P T E R

4

Decisions and Conditions

At the completion of this chapter, you will be able to . . .

1. Use block `If`s to control the flow of logic.
2. Understand and use nested `If`s.
3. Read and create flowcharts indicating the logic in a selection process.
4. Evaluate conditions using the relational operators.
5. Combine conditions using `And` and `Or`.
6. Test the Value property of option buttons and check boxes.
7. Perform validation on numeric fields.
8. Call event procedures from other procedures.
9. Create message boxes to display error conditions.
10. Apply the message box constants.
11. Debug projects using breakpoints, stepping program execution, and displaying intermediate results.

In this section you will learn to write projects that can take one action or another, based on a condition. For example, you may need to keep track of sales separately for different classes of employees, different sections of the country, or different departments. You may want to check the value entered by the user to make sure it is valid and display an error message for inappropriate values.

If Statements

A powerful asset of the computer is its ability to make decisions and to take alternate courses of action based on the outcome.

A decision made by the computer is formed as a question: Is a given condition true or false? If it is true, do one thing; if it is false, do something else.

If *the sun is shining* Then	(condition)
go to the beach	(action to take if condition is true)
Else	
go to class	(action to take if condition is false)
End If	(See Figure 4.1.)

Figure 4.1

The logic of an `If...Then...Else` *statement in flowchart form.*

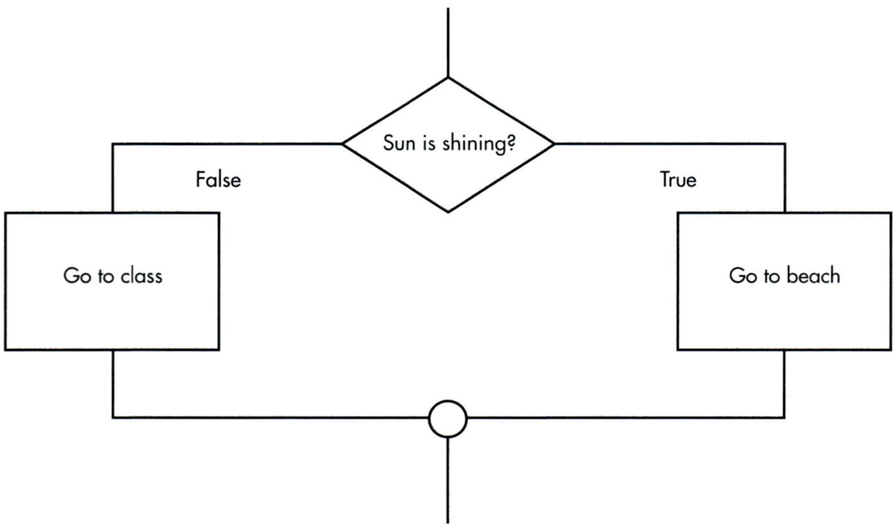

or

If *you don't succeed* Then	(condition)
try, try again	(action)
End If	(See Figure 4.2)

Figure 4.2

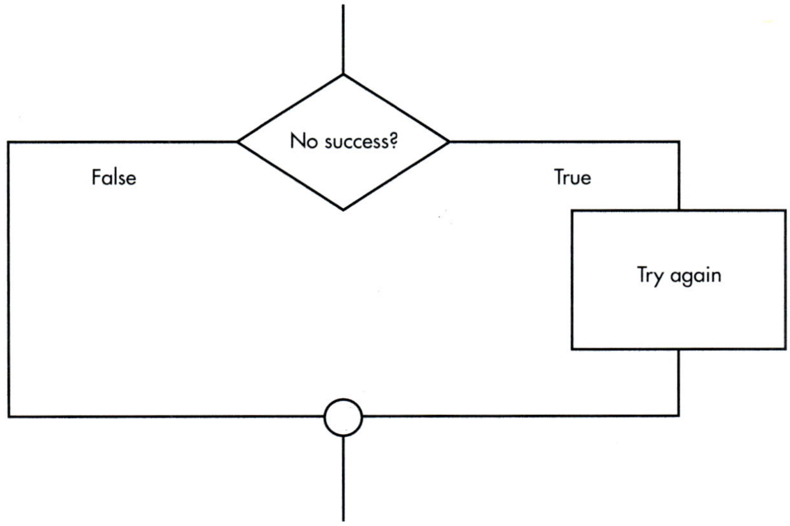

The logic of an `If` *statement without an* `Else` *action in flowchart form.*

Notice in the second example that no action is specified if the condition is not true.

In an `If` statement, when the condition is true, only the `Then` clause is executed. When the condition is false, only the `Else` clause, if present, is executed.

If...Then...Else Statement—General Form

```
If (condition) Then
   statement(s)
[ElseIf (condition) Then
   statement(s)]
[Else
   statements(s)]
End If
```

A block **`If...Then...Else`** must always conclude with **`End If`**. The word `Then` must appear on the same line as the `If` with nothing following `Then` (except a remark). `End If` and `Else` (if used) must appear alone on a line. The statements under the `Then` and `Else` clause are indented for readability and clarity.

Notice that the keyword `ElseIf` is all one word but that `End If` is two words.

If..Then..Else Statement—Examples

When the number of units in cUnits is less than 32, select the option button for *Freshman;* otherwise, make sure the button is unselected (Figure 4.3). Remember that when an option button is selected, the Value property has a Boolean value of True.

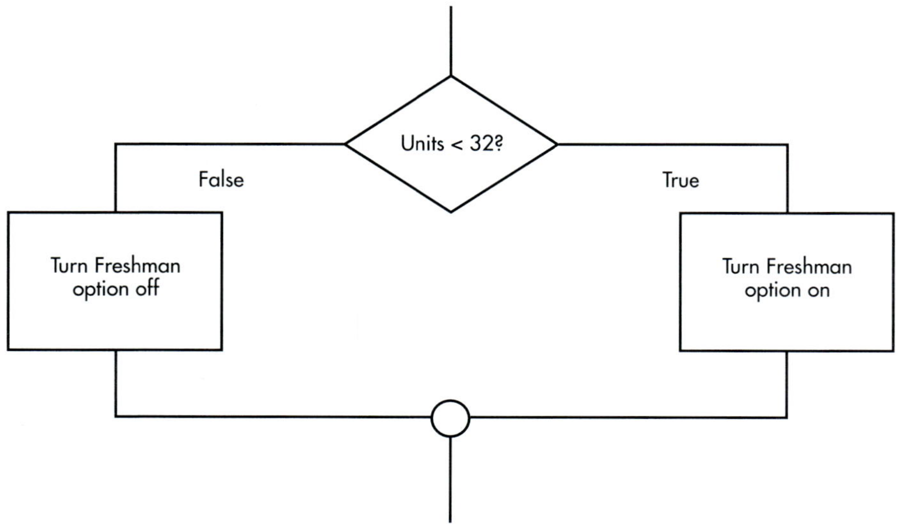

Figure 4.3

The `If` *statement logic in flowchart form. If the number of units is less than 32, the Freshman option button will be selected; otherwise, the Freshman option will be deselected.*

```
cUnits = Val(txtUnits.Text)

If cUnits < 32 Then
    optFreshman.Value = True
Else
    optFreshman.Value = False
End If
```

Tip

Always take the time to indent properly as you enter an `If` statement. You will save yourself debugging time; the indentation helps to visualize the intended logic.

Flowcharting If Statements

A flowchart is a useful tool for showing the logic of an `If` statement. It has been said that one picture is worth a thousand words. Many programmers find that a flowchart helps them organize their thoughts and design projects more quickly.

The symbols used in this text are a subset of the available flowcharting symbols. The diamond-shape symbol (called a *decision symbol*) represents a condition. The two branches from the symbol indicate which path to take when the condition evaluates True or False. (See Figure 4.4.)

Figure 4.4

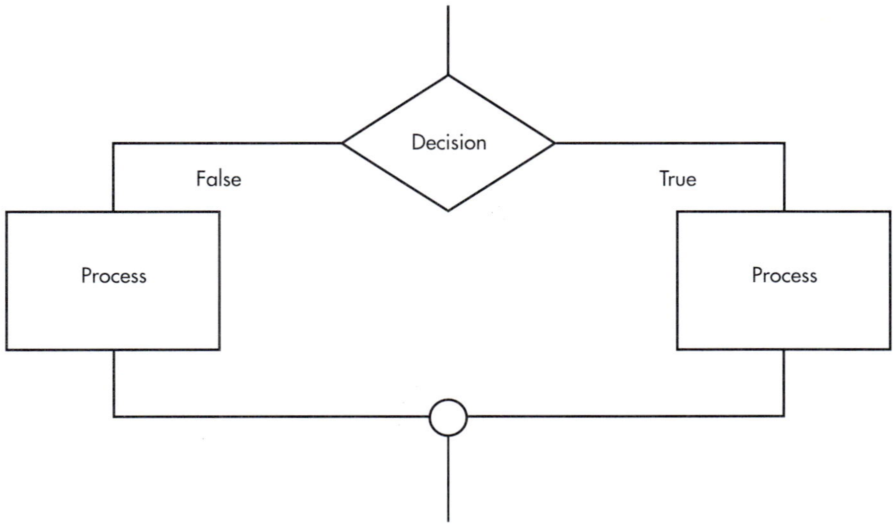

The flowcharting symbols used for program decisions and processes.

Conditions

The test in an `If` statement is based on a **condition**. To form conditions, six **relational operators** (Table 4.1) are used to compare values. The result of the comparison is either True or False.

Table 4.1

The six relational operators.

Symbol	Relation Tested	Examples
>	greater than	`Val(txtAmount.Text) > mcLIMIT` `frmMain.Height > mcSize`
<	less than	`Val(txtSales.Text) < 10000` `txtName.Text < stName`
=	equal to	`txtPassword.Text = "101"` `optButton1.Value = True`
<>	not equal to	`optButton1.Value <> True` `txtPassword.Text <> "101"`
>=	greater than or equal to	`Val(lblCorrect.Caption) >= 1000` `frmMain.Height >= 500`
<=	less than or equal to	`txtName1.Text <= txtName2.Text`

The conditions to be tested can be formed with numeric variables and constants, string variables and constants, object properties, and arithmetic expressions. However, it is important to note that comparisons must be made on like types; that is, strings can be compared only to other strings, and numeric values can be compared only to other numeric values, whether a variable, constant, property, or arithmetic expression.

Comparing Numeric Variables and Constants

When numeric values are involved in a test, an algebraic comparison is made; that is, the sign of the number is taken into account. Therefore, negative 20 is less than 10, and negative 2 is less than negative 1.

Even though an equal sign (=) means replacement in an assignment statement, in a relation test the equal sign is used to test for equality. For example, the condition

```
If Val(txtPrice.Text) = cMAX Then
```

means "Is the current numeric value stored in txtPrice.Text equal to the value stored in cMAX?"

Sample Comparisons

iAlpha	iBravo	iCharlie
5	4	−5

Condition	Evaluates
`iAlpha = iBravo`	False
`iCharlie < 0`	True
`iBravo > iAlpha`	False
`iCharlie <= iBravo`	True
`iAlpha >= 5`	True
`iAlpha <> iCharlie`	True

Comparing Strings

String variables can be compared to other string variables or string literals enclosed in quotation marks. The comparison begins with the left-most character and proceeds one character at a time from left to right. As soon as a character in one string is not equal to the corresponding character in the second string, the comparison is terminated, and the string with the lower ranking character is judged less than the other.

The determination of which character is less than another is based on the code used to store characters internally in the computer. The code, called the ***ASCII code*** (pronounced "ask-key"), has an established order (called the *collating sequence*) for all letters, numbers, and special characters. (ASCII stands for American Standard Code for Information Interchange.) Note in Table 4.2, that *A* is less than *B*, *L* is greater than *K*, and all numeric digits are less than all letters. Some special symbols are lower than the numbers and some are higher, and the blank space is lower than the rest of the characters shown.

Table 4.2

The ASCII collating sequence.

ASCII Code	Character
32	Space (blank)
33	!
34	"
35	#
36	$
37	%
38	&
39	' (apostrophe)
40	(
41	)
42	*
43	+
44	, (comma)
45	−
46	.
47	/
48	0
49	1
50	2
51	3
52	4
53	5
54	6
55	7
56	8
57	9
58	:
59	;

(continued)

ASCII Code	Character
60	<
61	=
62	>
63	?
64	@
65	A
66	B
67	C
68	D
69	E
70	F
71	G
72	H
73	I
74	J
75	K
76	L
77	M
78	N
79	O
80	P
81	Q
82	R
83	S
84	T
85	U
86	V
87	W
88	X
89	Y
90	Z
91	[
92	\
93	]

(continued)

ASCII Code	Character
94	^
95	_
96	‘
97	a
98	b
99	c
100	d
101	e
102	f
103	g
104	h
105	I
106	j
107	k
108	l
109	m
110	n
111	o
112	p
113	q
114	r
115	s
116	t
117	u
118	v
119	w
120	x
121	y
122	z
123	{
124	|
125	}
126	~
127	Del

txtPerson1.Text
JOHN

txtPerson2.Text
JOAN

The condition txtPerson1.Text < txtPerson2.Text evaluates False. The *A* in JOAN is lower ranking than the *H* in JOHN.

txtWord1.Text
HOPE

txtWord2.Text
HOPELESS

The condition txtWord1.Text < txtWord2.Text evaluates True. When one string is shorter than the other, it compares as if the shorter string is padded with blanks to the right of the string, and the blank space is compared to a character in the longer string.

lblCar1.Caption
300ZX

lblCar2.Caption
PORSCHE

The condition lblCar1.Caption < lblCar2.Caption evaluates True. When the number *3* is compared to the letter *P*, the *3* is lower, since all numbers are lower ranking than all letters.

Feedback 4.1

iCountOne	iCountTwo	iCountThree	txtFour.Text	txtFive.Text
5	5	−5	"Bit"	"Bite"

Determine which conditions will evaluate True and which ones will evaluate False.

1. iCountOne >= iCountTwo
2. iCountThree < 0
3. iCountThree < iCountTwo
4. iCountOne <> iCountTwo
5. iCountOne + 2 > iCountTwo + 2
6. txtFour.Text < txtFive.Text
7. txtFour.Text <> txtFive.Text
8. txtFour.Text > "D"
9. "2" <> "Two"
10. "$" <= "?"

Testing for True or False

You can use shortcuts when testing for True or False. Visual Basic evaluates the condition in an `If` statement. If the condition is a Boolean variable name, it holds the values True or False.

For example:

```
If bSuccessfulOperation = True Then ...
```

is equivalent to

```
If bSuccessfulOperation Then ...
```

Boolean variables hold the value 0 when False, and negative 1 when True. You can actually test *any* variable for True or False. Visual Basic considers any numeric variable with a value of 0 to be False; any other value will evaluate True. The variable or expression is referred to as an **implied condition.**

Examples

```
iCounter = 10
If iCounter Then ...      'Evaluates True

iTotal = 0
If iTotal Then ...        'Evaluates False
```

Comparing the Text Property of Text Boxes

When you compare the Text property of a text box with another value, you must be careful. The Text property behaves like a variant. That is, if you use it like a string, it acts like a string; but if you use it like a number, it acts like a number. However, sometimes your intentions are not clear, and sometimes you are using the Text property as numeric, but the user enters non-numeric data or no data at all.

Visual Basic compares one text box to another as strings and compares a text box to a numeric variable or constant with a numeric compare. You can force a numeric comparison on a Text property by using the `Val` function. You should always use the `Val` function on a numeric Text property when you need to compare or calculate. Remember, the `Val` function converts blank values to zero.

Examples

txtFirst.Text	txtSecond.Text	txtFirst.Text > txtSecond.Text	Val(txtFirst.Text) > Val(txtSecond.Text)
1	+1	True	False
2	100	True	False
+100	−100	False	True
0	(blank)	True	False

Comparing Uppercase and Lowercase Characters

When comparing strings, the case of the characters is important. An uppercase *Y* is not equal to a lowercase *y*. Since the user may type a name or word in uppercase, lowercase, or as a combination of cases, we must check all possibilities. The easiest way is to use the string function `Ucase` or `Lcase`, which returns the uppercase or lowercase equivalent of a string, respectively.

Ucase and Lcase—General Form

```
Ucase(string)
Lcase(string)
```

Ucase and Lcase—Examples

txtOne.Text Value	Ucase(txtOne.Text)	Lcase(txtOne.Text)
Basic	BASIC	basic
PROGRAMMING	PROGRAMMING	programming
Robert Jones	ROBERT JONES	robert jones
hello	HELLO	hello

An example of a condition using the `Ucase` function follows.

```
If Ucase(txtOne.Text) = "BASIC" Then
   'Do something
End If
```

Note that when you convert txtOne.Text to uppercase, you must compare it to an uppercase literal ("BASIC") if you want it to evaluate as True.

Compound Conditions

You can use **compound conditions** to test more than one condition. Create compound conditions by joining conditions with **logical operators**. The logical operators are `Or`, `And`, and `Not`.

Logical Operator	Meaning	Example
`Or`	If one condition or both conditions are true, the entire condition is true.	`lblNumber.Caption = 1 Or _` `lblNumber.Caption = 2`
`And`	Both conditions must be true for the entire condition to be true.	`txtNumber.Text > 0 And _` `txtNumber.Text < 10`
`Not`	Reverses the condition so that a true condition will evaluate false and vice versa.	`Not lblNumber.Caption = 0`

```
If optMale.Value = True And Val(txtAge.Text) < 21 Then
       miMinorMaleCount = miMinorMaleCount + 1
End If
If optJunior.Value = True Or optSenior.Value = True Then
       miUpperClassmanCount = miUpperClassmanCount + 1
End If
```

The first example requires that both the option button test and the age test be true for the count to be incremented. In the second example, only one of the conditions must be true.

One caution when using compound conditions: Each side of the logical operator must be a complete condition. For example,

```
optJunior.Value Or optSenior.Value = True
```

is incorrect.

Combining `And` and `Or`

You can create compound conditions that combine multiple `And` and `Or` conditions. When you have both an `And` and an `Or`, the `And` is evaluated before the `Or`. However, you can change the order of evaluation by using parentheses; any condition inside parentheses will be evaluated first.

For example, will the following condition evaluate True or False? Try it with various values for cSale, optDiscount, and txtState.Text.

```
If cSale > 1000 Or optDiscount.Value = True And Ucase(txtState.Text) <> "CA" Then
     '(Calculate the discount)
End If
```

cSale	optDiscount.Value	Ucase(txtState.Text)	Condition Evaluates
1500	False	CA	True
1000	True	OH	True
1000	True	CA	False
1500	True	NY	True
1000	False	CA	False

Using If Statements with Option Buttons and Check Boxes

In Chapter 2 you used the Click event for option buttons and check boxes to carry out the desired action. Now that you can use `If` statements, you should not take action in the Click events for these controls. Instead, use `If` statements to determine which options are selected.

To conform to good programming practice and make your programs consistent with standard Windows applications, place your code in the Click event of command buttons. For example, refer to the Visual Basic *Print* dialog box (Figure 4.5); no action will occur when you click on an option button or check box. Instead, when you click on the OK button, VB checks to see which options are selected.

Figure 4.5

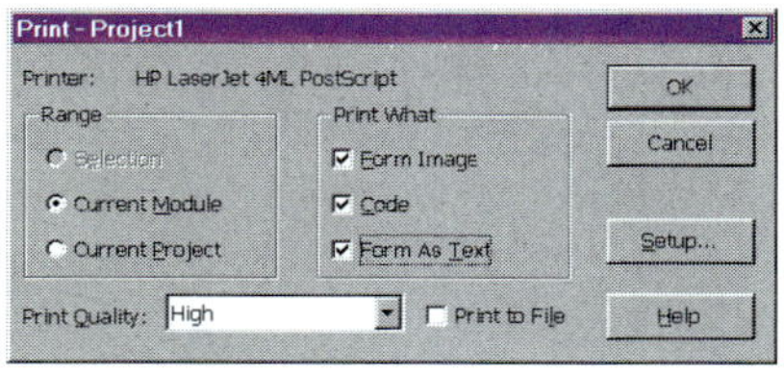

The Visual Basic Print *dialog box. When the user clicks OK, the program checks the state of all option buttons and check boxes.*

In an application such as the message formatter project in Chapter 2 (refer to Figure 2.18), you could add a Display command button and include code similar to the following:

```
If chkBlue.Value = True Then
    lblName.BackColor = vbBlue
End If
```

```
If optItalic.Value = True Then
    txtTitle.Font.Italic = True
Else
    txtTitle.Font.Italic = False
End If
```

A "Simple Sample"

Test your understanding of the use of the `If` statement by coding some short examples.

Test the Value of a Check Box

Create a small project that contains a check box, a label, and a command button. Name the command button cmdTest, the check box chkTest, and the label lblMessage. In the Click event for cmdTest, check the value of the check box. If the check box is currently checked, display "Check box is checked" in lblMessage.

```
Private Sub cmdTest_Click()
    'Test the value of the check box

    If chkTest.Value = Checked Then
       lblMessage.Caption = "Check box is checked"
    End If
```

Test your project. When it works, add an `Else` to the code that displays "Check box is not checked".

Test the Value of Option Buttons

Remove the check box from the previous project and replace it with two option buttons, named optFreshman and optSophomore and captioned "< 30 units" and ">= 30 units". Now change the `If` statement to display "Freshman" or "Sophomore" in the label.

```
If optFreshman.Value = True Then
    lblMessage.Caption = "Freshman"
Else
    lblMessage.Caption = "Sophomore"
End If
```

Can you modify the sample to work for Freshman, Sophomore, Junior, and Senior?

Nested If Statements

In many programs another `If` statement is one of the statements to be executed when a condition tests True or False. `If` statements that contain additional `If` statements are said to be ***nested*** **`If`** statements. The following example shows a nested `If` statement in which the second `If` occurs in the `Then` portion of the first `If` (Figure 4.6).

Figure 4.6

Flowcharting a nested `If` *statement.*

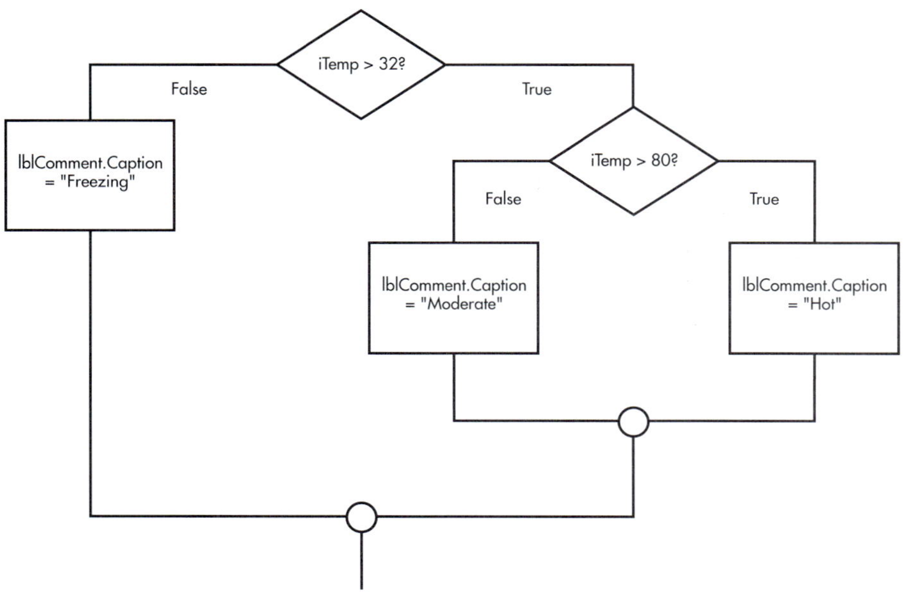

```
If iTemp > 32 Then
     If iTemp > 80 Then
         lblComment.Caption = "Hot"
     Else
         lblComment.Caption = "Moderate"
     End If
Else
     lblComment.Caption = "Freezing"
End If
```

To nest `If` statements in the `Else` portion, you may use either of the following approaches; however, your code is simpler if you use the second method (using `ElseIf...Then`).

```
If iTemp <= 32 Then
    lblComment.Caption = "Freezing"
Else
    If iTemp > 80 Then
        lblComment.Caption = "Hot"
    Else
     lblComment.Caption = "Moderate"
    End If
End If
```

```
If iTemp <= 32 Then
     lblComment.Caption = "Freezing"
ElseIf iTemp > 80 Then
     lblComment.Caption = "Hot"
Else
     lblComment.Caption = "Moderate"
End If
```

You may nest `Ifs` in both the `Then` and `Else`. In fact, you may continue to nest `Ifs` within `Ifs` as long as each `If` has an `End If`. However, projects become very difficult to follow (and may not perform as intended) when `Ifs` become too deeply nested (Figure 4.7.)

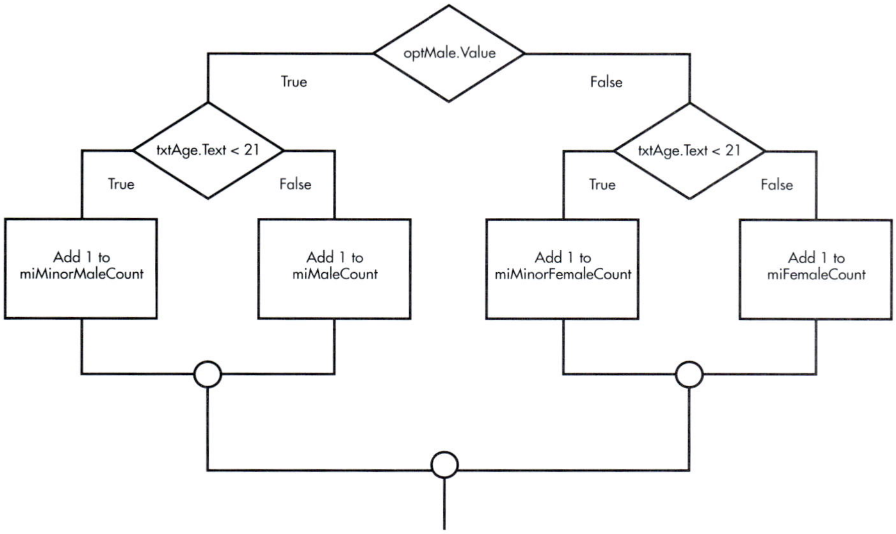

Figure 4.7

A flowchart of a nested `If` statement with `If`s nested on both sides of the original `If`.

```
If optMale.Value = True Then
     If txtAge.Text < 21 Then
          miMinorMaleCount = miMinorMaleCount + 1
     Else
          miMaleCount = miMaleCount + 1
     End If
Else
     If txtAge.Text < 21 Then
          miMinorFemaleCount = miMinorFemaleCount + 1
     Else
          miFemaleCount = miFemaleCount + 1
     End If
End If
```

Tip

Indentation can help you catch errors. Visual Basic always matches an `Else` with the last unmatched `If`, regardless of the indentation.

Feedback 4.2

Assume that `iFrogs` = 10, and `iToads` = 5, and `iPolliwogs` = 6. What will be displayed for each of the following statements?

1.
```
If iFrogs > iPolliwogs Then
     optFrogs.Value = True
     optToads.Value = False
Else
     optFrogs.Value = False
     optToads.Value = True
End If
```

2.
```
If iFrogs > iToads + iPolliwogs Then
    lblResult.Caption = "It's the frogs"
Else
    lblResult.Caption = "It's the toads and the polliwogs"
End If
```
3.
```
If iPolliwogs > iToads And iFrogs <> 0 Or iToads = 0 Then
    lblResult.Caption = "It's true"
Else
    lblResult.Caption = "It's false"
End If
```
4. Write the statements necessary to compare txtApples.Text and txtOranges.Text. Display in lblMost.Caption which has more, the apples or the oranges.
5. Write the Basic statements that will test the current value of cBalance. When cBalance is greater than 0, the check box for Funds Available called chkFunds should be selected, the cBalance set back to 0, and iCounter incremented by 1. When cBalance is 0 or less, chkFunds should not be selected (do not change the value of cBalance or increment the counter).

Input Validation

Careful programmers check the values entered into text boxes before beginning the calculations. Validation is a form of self-protection; it is better to reject bad data than to spend hours (and sometimes days) trying to find an error only to discover that the problem was caused by a "user error." Finding and correcting the error early can often keep the program from producing erroneous results or halting with a run-time error.

Checking to verify that appropriate values have been entered for a text box is called ***validation***. The validation may include checking the type of data, checking for specific values, or checking a range of values.

Checking the Data Type

You can make sure that data entered is truly numeric with Visual Basic's `IsNumeric` function. The `IsNumeric` function returns True or False to indicate the result of the value checking.

The IsNumeric Function—General Form

```
IsNumeric(expression)
```

The `IsNumeric` function tests whether the value is numeric and therefore can be used in a calculation. If numeric, the result will be True; if not, the result is False. This function can help avoid problems in procedures that contain calculations. If the data cannot be converted to a number, the calculation cannot be performed and a run-time error will occur. The only way the programmer can prevent the user from making this type of error is to check the contents of the field after the data has been entered.

The IsNumeric Function—Example

```
If IsNumeric(txtQuantity.Text) Then
     iQuantity = Val(txtQuantity.Text)
     lblDue.Caption = cPrice * iQuantity
End If
```

Checking for a Range of Values

Data validation may also include checking the reasonableness of a value. Assume you are using a text box to input the number of hours worked in a day. Even with overtime, the company does not allow more than 10 work hours in a single day. You could check the input for reasonableness with this code:

```
If Val(txtHours.Text) > 10 Then
        '.......
End If
```

So what should we do if the value is out of range? One solution is to display a message box to the user.

Message Boxes

A **message box** is a special type of Visual Basic window in which you can display a message to the user. You can display a message, an optional icon, a title bar caption, and command button(s) in a message box (Figure 4.8).

Validating input data is an appropriate time to use a message box. If we reject bad data, we need to tell the user why the desired action was not achieved.

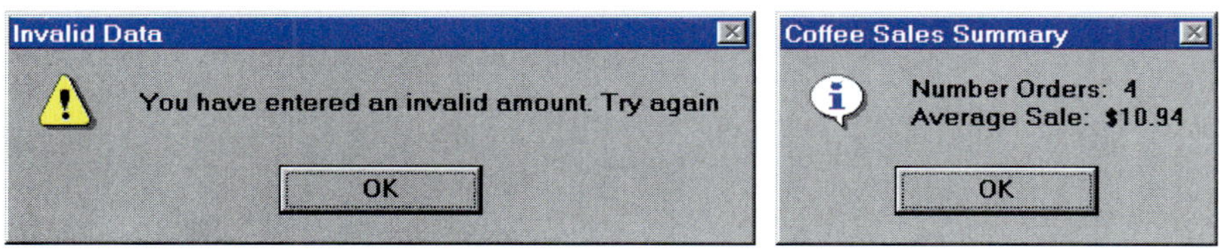

Figure 4.8

Two sample message boxes created with the `MsgBox` *statement.*

The MsgBox Statement—General Form

```
MsgBox "Message string" [, Buttons/icon][, "Caption of title bar"]
```

The *Message string* is the message you want to appear in the message box. The *Buttons* portion is optional; it determines the command buttons that will display and any icons that will appear. If you omit the *Caption of title bar,* the project name will appear in the message box title bar.

Usually you will display a message box in the `Else` clause of an `If` statement when checking the validity of data.

The MsgBox Statement—Example

```
If IsNumeric(txtQuantity.Text) Then
    iQuantity = Val(txtQuantity.Text)
    lblDue.Caption = cPrice * iQuantity
Else
    MsgBox "Please Enter a Numeric Value", vbOKOnly, "Error"
End If
```

Selecting the MsgBox Icon

For the button/icon entry, you can choose to use the numeric values in the following table, or to use the Visual Basic constant. For example, you can display the Warning Query icon with either of these statements:

```
MsgBox "Let this be a warning", vbQuestion, "Error"
```

or

```
MsgBox "Let this be a warning", 32, "Error"
```

Button/Icon	Value	Constant
OK button	0	vbOKOnly
Critical Message icon	16	vbCritical
Warning Query icon	32	vbQuestion
Warning Message icon	48	vbExclamation
Information Message icon	64	vbInformation

Note: MsgBox can be used as a statement, as explained here, which displays only an OK button. It can also be used as a function. When you use MsgBox as a function, you can choose the buttons to display (such as Yes, No, Cancel; or OK and Cancel). The function returns a value indicating which button was pressed. The MsgBox function is covered in Chapter 7.

Displaying a Message String

The message string you display may be a string literal enclosed in quotes or it may be a string variable. You may also want to concatenate several items, for example, combining a literal with a value from a variable. If the message you specify is too long for one line, Visual Basic will wrap it to the next line.

Combining Values into a Message String

You can concatenate a literal such as "Total Sales" with the value for the total sales:

```
Dim stMessageString As String

stMessageString = "Total Sales " & mcTotalSales
MsgBox stMessageString, vbOKOnly, "Sales Summary"
```

This example does not format the number. To remedy this condition, consider formatting the number before concatenating it to the string.

```
Dim stFormattedTotal  As String
Dim stMessageString   As String

stFormattedTotal = Format$(mcTotalSales, "Standard")
stMessageString = "Total Sales " & stFormattedTotal
MsgBox stMessageString, vbOKOnly, "Sales Summary"
```

Creating Multiple Lines of Output

If you want to display multiple lines of output, you can insert a line feed/carriage return code into the line. Use the Visual Basic intrinsic constant vbCRLF to determine line endings. You can concatenate this constant into a message string to set up multiple lines. This will allow you to determine the position of the line break, rather than rely on word wrap.

In this example, a second line is added to the MsgBox from the previous example.

```
Dim stFormattedTotal  As String
Dim stMessageString   As String

stFormattedTotal = Format$(mcTotalSales, "Standard")
stFormattedAvg = Format$(mcAverageSale, "Standard")
stMessageString = "Total Sales " & stFormattedTotal & vbCRLF & _
                  "Average Sale " & stFormattedAvg
MsgBox stMessageString, vbOKOnly, "Sales Summary"
```

Calling Event Procedures

If you wish to perform a set of instructions in more than one location, you don't have to duplicate the code. Write the instructions once, in an event procedure, and "call" the procedure from another procedure. When you **call** an event procedure, the entire procedure is executed and then execution returns to the statement following the call.

The Call Statement (No Arguments)—General Form

```
[Call] ProcedureName
```

Notice that the keyword `Call` is optional and rarely used.

The Call Statement—Examples

```
Call cmdCalculate_Click
cmdCalculate_Click  'Equivalent to previous statement
```

In the programming example that follows, you will accumulate individual items for one customer. When that customer's order is complete, you need to clear the entire order and begin an order for the next customer. Refer to the interface in Figure 4.9; notice the two command buttons: *Clear for Next Item* and *New Order*. The command button for next item clears the text boxes on the screen. The command button for a new order must clear the screen text boxes *and* clear the subtotal fields. Rather than repeat the instructions to clear the individual screen text boxes, we can call the event procedure for cmdNewOrder from the cmdClear_Click procedure.

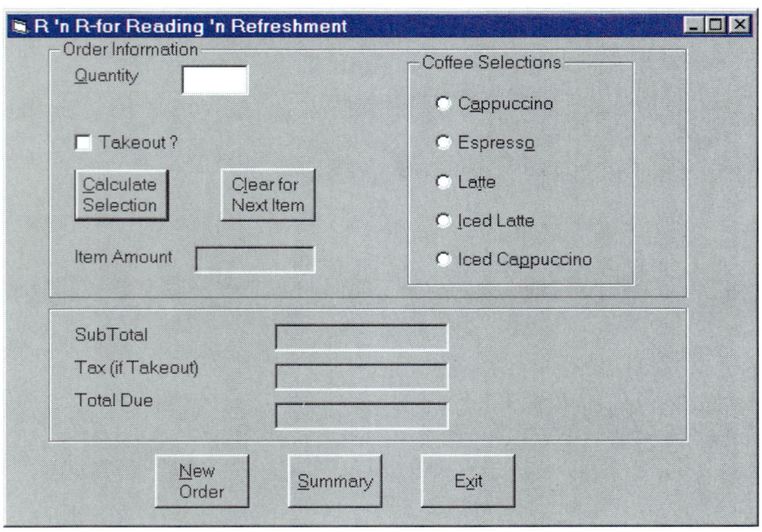

Figure 4.9

A form with command buttons that perform overlapping functions. The New Order button must do the same tasks as Clear for New Item.

```
Private Sub cmdNewOrder_Click()
     'Clear the current item and the current order

     cmdClear_Click 'call the procedure for the click event of cmdClear
     ... 'Continue with statements to clear subtotals
```

In the cmdNewOrder_Click procedure, all of the instructions in cmdClear_Click are executed. Then execution returns to the next statement following the call.

Your Hands-On Programming Example

Create a project for R 'n R—for Reading 'n Refreshment that calculates the amount due for individual orders and maintains accumulated totals for a summary. Have a check box for takeout items, which are taxable (8 percent); all other orders are nontaxable. Include option buttons for the five coffee selections—Cappuccino, Espresso, Latte, Iced Cappuccino, and Iced Latte. The prices for each will be assigned using these constants:

Cappuccino	2.00
Espresso	2.25
Latte	1.75
Iced (either)	2.50

Use a command button for Calculate This Item, which will calculate and display the amount due for each item. A button for Clear for Next Item will clear the selections and amount for the single item. Additional labels in a separate frame will maintain the summary information for the current order to include subtotal, tax, and total.

Buttons at the bottom of the form will be used for Next Order, Summary, and Exit. The Next Order button will clear the bill for the current customer and add to the totals for the summary. The button for Summary should display the average sale amount per customer and the number of customers.

Planning the Project

Sketch a form (Figure 4.10), which your users sign as meeting their needs.

Figure 4.10

The planning sketch of the form for the hands-on programming exercise.

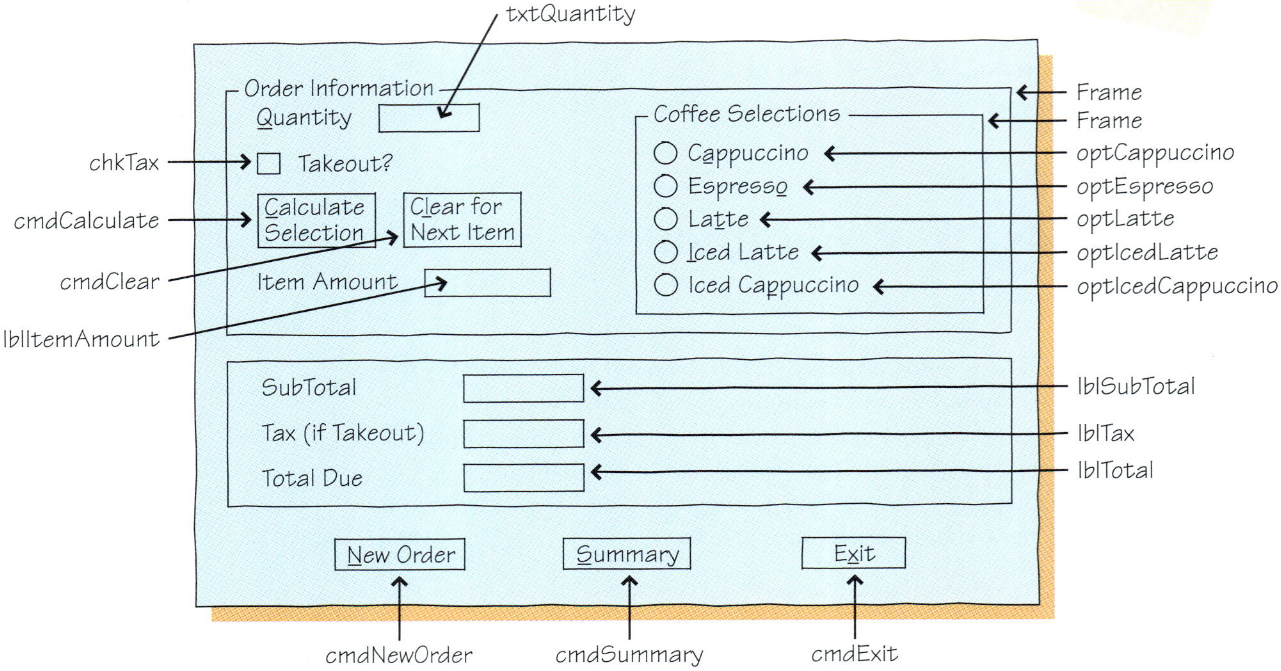

Plan the Objects and Properties

Plan the property settings for the form and each of the controls.

Object	Property	Setting
frmBilling	Name	frmBilling
	Caption	R 'n R—for Reading 'n Refreshment
Frame1	Caption	Order Information
Frame2	Caption	Coffee Selections
Frame3	Caption	(blank)
optCappuccino	Name	optCappuccino
	Caption	C&appuccino
optEspresso	Name	optEspresso
	Caption	Espress&o
optLatte	Name	optLatte
	Caption	La&tte
optIcedLatte	Name	optIcedLatte
	Caption	&Iced Latte

(continued)

Object	Property	Setting
optIcedCappuccino	Name	optIcedCappuccino
	Caption	Iced Ca&ppuccino
Label1	Caption	&Quantity
txtQuantity	Name	txtQuantity
	Text	(blank)
chkTax	Name	chkTax
	Caption	Takeout ?
Label2	Caption	Item Amount
Label3	Caption	SubTotal
Label4	Caption	Tax (if Takeout)
Label5	Caption	Total Due
lblItemAmount	Name	lblItemAmount
	Caption	(blank)
	BorderStyle	1 - FixedSingle
lblSubTotal	Name	lblSubTotal
	Caption	(blank)
	BorderStyle	1 - Fixed Single
lblTax	Name	lblTax
	Caption	(blank)
	BorderStyle	1 - Fixed Single
lblTotal	Name	lblTotal
	Caption	(blank)
	BorderStyle	1 - Fixed Single
cmdCalculate	Name	cmdCalculate
	Caption	&Calculate Selection
	Default	True
cmdClear	Name	cmdClear
	Caption	C&lear for Next Item
	Cancel	True
cmdNewOrder	Name	cmdNewOrder
	Caption	&New Order
cmdSummary	Name	cmdSummary
	Caption	&Summary
cmdExit	Name	cmdExit
	Caption	E&xit

Plan the Event Procedures

You need to plan the actions for five event procedures for the command.

Object	Procedure	Action
cmdCalculate	Click	Determine price per cup. Multiply price by quantity. Calculate tax if needed. Calculate total = subtotal + tax. Display the values.
cmdClear	Click	Clear the coffee selections. Clear the quantity and the item price. Disable the takeout check box. Set the focus to the quantity.
cmdSummary	Click	Display the average. Display the number of customers.
cmdNewOrder	Click	Clear the previous order. Accumulate total sales and count. Set subtotal and total due to 0. Enable takeout check box.
cmdExit	Click	Terminate the project.

Write the project

Follow the sketch in Figure 4.10 to create the form. Figure 4.11 shows the completed form.

Figure 4.11

The form for the hands-on programming exercise.

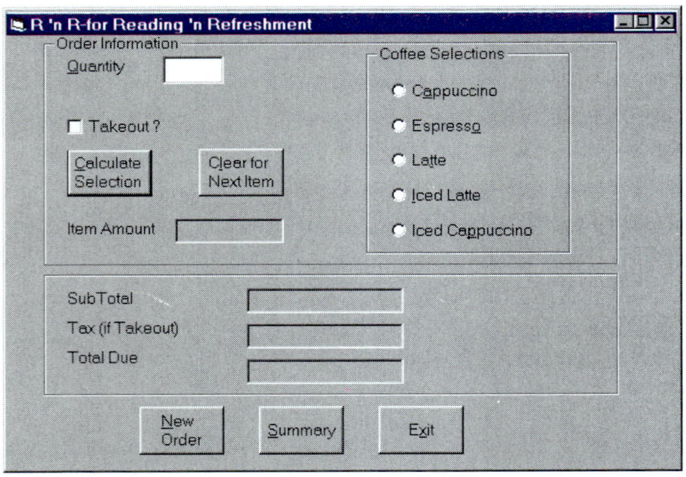

- Set the properties of each object as you have planned.
- Write the code. Working from the pseudocode, write each event procedure.
- When you complete the code, use a variety of data to thoroughly test the project. Make sure the tab order is set correctly so that the insertion point begins in txtQuantity.

The Project Coding Solution

```
'Program Name:    Billing
'Programmer:      A. Millspaugh
'Date:            July 1997
'Description:     This project calculates the amount due
'                 based on the customer selection
'                 and accumulates summary data for the day.
'Folder:          Ch0401

Option Explicit
Dim mcSubtotal                  As Currency
Dim mcTotal                     As Currency
Dim mcGrandTotal                As Currency
Dim miCustomerCount             As Integer
Const cCAPPUCCINO_PRICE         As Currency = 2
Const cESPRESSO_PRICE           As Currency = 2.25
Const cLATTE_PRICE              As Currency = 1.75
Const cICED_PRICE               As Currency = 2.5
```

```
Private Sub cmdCalculate_Click()
    'Calculate and display the current amounts, add to totals

    Dim cPrice                  As Currency
    Dim iQuantity               As Integer
    Dim cTax                    As Currency
    Dim cItemAmount             As Currency
    Const cTAX_RATE             As Currency = 0.08

    'Find the price
    If optCappuccino.Value = True Then
        cPrice = cCAPPUCCINO_PRICE
    ElseIf optEspresso.Value = True Then
        cPrice = cESPRESSO_PRICE
    ElseIf optLatte.Value = True Then
        cPrice = cLATTE_PRICE
    ElseIf optIcedCappuccino.Value = True Or _
            optIcedLatte.Value = True Then
        cPrice = cICED_PRICE
    Else
        MsgBox "Please Make Drink Selection", vbExclamation, "Oops"
    End If
```

```
    'Add the price times quantity to price so far
    If IsNumeric(txtQuantity.Text) Then
        iQuantity = Val(txtQuantity.Text)
        cItemAmount = cPrice * iQuantity
        mcSubtotal = mcSubtotal + cItemAmount
        If chkTax.Value = Checked Then
           cTax = mcSubtotal * cTAX_RATE
        End If
        mcTotal = mcSubtotal + cTax
        lblItemAmount.Caption = Format$(cItemAmount, "Currency")
        lblSubTotal.Caption = Format$(mcSubtotal, "Currency")
        lblTax.Caption = Format$(cTax, "Currency")
        lblTotal.Caption = Format$(mcTotal, "Currency")
    Else
        MsgBox "Quantity must be numeric", vbExclamation, "Oops"
        txtQuantity.SetFocus
    End If
End Sub
```

```
Private Sub cmdClear_Click()
   'Clear appropriate controls

   optCappuccino.Value = True   'Make first button selected to begin
   optEspresso.Value = False
   optLatte.Value = False
   optIcedLatte.Value = False
   optIcedCappuccino.Value = False
   lblItemAmount.Caption = ""
   chkTax.Enabled = False   'Allow change for new order only
   With txtQuantity
        .Text = ""
        .SetFocus
   End With
End Sub
```

```
Private Sub cmdExit_Click()
   'Terminate the project

   End
End Sub
```

```
Private Sub cmdNewOrder_Click()
   'Clear the current order and add to totals

   cmdClear_Click
   lblSubTotal.Caption = ""
   lblTax.Caption = ""
   lblTotal.Caption = ""

   'Add to Totals
   mcGrandTotal = mcGrandTotal + mcTotal
   mcSubtotal = 0
   mcTotal = 0   'reset for next customer
   miCustomerCount = miCustomerCount + 1
```

```
    'Clear appropriate display items and enable check box
    With chkTax
          .Enabled = True
          .Value = False
    End With
End Sub
```

```
Private Sub cmdSummary_Click()
    'Calculate the average and Display the totals

    Dim cAverage As Currency
    Dim stMessageString As String
    Dim stFormattedAvg As String

    If miCustomerCount > 0 Then
         If mcTotal <> 0 Then
            cmdNewOrder_Click   'Make sure last order is counted
         End If
         cAverage = mcGrandTotal / miCustomerCount

         'Format the numbers
         stFormattedAvg = Format$(cAverage, "Currency")
         'Concatenate the message string
         stMessageString = "Number Orders: " & miCustomerCount & vbCrLf & _
            "Average Sale: " & stFormattedAvg
         MsgBox stMessageString, vbInformation, "Coffee Sales Summary"
    Else
         MsgBox "No data to summarize", vbExclamation, "Coffee Sales Summary"
    End If
End Sub
```

Debugging Visual Basic Projects

One of the advantages of programming in the Visual Basic environment is the availability of debugging tools. You can use these tools to help find and eliminate logic and run-time errors. The debugging tools can also help you to follow the logic of existing projects to better understand how they work.

You can use the buttons in the toolbar or the *Debug* menu to access Visual Basic's debugging tools. (See Figure 4.12.) The debugging tools include the Debug window, single-stepping through a project, and watching the contents of variables and expressions.

Figure 4.12

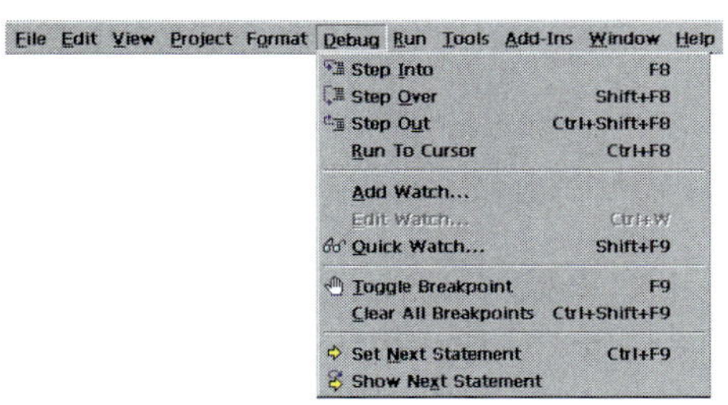

The debugging options on the Run *menu.*

Pausing Execution with the Break Button

You can click on the Break toolbar button to pause execution. This places the project into break time at the current line. The disadvantage of this method is that usually you prefer to break in the middle of a procedure. To choose the location of the break, you can force a break.

Forcing a Break

During the debugging process, often you want to stop at a particular location in code and watch what happens (which branch of an `If...Then...Else`; which procedures were executed; the value of a variable just before or just after a calculation). You can force the project to break by inserting a **breakpoint** in code.

```
If IsNumeric(txtQuantity.Text) Then
    lblDue.Caption = cPrice * txtQuantity.Text
Else
    MsgBox "Please Enter a Numeric Value", vbOKOnly, "Error"
End If
```

To set a breakpoint, place the cursor in the gray margin indicator area at the left edge of the Code window and click; the line will be highlighted in red and a large red dot will display in the margin indicator (Figure 4.13). You can also set a breakpoint by placing the cursor on the line before which you want to break and clicking on the Set Breakpoint button, by choosing *Toggle Breakpoint* from the *Run* menu, or by pressing F9, the keyboard shortcut. The breakpoint line will change to red (unless colors have been altered on your system).

Figure 4.13

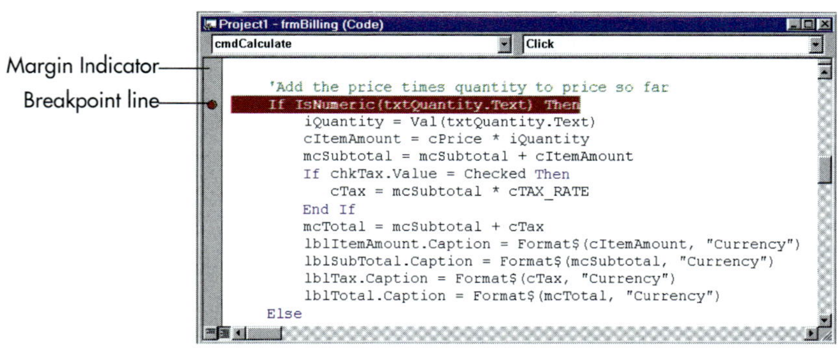

The highlighted line is set as a breakpoint. Note the dot in the gray margin indicator area.

After setting a breakpoint, start (or restart) program execution. When the project reaches the breakpoint, it will halt, display the line, and go into break time.

You can use *Toggle Breakpoint* again to turn off an individual breakpoint or clear all breakpoints from the *Run* menu.

Using the Immediate Window

The **Immediate window** is available at design time, run time, and break time. You can display the values of data or messages in the Immediate window while the project is executing. In break time you can use the Immediate window to view or change the current contents of variables or to execute lines of code. At design time you can view the window to see values from the previous run, but you cannot execute any code. You can display the window by selecting it from the *View* menu or use the shortcut Ctrl + G. You may want to move and resize the window to make it more visible. Figure 4.14 shows the Immediate window.

Figure 4.14

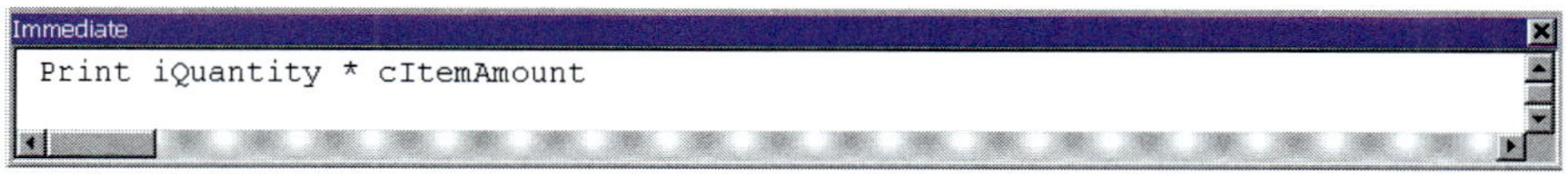

You can execute program statements in the Immediate window.

Checking the Current Values of Expressions

You can quickly check the current value of an expression, such as a variable, a control, a condition, or an arithmetic expression. During break time, display the Code window and point to the name of the expression that you want to view; a small label will pop up, similar to a ToolTip, which displays the current contents of the expression. If you want to view the contents of an expression of more than one word, such as a condition or arithmetic expression, highlight the entire expression and then point to the highlighted area; the current value will display. *Note:* For True/False values, Visual Basic displays 0 for False and −1 for True.

The steps for viewing the contents of a variable during run time are

1. Break the execution (using the *Run* menu, the toolbar button, or a breakpoint).
2. Click on the View Code button in the Project Explorer window or select *Code* from the *View* menu.
3. Point to the variable or expression you wish to view.

The current contents of the expression will pop up in a label (Figure 4.15).

Figure 4.15

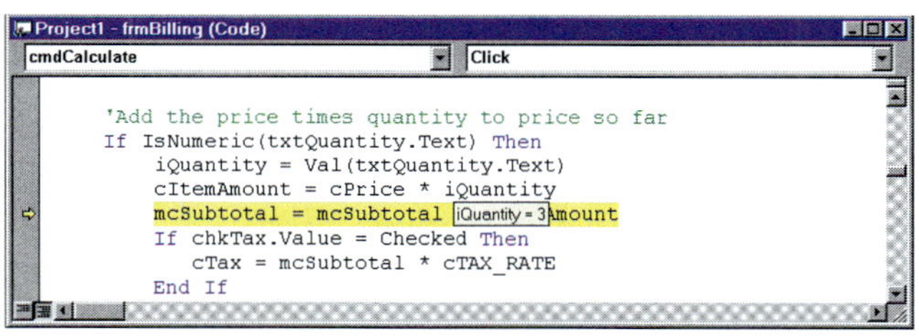

Point to a variable name, control name, condition, or arithmetic expression during break time to display the current value.

Stepping through Code

The best way to debug a project is to thoroughly understand what the project is doing every step of the way. Previously, this task was performed by following each line of code manually to understand its effect. You can now use the Visual Basic stepping tools to trace program execution line by line and see the progression of the program as it executes through your code.

You step through code at break time. You can use one of the techniques already mentioned to break execution or choose one of the stepping commands at design time; the program will begin running and immediately transfer to break time.

Two stepping commands on the *Debug* menu are *Step Into* and *Step Over.* You can also use the toolbar buttons for Step Into and Step Over or the keyboard shortcuts shown on the menu (refer to Figure 4.12).

These commands force the project to execute a single line at a time and to display the Code window with the current statement highlighted. As you execute the project, by pressing a command button, for example, the Click event occurs. Execution transfers to the click procedure, the Code window for that procedure appears on the screen, and you can follow line-by-line execution.

Step Into

Most likely you will use the **Step Into** command more than Step Over. When you choose Step Into (from the menu, the toolbar button, or F8), the next line of code is executed and the program pauses again in break time. If the line of code is a call to another procedure, the first line of code of the other procedure will be displayed.

To continue stepping through your program execution, continue choosing the Step Into command. When a procedure is completed, your form will display again, awaiting an event. You can click on one of your command buttons to continue stepping through code in an event procedure. If you want to continue execution without stepping, choose the Start command (from the menu, the toolbar button, or F5).

Step Over

The **Step Over** command also executes one line of code at a time. The difference between Step Over and Step Into occurs when your code has calls to other procedures. Step Over displays only the lines of code in the current procedure being analyzed; it does not display lines of code in the called procedures.

You can choose *Step Over* from the menu, from the toolbar button, or press Shift + F8. Each time you choose the command, one more program statement executes.

Debugging Step-by-Step Tutorial

In this exercise you will learn to set a breakpoint; pause program execution; single step through program instructions; display the current values in properties, variables, and conditions; and debug a Visual Basic project.

Test the Project

STEP 1: Open the debugging project on your student diskette. The project is found in the Ch04Debug folder.
STEP 2: Run the project.
STEP 3: Enter color Blue, quantity 100, and press Enter or click on the Calculate button.
STEP 4: Enter another color Blue, quantity 50, and press Enter. Are the totals correct?
STEP 5: Enter color Red, quantity 30, and press Enter.
STEP 6: Enter color Red, quantity 10, and press Enter. Are the totals correct?
STEP 7: Enter color White, quantity 50, and press Enter.
STEP 8: Enter color White, quantity 100, and press Enter. Are the totals correct?
STEP 9: Exit the project. You are going to locate and correct the errors in the red and white totals.

Break and Step Program Execution

STEP 1: Display the program code and click in the gray margin indicator area for the first calculation line in the cmdCalculate_Click event procedure:

```
cQuantity = Val(txtQuantity.Text)
```

A breakpoint will be set on the selected line. You screen should look like Figure 4.16.

Figure 4.16

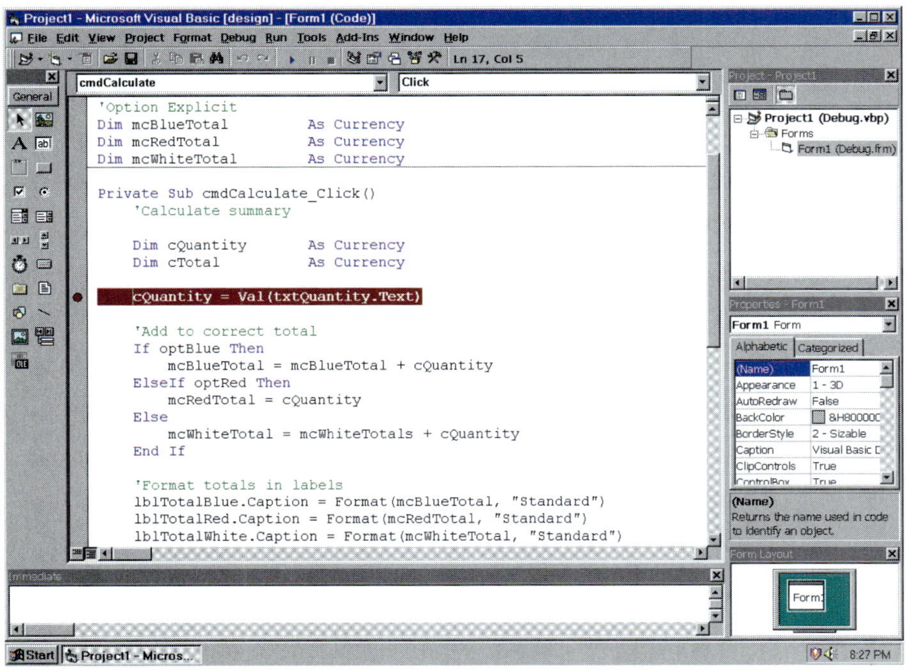

A program statement with a breakpoint set appears highlighted, and a dot appears in the gray margin indicator area.

STEP 2: Close the Code window.

STEP 3: Run the project, enter Red, quantity 30, and press Enter.

The project will transfer control to the cmdCalculate_Click procedure, stop when the breakpoint is reached, highlight the current line, and enter break time (Figure 4.17).

Note: The highlighted line has not yet executed.

Figure 4.17

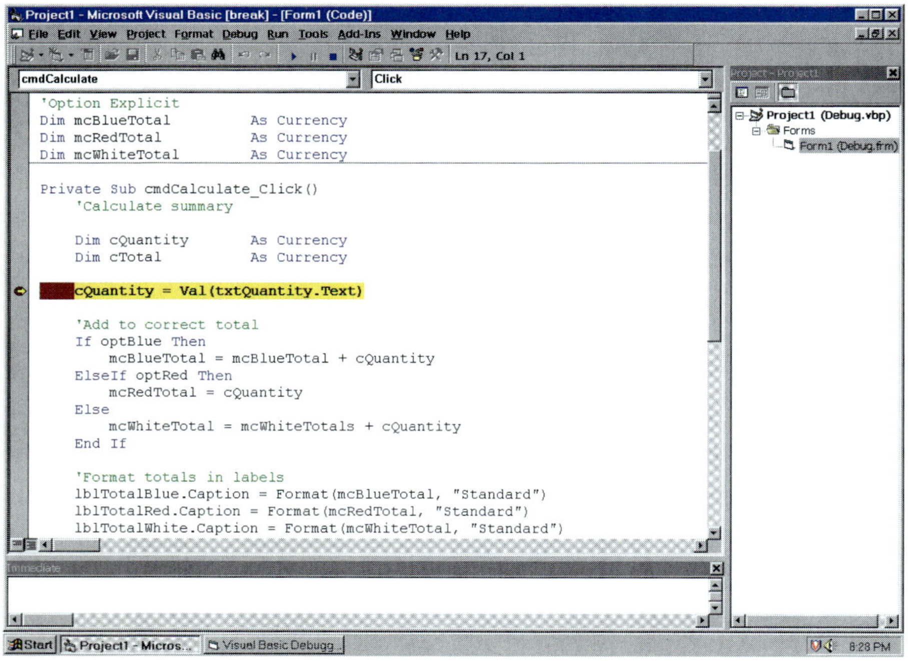

When a breakpoint is reached during project execution, Visual Basic enters break time, displays the Code window, and highlights the breakpoint line.

STEP 4: Press the F8 key, which causes VB to execute the current program statement (the assignment statement). F8 is the keyboard shortcut for *Debug/Step Into.*

The statement is executed and the highlight moves to the next statement (the `If` statement).

STEP 5: Press F8 again; the condition (`optBlue`) is tested and found to be False.

STEP 6: Continue pressing F8 and watch the order in which program statements execute.

View the Contents of Properties, Variables, and Conditions

STEP 1: Scroll up if necessary and point to `txtQuantity.Text` in the breakpoint line. The current contents of the Text property pops up (Figure 4.18).

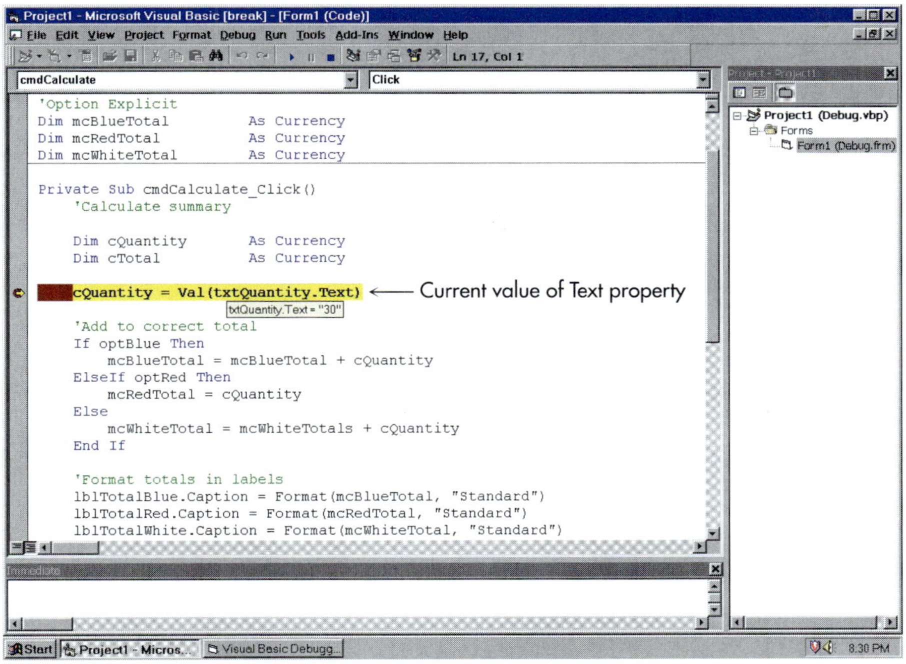

Figure 4.18

Point to a property reference in code, and the current content pops up.

STEP 2: Point to `cQuantity` and view the contents of that variable. Notice that the Text property is enclosed in quotes and the numeric variable is not.

STEP 3: Point to `optBlue` in the `If` statement; then point to `optRed`. The value that pops up is the current state of the Value property (the default property of an option button).

STEP 4: Point to `mcRedTotal` to see the current value of that total variable. This value looks correct, since you just entered 30, which was added to the total.

Continue Project Execution

STEP 1: Press F5, the keyboard shortcut for the Start command. The Start command continues execution.

If the current line is any line other than `Exit Sub`, execution continues and your form reappears. If the current line is `Exit Sub`, you must click on your project's Taskbar button (Figure 4.19) to make the form reappear.

Figure 4.19

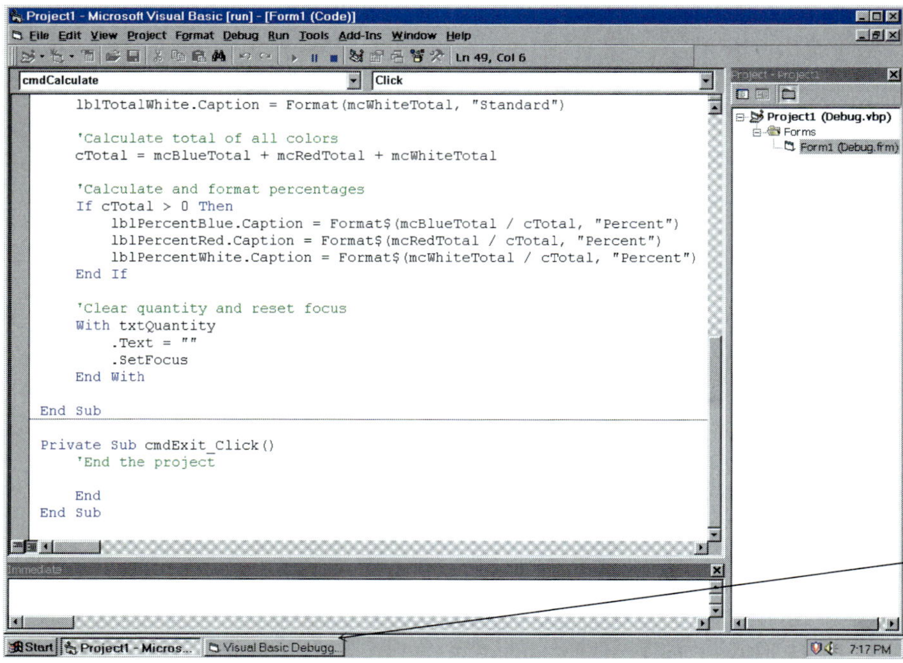

You may need to click on your project's Taskbar button to display the form during project execution.

STEP 2: Enter color Red and quantity 10. When you press Enter, program execution will again break at the breakpoint.

The 10 you just entered should be added to the 30 previously entered for Red, producing 40 in the Red total.

STEP 3: Use F8 to step through execution. Keep pressing F8 until the 10 is added to mcRedTotal. Display the current contents of the total. Can you see what the problem is?

Hint: mcRedTotal has only the current amount, not the sum of the two amounts. The answer will appear a little later; try to find it yourself first.

You will fix this error soon, after testing the White total.

Test the White Total

STEP 1: Press F5 to continue execution. If the form does not reappear, click the project's Taskbar button.

STEP 2: Enter color White, quantity 100, and press Enter.

STEP 3: When execution halts at the breakpoint, press F5 to continue.

STEP 4: Enter color White, quantity 50, and press Enter.

STEP 5: Press F8 several times when execution halts at the breakpoint until you execute the line that adds the 50 to the White total. Remember that the highlighted line has not yet executed; press F8 one more time, if necessary, to execute the addition statement.

STEP 6: Point to each variable name to see the current values (Figure 4.20). Can you see the problem?

Figure 4.20

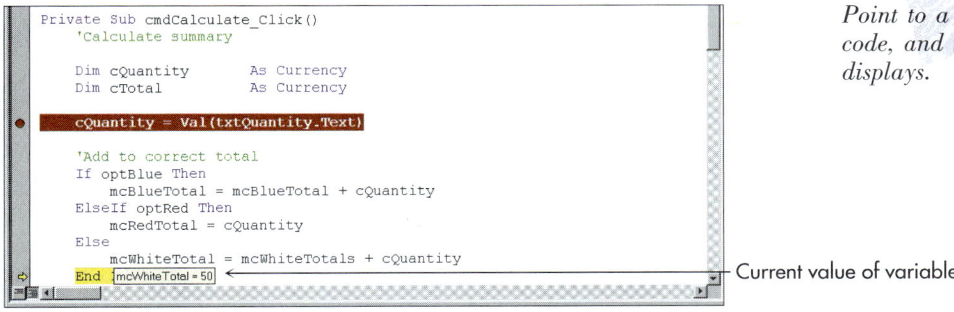

Point to a variable name in code, and its current value displays.

STEP 7: Identify all the errors. When you are ready to make the corrections, continue.

Correct the Red Total Error

STEP 1: Stop program execution by clicking on the End toolbar button (Figure 4.21).

Figure 4.21

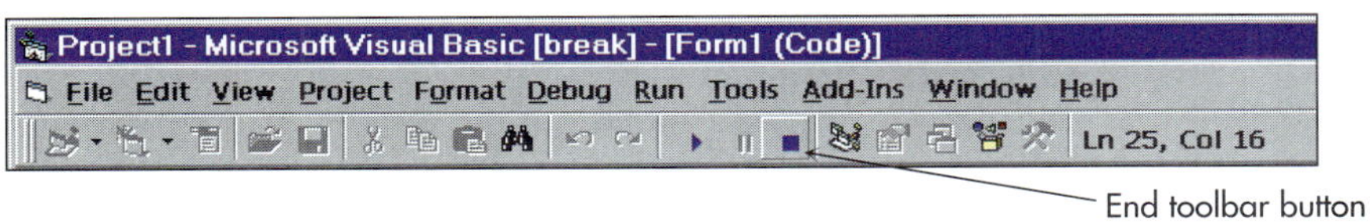

Click on the End toolbar button to halt project execution.

STEP 2: Locate this line:

```
mcRedTotal = cQuantity
```

This statement *replaces* the value of mcRedTotal with cQuantity rather than *adding* to the total.

STEP 3: Change the line to read

```
mcRedTotal = mcRedTotal + cQuantity
```

Correct the White Total Error

STEP 1: Locate this line:

```
mcWhiteTotal = mcWhiteTotals + cQuantity
```

Have you found the problem with this line? Look carefully at the spelling of the variable names. The compiler would find this error if the project included an `Option Explicit` statement.

STEP 2: First scroll up to the General Declarations section and remove the apostrophe from the `Option Explicit` statement.

STEP 3: Run the project again.

STEP 4: Enter color White and quantity 100; then press Enter.

The compiler displays a compile error message; click OK, and the Code window redisplays with the offending variable name highlighted (Figure 4.22).

Figure 4.22

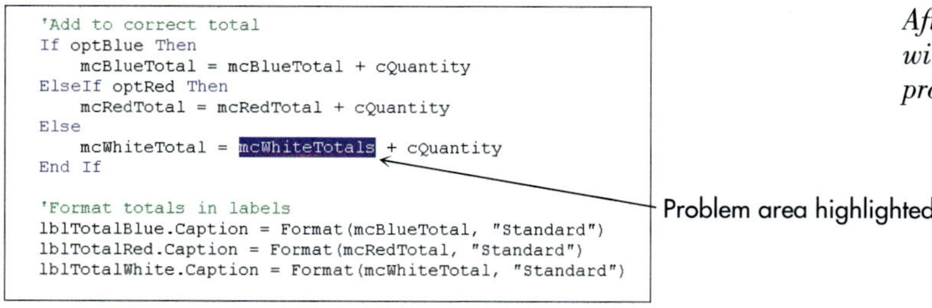

After a compile error, the Code window displays with the problem area highlighted.

STEP 5: Remove the s from `mcWhiteTotals`. The line should read:

```
mcWhiteTotal = mcWhiteTotal + cQuantity
```

STEP 6: Press F5 to continue project and execution. Remember that you already entered White and 100.

STEP 7: Press F5 to continue when the project halts at the breakpoint.

STEP 8: Enter White, 50, and Enter.

STEP 9: At the breakpoint, click on the breakpoint line, and select *Toggle Breakpoint* from the *Debug* menu to clear the breakpoint.

STEP 10: Press F5 to continue and check the total on the form. It should be correct now.

STEP 11: Test the totals for all three colors carefully and then click Exit.

Force a Run-Time Error

STEP 1: Display the code window and locate this line:

```
If cTotal > 0 Then
```

STEP 2: Type an apostrophe at the beginning of the line; then place another apostrophe on the `End If` line (Figure 4.23). This practice, called *commenting out* a statement, is a useful way to test program code.

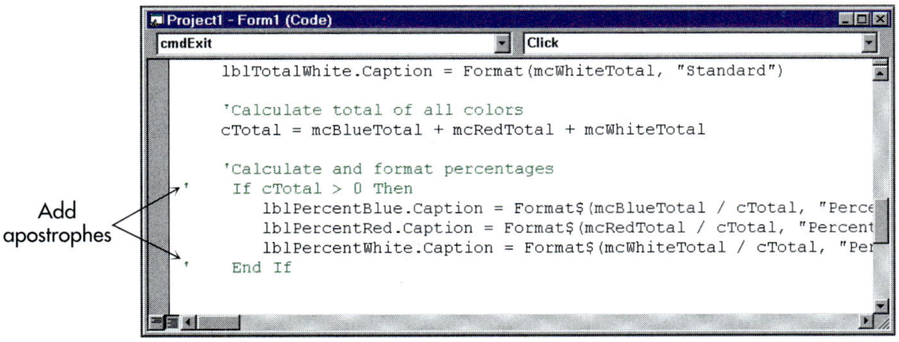

Figure 4.23

Convert statements to comments by typing an apostrophe at the beginning of the line. You can remove the apostrophes later to restore the lines.

STEP 3: Run the project. This time click the Calculate button without entering an Amount.

A run-time error will occur.

STEP 4: Click *Debug* on the error dialog box, and the Code window will display with the offending line highlighted.

STEP 5: Point to each variable name to see its value. Of course this error occurred because it is illegal to divide by zero.

STEP 6: Notice that the program is in break time. Click the End toolbar button to return to design time.

STEP 7: Remove the apostrophes from the `If` and `End If` lines.

STEP 8: Test the project carefully and thoroughly. If you have corrected all the errors, it should run correctly now.

Summary

1. Visual Basic uses the `If...Then...Else` statement to make decisions. An `Else` clause is optional and specifies the action to be taken if the condition is false. An `If...Then...Else` statement must conclude with an `End If`.
2. Flowcharts can help visualize the logic of an `If...Then...Else` statement.
3. The conditions for an `If` statement can be composed of the relational operators, which compare items for equality, greater than, or less than. The comparison of numeric values is based on the quantity of the number, while string comparisons are based on the ASCII code table.
4. The `Ucase` and `Lcase` functions can convert a text value to upper- or lowercase.
5. The `And` and `Or` logical operators may be used to combine multiple conditions. With the `And` operator, both conditions must be true for the entire condition to evaluate True. For the `Or` operator, if either or both conditions are true, the entire condition evaluates as True. When both `And` and `Or` are used in a condition, the `And` condition is evaluated before the `Or` condition.
6. The state of option buttons and check boxes should be tested with `If` statements in the event procedure for a command button, rather than coding event procedures for the option button or check box.
7. A nested `If` statement contains an `If` statement within either the true or false actions of a previous `If` statement. Nesting an `If` statement inside of another requires the use of the `End If` clause. An `Else` clause always applies to the last unmatched `If` regardless of indentation.
8. Data validation checks the reasonableness or appropriateness of the value in a variable or property. Since an error will occur if the data placed in a text box are not numeric, a popular validation tool is the `IsNumeric` function.
9. The MsgBox statement can be used to display a message to the person running the program. The programmer must supply the message and can optionally select an icon to display and enter a caption for the message box title bar.
10. One procedure can call another procedure.
11. A variety of debugging tools are available in Visual Basic. These include breaking program execution, displaying the current contents of variables, and stepping through code.

Key Terms

ASCII code *120*	implied condition *125*
breakpoint *144*	logical operator *126*
call *136*	message box *133*
compound condition *126*	nested `If` *129*
condition *119*	relational operator *119*
`End If` *117*	step into *146*
`If...Then...Else` *117*	step over *146*
Immediate window *145*	validation *132*

Review Questions

1. What is the general format of the statement used to code decisions in an application?
2. What is a condition?
3. Explain the purpose of relational operators and logical operators.
4. Differentiate between a comparison performed on numeric data and a comparison performed on string data.
5. How does Visual Basic compare the Text property of a text box?
6. Why would it be useful to include the `Ucase` function in a comparison?
7. Name the types of items that can be used in a comparison.
8. Explain a Boolean variable test for True and False. Give an example.
9. Give an example of a situation where nested `Ifs` would be appropriate.
10. When would you use a message box?
11. Give an example of three message box constants.
12. Define the term *validation.* When is it appropriate to do validation?
13. Define the term *checking a range.*
14. Explain the difference between Step Into and Step Over.
15. What steps are necessary to view the current contents of a variable during program execution?

Programming Exercises

4.1 Lynette Rifle owns an image consulting shop. Her clients can select from the following services at the specified regular prices: Makeover \$125, Hair Styling \$60, Manicure \$35, and Permanent Makeup \$200. She has distributed discount coupons that advertise discounts of 10 percent and 20 percent off the regular price. Create a project that will allow the receptionist to select a discount rate of 10 percent, 20 percent, or none, and then select a service. Display the price for the individual service in a label and have another label to display the total due after each visit is entered. Include command buttons for *Calculate*, *Clear*, *Print Form*, and *Exit*.

4.2 Modify project 4.1 to allow for sales to additional patrons. Include command buttons for *Next Patron* and *Summary*. When the receptionist clicks the *Summary* button, display the number of clients and the total dollar value for all services rendered in a summary message box.

4.3 Create a project to compute your checking account balance.
Form: Include option buttons to indicate the type of transaction—deposit, check, or service charge. A text box will allow the user to enter the amount of the transaction. Display the new balance in a label. Calculate the balance by adding deposits and subtracting service charges and checks. Include command buttons for *Calculate*, *Clear*, and *Exit*.

4.4 Add validation to project 4.3 by displaying a message box if the new balance would be a negative number. If there is not enough money to cover a check, do not deduct the check amount. Instead, display a message box with the message "Insufficient Funds" and deduct a service charge of $10.

4.5 Modify project 4.3 or 4.4 by adding a *Summary* command button that will display the total number of deposits, the total dollar amount of deposits, the number of checks, and the dollar amount of the checks. Do not include checks that were returned for insufficient funds, but do include the service charges.

4.6 Piecework workers are paid by the piece. Workers who produce a greater quantity of output are often paid at a higher rate.
Form: Use text boxes to obtain the person's name and the number of pieces completed. Include a *Calculate* command button to display the dollar amount earned. You will need a *Summary* button to display the total number of pieces, the total pay, and the average pay per person. A *Clear* button should clear the name and the number of pieces for the current employee.

Include validation to check for missing data. If the user clicks on the *Calculate* button without first entering a name and number of pieces, display a message box. Also, you need to make sure to not display a summary before any data are entered; you cannot calculate an average when no items have been calculated. You can check the number of employees in the Summary event procedure or disable the *Summary* command button until the first order has been calculated.

Pieces Completed	**Price Paid per Piece for All Pieces**
1–199	.50
200–399	.55
400–599	.60
600 or more	.65

4.7 Modify project 2.3 (the weather report) to treat option buttons the proper way. Do not have an event procedure for each option button; instead use a *Display* command button to display the correct image and message.

4.8 Modify project 2.2 (the flag viewer) to treat option buttons and check boxes in the proper way. Include a *Display* command button and check the settings of the option buttons and check boxes in the button's event procedure, rather than code event procedures for each option button and check box.

CASE STUDIES

VB Mail Order

Calculate the amount due for an order. For an order, the user should enter the following information into text boxes: customer name, address, city, state (two-letter abbreviation), and ZIP code. An order may consist of multiple items. For each item, the user will enter the product description, quantity, weight, and price into text boxes.

You will need command buttons for *Next Item*, *Update Summary*, *Print*, and *Exit*.

For the *Next Item* button, validate the quantity, weight, and price. Each must be present and numeric. For any bad data, display a message box. Calculate the charge for the current item and add the charge and weight into the appropriate totals. Do not calculate shipping and handling on individual items; rather, calculate shipping and handling on the entire order.

When the *Update Summary* button is clicked, calculate the sales tax, shipping and handling, and the total amount due for the order. Sales tax is 8 percent of the total charge and is charged only for shipments to a California address. Do not charge sales tax on the shipping and handling charges.

The shipping and handling charges depend on the weight of the products. Calculate the shipping charge as $.25 per pound and add that amount to the handling charge (taken from the following table).

Weight	Handling
Less than 10 pounds	$1.00
10 to 100 pounds	$3.00
Over 100 pounds	$5.00

Display the entire amount of the bill in labels titled *Dollar amount due*, *Sales tax*, *Shipping and handling*, and *Total amount due*.

Test Data

Description	Quantity	Weight	Price
Planter	2	3	19.95
Mailbox	1	2	24.95
Planter	2	3	19.95

Test Data Output

	Nontaxable	Taxable
Dollar Amount Due	$110.80	$110.80
Sales Tax	0.00	8.86
Shipping and Handling	5.75	5.75
Total Amount Due	116.55	125.41

VB Auto Center

Create a project that will be used to determine the total amount due for the purchase of a vehicle. You will need text boxes for the base price and the trade-in allowance. Check boxes will indicate if the buyer wants additional accessories: stereo system, leather interior, and/or computer navigation. A frame for the exterior finish will contain option buttons for Standard, Pearlized, or Customized Detailing.

Item	Price
Stereo System	425.76
Leather Interior	987.41
Computer Navigation	1,741.23
Standard	No additional charge
Pearlized	345.72
Customized Detailing	599.99
Tax Rate	8%

Have the trade-in allowance default to 0; that is, if the user does not enter a trade-in value, use 0 in your calculation. Validate the values from the text boxes, displaying a message box if necessary.

To calculate, add the price of selected accessories and finish to the base price and display the result in a label called *Subtotal*. Calculate the sales tax on the subtotal and display the result in a *Total* label. Then subtract any trade-in value from the total and display the result in an *Amount Due* label.

Include command buttons for *Calculate*, *Clear*, *Exit*, and *Print Form*. The Calculate button must display the total amount due after trade-in.

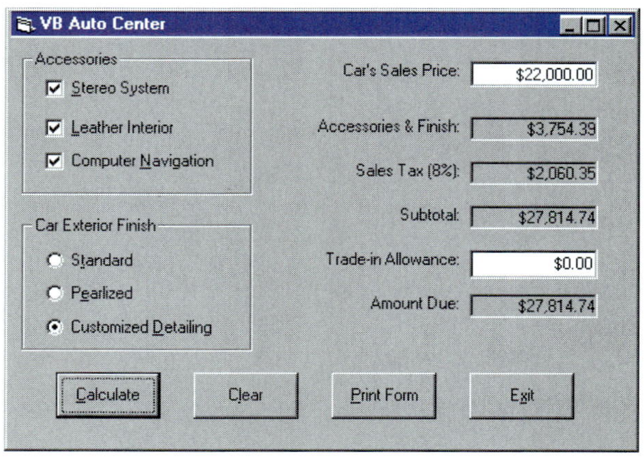

C H A P T E R

5

Menus, Sub Procedures, and Sub Functions

At the completion of this chapter, you will be able to . . .

1. Create menus and submenus for program control.

2. Display and use the Windows common dialog boxes.

3. Write reusable code in sub procedures and function procedures, and call the procedures from other locations.

4. Create an executable file that can be run from the Windows environment.

Menus

Undoubtedly you have used menus quite extensively while working with the computer. **Menus** consist of a menu bar with menu names, each of which drops down to display a list of menu commands. You can use menu commands in place of or in addition to command buttons to activate a procedure.

Menu commands are actually controls; they have properties and events. Each menu command has a Name property and a Click event, similar to a command button.

It is easy to create a menu for your form, using the Visual Basic menu editor. Your menu will appear across the top of the window and look like a standard Windows menu.

To use the menu editor, select *Menu Editor* from the *Tools* menu or click on the Menu Editor toolbar button (Figure 5.1).

Figure 5.1

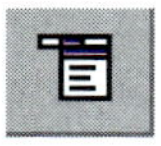

The Menu Editor toolbar button.

Defining Menus

You will use the Menu Editor window to set up your menus. Figure 5.2 shows the Menu Editor window with the various parts labeled.

Figure 5.2

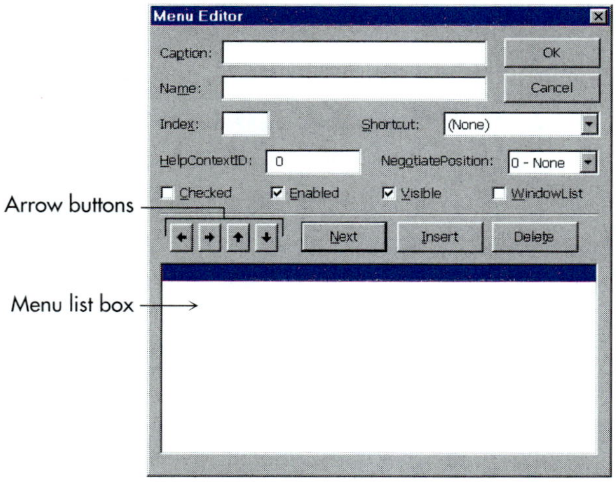

Define menus with the Menu Editor window.

The Caption

The Caption property holds the words you want to appear on the screen (just like the Caption property of a label or command button). Start creating a new menu by entering the Caption of the item you want for your first menu.

To conform to Windows standards, your first menu Caption should be File, with a keyboard access key. Use the ampersand (&) in the Caption to specify the key to use for keyboard access, as you learned in Chapter 2. For example, for File, the Caption should be &File.

The Name

The Name box indicates the name of the menu control, similar to other controls. The Name is required.

Naming Standards

The three-character prefix for a menu name is "mnu". Therefore, the name for the *File* menu should be mnuFile. For the commands on a menu use the prefix plus the name of the menu plus the name of the command. (You can abbreviate long names, if you do so consistently and clearly.) The name for the `Print` command on the `File` menu should be mnuFilePrint. The `Exit` command should be called mnuFileExit, which will trigger the mnuFileExit_Click event when the user selects it.

SubMenus

The drop-down list of commands below a menu name is called a *menu*. When a command on the menu has another list of commands that pops up, the new list is called a ***submenu***. A filled triangle to the right of the command indicates that a menu command has a submenu (Figure 5.3).

Figure 5.3

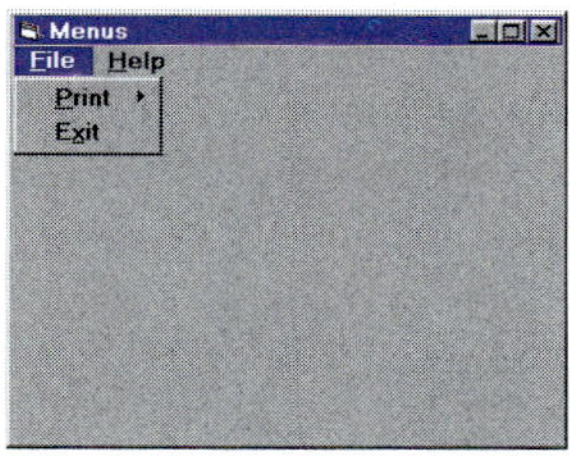

A filled triangle on a menu command indicates that a submenu will appear.

You specify menu names, menu commands, and submenu commands by their indentation levels. Menu names appear at the left of the list box; for a menu command, click on the Right arrow button to indent one level. For submenus, click on the Right arrow button again to indent two levels. The indentations show as dots (....) in the list box.

The Menu List Box

The menu list box contains a list of the menu items you have created and shows their indentation levels. You can move an item up or down, left or right by clicking on its name in the list box and clicking on one of the arrow buttons (refer to Figure 5.2).

```
&File
....E&xit
&Help
....&About
```

Separator Bars

When you have many commands in a menu, you should group the commands according to their purpose. You can create a **separator bar** in a menu, which draws a bar across the entire menu. To define a separator bar, type a single hyphen (-) for the Caption and give it a name. Even though you can never refer to the separator bar in code, and it does not have a Click event, you must still give it a unique name. Call your first separator bar mnuSep1, your second separator bar mnuSep2, and so on.

Creating a Menu—Step-by-Step

You are going to create a project with one form and a menu bar that contains these menu items:

```
File          Help
  Exit          About
```

STEP 1: Display the Menu Editor window (refer to Figure 5.2) by selecting *Menu Editor* from the *Tools* menu or clicking on the Menu Editor toolbar button (refer to Figure 5.1).

STEP 2: Type the Caption (&File) and Name (mnuFile) for the first menu (Figure 5.4).

Figure 5.4

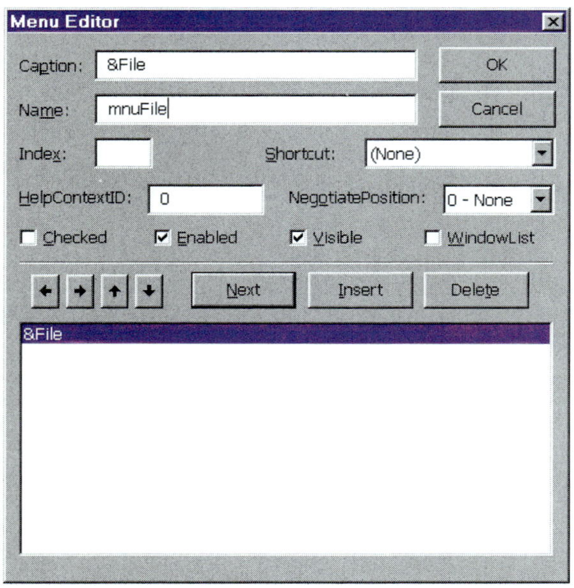

Type the Caption and Name for the first menu name.

STEP 3: Click on the *Next* button or press Enter; the text boxes will clear, and the name of your first menu appears in the menu list box (Figure 5.5).

Figure 5.5

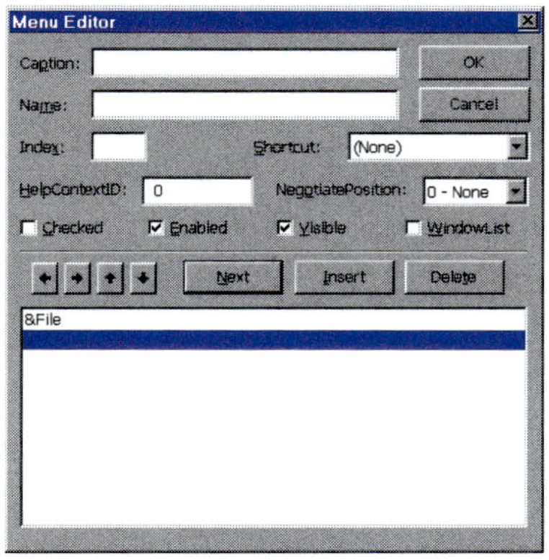

After entering the first menu name, the text boxes clear and the Caption of the first menu appears in the menu list box.

STEP 4: Click on the Right arrow button, which sets the indentation level for a menu command.

STEP 5: Click in the Caption text box to set the focus and then type the Caption and the Name for the Exit menu command (Figure 5.6).

Figure 5.6

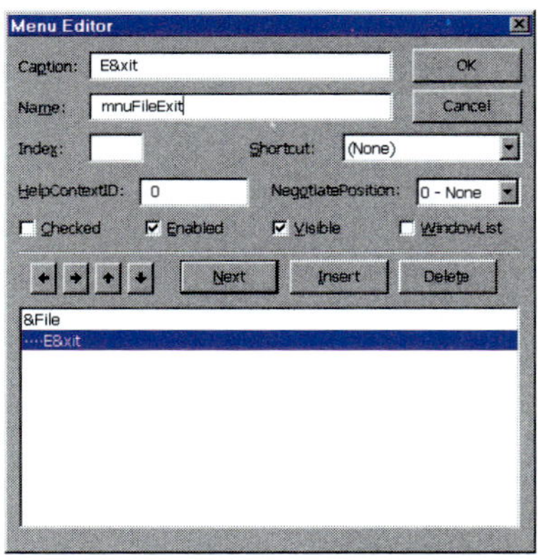

Type the Caption and Name for the Exit menu command.

STEP 6: Click on the Left arrow (outdent) button to return to the previous level.

STEP 7: Repeat the steps to create the *Help* menu and the *About* command indented below it (Figure 5.7).

Figure 5.7

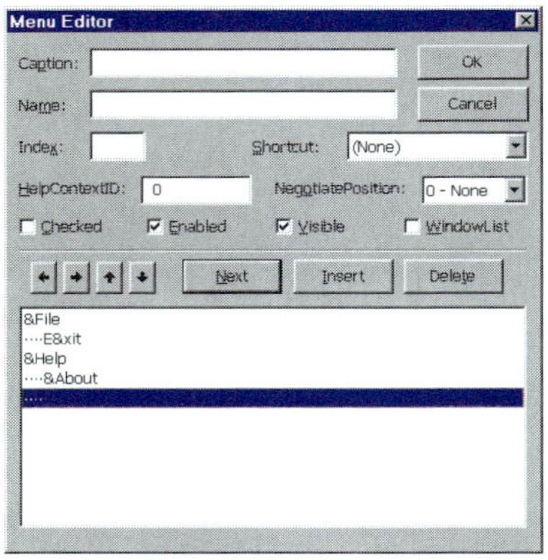

The completed menu appears in the menu list box.

STEP 8: Click OK when you are finished. The new menu will appear on your form.

Tip

You can rearrange the order of the menus and menu commands. Click on a name in the text box and click on the up and down arrows. Add or remove items using the Insert and Delete buttons.

Coding for Menu Commands

After you create your form's menu bar, it will appear on the form in design time. Just select any menu command, and the control's Click event procedure will appear in the Code window where you can write the code. For example, in design time, open your form's *File* menu and choose *Exit*. The Code window will open with the mnuFileExit_Click procedure displayed (assuming you have followed the suggested naming conventions and named the Exit command mnuFileExit).

STEP 9: Code the procedure for the Exit by pulling down the menu and clicking on the word *Exit*. Type in the remark and the *End* statement.

STEP 10: Use a MsgBox statement in the procedure for the Click event of the *About* on the *Help* menu. The Message string should say "Programmed by " followed by your name (Figure 5.8).

Figure 5.8

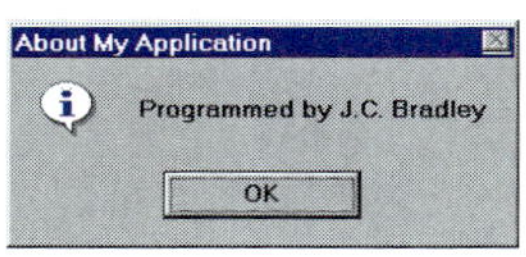

Display a message box for an About box.

Modifying a Menu

You can easily make changes to a menu bar you have created. With the form displaying in design time, display the Menu Editor window. Your complete menu will appear in the window.

You can click to select any menu item in the list box, and its information will appear in the top of the window where you can make modifications if desired. You can click on the Delete button to delete the selected item, or click Insert to insert a new blank line before the selection. To change the indentation level of any item, first select it and then click on the Left or Right arrow button. You can move an item up or down in the list by first selecting it and then clicking on the Up or Down arrow button.

Adding to your Sample Menu

To add a new menu and commands to the previous sample project, display the Menu Editor. Click on &Help in the list box and click the *Insert* button, which inserts a blank line in the list box above &Help (Figure 5.9). Add the following items to your menu, one at a time. (You must insert a new line for each item, including the separator bar.) Make sure to click the right arrow to indent each menu item, including the separator bar. Separator bars must also be indented.

Tip

If you receive the message "Cannot use separator bar as menu name for this control," check your separator bar. It must be indented.

Figure 5.9

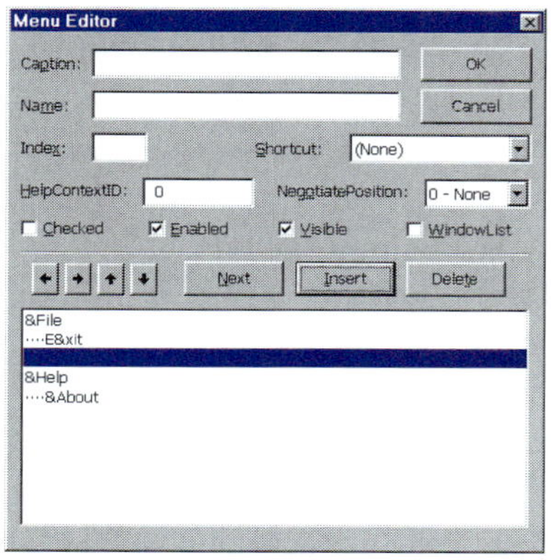

Click on the `Insert` *button to insert a blank line above &Help.*

```
&Edit
....&Color
....-
....&Font
```

Checked and Enabled

A menu command may contain a check mark beside it (**checked**), or it may be grayed (**disabled**). (See Figure 5.10.) An **enabled** menu item appears in black text and is available for selection, while the grayed out or disabled items are not available. A check mark placed next to a menu command usually indicates that the option is currently selected.

Figure 5.10

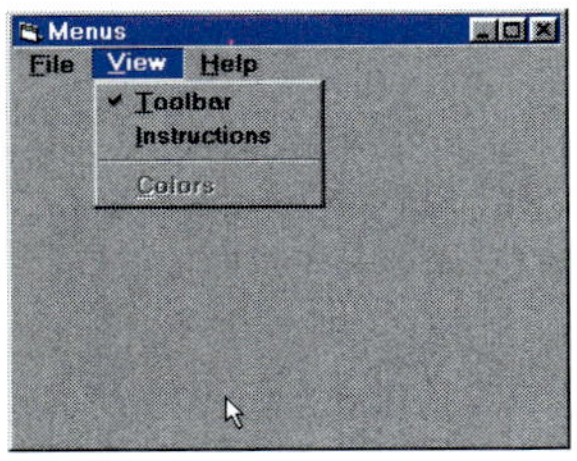

Menu commands can be disabled (grayed) or checked. A check mark usually indicates that the option is currently selected.

Check marks are often used on menu commands for options that can be toggled on and off. For example, for the option *Bold*, the check mark would indicate that Bold is currently selected. Choosing the *Bold* command a second time should remove the check mark and turn off the Bold option.

The check boxes in the Menu Editor for *Checked* and *Enabled* determine the beginning state for these options. By default, menu commands are enabled. If you wish the item to be grayed, the check box must be empty.

Toggling Check Marks On and Off

If you create a menu option that can be turned on and off, you should include a check mark to indicate the current state. You can set the initial state of the check mark in the Menu Editor (refer to Figure 5.2). In code you can change its state by setting the menu item's Checked property.

```
Private Sub mnuFormatBold_Click()
    If mnuFormatBold.Checked = True Then
        mnuFormatBold.Checked = False
        txtChangeable.Font.Bold = False
    Else
        mnuFormatBold.Checked = True
        txtChangeable.Font.Bold = True
    End If
End Sub
```

Standards for Windows Menus

When you write applications that run under Windows, you should make sure your programs follow the Windows standards. You should always include keyboard access keys; if you include keyboard shortcuts (Ctrl + key), stick with the standard keys, such as Ctrl + P for printing. Also follow the Windows standards for placing the *File* menu on the left end of the menu bar and ending the menu with an *Exit* command; if you have a *Help* menu, it belongs at the right end of the menu bar.

Plan your menus so that they look like other Windows programs unless your goal is to confuse people.

Common Dialog Boxes

You can use a set of predefined standard dialog boxes in your projects for such tasks as specifying colors and fonts, printing, opening, and saving. The **common dialog** control, which is a custom control, allows your project to use the dialog boxes that are provided as part of the Windows environment.

To use the common dialog control, you first place a control on your form (Figure 5.11). You cannot change the size of the control, and its location doesn't matter, since it will be invisible when your program runs. In code when you wish to display one of the standard dialog boxes, you will refer to properties and methods of the control. You don't need more than one common dialog control on your form, even if you plan to use several different dialog boxes; each time you refer to the control, you specify which dialog box you want. *Note:* Windows determines the size of the dialog boxes; you cannot modify their size.

Figure 5.11

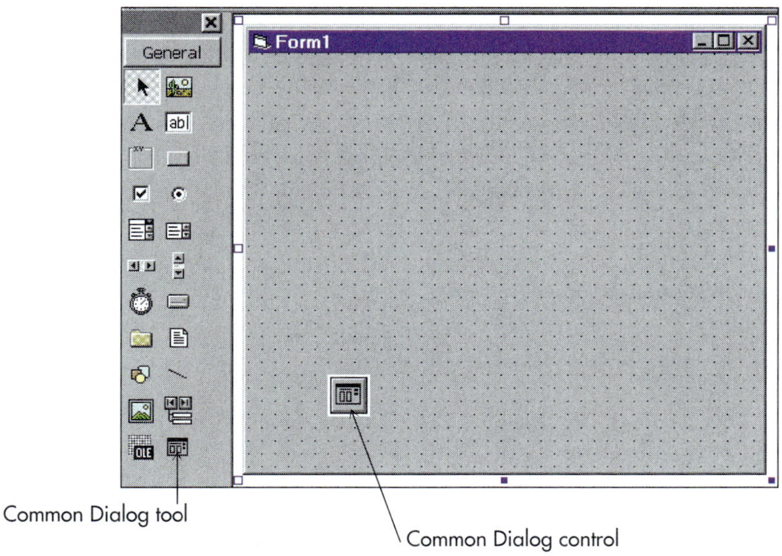

Use the common dialog tool in the toolbox to place a control on the form.

The common dialog control may not appear in your toolbox. It is a custom control, and you must add it to Visual Basic before you can use it. Custom controls are stored in files with an extension of .OCX. To use the common dialog, you must have Comdlg32.ocx in your Windows\System folder. Open the *Project* menu and choose *Components*; you should see *Microsoft Common Dialog Control 5.0* in the list (Figure 5.12). Make sure that a check appears next to the item, and its tool should appear in your toolbox.

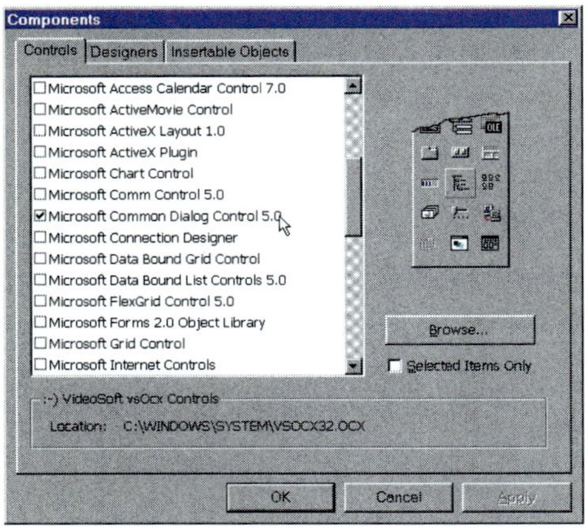

Figure 5.12

Select the common dialog control in the Components dialog box to make the Common Dialog tool appear in the toolbox.

When you name a common dialog control, use "dlg" as its three-character prefix.

Using a Common Dialog Box

Once you have placed a common dialog control on your form, you can display any of its dialog boxes at run time. In code you specify which box you want with the Show method.

Show Method—General Form

```
Object.ShowMethod
```

The method can be one of the following:

Dialog Box	Method
Open	ShowOpen
Save As	ShowSave
Color	ShowColor
Font	ShowFont
Print	ShowPrint

For example, assume you have a common dialog control called dlgCommon and a menu item named mnuEditColor. You could display the *Color* dialog box in the Click event for the menu command:

```
Private Sub mnuEditColor_Click()
    'Display the Color Dialog Box

    dlgCommon.ShowColor    'Display the Color dialog box
End Sub
```

The Windows dialog box for choosing colors (Figure 5.13) will appear when the user clicks on the *Color* menu option.

Figure 5.13

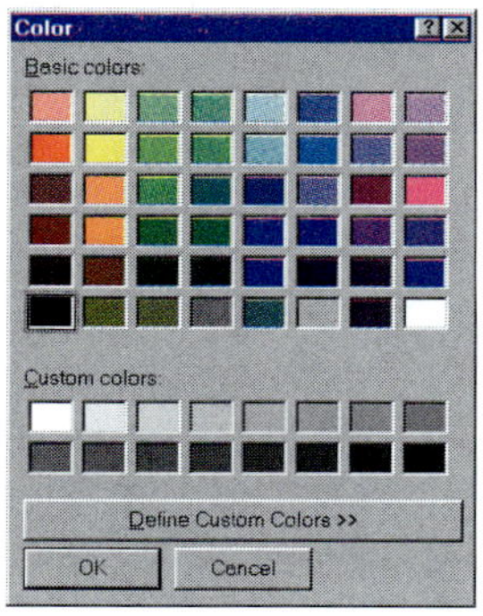

The Color common dialog box.

Using the Information from the Dialog Box

Just because you displayed the *Color* dialog box doesn't make the color of anything change. You must take care of that in your program code. What *does* happen is that the user's choices are stored in properties that you can access. You can assign these values to the properties of controls in your project.

Color Dialog Box

The color selected by the user is stored in the Color property. You can assign this property to another object, such as a control or the form.

```
frmMain.BackColor = dlgCommon.Color
```

Since Basic executes the statements in sequence, you would first display the dialog box with the ShowColor method. (Execution then halts until the user responds to the dialog box.) Then you can use the Color property:

```
Private Sub mnuEditColor_Click()
    'Display the Color dialog box

    dlgCommon.ShowColor
    'Assign dialog box color to the form
    frmMain.BackColor = dlgCommon.Color
End Sub
```

When the *Color* dialog box displays, it shows black as the default color. If you want to initialize the box to show the form's currently selected color when it appears, you must set the control's Flags property to cdlCCRGBInit and set its Color property before showing the dialog box.

```
Private Sub mnuEditColor_Click()
    'Select the color and set initial color
    With dlgCommon
        .Flags = cdlCCRGBInit           'Initialize the dialog box
        .Color = frmMain.BackColor      'Set initial color
        .ShowColor                      'Display dialog box
    End With

    'Assign dialog box color to the form
    frmMain.BackColor = dlgCommon.Color   'Set color of form
End Sub
```

Font Dialog Box

Before you can use the ShowFont method, you must set the Flags property of the control. This coding step installs the fonts to appear in the list box. The value of the Flags property may be cdlCFScreenFonts, cdlCFPrinterFonts, or cdlCFBoth. If you should forget to set the flags, an error will occur at run time that says "There are no fonts installed."

The Font properties for the common dialog control are different from those used for other controls. Instead of a group of properties for a Font object, each Font property is listed separately.

Font Object of Other Controls	Font Property of Common Dialog Control	Values
`Font.Bold`	`FontBold`	True or False (Boolean)
`Font.Italic`	`FontItalic`	True or False (Boolean)
`Font.Name`	`FontName`	System dependent
`Font.Size`	`FontSize`	Font dependent
`Font.StrikeThrough`	`FontStrikeThru`	True or False (Boolean)
`Font.Underline`	`FontUnderline`	True or False (Boolean)

Assign the FontName property before assigning the size and other attributes. The following code allows the user to change the font of a label.

```
Private Sub mnuEditFont_Click()
    'Display the Font dialog box

    With dlgCommon
        .Flags = cdlCFScreenFonts
        .ShowFont
    End With

    'Assign dialog box font to the label
    With lblEmployee.Font
        .Name = dlgCommon.FontName
        .Bold = dlgCommon.FontBold
    End With
End Sub
```

When the user clicks on the *Font* menu command, the *Font* dialog box appears on the screen (Figure 5.14).

Figure 5.14

The Font common dialog box.

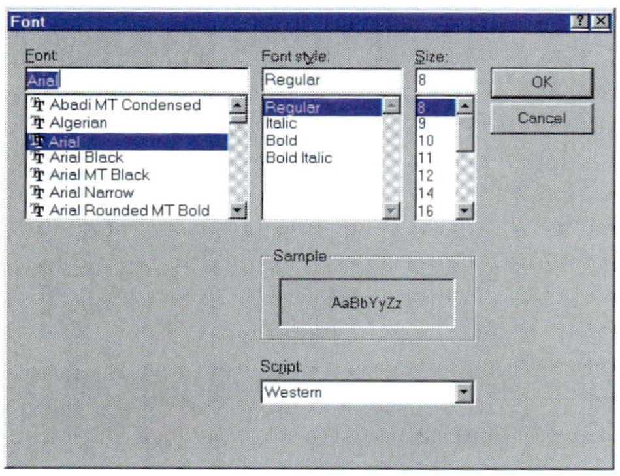

Setting Current Values

Before calling the common dialog box for colors or fonts, you should assign the existing values of the object properties that will be altered. This step will provide for the display of the current values in the dialog box. It also ensures that if the user selects the Cancel button, the property settings for the objects will remain unchanged.

```
Private Sub mnuEditFont_Click()
    'Display the Font common dialog box
'   and make the changes in the label settings

'Assign the current settings to the dialog box
With dlgCommon
     .FontName = lblEmployee.Font.Name
     .FontBold = lblEmployee.Font.Bold
     .FontItalic = lblEmployee.Font.Italic
     .FontSize = lblEmployee.Font.Size
End With
```

```
'Set the method for Font dialog box
With dlgCommon
      .Flags = cdlCFScreenFonts 'Specify screen fonts
      .ShowFont
End With

'Assign dialog box font to the label
With lblEmployee.Font
      .Bold = dlgCommon.FontBold
      .Italic = dlgCommon.FontItalic
      .Name = dlgCommon.FontName
      .Size = dlgCommon.FontSize
    End With
End Sub
```

Writing General Procedures

Often you will encounter programming situations in which multiple procedures perform the same operation. This condition can occur when the user can select either a command button or a menu option to do the same thing. Rather than retyping the code, you can write reusable code in a **general procedure** and call it from both event procedures.

Creating a New Sub Procedure

To add a new general procedure to a form:

STEP 1: Display the Code window for the form.
STEP 2: Select *Add Procedure* from the *Tools* menu.
STEP 3: Enter a name in the *Add Procedure* dialog box (Figure 5.15).

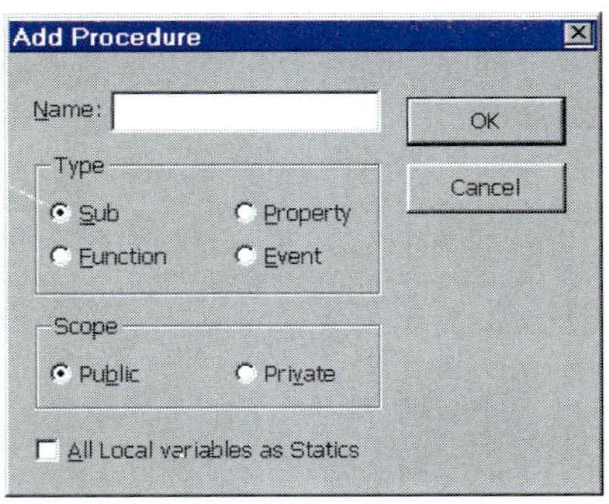

Figure 5.15

Use the Add Procedure dialog box to add a new general procedure to your form module.

STEP 4: Select *Private* for *Scope*. Choosing *Public* makes a procedure available from other project modules. *Note:* Leave the *Type* set to *Sub* for now.
STEP 5: Click OK.

In this example of a new general sub procedure, notice that the SelectColor sub procedure is not attached to any event.

```
Private Sub SelectColor()
    'Allow user to select a color

    dlgColor.ShowColor
End Sub
```

The coding of the new procedure is similar to the other procedures we have been coding, but is not yet attached to any event. Therefore, this code cannot be executed unless we specifically **call** the procedure from another procedure. To call a sub procedure, just give the procedure name, which in this case is SelectColor.

```
Private Sub cmdChangeMessage_Click()
    'Change the color of the message

    SelectColor
    lblMessage.ForeColor = dlgColor.Color
End Sub
```

```
Private Sub cmdChangeTitle_Click()
    'Change the color of the title

    SelectColor
    lblTitle.ForeColor = dlgColor.Color
End Sub
```

Passing Variables to Procedures

At times you may need to use the value of a variable in one procedure and also in a second procedure that is called from the first. In this situation you could declare the variable as module level, but that makes it visible to all other procedures. In order to keep the scope of a variable as narrow as possible, consider declaring the variable as local and passing it to any called procedures.

As an example, we will expand the capabilities of the previous ShowColor sub procedure to display the original color when the dialog box appears. Since the ShowColor procedure can be called from various locations, the original color must be passed to the procedure. Note that Visual Basic stores colors in Long Integer variables.

```
Private Sub SelectColor(lIncomingColor As Long)
    'Allow user to select a color

    With dlgColor
        .Flags = cdlCCRGBInit     'Initialize the Color dialog box
        .Color = lIncomingColor   'Set the initial color
        .ShowColor
    End With
End Sub
```

```
Private Sub cmdChangeMessage_Click()
    'Change the color of the message
    Dim lOriginalColor As Long

    lOriginalColor = lblMessage.ForeColor
    SelectColor lOriginalColor
    lblMessage.ForeColor = dlgColor.Color
End Sub
```

```
Private Sub cmdChangeTitle_Click()
    'Change the color of the title
    Dim lOriginalColor As Long

    lOriginalColor = lblTitle.ForeColor
    SelectColor lOriginalColor
    lblTitle.ForeColor = dlgColor.Color
End Sub
```

Notice that in this example the SelectColor procedure now has an argument inside the parenthesis. This specifies that when called, an argument must be supplied.

When a sub procedure definition names an argument, any call to that procedure must supply the argument. In addition, the argument value must be the same data type in both locations. Notice that in the two calling procedures (cmdChangeMessage_Click and cmdChangeTitle_Click), the variable lOriginalColor is declared as a Long Integer.

Another important point is that the *name* of the argument does not have to be the same in both locations. The ShowColor sub procedure will take whatever Long Integer value it is passed and refer to it as lIncomingColor inside the procedure.

You may specify multiple arguments in both the sub procedure header and the call to the procedure. The number of arguments, their sequence, and their data types must match in both locations! You will see some examples of multiple arguments in the sections that follow.

Function Procedures versus Sub Procedures

When you insert a new procedure, recall that you can choose to create a sub procedure or a function procedure (refer to Figure 5.15). Let's consider the difference between these two types of procedures. A **sub procedure** is a procedure that performs actions. A **function procedure** may perform an action, but it also returns a value (the **return value**) to the point from which it was called.

In the past we have used predefined functions, such as the `Format` function and the `Val` function. The `Format` function returns the formatted characters; the `Val` function returns the numeric value of the named argument.

As a programmer, you may need to calculate a value that will be needed in several different procedures or programs. You can write your own function that will calculate a value and call the function from the locations where it is needed. As an example we will create a function procedure called Commission, which calculates a salesperson's commission.

To create the new Commission function, follow the same steps as for creating a sub procedure. In the *Add Procedure* dialog box (refer to Figure 5.15), select the *Function* option button prior to selecting the OK command button.

When you insert a function procedure named Commission, your new Code window contains these statements:

```
Private Function Commission()
End Function
```

Notice that this procedure looks just like a sub procedure except that the word `Function` replaces the word `Sub` on both the first line and the last line.

Remember that functions also have arguments. You supply arguments to a function when you call the function by placing a value or values inside the parentheses.

When you write a function, you declare the argument(s) that the function needs. You give each argument an identifier and a data type. The name that you give an argument in the Function procedure header is the identifier that you will use inside the function to refer to the value of the argument.

Examples

```
Private Function Commission(cSalesAmount As Currency)
Private Function Payment(cRate As Currency, cTime As Currency, cAmount As Currency)
```

In the function procedure the argument list you enter establishes the number of arguments, their type, and their sequence. When using multiple arguments, the sequence of the arguments is critical, just as when you use the predefined Visual Basic functions.

The main difference between coding a function procedure and coding a sub procedure is that in a function you must set up the return value. This return value is placed in a variable that Visual Basic names with the same name as the function name. In the previous example the variable name is Commission. *Note:* Somewhere in the function, you *must* set the function name to a value.

You can also specify the data type of the return value by adding the As clause after the function name. Because the data type of the return value in this example is Currency, the function name has been changed to `cCommission`.

```
Private Function cCommission(cSalesAmount As Currency) As Currency
    'Calculate the sales commission

    If cSalesAmount < 1000 Then
        cCommission = 0
    ElseIf cSalesAmount <= 2000 Then
        cCommission = 0.15 * cSalesAmount
    Else
        cCommission = 0.2 * cSalesAmount
    End If
End Function
```

In another procedure in the project, you can call your function by using it in an expression.

Example

```
Dim cSales as Currency
If IsNumeric(txtSales.Text) Then
    cSales = Val(txtSales.Text)
    lblCommission.Caption = cCommission(cSales)
End If
```

Notice in the preceding example that the argument named in the function call does not have the same name as the argument named in the function definition. When the function is called, cSales is passed to the function and is assigned to the named argument, in this case cSalesAmount. As the calculations are done (inside the function), for every reference to cSalesAmount, the value of cSales is actually used.

In creating a function with multiple arguments such as a Payment function, the list of arguments is enclosed within the parentheses. The following example indicates that three arguments are needed in the call: The first argument is the interest rate, the second is the time, and the third is the loan amount. All three argument values will have a data type of currency, and the return value will be currency. Look carefully at the following formula and notice how the identifiers in the parentheses are used.

```
Private Function cPayment(cRate As Currency, cTime As Currency, _
       cAmt As Currency) As Currency
       'Calculate the monthly payment on an amortized loan

       cPayment = cAmt * (1 + cRate/12) ^ (cTime * 12) 'Set the _
                   return value of the function
End Function
```

To call this function from another procedure, use this statement:

```
cRate = Val(txtRate.Text)
cTime = Val(txtTime.Text)
cAmount = Val(txtAmount.Text)
lblPayment.Caption = cPayment(cRate, cTime, cAmount)
```

You can format the result, as well as pass the `Val` of the text boxes, by nesting functions:

```
lblPayment.Caption = Format$(cPayment(Val(txtRate.Text), _
      Val(txtTime.Text), Val(txtAmount.Text)), "Currency")
```

Feedback 5.1

You need to write a procedure to calculate and return the average of three integer values.

1. Should you write a sub procedure or a function procedure?
2. Write the first line of the procedure.
3. Write the calculation.
4. How is the calculated average passed back to the calling procedure?

Your Hands-On Programming Example

Modify the hands-on programming example from Chapter 4 by replacing some of the command buttons with menus. Use a function procedure to calculate the sales tax. You will need to move the constant for tax rate to the module level.

The project for R 'n R—for Reading 'n Refreshment calculates the amount due for individual orders and maintains accumulated totals for a summary. Have a check box for takeout items, which are taxable (8 percent); all other orders are nontaxable. Include option buttons for the five coffee selections—Cappuccino, Espresso, Latte, Iced Latte, and Iced Cappuccino. The prices for each will be assigned using these constants:

Cappuccino	2.00
Espresso	2.25
Latte	1.75
Iced (either)	2.50

Use a command button for Calculate Selection, which will calculate and display the amount due for each item. A button for Clear for Next Item will clear the selections and amount for the single item. Additional labels in a separate frame will maintain the summary information for the current order to include subtotal, tax, and total.

The Next Order menu will clear the bill for the current customer and add to the totals for the summary. The menu for Summary should display the total of all orders, the average sale amount per customer, and the number of customers.

The Edit menu contains options that duplicate the Calculate and Clear button. The Font and Color options change the contents of the subtotal, tax, and total labels.

The *About* selection on the *Help* menu will display a message box with information about the programmer.

```
File            Edit                      Help
  New Order       Calculate Selection       About
  Summary         Clear Item
  Exit            ______
                  Font
                  Color
```

Planning the Project

Sketch a form (Figure 5.16), which your users sign as meeting their needs.

Figure 5.16

A sketch of the form for the hands-on programming example.

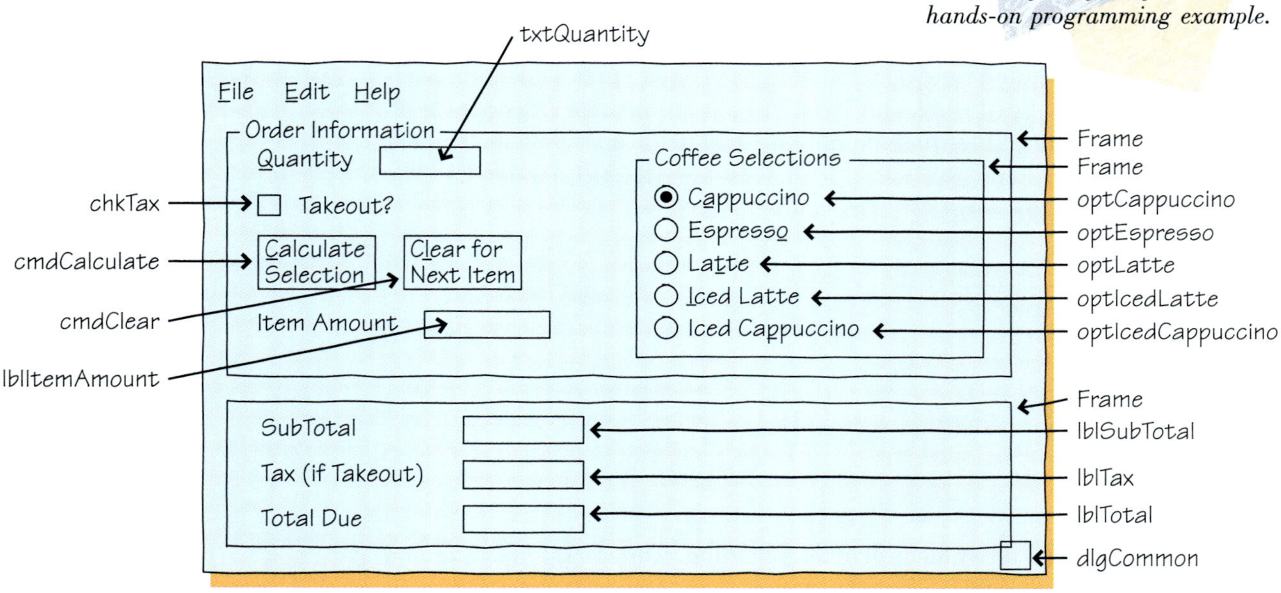

Plan the Objects and Properties

Plan the property settings for the form and each of the controls.

Object	Property	Setting
frmBilling	Name	frmBilling
	Caption	R 'n R—for Reading 'n Refreshment
Frame1	Caption	Order Information
Frame2	Caption	Coffee Selections
Frame3	Caption	(blank)
optCappuccino	Name	optCappuccino
	Caption	C&appuccino
	Value	True
optEspresso	Name	optEspresso
	Caption	Espress&o
optLatte	Name	optLatte
	Caption	La&tte
optIcedLatte	Name	optIcedLatte
	Caption	&Iced Latte
optIcedCappuccino	Name	optIcedCappuccino
	Caption	Iced Ca&ppuccino
Label1	Caption	Quantity
txtQuantity	Name	txtQuantity
	Text	(blank)
chkTax	Name	chkTax
	Caption	Takeout ?
Label2	Caption	Item Amount
Label3	Caption	SubTotal
Label4	Caption	Tax (if Takeout)
Label5	Caption	Total Due
lblItemAmount	Name	lblItemAmount
	Caption	(blank)
	BorderStyle	1 - FixedSingle
lblSubTotal	Name	lblSubTotal
	Caption	(blank)
	BorderStyle	1 - Fixed Single
lblTax	Name	lblTax
	Caption	(blank)
	BorderStyle	1 - Fixed Single

(continued)

Object	Property	Setting
lblTotal	Name	lblTotal
	Caption	(blank)
	BorderStyle	1 - Fixed Single
cmdCalculate	Name	cmdCalculate
	Caption	&Calculate Selection
	Default	True
cmdClear	Name	cmdClear
	Caption	C&lear for Next Item
	Cancel	True
mnuFile	Name	mnuFile
	Caption	&File
mnuFileNew	Name	mnuFileNew
	Caption	&New Order
mnuFileSummary	Name	mnuFileSummary
	Caption	&Summary
mnuFileExit	Name	mnuFileExit
	Caption	E&xit
mnuEdit	Name	mnuEdit
	Caption	&Edit
mnuEditCalc	Name	mnuEditCalc
	Caption	Calculate &Selection
mnuEditClear	Name	mnuEditClear
	Caption	C&lear Item
mnuSep1	Name	mnuSep1
	Caption	-
mnuEditFont	Name	mnuEditFont
	Caption	&Font
mnuEditColor	Name	mnuEditColor
	Caption	&Color
mnuHelp	Name	mnuHelp
	Caption	&Help
mnuHelpAbout	Name	mnuHelpAbout
	Caption	&About
dlgCommon	Name	dlgCommon

Plan the Event Procedures

You need to plan the actions for the command buttons, and the actions of the menu commands.

Object	Procedure	Action
cmdCalculate	Click	Determine price per cup. Multiply price by quantity. Call tax procedure if needed. Add quantity to item total. Display the values.
cmdClear	Click	Clear the coffee selections. Clear the quantity and the item price. Disable the takeout check box. Set the focus to the quantity.
mnuFileNew	Click	Clear the previous order. Accumulate total and count. Set subtotal and total to 0.
mnuFileSummary	Click	Display the Average. Display Total Sales. Display the number of customers.
mnuFileExit	Click	Terminate the project.
mnuEditCalc	Click	Call calculate command event.
mnuEditClear	Click	Call clear command event.
cFindTax	(call)	Calculate the sales tax.

Write the Project

Follow the sketch in Figure 5.16 to create the form. Figure 5.17 shows the completed form.

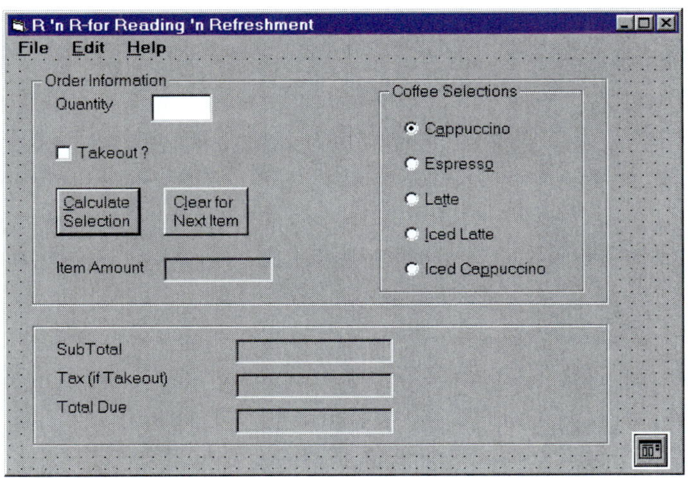

Figure 5.17

The form for the hands-on programming example.

- Set the properties of each object according to your plan.
- Write the code. Working from the pseudocode, write each event procedure.
- When you complete the code, use a variety of data to thoroughly test the project.

The Project Coding Solution

```
'Project Name:   Billing
'Programmer:     A. Millspaugh
'Date:           July 1997
'Description:    This project calculates the
'   amount due based on the customer selection
'   and accumulates summary data for the day.
'   The project incorporates menus and common dialog boxes.
'   The common dialog box allows the user to change
'   the color and font.
'Folder:         Ch0501

Option Explicit
Dim mcSubtotal                 As Currency
Dim mcTotal                    As Currency
Dim mcGrandTotal               As Currency
Dim miCustomerCount            As Integer
Const cCAPPUCCINO_PRICE        As Currency = 2
Const cESPRESSO_PRICE          As Currency = 2.25
Const cLATTE_PRICE             As Currency = 1.75
Const cICED_PRICE              As Currency = 2.5
Const mcTAX_RATE               As Currency = 0.08
```

```
Private Sub cmdCalculate_Click()
    'Calculate and display the current amounts; add to totals

    Dim cPrice             As Currency
    Dim iQuantity          As Integer
    Dim cTax               As Currency
    Dim cItemAmount        As Currency

    'Find the price
    If optCappuccino.Value = True Then
        cPrice = cCAPPUCCINO_PRICE
    ElseIf optEspresso.Value = True Then
        cPrice = cESPRESSO_PRICE
    ElseIf optLatte.Value = True Then
        cPrice = cLATTE_PRICE
    ElseIf optIcedCappuccino.Value = True Or _
            optIcedLatte.Value = True Then
       cPrice = cICED_PRICE
    Else
       MsgBox "Please Make Drink Selection", vbOKOnly, "Oops"
    End If

    'Add the price times quantity to price so far
    If IsNumeric(txtQuantity.Text) Then
        iQuantity = Val(txtQuantity.Text)
        cItemAmount = cPrice * iQuantity
        mcSubtotal = mcSubtotal + cItemAmount
        If chkTax.Value = Checked Then
            cTax = cFindTax(mcSubtotal) 'call a function procedure
        End If
        mcTotal = mcSubtotal + cTax
        lblItemAmount.Caption = Format$(cItemAmount, "Currency")
        lblSubTotal.Caption = Format$(mcSubtotal, "Currency")
        lblTax.Caption = Format$(cTax, "Currency")
        lblTotal.Caption = Format$(mcTotal, "Currency")
    Else
        MsgBox "Quantity must be numeric", vbExclamation, "Oops"
        txtQuantity.SetFocus
    End If
End Sub
```

```
Private Sub cmdClear_Click()
    'Clear appropriate controls

    optCappuccino.Value = True 'Make first button selected to begin
    optEspresso.Value = False
    optLatte.Value = False
    optIcedLatte.Value = False
    optIcedCappuccino.Value = False
    lblItemAmount.Caption = ""
    chkTax.Enabled = False 'Allow change for new order only
    With txtQuantity
        .Text = ""
        .SetFocus
    End With
End Sub
```

```
Private Sub mnuEditCalc_Click()
    'Call the Calculate event

    cmdCalculate_Click
End Sub
```

```
Private Sub mnuEditClear_Click()
    'Call the Clear command event

    cmdClear_Click
End Sub
```

```
Private Sub mnuEditColor_Click()
    'Change the color of the total labels

    dlgCommon.ShowColor
    lblSubTotal.ForeColor = dlgCommon.Color
    lblTax.ForeColor = dlgCommon.Color
    lblTotal.ForeColor = dlgCommon.Color
End Sub
```

```
Private Sub mnuEditFont_Click()
    'Change the font name for the subtotal labels

    dlgCommon.Flags = cdlCFScreenFonts 'Set up Font dialog box fonts
    dlgCommon.ShowFont
    lblSubTotal.Font.Name = dlgCommon.FontName
    lblTax.Font.Name = dlgCommon.FontName
    lblTotal.Font.Name = dlgCommon.FontName
End Sub
```

```
Private Sub mnuFileExit_Click()
    'Terminate the project

    End
End Sub
```

```
Private Sub mnuFileNew_Click()
    'Clear the current order and add to totals

    cmdClear_Click
    lblSubTotal.Caption = ""
    lblTax.Caption = ""
    lblTotal.Caption = ""

    'Add to Totals
    mcGrandTotal = mcGrandTotal + mcTotal
    mcSubtotal = 0
    mcTotal = 0 'reset for next customer
    miCustomerCount = miCustomerCount + 1

    'Clear appropriate display items and enable check box
    With chkTax
        .Enabled = True
        .Value = False
    End With
End Sub
```

```
Private Sub mnuFileSummary_Click()
    'Calculate the average and display the totals

    Dim cAverage As Currency
    Dim stMessageString As String
    Dim stFormattedAvg As String

    If miCustomerCount > 0 Then
        If mcTotal <> 0 Then
            mnuFileNew_Click 'Make sure last order is counted
        End If
        cAverage = mcGrandTotal / miCustomerCount

        'Format the numbers
        stFormattedAvg = Format$(cAverage, "Currency")
        'Concatenate the message string
        stMessageString = "Number of Orders: " & miCustomerCount & vbCr & _
            "Average Sale: " & stFormattedAvg
        MsgBox stMessageString, vbInformation, "Coffee Sales Summary"
    Else
        MsgBox "No data to summarize", vbExclamation, "Coffee Sales Summary"
    End If
End Sub
```

```
Private Sub mnuHelpAbout_Click()
    'Display a message box about the program

    MsgBox "R "n R Billing" & vbCrLf & vbCrLf _
        & "Programmed by A Millspaugh", vbOKOnly, "About R 'n R Billing"
End Sub
```

```
Public Function cFindTax(cAmount As Currency) As Currency
    'Calculate the sales tax

    cFindTax = cAmount * mcTAX_RATE
End Function
```

Programming Hints

Creating Executable Files

You can convert your project into an **executable file** that can be run from the Windows desktop. The resulting .EXE file contains the information from all your project's files, including the form files and the modules. The .EXE file will run much faster than the project runs in the VB environment.

After you create an .EXE file, the original project files are still intact and can be used to make any modifications. Any time you make changes in the original project files, you must re-create the .EXE file to incorporate the changes.

To create the .EXE file, select the *Make ...* command from the *File* menu. The *Make ...* menu choice displays the name of the current project. For example, Figure 5.18 show the menu for the chapter hands-on project, called Chap5Billing. Choose *Make Chap5Billing* from the *File* menu and the *Make Project* dialog box appears (Figure 5.18).

Figure 5.18

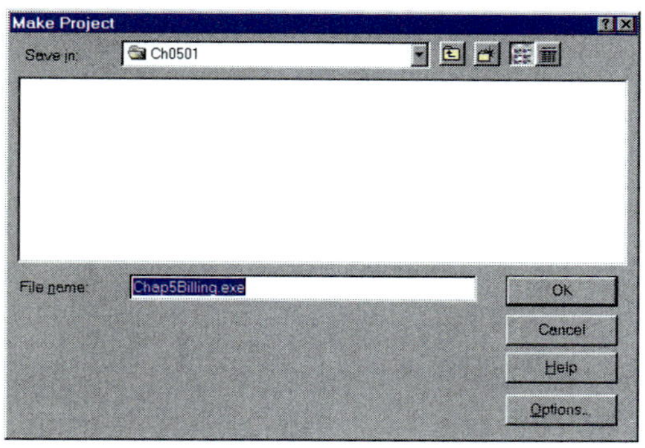

Use the Make Project dialog box to create an executable version of your project.

You will choose the location and name for your .EXE file. You can also set properties for your project by clicking on the *Options* button. In the *Project Properties* dialog box (Figure 5.19), you can specify the version number, company name, and an icon for your file.

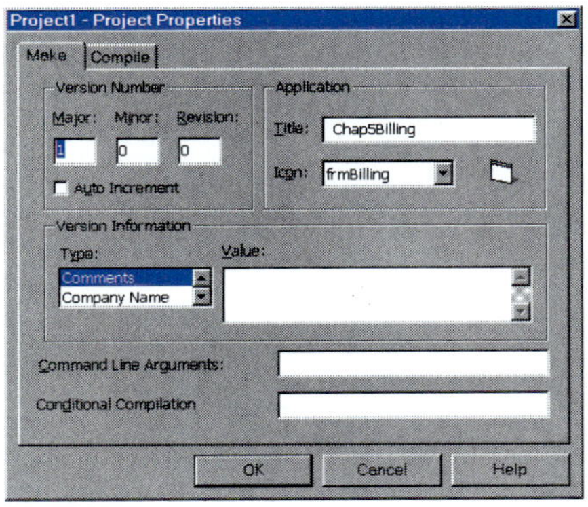

Figure 5.19

The Project Properties *dialog box allows you to specify version information, a company name, and an icon for your .EXE file.*

Summary

1. Menus are created in Visual Basic using the Menu Editor. The editor enables you to create menus, menu commands, and submenus, each with keyboard access keys.
2. The Caption and Name properties are required for each menu item.
3. In the Menu Editor, the order and level of menu items can be set and modified, as well as the initial settings of the Enabled and Checked properties.
4. Each menu command has a Click event. The code to handle selection of a menu command belongs in the command's Click event procedure.
5. Common dialog boxes allow Visual Basic programs to display the predefined Windows dialog boxes for *Print*, *Open*, *Save*, *Fonts*, and *Colors*. Since these dialog boxes are already a part of the operating environment, it is an unnecessary duplication of effort to have each programmer re-create them.
6. The programmer can write reusable code in general procedures. These procedures may be sub procedures or sub functions and may be called from any other procedure in the form module.
7. Sub procedures and sub functions can both perform an action. However, sub functions return a value and sub procedures do not. The value returned by a sub function will have a data type.
8. It is easy to convert a project to an .EXE file that can be run from the Windows environment. Use the *Make Project* command on the *File* menu.

Key Terms

call (procedure call) *173*
checked *165*
common dialog *167*
disabled *165*
enabled *165*
executable file *186*
function procedure *174*
general procedure *172*
menu *160*
return value *174*
separator bar *162*
sub procedure *174*
submenu *161*

Review Questions

1. Explain the difference between a menu and a submenu.
2. How can the user know if a menu command contains a submenu?
3. What is a separator bar and how is it created?
4. Explain the purpose of the Name and Caption properties of menu items.
5. What does the term *common dialog box* mean?
6. Name at least three types of common dialog boxes.
7. Why would you need procedures that are not attached to an event?
8. Code the necessary statements to produce a color dialog box and use it to change the background color of a form.
9. Explain the difference between a sub procedure and a function procedure.
10. What is a *return value*? How can it be used?
11. Give the steps required to convert a project into an .EXE file.

Programming Exercises

5.1 Modify project 4.6 (Piecework Pay) to replace command buttons with menus and add a function procedure.

This project will input the number of pieces and calculate the pay for multiple employees. It also must display a summary of the total number of pieces, the total pay, and the average pay for all employees.
Menu: The menu bar must have these commands:

```
File            Edit        Help
   Calc Pay        Clear       About
   Summary         ______
   Exit            Font
                   Color
```

Piecework workers are paid by the piece. Workers who produce a greater quantity of output may be paid at a higher rate.

Use text boxes to obtain the name and the number of pieces completed. The *Calc Pay* menu command calculates and displays the dollar amount earned. The *Summary* menu command displays the total number of pieces, the total pay, and the average pay per person in a message box. The *Clear* menu choice clears the name and the number of pieces for the current employee and resets the focus.

The *Color* and *Font* commands should change the color and font of the information displayed in the amount earned label.

Use a message box to display your name for the *About* option on the *Help* menu.

Use a function procedure to find the pay rate and return a value to the proper event procedure.

Pieces Completed	Price Paid per Piece for All Pieces
1 to 199	.50
200 to 399	.55
400 to 599	.60
600 or more	.65

5.2 Redo the checking account programming exercises from Chapter 4 (4.3, 4.4, and 4.5), using menus and sub procedures.
Menu:

```
File              Edit          Help
   Transaction       Clear         About
   Summary           ______
   Exit              Font
                     Color
```

Form: Use option buttons to indicate the type of transaction—deposit, check, or service charge. A text box will allow the user to enter the amount of the transaction. Display the balance in a label.

Include validation that displays a message box if the amount of the transaction is a negative number. If there is not enough money to cover a check, display a message box with the message "Insufficient Funds." Do not pay the check, but deduct a service charge of $10.

Use function procedures for deposits, checks, and service charges. The deposit function adds the deposit to the balance; the check function subtracts the transaction amount from the balance; the service charge function subtracts $10 from the balance.

The *Summary* menu command displays the total number of deposits and the dollar amount of deposits, the number of checks, and the dollar amount of the checks in a message box.

The *Clear* menu command clears the option buttons and the amount and resets the focus.

The *Color* and *Font* menu commands change the color and font of the information displayed in the balance label.

Use a message box to display your name as the programmer for the *About* option on the *Help* menu.

5.3 A salesperson earns a weekly base salary plus a commission when sales are at or above quota. Create a project that allows the user to input the weekly sales and the salesperson name, calculates the commission, and displays summary information.
Form: The form will have text boxes for the salesperson name and his or her weekly sales.
Menu:

```
File              Edit          Help
   Pay               Clear      About
   Summary           ______
   Exit              Font
                     Color
```

Use constants to establish the base pay, the quota, and the commission rate.

The *Pay* menu command calculates and displays in labels the commission and the total pay for that person. However, if there is no commission, do not display the commission amount (do not display a zero-commission amount).

Use a function procedure to calculate the commission. The function must compare sales to the quota. When the sales are equal to or greater than the quota, calculate the commission by multiplying sales by the commission rate.

Each salesperson receives the base pay plus the commission (if one has been earned). Format the dollar amounts to two decimal places; do not display a dollar sign.

The *Summary* menu command displays a message box containing total sales, total commissions, and total pay for all salespersons. Display the numbers with two decimal places and dollar signs.

The *Clear* menu command clears the name, sales, and pay for the current employee and then resets the focus.

The *Color* and *Font* menu commands should change the color and font of the information displayed in the amount earned label.

Use a message box to display your name as programmer for the *About* option on the *Help* menu.

Test Data: Quota = 1000; Commission rate = .15; and Base pay = 250.

Name	Sales
Sandy Smug	1,000.00
Sam Sadness	999.99
Joe Whiz	2,000.00

Totals should be:

Sales	$3,999.99
Commissions	450.00
Pay	1,200.00

5.4 The local library has a summer reading program to encourage reading. The staff keeps a chart with readers' names and bonus points earned. Create a project using a menu and a function procedure that will determine the bonus points.
Menu:

```
File            Edit       Help
  Points          Clear    About
  Summary         ______
  Exit            Font
                  Color
```

Form: Use text boxes to obtain the reader's name and the number of books read. Use a label to display the number of bonus points.

The *Points* menu command should call a function procedure to calculate the points using this schedule: the first three books are worth 10 points each. The next three books are worth 15 points each. All books over six are worth 20 points each.

The *Summary* menu command displays the average number of books read for all readers that session.

The *Clear* menu command clears the name, the number of books read, and the bonus points and then resets the focus.

The *Color* and *Font* menu commands change the color and font of the information displayed in the bonus points label.

Use a message box to display your name as programmer for the *About* option on the *Help* menu.

5.5 Modify project 2.2 (the flag viewer) to use a menu instead of option buttons, check boxes, and command buttons. Include check marks next to the name of the currently selected country and next to the selected display options.
Menu:

```
File      Country               Display
  Print     United States         Title
  Exit      Canada                Country Name
            Japan                 Programmer
            Mexico
```

CASE STUDIES

VB Mail Order

Modify the case study from Chapter 4 using menus and a function procedure. Refer to Chapter 4 for project specifications.

Use a function procedure to calculate the shipping and handling, based on the weight for an entire order. (Do not calculate shipping and handling on individual items—wait until the order is complete.)

Menu:

```
File            Edit               Help
Print Form        Next Item        About
Summary           Next Order
Exit              ______
                  Font
                  Color
```

VB Auto Center

Modify the case study project from Chapter 4 using menus and a function procedure. Refer to Chapter 4 for project specifications.

Use a function procedure to calculate the sales tax.

Menu:

```
File              Edit             Help
  Print Form        Calculate        About
  Exit              Clear
                    ________
                    Font
                    Color
```

C H A P T E R

6

Multiple Forms

At the completion of this chapter, you will be able to . . .

1. Create a project with multiple forms.
2. Use the Show and Hide methods to display and hide forms.
3. Create procedures that are accessible from multiple form modules.
4. Differentiate between variables that are global to a project and those visible only to a form.
5. Create an *About box* using a form.
6. Add a splash screen to your project.
7. Set the startup form or Sub Main to start project execution.

Multiple Forms

All the projects that you have created up to now have operated from a single form. It has probably occurred to you that the project could appear more professional if you could use different windows for different types of information. Consider the example in Chapter 5 in which summary information is displayed in a message box when the user presses the Summary button. You have very little control over the appearance of the message box. The summary information could be displayed in a much nicer format in a new window with identifying labels. Another window in Visual Basic is actually another form.

The first form a project displays is called the ***startup form***. You can add more forms to the project and display them as needed.

Creating New Forms

To add a new form to a project, select *Add Form* from the *Project* menu or click on the Form button on the toolbar (Figure 6.1). In the *Add Form* dialog box (Figure 6.2), you can select from a new form or an existing form. Notice in Figure 6.2 that VB provides several types of new forms that you can use; you will learn about some of these later in the chapter. For now, choose *Form* to add a regular new form.

Figure 6.1

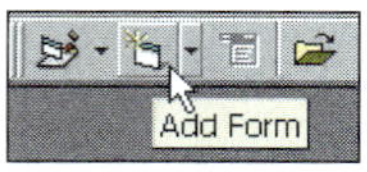

Add a new form to a project by clicking on the Add Form toolbar button.

Figure 6.2

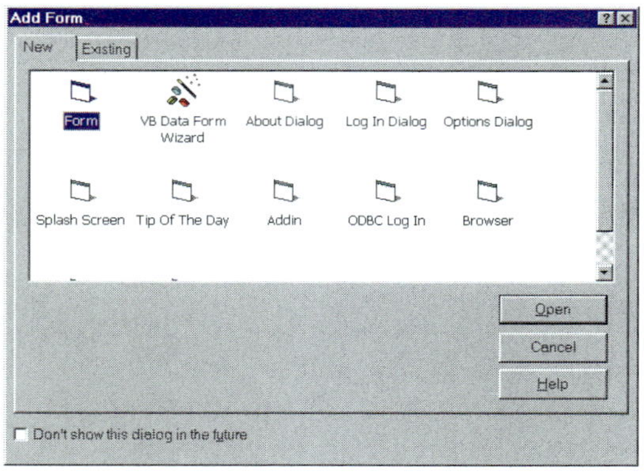

Select the type of new form you want in the Add Form dialog box.

Steps for adding a new form to a project:

STEP 1: Select *Add Form* from the *Project* menu.

STEP 2: In the dialog box select the *New* tab and indicate the type of form you want (Form, About, Splash).

STEP 3: Click on *Open*.

The new form will display on the screen and be added to the Project Explorer window (Figure 6.3).

Figure 6.3

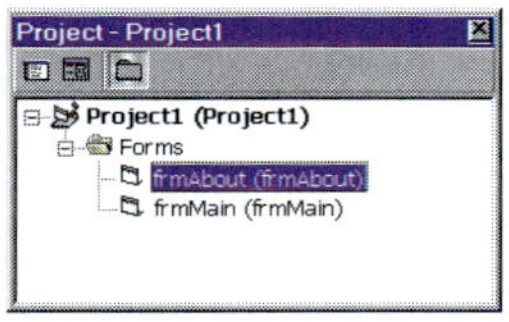

After adding a new form, the Project Explorer window shows the name of the new form.

If you want your newly created form to be the startup form (the one that appears when the project starts running), you will need to follow the steps for setting a startup form, which are found later in this chapter.

While in design time, you can switch between forms two ways. If you can see any part of the other form on the screen, just click on the form to make it active. You can also use the Project Explorer window. The Project Explorer window's View Form button and View Code button switch to the form or code of the module that is selected (highlighted). You can switch between forms by clicking on the form name in the Project Explorer window and clicking the View Form button, or by double-clicking on a form name.

Each form module is a separate file and a separate entity. The code that exists in one form module is not visible to any other form module. Note one exception: Any procedure declared with the `Public` keyword is callable from other modules in the project.

Adding and Removing Forms

The Project Explorer window shows the files that are included in a project. You can add new files and remove files from a project.

Adding Existing Form Files to a Project

Forms may be used in more than one project. You might want to use a form that you created for one project in a new project.

Each form is a separate module, which is saved as a separate file with an .FRM extension. All of the information for the form resides in the file, which includes the code procedures and the visual interface as well as all property settings for the controls.

To add an existing form to a project, use the *Add Form* command on the *Project* menu and select the *Existing* tab (Figure 6.4). You will need to supply the name of the form and the folder where it can be found.

Figure 6.4

Select the Existing *tab to add an existing form to a project.*

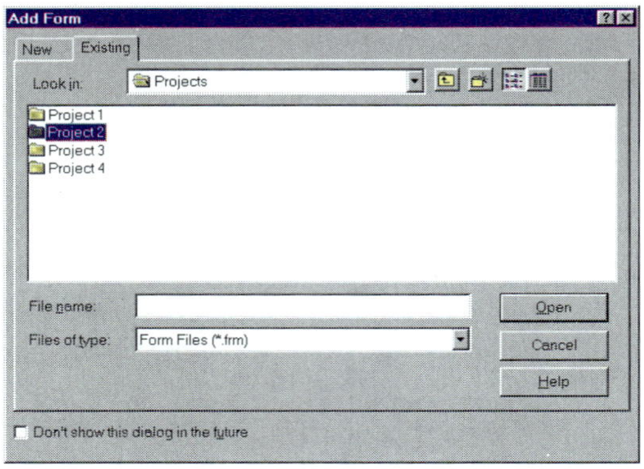

Steps for adding an existing form to a project:

STEP 1: Select *Add Form* from the *Project* menu.
STEP 2: In the *Add Form* dialog box, select the *Existing* tab and locate the folder and file desired.
STEP 3: Click on *Open*.

Removing Forms From a Project

If you want to remove a file from a project, select its name in the Project Explorer window. You can then either choose *Remove File* from the *Project* menu or right-click on the filename to display the Shortcut menu and choose *Remove Filename*.

The Hide and Show Methods

In code, you can display a form with the **`Show` method** and conceal a form with the **`Hide` method**. If both forms are the same size, the process of showing the second form will cover the first form on the screen. Use the `Hide` method when you want to make sure a form disappears.

The Show Method—General Form

```
FormName.Show [Style]
```

The FormName is the name of the form you wish to display. The optional *Style* determines whether the form will display modeless or modal. The values for Style can be 0 (for modeless) or 1 (for modal); the default is 0. You can also use the VB intrinsic constants: vbModal and vbModeless.

When you display a form as **modal**, the user must respond to the form in some way, usually by clicking a command button. No other program code can execute until the modal form has been responded to and hidden or unloaded. However, if you display a **modeless** form, the user may switch to another form in the project without responding to the form. *Note:* Even with a modal form, the user can switch to another application within Windows.

The Show Method—Examples

```
frmSummary.Show 1           'Display the summary form, modal style
frmSummary.Show vbModal     'Display the summary form, modal style
frmSummary.Show vbModeless  'Display the summary form, modeless style
frmSummary.Show             'Display the summary form, modeless style
```

When you choose whether to display a form as modal or modeless, you must be aware of an important difference in the way VB executes the statements. As you already know, code statements within a procedure execute one after another, in sequence. When you have a modal `Show` method in code, VB executes the `Show` and pauses; it does not execute any further statements until the user responds to the modal form. Conversely, when VB encounters a modeless `Show` method, it displays the form and continues execution; if additional statements follow the `Show`, they will be executed immediately, without waiting for response from the user. In most cases, you will want to display forms modally.

Recall the sample programs in Chapters 4 and 5, which display summary information in a message box. A nicer solution would be to display the summary data in a second form, called frmSummary. Replace the `MsgBox` statement in the cmdSummary_Click event procedure with this statement:

```
frmSummary.Show vbModal 'Display the summary form
```

The Form Load and Form Activate Events

The first time a form is displayed in a project, Visual Basic generates two events—a Form_Load and a Form_Activate. The Load event calls the form module into memory; the Activate event occurs after the Load event, just as control is passed to the form. Each subsequent time the form is shown, the Activate event occurs, but not the Load event. Therefore, if a form may be displayed multiple times, you may want to place initializing steps into the Form_Activate event procedure rather than into the Form_Load. Also, if you wish to set the focus in a particular place on the new form, place the SetFocus method in the Form_Activate procedure.

When you use a `Show` method, the size and location of the form depend upon the Left, Top, Height, and Width properties of the form being displayed. You can calculate these properties when the form is shown by placing the calculations in the Form_Activate event. If you would like to make your form fill the screen, see the hints for working with maximized forms in the "Programming Hints" at the end of this chapter.

Tip

To write code for the Form_Activate event, display the code window and choose *Form* in the *Object* box and *Activate* in the *Procedure* box.

Hiding a Form

The `Hide` method is very similar to the `Show` method but is used to remove a form from the screen.

The Hide Method—General Form

```
FormName.Hide
```

The Hide Method—Example

```
frmSummary.Hide
```

The Load and Unload Statements

When you work with multiple forms, you may also want to use the **Load** and **Unload** statements. Although you can explicitly load a form, in most cases the `Load` isn't necessary. When you `Show` a form, the `Load` is done automatically. The only time you will code a `Load` statement is when you want to load a form but not display it until later.

To remove a form from the screen, you can hide it or unload it. Hiding a form removes it from the screen, but the form still remains in memory and uses system resources. If you have many forms and you are sure you will not need a form again, it's best to unload it rather than to hide it.

The Load and Unload Statements—General Form

```
Load FormName
Unload FormName
```

The Load and Unload Statements—Examples

```
Load frmSummary
Unload frmSummary
```

Tip

You can quickly jump to another location in a project and then jump back to the same spot. Click on the name of a procedure or form where you want to jump and press Shift + F2. To jump back to the earlier spot, press Ctrl + Shift + F2.

The Me Keyword

You can refer to the current form by using the special keyword `Me`. `Me` acts like a variable and refers to the currently active form. You can use `Me` in place of the form name when coding form statements and methods.

The Me Keyword—Examples

```
Unload Me     'Unload the form that is currently executing code
Me.Hide       'Hide the form that is currently executing code
```

Referring to Objects on a Different Form

Each form is a separate module, with its own variables, objects, properties, and code. When your project has only one form, you can refer to any object and its properties in any procedure. But when you use multiple forms, the code in one module cannot "see" the objects in another module without some help. One way to reference an object in another form module is to expand the reference to include the name of the form:

```
FormName!ObjectName.Property
```

Using this technique, you can set the properties of objects in a form before displaying it.

Example

```
frmSummary!lblTotalAmount.Caption = mcTotal
frmSummary.Show vbModal
```

Consequently, you can use the same name for objects in two different forms. Although it may be confusing to have similarly named objects in multiple forms it is perfectly acceptable. An example is having an OK button in two forms, both named cmdOK. The two buttons would be referred to as frmStartup!cmdOK and frmSummary!cmdOK.

Note: Programmers have a language of their own. Just as you learned to say "dot" for the period ("Object dot Property"), if you want to speak like a programmer, you must call the exclamation point "bang." Therefore, to refer to a form's objects and properties, it's "FormName bang Object dot Property."

Standard Code Modules

When using multiple forms in a project, it is important for you to consider each sub procedure or function procedure that you create. If the procedure will be used in only one form, then it should be included in the code for that form module. If, in fact, you will need to use the procedure in multiple forms, write the procedure in a **standard code module.** A *standard code module* is a Basic file with the extension **.BAS**, which is added to the project. Standard code modules do not contain a form, only code.

Create a new standard code module by selecting the *Add Module* command on the *Project* menu. A new Code window titled *Module1* opens on the screen (Figure 6.5). Also note that Module1 is added to your Project Explorer window (Figure 6.6). Make sure that Module1 is highlighted in the Project Explorer window and choose *Save Module1* from the *File* menu to give the new file a name. It is a good idea to name this file the same as your project file unless you plan to use it for multiple projects. The file extension is .BAS by default.

Figure 6.5

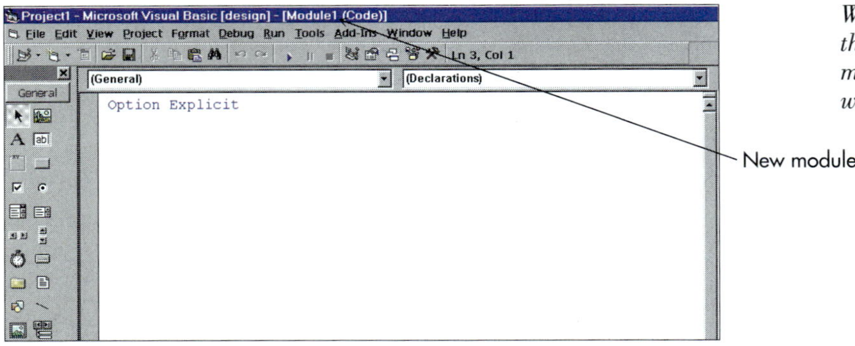

When you select Add Module *on the* Project *menu, a new code module opens in the Code window.*

Figure 6.6

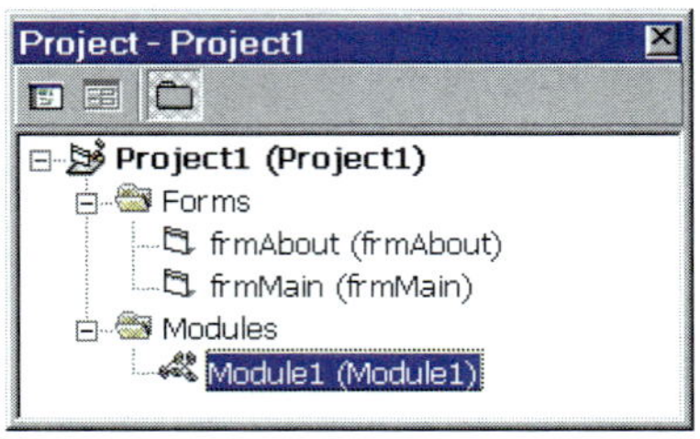

The new module, Module1, is added to the project in the Project Explorer window.

A standard code module has a General Declarations section and procedures, just like a form module. You can declare variables with the `Dim` statement in procedures or in the General Declarations section. Any `Dim`med variables or constants in the General Declarations section of a standard code module are visible to all the procedures in that module, but not to the procedures in the form module(s).

Variables and Constants in Multiple-Form Projects

When you have multiple modules in a project, the scope of the variables and constants becomes a little more complicated. The variables and constants can be local to a procedure; module level, which are available to all procedures in the module; or **global**, which are available to all procedures in all modules in the project.

Global Variables and Constants

If you want variables and constants to be accessible to more than one form in the project, they must be global variables. To declare global variables, use the **`Public`** statement in place of the `Dim` statement.

The Public Statement—General Form

```
Public Identifier [As DataType]
Public Const Identifier [As DataType] = Value
```

The format of the `Public` statement is similar to the `Dim` and `Const` statements. If the data type is omitted for a variable, the type defaults to variant. For a constant, if you omit the data type, Visual Basic selects the type most appropriate for the value.

It is important to know the scope of a variable when programming. A module-level variable or constant has a prefix of "m", and a public variable or constant has a prefix of "g" (for global; "p" refers to private). Any variable or constant without a scope prefix is assumed to be local to a procedure.

The Public Statement—Examples

```
Public gcGrandTotal As Currency
Public gPersonName 'Defaults to Variant data type
Public Const gsTAX_RATE As Single = .0825
Public Const gstCOMPANY = "R 'n R — for Reading and Refreshment" _
                          'Defaults to String data type
```

Note: Visual Basic also has a `Private` statement with the same syntax as the `Public` statement. Since all variables and constants are private by default, the `Private` statement is rarely used.

Static Variables

Another statement you can use to declare variables at the procedure level is the **`Static`** statement. Static variables retain their value for the life of the project, rather than being reinitialized for each call to the procedure. If you need to retain the value in a variable for multiple calls to a procedure, such as a running total, declare it as Static. (In the past we used module-level variables for this task. Using a static local variable is better than using a module-level variable because it is always best to keep the scope of a variable as narrow as possible.)

The Static Statement—General Form

```
Static Identifier [As DataType]
```

The format of the `Static` statement is the same as the format of the `Dim` statement. However, `Static` statements can appear only in procedures; `Static` statements never appear in the General Declarations section of a module.

The Static Statement—Examples

```
Static iPersonCount As Integer
Static cReportTotal As Currency
```

Static variables do not require a scope prefix, since all static variables are local.

Guidelines for Declaring Variables and Constants

When you declare variables and constants, select the location of the declaration carefully. These general guidelines will help you decide where to place declarations:

1. Place all local declarations (`Dim`, `Const`, `Static`) at the *top* of a procedure. Although Basic will accept declarations placed further down in the code, such placement is considered a poor practice. Your code will be easier to read, debug, modify, and maintain if you follow this guideline.
2. Use named constants for any value that doesn't change during program execution. It is far more clear to use named constants such as cMAXIMUM_RATE and stCOMPANY_NAME than to place the values into your code; and if in the future the values must be modified, having a constant name (at the top of your project) makes the task *much* easier.
3. Keep the scope of variables and constants as narrow as possible. Don't declare them all to be global or module level for convenience. There are books full of horror stories about strange program bugs popping up because the value of a variable was changed in an unknown location.
4. Consider making variables and constants local if possible.
5. If you need to keep the value of a variable for multiple executions of a procedure, but don't need the variable in any other procedure, make it Static.
6. If you need to use a variable both in a procedure and also in a second procedure called by the first procedure, declare the variable as local and pass it as an argument. (Refer to "Passing Variables to Procedures" in Chapter 5.)
7. If you need to use a variable in multiple procedures, such as to add to the variable in one procedure and to display it in another, use module-level variables. (Use a `Dim` statement in the General Declarations section of the module.)
8. If you need to use the value of a variable in multiple forms, you may still have two choices. Do you actually need to use the variable in the second form, or are you just displaying it in a control? Remember, you can assign a variable to a property in another form by specifying FormName!Object.Property.
9. Finally, if you really need the value of a variable in more than one form, make it global. Declare the variable with the `Public` statement in the General Declarations section of a standard code module. *Note:* Visual Basic allows you to use the `Public` statement in the General Declara-

tions section of *any* module, which means that you can declare global variables in any form module. Don't do it! Keep your `Public` declarations in a standard code module.

Feedback 6.1

For each of these situations, write the declaration statement and tell where it should appear. Assume the project will have multiple form modules and a standard code module. Be sure to give the proper prefixes to your identifiers.

1. The number of calories in a gram of fat (nine), to use in the calculations of a procedure.
2. The name of the person with the highest score, which will be determined in one procedure and displayed in a label on a different form. (The value must be retained for multiple executions of the procedure.)
3. The name of the company ("Bab's Bowling Service"), which will appear in several forms.
4. A total dollar amount to be calculated in one procedure of a form, added to a grand total in a procedure of a second form, and formatted and displayed in a third form.
5. A count of the number of persons entered using a single form. The count will be used to help calculate an average in a second form.
6. The formatted version of a dollar total, which will be displayed in a label in the next statement.
7. For each of these identifiers, tell the scope, data type, and whether it represents a variable or constant.
   (a) miLocations
   (b) gcPayment
   (c) cPayment
   (d) cPAYMENT
   (e) gstTEAM_NAME
   (f) stTeamName
   (g) mstTeamName
   (h) gstTeamName

An About Box

One type of additional form in a project is an **About box**, such as the one you find in most Windows programs in *Help/About.* Usually an About box gives the name and version of the project as well as information about the programmer or company. The About box may be displayed initially when the application begins or displayed when a specific event occurs (such as pressing a command button or selecting a menu command).

You can create your own About box by creating a new form and entering the information in labels. Of course, you may use any of the normal controls on this new form, but About boxes typically hold labels, an OK command button, and perhaps an image or shape controls for a logo. Figure 6.7 shows a typical About box.

Figure 6.7

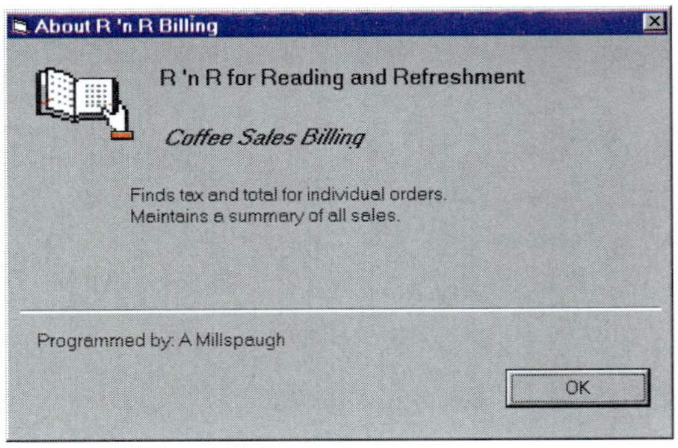

A typical About box containing labels, a line control, an image, and an OK command button.

You can also use VB's About Dialog template to create a new About box. Choose *Add Form* from the *Project* menu and on the *New* tab select *About Dialog* (Figure 6.8). A new form is added to your project with controls you can modify (Figure 6.9). You can change the captions and image by setting the properties as you would on any other form. Once you create the form in your project, it is yours and may be modified as you please.

Figure 6.8

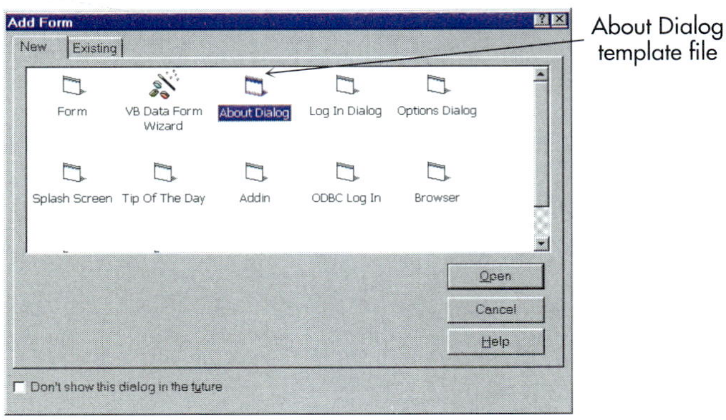

Select About Dialog from the New tab of the Add Form dialog box.

Figure 6.9

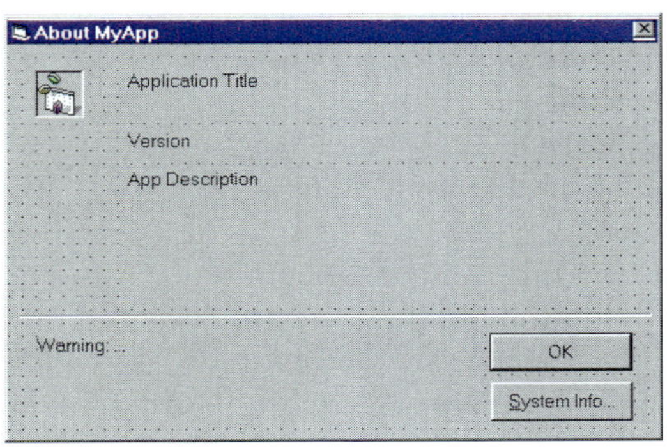

A new form created with the About Dialog template.

A Splash Screen

Perhaps you have noticed the logo or window that often appears while a program is loading, such as the one in Figure 6.10. This initial form is called a **splash screen**. Professional applications use splash screens to tell the user that the program is loading and starting. It can make a large application appear to load and run faster, since something appears on the screen while the rest of the application loads.

Figure 6.10

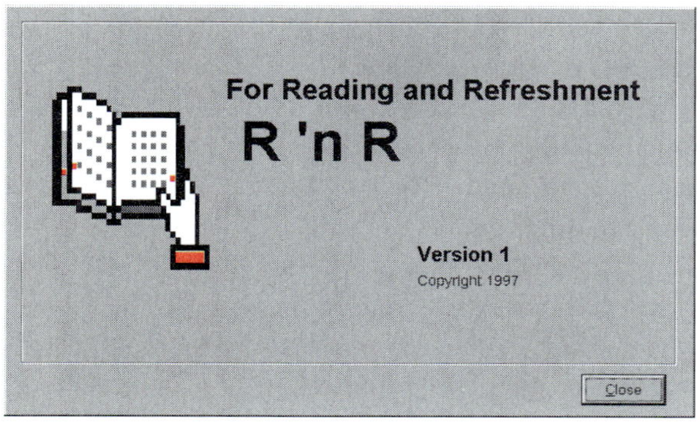

A splash screen.

You can create your own splash screen or use the splash screen template included with VB5 (Figure 6.11). In the *Add Form* dialog box (refer to Figure 6.8), choose *Splash Screen* to add the new form; then modify the form to fit your needs. In the case of this splash screen, you will need to make major modifications to all the labels and to the code.

New to VB 5!

Figure 6.11

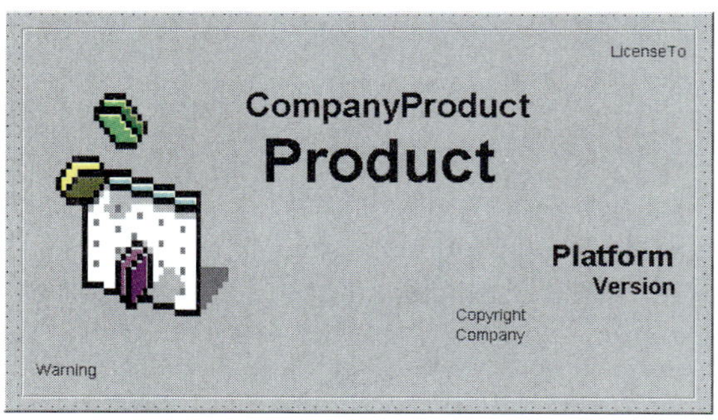

A new form created with the Splash Screen form template.

When you use this style of splash screen, your project does not display the main form as a startup form. Instead, when you run the project, execution begins with a sub procedure named Main, which is located in your .BAS file.

Tip

To switch from one form to another in design time, use the Project Explorer window. Double-click on a form name to display the form. Or click on a form name and then click either the View Object or the View Code button.

Using Sub Main for Startup

A project may begin execution by displaying a startup form or by executing a procedure called Main, which you will code in your standard code module. You will use a Main sub procedure when you have tasks that should be done before the first form loads, such as when you want to display a splash screen while the main form loads.

When you begin execution with a Main sub procedure, you must explicitly load and/or show each form. In the following example, the splash screen is displayed as modeless, so that the `Load` statement in the next statement will execute. In the `Load` statement, the project's main form is loaded but not shown. The last actions performed by the form module will be to unload the splash screen and show the main form.

You have some choices about when to unload the splash screen and show the main form. In a large application, where it may take several seconds to load the main form, the logic is usually set up to exit the splash screen as soon as the main form finishes loading. In a small application, such as the ones we are writing in this text, the main form loads so quickly that the splash screen disappears before you can see it. We will place a Close button on the splash screen rather than have the form disappear automatically. You might also consider using a Timer control to close the form after an interval of time. See Chapter 13 or Visual Basic Help for information on the Timer control.

Coding the Standard Code Module

This code goes in the standard code module (.BAS file):

```
Sub Main()
    'Display the splash screen while the main form loads

    frmSplash.Show vbModeless 'Display the splash form
    Load frmMain              'Load the main form
End Sub
```

Coding the Splash Screen Event Procedure

The following code goes in the cmdClose_Click event procedure of the splash screen form. *Note:* If you started with the VB Splash Screen template, first remove all code that appeared automatically, add a cmdClose command button, and add this procedure:

```
Private Sub cmdClose_Click()
    'Unload splash screen and show the main form

    Unload Me                 'Unload the splash screen form
    frmMain.Show vbModal      'Show the main form
End Sub
```

Setting the Startup Form or Procedure

The startup form by default is the first form created in a project. However, you can select a different form to be the startup form, or you can specify that your Main sub procedure should begin when the project is run. In the *Project Properties* dialog box (Figure 6.12), you can choose one of the project's forms or *Sub Main.*

Figure 6.12

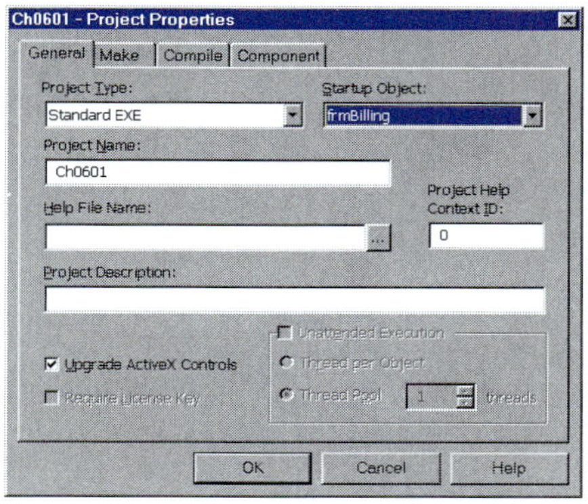

Set the startup form or procedure in the Project Properties dialog box.

To change the startup option:

STEP 1: Select *Project Properties* from the *Project* menu (or right-click on project name in the Project Explorer window and choose *Project Properties*).

STEP 2: In the *Project Properties* dialog box, click on the *General* tab.

STEP 3: Drop down the list for *Startup Object* (Figure 6.13) and select the desired form or the *Sub Main* procedure.

Figure 6.13

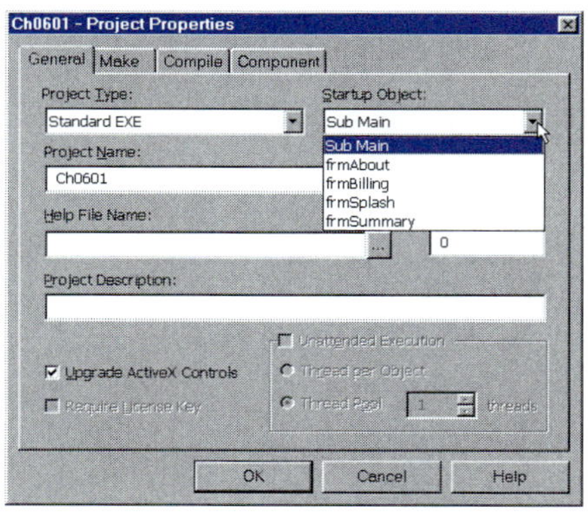

Drop down the Startup Object list to select a startup form or Sub Main.

STEP 4: Click OK.

Your Hands-On Programming Example

Modify the hands-on project from Chapter 5 to include multiple forms. This version of the project requires four forms: frmBillling, frmAbout, frmSplash, and frmSummary.

frmBilling: Add the frmBilling form from Chapter 5 to a new project. Do a ***Save As***, create a new folder, and save the form into the new folder. This step will create a copy of the Chapter 5 form which you can modify for this project.

frmAbout: Replace the MsgBox About Box from Chapter 5 with a new form using the About Dialog template. Delete all of the code attached to the new form file. Delete the command button for system information from the form. (You may want to test this command on your own.)

frmSplash: Create a splash screen using the Splash Screen template. Customize the label captions and the image and delete all of the code attached to the new form file.

frmSummary: Replace the summary labels from the main form (frmBilling) with a separate form for the summary.

Startup Object: Create a standard code module with a Main sub procedure. Set the form properties Startup Object to Sub Main.

Reviewing the project requirements:

frmBilling: The user enters the number of items, selects the coffee type from option buttons, and selects the check box for taxable items. The price for each coffee is calculated according to these prices:

Cappuccino	2.00
Espresso	2.25
Latte	1.75
Iced (either)	2.50

The Calculate Selection command button calculates and displays the amount due for each item, adds the current item to the order, and calculates and displays the order information in labels. The Clear for Next Item button clears the selections and amount for the single item.

The *Next Order* menu command clears the bill for the current customer and add to the totals for the summary. The *Summary* menu command shows the summary form that displays the total of all orders, the average sale amount per customer, and the number of customers.

The *Edit* menu contains options that duplicate the Calculate and Clear buttons. The *Font* and *Color* options change the contents of the subtotal, tax, and total labels.

The *About* selection on the *Help* menu displays the About form, which contains information about the program and the programmer.

```
File              Edit                    Help
    New Order         Calculate Amount        About
    Summary           Clear Item
    Exit              ___
                      Font
                      Color
```

Planning the Project

Sketch the four forms (Figure 6.14). Your user checks the sketches and signs off the design.

Figure 6.14

Sketches of the four forms for the hands-on programming example.

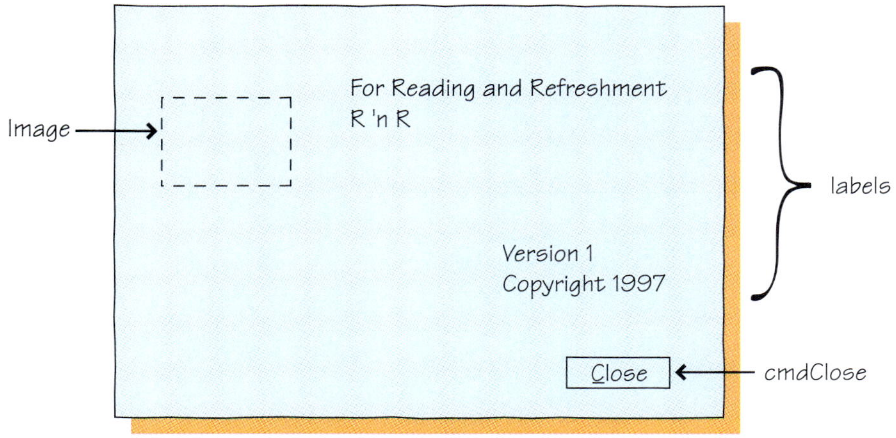

(a) frmSplash

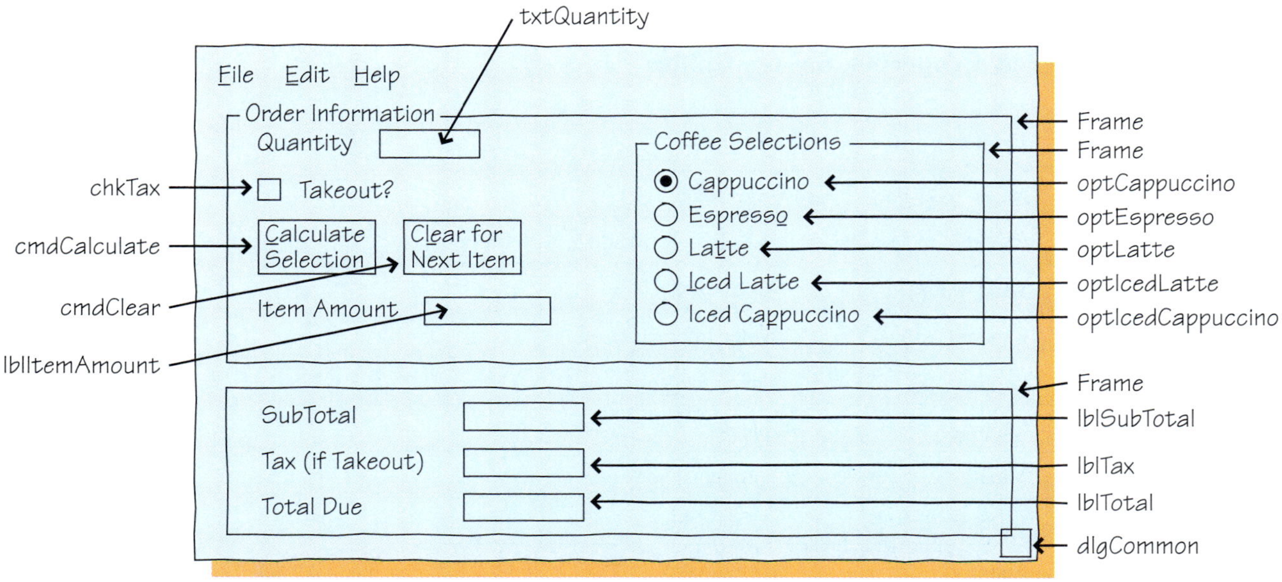

(b) frmBilling

Figure 6.14

Continued

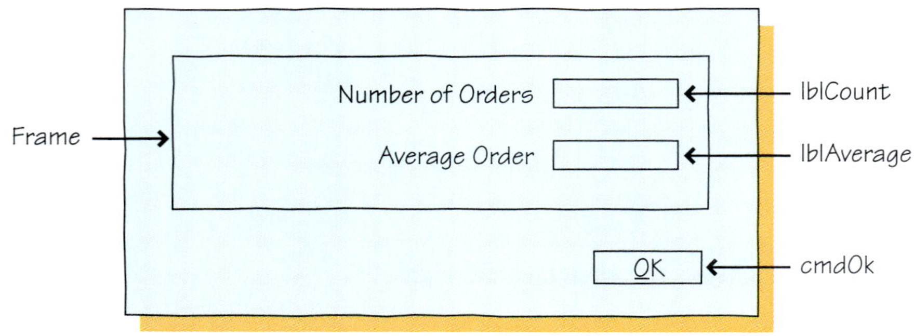

(c) frmSummary

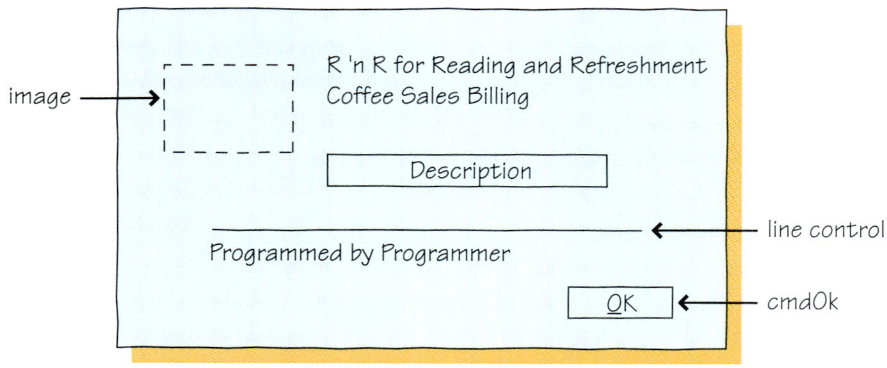

(d) frmAbout

The next step is to plan the property settings for each of the forms and the controls. *Note:* The frmBilling user interface is unchanged from Chapter 5.

frmBilling

Plan the Objects and Properties for frmBilling

Object	Property	Setting
frmBilling	Name	frmBilling
	Caption	R 'n R—for Reading 'n Refreshment
	WindowState	Maximized
Frame1	Caption	Order Information
Frame2	Caption	Coffee Selections
Frame3	Caption	(blank)
optCappuccino	Name	optCappuccino
	Caption	C&appuccino
optEspresso	Name	optEspresso
	Caption	Espress&o

(continued)

Object	Property	Setting
optLatte	Name	optLatte
	Caption	La&tte
optIcedLatte	Name	optIcedLatte
	Caption	&Iced Latte
optIcedCappuccino	Name	optIcedCappuccino
	Caption	Iced Ca&ppuccino
Label1	Caption	Quantity
txtQuantity	Name	txtQuantity
	Text	(blank)
chkTax	Name	chkTax
	Caption	Takeout ?
Label2	Caption	Item Amount
Label3	Caption	SubTotal
Label4	Caption	Tax (if Takeout)
Label5	Caption	Total Due
lblItemAmount	Name	lblItemAmount
	Caption	(blank)
	BorderStyle	1 - FixedSingle
lblSubTotal	Name	lblSubTotal
	Caption	(blank)
	BorderStyle	1 - Fixed Single
lblTax	Name	lblTax
	Caption	(blank)
	BorderStyle	1 - Fixed Single
lblTotal	Name	lblTotal
	Caption	(blank)
	BorderStyle	1 - Fixed Single
cmdCalculate	Name	cmdCalculate
	Caption	&Calculate Selection
	Default	True
cmdClear	Name	cmdClear
	Caption	C&lear for Next Item
	Cancel	True
mnuFileNew	Name	mnuFileNew

(continued)

Object	Property	Setting
	Caption	&New Order
mnuFileSummary	Name	mnuFileSummary
	Caption	&Summary
mnuFileExit	Name	mnuFileExit
	Caption	E&xit
mnuEditCalc	Name	mnuEditCalc
	Caption	&Calculate Selection
mnuEditClear	Name	mnuEditClear
	Caption	C&lear Item
mnuEditFont	Name	mnuEditFont
	Caption	&Font
mnuEditColor	Name	mnuEditColor
	Caption	&Color
mnuHelpAbout	Name	mnuHelpAbout
	Caption	&About

Plan the Event Procedures for frmBilling

Plan the actions for the event procedures for the menu commands and command buttons.

Object	Procedure	Action
cmdCalculate	Click	Determine price per cup. Multiply price by quantity. Call tax procedure if needed. Add quantity to item total. Display the values.
cmdClear	Click	Clear the coffee selections. Clear the quantity and the item price. Disable the takeout check box. Set the focus to the quantity.
mnuFileNew	Click	Clear the previous order. Accumulate total and count. Set subtotal and total to 0.
mnuFileSummary	Click	Display the Average. Display Total Sales. Display the number of customers.
mnuFileExit	Click	Terminate the project.
mnuEditCalc	Click	Call calculate command event.
mnuEditClear	Click	Call clear command event.
cFindTax	(call)	Calculate the sales tax.

frmSplash

Plan the Objects and Properties for frmSplash

Object	Property	Setting
frmSplash	Name	frmSplash
	Caption	(blank)
	ControlBox	False (Already set by the form template)
	MaxButton	False (Already set by the form template)
	MinButton	False (Already set by the form template)
All labels	Caption	Program information (*Note:* Student information goes here.)
cmdClose	Name	cmdClose
	Caption	&Close

Plan the Event Procedures for frmSplash

Object	Procedure	Action
cmdClose	Click	Unload the splash form. Show the main form.

frmAbout

Plan the Objects and Properties for frmAbout

Object	Property	Setting
frmAbout	Name	frmAbout
	Caption	About R 'n R Billing
	MaxButton	False (Already set by the form template)
	MinButton	False (Already set by the form template)
All labels	Caption	Program and programmer information
cmdOK	Name	cmdOK
	Caption	&OK

Plan the Event Procedures for frmAbout

Object	Procedure	Action
cmdOK	Click	Hide the About form.

frmSummary

Plan the Objects and Properties for frmSummary

Object	Property	Setting
frmSummary	Name	frmSummary
	Caption	Coffee Sales Summary
Frame1	Caption	Program and programmer information (*Note:* Student information goes here.)
Label1	Name	Label1
	Caption	Number of Orders
Label2	Name	Label2
	Caption	Average Order
lblCount	Name	lblCount
	Caption	(blank)
	Alignment	Right Justify
lblAverage	Name	lblAverage
	Caption	(blank)
	Alignment	Right Justify
cmdOK	Name	cmdOK
	Caption	&OK

Plan the Event Procedures for frmSummary

Object	Procedure	Action
cmdOK	Click	Hide the Summary form.

Form	Activate	If Count > 0 then
		  Calculate Average = Total / Count
		Else
		  Average = 0
		End If
		Format and display Count and Average.

Standard Code Module

Plan the Procedures for the Standard Code Module

Procedure	Action
Main	Show the Splash screen. Load frmBilling.

Write the Project

After completing the planning steps, create the forms following the sketches in Figure 6.14. Figure 6.15 shows the completed forms.

Figure 6.15

The four forms for the hands-on programming example are frmSplash, frmBilling, frmSummary, and frmAbout.

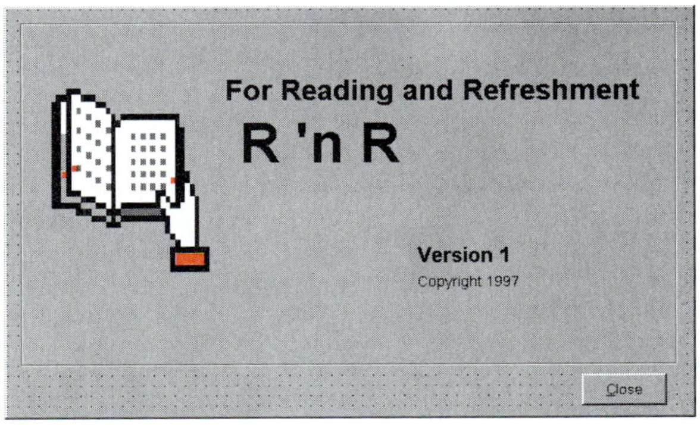

(a) *frmSplash*

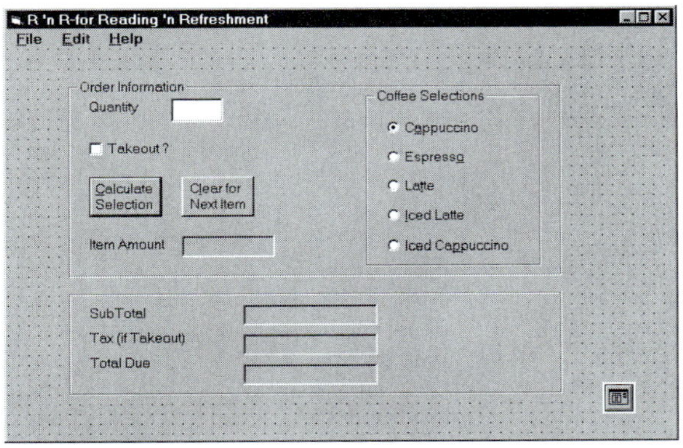

(b) *frmBilling*

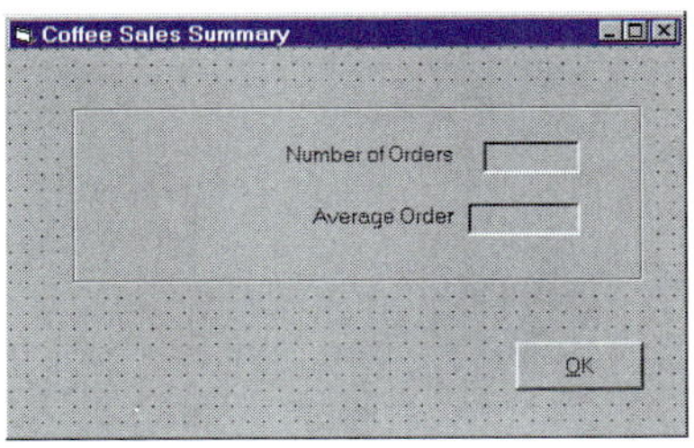

(c) *frmSummary*

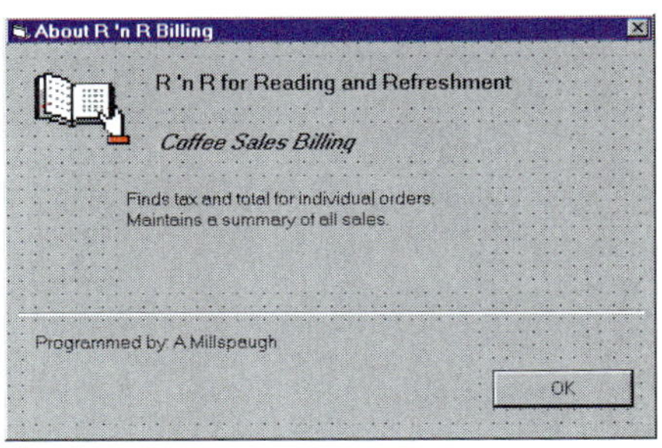

(d) *frmAbout*

frmBilling:

STEP 1: Begin a new project.

STEP 2: Point to *Form1* in the Project Explorer window, right-click to display the shortcut menu, and select *Remove Form1.*

STEP 3: Select *Add Form* from the *Project* menu and click on the *Existing* tab.

STEP 4: Locate frmBilling in the Ch0501 folder (or wherever you placed the hands-on project from Chapter 5). Click on *Open.*

STEP 5: Click on *frmBilling* in the Project Explorer window and select *Save frmBilling.frm As* from the *File* menu. Open the *Save In* list and select the location you want for a new folder and then click on the *Create New Folder* button. Name your new folder *Ch0601.*

STEP 6: Double-click on your new folder so that it appears in the *Save In* box, check the filename, and click *Save.* Your Project Explorer window should resemble Figure 6.16.

Figure 6.16

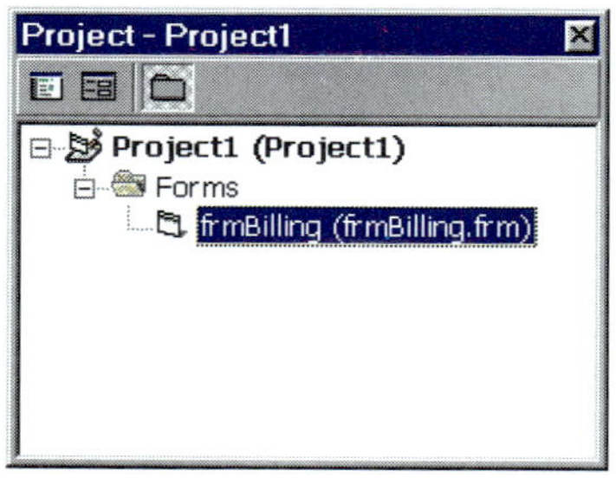

The Project Explorer window shows the newly added form in the project.

STEP 7: Make the planned changes to the mnuFileSummary_Click and mnuHelpAbout_Click event procedures, as well as changes to global variables used for the summary.

Note: If you wish you can continue adding forms to your project and return later to the steps that modify the forms and code.

frmAbout:

STEP 1: Select *Add Form* from the *Project* menu and click on the *New* tab.

STEP 2: Double-click on *About Dialog.*

STEP 3: Set the form's properties to match the plans detailed earlier.

STEP 4: Choose *Save frmAbout As* from the *File* menu, check the folder and filename, and save the new form.

STEP 5: Modify the label captions on the form to match your planning sketch.

STEP 6: Add the OK command button.

STEP 7: Switch to the code window and delete all code there except `Option Explicit`.

STEP 8: Write the code for frmAbout.

frmSplash:

STEP 1: Select *Add Form* from the *Project* menu and click on the *New* tab.

STEP 2: Double-click on *Splash Screen.*

STEP 3: Set the form's properties to match the plans detailed earlier.

STEP 4: Choose *Save frmSplash As* from the *File* menu, check the folder and filename, and save the new form.
STEP 5: Modify the label captions on the form to match your planning sketch.
STEP 6: Add the Close command button.
STEP 7: Switch to the code window and delete all code there except `Option Explicit`.
STEP 8: Write the code for frmSplash.

frmSummary:

STEP 1: Select *Add Form* from the *Project* menu and click on the *New* tab.
STEP 2: Double-click on *Form*.
STEP 3: Set the form's properties to match the plans detailed above.
STEP 4: Choose *Save Form1 As* from the *File* menu, check the folder, change the filename to *frmSummary*, and save the new form.
STEP 5: Create the controls on the form to match your planning sketch.
STEP 6: Set the properties for the controls.
STEP 7: Write the code for frmSummary.

Standard Code Module:

STEP 1: Select *Add Module* from the *Project* menu and click on the *New* tab.
STEP 2: Double-click on *Module*.
STEP 3: Choose *Save Module1 As* from the *File* menu, check the folder, change the filename to *Ch0601*, and save the new code module. Your Project Explorer window should look like Figure 6.17.

Figure 6.17

The completed project should show all four forms and the standard code module.

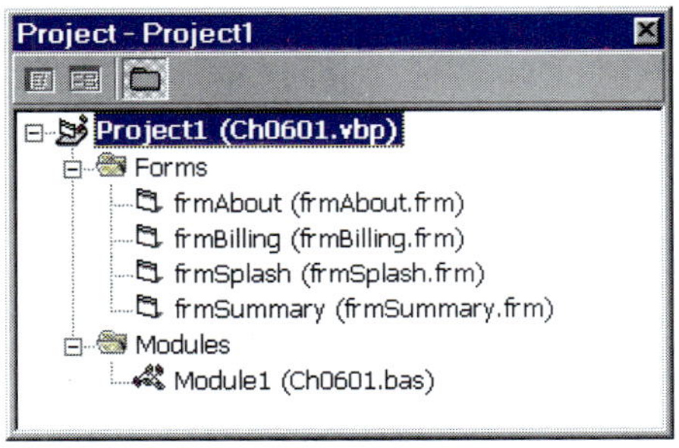

STEP 4: Write the code for the standard code module, which includes declarations for the global variables and the Main sub procedure.

Set the Startup Object:

STEP 1: Select *Project Properties* from the *Project* menu (or right-click on project name in the Project Explorer window and choose *Project Properties*).
STEP 2: In the *Project Properties* dialog box, click on the *General* tab.
STEP 3: Drop down the list for *Startup Object* and select *Sub Main*. The Main sub procedure displays frmSplash and loads frmBilling.
STEP 4: Click on OK.

Write the Code

frmBilling

```
'Program Name:      Billing
'Programmer:        A. Millspaugh
'Date:              July 1997
'Description:       This project calculates the
'                   amount due based upon the customer selection
'                   and accumulates summary data for the day.
'                   The project incorporates menus, common dialog
'                   boxes, and multiple forms.
'Folder:            Ch0601

Option Explicit
Dim mcSubtotal                  As Currency
Dim mcTotal                     As Currency
Const cCAPPUCCINO_PRICE         As Currency = 2
Const cESPRESSO_PRICE           As Currency = 2.25
Const cLATTE_PRICE              As Currency = 1.75
Const cICED_PRICE               As Currency = 2.5
Const mcTAX_RATE                As Currency = 0.08
```

```
Private Sub cmdCalculate_Click()
    'Calculate and display the current amounts, add to totals

    Dim cPrice          As Currency
    Dim iQuantity       As Integer
    Dim cTax            As Currency
    Dim cItemAmount     As Currency

    'Find the price
    If optCappuccino.Value = True Then
        cPrice = cCAPPUCCINO_PRICE
    ElseIf optEspresso.Value = True Then
        cPrice = cESPRESSO_PRICE
    ElseIf optLatte.Value = True Then
        cPrice = cLATTE_PRICE
    ElseIf optIcedCappuccino.Value = True Or _
        optIcedLatte.Value = True Then
    cPrice = cICED_PRICE
    Else
        MsgBox "Please Make Drink Selection", vbOKOnly, "Oops"
    End If

    'Add the price times quantity to running total
    If IsNumeric(txtQuantity.Text) Then
        iQuantity = Val(txtQuantity.Text)
        cItemAmount = cPrice * iQuantity
        mcSubtotal = mcSubtotal + cItemAmount
        If chkTax.Value = Checked Then
           cTax = cFindTax(mcSubtotal) 'Call a function procedure
```

```
    End If
        mcTotal = mcSubtotal + cTax
        lblItemAmount.Caption = Format$(cItemAmount, "Currency")
        lblSubTotal.Caption = Format$(mcSubtotal, "Currency")
        lblTax.Caption = Format$(cTax, "Currency")
        lblTotal.Caption = Format$(mcTotal, "Currency")
    Else
        MsgBox "Quantity must contain a number", vbExclamation, "Oops"
        txtQuantity.SetFocus
    End If
End Sub
```

```
Private Sub cmdClear_Click()
    'Clear appropriate controls

    optCappuccino.Value = True     'Make first button selected to begin
    optEspresso.Value = False
    optLatte.Value = False
    optIcedLatte.Value = False
    optIcedCappuccino.Value = False
    lblItemAmount.Caption = ""
    chkTax.Enabled = False         'Allow change for new order only
    With txtQuantity
        .Text = ""
        .SetFocus
    End With
End Sub
```

```
Private Sub mnuEditCalc_Click()
    'Call the Calculate event

    cmdCalculate_Click
End Sub
```

```
Private Sub mnuEditClear_Click()
    'Call the Clear command event

    cmdClear_Click
End Sub
```

```
Private Sub mnuEditColor_Click()
    'Change the color of the total labels

    dlgCommon.ShowColor
    lblSubTotal.ForeColor = dlgCommon.Color
    lblTax.ForeColor = dlgCommon.Color
    lblTotal.ForeColor = dlgCommon.Color
End Sub
```

```
Private Sub mnuEditFont_Click()
    'Change the font name for the subtotal labels
    dlgCommon.Flags = cdlCFScreenFonts 'Set up Font dialog box fonts
    dlgCommon.ShowFont
    lblSubTotal.Font.Name = dlgCommon.FontName
    lblTax.Font.Name = dlgCommon.FontName
    lblTotal.Font.Name = dlgCommon.FontName
End Sub
```

```
Private Sub mnuFileExit_Click()
    'Terminate the project

    End
End Sub
```

```
Private Sub mnuFileNew_Click()
    'Clear the current order and add to totals

    cmdClear_Click
    lblSubTotal.Caption = ""
    lblTax.Caption = ""
    lblTotal.Caption = ""

    'Add to Totals
    gcGrandTotal = gcGrandTotal + mcTotal
    mcSubtotal = 0    'Reset totals for next order
    mcTotal = 0
    giCustomerCount = giCustomerCount + 1

    'Clear and enable tax check box
    With chkTax
        .Enabled = True
        .Value = False
    End With
End Sub
```

```
Private Sub mnuFileSummary_Click()
    'Load and display the summary information

    If mcTotal <> 0 Then
        mnuFileNew_Click 'Make sure last order is counted
    End If
    frmSummary.Show vbModal
End Sub
```

```
Private Sub mnuHelpAbout_Click()
    'Display a message box about the program

    frmAbout.Show vbModal
End Sub
```

```
Public Function cFindTax(cAmount As Currency) As Currency
    'Calculate the sales tax

    cFindTax = cAmount * mcTAX_RATE
End Function
```

frmAbout

```
'Module:         frmAbout
'Description:    Display information about the program and the
'                programmer.
'Folder:         Ch0601

Option Explicit
```

```
Private Sub cmdOK_Click()
    'Hide the form

    Me.Hide
End Sub
```

frmSplash

```
'Module:         frmSplash
'Description:    Splash screen to display while main form loads.
'Folder:         Ch0601

Option Explicit
```

```
Private Sub cmdClose_Click()
    'Unload the form and display the main form

    Unload Me                 'Close the Splash form
    frmBilling.Show vbModal  'Display the Billing form
End Sub
```

frmSummary

```
'Module:         frmSummary
'Description:    Display summary information on a separate form
'Folder:         Ch0601

Option Explicit
```

```
Private Sub cmdOK_Click()
    'Return to the main form

    Me.Hide
End Sub
```

```
Private Sub Form_Activate()
    'Calculate the average and display the totals
    Dim cAverage As Currency

    If giCustomerCount > 0 Then
        cAverage = gcGrandTotal / giCustomerCount
    Else
        cAverage = 0
    End If
    lblCount.Caption = giCustomerCount
    lblAverage.Caption = Format$(cAverage, "Currency")
End Sub
```

Standard Code Module

```
'Module:         ch0601.BAS
'Programmer:     A Millspaugh
'Date:           March 1997
'Description:    Code module to declare the global variables
'                and the Main procedure, which displays the
'                splash screen.
'Folder:         CH0601

Public gcGrandTotal          As Currency
Public giCustomerCount       As Integer

Sub Main()
    'Display a splash screen while the main form is being loaded

    frmSplash.Show vbModeless        'Show the splash screen
    Load frmBilling                  'Load the main form
End Sub
```

Programming Hints

Here are some useful tips for working with maximized forms.

Working with Maximized Forms

Until this point all of our forms have been smaller than the full screen. If you want your application's form to fill the entire screen, these techniques can help you in designing and running your project.

Design-Time Tips

Make your form run maximized by setting its WindowState property to *2-Maximized.* To work on the form in design time, click on the form's Maximize button, which will make it larger. You can use the Form window's scroll bars to view the entire area of the form.

You can close the extra windows on the screen or undock them so that they float on top of your form. The borders of each window are resizable, and you can hide the toolbar. Figure 6.18 shows one possible screen setup for working on a maximized form.

The keyboard shortcut for the Code window is F7. Of course, you can always double-click on a control to display the Code window, if you prefer.

Figure 6.18

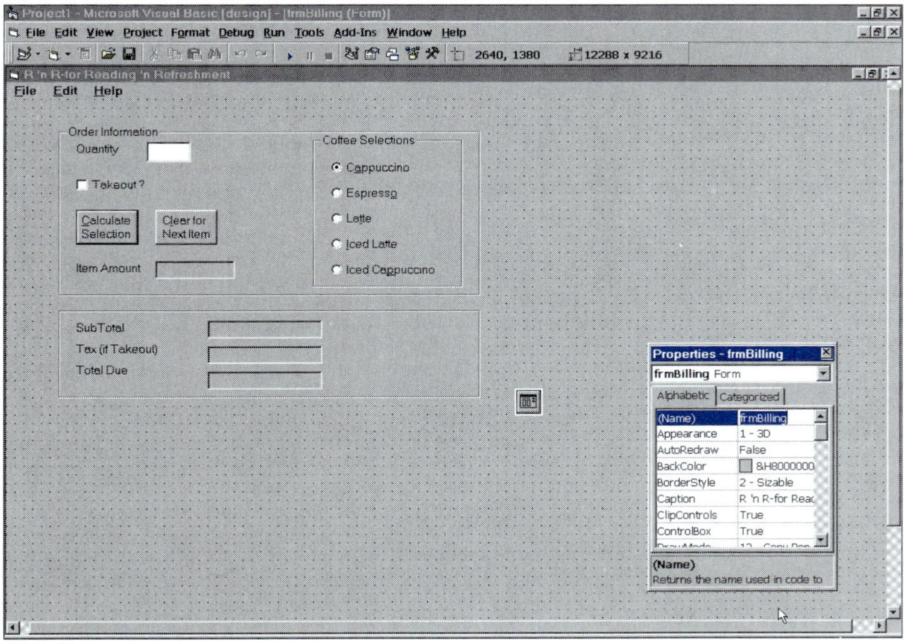

Modify the screen layout to make it easier to work on maximized forms. Here is one possible layout.

Stopping Execution with a Maximized Form

To stop program execution, it is best to have a working Exit command button, but even if you don't, you can still stop your program. Click on your form's Close box, which exits the program, or click on the form's Restore button, which will make it smaller so you have access to the Visual Basic toolbar buttons and menu bar.

Summary

1. Projects may need more than one form—there is virtually no limit to the number of forms that can be used within a single project. Add forms by clicking the Form toolbar button or the *Add Form* command on the *Project* menu.
2. The first form displayed when a project runs is called the startup form.
3. Forms used for one project can be added to another project. Forms can also be removed from a project.
4. The Show and Hide methods are used to display a form or remove one from the screen.
5. A form displayed as modal requires the user to respond to the form; it must be closed or unloaded before any execution continues. When a form is displayed as modeless, the user can switch to another form without closing the modeless form.

6. The `Load` statement loads a form but does not show it. The `Unload` statement hides a form, removes it from memory, and releases any system resources used by the form.
7. The `Me` keyword refers to the current active form. `Me` can be used to hide or unload the active form.
8. To refer to an object in a different form, use the form name, an exclamation point, and the object name.
9. A standard code module contains global declarations and procedures that may be used by multiple forms. To add a standard code module use the *Add Module* command on the *Project* menu; the file will have a .BAS extension.
10. Global variables, which are visible to all forms within a project, are declared using the keyword `Public`. The `Public` statement can appear only in the General Declarations section of a module and *should* be placed in a standard code module.
11. Variables declared with the keyword `Static` retain their values for multiple calls to the procedure in which they are defined.
12. An About box, which typically contains information about the version of an application and the programmer and copyrights, may be created by adding a new form. VB5 has an About Dialog template form that can be used to create an About box.
13. A splash screen may be displayed while a program loads. VB5 provides a splash screen template that may be used to create a new splash screen form.
14. Program execution can start with a startup form or from a sub procedure called *Main*. Use a Sub Main to display a splash screen.

Key Terms

About box *203*
.BAS file extension *199*
global *200*
`Hide` method *196*
`Load` statement *198*
`Me` *198*
modal *196*
modeless *196*
`Public` *200*
`Show` method *196*
splash screen *205*
standard code module *199*
startup form *194*
`Static` *201*
`Unload` statement *198*

Review Questions

1. What does the phrase *standard code module* mean?
2. Discuss the difference between declaring a variable in the General Declarations section of a standard code module and declaring a variable in the General Declarations section of a form code module.
3. List some of the items generally found in an About box.
4. What is the purpose of a splash screen?

5. What is the term used for the first form to display in a project?
6. How can you choose a different form as the startup form after the project has been created?
7. Explain how to include an existing form in a new project.

Programming Exercises

6.1 Modify project 5.5 (the flag viewer) to include a splash screen and an About form.

Menus:

```
File      Country              Display            Help
  Print     United States        Title               About
  Exit      Canada               Country Name
            Japan                Programmer
            Mexico
```

6.2 Create a project that will produce a summary of the amounts due for Pat's Auto Repair Shop. Display a splash screen first; then display the main form.

The main form menus:

```
File        Process                  Help
  Exit        Job Information           About
```

Job Information command:

The Job Information menu command will display the Job Information form.

The Job Information form:

The Job Information form must have text boxes for the user to enter the job number, customer name, amount charged for parts, and the hours of labor. Include labels for Parts, Labor, SubTotal, Sales Tax, and Total.

Include command buttons for Calculate, Print, Clear, and OK.

The Calculate button finds the charges and displays them in labels. The tax rate and the hourly labor charge should be set up as named constants so that they can be easily modified if either changes. Current charges are $30 per hour for labor and 8 percent (.08) for the sales tax rate. Sales tax is charged only on parts, not on labor.

The Print button prints the current contents of the form.

The Clear button clears the text boxes and resets the focus in the first text box.

The OK button hides the Job Information form and displays the main form.

6.3 Modify project 6.2 so that summary information is maintained for the total dollar amount for parts, labor, sales tax, and total for all customers.

Add a *Summary* command under the *Process* menu with a separator bar between the two menu commands. When the user selects the *Summary* command, display the summary information in a Summary form. The Summary form should have an OK button that hides the Summary form and returns the user to the main form.

6.4 A battle is raging over the comparative taste of Prune Punch and Apple Ade. Each taste tester rates the two drinks on a scale of 1 to 10 (10 being best). The proof of the superiority of one over the other will be the average score for the two drinks.

Display a splash screen and then the main form.

The main form menus:

```
File              Help
   New Tester        About
   Summary
   ___________
   Exit
```

New Tester command:

The *New Tester* command displays a form that inputs the test results for each drink. The form contains an OK button and a Cancel button.

When the user clicks the OK button, add the score for each type of drink to the drink's total, clear the text boxes, and reset the focus. Leave the form on the screen in case the next tester is ready to enter scores. If either score is blank when the OK button is pressed, display a message in a message box and reset the focus to the box for the missing data.

The Cancel button returns to the startup form without performing any calculation.

Summary command:

The *Summary* command displays a form that contains the current results of the taste test. It should display the winner, the total number of taste testers, and the average rating for each drink. The form contains an OK button that returns to the startup form. (The user will be able to display the summary at any time and as often as desired.)

The About form:

The About form should display information about the program and the programmer. Include an OK button that returns the user to the main form.

CASE STUDIES

VB Mail Order

Modify the VB Mail Order project from Chapter 5 to include a splash screen, an About form, and a summary form. Include an image on both the splash form and the About form.

VB Auto Center

Create a project that uses three forms. Add the form from the Chapter 5 case study and create a splash screen and an About form.

The splash screen:

Display a splash screen and then the main form.

The About form:

Include an image and identifying information about the program and programmer.

The main form:

The main form should display "Valley Boulevard Auto Center—Meeting all your vehicle's needs" and appropriate image(s).

The main form menus:

```
File              Edit          Help
   Input Sale        Color         About
   Exit              Font
```

The Color and Font commands should allow the user to change the large label on the form.

The Input Sale command should display the form from Chapter 5. You will need to modify the Chapter 5 form to hide itself rather than to terminate execution.

C H A P T E R

7

Lists, Loops, and Printing

At the completion of this chapter, you will be able to . . .

1. Create and use list boxes and combo boxes.
2. Enter items into list boxes using the Properties window and the AddItem method.
3. Determine which item in a list is selected.
4. Use the ListCount property to determine the number of items in a list.
5. Display a selected item from a list.
6. Differentiate among the available types of combo boxes.
7. Use `Do/Loops` and `For/Next` statements to iterate through a loop.
8. Use the `MsgBox` function to determine the button pressed by the user.
9. Use the string functions `Left`, `Right`, and `Mid` to refer to part of a string and use the `Len` function to count the number of characters in a string.
10. Send information to the printer using the `Print` method.
11. Control the format of printing using commas, semicolons, the `Tab` function, and the `Spc` function.

You may want to offer the user a list of items from which to choose. You can use the Windows list box and combo box controls to display lists on a form. You may choose to add items to a list during design time, during run time, or perhaps during a combination of both. Several styles of list boxes are available; the style you use is determined by design and space considerations, as well as whether or not you will allow the user to add items to the list.

List Boxes and Combo Boxes

Both **list box controls** and **combo box controls** allow you to have a list of items from which the user can make a selection. Figure 7.1 shows the toolbox tools for creating the controls; Figure 7.2 shows several types of list boxes and combo boxes, including simple list boxes, **simple combo boxes**, **dropdown combo boxes**, and **dropdown lists**. The list boxes on the left of the form in Figure 7.2 are all created with the List box tool; the boxes on the right of the form are created with the Combo box tool. Notice the three distinct styles of combo boxes.

Figure 7.1

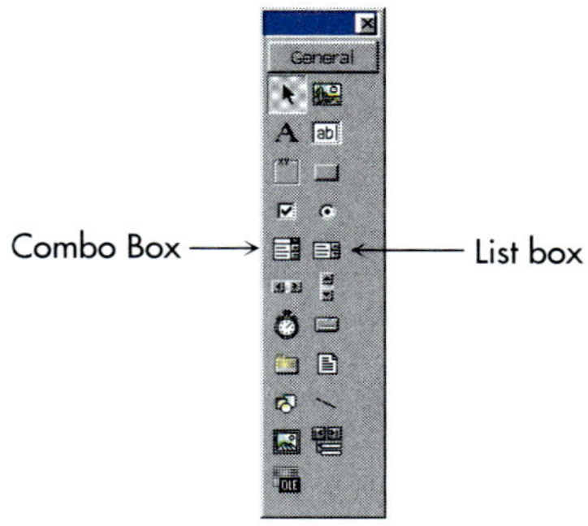

Use the list box tool and the combo box tool to create list boxes and combo boxes on your forms.

Figure 7.2

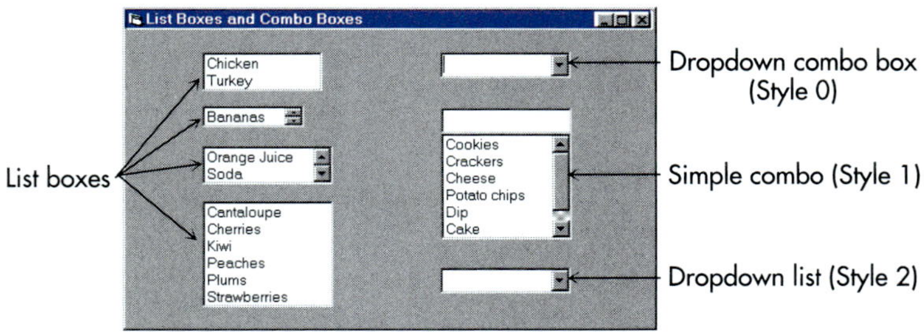

Various styles of list box controls and combo box controls.

List boxes and combo boxes have most of the same properties and operate in a similar fashion. One exception is that a combo box control has a Style property, which determines whether or not the list box also has a text box for user entry and whether or not the list will drop down (refer to figure 7.2). The second exception is that combo boxes have a Text property and list boxes do not.

Both list boxes and combo boxes have a great feature. If the list has more items than can be seen at one time, given the size of the box, VB automatically adds a scroll bar. You do not have to be concerned with the location of the scroll box in the scroll bar; the scrolling is handled automatically.

When you add a list box to a form, choose the style according to the space you have available and how you want the box to operate. Do you want the user to select from an existing list? If so, use a simple list box or a dropdown list (combo box Style 2). Do you want the user to be able to type a new entry if necessary? In this case, use one of the two styles with an added text box: the dropdown combo box (Style 0) or the simple combo box (Style 1).

When you create a list box or combo box at design time, you determine the size of the control. There is no Caption property, so for list boxes Visual Basic displays the Name property in the control during design time. For combo boxes, the Text property displays. Don't spend any time trying to make a list box or dropdown list (combo box style 2) appear empty during design time; the box will appear empty at run time. Dropdown combo boxes and simple combos (styles 0 and 1) have a Text property, which you can set or remove at design time.

When you name list boxes and combo boxes, use "lst" as the list box prefix and "cbo" as the prefix for combo boxes.

Filling the List

You can use several methods to fill a list box and combo box. If you know the list contents at design time and the list never changes, you can define the list items in the Properties window. If you must add items to the list during program execution, you will use the AddItem method in an event procedure. In Chapter 9 you will learn to fill a list from a data file on disk. This method allows the list contents to vary from one run to the next.

Using the Properties Window

The List property holds the list of items for a list box or combo box. To define the List property at design time, select the control and scroll the Properties window to the List property (Figure 7.3). Click on the down arrow to drop down the empty list and type your first list item. Then press Ctrl + Enter to move to the next list item. Continue typing items and pressing Ctrl + Enter until you are finished (Figure 7.4). On the last list item, do not press Ctrl + Enter, or you will have an extra (blank) item on the list. Press Enter or click anywhere off the list to complete the operation.

Figure 7.3

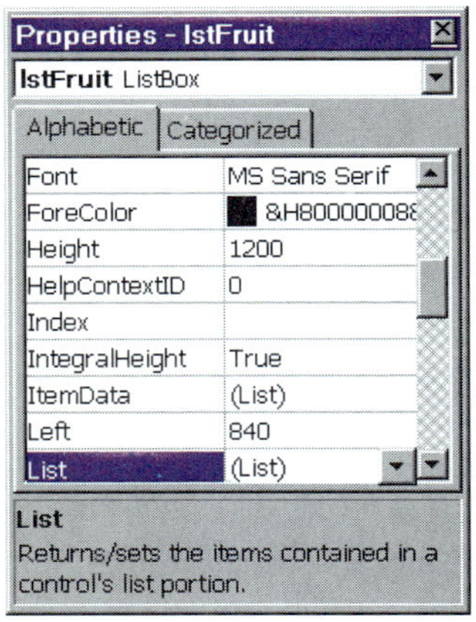

Select the List property of a list box to enter the list items.

Figure 7.4

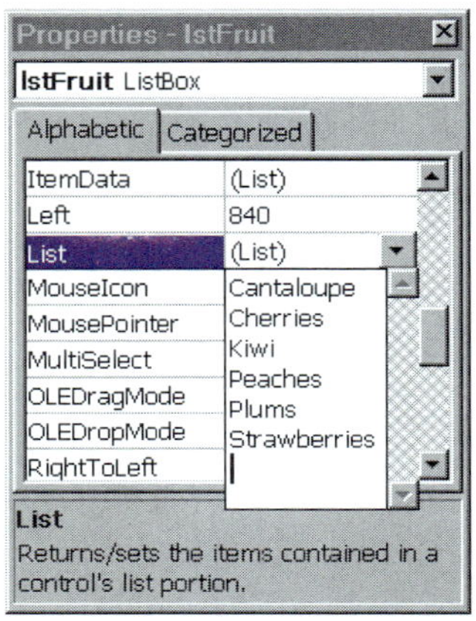

Type each list item and press Ctrl + Enter.

Using the AddItem Method

To add an item to a list box at run time, use the **AddItem method**. You may choose to add to a list the contents of the text box at the top of a combo box, a variable, a constant, or the property of another control.

The AddItem Method—General Form

```
Object.AddItem Value [, Index]
```

Value is the value to add to the list. If the value is a string literal, enclose it in quotation marks.

The optional *Index* specifies the position within the list to place the new item; the first element in the list has an Index of 0.

When you omit the Index, the new item generally goes at the end of the list. However, you can alter that by setting the control's **Sorted property** to True. Then the new item will be placed alphabetically in the list.

The AddItem Method—Examples

```
lstSchools.AddItem "Harvard"
lstSchools.AddItem "Stanford"
lstSchools.AddItem txtSchools.Text
cboMajors.AddItem cboMajors.Text
cboMajors.AddItem stMajor
```

When the user types a new value in the text box portion of a combo box, that item is not automatically added to the list. If you want to add the newly entered text to the list, use the AddItem method:

```
cboCoffee.AddItem cboCoffee.Text
```

Clearing the List

In addition to adding items during run time, you can also clear all items from a list. Use the **Clear method** to empty a combo box or list box.

The Clear Method—General Form

```
Object.Clear
```

The Clear Method—Examples

```
lstSchools.Clear
cboMajors.Clear
```

The ListIndex Property

When a project is running and the user selects (highlights) an item from the list, the index number of that item is stored in the **ListIndex property** of the list box. Recall that the ListIndex of the first item in the list is 0. If no list item is selected, the ListIndex property is set to negative 1.

You can use the ListIndex property to select an item in the list or deselect all items in code.

Example

```
lstCoffeeTypes.ListIndex = 3     'Select the fourth item in list
lstCoffeeTypes.ListIndex = -1    'Deselect all items in list
```

The ListCount Property

The application uses the **ListCount property** of a list box or combo box to store the number of items in the list. We will use the ListCount property later in this chapter to process each element in the list. ListCount is also handy when you need to display the count at some point in your project.

Remember, ListCount is always one more than the highest ListIndex, since ListIndex begins with 0. For example, if there are 20 items in a list, ListCount is 20 and the highest ListIndex is 19.

Example

```
iTotalItems = lstItem.ListCount
```

The List Property

If you need to display one item from a list, you can refer to one element of the **List property**. The List property of a list box or combo box holds the text of all of the list elements. You specify which element you want by including an index. This technique can be useful if you need to display a list item in a label on another form. Later in this chapter we will use the List property to send the contents of the list box to the printer.

Using the List Property—General Form

```
Object.List(Index) [ = Value]
```

The index of the first list element is 0, so the highest index is ListCount negative 1.

You can retrieve the value of a list element or set an element to a different value.

Using the List Property—Examples

```
lstSchools.List(5) = "University of California"
lblMyMajor.Caption = cboMajors.List(iIndex)
lblSelectedMajor.Caption = cboMajors.List(cboMajors.ListIndex)
```

To refer to the currently selected element of a list, you must combine the List property and the ListIndex property:

```
stSelectedFlavor = lstFlavor.List(lstFlavor.ListIndex)
```

Removing an Item from a List

Earlier you learned how to clear all the elements from a list. However, you might want to remove individual elements from a list. To remove an element from the list, use the **RemoveItem method**.

The RemoveItem Method—General Form

```
Object.RemoveItem Index
```

The Index is required; it specifies which element to remove. The Index of the first list element is 0, and the Index of the last element is ListCount negative 1.

The RemoveItem Method—Examples

```
lstNames.RemoveItem 0          'Remove the first name from the list
cboSchools.RemoveItem iIndex   'Remove the element in position iIndex
cboCoffee.RemoveItem cboCoffee.ListIndex   'Remove the currently selected item
```

List Box and Combo Box Events

Later in the chapter we will perform actions in event procedures for events of list boxes and combo boxes. Some useful events are the Change, GotFocus, and LostFocus. *Note:* Although we haven't used these events up until this point, many other controls have these same events. For example, you can code event procedures for the Change event of text boxes.

The Change Event

As the user types text into the text box portion of a combo box (styles 0 and 1), the Change event occurs. Each keystroke generates another change event. This event will be used later to match the characters typed to the elements in the list. A list box does not have a Change event because it does not have a text box associated with it.

The GotFocus Event

When a control receives the focus, a GotFocus event occurs. As the user tabs from control to control, a GotFocus event fires for each control. Later you will learn to make any existing text appear selected when the user tabs to a text box or the text portion of a combo box.

The LostFocus Event

You can also write code for the LostFocus event of a control. The LostFocus event fires as the control loses the focus. Often LostFocus event procedures are used for validating input data.

Feedback 7.1

Describe the purpose of each of the following methods or properties for a list box control.

1. ListCount
2. ListIndex
3. List
4. AddItem
5. Clear
6. RemoveItem
7. Sorted

Do/Loops

Until now, there has been no way to repeat the same steps in a procedure without calling them a second time. The computer is capable of repeating a group of instructions many times without calling the procedure for each new set of data. The process of repeating a series of instructions is called *looping*. The group of repeated instructions is called a ***loop***. An **iteration** is a single execution of the statement(s) in the loop. In this section you will learn about the `Do/Loop`. Later in this chapter you will learn about another type of loop—a `For/Next` loop.

A `Do/Loop` terminates based on a condition that you specify. Execution of a `Do/Loop` continues *while* a condition is True or *until* a condition is True. You can choose to place the condition at the top or the bottom of the loop. Use a `Do/Loop` when the exact number of iterations is unknown.

Align the **`Do`** and **`Loop` statements** with each other and indent the lines of code to be repeated in between.

The Do and Loop Statements—General Form

```
Do {While | Until} Condition
  'statements in loop
Loop

or

Do

  'statements in loop
Loop {While | Until} Condition
```

The first form of the `Do/Loop` tests for completion at the top of the loop. With this type of loop, also called a ***pretest***, the statements inside the loop may never be executed if the terminating condition is True the first time it is tested.

Example

```
iTotal = 0
Do Until iTotal = 0
    'statements in loop
Loop
```

Since iTotal is zero the first time the condition is tested, the condition is True and the statements inside the loop will not execute. Control will pass to the statement following the `Loop` statement.

The second form of the `Do/Loop` tests for completion at the bottom of the loop, which means that the statements in the loop will *always* be executed at least once. This form of loop is sometimes called a ***posttest***. Changing the example to a posttest, you can see the difference.

```
iTotal = 0
Do
    'statements in loop
Loop Until iTotal = 0
```

In this case the statements inside the loop will be executed at least once. Assuming the value for iTotal does not change inside the loop, the condition (iTotal = 0) will be True the first time it is tested and control will pass to the first statement following the `Loop` statement. Figure 7.5 shows flowcharts of pretest and posttest loops, using both `While` and `Until`.

Figure 7.5

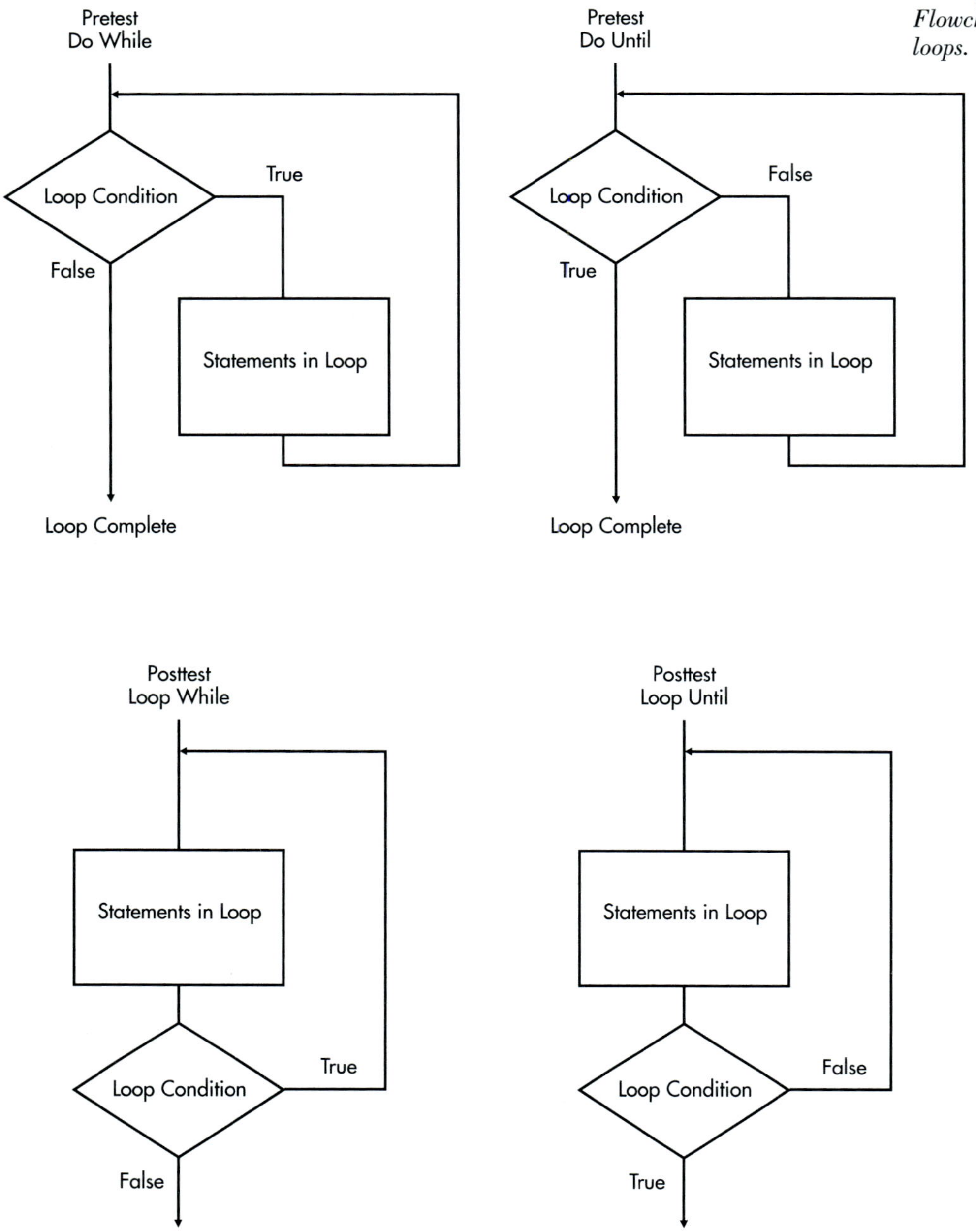

Flowcharts of pretest and posttest loops.

The Do and Loop Statements—Examples

```
Do Until iItemIndex = lstItems.ListCount - 1
       'Statements in loop

Loop

Do While cAmount >= 10 And cAmount <= 20
       'Statements in loop

Loop

Do
       'Statements in loop
Loop Until iTotal > 0
```

The Boolean Data Type Revisited

In Chapter 2 you learned about the Boolean data type, which holds only the values True or False. You will find Boolean variables very useful when setting and testing conditions for a loop. You can set a Boolean variable to True when a specific circumstance occurs, and then write a loop condition to continue until the variable is True.

An example of using a Boolean variable is when you want to search through a list for a specific value. The item may be found or not found, and you want to quit looking when a match is found.

Using a Boolean variable is usually a three-step process. First you must dimension a variable and set its initial value (or use the default VB setting of False). Then, when a particular situation occurs, set the variable to True. A loop condition can then check for True.

```
Dim bItemFound as Boolean
bItemFound = False
Do Until bItemFound        'Checks for True
    ...
```

A Boolean variable is always in one of two states—True or False. Many programmers refer to Boolean variables as *switches* or *flags*. Switches have two states: on or off; flags are considered either up or down.

Using a Do/Loop with a List Box

This small example combines a Boolean variable with a **Do/Loop**. Inside the loop each element of the list is compared to txtNewItem for a match. The loop will terminate when a match is found or when all elements have been tested. Follow through the logic to see what happens when there is a match, when there isn't a match, when the match occurs on the first list element, and when the match occurs on the last list element.

```
Private Sub cmdFind_Click()
    'Look for a match between the text box and list elements

    Dim bItemFound As Boolean
    Dim iItemIndex As Integer

    bItemFound = False
    iItemIndex = 0
    Do Until bItemFound Or iItemIndex = lstItems.ListCount
        If txtNewItem.Text = lstItems.List(iItemIndex) Then
            bItemFound = True
        End If
        iItemIndex = iItemIndex + 1
    Loop
    If bItemFound Then
        MsgBox "Item is in the list", vbInformation, "Item match"
    Else
        MsgBox "Item is not is the list", vbInformation, "Item no match"
    End If
End Sub
```

Feedback 7.2

Explain the purpose of each line of the following code:

```
bItemFound = False
iItemIndex = 0
Do Until bItemFound Or iItemIndex = lstItems.ListCount
    If txtNewItem.Text = lstItems.List(iItemIndex) Then
        bItemFound = True
    End If
    iItemIndex = iItemIndex + 1
Loop
```

For/Next Loops

When you want to repeat the statements in a loop a specific number of times, the **For/Next loop** is ideal. The For/Next loop uses the **`For`** and **`Next`** statements and a counter variable, called the ***loop index***. The loop index determines the number of times the statements inside the loop will be executed.

```
Dim iLoopIndex as Integer
Dim iMaximum as Integer
iMaximum = lstSchools.ListCount - 1

For iLoopIndex = 0 To iMaximum
    'The statements inside of the loop are indented
    ' and referred to as the body of the loop
Next iLoopIndex
```

When the `For` statement is reached during program execution several things occur. The loop index, iLoopIndex, is established as the loop counter and is initialized to 0. The final value for the loop index is set to the value of iMaximum, which was assigned the value of lstSchools.ListCount − 1 in the previous statement.

Execution is now "controlled by" the `For` statement. After the value of iLoopIndex is set, it is tested to see if iLoopIndex is greater than iMaximum. If not, the statements in the body of the loop are executed. The `Next` statement causes the iLoopIndex to be incremented by one. The control passes back to the `For` statement. Is the value of iLoopIndex greater than iMaximum? If not, the loop is again executed. When the test is made and the loop index is greater than the final value, control passes to the statement immediately following the `Next`.

A counter-controlled loop generally has three elements (see Figure 7.6 for a flowchart of loop logic).

1. Initialize the counter.
2. Increment the counter.
3. Test the counter to determine when it is time to terminate the loop.

Figure 7.6

A flowchart of the logic of a `For/Next` *loop.*

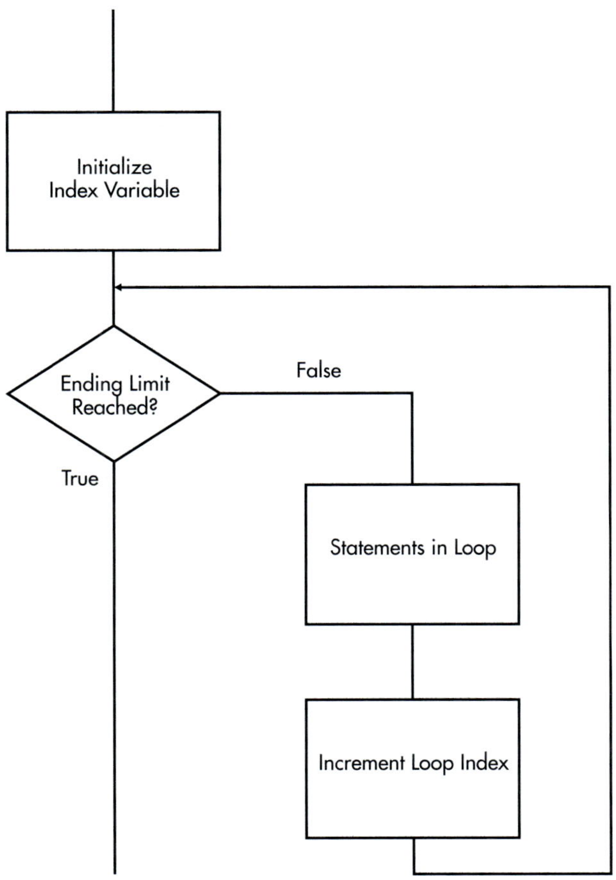

The For and Next Statements—General Form

```
For LoopIndex = InitialValue To TestValue [Step Increment]
    ::
     ::(Body of loop)
    ::
Next [LoopIndex]
```

LoopIndex must be a numeric variable; InitialValue and TestValue may be constants, variables, numeric property values, or numeric expressions. The optional word `Step` may be included, along with the value to be added to the loop index for each iteration of the loop. When the `Step` is omitted, the increment is assumed to be 1.

The For and Next Statements—Examples

```
For iIndex = 2 To 100 Step 2
For iCount = iStart To iEnding Step iIncrement
For iCounter = 0 To cboCoffeeType.ListCount - 1
For iNumber = (iNumberCorrect - 5) To iTOTAL_POSSIBLE
For cRate = .05 To .25 Step .05
For iCountDown = 10 To 0 Step -1
```

Each `For` statement has a corresponding `Next` statement, which must follow the `For`. All statements between the `For` and `Next` are considered to be the body of the loop and will be executed the specified number of times.

The first example `For` statement will count from 2 to 100 by 2. The statements in the body of the loop will be executed 50 times—first with iIndex = 2, next with iIndex = 4, next with iIndex = 6, and so forth.

When the comparison is done, the program checks for *greater than* the test value—not equal to. When iIndex = 100 in the preceding example, the body of the loop will be executed one more time. Then, at the `Next` statement, iIndex will be incremented to 102, the test made, and control will pass to the statement following the `Next`. If you were to display the value of iIndex *after completion* of the loop, its value would be 102.

Negative Increment or Counting Backward

You may use a negative number for the `Step` increment. This has the effect of decreasing the loop index rather than increasing it. When the `Step` is negative, Basic will test for *less than* the test value instead of greater than.

```
'Count Backwards
For iCount = 10 To 1 Step -1

Next iCount
```

Tip

Use a `For/Next` loop when you know the number of iterations needed for the loop. Use a `Do/Loop` when the loop should end based on a condition.

Conditions Satisfied before Entry

At times the final value will be reached before entry into the loop. In that case the statements in the body of the loop will not be executed at all.

```
'An unexecutable loop
iFinal = 5
For iIndex = 6 to iFinal
    'The execution will never reach here
Next iIndex
```

Altering the Values of the Loop Control Variables

Once a `For` loop has been entered, the values for InitialValue, TestValue, and Increment have already been set. Changing the value of these control variables within the loop will have no effect on the number of iterations of the loop. Many texts admonish against changing the values within the loop. However, Visual Basic just ignores you if you try.

```
'Bad Example—Changing the Control Variable
iFinal = 10
iIncrease = 2
For iIndex = 1 to iFinal Step iIncrease
    iFinal = 25
    iIncrease = 5
Next iIndex
```

If you tried this example and displayed the values of iIndex, you would find that the final value will remain 10 and the increment value will be 2.

The value that you *can* change within the loop is the LoopIndex. This practice is considered poor programming.

```
'Poor Programming
For iIndex = 1 To 10 Step 1
    iIndex = iIndex + 5
Next iIndex
```

Endless Loops

Changing the value of a LoopIndex variable is not only considered a poor practice but also may lead to an endless loop. Your code could get into a loop that is impossible to exit. Consider the following example; when will the loop end?

```
'More Poor Programming
For iIndex = 1 To 10 Step 1
    iIndex = 1
Next iIndex
```

Exiting For/Next Loops

In the previous example of an endless loop, you will have to break the program execution manually. You can click on your form's close box, or use the Visual Basic menu bar or toolbar to stop the program. If you can't see the menu bar or toolbar, you can usually move or resize your application's form to bring it into view. If you prefer, press Ctrl + Break to enter break time; you may want to step program execution to see what is causing the problem.

Usually, `For/Next` loops should proceed to normal completion. However, on occasion you may need to terminate a loop before the loop index reaches its final value. Visual Basic provides an `Exit For` statement for this situation. Generally the `Exit For` statement is part of an `If` statement.

The Exit For Statement—General Form

```
Exit For
```

The Exit For Statement—Example

```
For iLoopIndex = 1 to 10
    If txtInput.Text = "" Then   'Nothing was entered into the Input textbox
        MsgBox "You must enter something"
        Exit For
    End If
    ...                          'Statements in loop
Next iLoopIndex
```

Feedback 7.3

1. Identify the statements that are correctly formed and those that have errors. For those with errors, state what is wrong and how to correct it.
   (a) `For cIndex = 3.5 To 6, Step .5`
       `Next cIndex`
   (b) `For iIndex = iBegin To iEnd Step iIncrement`
       `Next iEnd`
   (c) `For 4 = 1 To 10 Step 2`
       `Next For`
   (d) `For iIndex = 100 To 0 Step -25`
       `Next iIndex`
   (e) `For iIndex = 0 To -10 Step -1`
       `Next iIndex`
   (f) `For iIndex = 10 To 1`
       `Next iIndex`

2. How many times will the body of the loop be executed for each of these examples? What will be the value of the loop index *after* normal completion of the loop?
   (a) `For iCounter = 2 To 11 Step 3`
   (b) `For iCounter = 10 To 1 Step -1`
   (c) `For cCounter = 3 To 6 Step .5`
   (d) `For iCounter = 5 To 1`
   (e) `For iCounter = 1 To 3`

Using the MsgBox Function

You have been using the `MsgBox` statement to display messages since Chapter 4. In each case the box displayed only an OK button. You can also use the **`MsgBox` function** to display a dialog box with more than one button; the function returns a value to indicate which button was pressed.

Consider a message box that asks if you really want to clear a combo box. You need to display Yes and No buttons and then be able to determine which button the user clicked. Figure 7.7 illustrates a message box with Yes and No buttons.

Figure 7.7

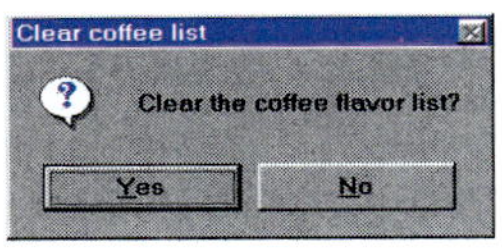

Display a message box with more than one button and check which button was clicked with the `MsgBox` *function.*

The MsgBox Function—General Form

```
MsgBox(Prompt [, Buttons] [, Title])
```

The MsgBox Function—Example

```
Dim iResponse As Integer
iResponse = MsgBox("Do you wish to continue?", vbYesNo + vbQuestion, "Title")
If iResponse = vbYes Then       '...Continue processing

If MsgBox(stMsg, vbOKCancel) = vbOK Then
    ClearList
Else
    CancelOperation
End If
```

Function Return Values

The `MsgBox` function returns a value that can be tested in a condition using the value (numbers 1 through 7) or the associated intrinsic constant.

Return Values

Constant	Value	Button Pressed
vbOk	1	OK
vbCancel	2	Cancel
vbAbort	3	Abort
vbRetry	4	Retry
vbIgnore	5	Ignore
vbYes	6	Yes
vbNo	7	No

Specifying the Buttons and/or Icons to Display

You can specify which buttons to display by using numbers or the Visual Basic intrinsic constants. If you want to choose the buttons and an icon, use a plus sign to add the two values together.

Button and Icon Values

Buttons to Display	Value	Constant
OK	0	vbOKOnly
OK and Cancel	1	vbOKCancel
Abort, Retry, and Ignore	2	vbAbortRetryIgnore
Yes, No, and Cancel	3	vbYesNoCancel
Yes and No	4	vbYesNo
Retry and Cancel	5	vbRetryCancel

Icons to Display	Value	Constant
Critical Message	16	vbCritical
Warning Query	32	vbQuestion
Warning Message	48	vbExclamation
Information Message	64	vbInformation

To display Yes, No, and Cancel buttons along with a question mark icon, use one of these statements:

```
iResponse = MsgBox(stMsg, vbYesNoCancel + vbQuestion, "Good Question")
iResponse = MsgBox(stMsg, 3 + 32, "Good Question")
iResponse = MsgBox(stMsg, 35, "Good Question")
```

MsgBox Example

Earlier you learned to use the `Clear` method to clear the contents of a list box or combo box. In this example we will give the user a chance to confirm whether or not to really clear the list. (Refer to Figure 7.7 for the message box displayed by this procedure.)

```
Private Sub mnuEditClear_Click()
    'Clear the coffee list
    Dim iResponse As Integer

    iResponse = MsgBox("Clear the coffee flavor list?", _
        vbYesNo + vbQuestion, "Clear coffee list")
    If iResponse = vbYes Then
        cboCoffee.Clear
    End If
End Sub
```

Using String Functions

When you need to look at part of a string, rather than the entire string, Visual Basic provides the **Left**, **Right**, and **Mid functions** that return the specified section of a string.

The Left, Right, and Mid Functions—General Form

```
Left(StringExpression, NumberOfCharacters)
Right(StringExpression, NumberOfCharacters)
Mid(StringExpression, StartPosition, [NumberOfCharacters])
```

StringExpression in each of these statements may be a string variable, string literal, or text property. NumberOfCharacters and StartPosition are both numeric and may be variables, literals, or numeric expressions. In the `Mid` function, if you omit the NumberOfCharacters argument, the function returns all characters starting with StartPosition.

The Left, Right, and Mid Functions—Examples

```
Left(txtName.Text , 5)     'Returns first 5 characters
Right(stLongString, 1)     'Returns last 1 character
Mid("Mad Hatter", 5, 3)    'Returns 3 characters beginning with character 5
Mid(stProductID, 4)        'Returns all characters beginning with character 4
```

Examples Using Left, Right, and Mid Functions

```
Dim stExample As String
stExample = "It's a wonderful life"
lblMessage.Caption = Left(stExample, 1)      'Returns "I"
lblMessage.Caption = Left(stExample, 6)      'Returns "It's a"
lblMessage.Caption = Left(stExample, 21)     'Returns "It's a wonderful life"
lblMessage.Caption = Left(stExample, 50)     'Returns "It's a wonderful life"
lblMessage.Caption = Right(stExample, 1)     'Returns "e"
lblMessage.Caption = Right(stExample, 4)     'Returns "life"
lblMessage.Caption = Mid(stExample, 8, 9)    'Returns "wonderful"
lblMessage.Caption = Mid(stExample, 8)       'Returns "wonderful life"

If Left(txtDirection.Text, 1) = "N" Then
    lblDirection.Caption = "North"
End If
```

The Len Function

You can use the **Len function** to determine the length of a string expression. You may need to know how many characters the user has entered or how long a list element is.

The Len Function—General Form

```
Len(StringExpression)
```

The value returned by the `Len` function is an integer count of the number of characters in the string.

The Len Function—Examples

```
Len("Visual Basic")     'Returns 12
Len(txtEntry.Text)      'Returns the number of characters in the text box
Len(stSelection)        'Returns the number of characters in the string variable

If Len(txtName.Text) = 0 Then
    MsgBox "Enter a name", vbInformation, "Data Missing"
End If
```

You can combine the Len function with two new properties of text boxes and the text portion of a combo box—the SelStart and SelLength properties. The SelStart property sets or returns the position of the first selected character; the SelLength property sets or returns the number of selected characters. You can make the current contents of a text box or the Text property of a combo box appear selected when the user tabs into the control and it receives the focus.

```
Private Sub txtName_GotFocus()
    'Select the current entry

    With txtName
        .SelStart = 0                      'Begin selection at start
        .SelLength = Len(txtName.Text)     'Select the number of characters
    End With
End Sub
```

Selecting Entries in a List Box

When a list box has a very large number of entries, you can help the user by selecting the matching entry as he types in a text box. This method is similar to the way the Help Topics list in Visual Basic works. For example, when you type *p* the list quickly scrolls and displays words beginning with *p*. Then if you next type *r*, the list scrolls down to the words that begin with *pr*, and the first such word is selected. If you type *i* next, the first word beginning with *pri* is selected. This small example implements this feature. See if you can tell what each statement does.

```
Private Sub txtCoffee_Change()
    'Locate first matching occurrence in the list

    Dim iIndex As Integer
    Dim bFound As Boolean

    Do While Not bFound And iIndex < lstCoffee.ListCount
        If UCase(Left(lstCoffee.List(iIndex), Len(txtCoffee.Text))) = _
            UCase(txtCoffee.Text) Then
            lstCoffee.ListIndex = iIndex
            bFound = True
        End If
        iIndex = iIndex + 1
    Loop
End Sub
```

Sending Information to the Printer

So far, any printed output has been done with the PrintForm method. When you print using PrintForm, all output is produced as a graphic, which does not produce attractive text. In addition to printing forms, you will need to create reports or print small bits of information on the printer. You can use VB's **Print method** to print text on a Form, on the Printer object, or in the Debug window.

Visual Basic was designed to run under Windows, which is a highly interactive environment. It is extremely easy to create forms for interactive programs, but not easy at all to print on the printer. Most professional programmers using Visual Basic use a separate utility program to format printer reports. The VB Professional Edition and Enterprise Edition include an add-in utility called Crystal Reports. Newer versions of Crystal Reports and several other printing utilities may be purchased separately.

Printing to the Printer

You can send output to the printer using `Printer.Print` (Object.Method). Visual Basic sets up a Printer object in memory for your output. When your job terminates or it receives an `EndDoc` or `NewPage` method, VB actually sends the contents of the Printer object to the printer.

Formatting Lines

The format of a print line uses punctuation from earlier versions of Basic, the comma and semicolon, as well as a `Tab` function and a `Spc` function. When a line of output contains multiple items to be printed, the items will be separated by commas or semicolons. The list of items may contain literals, variables, or the contents of objects.

When you print on the printer, it is important to consider the font being used. Normally, printing is done with proportional fonts, which means that the amount of space for one character varies with the character. For example, a *w* takes more space than an *i*. You can use a fixed-pitch font, such as Courier, if you want every character to take the same amount of space.

Commas

Consider that the output page has preset tab settings with the line being divided into five columns. Each column is referred to as a **print zone**. Use a comma to advance the output to the next print zone.

The statement

```
Printer.Print ,"R 'n R"
```

prints the "R 'n R" in the second print zone. You can use two commas to advance two print zones:

```
Printer.Print "Name", ,"Phone"
```

The string literal "Name" is printed in print zone 1 and "Phone" is placed in print zone 3. Note that the line prints as though print zone 2 had an empty string literal.

The only way to control the size of a print zone is to change the font size. The width of a print zone is 14 characters, based on the average size of a character for the font being used. That means if you use many narrow characters, such as *i* and *t*, more than 14 characters will fit, but if you are printing many wide characters, such as *w* and *m*, fewer than 14 characters will print in a print zone. Therefore, you may find that some items you print exceed the width of the print zone.

Conceptually, print zones resemble tab stops in a word processor. Each time a comma is encountered, it means "Jump to the next tab stop." Sometimes you may print a string that extends further than you expected (past the beginning of the next print zone). Then the next comma jumps to the following print zone, perhaps causing your columns to align improperly. In the following example the label will be placed in print zone 4.

```
Printer.Print "The average amount of sales for the current month is ", _
              lblSales.Caption
```

When the number of print zones exceeds the number for a single line, the output will automatically wrap to the next line on the printed page.

```
Printer.Print 1, 2, 3, 4, 5, 6
```

will output as

```
1                    2                    3                    4                    5
6
```

Semicolons

If you need to separate items without advancing to the next print zone, use a semicolon between the two items. If you leave spaces between items, VB adds a semicolon in the code for you. If the value of txtName.Text is "Mary" the line of code

```
Printer.Print "Name:  "; txtName.Text
```

will output as

```
Name:  Mary
```

Note that the number of spaces left inside the string literal will print out exactly as indicated. If you do not put spaces inside the quotes, you may well end up with one item printing right next to the previous one. The semicolon does not provide spacing on the output, only a means of listing items to print.

Trailing Commas and Semicolons

If the last character on a line of output is a comma or semicolon, the next `Print` method will continue on the same line without advancing the line.

```
Printer.Print "First this ",
Printer.Print "Then this"
```

will output as

```
First this    Then this
```

The print zone rule is still in effect because the first **Print** method ended with a trailing comma.

```
Printer.Print "First this ";
Printer.Print "Then this"
```

will output as

```
First this Then this
```

Printing Blank Lines

When you want to print a blank line on your printed report, use a **Print** method without any item to print:

```
Printer.Print   'Print a blank line
```

The Tab Function

Creating program output that is pleasing, properly spaced, and correctly aligned can be a difficult task. VB has functions to assist in the formatting process.

You can control the placement of variables and constants on a printed line by using the **Tab function**. In the **Tab** function you specify the column position where you want the output to appear. (*Note:* Basic uses the average character width to determine the column position.) The value of the column position argument must be numeric (fractional values will be rounded up), but it may be a constant, a variable, or a numeric expression (calculation).

The column position is absolute, meaning that the 1st position on the line is **Tab(1)** and the 20th position is **Tab(20).**

The Tab Function—General Form

```
Tab(Position)
```

The Tab Function—Examples

```
Printer.Print Tab(20); "R 'n R—for Reading 'n Refreshment"
Printer.Print Tab(10); "Name"; Tab(30); "Pay"
Printer.Print Tab(iCOLUMN1); txtName.Text; Tab(iCOLUMN2); cPay
```

If you try to tab to a column that precedes the previous output on the line, the `Tab` will advance to the specified column position on the next line. Do not use a comma following a `Tab` function; after tabbing to the specified position, it will still advance to the next print zone, destroying the effect of your `Tab`.

The Spc Function

Another function that controls horizontal spacing on the line is the `Spc` (space) function. The **`Spc` function** differs from the `Tab` in that you specify the number of spaces on the line that you want to advance *from the last item printed.*

The Spc Function—General Form

```
Spc(NumberOfCharacters)
```

The Spc Function—Examples

```
Printer.Print Tab(20); "Name"; Spc(5); "Phone"; Spc(5); "Address"
```

Notice that you can combine `Tab` and `Spc` on one print line.

Aligning String and Numeric Data

VB handles spacing for string and numeric data a little differently. String values print with no extra spacing between items. For example, the statement

```
Printer.Print "Sweet"; "Pea"
```

prints as

```
SweetPea
```

Numeric data prints with additional spacing. VB allows one space before each number for a sign. For negative values, a minus sign appears in the position; for positive values, the space remains blank. VB also adds a space following each numeric value. The statement

```
Printer.Print 1; 2; 3; -1; -2; -3
```

outputs this line

```
 1  2  3 -1 -2 -3
```

If you combine string and numeric data you must be aware of the difference in the spacing. This example combines string and numeric data using print zones.

```
Printer.Print "Item", "Quantity"
Printer.Print "Scissors", 10
Printer.Print "Rocks", -2
Printer.Print "Porcupines", 1
```

The output from these statements appears aligned like this:

```
Item         Quantity
Scissors      10
Rocks        -2
Porcupines    1
```

Selecting the Font

Changing the font of printed output is similar to changing the font of a control. The Printer object has a Font property, which refers to the Font object. However, you cannot use the Properties window and *Font* dialog box to change the Font properties; you must change properties in code. When you change the font name, make sure you enter a font name supported by the target printer, spelled correctly. *Hint:* Display the *Font* dialog box for a control and make a note of the available font names. If you aren't sure which fonts are supported by your printer, stick with TrueType fonts (such as Arial and Times New Roman), which should work on any printer properly installed in Windows.

Examples

```
Printer.Font.Name = "Times New Roman"
Printer.Font.Size = 12
```

You need to change the font name and size only once, before the first item you print.

Terminating the Page or the Job

The `NewPage` method sends the current page to the printer and clears the printer object in memory so you can begin a new page. The `EndDoc` method sends the current page to the printer and terminates the printer job. *Note:* When your program terminates, Visual Basic automatically sends an `EndDoc`.

```
Printer.NewPage      'Send page and begin a new page
Printer.EndDoc       'Send page and terminate the print job
```

Use the `NewPage` or `EndDoc` methods after sending the information to the printer.

Example

```
Private Sub Form_Click()
    Printer.Print
    Printer.Print Tab(13); "Monthly Sales Summary"
    Printer.Print
    Printer.Print
    Printer.Print Tab(10); "Sales"; Tab(30); "Returns"
    Printer.Print Tab(10); "=============================="
    Printer.Print
    Printer.Print Tab(10); Format(mcSalesTotal, "currency"); _
                  Tab(30); Format(mcReturnsTotal, "currency")
    Printer.EndDoc
End Sub
```

Printing the Contents of a List Box

You can combine the techniques for printing, a loop, and the list box properties to send the contents of a list box to the printer. You know how many iterations to make, using the ListCount property. The List property allows you to print out the actual values from the list.

```
Private Sub mnuFilePrintAll_Click()
    'Print the contents of the coffee flavors
    'combo box on the printer

    Dim iIndex As Integer
    Dim iFinalValue As Integer
    iFinalValue = cboCoffee.ListCount - 1 'List index starts at 0
    For iIndex = 0 To iFinalValue
        Printer.Print cboCoffee.List(iIndex)
    Next iIndex
    Printer.EndDoc
End Sub
```

Aligning Decimal Columns

When the output to the printer includes numeric data, the alignment of the decimal points is important. One solution you may wish to use incorporates the `Len` function.

To right align numeric output:

STEP 1: Assign the formatted value to a string variable.
STEP 2: Determine the column position for the `Tab` at the position where you want the formatted value to *end*.
STEP 3: Tab the difference between the `Tab` position and the length of the formatted string variable.
STEP 4: Print the formatted value.

For example, if you want to right align a column for total pay on a printed report, you can use the following code:

```
Dim stFormattedNumber As String

stFormattedNumber = Format$(cTotalPay, "Currency")
Printer.Print Tab(10); stName ; Tab(50 - Len(stFormattedNumber)); _
              stFormattedNumber
```

The formatted cTotalPay will print right aligned at column 50.

Feedback 7.4

What will print for each of these code segments? Try to determine the results by hand; then enter them into the computer to verify your results.

1. ```
   Printer.Print "Half a loaf ";
   Printer.Print "Is better than none"
   ```
2. ```
   Printer.Print "Half, ", "My Eye"
   ```
3. ```
   Printer.Print "Hawks"; 0, "Doves"; 0
   ```
4. ```
   Printer.Print 1,
   Printer.Print 2,
   Printer.Print 3,
   Printer.Print 4,
   Printer.Print 5,
   Printer.Print 6
   ```
5. ```
   Printer.Print 1, 2, 3, 4, 5, 6
   ```
6. ```
   Printer.Print Tab(10); 3; Tab(20); 5
   ```
7. ```
   Printer.Print Spc(10); 3; Spc(20); 5
   ```

Your Hands-On Programming Example

Create a project for R 'n R—for Reading 'n Refreshment that contains a dropdown combo box of the coffee flavors and a list box of the syrup flavors. Adjust the size of the boxes as needed when you test the project. The controls should have labels above them containing the words *Coffee* and *Syrup*. Enter the initial values for the syrup flavors and coffee flavors in the Properties window. The user will be able to add more coffee flavors to the list at run time.
   ```

Coffee Flavors	Syrup Flavors
Espresso Roast	Chocolate
Jamaica Blue Mountain	Irish Cream
Kona Blend	Hazelnut
Chocolate Almond	Orange
Vanilla Nut	

Include one menu item to print all the flavors on the printer and another to print only a selected item from each list. These two menu print commands belong on the *File* menu along with the *Exit* command. Use a separator bar between the *Print*s and the *Exit*.

Include an *Edit* menu with commands to *Add coffee flavor*, *Remove coffee flavor*, *Clear coffee list*, and *Display coffee count*.

Add the About form from Chapter 6 into your project and add a *Help* menu with an *About* command.

After you have completed the project, try using different styles for the combo box and rerun the project. As an added challenge, modify the add coffee flavor routine so that duplicates are not allowed.

Planning the Project

Sketch a form (Figure 7.8), which your users sign off as meeting their needs.

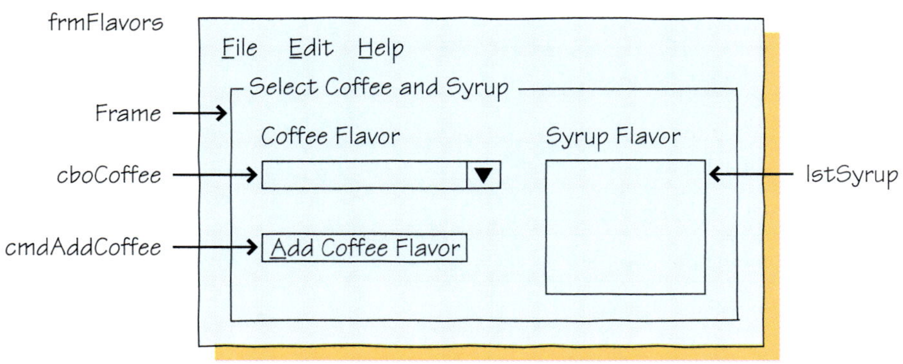

Figure 7.8

A sketch of the main form for the hands-on project.

Plan the Objects and Properties

Object	Property	Setting
frmFlavors	Name	frmFlavors
	Caption	R 'n R—for Reading 'n Refreshment
Frame1	Name	Frame1
	Caption	Select Coffee and Syrup
Label1	Caption	Coffee Flavor
Label2	Caption	Syrup Flavor
cboCoffee	Name	cboCoffee
	Style	0 - Dropdown combo
	Text	(blank)
	List	Chocolate Almond Espresso Roast Jamaica Blue Mtn. Kona Blend Vanilla Nut
	Sorted	True
lstSyrup	Name	lstSyrup
	Sorted	True
	List	Chocolate Hazelnut Irish Creme Orange
cmdAddCoffee	Name	cmdAddCoffee
	Caption	&Add to Coffees
mnuFile	Name	mnuFile
	Caption	&File
mnuFilePrintSelect	Name	mnuFilePrintSelect
	Caption	Print &Selected Flavors
mnuFilePrintAll	Name	mnuFilePrintAll
	Caption	Print &All Flavors
mnuSep	Name	mnuSep
	Caption	-
mnuEdit	Name	mnuEdit
	Caption	&Edit
mnuEditAdd	Name	mnuEditAdd
	Caption	&Add coffee flavor

(continued)

Object	Property	Setting
mnuEditRemove	Name	mnuEditRemove
	Caption	&Remove coffee flavor
mnuEditClear	Name	mnuEditClear
	Caption	&Clear coffee list
mnuEditCount	Name	mnuEditCount
	Caption	Count coffee &list
mnuFileExit	Name	mnuFileExit
	Caption	E&xit
mnuHelp	Name	mnuHelp
	Caption	&Help
mnuHelpAbout	Name	mnuHelpAbout
	Caption	&About

Plan the Event Procedures

Main Form

Procedure	Actions

cmdAddCoffee	If text box in cboCoffee not empty then
	  Add contents of cboCoffee text box to list
	  Clear the text box in cboCoffee.
	Else
	  Display error message.
	End If
	Set the focus to cboCoffee.

mnuFilePrintSelect	If both coffee and syrup selected
	  Print only selected items.
	Else
	  Display error message.
	End If

mnuFilePrintAll	Print title and headings. Use a loop to send all flavor names to the printer.
mnuFileExit	Terminate the Project.
mnuEditAdd	Call cmdAddCoffee_Click.

mnuEditRemove	If coffee flavor selected then
	  Remove selected item.
	Else
	  Display error message.
	End If

mnuEditClear	Clear the coffee list.
mnuEditCount	Display list count in message box.
mnuHelpAbout	Display the About box.

About Form

Procedure	Action
cmdOK	Hide the About box.

Write the Project

- Follow the sketch in Figure 7.8 to create the form. Figure 7.9 shows the completed form.

Figure 7.9

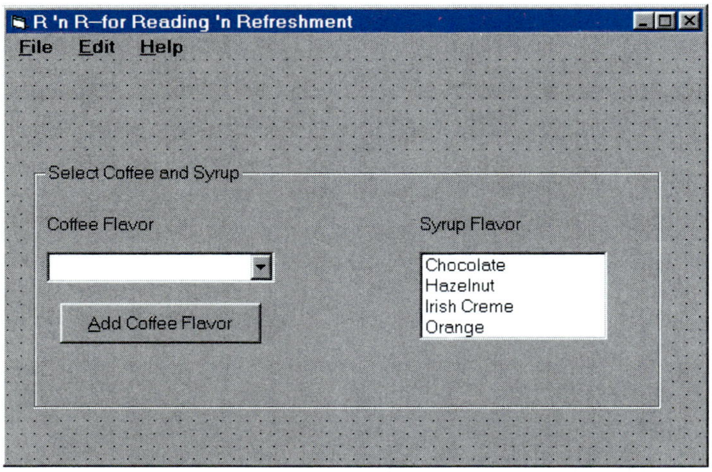

The form for the hands-on project.

- Set the properties of each object as you have planned.
- Write the code. Working from the pseudocode, write each event procedure.
- When you complete the code, use a variety of data to thoroughly test the project.

The Project Coding Solution

Main Form

```
'Module:        frmFlavors
'Programmer:    A. Millspaugh
'Date:          July 1997
'Description:   Print the selected flavor of coffee and syrup
'               or print a list of all of the coffee flavors.
'Folder:        Ch0701

Option Explicit
```

```
Private Sub cmdAddCoffee_Click()
    'Add a new coffee flavor to the coffee list

    If cboCoffee.Text <> "" Then
        With cboCoffee
            .AddItem cboCoffee.Text
            .Text = ""
        End With
    Else
        MsgBox "Enter a coffee name to add", vbExclamation, "Missing data"
    End If
    cboCoffee.SetFocus
End Sub
```

```
Private Sub mnuEditAdd_Click()
    'Add a new coffee to list

    cmdAddCoffee_Click
End Sub
```

```
Private Sub mnuEditClear_Click()
    'Clear the coffee list

    cboCoffee.Clear
End Sub
```

```
Private Sub mnuEditCount_Click()
    'Display a count of the coffee list

    MsgBox "The number of coffee types is " & cboCoffee.ListCount
End Sub
```

```
Private Sub mnuEditRemove_Click()
    'Remove the selected coffee from list

    If cboCoffee.ListIndex <> -1 Then
        cboCoffee.RemoveItem cboCoffee.ListIndex
    Else
        MsgBox  "First select the coffee to remove", vbInformation, _
                "No selection made"
    End If
End Sub
```

```
Private Sub mnuHelpAbout_Click()
    'Display frmAbout

    frmAbout.Show
End Sub
```

```
Private Sub mnuFileExit_Click()
    'Terminate the project

    End
End Sub
```

```
Private Sub mnuFilePrintAll_Click()
    'Print the contents of the coffee flavors
    'combo box on the printer

    Dim iIndex          As Integer
    Dim iFinalValue     As Integer

    Printer.Print                           'Blank line
    Printer.Print Tab(20); "Coffee Flavors"
    Printer.Print                           'Blank line
    iFinalValue = cboCoffee.ListCount - 1
    'List index starts at 0
    For iIndex = 0 To iFinalValue
        Printer.Print Tab(20); cboCoffee.List(iIndex)
    Next iIndex
    Printer.EndDoc
End Sub
```

```
Private Sub mnuFilePrintSelect_Click()
    'Send the current selection of coffee flavor
    ' and syrup flavor to the printer

    If cboCoffee.ListIndex <> -1 And lstSyrup.ListIndex <> -1 Then
        Printer.Print   'Blank line
        Printer.Print Tab(15); "Coffee Selection"
        Printer.Print   'Blank line
        Printer.Print Tab(10); "Coffee Flavor: "; _
                      cboCoffee.List(cboCoffee.ListIndex)
        Printer.Print   'Blank line
        Printer.Print Tab(10); "Syrup Flavor: "; _
                      lstSyrup.List(lstSyrup.ListIndex)
        Printer.EndDoc
    Else
        MsgBox "Make a selection for coffee and syrup.", vbExclamation, _
               "Missing Data"
    End If
End Sub
```

About Form

```
'Module:        frmAbout
'Programmer:    A. Millspaugh
'Date:          July 1997
'Description:   Display information about the program
'               and the programmer
'Folder:        Ch0701
Option Explicit
```

```
Private Sub cmdOK_Click()
    'Returns to the main form

    frmAbout.Hide
End Sub
```

Summary

1. List boxes and combo boxes hold lists of values. The three styles of combo boxes are simple combo boxes, dropdown combo boxes, and dropdown lists.
2. The size of a list box or combo box is determined at design time. If all of the items will not fit into the box, VB automatically adds scroll bars.
3. Initial values for the items in a list can be entered in the List property in the Properties window. At run time, items are added to lists using the AddItem method.
4. The `Clear` method may be used to remove the contents of a list box.
5. The ListIndex property can be used to select an item in the list or to determine which item is selected.
6. The ListCount property holds the number of elements in the list.
7. The List property holds all of the elements of the list. The individual elements can be referenced by using an index.
8. The RemoveItem method removes one element from a list.
9. Code can be written for several events of list boxes and combo boxes. Combo boxes have a Change event; both combo boxes and list boxes have GetFocus and LostFocus events.
10. A loop allows a statement or series of statements to be repeated. `Do/Loops` continue to execute the statements in the loop until a condition is met.
11. `Do/Loops` can have the condition test at the top or the bottom of the loop and can use a `While` or `Until` to test the conditon.
12. A `Do/Loop` can be used to locate a selected item in a combo box.
13. A loop index controls `For/Next` loops; the index is initialized to a starting value. After each iteration the loop index is incremented by the `Step` value, which defaults to 1. The loop is terminated when the loop index reaches the ending value.
14. The `Left`, `Right`, and `Mid` functions return a part of a string.
15. The `Len` function returns the number of characters in a string.
16. The `Printer.Print` statement sends lines of text to the printer, rather than printing the graphical form.
17. The `Print` method uses commas, semicolons, and the `Spc` function to control spacing. The `Tab` function can be used to align columns of information.

18. By default, the `Print` method uses proportional fonts, which allow a variable amount of space for a character, depending on the character width. Judging the number of characters in a print zone or the amount of space text will require using proportional fonts is difficult.
19. Aligning columns of numbers is difficult because print zones and the `Tab` function left align values. Numbers can be right aligned with the assistance of the `Len` function.

Key Terms

Review Questions

1. What is a list box? a combo box?
2. Name and describe the three styles of combo boxes.
3. How can you make scroll bars appear on a list box or combo box?
4. Explain the purpose of the ListIndex property and the ListCount property.
5. When and how is information placed inside a list box or a combo box?
6. In what situation would a loop be used in a procedure?
7. Explain the difference between a pretest and a posttest in a `Do/Loop`.
8. Explain the differences between a `Do/Loop` and a `For/Next` loop.
9. What are the steps in processing a `For/Next` loop?
10. Discuss how and when the values of the loop index change throughout the processing of the loop.
11. What is the purpose of `Printer.Print`?
12. How do the `Left`, `Right`, and `Len` functions operate?
13. How do you control the horizontal spacing of printer output?

Programming Exercises

7.1 Create a project for obtaining student information.
Startup form controls are as follows:
- Text boxes for entering the name and units completed.
- Option buttons for Freshman, Sophomore, Junior, and Senior.
- Check box for Dean's List.
- Use a list box for the following majors: Accounting, Business, Computer Information Systems, and Marketing.
- A simple combo for name of high school—initially loaded with Franklin, Highland, West Highland, and Midtown. If the user types in a new school name, it should be added to the list.
- Print command button that will print the data from the form. Send the output to the printer, nicely formatted. (Do not use PrintForm.)
- An OK (for Enter) button that will clear the entries from the form and reset the focus. Set the button's Default property to True.

Menu: The *File* menu will have an option for *Print Schools* and *Exit*. The *Help* menu will have an option for the *About* box.
Note: Print your name at the top of the printer output for the schools.

7.2 R 'n R—for Reading 'n Refreshment needs a project that contains a form for entering book information.
Form Controls:
- Text boxes for author and title.
- Option buttons for type: fiction or nonfiction.
- Dropdown list for Subject that will include: Best-Seller, Fantasy, Religion, Romance, Humor, Science Fiction, Business, Philosophy, Education, Self-Help, and Mystery.
- List box for Shelf Number containing RC-1111, RC-1112, RC-1113, and RC-1114.
- Print command button that will print the data from the form. (Do not use PrintForm.)
- An OK (for Enter) button that will clear the entries from the form and reset the focus. Set the Default property to True.

Menu: The *File* menu will have an option for *Print Subjects* and *Exit*. The *Help* menu will have an option for the *About* box.
Note: Print your name at the top of the printer output for the subjects.

7.3 Create a project to input chartering information about yachts and print a summary report showing the total revenue and average hours per charter.
Startup Form:
The startup form will contain a menu. The *File* menu will contain commands for *New Charter*, *Print Summary*, *Print Yacht Types*, and *Exit*. Place separator bars before *Print Summary* and after *Print Yacht Types*. The *Edit* menu should have commands for *Add Yacht Type*, *Remove Yacht Type*, and *Display Count of Yacht Types*. The *Help* menu will contain an *About* command.

New Charter Form:

- The new charter form will contain text boxes for responsible party and hours chartered.
- A dropdown combo box will contain the type of yacht: Ranger, Wavelength, Catalina, Coronado, Hobie, C & C, Hans Christian, and Excalibur. Any items that are added to the text box during processing must be added to the list.
- Another dropdown list will contain size: 22, 24, 30, 32, 36, 38, 45. (No new sizes can be entered at run time.)
- An OK command button will add to the totals, print a line on the summary report (do not end the page), and return to the startup form. The print line will contain the yacht type, size, responsible party, hours chartered, and total revenue for the hours chartered. The calculations will require price per hour—use the following chart:

Size	Hourly Rate
22	95.00
24	137.00
30	160.00
32	192.00
36	250.00
38	400.00
45	550.00

A Cancel command button will return to the startup form with no calculations.

Set the Default property of the OK button to True; set the Cancel property of the Cancel button to True.

Summary Report: The summary report will print the summary information and send the report to the printer. The summary information will include *Total Revenue* and *Average Hours Chartered.*

7.4 Create a project that contains a list box with the names of the United States and territories. When the user types the first letters of the state into a text box, set the ListIndex property of the list box to display the appropriate name.

Alabama
Alaska
American Samoa
Arizona
Arkansas
California
Colorado
Connecticut
Delaware
District of Columbia
Florida
Georgia
Guam
Hawaii
Idaho
Illinois
Indiana
Iowa
Kansas
Kentucky
Louisiana
Maine
Maryland
Massachusetts
Michigan
Minnesota
Mississippi
Missouri
Montana
Nebraska
Nevada
New Hampshire
New Jersey
New Mexico

(continued)

New York
North Carolina
North Dakota
Ohio
Oklahoma
Oregon
Pennsylvania
Puerto Rico
Rhode Island
South Carolina
South Dakota
Tennessee
Texas
Trust Territories
Utah
Vermont
Virgin Islands
Virginia
Washington
West Virginia
Wisconsin
Wyoming

7.5 Generate mailing labels with an account number for catalog subscriptions. The project will allow the user to enter Last Name, First Name, Street, City, State, and the ZIP Code, and Expiration Date for the subscription. A dropdown list box will contain the names of the catalogs: *Odds and Ends, Solutions, Camping Needs, ToolTime, Spiegel, The Outlet,* and *The Large Size.*

Use validation to make sure there are entries in the Last Name, ZIP code, and Expiration Date fields.

The account number will consist of the first two characters of the last name, the first three digits of the ZIP code, and the expiration date. Display the account number in a label on the form when the user clicks on the *Display Account Number* button or menu option.

The menu or command buttons for the project should have options for Print Label, Display Account Number, Exit, and Clear.

The *Print label* menu command will print the label using the following format:

First Name Last Name Account Number
Street
City, State ZIP Code

7.6 Maintain a list of bagel types for Bradley's Bagels. Use a dropdown combo box to hold the bagel types and use command buttons or menu choices to Add Bagel Type, Remove Bagel Type, Clear Bagel List, Print Bagel List, Display Bagel Type Count, and Exit. Keep the list sorted in alphabetic order.

Do not allow a blank type to be added to the list. Display an error message if the user selects Remove without first selecting a bagel type.

Before clearing the list, display a message box to confirm the operation.

Here are some suggested bagel types. You can make up your own list.

Plain	Poppy seed
Egg	Sesame seed
Rye	Banana nut
Salt	Blueberry

CASE STUDIES

VB Mail Order

Modify your project from Chapter 6 by adding a dropdown combo box to the New Item form. The combo box will contain the names of the catalogs: *Odds and Ends, Solutions, Camping Needs, ToolTime, Spiegel, The Outlet,* and *The Large Size.*

Add a *Print Catalog List* to your menu on the startup form and remove the *Print* that uses a `PrintForm` from the menu.

When the user begins a new order, print the *Bill To* section and the invoice headings on the printer.

Print one line for each item when the OK button is pressed on the New Item form; do not use the `EndDoc` method until after the summary information has been printed in the PrintInvoice event.

Note: You may want to disable the *Print Catalog List* menu option while an invoice is in progress. Set `mnuFilePrintCatalogList.Enabled = False` when you begin an invoice, and reset it to True after an invoice is complete.

```
Bill To:    Customer Name
            Customer Street Address
            Customer City, State, Zip
Catalog Name   Description   Quantity   Each Price

Total Price
Tax
Shipping and Handling
Total Due
```

VB Auto Center

Create a project for the car wash located at VB Auto Center.

The form will contain three list box or combo box controls that do not permit the user to add items at run time. The first list will contain the names of the packages available for detailing a vehicle: Standard, Deluxe, Executive, or Luxury.

The contents of the other two lists will vary depending upon the package selected. Display one list for the interior work and one list for the exterior work. Store the descriptions of the items in string constants. The list for the interior and exterior must be cleared and new items added each time a selection is made from the package list.

Use a dropdown list to allow the user to select the fragrance. The choices are Hawaiian Mist, Baby Powder, Pine, Country Floral, Pina Colada, and Vanilla.

Include menu commands for *Print*, *Clear*, and *Exit*. The printout will contain the package name, the interior and exterior items being formed, and the fragrance selected. Use a `For/Next` loop when printing the interior and exterior lists.

	Item Description	S	D	E	L
Exterior	Hand Wash	✓	✓	✓	✓
	Hand Wax		✓	✓	✓
	Check Engine Fluids			✓	✓
	Detail Engine Compartment				✓
	Detail Under Carriage				✓
Interior	Fragrance	✓	✓	✓	✓
	Shampoo Carpets		✓	✓	✓
	Shampoo Upholstery				✓
	Interior Protection Coat (dashboard and console)				
	Scotchgard™				✓

Note: S—Standard; D—Deluxe; E—Executive; L—Luxury

C H A P T E R

8

Arrays

At the completion of this chapter, you will be able to ...

1. Set up and use a control array.
2. Code selection logic using a `Select Case` statement.
3. Establish an array of variables and refer to individual elements in the array with variable subscripts.
4. Use the `For Each/Next` to traverse the array.
5. Create user-defined data types for multiple fields of related data.
6. Accumulate totals using arrays.
7. Distinguish between direct access and indirect access of a table.
8. Combine the advantages of list box controls with arrays.
9. Coordinate lists and arrays using the ItemData property.
10. Store data in multidimensional arrays.

Control Arrays

When you plan to include a group of option buttons or check boxes on a form, it often makes sense to create a control array. A ***control array*** is a group of controls that all have the same name. All controls in an array must be the same class. An advantage of using a control array, rather than independent controls, is that the controls share one Click event. In the array's Click event, you can use a Case structure (discussed in the next section) to determine which button or box is selected.

For an example, assume that you are using a group of five option buttons to allow the user to choose a color. After creating the five buttons (Figure 8.1), begin setting the properties by setting the Name property. Name the first option button *optColor*. Then change the Name property of the second option button to *optColor* also (Figure 8.2); a message box will appear (Figure 8.3), asking if you want to create a control array.

Figure 8.1

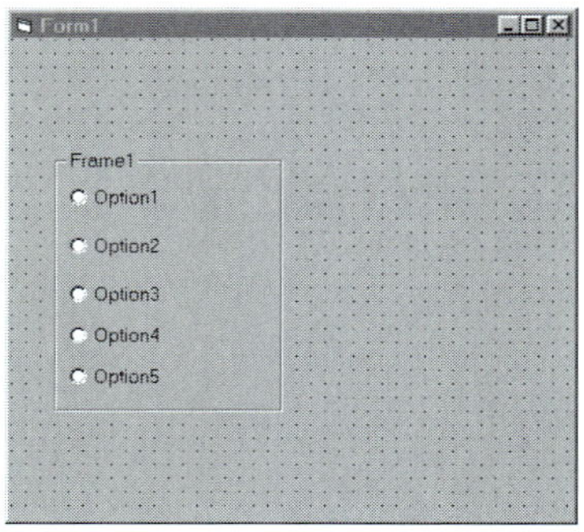

The five option buttons allow the user to choose the color.

Figure 8.2

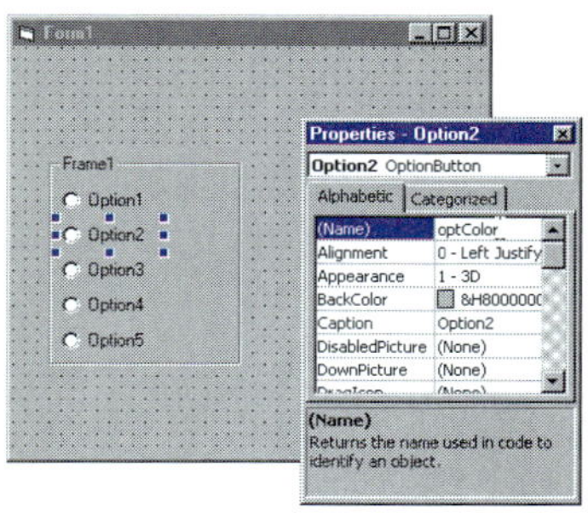

Set the name of the first button to optColor.

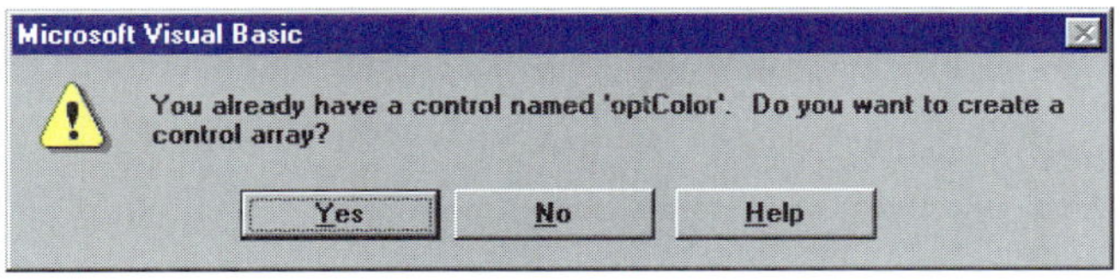

Figure 8.3

After naming a second control with the same name, this dialog box appears. Select Yes to create a control array.

After you select Yes, the name in the top of the Properties window becomes *optColor(0)* for the first control and *optColor(1)* for the second. The number inside the parentheses is called an ***index*** and is used to refer to the specific control within the array. All subsequent controls given the same name will automatically have an index attached.

The option buttons in Figure 8.1 are named optColor(0), optColor(1), optColor(2), optColor(3), and optColor(4).

The Case Structure

In Chapter 4 you used the `If` statement for testing conditions and making decisions. Whenever you want to test a single variable or expression for multiple values, the Case structure provides a flexible and powerful solution. Any program decisions that you can code with a Case structure can also be coded with nested `If` statements, but usually the Case structure is simpler and clearer.

The Select Case Statement—General Form

```
Select Case expression
    Case constant list
        [statement(s)]
    [Case constant list
        [statement(s)]]

.
.
.
    [Case Else]
        [statement(s)]
End Select
```

The expression in a Case structure is usually a variable or property you wish to test.

The constant list is the value that you want to match; it may be a numeric or string constant or variable, a range of values, a relational condition, or a combination of these.

There is no limit to the number of statements that can follow a `Case` statement.

The Select Case Statement—Example

```
Select Case iScore
    Case Is >= 100
        lblMessage1.Caption = "Excellent Score"
        lblMessage2.Caption = "Give yourself a pat on the back"
    Case 80 To 99
        lblMessage1.Caption = "Very Good"
        lblMessage2.Caption = "You should be proud"
    Case 60 To 79
        lblMessage1.Caption = "Satisfactory Score"
        lblMessage2.Caption = "You should have a nice warm feeling"
    Case Else
        lblMessage1.Caption = "Your score shows room for improvement"
        lblMessage2.Caption = ""
End Select
```

This example shows a combination of relational operators and constant ranges. Two points that were illustrated must be noted here:

When using a relational operator (e.g., `Is >= 100`) the word `Is` must be used.

To indicate a range of constants, use the word `To` (e.g., `80 To 99`).

The elements used for the constant list may have any of these forms:

constant [,*constant*...]	Case 2, 5, 9
constant To *constant*	Case 25 To 50
Is *relational-operator constant*	Case Is < 10

When you want to test for a string value, you must include quotation marks around the literals.

Example

```
Select Case txtTeamName.Text
      Case "Tigers"
            (Code for Tigers)
      Case "Leopards"
            (Code for Leopards)
      Case "Cougars", "Panthers"
            (Code for Cougars and Panthers)
      Case Else
            (Code for any nonmatch)
End Select
```

Note that in the previous example, the capitalization must also match exactly. A better solution would be

```
Select Case Ucase(txtTeamName.Text)
      Case "TIGERS"
              (Code for Tigers)
      Case "LEOPARDS"
              (Code for Leopards)
      Case "COUGERS", "PANTHERS"
              (Code for Cougars and Panthers)
      Case Else
              (Code for any nonmatch)
End Select
```

Although the `Case Else` clause is optional, generally you will want to include it in `Select Case` statements. The statements you code beneath `Case Else` will execute only if none of the other `Case` conditions is matched. This clause will provide checking for any invalid or unforeseen values of the expression being tested. If the `Case Else` clause is omitted and none of the `Case` conditions is True, the program will continue execution at the statement following the `End Select`.

If more than one `Case` value is matched by the expression, only the statements in the first matching `Case` clause will be executed.

Testing Option Buttons with the Case Structure

The Case structure is ideal for testing which option button in a control array is selected. When the user selects one of the option buttons, their common Click event occurs. Notice in the following example that Visual Basic passes Index as an argument to the event procedure. Index holds the number of the selected button (0, 1, 2, 3, or 4). You can use the value of Index in a `Select Case` statement.

Note: The argument inside the parentheses, "Index as Integer," means that Visual Basic is passing a variable called *Index*, with a data type of integer.

Example

```
Private Sub optColor_Click(Index As Integer)
     'Set the color to match the selected option button

     Select Case Index
          Case 0          'First button is selected
               lblMessage.ForeColor = vbBlue
          Case 1          'Second button is selected
               lblMessage.ForeColor = vbBlack
          Case 2          'Third button is selected
               lblMessage.ForeColor = vbRed
          Case 3          'Fourth button is selected
               lblMessage.ForeColor = vbWhite
          Case 4          'Fifth button is selected
               lblMessage.ForeColor = vbYellow
     End Select
End Sub
```

As you know, making changes occur for the Click event of an option button violates one of the standards for Windows programming. The color should actually be changed in the Click event for a command button. However, the option button's Index is not available in the command button's Click event. Therefore, the best practice is to set up a module-level variable to hold the selection. In the Click event for the option button, set the value of the variable; in the Click event for the command button, check the value of the variable.

Example

```
'General Declarations
    Option Explicit
    Dim mlSelectedColor As Long   'The color constants are long integers
```

```
Private Sub cmdDisplay_Click()
    'Change the color of the label

    lblMessage.ForeColor = mlSelectedColor
End Sub
```

```
Private Sub optColor_Click(Index As Integer)
    'Save color selection

    Select Case Index
        Case 0    'Blue button is selected
            mlSelectedColor = vbBlue
        Case 1    'Black button is selected
            mlSelectedColor = vbBlack
        Case 2    'Red button is selected
            mlSelectedColor = vbRed
        Case 3   'White button is selected
            mlSelectedColor = vbWhite
        Case 4   'Yellow button is selected
            mlSelectedColor = vbYellow
    End Select
End Sub
```

Feedback 8.1

1. Convert the following `If` statement to a `Select Case`.

```
If iTemp <= 32 Then
    lblComment.Caption = "Freezing"
ElseIf iTemp > 80 Then
    lblComment.Caption = "Hot"
Else
    lblComment.Caption = "Moderate"
End If
```

2. Convert the following to a `Select Case` in the Click event procedure for optCoffee.

```
If optCoffee(0).Value = True Then
    cPrice = 2
ElseIf optCoffee(1).Value = True Then
    cPrice = 2.25
ElseIf optCoffee(2).Value = True Then
    cPrice = 1.75
ElseIf optCoffee(3).Value = True
    cPrice = 2.5
End If
```

3. Add a clause to the previous `Select Case` to display a message box if no option button is selected.

Single-Dimension Arrays

You have just seen how you can set up an array of controls in which several controls have the same name. Now you will find similar advantages to creating and using an array of variables.

A variable array can contain a list of values, similar to a list box or a combo box. In fact, Visual Basic actually stores the List property of a list box or a combo box in an array. You can think of an array as a list box without the box. Any time you need to keep a series of variables for later processing, such as reordering, calculating, or printing, you need to set up an array.

Consider an example that has a form for entering product information, one product at a time. After the user has entered many products, you will need to calculate some statistics and perhaps use the information in different ways. Of course, each time the user enters the data for the next product, the previous contents of the text boxes are replaced. You could assign the previous values to variables, but they also would be replaced for each new product. Another approach might be to create multiple variables, such as stProduct1, stProduct2, stProduct3, and so on. This approach might be reasonable for a few entries, but what happens when you need to store 50 or 500 products?

When you need to store multiple values, use an array. An **array** is a series of individual variables, all referenced by the same name. Sometimes arrays are referred to as **tables** or **subscripted variables**. When you use a control array, the individual controls are referenced as optCoffee(0) or optCoffee(1). The same notation is used with variable arrays. Therefore, in an array for storing names, you may have stName(0), stName(1), stName(2), and so on.

Each individual variable is called an **element** of the array. The individual elements are treated the same as any other variable and may be used in any statement, such as an assignment or a `Printer.Print`. The **subscript** (which may also be called an *index*) inside the parentheses is the position of the element within the array. Figure 8.4 illustrates an array of 10 elements with subscripts from 0 to 9.

Figure 8.4

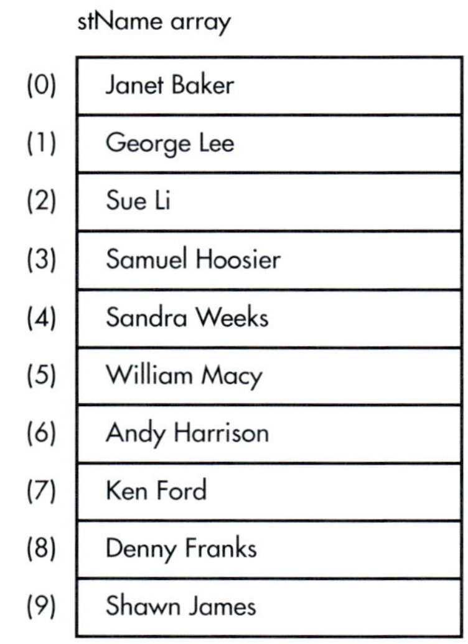

An array of string variables with 10 elements. Subscripts are 0 through 9.

Subscripts

The real advantage of using an array is not realized until you use variables for subscripts in place of the constants.

```
stName(iIndex) = ""
Printer.Print stName(iIndex)
```

Subscripts may be constants, variables, or numeric expressions. Although the subscripts must be integers, Visual Basic will round any noninteger subscript.

A question has probably occurred to you by now—how many elements are there in the stName array? The answer is that you must specify the number of elements in a `Dim` statement.

The Dim Statement for Arrays—General Form

```
Dim ArrayName( [LowerSubscript To] UpperSubscript) [As Datatype]
```

The Dim Statement for Arrays—Examples

```
Dim stName(0 to 25) As String
Dim cBalance(10) As Currency
Dim iCollected(iCount) As Integer
Public gstProduct(1 To 100) As String
Dim miValue(-10 To 10) As Integer
```

The `Dim` statement allocates storage for the specified number of elements and initializes each numeric variable to 0. In the case of string arrays, each element is set to an empty string (zero characters). It is not necessary to specify the lower subscript value. If no value is set for the lower subscript, then the lowest subscript is 0.

Arrays can be dimensioned with empty parentheses, such as

```
Dim gstCustomer() As String
```

An array dimensioned in this way is referred to as a *dynamic array*, because the number of elements may change during program execution by using the `Redim` statement. All other arrays are *static arrays*. Each static array may be dimensioned only once in a project. Any attempt to change the size of a static array after its first use causes the following error message: *Array already dimensioned.* This text treats all arrays as static.

More on Subscripts

A subscript must reference a valid element of the array. If a list contains 10 names, it wouldn't make sense to ask: What is the 15th name on the list? or What is the 2½th name on the list? Visual Basic rounds fractional subscripts and gives the error message: *Subscript out of range* for invalid subscripts.

Feedback 8.2

```
Dim stName(20) As String
Const iValue As Integer = 10
```

After execution of the preceding statements, which of the following are valid subscripts?

1. `stName(20)`
2. `stName(iValue)`
3. `stName(iValue * 2)`
4. `stName(iValue * 3)`
5. `stName(0)`
6. `stName(iValue - 20)`
7. `stName(iValue / 3)`
8. `stName(iValue / 5 - 2)`

For Each/Next Statements

When you use an array, you need a way to reference each element in the array. `For/Next` loops, which you learned to use in Chapter 7, work well to traverse the elements in an array. Another handy loop construct is the **`For Each`** and **`Next`**. The significant advantage of using the `For Each/Next` is that you don't have to manipulate the subscripts of the array.

The For Each and Next Statements—General Form

```
For Each ElementName In ArrayName
    statement(s) in loop
Next [ElementName]
```

Visual Basic automatically references each element of the array, assigns its value to ElementName, and makes one pass through the loop. If the array has 12 elements, for example, the loop will execute 12 times. The variable used for ElementName must be a variant data type.

In the following examples assume that the arrays stName and iTotal have already been dimensioned and that they hold data.

The For Each and Next Statements—Examples

```
Dim vOneName As Variant
For Each vOneName In stName
    Printer.Print vOneName    'Print one element of the array
Next vOneName

Dim vTotal As Variant
For Each vTotal In iTotal
    vTotal = 0                'Set one element of the array to zero
Next vTotal
```

The `For Each` loop will execute if the array has at least one element. All the statements within the loop are executed for the first element. If the array has more elements, the loop continues to execute until all the elements are processed. When the loop finishes, execution of code continues with the line following the `Next` statement.

Note: You may use an `Exit For` statement within a loop to exit early, just as in a `For/Next` loop.

Initializing an Array Using For Each

Although all numeric variables are initially set to 0, it is sometimes necessary to reinitialize variables. To zero out an array, each individual element must be set to 0.

```
For Each vTotal In iTotal
    vTotal = 0  'Set value of each element to 0
Next vTotal
```

User-Defined Data Types

You have been using the Visual Basic data types, such as integer, string, and currency, since Chapter 3. You can also define your own data types by combining multiple fields of data into a single unit. A **user-defined data type** can be used to combine several fields of related information. For example, an Employee data type may contain last name, first name, Social Security number, street, city, state, ZIP code, date of hire, and pay code. A Product data type might contain a description, product number, quantity, and price. The fields can be combined into a user-defined data type using the **Type** and **End Type statements.**

The Type Statement—General Form

```
Type NameOfNewDataType
     List of fields
End Type
```

The Type Statement—Examples

```
Type Employee
     stLastName                As String
     stFirstName               As String
     stSocialSecurityNumber    As String
     stStreet                  As String
     stState                   As String
     stZipCode                 As String
     dHireDate                 As Date
     iPayCode                  As Integer
End Type

Type Product
     stDescription             As String
     stProductNumber           As String
     iQuantity                 As Integer
     cPrice                    As Currency
End Type

Private Type SalesDetail
     cSales(7)                 As Currency
End Type
```

Once you have created your own data type, you may use it to declare variables just as you use any other data type.

```
Dim Widget As Product
Dim Inventory(1 To 100) As Product
Dim HomeFurnishings As SalesDetail
Dim Housewares As SalesDetail
Dim Office As Employee
Dim Warehouse As Employee
```

`Type` statements can appear only at the module level in the General Declarations section of a standard code module or a form module. When placed in a standard code module, they are `Public` by default. If `Type` statements are placed at the module level of a form, *they must be declared as Private.*

Example of a `Type` statement in a form module:

```
'General Declarations section
Option Explicit
Private Type Item
    iCount          As Integer
    stDescription   As String
End Type
```

Accessing Information with User-Defined Data Types

Each field of data within a user-defined type is referred to as an *element* of the data type. To access the elements use the dot notation similar to that used for objects: Specify Variable.Element.

```
Widget.stDescription
Widget.iQuantity
Widget.cPrice
Inventory(iIndex).stDescription
Inventory(iIndex).iQuantity
HomeFurnishings.cSales(iIndex)
Office.stLastName
Item.iCount
```

Notice the use of indexes in the preceding examples. Each example was taken from the preceding `Type` and `Dim` statements. A variable that is not an array, such as Widget, does not need an index. However, for Inventory, which was dimensioned as an array of 100, you must specify not only *which* Inventory item but also the element within the data type. HomeFurnishings is a different situation: The variable was dimensioned as a single variable (not an array). Now look back at the `Type` statement for SalesDetail on the preceding page; there are eight elements in the data type. Therefore, you must use an index on the element within the data type.

Note: You could even declare an array of a data type that includes an array. This type of array requires an index on the variable name and another index on the element name.

Example

```
Dim Clothing(3) as SalesDetail
```

The following line references one element:

```
Clothing(iClothingIndex).cSales(iSalesIndex)
```

You specify the type name in the dimension, but you do not refer to the type name anywhere else in the program. This syntax is consistent with using the built-in data types such as currency and integer; we don't usually use the type names anywhere beyond the declaration.

Note: The `For Each` statement cannot be used with an array of user-defined `Types`. No problem; just use `For/Next` and keep track of the number of elements used.

Feedback 8.3

(Don't forget, subscripts start at zero unless declared otherwise.)

1. Write a `Type` statement to hold student data containing last name, first name, student number, number of units completed, and GPA. The new data type should be called StudentInfo.
2. Declare an array of 100 students that will use the user-defined data type for student information.
3. Code the `Type` statement for a data type called Project containing project name, form name (up to 10), and the folder name.
4. Declare a variable called MyProject with a data type of Project.
5. Declare an array (with 100 elements) called OurProjects with a data type of Project.

Using Array Elements for Accumulators

Array elements are regular variables and perform in the same ways as all variables used so far. You may use the subscripted variables in any way you choose, such as for counters or total accumulators.

To demonstrate the use of array elements as total accumulators, eight totals will be accumulated. For the example, eight scout troops are selling raffle tickets. A separate total must be accumulated for each of the eight groups. Each time a sale is made, the number of tickets must be added to the correct total. The statement

```
Dim iTotal(1 To 8) As Integer
```

declares the eight accumulators.

Adding to the Correct Total

Assume that your user inputs a group number into txtGroup.Text and the number of tickets sold into txtSale.Text. The sales may be input in any order, with multiple sales for each group. Your problem is to add each ticket count to the correct total (1 to 8).

You will use the group number as the subscript to add to the correct total. If the first sale of 10 tickets is for group 4, the 10 must be added to the group 4 total. (Figure 8.5 shows the form and the variables used for this example.)

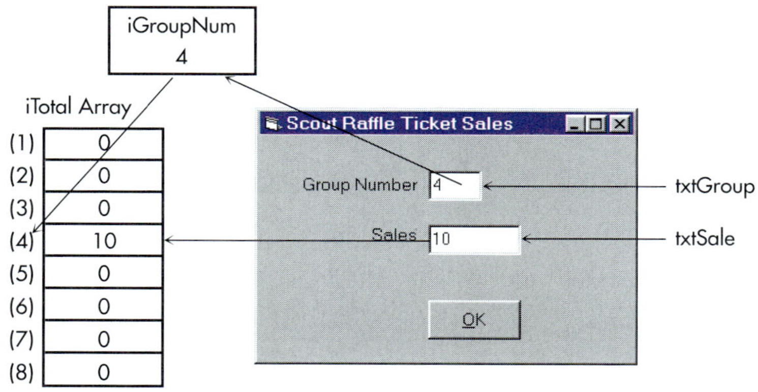

Figure 8.5

The group number entered in the txtGroup text box is used as a subscript to determine the correct iTotal array element to which to add.

```
iGroupNum = Val(txtGroup.Text)
cSale = Val(txtSale.Text)
iTotal(iGroupNum) = iTotal(iGroupNum) + cSale
```

Of course, there is always the danger that the user will enter an incorrect group number. Since it is undesirable for the user to get the error message *Subscript out of range*, the group number must be validated.

```
iGroupNum = Val(txtGroup.Text)
If iGroupNum >= 1 And iGroupNum <= 8 Then
    cSale = Val(txtSale.Text)
    iTotal(iGroupNum) = iTotal(iGroupNum) + cSale
Else
    MsgBox "Please Enter a Valid Group Number (1-8)", vbExclamation, "Data error"
End If
```

Using the group number as an index to the array is a technique called **direct reference**. The groups are assigned numbers from one to eight, which match the subscripts of the array.

Table Lookup

Things don't always work out so neatly as having sequential group numbers that can be used to access the table directly. Sometimes you will have to do a little work to find (**lookup**) the correct value. Reconsider the eight scout troops and their ticket sales. Now the groups are not numbered 1 to 8, but 101, 103, 110, 115, 121, 123, 130, and 145. The group number and the number of tickets sold are still input and the number of tickets must be added to the correct total. But now you must do one more step—determine to which array element to add the ticket sales.

The first step in the project is to establish a user-defined type with the group numbers and totals and then dimension an array of the new type. Before any processing is done, load the group numbers into the table.

Place the following statements in the General Declarations section of a form module:

```
Private Type GroupInfo
    iNumber As Integer
    iTotal As Integer
End Type
Dim mGroup(1 To 8) As GroupInfo
```

Then initialize the values of the array elements by placing these statements into the Form_Load procedure:

```
mGroup(1).iNumber = 101
mGroup(2).iNumber = 103
mGroup(3).iNumber = 110
```

etc.

During program execution the user still enters the group number and the number of tickets sold into text boxes.

The technique used to find the subscript is called a *table lookup*. In this example the object is to find the element number (1 to 8) of the group number and use that element number as a subscript to the total table. If the user enters the third group number (110), the sale is added to the third total. If the seventh group number (130) is entered, the sale is added to the seventh total, and so on. Hence, you need a way, given the group number in txtGroup.Text, to find the corresponding subscript of the mGroup array.

When Visual Basic executes the statement

```
mGroup(iGroupNum).iTotal = mGroup(iGroupNum).iTotal + cSale
```

the value of iGroupNum must be a number in the range 1 to 8. The task for the lookup operation is to find the number to place in iGroupNum, based on the value of txtGroup.Text. Figure 8.6 shows the variables used for the lookup. Figure 8.7 shows the flowchart of the lookup logic.

Figure 8.6

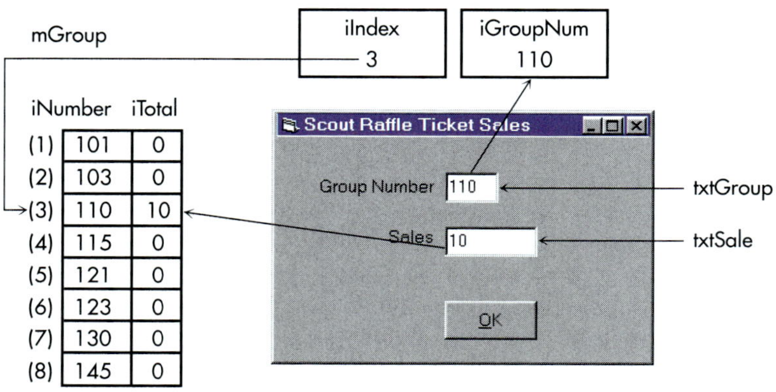

A lookup operation: The group number is looked up in the mGroup array; the correct subscript is found and used to add the sale to the correct iTotal.

Figure 8.7

A flowchart of the logic of a lookup operation.

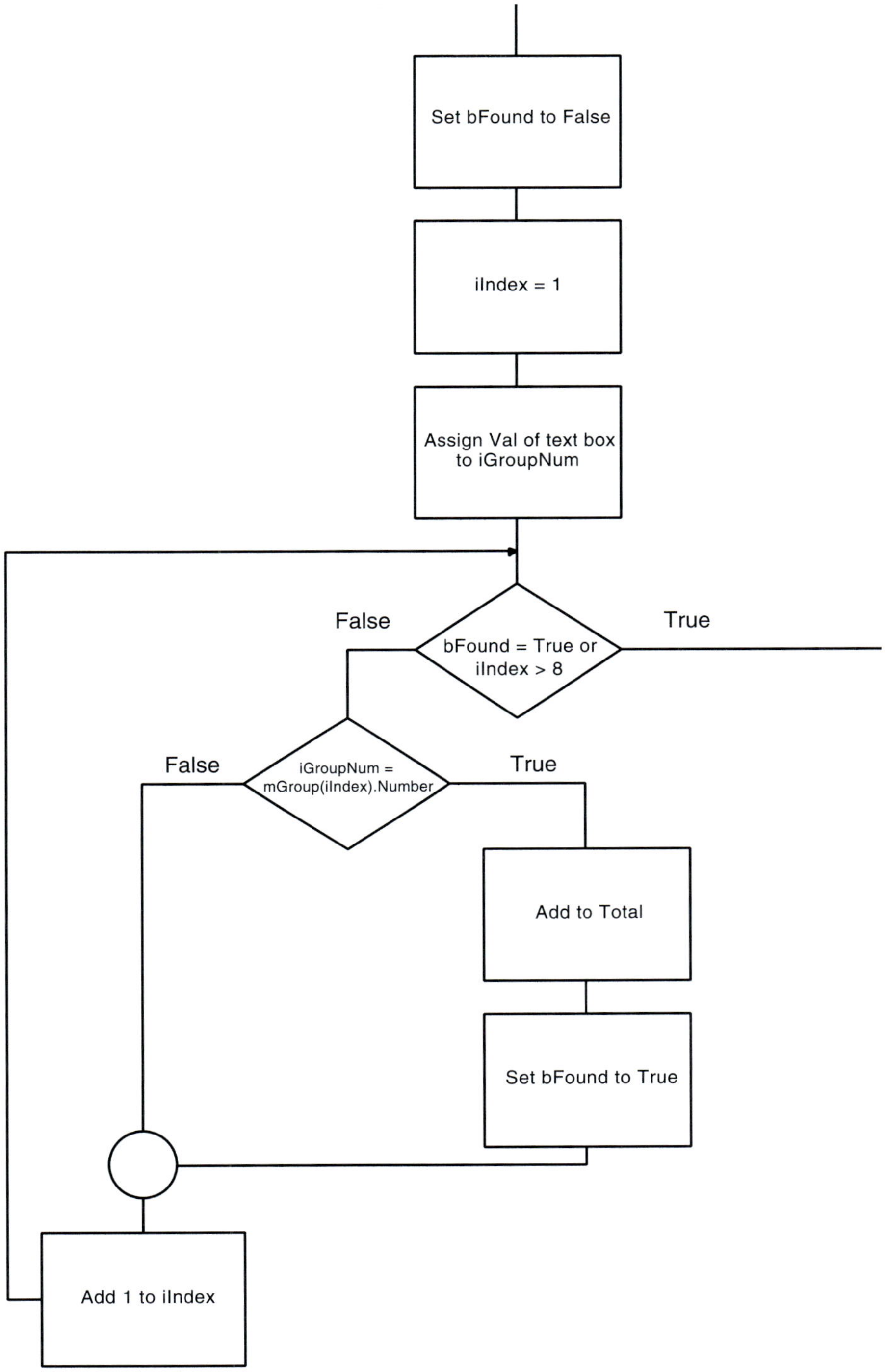

Coding a Table Lookup

For a table lookup, you will find that a `Do/Loop` works better than `For Each`. As you compare to each element in the array and eventually find a match, you need to know the subscript of the matching element.

```
Dim iGroupNum As Integer
Dim iIndex    As Integer
Dim cSale     As Currency
Dim bFound    As Boolean

bFound = False
iIndex = 1
iGroupNum = Val(txtGroup.Text)
Do Until bFound Or iIndex > 8
    If iGroupNum = mGroup(iIndex).iNumber Then
        cSale = Val(txtSale.Text)
        mGroup(iIndex).iTotal = mGroup(iIndex).iTotal + cSale
        bFound = True
    End If
    iIndex = iIndex + 1
Loop
```

Once again, you should do some form of validation. If the user enters an invalid group number, you should display a message box. You can check the value of the Boolean variable bFound after completion of the loop to determine whether the loop terminated because of a match or without a match.

```
If bFound = False Then 'No match was found
    MsgBox "Invalid group number—Sale not added to a total", vbInformation, _
           "Data error"
End If
```

The table-lookup technique will work for any table, numeric or string. It isn't necessary to arrange the fields being searched in any particular sequence. The comparison is made to one item in the list, then the next, and the next—until a match is found. In fact, you can save processing time by arranging the table with the most-often-used entries at the top so that fewer comparisons must be made.

Using List Boxes with Arrays

In the previous example of a lookup, the user had to type some information into a text box, which was used to look up the information in an array. A more efficient and friendly solution might be to substitute a list box for the text box. You can store the eight group numbers in a list box and allow the user to select from the list.

The initial List property can contain the values 101, 103, 110, 115, 121, 123, 130, and 145.

You have probably already realized that you can use the ListIndex property to determine the array subscript. Remember that the ListIndex property holds the position or index of the selected item from the list. You could then use this index with one minor change to access the group total. Recall that the ListIndex property always begins with 0. If you plan to coordinate an array and a list, dimension the array with elements beginning with zero. For this example, we'll change the dimension in the General Declarations section to

```
Dim miTotal(0 to 7) As Integer
```

In place of the lookup operation, we can use this code:

```
Dim iGroupNum As Integer
Dim cSale     As Currency

iGroupNum = lstGroup.ListIndex

If iGroupNum >= 0 And iGroupNum <= 7 Then
    cSale = Val(txtSale.Text)
    miTotal(iGroupNum) = miTotal(iGroupNum) + cSale
Else
    MsgBox "You must select a group number from the list", _
           vbInformation, "Data error"
End If
```

The ItemData Property

Visual Basic offers another handy property for list boxes and combo boxes that can be a big help when working with indexes. A problem can arise when you use the ListIndex of the items in the list as an array subscript. What happens if you sort the data in the list? The ListIndex of each list element could be different than it was previously, which means the position in the array would be incorrect. The **ItemData property** can associate a specific number with each item in the list. Each element of the List property can have a corresponding ItemData that does not change when the list is sorted.

You can set initial values for the ItemData property, just as you set initial values for the List property. If you add an item to the list during run time, you can also add a corresponding value to the ItemData property.

The ItemData Property—General Form

```
Object.ItemData(Index) [= number]
```

In this next example, we'll use a combo box for a list of names and a corresponding array holding the phone numbers for each name in the list.

The array of phone numbers will have the same positions as the original list of names. When the data is first entered into the list, the ItemData property must also be assigned. The ListIndex and the ItemData properties match when first entered.

cboName.List	cboName.ItemData	cboName.ListIndex	stPhone()
Jones, Bill	0	0	111-1111
Lee, Brian	1	1	222-2222
Platt, Cece	2	2	333-3333
Adams, Keith	3	3	444-4444
Lopex, Ana	4	4	555-5555

Notice that after the sort the ItemData property stayed with the associated list item. The ListIndex still represents the position within the array.

cboName.List	cboName.ItemData	cboName.ListIndex
Adams, Keith	3	0
Jones, Bill	0	1
Lee, Brian	1	2
Lopex, Ana	4	3
Platt, Cece	2	4

You can use the ItemData property to access the proper array element.

```
Dim iIndex As Integer
iIndex = cboName.ItemData(cboName.ListIndex) 'Save position number of current
                                              selection
If iIndex <> -1 Then                          'If a selection is made
    lblPhone.Caption = stPhone(iIndex)        'Assign corresponding array element to
                                              label
Else
    MsgBox "Please select a name from the list", vbExclamation, "Data error"
End If
```

Using Nonsequential ItemData Values

The values that are placed in the ItemData property do not need to be in sequence. In our earlier scouting example, we could give names to the groups and have those names associated with the group numbers 101, 103, 110, 115, 121, 123, 130, and 145.

lstGroupName.List	lstGroupName.ItemData
Eagles	101
Bats	103
Wolves	110
Tigers	115
Bears	121
Mountain Lions	123
Panthers	130
Cobras	145

The value stored in the ItemData property is a long integer, but it may hold any numeric value you wish. Using ItemData is an easy way to assign such things as a product number to a description.

Adding Items with ItemData to a List

You learned in Chapter 7 to use the AddItem method to add a new item to a list box or combo box. If you want to store an ItemData property for the new list item, you must include an additional step. Assume that the user enters a new group name and number (using the previous scout group example), using txtGroupName and txtGroupNumber. You can use the AddItem method to add the group name. But then you must know the index of the new item in order to add the corresponding ItemData.

If your list is unsorted, the new item is always last—in the highest ListIndex position. (Remember that the highest ListIndex is one less than ListCount.) Therefore, these statements will add the group name and number to corresponding positions in the list:

```
lstGroupName.AddItem txtGroupName.Text
lstGroupName.ItemData(lstGroupName.ListCount - 1) = txtGroupNumber.Text
```

However, if your list is sorted, the AddItem method adds the new item alphabetically in the list. You can determine the index of the new item using the **NewIndex property**, which VB sets to the index of the new item.

```
lstGroupName.AddItem txtGroupName.Text
lstGroupName.ItemData(lstGroupName.NewIndex) = txtGroupNumber.Text
```

Note that you can use the second method (using the NewIndex property) for an unsorted list as well as a sorted list.

Multidimensional Arrays

You may need to use two subscripts to identify tabular data, where data are arranged in rows and columns.

Many applications of two-dimensional tables quickly come to mind—insurance rate tables, tax tables, addition and multiplication tables, postage rates, foods and their nutritive value, population by region, rainfall by state.

To define a two-dimensional array or *table*, the `Dim` statement specifies the number of rows and columns in the array. The **row** is horizontal and the **column** is vertical. The following table has three rows and four columns:

The Dim Statement for Two-Dimensional Arrays—General Form

```
Dim ArrayName([LowerLimit To] UpperLimit, [LowerLimit To] UpperLimit) As Datatype
```

The Dim Statement for Two-Dimensional Arrays—Examples

```
Dim stName(2, 3) As String
Dim stName(0 To 2, 0 To 3) As String
```

Either of these two statements establishes an array of 12 elements, with three rows and four columns. You must always use two subscripts when referring to individual elements of the table. Specify the row with the first subscript and the column with the second subscript.

(0,0)	(0,1)	(0,2)	(0,3)
(1,0)	(1,1)	(1,2)	(1,3)
(2,0)	(2,1)	(2,2)	(2,3)

The elements of the array may be used in the same ways as any other variable—in accumulators, counts, reference fields for lookup; in statements like assignment and printing; and as conditions. Some valid references to the table include

```
stName(1, 2) = "Value"
stName(iRowIndex, iColIndex) = "Value"
lblDisplay.Caption = stName(1, 2)
Printer.Print stName(iRowIndex, iColIndex)
```

Invalid references for the stName table would include any value greater than 2 for the first subscript or greater than 3 for the second subscript.

Initializing Two-Dimensional Arrays

Although numeric array elements are initially set to 0 and string elements are set to empty strings, many situations require that you initialize arrays to 0 or some other value. You can use nested `For/Next` loops or `For Each/Next` to set each array element to an initial value.

Nested For/Next Example

The assignment statement in the inner loop will be executed 12 times, once for each element of stName.

```
Dim iRow   As Integer
Dim iCol   As Integer

For iRow = 1 To 3
    For iColumn = 1 To 4
        stName(iRow, iColumn) = ""    'Initialize each element
    Next iColumn
Next iRow
```

For Each/Next Example

You can also perform the initialization with a `For Each` statement, which initializes all 12 elements.

```
Dim vName As Variant
For Each vName In stName
    vName = ""                        'Initialize each element
Next vName
```

Printing a Two-Dimensional Table

When you want to print the contents of a two-dimensional table, you can also use a `For Each/Next` loop.

```
Dim vName As Variant
For Each vName In stName
    Printer.Print vName
Next vName
```

If you wish to print an entire row in one line, use a `For/Next` loop and set up the print statements for multiple elements.

```
For iRowIndex = 0 To 2
 Printer.Print stName(iRowIndex, 0); Tab(15); stName(iRowIndex, 1); _
  Tab(30); stName(iRowIndex, 2); Tab(45); stName(iRowIndex, 3)
Next iRowIndex
```

Summing a Two-Dimensional Table

You can find the sum of a table in various ways. You may sum either the columns or the rows of the table; or, as in a cross-foot, you may sum the figures in both directions and double-check the totals.

To sum the array in both directions, each column needs one total field and each row needs one total field. Two one-dimensional arrays will work well for the totals. Figure 8.8 illustrates the variables used in this example.

Figure 8.8

Two one-dimensional arrays hold totals for the two-dimensional array.

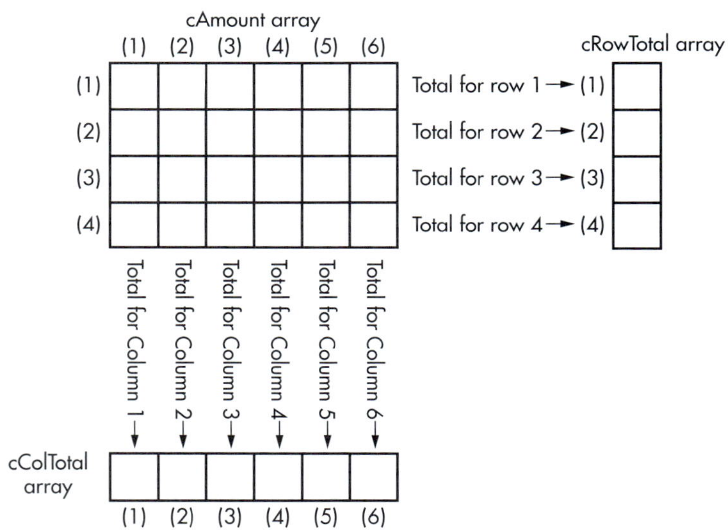


```
Dim cAmount(1 To 4, 1 To 6) As Currency
Dim cRowTotal(1 To 4) As Currency
Dim cColTotal(1 To 6) As Currency
Dim iRowIndex As Integer
Dim iColIndex As Integer

For iRowIndex = 1 To 4
 For iColIndex = 1 To 6
    cRowTotal(iRowIndex) = cRowTotal(iRowIndex) _
     + cAmount(iRowIndex, iColIndex)
    cColTotal(iColIndex) = cColTotal(iColIndex) _
     + cAmount(iRowIndex, iColIndex)
 Next iColIndex
Next iRowIndex
```

Feedback 8.4

Write VB statements to do the following:

1. Dimension a table called cTemperature with five columns and three rows.
2. Set each element in the first row to 0.
3. Set each element in the second row to 75.
4. For each column of the table, add together the elements in rows 1 and 2, placing the sum in row 3.
5. Print the entire table.

Lookup Operation for Two-Dimensional Tables

When you look up items in a two-dimensional table, you can use the same techniques discussed with single-dimensional arrays—direct reference and table lookup. The limitations are the same.

1. To use a direct reference, row and column subscripts must be readily available. For example, you can tally the hours used for each of five machines (identified by machine numbers 1 to 5) and each of four departments (identified by department numbers 1 to 4).

```
iRowIndex = Val(txtMachine.Text)
iColIndex = Val(txtDepartment.Text)
cHours = Val(txtHours.Text)
MachineTotal(iRowIndex, iColIndex) = MachineTotal(iRowIndex, iColIndex) + cHours
```

2. A table lookup is the most common lookup technique.

Many two-dimensional tables used for lookup require additional one-dimensional arrays or lists to aid in the lookup process. For an example, use a shipping rate table (Figure 8.9) to look up the rate to ship a package. The shipping rate depends on the weight of the package and the zone to which it is being shipped. You could design the project with the weight and zones in dropdown list boxes, or you could use a text box and let the user input the data.

Figure 8.9

This shipping rate table in a two-dimensional array can be used to look up the correct shipping charges.

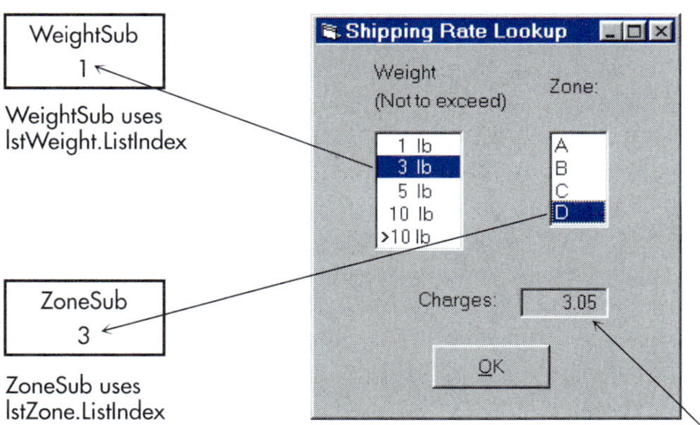

Weight (Not to exceed)	Zone A	Zone B	Zone C	Zone D
1 lb	1.00	1.50	1.65	1.85
3 lb	1.58	2.00	2.40	3.05
5 lb	1.71	2.52	3.10	4.00
10 lb	2.04	3.12	4.00	5.01
>10 lb	2.52	3.75	5.10	7.25

Using List Boxes

In this example a list box holds the weight limits, and another list holds the zones. The values for the two lists are set with the List and ItemData properties at design time. The five-by-four rate table is two dimensional, and the values are preloaded. The best way to preload values is to load the values from a data file, which is discussed in Chapter 9. The other alternative is to assign the values in the Form_Load procedure of the startup form.

```
Dim mcRate(0 to 4, 0 to 3) As Currency   'Module-level array for lookup
Dim iWeightSub   As Integer
Dim iZoneSub     As Integer
iWeightSub = lstWeight.ListIndex
iZoneSub = lstZone.ListIndex

If iWeightSub <> -1 And iZoneSub <> -1 Then
    lblShipping.Caption = mcRate(iWeightSub, iZoneSub)
Else
    MsgBox "Please select the weight and zone from the proper lists."
End If
```

Using Text Boxes

If you are using text boxes for data entry rather than list boxes, the input requires more validation. Both the weight and zone entries must be looked up before the correct rate can be determined. The valid zones and weight ranges will be stored in two separate one-dimensional arrays. The first step in the project is to establish and fill the two arrays. The five-by-four rate table is two dimensional, and the values should be preloaded, as in the previous example.

```
Dim mcRate(0 to 4, 0 to 3) As Currency    'Module-level array for lookup
Dim iWeight(0 To 4) As Integer
Dim stZone(0 to 3)  As String
Dim iWeightSub      As Integer
Dim iZoneSub        As Integer
Dim iIndex          As Integer
Dim iWeightInput    As Integer
Dim bWeightFound    As Boolean
Dim bZoneFound      As Boolean
```

```
'Look up the weight to find the iWeightSub

iWeightInput = Val(txtWeight.Text)
bWeightFound = False
iIndex = 0
Do Until bWeightFound or iIndex > 4
    If iWeightInput <= iWeight(iIndex) Then
        iWeightSub = iIndex
        bWeightFound = True
    End If
    iIndex = iIndex + 1
Loop
If Not bWeightFound Then
    iWeightSub = 4
End If

'Look up the zone to find the iColIndex
bZoneFound = False
iIndex = 0
Do Until bZoneFound or iIndex > 3
    If txtZone.Text = stZone(iIndex) Then
        iZoneSub = iIndex
        bZoneFound = True
    End If
    iIndex = iIndex + 1
Loop

'Display the appropriate rate
If (iWeightSub >= 0 And iWeightSub <= 4) And _
        (iZoneSub >= 0 And iZoneSub <= 3) Then
    lblShipping.Caption = mcRate(iWeightSub, iZoneSub)
Else
    MsgBox "Invalid zone or weight entered", vbExclamation, "Invalid data"
End If
```

Your Hands-On Programming Example

Create a project for R 'n R—for Reading 'n Refreshment that determines the price per pound for bulk coffee sales. The coffees are divided into categories: regular, decaf, and special blend. The prices are set by the ¼ pound, ½ pound, and full pound. Use a Find Price command button to search for the appropriate price based on the selections.

	Regular	Decaf	Blend
¼ pound	2.60	2.90	3.25
½ pound	4.90	5.60	6.10
Full pound	8.75	9.75	11.25

Create a user-defined data type that contains the coffee type, amount, and price. Set up a variable called mTransaction that is an array of 20 elements of your data type. Each time the Find Price button is pressed, add the data to the array.

When the Exit button is pressed, print appropriate headings and the data from the mTransaction array.

Planning the Project

Sketch a form (Figure 8.10), which your users sign off as meeting their needs.

Figure 8.10

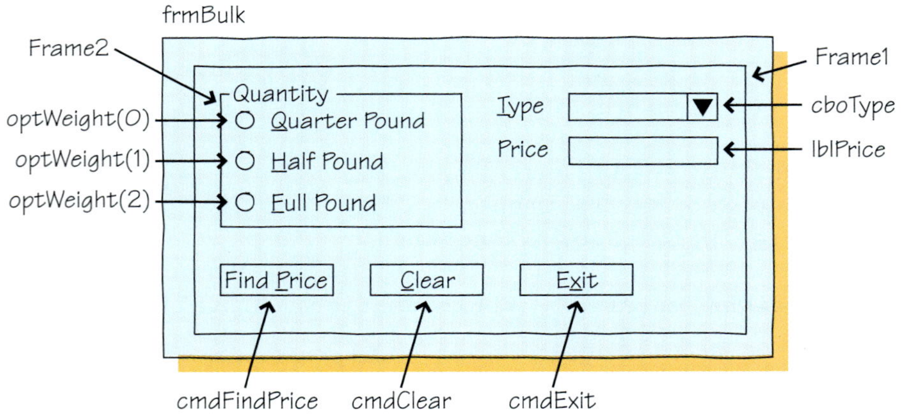

A planning sketch of the form for the hands-on programming example.

Plan the Objects and Properties

Object	Property	Setting
frmBulk	Name	frmBulk
	Caption	R 'n R—for Reading 'n Refreshment
Frame1	Caption	(blank)
Frame2	Caption	Quantity
Label1	Caption	Type
Label2	Caption	Price
lblPrice	Name	lblPrice
	Caption	(blank)
cboType	Name	cboType
	List	Regular
		Decaffeinated
		Special Blend
	ItemData	0
		1
		2
	Sorted	True
	Style	2 - Dropdown list
optWeight	Name	optWeight
	Caption	Quarter pound
optWeight	Name	optWeight
	Caption	Half pound
optWeight	Name	optWeight
	Caption	Full pound
cmdFindPrice	Name	cmdFindPrice
	Caption	Find &Price
cmdClear	Name	cmdClear
	Caption	&Clear
cmdExit	Name	cmdExit
	Caption	E&xit

Plan the Event Procedures

You need to plan the actions for the event procedures and the Form_Load event.

Procedure	Actions
Form_Load	Create and load the price table.
cmdFindPrice	Look up the price in the table. Display the price in the label. Store type, quantity, and price in the array.
cmdClear	Erase the price. Set list box indexes to −1.
cmdExit	Print the Transaction array. Terminate the project.

Write the Project

- Follow the sketch in Figure 8.10 to create the form. Figure 8.11 shows the completed form.

Figure 8.11

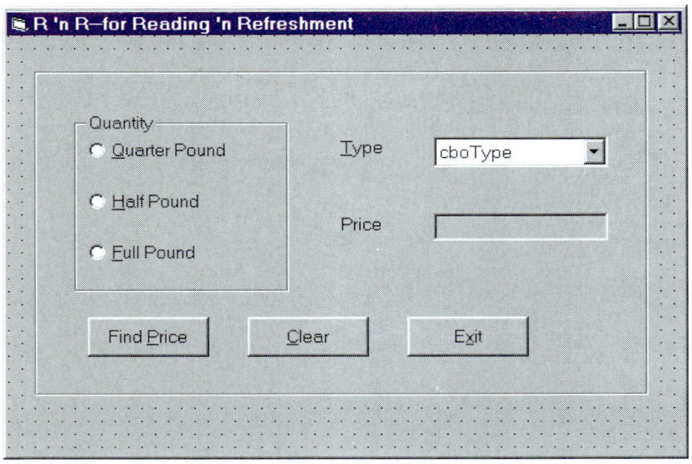

The form for the hands-on programming example.

- Set the properties of each object, according to your plan.
- Write the code. Working from the pseudocode, write each event procedure.
- When you complete the code, use a variety of data to thoroughly test the project.

The Project Coding Solution

```
'Module:        frmBulk
'Programmer:    A. Millspaugh
'Date:          July 1997
'Description:   Look up the price for bulk coffee
'               based on quantity and type.
'Folder:        Ch0801

Option Explicit
Dim mcPrice(0 To 2, 0 To 2) As Currency    'Table to store coffee prices

Private Type CoffeeSale
    stType As String
    stQuantity As String
    cPrice As Currency
End Type

Dim mTransaction(20)         As CoffeeSale          'Store transactions for report
Dim miNumberTransactions     As Integer
Dim mlWeight                 As Long
```

```
Private Sub cmdClear_Click()
    'Remove the selection from the lists and
    '    clear the price
    Dim iIndex As Integer

    cboType.ListIndex = -1   'Clear selection
    lblPrice.Caption = ""
    mlWeight = 0
    For iIndex = 0 To 2
        optWeight(iIndex).Value = False
    Next iIndex
End Sub
```

```
Private Sub cmdExit_Click()
    'Print report and terminate the project

    Dim iIndex          As Integer
    Dim stPrintPrice    As String
```

```
    Printer.Print Tab(45); "Sales Report"
    Printer.Print ""
    Printer.Print Tab(15); "Type"; Tab(40); "Quantity"; Tab(60); "Price"
    Printer.Print ""
    For iIndex = 0 To miNumberTransactions - 1
        stPrintPrice = Format$(mTransaction(iIndex).cPrice, "Currency")
        Printer.Print Tab(10); mTransaction(iIndex).stType; _
            Tab(35); mTransaction(iIndex).stQuantity; _
            Tab(65 - Len(stPrintPrice)); stPrintPrice
    Next iIndex
    End
End Sub
```

```
Private Sub cmdFindPrice_Click()
    'Lookup the price using the quantity and type

    Dim iRow     As Integer
    Dim iCol     As Integer
    Dim cPrice   As Currency

    iRow = mlWeight
    If miNumberTransactions <= 20 Then        'Allow only 20 transactions
        If cboType.ListIndex <> -1 Then
            iCol = cboType.ListIndex
            Select Case mlWeight
                Case 0
                   mTransaction(miNumberTransactions).stQuantity = "Quarter Pound"
                Case 1
                   mTransaction(miNumberTransactions).stQuantity = "Half Pound"
                Case 2
                   mTransaction(miNumberTransactions).stQuantity = "Full Pound"
                Case Else
                   'Default to quarter pound
                   mTransaction(miNumberTransactions).stQuantity = "Quarter Pound"
            End Select
            cPrice = mcPrice(iRow, iCol)
            lblPrice.Caption = Format$(cPrice, "Currency")
            mTransaction(miNumberTransactions).stType = cboType.List(iCol)
            mTransaction(miNumberTransactions).cPrice = cPrice
            miNumberTransactions = miNumberTransactions + 1
        Else
            MsgBox "Select a type and quantity", vbExclamation, "Entry Error"
        End If
    End If
End Sub
```

```
Private Sub Form_Load()
    'Load prices into the table

    mcPrice(0, 0) = 2.6
    mcPrice(0, 1) = 2.9
    mcPrice(0, 2) = 3.25
    mcPrice(1, 0) = 4.9
    mcPrice(1, 1) = 5.6
    mcPrice(1, 2) = 6.1
    mcPrice(2, 0) = 8.75
    mcPrice(2, 1) = 9.75
    mcPrice(2, 2) = 11.25
End Sub
```

```
Private Sub optWeight_Click(Index As Integer)
    'Find the selected weight

    mlWeight = Index
End Sub
```

Programming Hints

The Array Function

As you saw in the earlier programming example, initializing an array at run time is somewhat tedious (refer to the Form_Load procedure in the hands-on programming example). Visual Basic provides another method of initializing an array that uses a variant variable. You declare the variable to be an array and assign a list of values to it with the `Array` function.

The Array Function—General Form

```
Variable = Array(list of values)
```

The Array Function—Examples

```
vNames = Array("Ann", "Mary", "Jorge", "Peter")
vCodes = Array(45, 76, 53, 24)
```

The values within the array are accessed with the same subscript notation as a dimensioned array.

```
Dim vMonth As Variant
vMonth = Array("Jan", "Feb", "Mar", "Apr", "May", "Jun", "Jul", "Aug", _
  "Sep", "Oct", "Nov", "Dec")
```

After the previous declaration and assignment, the statement

```
Printer.Print vMonth(4)
```

would print *May*. (As usual, the subscripts start at 0.)

Summary

1. A series of controls with the same name is called a control array. Each individual control is referenced using an index, which is its position number within the array.
2. The controls in a control array share one event procedure.
3. A `Select Case` statement may be used when an expression is being tested for many different values or ranges of values. The statement also includes a `Case Else` for the situation that none of the values specified was a match.
4. A series of variables with the same name is called an array. The individual values are referred to as elements, and each element is accessed by its subscript, which is a position number.
5. A special form of the `For` loop called `For Each` is available for working with arrays. The `For Each` eliminates the need for the programmer to manipulate the subscripts of the array.
6. In addition to the existing data types, programmers may use the `Type` statement to combine fields and create user-defined data types. `Type` statements must appear in the General Declarations section of a module.
7. Arrays can be used like any other variables; they can be used to accumulate a series of totals or store values for a lookup procedure.
8. The information in arrays may be accessed directly by subscript, or a table lookup may be used to determine the correct table position.
9. List box and combo box controls have an ItemData property that can be used to assign a numeric value to each item in the list.
10. Arrays may be multidimensional. A two-dimensional table contains rows and columns and is processed similarly to a one-dimensional array. Access of a multidimensional array frequently requires the use of nested loops.

Key Terms

array *277*
column *292*
control array *272*
direct reference *285*
element *277*
`For Each` and `Next` *279*
index *273*
ItemData property *289*
lookup *285*
NewIndex property *291*
row *292*
subscript *277*
subscripted variable *277*
table *277*
`Type/End Type` statements *281*
user-defined data type *281*

Review Questions

1. Define the following terms:
   (a) array
   (b) element
   (c) subscript
   (d) control array
   (e) subscripted variable
2. Describe the logic of a table lookup.
3. Name some situations in which it is important to perform validation when working with subscripted variables.
4. Why would a list box control need both a ListIndex property and an ItemData property?
5. Compare a two-dimensional table to an array of a user-defined data type.
6. When initializing values in a two-dimensional table, what statements should be used?

Programming Exercises

8.1 (*Array of user-defined type*) Create a project to analyze an income survey. The statistics for each home include an identification code, the number of members in the household, and the yearly income. A menu will contain *File*, *Reports*, and *Help*. The *File* menu will contain *Enter Data* and *Exit*. As the data are entered, they should be assigned from the text boxes to the elements of a user-defined type.

The reports for the project will be sent to the printer and include the following:

(a) A three-column report displaying the input data.
(b) A listing of the identification number and income for each household that exceeds the average income.
(c) The percentage of households having incomes below the poverty level.

Test Data

Poverty Level: 8000 for a family of one or two, plus 2000 for each additional member.

ID Number	Annual Income	Number of Persons
2497	12500	2
3323	13000	5
4521	18210	4
6789	8000	2
5476	6000	1
4423	16400	3
6587	25000	4
3221	10500	4
5555	15000	2
0085	19700	3
3097	20000	8
4480	23400	5
0265	19700	2
8901	13000	3

Check Figures

Households exceeding average income:
You should have 7 entries on the list.
Households below poverty level:
21.43%

8.2 (*Two-dimensional table*) Modify project 8.1 to assign the data to a multidimensional array rather than use an array of user-defined types.

8.3 Create a project to keep track of concert ticket sales by your club. Ticket prices are based on the section of the auditorium in which the seats are located. Your program should calculate the price for each sale, accumulate the total number of tickets sold in each section, display the ticket price schedule, and print a summary of all sales.

The form will contain a sorted list box of the sections for seating and use an ItemData property to store the ticket price subscript.

Section	Price
Orchestra	40.00
Mezzanine	27.50
General	15.00
Balcony	10.00

Special Consideration: Do not allow the user to receive a subscript-out-of-range error message.

8.4 (*Array of a user-defined type*) Create a project that will allow a user to look up state names and their two-letter abbreviations. The user will have the options to *Look up the Abbreviation* or to *Look up the State Name*. In the event that a match cannot be found for the input, print an appropriate error message.

Use an option button control array and a `Select Case` to determine which text box (state name or abbreviation) should have the focus and which should be disabled.

Data

AL	Alabama
AK	Alaska
AS	American Samoa
AZ	Arizona
AR	Arkansas
CA	California
CO	Colorado
CT	Connecticut
DE	Delaware
DC	District of Columbia
FL	Florida
GA	Georgia
GU	Guam
HI	Hawaii
ID	Idaho
IL	Illinois
IN	Indiana
IA	Iowa
KS	Kansas
KY	Kentucky
LA	Louisiana
ME	Maine
MD	Maryland
MA	Massachusetts
MI	Michigan
MN	Minnesota

(*continued*)

MS	Mississippi
MO	Missouri
MT	Montana
NE	Nebraska
NV	Nevada
NH	New Hampshire
NJ	New Jersey
NM	New Mexico
NY	New York
NC	North Carolina
ND	North Dakota
OH	Ohio
OK	Oklahoma
OR	Oregon
PA	Pennsylvania
PR	Puerto Rico
RI	Rhode Island
SC	South Carolina
SD	South Dakota
TN	Tennessee
TX	Texas
TT	Trust Territories
UT	Utah
VT	Vermont
VA	Virginia
VI	Virgin Islands
WA	Washington
WV	West Virginia
WI	Wisconsin
WY	Wyoming

8.5 (*Two-dimensional table*) Create a project that looks up the driving distance between two cities. Use two dropdown lists that contain the names of the cities. Label one list *Departure* and the other *Destination*. Use a command button to calculate distance.

Store the distances in a two-dimensional table.

	Boston	Chicago	Dallas	Las Vegas	Los Angeles	Miami	New Orleans	Toronto	Vancouver	Washington DC
Boston	0	1004	1753	2752	3017	1520	1507	609	3155	448
Chicago	1004	0	921	1780	2048	1397	919	515	2176	709
Dallas	1753	921	0	1230	1399	1343	517	1435	2234	1307
Las Vegas	2752	1780	1230	0	272	2570	1732	2251	1322	2420
Los Angeles	3017	2048	1399	272	0	2716	1858	2523	1278	2646
Miami	1520	1397	1343	2570	2716	0	860	1494	3447	1057
New Orleans	1507	919	517	1732	1858	860	0	1307	2734	1099
Toronto	609	515	1435	2251	2523	1494	1307	0	2820	571
Vancouver	3155	2176	2234	1322	1278	3447	2734	2820	0	2887
Washington DC	448	709	1307	2420	2646	1057	1099	571	2887	0

8.6 *(Two-dimensional table)* Create a project in which the user will complete a 10-question survey. Create a form containing labels with each of the questions and a group of option buttons for each question with the following responses: Always, Usually, Sometimes, Seldom, and Never.

Use a two-dimensional array to accumulate the number of each response for each question.

Have a menu or command option that will print an item analysis on the printer that shows the question number and the count for each response.

Sample of partial output:

Question	Always	Usually	Sometimes	Seldom	Never
1	5	2	10	4	6
2	2	2	10	2	1
3	17	0	10	0	0

CASE STUDIES

VB Mail Order

Create a project that will calculate shipping charges from a two-dimensional table of rates. The rate depends on the weight of the package and the zone to which it will be shipped. The Wt. column specifies the maximum weight for that rate. All weights over 10 pounds use the last row.

Wt.	Zone	A	B	C	D
1		1.00	1.50	1.65	1.85
3		1.58	2.00	2.40	3.05
5		1.71	2.52	3.10	4.00
10		2.04	3.12	4.00	5.01
>10		2.52	3.75	5.10	7.25

VB Auto Center

VB Auto sells its own brand of spark plugs. In order to cross-reference to major brands, it keeps a table of equivalent part numbers. VB Auto wants to computerize the process of looking up part numbers in order to improve its customer service.

The user should be able to enter the part number and brand and look up the corresponding VB Auto part number. You may allow the user to select the brand (Brand A, Brand B, or Brand X) from a list or from option buttons.

You can choose from two alternate approaches for the lookup table. Either store the part numbers in a two-dimensional table or in an array of user defined types. In either case, use the part number and brand entered by the user; look up and display the VB Auto part number.

VB Auto	Brand A	Brand C	Brand X
PR214	MR43T	RBL8	14K22
PR223	R43	RJ6	14K24
PR224	R43N	RN4	14K30
PR246	R46N	RN8	14K32
PR247	R46TS	RBL17Y	14K33
PR248	R46TX	RBL12-6	14K35
PR324	S46	J11	14K38
PR326	SR46E	XEJ8	14K40
PR444	47L	H12	14K44

CHAPTER

9

Data Files

At the completion of this chapter, you will be able to . . .

1. Create data files.
2. Read and write records to disk.
3. Determine the appropriate locations for data file–related code.
4. Understand the significance of a `Close` statement.
5. Differentiate between sequential and random files.
6. Trap user errors and handle errors to avoid run-time errors.
7. Incorporate fixed-length strings into user-defined data types.
8. Read and write random files.
9. Perform add, delete, and edit operations on random files.
10. Allow the user to input data using the `InputBox` function.

Data Files

In all of your projects so far, the user has entered information through text boxes. Although this input method is satisfactory for many applications, some situations require large quantities of data or information to be processed week after week.

Many computer applications require data to be saved from one run to the next. Some examples are personal tasks, such as budgeting, mailing lists, and sports-team records, and business applications, such as inventory records, customer files, and master files. This chapter deals with methods to store and access **data files** on disk.

Data Files and Project Files

In computer terminology anything that you store on a diskette or hard disk is given its own unique name and called a **file**. Each of your Visual Basic projects requires multiple files—for the forms, standard code modules, and project information. However, the files you will create now are different; they contain actual data, such as names and addresses, inventory amounts, and account balances.

Data File Terminology

The entire collection of data is called a file. The file is made up of **records**—one record for each entity in the file. Each record can be broken down further into **fields** (also called ***data elements***). For example, in an employee file, the data for one employee are one record. In a name and address file, the data for one person are a record.

In the name and address file, each person has a last name field, a first name field, address fields, and a phone number field. Each field in a record pertains to the same person. Figure 9.1 illustrates a name and address file.

Figure 9.1

The rows in this data file represent records; the columns represent fields.

Last Name	First Name	Street	City	State	Zip	Phone	Email
Maxwell	Harry	795 W. J Street	Ontario	CA	91764	909-555-1234	
Helm	Jennifer	201 Cortez Way	Pomona	CA	91766	818-555-2222	JHelm@ms.org
Colton	Craig	1632 Granada Place	Pomona	CA	91766	909-555-3333	

A record

A field

The data stored in files is nearly always entered in an organized manner. Records may be stored in account number order, alphabetically by name, by date, or by the sequence in which they are received. One field in the record is the organizing factor for the file (such as account number, name, or date). This field, which is used to determine the order of the file, is called the ***record key***, or ***key field.***

A key field may be either a string or numeric field. In an employee file, if the records are in order by an employee number, then the employee number is the key field. If the order is based on employee name, then the name is the key field, although key fields are normally unique data items.

File Organizations

The manner in which data are organized, stored, and retrieved is called the *file organization*. Two common file organizations are *sequential* and *random*. In this chapter you will learn to read and write both sequential and random files.

Opening and Closing Data Files

Three steps are necessary to process data files:

1. *Open* the file. Before any data may be placed on the disk or read from the disk, the file must be opened. Generally you will open the file in the Form_Load procedure.
2. *Read* or *write* the data records. You will read or write in a save procedure associated with the data entry form.
3. *Close* the file. You must always close a file when you are finished with it.

The Open Statement—General Form

```
Open "FileName" For {Input | Output | Append | Random} As #FileNumber [Len = RecLength]
```

The elements shown in the braces are the **file mode**, indicating the way in which a file will be accessed. The braces indicate that a choice may be made, but that the entry is required. The first three choices are used for sequential files. The FileNumber may be from 1 to 511. The record length can be up to 32,767 characters.

The Open Statement—Examples

```
Open "A:\DataFile.Dat" For Output As #1
Open "C:\VB5\CH0701\Names" For Input As #2
```

The first example opens a file called *DataFile.Dat* as an output file, calling it file #1. The second example opens a file in the C: drive called *Names* as an input file, calling it file #2.

File Mode	Description
Output	Data are output from the project and written on the disk. New data is written at the beginning of the file, overwriting any existing data.
Input	Data are input into the project from the disk. This mode reads data previously stored on the disk.
Append	Data are output from the project and written on the disk. The new data are added to the end of the file.
Random	Data can be input or output and records may be accessed in any order.

Remember that a data file must always be opened prior to being used. When a data file is opened, the following actions are taken:

1. The directory is checked for the named file. If the file does not exist, a directory entry is created for this file, with the exception of Input mode, which will cause an error message if the file does not exist.
2. For sequential files a **buffer** is established in memory. A buffer is simply an area of main storage. As the program instructs Visual Basic to write data on the disk, the data are actually placed in the buffer. When the buffer is filled, the data are physically written to the disk. The size of the buffer for a random file is the number specified in the `Len =` clause of the `Open` statement.
3. A **file pointer** is created and set to the beginning of the file for all modes except Append, in which it is set to the end of the file. The pointer is always updated to indicate the current location in the file.
4. The file is given a **file number** for future reference. Each file used in a project must be assigned a unique number; however, the numbers need not begin with 1. After a file is closed, the number may be reused for a different file.

The Close Statement—General Form

```
Close [#filenumber...]
```

The Close Statement—Examples

```
Close #1
Close #1, #2
Close
```

The `Close` statement terminates processing of a disk file. When used without a file number, all open files are closed. The `Close` statement performs many housekeeping tasks:

1. Physically writes the last partially filled buffer on the disk (sequential files only). The `Write` statement places data in the buffer, and the data are written to the disk when the buffer is filled. Generally, the buffer will contain data when the project terminates. Those data must be written to the disk.
2. Writes an end-of-file mark (**EOF**) at the end of the file.
3. Releases the buffer.
4. Releases the file number.

Note: Executing an `End` statement will automatically close all open files, but you should not rely on this technique. A good rule is to always explicitly `Close` every file that has been opened in the project.

The FreeFile Function

When you open a file, you must assign a file number to each file. For a small project with one or two data files, most programmers assign #1 and #2. But in a larger project, selecting a file number can be a problem. If your code will be part of a larger project with code from other programmers and other libraries, you must make sure to avoid any conflicting file numbers. To solve this problem, you can allow the system to assign the next available file number. Use the `FreeFile` function to assign the next available file number to your file, and you will never have conflicts.

```
Dim iFileNumber As Integer
iFileNumber = FreeFile 'Get next available file number
Open "FILE.DAT" For Output As #iFileNumber
```

Viewing the Data in a File

When you wish to look at the data in your file, use the Notepad or Wordpad application available in Windows Accessories (or any other text editor). Sequential files appear as text, with commas separating the fields. When viewing random data files, you may notice some strange characters appearing in your file; these represent numeric fields. Numeric data types such as integer, single, and currency are stored in 2 or 4 bytes that can be reread by a project but look cryptic when displayed by a text editor. When you finish viewing your data file, make sure to exit without saving.

Sequential File Organization

Sequential files contain data elements that are stored one after another in sequence. When you read the data from the disk, it must be read in the same sequence in which it was written. In order to read any particular element of data, all preceding elements must first be read.

As data elements are written on disk, string fields are enclosed in quotation marks and the fields are separated by commas. Records are generally terminated by a carriage return character.

A sequential name and address file on the disk might look like this:

"Maxwell", "Harry", "795 W. J. Street", "Ontario", "CA", "91764"<CR>
"Helm", "Jennifer", "201 Cortez Way", "Pomona", "CA", "91766"<CR>
"Colton", "Craig", "1632 Granada Place", "Pomona", "CA", "91766"<EOF>

Writing Data to a Sequential Disk File

Use the **`Write #` statement** to place data into a sequential data file. Before the `Write #` statement can be executed, the file must be opened in either Output mode or Append mode. Remember that for Append mode, the file pointer is placed at the end of the file. If there are no records, the beginning of the file *is* the end of the file. In Output mode, the pointer is placed at the beginning of the file. Use Output mode when you wish to create a new file or write over old data.

The list of fields to write may be string expressions, numeric expressions, or both and may be separated by commas or semicolons.

The Write Statement—General Form

```
Write #FileNumber, ListOfFields
```

The Write Statement—Examples

```
Write #1, txtAccount.Text, txtDescription.Text, txtPrice.Text
Write #2, stAccount
Write #iFileNum, miCount; miQuantity; mcTotal
```

The `Write #` statement outputs data fields to the disk. As the elements are written on disk, commas are written between elements, string data are enclosed in quotation marks, and a carriage return and a line feed are inserted after the last element.

Creating a Sequential Data File

Sequential files are most commonly used to store small quantities of data that will rarely change. A common use of the sequential file is to store the information from a list box from one run to the next. In Chapter 7 your project added, removed, and cleared items from a list. These changes were not saved, so on the next execution of the project, the list reverted to its original contents stored in the List property of the control. The following save procedure writes the contents of a list box to a sequential file:

```
Private Sub mnuFileSave_Click()
    'Save the list box contents to a sequential file
    Dim iIndex   As Integer
    Dim iMaximum As Integer

    Open "Coffee.Dat" For Output As #1
    iMaximum = cboCoffee.ListCount - 1
    For iIndex = 0 To iMaximum
        Write #1, cboCoffee.List(iIndex)
    Next iIndex
    Close
End Sub
```

After execution of this procedure, the Coffee.Dat file on disk will hold the elements from the list box. VB automatically writes a carriage return at the end of each `Write #` statement and an EOF mark (end-of-file) at the end of the file.

Disk file contents

"Chocolate Almond"<CR>"Espresso Roast"<CR>
"Jamaica Blue Mtn."<CR>"Kona Blend"<CR> "Vanilla Nut"<EOF>

Reading the Data in a Sequential File

When you want to read a sequential file from the disk, you must open it for input. A successful `Open` sets the file pointer to the beginning of the file. After you have opened the file in Input mode, you can read the records using the **`Input #` statement**. One word of warning: Recall that if you open a file for input and it does not exist, a run-time error occurs and the program terminates. Later in this chapter you will learn to check for errors and avoid the error message.

The Input # Statement—General Form

```
Input #FileNumber, ListOfFields
```

The Input # Statement—Examples

```
Input #1, lblName.Caption, lblStreet.Caption, lblCity.Caption, lblZipCode.Caption
Input #2, stAccount
Input #iFileNum, iSavedCount, iSavedQuantity, cSavedTotal
```

The FileNumber named on the **`Input #` statement** must be the number of a previously opened data file. The fields named should be separated by commas. It doesn't matter what variable names were used when the data were written to the disk. When the data elements are read from the disk, they may be called by the same variable names or by completely different ones.

If you plan to load a list box from the data stored in a sequential file, the `Open` in the Form_Load must be followed by a loop that adds the data to the list. The loop will terminate when the end-of-file marker is read.

Finding the End of a Data File

When reading data from the disk, you must know when to stop. Recall that closing the file created an EOF mark. You can read until the EOF mark has been reached. (Attempting to read past the EOF mark causes a run-time error.)

The EOF(N) Function—General Form

```
EOF(FileNumber)
```

The `EOF(n)` function returns True when the EOF mark is read on the last good record. You can test for EOF using an `If` statement, but a better solution is to use a loop that continues until the condition is True. This example uses a `Do/Loop`:

```
Do Until EOF(1)                            'Continue processing until EOF condition is True
    Input #1, stCoffeeFlavor               'Read a record from the data file
    cboCoffee.AddItem stCoffeeFlavor       'Assign the variables to the list boxes
Loop
```

Feedback 9.1

1. Write the Visual Basic statements to
   (a) Open a sequential file called Vendor.dat for Output.
   (b) Write the items in the lstVendor list box to the Vendor.dat file.
   (c) Close the Vendor.dat file.
   (d) Open the Vendor.dat file so it can be used to read the records.
   (e) Read the records from the disk file into a list box.
2. What function is used to find the end of the file?

Trapping Program Errors

You have already learned to use `If` statements to test field values and shield the user from nasty run-time errors. When you start coding for data files, you will find that some problems cannot be avoided but must be anticipated. One such case is opening a data file for input when the file does not exist. It may be that the user has not inserted the proper disk containing the file or has selected an incorrect option.

When a run-time error occurs, Visual Basic generates an error number and checks it against a table of error codes. You can intercept the error number and take action without terminating the project. The statements used in this **error-trapping** process are the **`On Error` statement** and the Err object.

For you to trap errors, you must:

1. Turn on the error-handling feature using the **`On Error` statement**.
2. Create error-handling code routines, which are set off from your other code with line labels.
3. Determine how and where the program is to continue after the error is taken care of.

The On Error Statement

You must place an `On Error` statement at the beginning of any procedure where errors might occur, such as before opening a sequential file for input. The following procedure has minimal error trapping. The individual statements and options will be explained in the sections that follow.

```
Private Sub Form_Load()
    'Open the file

    On Error Go To HandleErrors          'Turn on error trapping
    Open "A:\datafile.txt" For Input As #1

Form_Load_Exit:
    Exit Sub

HandleErrors:                            'Error-handling routine
    'Code here to determine cause of error and display message
    Resume
End Sub
```

You may not want to add error-handling statements until you have tested and debugged your project (assuming the possibility that your projects don't always run perfectly the first time you test them). You want your error-handling code to trap user errors, not any programming errors. You may want to include the error-handling statements but remark them out while debugging. An alternative is to set the environment to disable error handlers while you complete your normal debugging. Choose *Options* on the *Tools* menu. On the *General* tab select *Break on All Errors* and then click OK.

Although there are three forms of the `On Error` statement, you will want to use form 1 and form 3 in most of your work. Form 1 turns on error trapping, and form 3 turns it off. Anytime error trapping is turned off, the project is subject to terminating with an `Error` dialog box.

The On Error Statement—General Form 1

```
On Error Go To LineLabel
```

The `On Error Go To` specifies the label of the line where your error-handling code begins. A **line label** is a name (following identifier naming conventions) on a line by itself and followed by a colon. The error-handling code must be in the same procedure as the `On Error` statement.

The On Error Statement—General Form 2

```
On Error Resume Next
```

Using the `Resume Next` option of error handling causes execution to skip the line that generated the error and continue execution with the following line of code.

The On Error Statement—General Form 3

```
On Error Go To 0
```

The `Go To 0` option of the `On Error` turns off error handling. Any error that occurs after this statement executes will cause a run-time error.

The Err Object

The **Err object** holds information about an error that has occurred. You can check the properties of the Err object to determine the error number and a description of the error. The name of the object or application that caused the error is stored in the **Source property**. The **Number property** contains the error number (ranging from 0 to 65,535), which is described in the **Description property**.

You don't need to define or include the Err object. It has global scope and is automatically a part of your project, similar to the Printer object.

If you transfer execution of your project to another procedure or execute a `Resume` statement, the properties of the Err object are cleared. If you will need these values for further processing, make sure to assign them to variables before performing any action that causes them to clear.

The Err.Number Property

The following table includes a partial list of errors. The complete list of errors may be found in VB Help under the heading *Trappable Errors.*

Err.Number	Err.Description
7	Out of memory
9	Subscript out of range
11	Division by zero
13	Type mismatch
52	Bad file name or number
53	File not found
54	Bad file mode
58	File already exists
61	Disk full
67	Too many files
68	Device unavailable
70	Permission denied
71	Disk not ready
75	Path/file access error
76	Path not found
482	Printer error

Raising Error Conditions

You can use the `Raise` method to set the error code, effectively "turning on" an error, or making it occur. This may be necessary when an error that occurs is not among those that you anticipated and coded for; you may want to turn on the error so that the system handles the error and displays a dialog box for the user.

```
Err.Raise Number:=71
Err.Raise Err
```

The full `Raise` method allows several arguments—only the error number is required.

The Raise Method—General Form

```
Object.Raise Number:=NumericValue
Err.Raise Err              'Raise the previous unhandled error
```

The numeric value that you assign may be a constant, a named constant, or a variable.

The Raise Method—Examples

```
Err.Raise Number:=76
Err.Raise Number:=iPATH_NOT_FOUND
```

Coding Error-Handling Routines

The code that you use to handle errors begins with a line label. Assuming that you have used the statement:

```
On Error Go To HandleErrors
```

your error-handling code begins with the line label:

```
HandleErrors:
```

A line label follows the rules for naming identifiers and is followed by a colon. It must appear on a line by itself and will begin in column 1. If you attempt to insert spaces or a tab before the line label, they are deleted by the editor.

```
HandleErrors:
    'Check to make sure the user put a disk in the drive
    Dim stMsg          As String
    Dim iResponse      As Integer
    Const iERR_NODISK  As Integer = 71
    stMsg = "Make sure there is a disk in the drive"

    If Err.Number = iERR_NODISK Then               'Check for Err 71
        iResponse = MsgBox(stMsg, vbOKCancel)   'Returns button pressed
        If iResponse = vbOK Then                'OK button pressed
            Resume                              'Try again
        Else
            mnuFileExit_Click                   'Exit the project
        End If
    Else                                        'Any other error
        Err.Raise Err                           'Cancel with error message
    End If
```

The previous example includes a routine that continues execution if the error is solved and also handles the situation for any unsolved errors.

Using Select Case to Check for Errors

You will probably find the `Select Case` statement very handy when you have a series of errors to check.

```
Select Case Err.Number
    Case 53                   'File not found
        'Code to handle File not found error
    Case 71                   'Disk not ready
        'Code to handle Disk not ready error
    Case 76                   'Path not found
        'Code to handle Path not found error
    Case Else                 'All other errors
        Err.Raise Err         'Make the error re-appear
End Select
Resume
```

The Resume Statement

When you have resolved the problem causing an error, your program should continue execution, if possible. This is accomplished with the **Resume statement**. You can choose to continue with the statement that caused the error, with the statement following the one causing the error, or at a specified location in the code.

The Resume Statement—General Form 1

```
Resume
```

If you use the `Resume` statement in the procedure that originally generated the error, execution of the project continues with the line of code that caused the error to occur. If the error-handling routine calls a different procedure that contains a `Resume`, execution continues with the statement that called the second procedure.

The Resume Statement—General Form 2

```
Resume Next
```

Using the `Next` option of `Resume` continues execution with the statement immediately following the line that caused the error (assuming that the `Resume Next` appears in the same procedure as the line of code causing the error). Similar to form 1, if you call another procedure from the error-handling routine, `Resume Next` continues execution at the line following the call.

The Resume Statement—General Form 3

```
Resume LineLabel
```

Execution continues at the line label, which *must be in the same procedure* as the `Resume`.

Tip

Make sure that you cannot reach a Resume statement without an error occurring. This condition causes an error that generates the message *Resume without an Error*.

Handling Errors

Your error-handling routine should do *something* to handle each error:

- If you identify the error type and the user can correct the problem (such as insert the correct diskette in the drive), use `Resume`, which will reexecute the statement that caused the error. If another error occurs, it will return to the error handler.
- If you identify the error type and execution can proceed without the error-causing statement, use `Resume Next`.
- If you prefer to check in-line for a particular type of error (following the `Open`, for example), use `Resume Next`.
- If the error number is unexpected or unidentified, raise the error again so that Visual Basic will handle it. The system error message will display for the user.
- If you want to exit the current procedure and continue project execution, use `Resume` *`LineLabel`*. Make sure to code a line label before your `Exit Sub` statement. For an example, see the following section describing the `Exit Sub` statement.
- If you want to end your project execution without displaying the system error message, call your exit procedure code (e.g., mnuFileExit_Click or cmdExit_Click).
- If you want to turn off error trapping, use `On Error Go To 0`. (Any further error will cause a run-time error and display the system error message to the user.)

The Exit Function and Exit Sub Statements

The statements in your procedure execute sequentially. In order to include an error-handling routine that will not execute accidentally (when no error occurs), you must exit the procedure before the line label. Precede the error-handling line label with an **`Exit Sub`** or **`Exit Function` statement** (depending on whether the code is in a sub procedure or a function procedure). The `Exit Sub` or `Exit Function` causes execution to exit the procedure immediately.

You can simplify your error-handling code if you adopt the following pattern for any procedure with error trapping:

1. Include an `On Error` statement at the top of any procedure that might require error handling.
2. Code a line label just before the `Exit Sub` statement. Name the line label the same as the procedure name, plus an underscore and Exit. Example: mnuFileSave_Click_Exit.
3. After the `Exit Sub` statement, code your error-handling routine.

```
Private Sub Form_Load()
    'Template for procedure that includes error handling

    On Error Go To HandleErrors            'Turn on error trapping
    Open "A:\Filename.txt" For Input As #1

Form_Load_Exit:
    Exit Sub

HandleErrors:                              'Error-handling routine
    'Code here to determine cause of error and display message

    Select Case Err.Number
        Case n
            'Code to handle error
        Case n
            'Code to handle error
        Case Else
            'Code to handle any other errors
    End Select
    Resume
End Sub
```

Here is an error-handling sub procedure to handle any errors that occur when opening a sequential file for input.

```
Private Sub Form_Load()
    'Load the Coffee list
    Dim stCoffee As String

    On Error GoTo HandleErrors
    Open "Coffee.Dat" For Input As #1
    Do Until EOF(1)
      Input #1, stCoffee
      cboCoffee.AddItem stCoffee
    Loop
    Close #1

Form_Load_Exit:
    Exit Sub

HandleErrors:
    Dim iResponse As Integer
```

```
    Select Case Err.Number
       Case 53, 76                    'File or path not found
           iResponse = MsgBox("Create a new file?", _
               vbYesNo + vbQuestion, "File not Found")
           If iResponse = vbYes Then
               Resume Form_Load_Exit
           Else
               mnuFileExit_Click
           End If
       Case 71                        'Disk not ready
           iResponse = MsgBox("Disk not ready. Retry?", _
               vbRetryCancel + vbQuestion, "Disk Error")
           If iResponse = vbRetry Then
               Resume                       'Try again
           Else
               mnuFileExit_Click            'Exit project
           End If
       Case Else                      'All other errors should cancel execution
           Err.Raise Err
    End Select
    Resume
End Sub
```

Feedback 9.2

What is the purpose of the following statements?

1. `On Error Go To 0`
2. `On Error Go To WhatToDo`
3. `Err.Raise Number:=53`
4. `Resume`
5. `Resume Next`

Sequential File Programming Example

This programming example is based on the hands-on example at the end of Chapter 7, which contains a dropdown combo box with the flavors of coffee (Figure 9.2). The user can add new flavors to the list, remove items from the list, or clear the list. However, in Chapter 7 those changes were not saved from one program run to the next. If you wish to allow the user to update the list of flavors, the data should be stored in a data file. For each program run, the list will be loaded from the data file during the Form_Load procedure of the startup form. If the flavors file does not yet exist, the program skips over loading the combo box to allow the user to add coffee flavors and create the file.

Figure 9.2

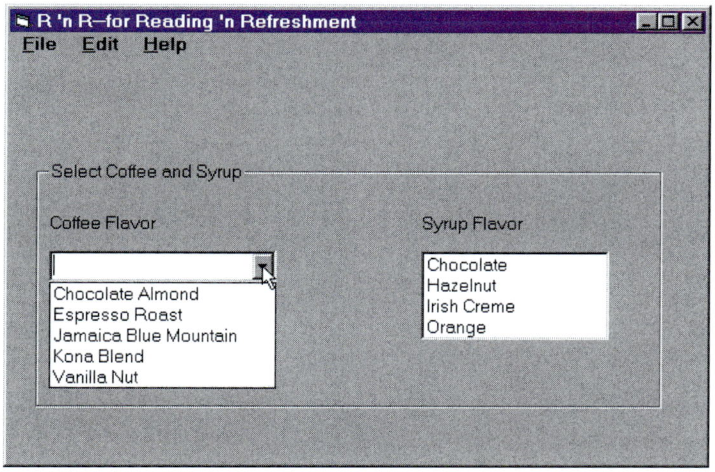

The dropdown combo box from Chapter 7. Users can add new flavors, delete flavors, and clear the list.

The user can choose to save the coffee list into a disk file by selecting a menu choice. Also, when the *Exit* menu choice is selected, if any changes have been made to the list, the project prompts the user to save the file. A Boolean variable is used to determine if any changes have been made since the file was last saved.

Notice that this example is only a partial program, showing the changes made to the hands-on example program from Chapter 7. Only a few procedures are changed.

```
'Module:        frmFlavors
'Programmer:    A. Millspaugh
'Date:          August 1997
'Description:   Print the selected flavor of coffee and syrup
'               or print a list of all of the coffee flavors.
'Folder:        Ch0901

Option Explicit
Dim mbUnsavedChange As Boolean

Private Sub cmdAddCoffee_Click()
    'Add a new coffee flavor to the coffee list

    If cboCoffee.Text <> "" Then
        With cboCoffee
            .AddItem cboCoffee.Text
            .Text = ""
        End With
        mbUnsavedChange = True
    Else
        MsgBox "Enter a coffee name to add", vbExclamation, "Missing data"
    End If
    cboCoffee.SetFocus
End Sub
```

```
Private Sub Form_Load()
    'Load the coffee list
    Dim stCoffee As String

    On Error GoTo HandleErrors
    Open "Coffee.Dat" For Input As #1
    Do Until EOF(1)
      Input #1, stCoffee
      cboCoffee.AddItem stCoffee
    Loop
    Close #1

Form_Load_Exit:
    Exit Sub

HandleErrors:
    Dim iResponse As Integer

    Select Case Err.Number
        Case 53, 76                         'File or path not found
            iResponse = MsgBox("Create a new file?", _
                vbYesNo + vbQuestion, "File not Found")
            If iResponse = vbYes Then
                Resume Form_Load_Exit       'Exit the procedure
            Else
                mnuFileExit_Click           'Exit the project
            End If
        Case 71                             'Disk not ready
            iResponse = MsgBox("Disk not ready. Retry?", _
                vbRetryCancel + vbQuestion, "Disk Error")
            If iResponse = vbRetry Then
                Resume                      'Try again
            Else
                mnuFileExit_Click           'Exit project
            End If
        Case Else                  'All other errors should cancel execution
            Err.Raise Err
    End Select
End Sub
```

```
Private Sub mnuEditClear_Click()
    'Clear the coffee list
    Dim iResponse As Integer

    iResponse = MsgBox("Clear the coffee flavor list?", _
        vbYesNo + vbQuestion, "Clear coffee list")
    If iResponse = vbYes Then
        cboCoffee.Clear
        mbUnsavedChange = True
    End If
End Sub
```

```
Private Sub mnuEditRemove_Click()
    'Remove the selected coffee from list

    If cboCoffee.ListIndex <> -1 Then
        cboCoffee.RemoveItem cboCoffee.ListIndex
        mbUnsavedChange = True
    Else
        MsgBox "First select the coffee to remove", vbInformation, _
        "No selection made"
    End If
End Sub
```

```
Private Sub mnuFileSave_Click()
    'Save the list box contents to a sequential file
    Dim iIndex   As Integer
    Dim iMaximum As Integer

    Open "Coffee.Dat" For Output As #1
    iMaximum = cboCoffee.ListCount - 1
    For iIndex = 0 To iMaximum
        Write #1, cboCoffee.List(iIndex)
    Next iIndex
    Close #1
    mbUnsavedChange = False
End Sub
```

```
Private Sub mnuFileExit_Click()
    'Terminate the project
    Dim iResponse As Integer

    If mbUnsavedChange = True Then
        iResponse = MsgBox("Coffee list has changed. Save the list?", _
            vbYesNo + vbQuestion, "Coffee List Changed")
        If iResponse = vbYes Then
            mnuFileSave_Click
        End If
    End If
    End
End Sub
```

The previous procedures are a partial program listing that demonstrate loading a combo box from a sequential file. Notice that the error handling in the Form_Load procedure traps for any error on the `Open`. If there is no error, the combo box is loaded with a `Do/Loop`.

If error number 53 or 76 occurs (File not found or Path not found), a message box asks the user whether or not to create the file. An answer of No terminates the program, but a Yes continues execution without attempting the read.

The user can enter new flavors during program execution, remove flavors, or clear the list. If any changes are made to the list, the Boolean variable mbUnsavedChange is set to True. When the project exits, if mbUnsavedChange is True, the user is prompted to save the list.

Random Data Files

The primary difference between sequential files and random files is that you may read and write the data in any order in a **random file**. With sequential files, you must always start at the beginning of the file and proceed in order through the file. Random files offer greater speed as well as the capability for random access.

You can visualize random files as a table in which each entry may be referenced by its relative position. Each entry in a file is one record, which is referred to by its record number. Any record in the file may be read or written without accessing the preceding records. Figure 9.3 illustrates the table concept of random files.

Figure 9.3

	Last Name Field	First Name Field	Phone Number Field
(1)			
(2)			
(3)			
(4)			
(5)			
(6)			
(7)			
(8)			
....			

Layout of a random file. Each record consists of a Last Name field, a First Name field, and a Phone Number field.

All records in a random file are exactly the same size. The fields within the record are fixed in length and position. That is, if the name takes the first 30 bytes (characters) in one record, every record will allocate the first 30 bytes for the name. This scheme is a departure from sequential files with their variable length fields and records. Before reading or writing a random file, the record structure or layout must be defined. The `Type/End Type` statements set up record structures. The only modification you will need is to use fixed-length strings.

Fixed-Length Strings

String variables may be variable length or fixed length. Until this point, all strings have been variable length. But for random files you will need to specify fixed-length strings. You can define a specific number of characters for elements of user-defined data types and dimension fixed-length single variables and arrays.

If the value you store in a field is less than its specified length, the extra positions are filled with spaces. If you assign a value that is longer than the fixed length, the extra characters are truncated (chopped off) when the value is stored in the fixed-length string.

To specify the string length, add an asterisk (*) followed by the size to the string declaration.

```
Dim stName          As String * 30

Type FullName
     stLastName     As String * 20
     stFirstName    As String * 20
End Type
```

Defining a Record for a Random File

To define a record for a random file, first set up its structure with a `Type` statement. Then dimension a record variable of the data type.
Note: You can code `Type` statements in a standard code module or the General Declarations section of a form module. In a form module you must specify `Private`.

```
Private Type MemberStructure
     stLastName        As String * 20
     stFirstName       As String * 20
     stPhone           As String * 12
End Type
Dim mMemberRecord      As MemberStructure
```

Opening a Random File

The `Open` statement for a random file is the same as for sequential files, using a file mode of Random. This mode allows you to input and output to the same file without closing and reopening it.

```
Open "b:\Data\Names.txt" For Random As #1 Len = 52
Open "A:MEMBERS.DAT" For Random As #2 Len = Len(mMemberRecord)
```

For a random file, the `Len` (length) entry refers to the length of a single record. In the second example, the second `Len` is actually the `Length` function that returns the size in bytes of the item enclosed in parentheses. The item in parentheses is the name used for the record variable you declared.

Reading and Writing a Random File

The input/output statements that you will be using for a random file differ from those used for sequential files. When accessing a random file, the data are handled a record at a time. The statements used are `Get` and `Put`, which include the record position in the file and the name of the variable defined as the record.

You can `Get` and `Put` records in a random file in any order you choose. That is, you may first write record #5, then #1, then #20, or any other order. When record #5 is written in the file, VB skips enough space for four records and writes in the fifth physical location. Record positions 1 to 4 are skipped until such time as records are written in those locations. See the diagram in Figure 9.4.

Figure 9.4

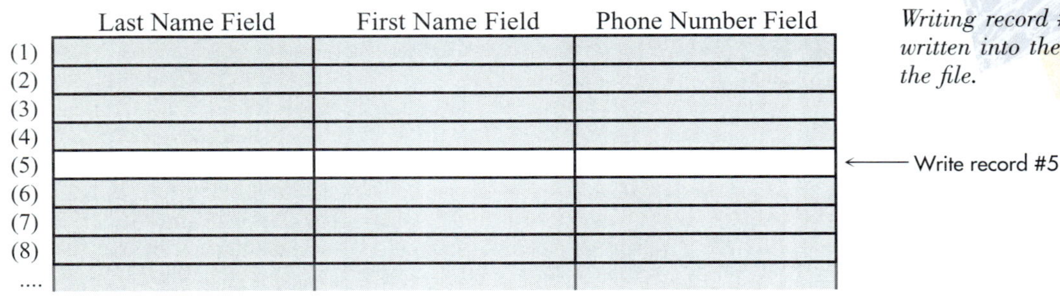

Writing record # 5. The record is written into the fifth location in the file.

The record numbers start at record 1. This rule will probably feel strange to you, since you are used to arrays and lists beginning with an index of 0. If you attempt to `Get` or `Put` a record number of zero, you receive a *Bad Record Number* error.

The Get Statement—General Form

```
Get [#]FileNumber, [RecordNumber], RecordName
```

The Get Statement—Examples

```
Get #2, RecNumber, mMemberRecord
Get #1, iRecordNumber, mInventoryRecord(iRecordNumber)
Get #2, iCustomerNumber, gCustomerRecord(iIndex)
Get #3, 4, AccountRecord
Get #1,, mMemberRecord
```

The **`Get` statement** reads data from a random disk file and places the data into the record-name variable. This variable should be one declared with a user-defined data type. If the variable is an array, the appropriate subscript number must be included.

When you omit the record number, the *next* record (after the last `Get` or `Put` that was processed) is read from the file. Either a variable or a constant may be used for the record number. Generally you will want to use a variable to allow selection of any record in the file.

The Put Statement—General Form

```
Put [#]FileNumber, [RecordNumber], RecordName
```

The Put Statement—Examples

```
Put #2, RecNumber, mMemberRecord
Put #1, iRecordNumber, mInventoryRecord(iRecordNumber)
Put #2, iCustomerNumber, gCustomerRecord(iIndex)
Put #3, 4, AccountRecord
Put #1, , mMemberRecord
```

The **`Put` statement** takes the contents of the specified record and writes it on the disk. The record number determines the relative location within the file for the record. If the record number is omitted, the record will be placed in the *next* location from the last `Get` or `Put`. Note that the next location is likely not the end of the file. Be careful not to write over other data by accident. If you wish to add a record to the end of the file, add 1 to the current number of records and `Put` the record at that position.

Accessing Fields in a Random Record

The `Get` and `Put` statements always read or write an entire record. In order to access the individual fields within the record, the elements must be referenced by the record name, a period, and the element name that is defined with the `Type` statement.

```
Get #1, iRecordNumber, mMemberRecord
lstName.AddItem mMemberRecord.LastName
```

Finding the End of a Random File

To find the end of a random file, use the **`LOF` function** (length of file) rather than the `EOF` function. The `LOF` function returns the size of the file in bytes. Although `EOF` can sometimes be used, problems can occur if records are written randomly and any gaps exist in the file.

The FileNumber entry is the file number from a currently open file.

To determine the highest record number in the file, divide the return value of the `LOF` function by the size of one record (the name dimensioned using the user-defined data type).

The LOF Function—General Form

```
LOF(FileNumber)
```

The LOF Function—Example

```
iNumberRecords = LOF(1) / Len(mMemberRecord)
```

You can use the LOF function to find out how may records are in the file prior to using a For/Next loop that might load the data into a table or list.

```
'Read a random file and store member names into a list box
Dim iNumberRecords As Integer
Dim iIndex As Integer 'Index for the loop

iNumberRecords = LOF(1) / Len(mMemberRecord)
For iIndex = 1 To iNumberRecords
    Get #1, iIndex, mMemberRecord
    lstNames.AddItem mMemberRecord.LastName
Next iIndex
```

When you are adding to the end of the file, you can use a calculation to find the next record number.

```
iRecordNumber = LOF(1) / Len(mMemberRecord) + 1
Put #1, iRecordNumber, mMemberRecord
```

The Seek Function

At times you may need to determine the position of the file pointer within the file. The **Seek function** returns the current location of the pointer. For a sequential file, the current byte number is returned. For a random file, Seek returns the position (record number) of the *next* record in the file.

The Seek Function—General Form

```
Seek(FileNumber)
```

FileNumber is the file number of a currently open file.

The Seek Function—Example

```
iNextRecord = Seek(1)
```

Using a List Box to Store a Key Field

When you Get or Put a record in a random file, you need to know the record number. However, keeping track of record numbers is inconvenient. Who wants to remember record numbers?

A slick visual solution to the record number problem is to display the name or identifying information in a list box. The list box can have its Sorted property set to True, which makes it easy for the user to find the desired record. Each name's corresponding ItemData property can hold the record number. When the user selects a record from the list, you can use the number stored in ItemData to retrieve the correct record. Figure 9.5 illustrates using a list box for record selection.

Figure 9.5

List box List property	ItemData property
Brooks, Barbara	5
Chen, Diana	3
Dunning, Daniel	1
Khan, Brad	6
Lester, Les	2
Nguyen, Ahn	4
Potter, Pete	8
Stevens, Roger	7

User selects this name from list. (Khan, Brad)

Program reads record 6 from file.

The list box holds customer names in the List property and corresponding record numbers in the ItemData property.

The following code segment concatenates a first and last name, adds to the list box, and then assigns the record number to the ItemData property.

```
Public Sub AddtoList(iIndex As Integer)
    'Add to the list box and the ItemData
    Dim StName As String

    stName = Trim(gEmployee.stLastName) & ", " & gEmployee.stFirstName
    lstEmployee.AddItem stName
    lstEmployee.ItemData(lstEmployee.NewIndex) = iIndex
End Sub
```

When concatenating fixed-length strings the entire string length, including the spaces, is used. You can use a trim function to avoid printing the extra spaces.

Trimming Extra Blanks from Strings

The **Trim**, **LTrim**, and **RTrim functions** remove extra blank characters in a string. When you have fixed-length strings, such as the fields in a random file, the strings are likely padded with extra spaces. The LTrim function removes extra spaces at the left end of the string; RTrim removes extra spaces on the right, and Trim removes extra spaces from both the left and right ends of the string.

The Trim, LTrim, and RTrim Functions—General Form

```
Trim(StringExpression)
LTrim(StringExpression)
RTrim(StringExpression)
```

The Trim, LTrim, and RTrim functions return a string with the extra spaces removed.

The Trim, LTrim, and RTrim Functions—Examples

```
Trim(" Harry Rabbit ")      'Returns "Harry Rabbit"
LTrim(" Harry Rabbit ")     'Returns "Harry Rabbit "
RTrim(" Harry Rabbit ")     'Returns " Harry Rabbit"
```

Navigating through a Random File

When displaying information from a file, you should allow your user to move through the records within the file. Common options for navigation are First, Last, Previous, and Next. The First button or command displays the first record from the file, and Last displays the last record. Previous and Next move one record in the desired direction.

Since we are using a sorted list box to control the sequence of the records, the option for Next takes you to the data for the next item in the list box. This task is easy to accomplish by using the properties of the list box. ListIndex indicates the currently selected record. You can move to the next or previous record by adding or subtracting 1 to/from the ListIndex property. Make sure that the result of the calculation will be a valid record number, not less than one and not exceeding the record count. Figure 9.6 illustrates using the list box for navigation.

Figure 9.6

ListIndex property	List box List property	ItemData property
(0)	Brooks, Barbara	5
(1)	Chen, Diana	3
(2)	Dunning, Daniel	1
(3)	Khan, Brad	6
(4)	Lester, Les	2
(5)	Nguyen, Ahn	4
(6)	Potter, Pete	8
(7)	Stevens, Roger	7

When record 6 displays, the ListIndex property is 3.

Add 1 to ListIndex, then read record 2.

The list box ItemData property holds the record number. To move through the file sequentially, use the ListIndex property to determine the next customer and then use the ItemData property to read the correct record.

Coding the Navigation Buttons

```
Private Sub cmdPrevious_Click()
    'Display the previous record from sorted list

    If frmMain!lstEmployee.ListIndex < 1 Then
        cmdLast_Click          'Go to end of file when at beginning
    Else
        'Subtract one from the list box ListIndex
        frmMain!lstEmployee.ListIndex = frmMain!lstEmployee.ListIndex - 1
        ReadRecord             'Read the new record based on the ItemData property
    End If
End Sub
```

```
Private Sub cmdNext_Click()
    'Display the next record from sorted list

    If frmMain!lstEmployee.ListIndex < frmMain!lstEmployee.ListCount - 1 Then
        'Add one to the list box ListIndex
        frmMain!lstEmployee.ListIndex = frmMain!lstEmployee.ListIndex + 1
        ReadRecord             'Read the new record based on the ItemData property
    Else
        cmdFirst_Click         'Go to beginning of file when at end
    End If
End Sub
```

You can find the first and last record using list box properties. Remember that the ListIndex of the first record is 0. The ListIndex of the last record is one less than the ListCount.

```
Private Sub cmdFirst_Click()
    'Display the first record from sorted list

    frmMain!lstEmployee.ListIndex = 0
    ReadRecord                'Read the new record, based on the ItemData property
End Sub
```

```
Private Sub cmdLast_Click()
    'Display the last record from sorted list

    frmMain!lstEmployee.ListIndex = frmMain!lstEmployee.ListCount - 1
    ReadRecord                'Read the new record, based on the ItemData property
End Sub
```

Navigation during an Add or Delete

If the user is allowed to click on the navigation button when an Add or Delete operation is in progress, a problem can arise. You can avoid this problem by disabling the navigation buttons during an Add or Delete. You will need to enable the buttons during an Update or Browse operation.

```
Private Sub DisableNavigation()
    'Disable the navigation commands

    cmdLast.Enabled = False
    cmdFirst.Enabled = False
    cmdPrevious.Enabled = False
    cmdNext.Enabled = False
End Sub
```

```
Private Sub EnableNavigation()
    'Enable the navigation commands

    cmdLast.Enabled = True
    cmdFirst.Enabled = True
    cmdPrevious.Enabled = True
    cmdNext.Enabled = True
End Sub
```

Locking the Contents of Controls

Another technique for keeping the user out of trouble is to lock text boxes when you don't want to allow any changes. Although you can set the Enable property of a text box to False, the contents will display as grayed. A better approach is often to set its Locked property to True. If you lock text boxes, make sure to unlock them again when you *do* want to allow changes.

```
txtLastName.Locked = True
txtFirstName.Locked = True
txtStreet.Locked = True
```

Updating a Random File

A file update generally consists of routines to add records, update records, delete records, and browse through records. The procedures for these options might be selected from a command button or a menu command.

Each routine must display the fields from the file, so we will use one form and refer to it as the *data form.* This form will contain text boxes for each of the fields of a record along with the appropriate labels. (Figure 9.7 shows the data form for the random file update in the hands-on programming example.)

Figure 9.7

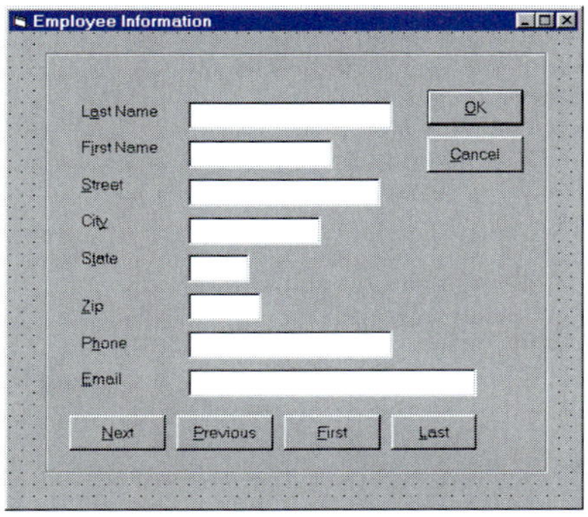

The data entry form for the hands-on programming example.

Adding and Editing Records

When the user wants to add a record, all of the text boxes must be cleared. After the data are entered, the record will be written to the disk file. The record will be written at the end of the file. The list box must be updated and the record number stored in the ItemData property for the list. It is a good idea to set the current ListIndex to the new record.

```
miIndex = LOF(1) / Len(gEmployee) + 1   'Find next available record number
gEmployee.stDeleted = "N"
SaveData                                'Send text box fields to record variables
WriteRecord                             'Write record variable in file
frmMain.AddtoList (miIndex)             'Add entry to list box on main form
frmMain!lstEmployee.ListIndex = frmMain.lstEmployee.NewIndex   'Set ListIndex
```

An alternative approach would be to search through the records in the file to find the location of a deleted record. You could add a new record in the location of the deleted record. For this example we will add all new records at the end of the file.

Deleting a Record

You can delete a record from a random file in several ways. A common method is to mark a record in some way to indicate that the record is deleted rather than to actually remove it. If you were to actually remove a record, you would also have to move forward all of the remaining records. That would take time and also change the record numbers. (Often the record number is used as a form of identification.)

One technique is to write some special character in a field of the record to indicate that the record has been deleted. A drawback of this method is that the data in the record cannot be recovered later, if you want to add undelete routines.

Another more popular method is to add a special field to the record description. The field, commonly called a *delete flag* or *delete code*, holds one of two values, such as *Y* and *N*; or *A* for *active* and *D* for *deleted*; or True/False values. We will use this approach.

In the following data type, the field stDeleted indicates whether a record is deleted. A *Y* in stDeleted means that the record is deleted. When a record is added, *N* is placed in the field.

```
Type PersonalInfo
    stLastName  As String * 15
    stFirstName As String * 10
    stStreet    As String * 20
    stCity      As String * 15
    stState     As String * 2
    stZip       As String * 5
    stPhone     As String * 15
    stEmail     As String * 25
    stDeleted   As String * 1
End Type
Public gEmployee As PersonalInfo
```

To mark a record as deleted, store a *Y* in the stDeleted field.

```
gEmployee.stDeleted = "Y"
```

When records are loaded into the list box, only those without the *Y* will be loaded.

```
If gEmployee.stDeleted <> "Y" Then
    AddtoList (iIndex)
End If
```

Keep the List Box Up-to-Date

Whenever a record is deleted from the file, the list box must also be updated. Use a `RemoveItem` method to delete the reference to the deleted record from the list. The next code segment puts together the steps for deletion.

```
'Set the record number to match the list box ItemData property
miIndex = frmMain!lstEmployee.ItemData(frmMain!lstEmployee.ListIndex)
gEmployee.stDeleted = "Y"        'Set the delete field to indicate deleted record
WriteRecord                      'Write the record back into the file
'Remove the current list element from the list box
frmMain!lstEmployee.RemoveItem frmMain!lstEmployee.ListIndex
```

Confirm the Deletion

You may want to verify that the record is really to be deleted. If you do so, make sure to offer a Cancel button.

The Read and Write Procedures

Good programming technique uses a single procedure for reading a file and one for writing to the data file. Write a procedure to write a record and call it from any location that needs a write. Then code a single procedure to read a record and call it as needed. The following code segment writes a record in the file:

```
Private Sub WriteRecord()
    'Write to disk

    Put #1, miIndex, gEmployee
End Sub
```

Notice that for this procedure to work correctly, miIndex must be set to the record number, and gEmployee must have the fields for the record.

The Read procedure is very much the same, but it must find which record to read by checking the selection in the list box. Notice that the ItemData property is used to get the record number, miIndex. After the record is read, the data is displayed.

```
Private Sub ReadRecord()
    'Use ItemData to directly access record in the file

    'Set the record number to the current ItemData
    miIndex = frmMain!lstEmployee.ItemData(frmMain!lstEmployee.ListIndex)
    Get #1, miIndex, gEmployee       'Read the record
    DisplayData                      'Move fields into text boxes to display
End Sub
```

Feedback 9.3

1. Write the `Type` statement called *Inventory*, which contains 30 characters for a description, 5 characters for a part number, a price (currency), and a quantity (integer).
2. Declare a variable called *InventoryRecord* that will use the Inventory data type.
3. Write the statement to open a random file using the disk file Inventory.Dat on the C: drive.
4. Write the statement(s) to find the number of records in the Inventory.Dat file.
5. Write the statement to write one record to the Inventory.Dat file using a record number called *iRecordNumber*.

6. What value is returned by the `Seek` function if the current record is record # 5?
7. Write the statement to read one record from the Inventory.Dat file.

Your Hands-On Programming Example

The employee file for R 'n R will be maintained using a random file. Create a project with two forms: a main form and a data form.

The main form will have a list box of employee names and command buttons for Add, Delete, Update, and Browse. When the user clicks on one of the command buttons, the data form will display, set for the correct action.

The data form for the file will display the fields in text boxes and provide OK and Cancel buttons for changes to the file. The data form will also include navigation buttons (First, Last, Next, and Previous), which are enabled for the Update and Browse options, but disabled for the Add and Delete options.

The project will use the list box on the main form for navigation. The user selects a record by the employee name, and the correct record is read from the file. The list box ItemData property holds the record number for the random reads. Refer to Figure 9.5 for an illustration of the list box.

Add option

Display the data form with the fields empty. When the user clicks the OK button, save the record in the next-available record position.

Delete option

Display the data form with the selected record displayed. The user can then choose OK to delete the record or to cancel the operation.

Update option

Display the data form with the selected record displayed. The user can then choose OK to save any change or to cancel the operation.

Browse option

Display the data form with the text boxes locked. The user can use the navigation buttons to move through the file, but cannot make any changes.

Planning the Project

Sketch a main form (Figure 9.8*a*) and a data form (Figure 9.8*b*), which your users sign off as meeting their needs.

Figure 9.8

Sketches of the two forms for the hands-on programming example: (a) The main form and (b) the data entry form.

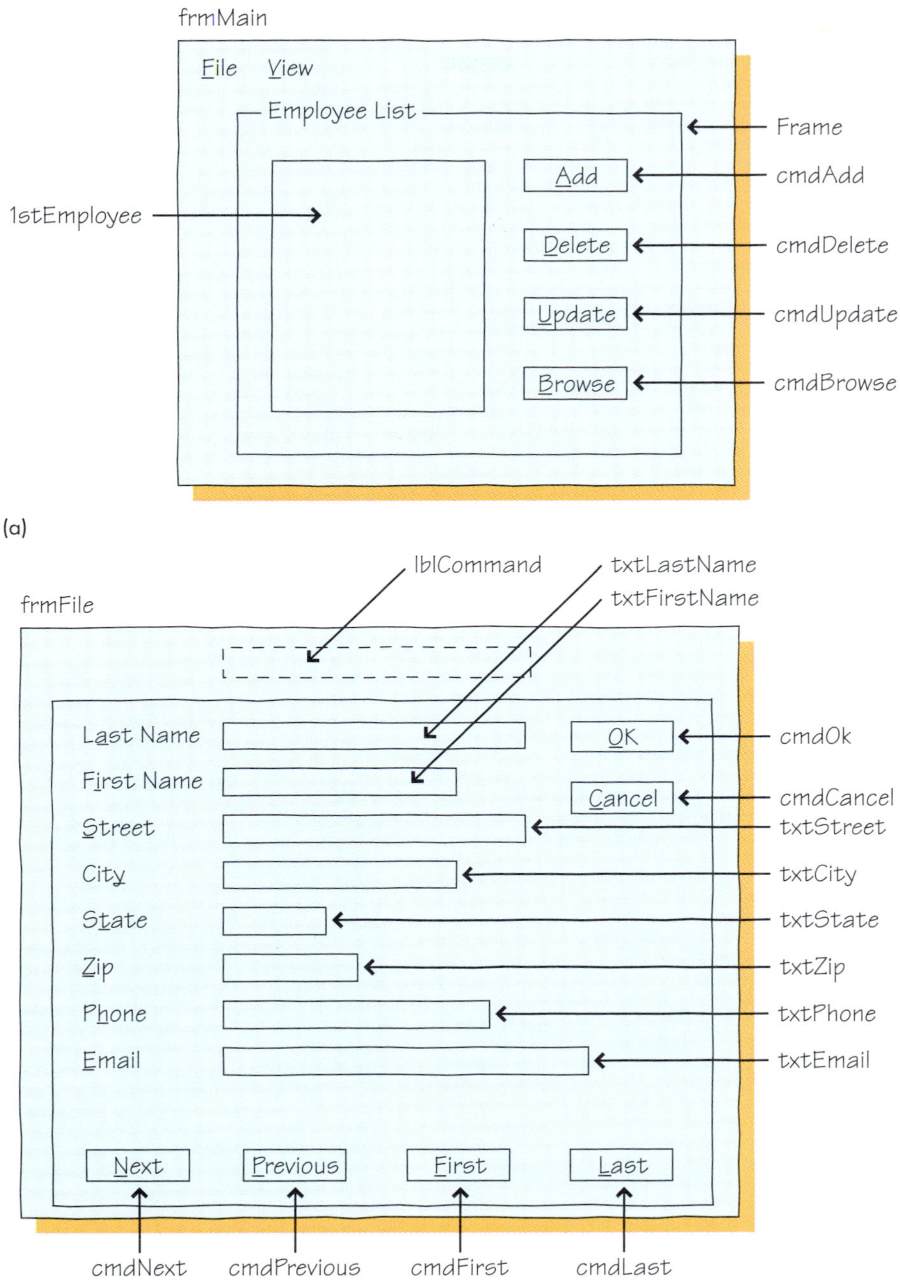

(a)

(b)

Plan the Objects and Properties: Main Form

Object	Property	Setting
frmMain	Name	frmMain
	Caption	R 'n R—for Reading 'n Refreshment
Frame1	Name	Frame1
	Caption	Employee List
lstEmployee	Name	lstEmployee
	Sorted	True
cmdAdd	Name	cmdAdd
	Caption	&Add
cmdDelete	Name	cmdDelete
	Caption	&Delete
cmdUpdate	Name	cmdUpdate
	Caption	&Update
cmdBrowse	Name	cmdBrowse
	Caption	&Browse
mnuFile	Name	mnuFile
	Caption	&File
mnuFileExit	Name	mnuFileExit
	Caption	E&xit
mnuView	Name	mnuView
	Caption	&View
mnuViewEmployee	Name	mnuViewEmployee
	Caption	&Employee File

Plan the Event Procedures: Main Form

Procedure	Actions

Form_Load	If file not empty Then
	  Open the file.
	  Load the list box.
	Else
	  Prompt user for new file.
	End If

cmdAdd	Set the Action flag for Add. Display the data form.

(continued)

Procedure	Actions

cmdDelete	If employee selected Then
	Set the Action flag for Delete.
	Display the data form.
	Else
	Display error message.
	End If

cmdUpdate	If employee selected Then
	Set the Action flag for Update.
	Display the data form.
	Else
	Display error message.
	End If

cmdBrowse	Set the Action flag for Browse. Display the data form.
mnuFileExit	Close the file. Terminate the project.
MnuViewEmployee	Set Action flag for Browse. Display the data form.
AddtoList	Concatenate first and last name Add name to list box. Set ItemData to record number.

Plan the Objects and Properties: Data Form

Object	Property	Setting
frmFile	Name	frmFile
	Caption	Employee Information
lblCommand	Name	lblCommand
	Caption	(blank)
Frame1	Caption	Employee List
Label1	Caption	L&ast Name
Label2	Caption	F&irst Name
Label3	Caption	&Street
Label4	Caption	Cit&y
Label5	Caption	S&tate
Label6	Caption	&Zip
Label7	Caption	P&hone
Label8	Caption	&Email
txtLastName	Name	txtLastName
	Text	(blank)

(continued)

Object	Property	Setting
txtFirstName	Name	txtFirstName
	Text	(blank)
txtStreet	Name	txtStreet
	Text	(blank)
txtCity	Name	txtCity
	Text	(blank)
txtState	Name	txtState
	Text	(blank)
txtZip	Name	txtZip
	Text	(blank)
txtPhone	Name	txtPhone
	Text	(blank)
txtEmail	Name	txtEmail
	Text	(blank)
cmdOK	Name	cmdOK
	Caption	&OK
	Default	True
cmdCancel	Name	cmdCancel
	Caption	&Cancel
	Default	True
cmdNext	Name	cmdNext
	Caption	&Next
cmdPrevious	Name	cmdPrevious
	Caption	&Previous
cmdFirst	Name	cmdFirst
	Caption	&First
cmdLast	Name	cmdLast
	Caption	&Last

Plan the Event Procedures: Data Form

Procedure	Actions
Form_Activate	Case Add Set label to Add. Clear text boxes.

(continued)

Procedure	Actions
	Disable navigation buttons. Set the focus. Case Delete Set label to Delete. Read a record. Disable navigation buttons. Lock controls. Case Update Set label to Update. Read a record. Enable navigation buttons. Unlock controls. Case Browse Set label to Browse. Lock controls. Enable navigation buttons. cmdFirst_Click.
Write Record	Save to disk.
Read Record	Get record number from ItemData. Get record from disk. Display data fields.
ClearTextBoxes	Clear the contents of text boxes.
DisableNavigation	Set Enable to False for navigation command buttons.
EnableNavigation	Set Enable to True for navigation command buttons.
DisplayData	Transfer data from record to text boxes.
SaveData	Transfer data from text boxes to record.
LockTheControls	Set Locked to True for the text boxes.
UnlockTheControls	Set Locked to False for the text boxes.
CmdOK	Case Add Save record. Add to list box. Case Delete Set Deleted to Y. Save record. Delete from list box. Case Update Save record. Change list box. End Select Hide the data form.
cmdCancel	Hide the data form.

cmdNext	If not on last record Then
	Add one to list index.
	Read the record.
	Else
	Go to first record.
	End If

(continued)

Procedure	Actions

cmdPrevious	If on first record Then
	 Go to last record.
	Else
	 Subtract one from list index.
	 Read the record.
	End If

cmdFirst	Set ListIndex to zero. Read the first record.
cmdLast	Set ListIndex to last record. Read the last record.

Write the Project

- Follow the sketches in Figure 9.8 to create the forms. Figure 9.9 shows the completed forms.

Figure 9.9

The two forms for the hands-on programming example: (a) The main form and (b) the data entry form.

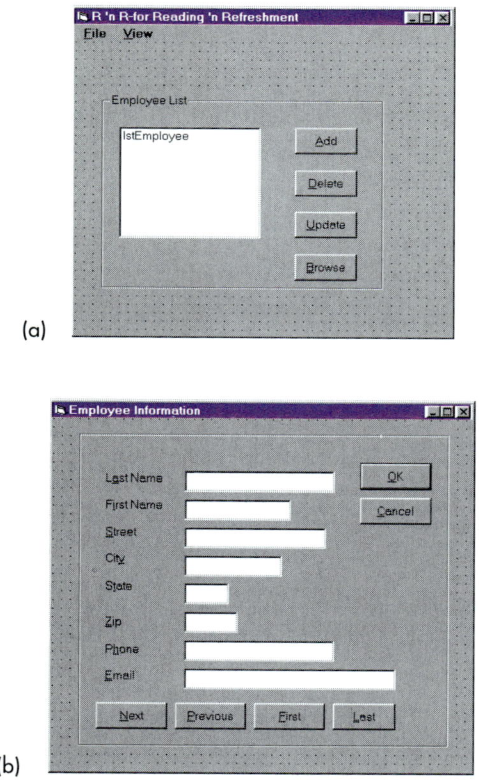

- Set the properties of each of the objects according to your plan.
- Write the code. Working from the pseudocode, write each event procedure.
- When you complete the code, use a variety of data to thoroughly test the project.

The Project Coding Solution

Standard Code Module

```
'Module        Filetype.bas
'Programmer:   A. Millspaugh
'Date:         Aug 1997
'Description:  Define the record
'Folder:       Ch0902

Option Explicit
Type PersonalInfo
    stLastName  As String * 15
    stFirstName As String * 10
    stStreet    As String * 20
    stCity      As String * 15
    stState     As String * 2
    stZip       As String * 10
    stPhone     As String * 15
    stEmail     As String * 25
    stDeleted   As String * 1
End Type

Public gEmployee          As PersonalInfo
Public gstFileAction      As String
```

Main Form: frmMain

```
'Form          FrmMain
'Programmer:   A. Millspaugh
'Date:         Aug 1997
'Description:  This project uses a random file to store employee
'              information. It stores employee names in a list box
'              and allows file updating and browsing.
'Folder:       Ch0902

Private Sub cmdAdd_Click()
    'Display a blank form for an add

    gstFileAction = "A"
    frmFile.Show vbModal
End Sub
```

```
Private Sub cmdBrowse_Click()
    'Look at the file

    gstFileAction = "B"
    frmFile.Show vbModal
End Sub
```

```
Private Sub cmdDelete_Click()
    'Display and delete the selected item from list

    If lstEmployee.ListIndex <> -1 Then
        gstFileAction = "D"
        frmFile.Show vbModal
    Else
        MsgBox "Select record to Delete", vbOKOnly + vbInformation, "Delete"
    End If
End Sub
```

```
Private Sub cmdUpdate_Click()
    'Display the selected item from list

    If lstEmployee.ListIndex <> -1 Then
        gstFileAction = "U"
        frmFile.Show vbModal
    Else
        MsgBox "Select record to update", _
          vbOKOnly + vbInformation, "Update"
    End If
End Sub
```

```
Private Sub Form_Load()
    'Read the file and store in the sorted list box.
    'Store the random record number into ItemData.

    Dim iIndex    As Integer
    Dim iResponse As Integer

    On Error GoTo HandleErrors
    Open "a:\Employee.Dat" For Random As #1 Len = Len(gEmployee)
    If LOF(1) / Len(gEmployee) > 0 Then   'If file not empty
        For iIndex = 1 To LOF(1) / Len(gEmployee)
            Get #1, iIndex, gEmployee
            If gEmployee.stDeleted <> "Y" Then
                AddtoList (iIndex)
            End If
        Next iIndex
    Else
        iResponse = MsgBox("File is empty. Create new file?", _
            vbYesNo + vbQuestion, "No File")
        If iResponse = vbNo Then
            mnuFileExit_Click    'Exit project
        End If
    End If

Form_Load_Exit:
    Exit Sub
```

```
HandleErrors:
    If Err.Number = 71 Then
        iResponse = MsgBox("No disk. Retry?", _
            vbRetryCancel + vbQuestion, "No Disk in Drive")
        If iResponse = vbRetry Then
            Resume                  'Try again
        Else
            mnuFileExit_Click       'Exit project
        End If
    Else
        On Error GoTo 0             'Turn off error handling
    End If
End Sub
```

```
Private Sub mnuFileExit_Click()
    'Terminate the project

    Close #1
    End
End Sub
```

```
Private Sub mnuViewEmployee_Click()
    'Display the Employee file form

    gstFileAction = "B"             'Browse
    frmFile.Show vbModal
End Sub
```

```
Public Sub AddtoList(iIndex As Integer)
    'Add to the list box and the ItemData
    Dim stName As String

    stName = Trim(gEmployee.stLastName) & ", " & gEmployee.stFirstName
    lstEmployee.AddItem stName
    lstEmployee.ItemData(lstEmployee.NewIndex) = iIndex
End Sub
```

Data Entry Form: frmFile

```
'Form:           frmFile
'Programmer:     A. Millspaugh
'Date:           Aug 1997
'Description:    Obtain and display data for the employee file
'Folder:         Ch0902

Option Explicit
Dim miIndex As Integer
```

```
Private Sub cmdCancel_Click()
    'Return to main form with no action

    frmFile.Hide
End Sub
```

```
Private Sub DisplayData()
    'Transfer from record to text fields

    txtLastName.Text = gEmployee.stLastName
    txtFirstName.Text = gEmployee.stFirstName
    txtStreet.Text = gEmployee.stStreet
    txtCity.Text = gEmployee.stCity
    txtState.Text = gEmployee.stState
    txtZip.Text = gEmployee.stZip
    txtPhone.Text = gEmployee.stPhone
    txtEmail.Text = gEmployee.stEmail
End Sub
```

```
Private Sub SaveData()
    'Transfer from text fields to data record

    gEmployee.stLastName = txtLastName.Text
    gEmployee.stFirstName = txtFirstName.Text
    gEmployee.stStreet = txtStreet.Text
    gEmployee.stCity = txtCity.Text
    gEmployee.stState = txtState.Text
    gEmployee.stZip = txtZip.Text
    gEmployee.stPhone = txtPhone.Text
    gEmployee.stEmail = txtEmail.Text
End Sub
```

```
Private Sub cmdFirst_Click()
    'Display the first record from sorted list

    frmMain!lstEmployee.ListIndex = 0
    ReadRecord
End Sub
```

```
Private Sub cmdLast_Click()
    'Display the last record from sorted list

    frmMain!lstEmployee.ListIndex = frmMain!lstEmployee.ListCount - 1
    ReadRecord
End Sub
```

```
Private Sub cmdNext_Click()
    'Display the next record from sorted list
```

```
    If frmMain!lstEmployee.ListIndex < frmMain!lstEmployee.ListCount - 1 Then
        frmMain!lstEmployee.ListIndex = frmMain!lstEmployee.ListIndex + 1
        ReadRecord
    Else
        cmdFirst_Click
    End If
End Sub
```

```
Private Sub cmdOK_Click()
    'Choose action depending upon the command
    Dim stName As String

    Select Case gstFileAction
    Case "A"
        miIndex = LOF(1) / Len(gEmployee) + 1
        gEmployee.stDeleted = "N"
        SaveData
        WriteRecord
        frmMain.AddtoList (miIndex)
        frmMain!lstEmployee.ListIndex = frmMain!lstEmployee.NewIndex
    Case "D"
        miIndex = frmMain!lstEmployee.ItemData(frmMain!lstEmployee.ListIndex)
        gEmployee.stDeleted = "Y"
        WriteRecord
        frmMain!lstEmployee.RemoveItem frmMain!lstEmployee.ListIndex
    Case "U"
        SaveData
        miIndex = frmMain!lstEmployee.ItemData(frmMain!lstEmployee.ListIndex)
        WriteRecord
        'Change name in list box if needed
        frmMain!lstEmployee.RemoveItem frmMain!lstEmployee.ListIndex
        frmMain.AddtoList (miIndex)
    Case "B"
        UnlockTheControls
    End Select

    'Return to main form
    frmFile.Hide
End Sub
```

```
Private Sub cmdPrevious_Click()
    'Display the previous record from sorted list

    If frmMain!lstEmployee.ListIndex < 1 Then
        cmdLast_Click
    Else
        frmMain!lstEmployee.ListIndex = frmMain!lstEmployee.ListIndex - 1
        ReadRecord
    End If
End Sub
```

```
Private Sub DisableNavigation()
    'Disable the navigation commands

    cmdLast.Enabled = False
    cmdFirst.Enabled = False
    cmdPrevious.Enabled = False
    cmdNext.Enabled = False
End Sub
```

```
Private Sub ReadRecord()
    'Use ItemData to directly access record in the file

    miIndex = frmMain!lstEmployee.ItemData(frmMain!lstEmployee.ListIndex)
    Get #1, miIndex, gEmployee
    DisplayData
End Sub
```

```
Private Sub WriteRecord()
    'Write to disk

    Put #1, miIndex, gEmployee
End Sub
```

```
Private Sub ClearTextBoxes()
    'Clear all of the text boxes

    txtLastName.Text = ""
    txtFirstName.Text = ""
    txtStreet.Text = ""
    txtCity.Text = ""
    txtState.Text = ""
    txtZip.Text = ""
    txtPhone.Text = ""
    txtEmail.Text = ""
End Sub
```

```
Private Sub Form_Activate()
    'Set up the form and set the focus to the name field

    Select Case gstFileAction
        Case "A"
            lblCommand.Caption = "Add a Record"
            ClearTextBoxes
            DisableNavigation
            UnlockTheControls
            txtLastName.SetFocus
        Case "D"
            ReadRecord
            lblCommand.Caption = "Delete this record?"
            DisableNavigation
            LockTheControls
```

```
        Case "U"
            ReadRecord
            lblCommand.Caption = "Update"
            EnableNavigation
            UnlockTheControls
        Case "B"
            lblCommand.Caption = "Browse"
            LockTheControls
            EnableNavigation
            cmdFirst_Click
    End Select
End Sub
```

```
Private Sub LockTheControls()
    'Lock the text boxes so no edits can be made

    txtLastName.Locked = True
    txtFirstName.Locked = True
    txtStreet.Locked = True
    txtCity.Locked = True
    txtState.Locked = True
    txtZip.Locked = True
    txtPhone.Locked = True
    txtEmail.Locked = True
End Sub
```

```
Private Sub UnlockTheControls()
    'Unlock the text boxes

    txtLastName.Locked = False
    txtFirstName.Locked = False
    txtStreet.Locked = False
    txtCity.Locked = False
    txtState.Locked = False
    txtZip.Locked = False
    txtPhone.Locked = False
    txtEmail.Locked = False
End Sub
```

```
Private Sub EnableNavigation()
    'Enable the navigation commands

    cmdLast.Enabled = True
    cmdFirst.Enabled = True
    cmdPrevious.Enabled = True
    cmdNext.Enabled = True
End Sub
```

Programming Hints

The InputBox Function

When you need to request input from the user, you can always use a text box, either on the current form or on a new form. Visual Basic also provides a quick and easy way to pop up a new form that holds a text box, using the `InputBox` function.

The `InputBox` function is similar to `MsgBox`. In the input box you can display a message, called the *prompt*, and allow the user to type input into the text box (Figure 9.10).

Figure 9.10

The InputBox function produces a dialog box with a prompt and a text box for entering program input.

The InputBox Function—General Form

```
VariableName = InputBox("Prompt" [, "Title"] [, Default] [, XPos] [, YPos])
```

The prompt must be enclosed in quotation marks and may include NewLine characters (`vbCrLf`) if you want the prompt to appear on multiple lines. The Title displays in the title bar of the dialog box; if the Title is missing, the project name appears in the title bar. Any value you place in *Default* appears in the text box when it is displayed; otherwise, the text box is empty. (If *Default* is a string, it must be enclosed in quotation marks.) *XPos* and *YPos*, if present, define the measurement in twips for the left edge and top edge of the box.

The InputBox Function—Examples

```
stName = InputBox("Enter your name.")
iQuantity = InputBox("How many do you want?", "Order Quantity")
```

Using the InputBox to Randomly Retrieve a Record

You will find the input box to be a great tool when you need to retrieve a record from a random file. Many applications use the record number as a method of identification, such as customer number or product number. If you request this number, you can read the correct record in the random file directly.

```
Dim iRecordNumber As Integer
iRecordNumber = Val(InputBox("Enter Customer Number"))
If iRecordNumber >= 0 And iRecordNumber <= LOF(1) / Len(Customer) Then
    Get #1, iRecordNumber, Customer
Else
    MsgBox "Invalid Customer Number"
End If
```

Summary

1. A data file is made up of records, which can be further broken down into fields or data elements. The field used for organizing the file is the key field.
2. An `Open` statement is needed to access data files. The `Open` allows modes for Input, Output, Append, and Random. A FileNumber is associated with a file at the time the file is opened.
3. A `Close` statement should be used prior to the termination of a program that uses data files.
4. The `FreeFile` function can be used to find the next available file number.
5. Sequential files use the `Write #` and `Input #` statements for writing and reading records. Each field to be written or read is listed in the statement.
6. The records in a sequential file must be accessed in order, and the file is either input or output, not both. With a random file the records may be accessed in any order and may be read or written without closing the file.
7. The `EOF` function returns True when the end of a file is reached.
8. The `On Error` statement allows the programmer to test for known error situations and handle errors without the application aborting. An example of the type of error that can be found through error trapping is the failure of the user to place a disk in the disk drive.
9. The Err object holds the error number and description of the current error.
10. The `Resume` statement continues execution after an error condition.
11. Random file access uses fixed-length records and requires the string fields to be a specified length. Use the `Type` statement to define the record structure for a random file.
12. The `Get` and `Put` statements read and write records in a random file.
13. A file update program allows the user to make changes to the data file, such as adding a record, changing the contents of a record, and deleting a record.
14. The `LOF` function returns the length of a random file in bytes. You can use the result to calculate the number of records in the file and the record number of the next available record.
15. You can use list box to allow the user to select a record from a random file. The ItemData property of the list box is set to the record number so that random reads can retrieve the correct record.

16. The `Trim`, `LTrim`, and `RTrim` functions remove extra spaces from fixed-length strings.
17. The input box is similar to a message box; it allows the user to enter information that can be returned to the project.

Key Terms

Review Questions

1. What is the difference between a Visual Basic project file and a data file?
2. Explain what occurs when an `Open` statement is executed.
3. List and explain the file modes for data files.
4. What is the significance of a file number?
5. Differentiate between the Output and Append modes.
6. What is the format for the statements to read and write sequential files?
7. When would an `On Error` statement be used?
8. Explain the function and use of the Err object.
9. Differentiate between a random file and a sequential file.
10. What does *updating a data file* mean?
11. Give examples for using the `InputBox` function.
12. What function can be used to determine an available file number?

Programming Exercises

9.1 (*Sequential file*) Rewrite project 8.4 using a sequential file to store the state names and abbreviations. You will need two projects. The first will allow the typist to enter the state name and the abbreviation in text boxes and store them in a sequential file. The second project will perform the functions specified in 8.4.

9.2 Create a *sequential file* for employee information and call it *employee.dat*. Each record will contain fields for first name, last name, Social Security number, and hourly pay rate.

Write a project to process payroll. The application will load the employee data into an array of user-defined types from the sequential file with an extra field for the pay. The form will contain labels for the information from the array and display one record at a time.

A command button called *FindPay* will use a `For Next` loop to process the array. First you will display an input box for the number of hours worked, calculate the pay, and add to the totals. Then you will display the labels for the next employee. (Place the pay into the extra field in the array.)

The Exit button will print a report on the printer and terminate the project. (Print the array.)

Processing: Hours over 40 will receive time-and-a-half pay. Accumulate the total number of hours worked, the total number of hours of overtime, and the total amount of pay.

Sample Report

Ace Industries

Employee Name	Hours Worked	Hours Overtime	Pay Rate	Amount Earned
Janice Jones	40	0	5.25	210.00
Chris O'Connel	35	0	5.35	187.25
Karen Fisk	45	5	6.00	285.00
Tom Winn	42	2	5.75	247.25
Totals	162	7		929.50

9.3 (*Sequential file*) Modify project 7.6 to store the list box for Bradley's Bagels in a sequential file. Load the list during the Form Load and then close the file. Be sure to use error checking in case the file does not exist.

In the exit procedure, prompt the user to save the bagel list back to the disk.

9.4 (*Random file*) Create a project that stores and updates personal information for a little electronic "Black Book." The fields in the file should include

Last name	Street
First name	City
	State
Birthday	ZIP code
Phone number—home	Phone number—work
Phone number—pager	E-mail address

9.5 Create a *random file* project that stores and updates student information. Use a list box to display the student names, and store record numbers in the ItemData property, similar to the chapter hands-on example project.

The fields include

Name
Major—use a dropdown combo box to list available majors.
Class level—use option buttons for Freshman, Sophomore, Junior, and Senior.
Dean's list—use a check box.

CASE STUDIES

VB Mail Order

Modify the project created in Chapters 6 and 7 to include a sequential file to store catalog names and a random file to store customer information.

The list of catalog names must be stored in a sequential file and loaded into a dropdown combo box during the initial processing. Any catalogs that are added during execution of the program must be written to the disk. (If the file does not yet exist, either write another project to create it or allow the user to create it using the combo box and the Add button.)

When customer information is processed, allow the user to select the customer name from a list box or type in the customer number. The remaining controls for customer information will be changed from text boxes to labels. The information displayed in these labels will be found through a search of the random file. You may use techniques similar to the ones used to search an array, or you may load the file into an array or list box and search it.

You must create the customer random file and provide routines to update the records. Fields include name, street, city, state, and ZIP. The customer number is the record number, which you can use to directly reference a record when the user enters the number.

VB Auto Center

Create a project that maintains a random file for vehicle inventory. The fields contained in each record should be an inventory ID number, manufacturer, model name, year, vehicle ID number, and cost value.

Hint: Refer to the hands-on programming example in this chapter for ideas for the data entry screen, menus, and command buttons.

C H A P T E R

10

Accessing Database Files

At the completion of this chapter, you will be able to . . .

1. Use database terminology correctly.

2. Differentiate between the data control and data-bound controls.

3. Create a project to view an existing database table.

4. Set up a lookup table for a database field.

5. Change records, add new records, and delete records in a database table.

6. Write code to help prevent user errors.

Visual Basic and Database Files

You can use Visual Basic to write projects that view and update database files. You can use the data control in the Learning Edition to create database applications with very little coding. However, if you want to use the more advanced features, including creating new databases and modifying the structure of existing database tables, you will need the Professional Edition or Enterprise Edition of Visual Basic. The applications in this text can be done with the Standard Edition or the Learning Edition.

Database Formats Supported by Visual Basic

Visual Basic directly supports database files in several formats. The native format is Microsoft Access, using the Jet database engine. However, by setting just one property, the VB Standard Edition and Learning Edition can access files created with dBASE III, dBASE IV, dBASE 5.0, Excel, FoxPro, Lotus, Paradox, or text files. With the Professional Edition and Open DataBase Connectivity (ODBC), you can use many other database formats, such as SQL Server, Oracle, and DB2.

Database Terminology

In order to use database files, you must understand the standard terminology of relational databases. Although there are various definitions of standard database terms, we will stick with those used by Access.

An Access **file** (with an .MDB extension) can hold multiple **tables**. Each table can be viewed as a spreadsheet—with **rows** and **columns**. Each row in a table represents the data for one item, person, or transaction and is called a ***record***. Each column in a table is used to store a different element of data, such as an account number, a name, address, or numeric amount. The elements represented in columns are called ***fields***. You can think of the table in Figure 10.1 as consisting of rows and columns or of records and fields.

Figure 10.1

A database table consists of rows (records) and columns (fields).

ISBN	Title	Author	Publisher
0-15-500139-6	Business Programming in C	Millspaugh, A. C.	The Dryden Press
0-446-51652-X	Bridges of Madison County	Waller, Robert James	Warner Books
0-451-16095-9	The Stand	King, Stephen	Signet
0-517-59905-8	How to Talk to Anyone, Anytime, Anywhere	King, Larry	Crown
0-534-26076-4	A Quick Guide to the Internet	Bradley, Julia Case	Integrated Media Group
0-670-85332-1	How to Be Hap-Hap-Happy Like Me	Markoe, Merrill	Viking
0-671-66398-4	Seven Habits of Highly Effective People	Covey, Stephen R.	Fireside
0-697-12897-0	QuickBasic and QBasic Using Modular Structure	Bradley, Julia Case	B & E Tech
0-697-21361-7	Desktop Publishing Using PageMaker 5.0	Bradley, Julia Case	B & E Tech
0-8007-1213-7	Secrets of Closing the Sale	Ziglar, Zig	Revell
1-55615-484-4	Code Complete	McConnell, Steve	Microsoft Press

Record or row

Field or column

Most tables use a **key field** (or combination of fields) to identify each record. The key field is often a number, such as employee number, account number, identification number, or Social Security number; or it may be a text field, such as last name, or a combination, such as last name and first name.

Any time a database table is open, one record is considered the **current record**. As you move from one record to the next, the current record changes.

Creating Database Files for Use by Visual Basic

Although you cannot create a new database file with the VB Standard Edition or Learning Edition, you have other options. You can use Access to create the database, or you can use the Visual Data Manager add-in application that comes with Visual Basic.

You can run the VB Visual Data Manager by selecting *Visual Data Manager* from the *Add-Ins* menu (Figure 10.2). The VisData application window opens (Figure 10.3); you can create a new file or open and modify an existing database file. The application is quite straightforward; you can use Help if you need instructions.

Figure 10.2

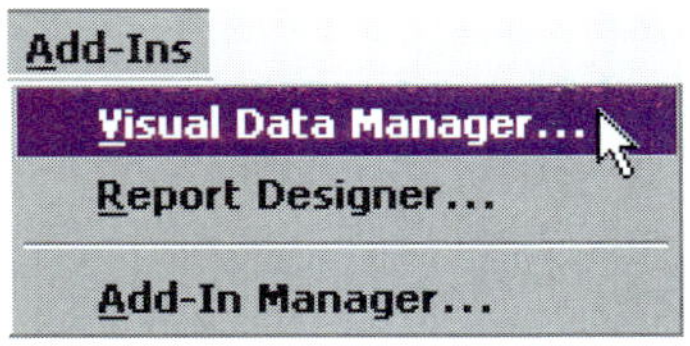

Select Visual Data Manager from the Add-Ins menu to run the VB Visual Data Manager.

Figure 10.3

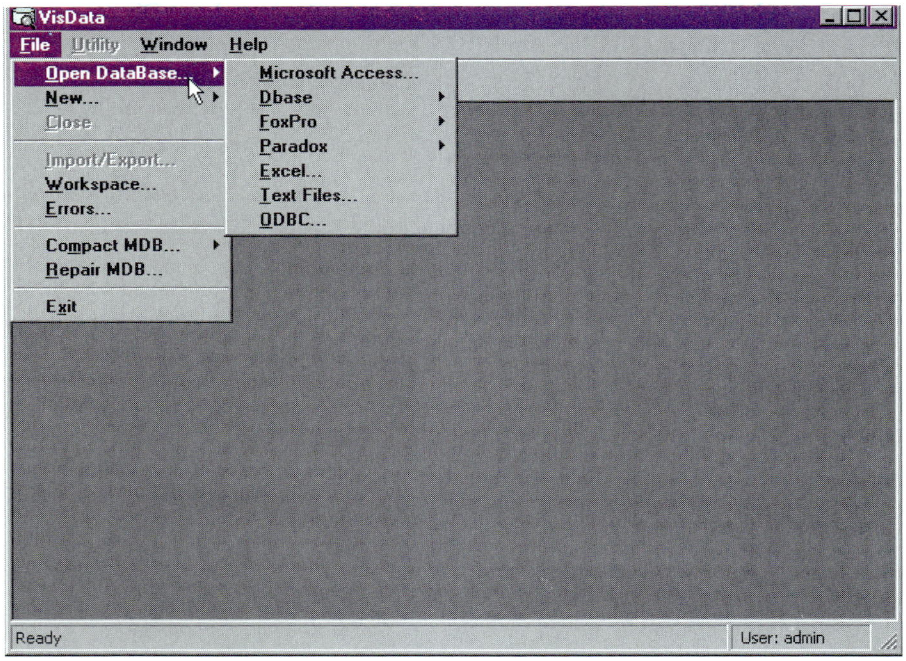

Create a new database or modify an existing one using the Visual Data Manager window.

Using the Data Control

You will find programming with the Visual Basic data control quite easy and powerful. Figure 10.4 shows the toolbox tool for creating a data control, and Figure 10.5 shows a data control on a form.

Figure 10.4

The toolbox tool for the data control.

Figure 10.5

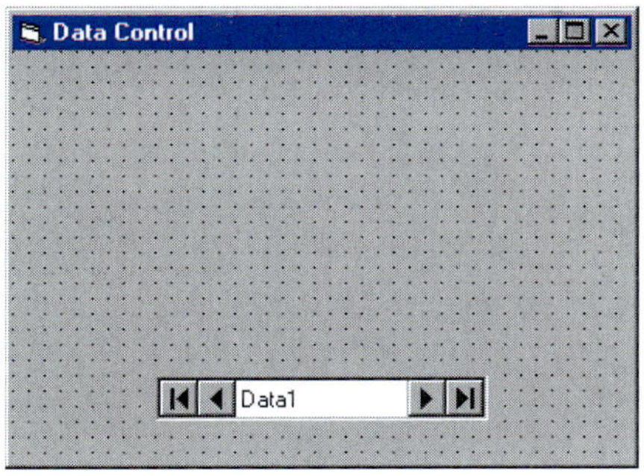

A data control on a form.

The Data Control and Data-Bound Controls

Using a data control is a two-step process. First you place a data control on a form and set the properties to link it to a database file and table. Then you create the controls, such as labels and text boxes, to display the actual data. Each control is bound to a particular field in the table. In this example, the label is called a ***data-bound*** control and will automatically display the contents of the bound field when the project runs. Figure 10.6 shows a form with a data control and two data-bound labels.

Figure 10.6

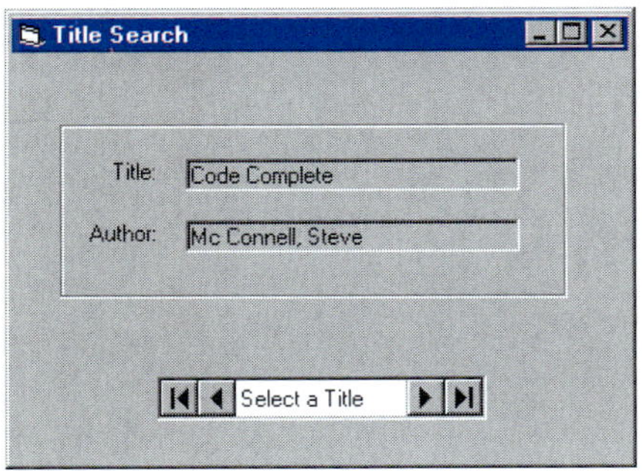

The data control binds the form to a database table. The data-bound labels each display a field from the table.

Microsoft also uses the term *data aware* for controls that can be bound to a database table. You might say that labels are data aware; therefore, you can use a label to create a data-bound control. The standard data-aware controls are labels, text boxes, check boxes, list boxes, combo boxes, images, picture boxes, data-bound list boxes, data-bound combo boxes, and data-bound grids.

A data control generally links one form with one table. If you want to have data-bound controls on a second form, you must place a data control on that form. You may place more than one data control on a single form when you wish to reference more than one table.

Properties of the Data Control

After you place a data control on a form, you must set its properties (Figure 10.7). By default, the Name and Caption are set to Data1. First change the Name property, using "dat" as its three-character prefix. The Caption appears inside the control (refer to Figure 10.6).

Figure 10.7

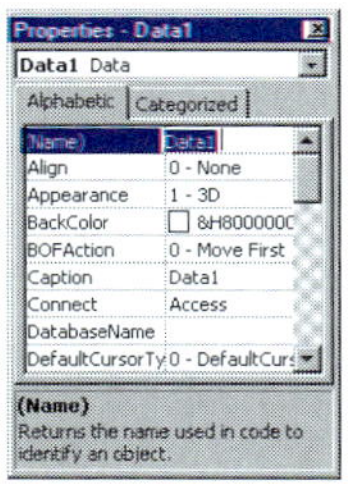

Set the properties for a data control in the Properties window.

Set the **Connect property** of the data control to the type of database file (Figure 10.8). Access is the default, but you can choose dBASE III, IV, or 5.0; Excel 3.0, 4.0, 5.0, or 8.0; FoxPro 2.0, 2.5, 2.6, or 3.0; Lotus WK1, WK3, or WK4; Paradox 3.*x*, 4.*x*, or 5.*x*; or text.

Figure 10.8

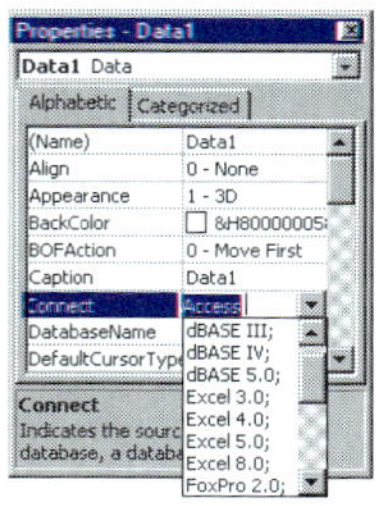

Set the Connect property to the type of database you plan to use.

Then set the **DatabaseName property**. Although you can type the path and filename into the Settings box, the easy way is to click on the Settings button and open the *DatabaseName* dialog box (Figure 10.9). After you have specified the filename, the next step is to select the name of the table from within the file.

Figure 10.9

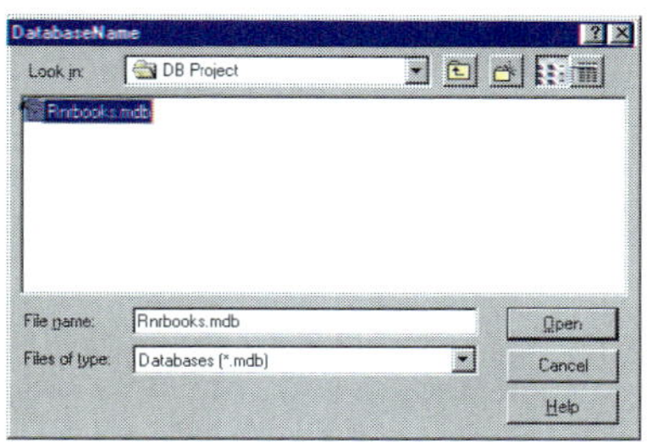

Select the database file in the DatabaseName dialog box.

Set the **RecordSource property**. When you click on the Settings button, a list appears with the names of the tables and queries in the database file (Figure 10.10). *Note:* A query is a named subset of the data in one or more tables and is sometimes referred to as a *view*. You can set the RecordSource of the data control to any table or query named in the database file.

Figure 10.10

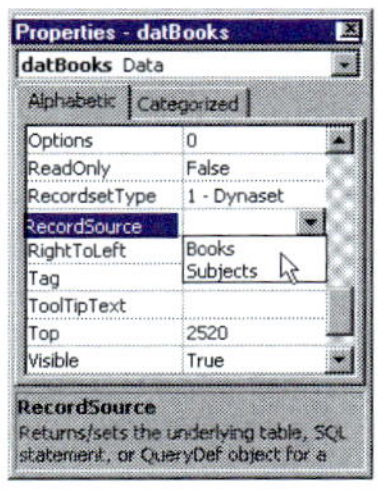

Select the table name for the RecordSource property.

If you don't want the user to be able to change the data in the table, set the ReadOnly property to True. Otherwise, any changes made to the data on the screen are automatically saved in the file.

After setting the properties for the data control, you are ready to set the properties for the data-bound controls.

Properties of Data-Bound Controls

Place the controls that you want to display in the database fields on the form and then change their properties. Use labels for any fields you don't want the user to be able to change; use text boxes if the field content is user updatable. Use check boxes for fields with a True/False or Yes/No value; the check box will display a check mark for True or Yes and remain blank for False or No.

After setting the Name and Text or Caption properties of your text boxes or labels, set the two properties that bind the control to a particular field in a table.

First set the **DataSource property** of the text box or label to point to the data control. Click on the down arrow in the Settings box to drop down the list of data controls on the form (Figure 10.11). Once you have selected the data control, VB knows the name of the file and table. Next you specify the particular field to bind to the control.

Figure 10.11

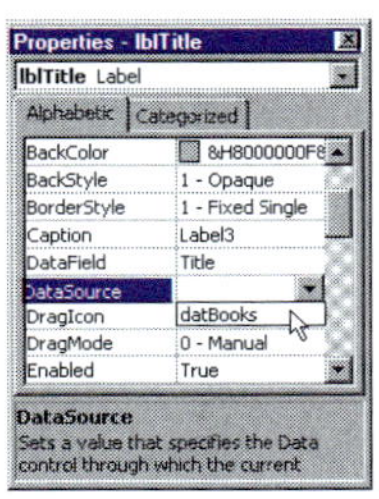

Select the name of the data for the data-bound control's DataSource property.

Set the **DataField property** by clicking on the down arrow in the Settings box. The list of fields in the selected table will appear (Figure 10.12). After choosing the field name for one of your data-bound controls, set the DataSource and DataField properties for the rest of your controls.

Figure 10.12

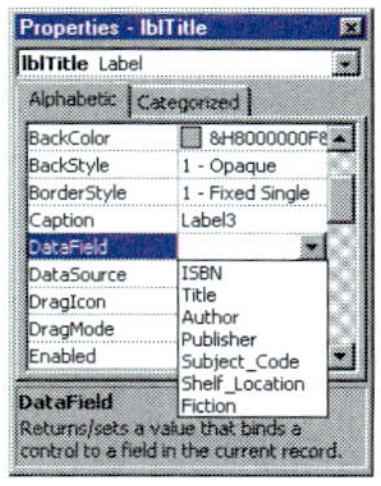

Set the DataField property to the name of the field to bind to the control.

That's all there is to it. Once you have bound the table and fields to the controls on your form, you are ready to run the application. With no code at all, the fields will fill with data when your project begins. You can use the navigation buttons on the data control to move from one record to the next.

Viewing a Database File—Step-by-Step

In this step-by-step tutorial, you will create a simple project to display the data from the Books table for R 'n R—for Reading 'n Refreshment. The only code required is for the Exit procedure.

Design and Create the Form

Figure 10.13 shows the user interface for this project.

Figure 10.13

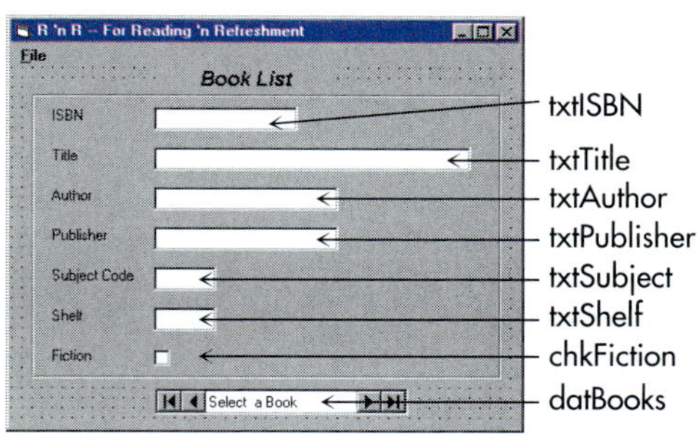

The user interface for the database step-by-step tutorial.

The Form

STEP 1: Create a new form large enough to hold the controls (see Figure 10.13).

The Controls

STEP 1: Click on the data control tool and draw a data control along the bottom of the form.
STEP 2: Create a large frame to hold the labels and text boxes; then delete the frame's Caption property.
STEP 3: Create labels that describe the data and the form title (Book List).
STEP 4: Create the controls to hold the data. Use text boxes for ISBN, Title, Author, Publisher, Subject Code, and Shelf; use a check box for Fiction.

The Menu

STEP 1: Open the Menu Editor window and create a *File* menu with an *Exit* command. Name the menu mnuFile and the command mnuFileExit.

Set the Properties for the Data Control

STEP 1.:Select the data control and display the Properties window.
STEP 2: Change the Name property to datBooks.
STEP 3: Change the Caption property to Select a Book.
STEP 4: Click on the Settings button for the DatabaseName property to display the *DatabaseName* dialog box.
STEP 5: Change the drive and directory as necessary to locate the database file called RnrBooks.mdb. It was supplied on your student diskette and may be installed on the local hard drive or network. (Consult your instructor or lab technician if you can't find it.) Click OK after selecting the filename.
STEP 6: Scroll to the RecordSource property and click the down arrow in the Settings box. The list of tables should appear; click on *Books*.
STEP 7: Change the ReadOnly property to True.

Set the Properties for the Data-Bound Controls

STEP 1: Select the text box to hold the ISBN number; switch to the Properties window.
STEP 2: Set the following properties:
STEP 3: Click on the Settings down arrow for the DataSource property and select datBooks (the name of the data control).

Name	txtISBN
Caption	(blank)

STEP 4: Click on the Settings down arrow for the DataField property; the list of fields in the Books table appears. Click on ISBN.

STEP 5: Set the properties for the rest of the data-bound controls.

Object	Property	Setting
txtTitle	Name	txtTitle
	Text	(blank)
	DataSource	datBooks
	DataField	Title
txtAuthor	Name	txtAuthor
	Text	(blank)
	DataSource	datBooks
	DataField	Author
txtPublisher	Name	txtPublisher
	Text	(blank)
	DataSource	datBooks
	DataField	Publisher
txtSubject	Name	txtSubject
	Text	(blank)
	DataSource	datBooks
	DataField	Subject_Code
txtShelf	Name	txtShelf
	Text	(blank)
	DataSource	datBooks
	DataField	Shelf_Location
chkFiction	Name	chkFiction
	Caption	(blank)
	DataSource	datBooks
	DataField	Fiction

Write the Code

The coding for this project will surprise you. All you need are a few remarks and an Exit procedure.

STEP 1: Select the *Exit* command from the *File* menu to open the mnuFileExit_Click procedure.
STEP 2: Type the following code:

```
'Exit the project

End
```

STEP 3: Switch to the General Declarations section and type the remarks:

```
'Program Name: R 'n R Book List Database
'Programmer:   Your Name
'Date:         Today's date
'Purpose:      Display book information in the
'              R 'n R Book database
'Folder:       Ch1001
```

STEP 4: Save your form and project. You will use them again later in this chapter.

Run the Project

STEP 1: Start the project running. You should see your form on the screen filled with the data for the first record. (Maybe a "Wow" is in order?)
STEP 2: Try the navigation buttons on the data control: Click on the arrows for Move Next, Move Previous, Move First, and Move Last (Figure 10.14).

Figure 10.14

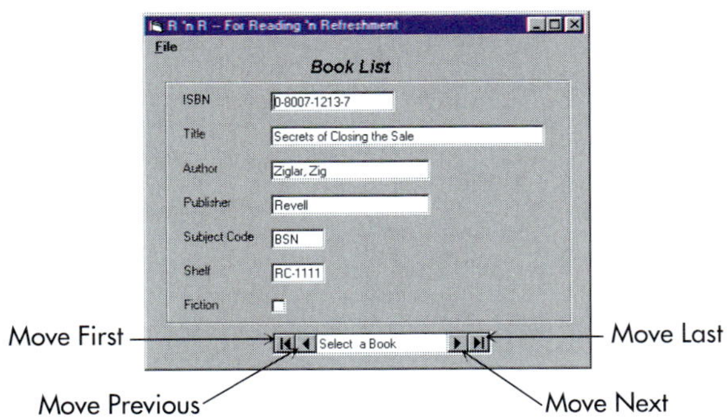

Click on the navigation buttons to display different records.

Feedback 10.1

Use this information to fill in the answers to the following questions.

Database name:	Classes.mdb
Table name:	Teachers
Field name:	Name
Data control name:	datClasses
Text box name:	txtTeacher

You want to display the name field in txtTeacher. How should these properties be set?

1. datClasses.DatabaseName
2. datClasses.RecordSource
3. txtTeacher.DataSource
4. txtTeacher.DataField
5. txtTeacher.Text

Navigating the Database in Code

The navigation buttons on the data control can be used to move from record to record, or you can make the data control invisible and provide the navigation in code. You can use the **Recordset object** to manipulate the database.

The Recordset Object

When you set the RecordSource property of a data control to the name of a table or query, you are defining a new object called a *Recordset.* The Recordset object has its own set of properties and methods, which you can use to move from record to record, check for the beginning or end of the file, and search for records to match a condition (covered in Chapter 11).

When you refer to the Recordset object, you must first name the data control:

```
DataControl.Recordset.Property
DataControl.Recordset.Method
```

Using the MoveNext, MovePrevious, MoveFirst, and MoveLast Methods

The `MoveNext`, `MovePrevious`, `MoveFirst`, and `MoveLast` methods provide the same functions as the data control buttons. Each method is applied to the Recordset object created by the data control.

```
datBooks.Recordset.MoveNext       'Move to the next record
datBooks.Recordset.MoveLast       'Move to the last record
datBooks.Recordset.MovePrevious   'Move to the previous record
datBooks.Recordset.MoveFirst      'Move to the first record
```

Checking for BOF and EOF

Two handy properties of the Recordset object are **BOF** (beginning of file) and **EOF** (end of file). The BOF property is automatically set to True when the record pointer is before the first record in the Recordset. This condition happens when the first record is current and the user chooses MovePrevious. The BOF property is also True if the Recordset is empty (contains no records).

The EOF property is similar to BOF; it is True when the record pointer moves beyond the last record in the Recordset and when the Recordset is empty.

When you are doing your own navigation in code, you need to check for BOF and EOF so that run-time errors do not occur. If the user clicks MoveNext when on the last record, what do you want to do? Have the program cancel with a run-time error? display a message? wrap around to the first record? keep the record pointer on the last record? (The last approach matches the action of the navigation buttons on the data control.)

In the examples that follow, we will use the wrap around method. If the user clicks on the MoveNext button from the end of the table, the first record becomes the active record.

```
Private Sub cmdNext_Click()
    'Move to the next record

    datBooks.Recordset.MoveNext
    If datBooks.Recordset.EOF Then
        datBooks.Recordset.MoveFirst
    End If
End Sub
```

Just as with any other object reference in Visual Basic, you can use the `With/End With` statements to refer to the Recordset object. This style of coding not only simplifies the VB code but also makes a project run a little faster.

```
Private Sub cmdNext_Click()
    'Move to the next record

    With datBooks.Recordset
        .MoveNext
        If .EOF Then
            .MoveFirst
        End If
    End With
End Sub
```

Using List Boxes and Combo Boxes as Data-Bound Controls

Beginning with release 4.0 of Visual Basic, list boxes and combo boxes are data aware. You can see the value of using data-bound lists when you have a list of acceptable values for a field. The user can select an item from the list when updating records or adding new ones.

Setting Up a Lookup Table for a Field

To set up a lookup table of acceptable values for a field, use a combo box. You can bind the combo box to a field in the database *and* specify initial values for the List property. Figure 10.15 shows a combo box as a data-bound control, displaying the Subject field from the database. When the user selects a subject from the dropdown combo box, the field's contents are updated to the new value. (In the following example, we set the ReadOnly property of the database to False so that changes can actually occur.)

Figure 10.15

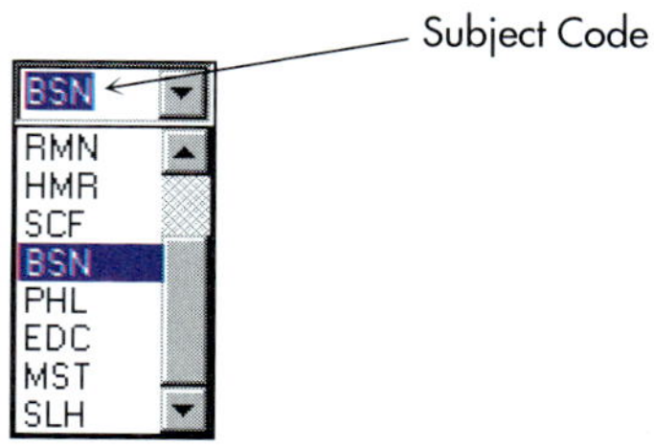

The List property of the combo box shows the acceptable choices for the field. Select an entry from the list to change the contents of the field.

Adding a Lookup Table and Navigation—Step-by-Step

For this step-by-step example, we add navigation buttons and two lookup combo boxes to the previous programming example.

Modify the User Interface

STEP 1: Open the previous program example.

STEP 2: Resize the form and add four command buttons for navigation. (See Figure 10.16.)

Figure 10.16

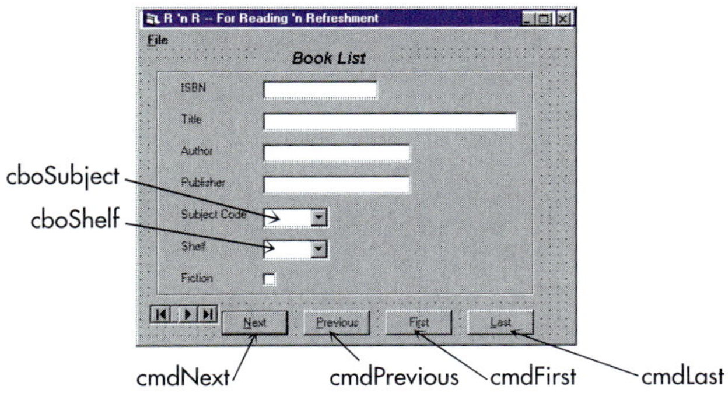

Add the four command buttons to use for navigation.

STEP 3: Delete the text box for Subject Code and add a combo box in its place.
STEP 4: Delete the text box for Shelf and add a combo box in its place.

Change the Properties

STEP 1: Set the properties of the four command buttons.

Object	Property	Setting
cmdNext	Name	cmdNext
	Caption	&Next
	Default	True
cmdPrevious	Name	cmdPrevious
	Caption	&Previous
cmdFirst	Name	cmdFirst
	Caption	Fi&rst
cmdLast	Name	cmdLast
	Caption	&Last

STEP 2: Change the Visible property of the data control to False.
STEP 3: Change the ReadOnly property of the data control to False.
STEP 4: Change the Locked property of txtISBN to True. This setting prevents the user from changing the ISBN, which is the key field for the table.
STEP 5: Set the properties of the two combo boxes as described in the following table.

Object	Property	Setting
cboSubject	Name	cboSubject
	Text	(blank)
	DataSource	datBooks
	DataField	Subject_Code
	List	BSS (Ctrl + Enter after each) FNT RLG RMN HMR SCF BSN PHL EDC MST SLH
cboShelf	Name	cboShelf
	Text	(blank)
	DataSource	datBooks
	DataField	Shelf_Location
	List	RC-1111 (Ctrl + Enter after each) RC-1112 RC-1113 RC-1114

Reset the Tab Order for the Controls

STEP 1: Click on the text box for the ISBN (txtISBN) on the form, switch to the Properties window, and change the TabIndex to 0.

STEP 2: Click on the second text box on the form (txtTitle), and the TabIndex property for txtTitle should appear in the Properties window. Change it to 1.

STEP 3: Click on the next text box (txtAuthor) and change its TabIndex property to 2.

STEP 4: Click on the next text box (txtPublisher) and change its TabIndex property to 3.

STEP 5: Click on the combo box for subject (cboSubject) and change its TabIndex property to 4.

STEP 6: Set the TabIndex properties for the rest of the controls.

cboShelf	5
chkFiction	6
cmdNext	7
cmdPrevious	8
cmdFirst	9
cmdLast	10

Write the Code

STEP 1: Change the remarks in the General Declarations section to reflect the changes.

STEP 2: Add coding for each command button. See the following listing for help.

```
'Program Name: R 'n R Book List Database
'Programmer:   J.C. Bradley
'Date:         August 1997
'Purpose:      Display and update book information in the
'              R 'n R Book database, using buttons for
'              navigation and combo boxes for field lookup
'Folder:       Ch1002
```

```
Private Sub cmdFirst_Click()
    'Move to first record

    datBooks.Recordset.MoveFirst
End Sub
```

```
Private Sub cmdLast_Click()
    'Move to last record

    datBooks.Recordset.MoveLast
End Sub
```

```
Private Sub cmdNext_Click()
    'Move to next record

    With datBooks.Recordset
        .MoveNext
        If .EOF Then
            .MoveFirst
        End If
    End With
End Sub
```

```
Private Sub cmdPrevious_Click()
    'Move to previous record

    With datBooks.Recordset
        .MovePrevious
        If .BOF Then
            .MoveLast
        End If
    End With
End Sub
```

```
Private Sub mnuFileExit_Click()
    'Exit the project

    End
End Sub
```

Testing the Navigation and Lookup Tables

Save the project; then test it. Try each of your navigation buttons. Make sure that you can move forward and backward and that the project properly handles moving before the first record and after the last.

As you move from record to record, notice the contents of the two lookup combo boxes. Try selecting a new subject for a record; then move to the next record. Move back to the changed record, and you will see that the change has been made. *Caution:* All changes you make to the data records are permanently saved when you move to another record or exit the database. You do not have an option to abandon changes; all changes are recorded in the file.

Updating a Database File

As you saw in the previous example, a project that displays data from a database allows updates automatically. If you don't want the user to change the data, you must set the ReadOnly property of the data control to True. You can also keep the user from making changes to the data by displaying fields in labels rather than in text boxes.

The Recordset object has an **`Update` method**, which you can use to save any changes in the data. Most of the time, updating is automatic, since Visual Basic automatically executes the `Update` method any time the user clicks one of the navigation buttons or one of the `Move` methods executes.

Adding Records

When you want to add new records to a database, you have a couple of choices. If you are using the data control's navigation buttons (rather than your own code for navigation), you can allow Visual Basic to do the adds automatically. Set the data control's EOFAction property to 2-AddNew. When the user moves to the end of the table and clicks the arrow for Next Record, an *Add* operation begins. The data in all bound controls are cleared so that new data can be entered. Then, when the user clicks one of the arrow buttons, the `Update` method is automatically executed and the new record is written in the file.

You need a different approach when you use code to accomplish record navigation. Assume that you have a command button or menu choice to add a new record. In the Click event for the command button, use the Recordset's **`AddNew` method:**

```
datBooks.Recordset.AddNew
```

When this statement executes, all bound controls are cleared so that the user can enter the data for the new record. After the data fields are entered, the new record must be saved in the file. You can explicitly save it with an `Update` method; or, if the user moves to another record, the `Update` method is automatically executed.

```
datBooks.Recordset.Update
```

You may want to use two buttons for adding a new record—an Add button and a Save button. For the Add button, use an `AddNew` method; for the Save button, use the `Update` method.

When adding new records, some conditions can cause errors to occur. For example, if the key field is blank on a new record, a run-time error halts program execution. See "Preventing Errors" later in this chapter for some solutions.

In the sample project for this chapter, the Locked property for txtISBN will have to be set to False. If you are going to allow adds, the user must be able to enter a new key field. (You might also consider setting the Locked property to False during an Add operation and True the rest of the time.)

Deleting Records

The **`Delete` method** deletes the current record. The user should display the record to delete and click a Delete command button or menu choice. When a record is deleted, the current record is no longer valid. Therefore, a `Delete` method must be followed by a `MoveNext` (or any other `Move`) method.

```
With datBooks.Recordset
    .Delete
    .MoveNext
End With
```

But what if the record being deleted is the last record in the table? Remember that if the navigation buttons are used to navigate, moving beyond EOF just resets the current record to the last record. No problem. However, if you are using event procedures for navigation, you must take care of this situation. If a `MoveNext` causes an EOF condition, then the program should do a `MovePrevious`.

```
Private Sub cmdDelete_Click()
    'Delete the current record

    With datBooks.Recordset
        .Delete           'Delete the current record
        .MoveNext         'Move to the following record
        If .EOF Then      'If last record deleted
            .MovePrevious
        End If
    End With
End Sub
```

Did you find another problem with this code? Stop and look at the preceding delete routine a moment. What will happen if the user deletes the *only* record in the Recordset?

Did you spot the problem? If the user deletes the last and only record in the Recordset, you must check for both EOF and BOF.

```
Private Sub cmdDelete_Click()
    'Delete the current record

    With datBooks.Recordset
        .Delete           'Delete the current record
        .MoveNext         'Move to the following record
        If .EOF Then      'If last record deleted
            .MovePrevious
            If .BOF Then 'If BOF and EOF true, no records remain
                MsgBox "The recordset is empty.", vbInformation, "No records"
                'Take any other desired action for empty recordset
            End If
        End If
    End With
End Sub
```

Preventing Errors

It is considered very poor programming style to allow your users to get run-time errors. Catching errors before they can cancel a program is called ***error trapping***. In Chapter 9 you learned to use the `On Error` statement for error trapping with data files; in Chapter 11 you will learn to use error trapping and validation with the data control.

In the meantime you can do some simple things to prevent user errors, such as disabling command buttons. In Chapter 9 you learned to disable navigation buttons during an Add or a Delete operation. Those techniques can keep a user out of trouble in a database Recordset also.

Protecting an Add Operation

When the user clicks on the Add button, the cmdAdd_Click event will occur:

```
Private Sub cmdAdd_Click()
    'Add a new record

    datBooks.Recordset.AddNew    'Clear out fields for new record
End Sub
```

Once the Add operation starts, you want the user to fill in the text boxes for the new record and click on *Save*. However, if the user clicks on one of the navigation buttons first, any data that she has already entered in the text boxes is saved automatically. How can the user be forced to click on *Save*? How can she be allowed to cancel the operation?

Limiting User Actions

The best way to avoid errors is to avoid any extra options that can cause trouble. Once the Add begins, the user should have two choices only: *Save* or *Cancel*. The navigation buttons and the *Delete* button should be disabled. Figure 10.17 illustrates a data form used for updating; Figure 10.18 shows the same form during an Add operation with only two buttons available.

Figure 10.17

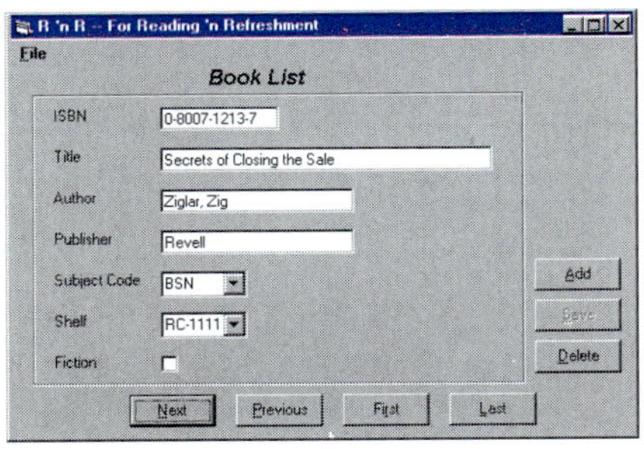

The update form as it appears before the user clicks on Add.

Figure 10.18

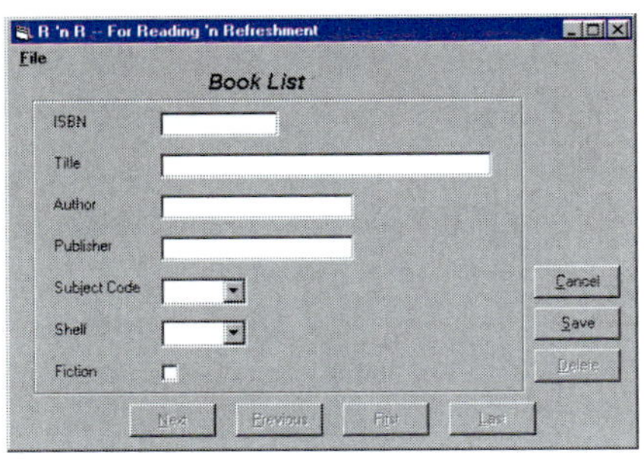

The update form as it appears during the Add operation. The Caption on the Add button changes to Cancel.

In the following example, when the user clicks on the Add button, several actions occur:

1. An `AddNew` method clears the bound controls to await entry of new data.
2. The focus is set in the first text box.

3. The navigation buttons and the *Delete* button are disabled.
4. The *Save* button is enabled.
5. The caption of the *Add* button changes to *Cancel*, which gives the user only two choices: *Save* or *Cancel*.

Sharing the Functions of a Command Button

Sometimes the best technique is to have one command button perform different actions, depending on the situation. Notice in Figures 10.17 and 10.18 that the *Save* button becomes the *Cancel* button during an Add operation. Of course, this isn't the only solution: You could create a separate Cancel button and disable it.

To make a command button perform more than one action, you must change its Caption when appropriate. Then in the button's Click event, check the Caption before responding to the event.

Tip

A good programming practice is to disable buttons when they shouldn't be used. It is not good practice to make them invisible and suddenly appear.

```
Private Sub cmdAdd_Click()
    'Add a new record or cancel an add

    If cmdAdd.Caption = "&Add" Then
        'Code to handle Add
        cmdAdd.Caption = "&Cancel"    'Change the button's Caption
    Else                              'A Cancel action is selected
        'Code to handle Cancel
        cmdAdd.Caption = "&Add"       'Reset the button's Caption
    End If
End Sub
```

Coding the New Add Procedure

The new cmdAdd_Click event performs two distinct operations: Add or Cancel. A new statement, the **`CancelUpdate` method**, also appears in the Cancel operation. `CancelUpdate` does what it sounds like—it cancels the Add and returns to the record that was active before the Add started.

```
Private Sub cmdAdd_Click()
    'Add a new record

    If cmdAdd.Caption = "&Add" Then
        datBooks.Recordset.AddNew       'Clear out fields for new record
        txtISBN.SetFocus
        DisableButtons                  'Disable navigation
        cmdSave.Enabled = True          'Enable the Save button
        cmdAdd.Caption = "&Cancel"      'Allow a Cancel option
    Else                                'A Cancel action is selected
        datBooks.Recordset.CancelUpdate 'Cancel the Add
        EnableButtons                   'Enable navigation
        cmdSave.Enabled = False         'Disable the Save button
        cmdAdd.Caption = "&Add"         'Reset the Add button
    End If
End Sub
```

Procedures to Disable and Enable Buttons

These two new general procedures simplify the disable/enable operations.

```
Private Sub DisableButtons()
    'Disable navigation buttons

    cmdNext.Enabled = False
    cmdPrevious.Enabled = False
    cmdFirst.Enabled = False
    cmdLast.Enabled = False
    cmdDelete.Enabled = False
End Sub

Private Sub EnableButtons()
    'Enable navigation buttons

    cmdNext.Enabled = True
    cmdPrevious.Enabled = True
    cmdFirst.Enabled = True
    cmdLast.Enabled = True
    cmdDelete.Enabled = True
End Sub
```

The Save Procedure

When the user clicks on Save, you must first save the new record by executing the `Update` method. Then reset the controls to their "normal" state.

```
Private Sub cmdSave_Click()
    'Save the current record

    datBooks.Recordset.Update
    EnableButtons
    cmdSave.Enabled = False
    cmdAdd.Caption = "&Add"
End Sub
```

Your Hands-On Programming Example

This example displays and maintains a database table to keep track of books for R 'n R—for Reading 'n Refreshment. This project puts together all the examples shown in this chapter. If you have completed the second example, you can just add the buttons and coding for Add, Cancel, Save, and Delete and change the Locked property for txtISBN.

Planning the Project

Sketch the modified form (Figure 10.19). Your user checks it over and approves the design.

Figure 10.19

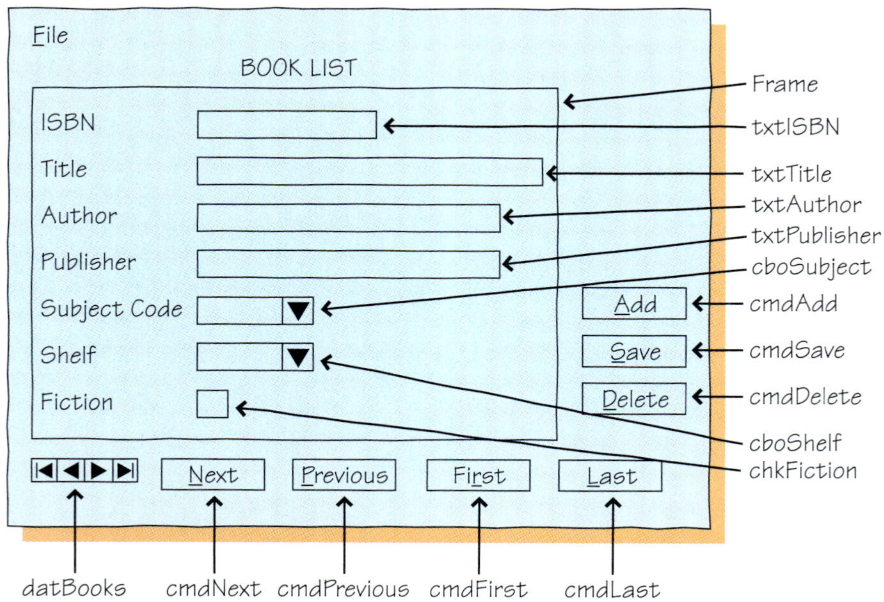

The planning sketch of the data entry form for the hands-on programming example.

Plan the Objects and Properties

Object	Property	Setting
frmBookData	Name	frmBookData
	Caption	R 'n R—for Reading 'n Refreshment
datBooks	Name	datBooks
	Caption	Select a Book
	Connect	Access
	DatabaseName	RNRBOOKS.MDB
	RecordSource	Books
	Read Only	False
	Visible	False
Frame1	Caption	(blank)
Label1	Caption	ISBN

Object	Property	Setting
Label2	Caption	Title
Label3	Caption	Author
Label4	Caption	Subject Code
Label5	Caption	Shelf
Label6	Caption	Fiction
txtISBN	Name	txtISBN
	Text	(blank)
	DataSource	datBooks
	DataField	ISBN
	Locked	False
txtTitle	Name	txtTitle
	Text	(blank)
	DataSource	datBooks
	DataField	Title
txtAuthor	Name	txtAuthor
	Text	(blank)
	DataSource	datBooks
	DataField	Author
txtPublisher	Name	txtPublisher
	Text	(blank)
	DataSource	datBooks
	DataField	Publisher
cboSubject	Name	cboSubject
	Text	(blank)
	DataSource	datBooks
	DataField	Subject_Code
	List	BSS FNT RLG RMN HMR SCF BSN PHL EDC MST SLH

(continued)

Object	Property	Setting
cboShelf	Name	cboShelf
	Text	(blank)
	DataField	Shelf_Location
	List	RC-1111 RC-1112 RC-1113 RC-1114
chkFiction	Name	chkFiction
	Caption	(blank)
	DataSource	datBooks
	DataField	Fiction
cmdAdd	Name	cmdAdd
	Caption	&Add
cmdSave	Name	cmdSave
	Caption	&Save
	Enabled	False
cmdDelete	Name	cmdDelete
	Caption	&Delete
cmdNext	Name	cmdNext
	Caption	&Next
	Default	True
cmdPrevious	Name	cmdPrevious
	Caption	&Previous
cmdFirst	Name	cmdFirst
	Caption	Fi&rst
cmdLast	Name	cmdLast
	Caption	&Last
mnuFile	Name	mnuFile
	Caption	&File
mnuFileExit	Name	mnuFileExit
	Caption	E&xit

Plan the Code Procedures

Plan the actions for the event procedures and the general procedures.

Procedure	Actions
mnuFileExit_Click	Terminate the project.

cmdAdd_Click	If button caption = "Add" Then
	AddNew record.
	Set the focus in txtISBN.
	Disable buttons.
	Enable the Save button.
	Set Add button caption to "Cancel."
	Else
	CancelAdd method.
	Enable buttons.
	Disable the Save button.
	Set button caption to "Add."
	End If

cmdDelete_Click	Delete record.
	Move to next record.
	If EOF Then
	Move to the previous record.
	If BOF Then (no records in recordset)
	Display message.
	Disable buttons.
	End If
	End If

cmdSave_Click	Update record. Enable buttons. Disable the Save button. Set cmdAdd caption to "Add."

cmdNext_Click	Move to next record.
	If EOF Then
	Move to first record.
	End If

cmdPrevious_Click	Move to previous record
	If BOF Then
	Move to last record.
	End If

cmdFirst_Click	Move to first record.
cmdLast_Click	Move to last record.

Write the Project

- Follow the sketch in Figure 10.19 to create the form. Figure 10.20 shows the completed form. If you have done the preceding step-by-step examples in this chapter, you can just modify the previous project.

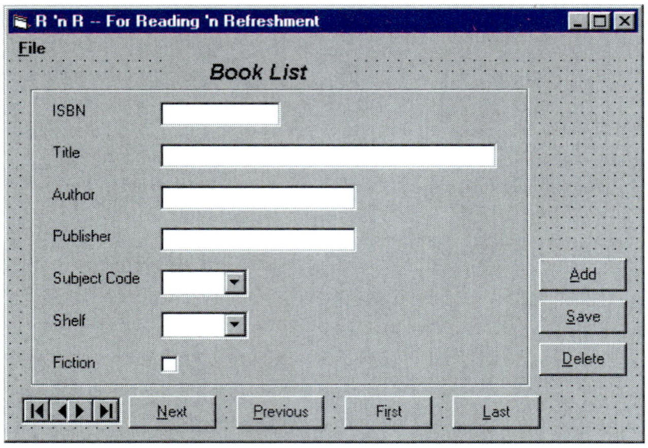

Figure 10.20

The data entry form for the hands-on programming example.

- Set the properties of each of the objects, as you have planned.
- Write the code. Working from the pseudocode, write each procedure.
- Thoroughly test the project. Make sure to try every option, including canceling an Add and deleting the last record in a table.

The Project Coding Solution

```
'Program Name:    R 'n R Book List Database
'Programmer:      J.C. Bradley
'Date:            August 1997
'Purpose:         Display and update book information in the
'                 R 'n R Book database, using buttons for
'                 navigation and combo boxes for field lookup
'Folder:          Ch1003
```

```
Private Sub cmdAdd_Click()
     'Add a new record

     If cmdAdd.Caption = "&Add" Then
         datBooks.Recordset.AddNew          'Clear out fields for new record
         txtISBN.SetFocus
         DisableButtons                     'Disable navigation
         cmdSave.Enabled = True             'Enable the Save button
         cmdAdd.Caption = "&Cancel"         'Allow a Cancel option
     Else
         datBooks.Recordset.CancelUpdate    'Cancel the Add
         EnableButtons                      'Enable navigation
         cmdSave.Enabled = False            'Disable the Save button
         cmdAdd.Caption = "&Add"            'Reset the Add button
     End If
End Sub
```

```
Private Sub cmdDelete_Click()
    'Delete the current record

    With datBooks.Recordset
        .Delete         'Delete the current record
        .MoveNext       'Move to the following record
        If .EOF Then    'If last record deleted
            .MovePrevious
            If .BOF Then            'If BOF and EOF true, no records remain
                MsgBox "The recordset is empty.", vbInformation, "No records"
                DisableButtons
            End If
        End If
    End With
End Sub
```

```
Private Sub cmdFirst_Click()
    'Move to first record

    datBooks.Recordset.MoveFirst
End Sub
```

```
Private Sub cmdLast_Click()
    'Move to last record

    datBooks.Recordset.MoveLast
End Sub
```

```
Private Sub cmdNext_Click()
    'Move to next record

    With datBooks.Recordset
        .MoveNext
        If .EOF Then
            .MoveFirst
        End If
    End With
End Sub
```

```
Private Sub cmdPrevious_Click()
    'Move to previous record

    With datBooks.Recordset
        .MovePrevious
        If .BOF Then
            .MoveLast
        End If
    End With
End Sub
```

```
Private Sub cmdSave_Click()
    'Save the current record

    datBooks.Recordset.Update
    EnableButtons
    cmdSave.Enabled = False
    cmdAdd.Caption = "&Add"
End Sub
```

```
Private Sub mnuFileExit_Click()
    'Exit the project

    End
End Sub
```

```
Private Sub DisableButtons()
    'Disable navigation buttons

    cmdNext.Enabled = False
    cmdPrevious.Enabled = False
    cmdFirst.Enabled = False
    cmdLast.Enabled = False
    cmdDelete.Enabled = False
End Sub
```

```
Private Sub EnableButtons()
    'Enable navigation buttons

    cmdNext.Enabled = True
    cmdPrevious.Enabled = True
    cmdFirst.Enabled = True
    cmdLast.Enabled = True
    cmdDelete.Enabled = True
End Sub
```

Programming Hints

1. If you have trouble with your project running correctly, try single-stepping through the execution. Place a breakpoint at the top of a suspect procedure and begin execution. When the program halts at the breakpoint, press F8 (the shortcut for Step) repeatedly and watch the execution. While the project is in break time, you can highlight any expression in code and wait a second; the current value of the expression will display.
2. You can look up all properties, events, and methods for the data control in the Object Browser (Figure 10.21). Select *Object Browser* from the *View* menu, drop down the */Project/Library* list, and choose *VB*; then select *Data*.

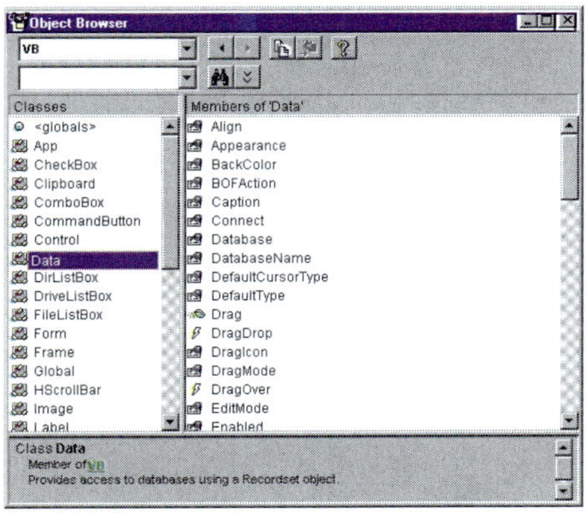

Figure 10.21

Look up the properties and methods for the data control in the Object Browser.

Summary

1. Microsoft Access is Visual Basic's native format for database files.
2. In database terminology a *file* consists of *tables*, which consist of *rows* or *records*, which consist of *columns* or *fields*. Each record is identified by its *key* field. One record is always the *current* record.
3. A data control placed on a form links to a database file and a particular table within that file. Data-bound controls link to a data control for the table name and to a particular field within the table.
4. Data-aware controls (those that can become data bound) are labels, text boxes, check boxes, list boxes, combo boxes, images, picture boxes, data-bound list boxes, and data-bound grids.
5. Set the Connect, DatabaseName, and RecordSource properties of a data control to link it to a database table.
6. Set the DataSource and DataField properties of data-aware controls to bind them to a field in a database table.
7. The Recordset object defined by the data control has its own properties and methods. Use the `MoveNext`, `MovePrevious`, `MoveFirst`, and `MoveLast` methods to navigate the database. The BOF and EOF properties indicate the beginning or end of file.
8. A combo box can be used as a data-bound control, and its List property can hold the possible choices for the field.
9. Any data that the user changes on the screen is automatically written into the file unless the ReadOnly property is set to True.
10. The `AddNew` method clears the fields on the screen to allow the user to add a new record. After the Add, an `Update` method is needed; however, an `Update` occurs automatically when the user moves to another record.
11. The `Delete` method removes a record from the table. A `Move` must be executed after a `Delete`, because the current record is no longer valid.
12. To protect the user from making errors, you can disable and enable buttons. During an Add operation, the user have only the options to Save or to Cancel. A `CancelUpdate` method cancels an Add operation.

Key Terms

`AddNew` method *378*
BOF *373*
`CancelUpdate` method *382*
column *326*
Connect property *366*
current record *363*
DatabaseName property *366*
data-bound control *365*
DataField property *368*
DataSource property *367*
`Delete` method *379*
EOF *373*
error trapping *380*
field *362*
file *362*
key field *363*
record *362*
Recordset object *372*
RecordSource property *367*
row *362*
table *362*
`Update` method *378*

Review Questions

1. Assume you have a database containing the names and phone numbers of your friends. Describe how the terms *file, table, row, column, record, field,* and *key* apply to your database.
2. Explain the difference between a data control and a data-bound control.
3. Which controls can be data bound?
4. Explain how the BOF and EOF properties are set and how they might be used in a project.
5. What properties must be set for a combo box in order for it to be bound to a field in a database and display a dropdown list of the choices for that field?
6. What steps are needed to add a new record to a database?
7. What steps are needed to delete a record from a database?
8. What steps are needed to change the data in a database record?
9. How can you check for the user deleting the only record in a Recordset?

Programming Exercises

10.1 The Rnrbooks.mdb database file holds two tables: the Books table used in this chapter and the Subjects table. The Subjects table has only two fields: the Subject Code (the key) and the Subject Name. Write a project that will display the Subjects table. Include command buttons for record navigation, make the data control invisible, and set the table to ReadOnly.

10.2 Write a project to maintain the Subjects table described in project 10.1. Use the (visible) data control for record navigation. Set the EOFAction property of the data control to 2-AddNew. Include command buttons for Add, Delete, and Exit.

10.3 Write a project to maintain the Subjects table described in project 10.1. Use menu choices rather than command buttons for the following program functions:

Menus

File	Record	Help
Exit	Next	About
	Previous	
	First	
	Last	
	————	
	Add New	
	Delete Current	

Give each menu command a keyboard shortcut (in the Menu Editor) if you wish, to make selecting a command quicker.

Include two command buttons on the form—a Save button and a Cancel button, which are both disabled most of the time. When the user chooses Add New, make the Save and Cancel buttons enabled. If the user clicks on Save, update the record; a click on Cancel cancels the Add operation. After either a Save or Cancel, make both buttons disabled again.

Make the Save button the default button. Set the Cancel property to True on the Cancel button.

Disable the menu options for navigation, Add, and Delete when an Add is in progress.

10.4 Write a project to display the Publishers table from the Biblio.mdb database that comes with Visual Basic. (Biblio.mdb should be stored in the VB directory.) Include command buttons for record navigation and hide the data control. Do not allow the user to change the data.

Hint: Copy the Biblio.mdb file to the directory where your project will be stored before setting the properties for the data control.

Fields in the Publishers table
PubID (Publisher Identification—key field)
Name
Company Name
Address
City
State
ZIP
Telephone
Fax

Note: The Biblio.mdb database included with VB4 was 288 KB, small enough to easily fit on a diskette. The version included with VB5 is 3.5 MB—too large for a diskette. The older version is included on your Student Diskette. The two versions of the file have the same structure; the size difference is due to the large number of records added to the newer version.

10.5 Write a project to maintain the Publishers table described in project 10.4. Allow Adds and Deletes to the database. On an Add, disable the navigation and Delete buttons so that the only options are Save or Cancel.

Hint: Copy the Biblio.mdb file to the directory where your project will be stored before setting the properties for the data control. See the note in Exercise 10.4 about the file size.

CASE STUDIES

VB Mail Order

VB Mail Order Assignment 1—Display Only

Create a project to display the VB Mail Order Customer table from the Vbmail.mdb database on your student diskette. Set the database ReadOnly property to True so that the user cannot change the data.

Make the data control invisible; instead, include command buttons for Next, Previous, First, and Last.

VB Mail Order Assignment 2—Display and Update

Create a project to display and maintain the customer table. See project 10.3 for a list of the menu choices.

Allow adds and deletions to the database through menu selections. During an Add, allow the user to Save or to Cancel only.

Fields

Customer ID
LastName
FirstName
Address
City
State
ZipCode

VB Auto Center

VB Auto Center Assignment 1—Display Only

Create a project to display the VB Auto Center Vehicle table from the Vbauto.mdb database on your student diskette. Set the database ReadOnly property to True so that the user cannot change the data.

Make the data control invisible; instead, include command buttons for Next, Previous, First, and Last.

VB Auto Center Assignment 2—Display and Update

Create a project to display and maintain the Auto Center Vehicle table. See project 10.3 for a list of the menu choices.

Allow adds and deletions to the database through menu selections. During an Add, allow the user to Save or to Cancel only.

Fields

InventoryID
Manufacturer
ModelName
Year
VehicleID
CostValue

C H A P T E R

11

Advanced Data Handling—Grids, Validation, Selection, and SQL

At the completion of this chapter, you will be able to . . .

1. Write a database application using the DB Grid control.
2. Improve database validation techniques with error-trapping techniques.
3. Find records that meet a specific criterion using both the `Find` and the `Seek` methods.
4. Differentiate among tables, dynasets, and snapshot recordsets.
5. Reorder table type recordsets using indexes.
6. Create a new dynaset using Structured Query Language (SQL).

Displaying Data in Grids

In Chapter 10 you learned to display database tables in bound controls, such as labels, text boxes, check boxes, and list boxes. Another good way to display data is in **grids**, which present tables in rows and columns similar to a spreadsheet.

Visual Basic comes with two grid controls: the DBGrid and the MSFlexGrid. In addition, many companies sell powerful grid controls that you can include in your project. In the following example, you will create a simple application using Microsoft's DBGrid control.

A Grid Control—Step-by-Step

This step-by-step tutorial shows you how to create an application that displays the Books table for R 'n R. Although the application is quite simple, it does allow the user to add, change, and delete data records. You also learn how to display the record number and record count. Figure 11.1 shows the completed form.

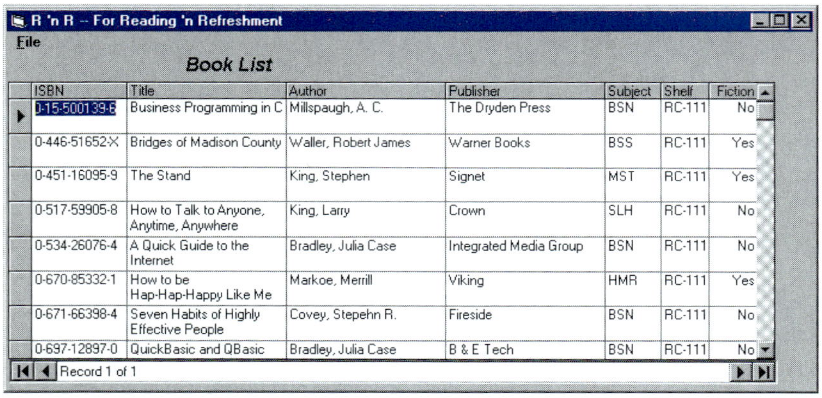

Figure 11.1

The completed form using the grid control.

Create The Form and Controls

STEP 1: Begin a new project and widen the form. You may want to close the Project Explorer and Form Layout windows and float the Properties window to allow room to work on the wide form (Figure 11.2).

Figure 11.2

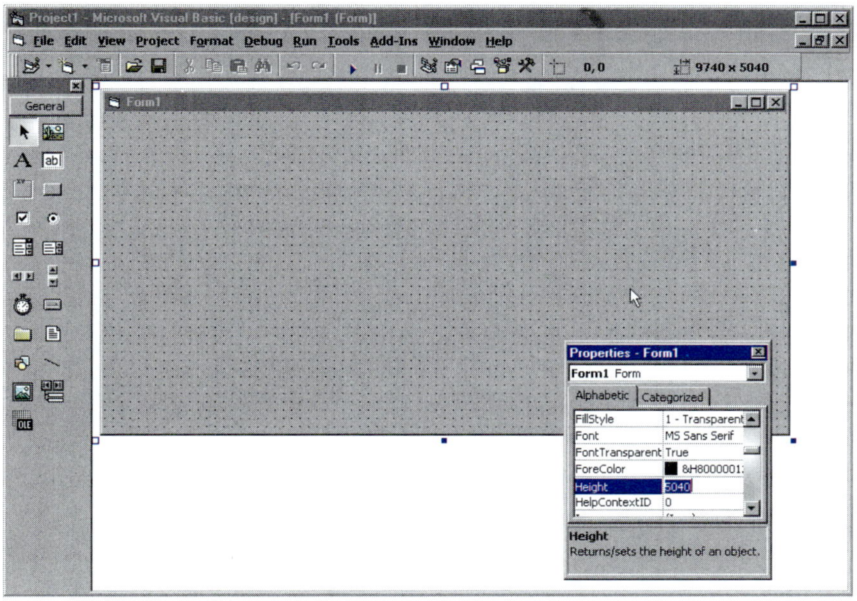

Modify the screen layout to work on a wide form.

STEP 2: Add a data control along the bottom of the form. Set the control's Name property to *datBooks* and its DatabaseName property to *Rnr-Books.mdb*. (This file should be on your student diskette.) Set the RecordSource property to *Books* and verify that the RecordsetType is *1 - Dynaset*.

STEP 3: Select *Project/Components* to display the *Components* dialog box. Then locate *Microsoft Data Bound Grid Control,* select it, and close the dialog box. You should see the new tool in the toolbox (Figure 11.3).

Figure 11.3

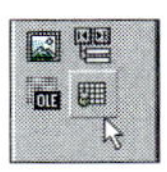

Add the DB Grid control to your toolbox.

STEP 4: Click on the DBGrid tool and draw a large grid on the form (Figure 11.4). Then, using the Properties window, change the control's Name property to *dbgBooks* and its DataSource property to *datBooks*.

Figure 11.4

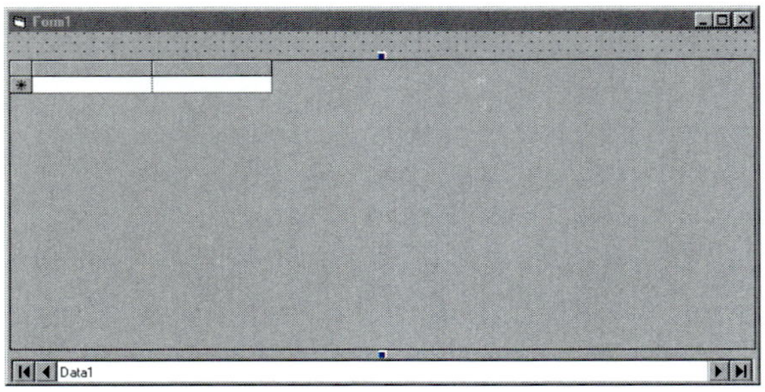

Draw a large grid control on your form.

STEP 5: Create the menu bar. It should have a *File* menu with only an *Exit* command.

STEP 6: Create the large label at the top of the form with the form's title: *Book List.* Change the font and size to something you like.

Set the Properties of the Form

STEP 1: Set the form's Name property to *frmBookGrid* and its Caption property to *R 'n R—For Reading and Refreshment.*

Set the Properties of the Grid

STEP 1: Point to the grid control and right-click to display the shortcut menu. Select *Retrieve Fields* and watch as the grid changes to display all the fields from the Books table. One column is set up for each field, with the field name at the top of the column as a caption.

We are going to set more properties to improve the display of the table, but at this point the application will work. We'll make a quick test before setting the rest of the properties.

STEP 2: Start the project running. You should see the grid fill with data. Scroll to the right and view all the fields. You can also scroll down to see more records.

Next we will resize the columns, change captions for some columns, fix the display format of the Yes/No field (Fiction), and make the long titles and names wrap to a second line.

STEP 3: Stop program execution, point to the grid control, and right-click to display the shortcut menu. Select *Properties* (Figure 11.5), and the custom *Property Pages* dialog box appears (Figure 11.6). Although you can change the properties in the regular Properties window, the process is much easier from this custom dialog box.

Figure 11.5

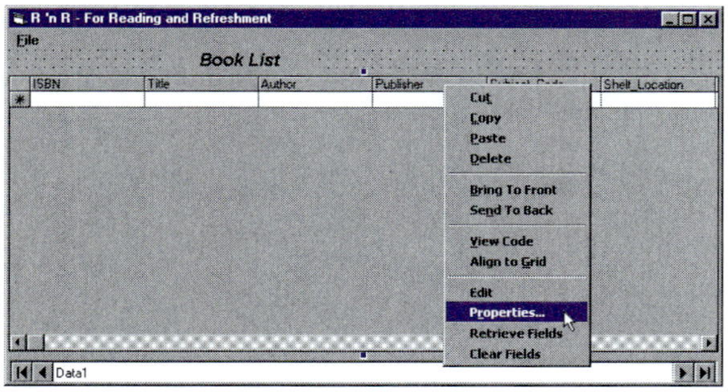

Right-click on the grid control to display the shortcut menu; select Properties.

Figure 11.6

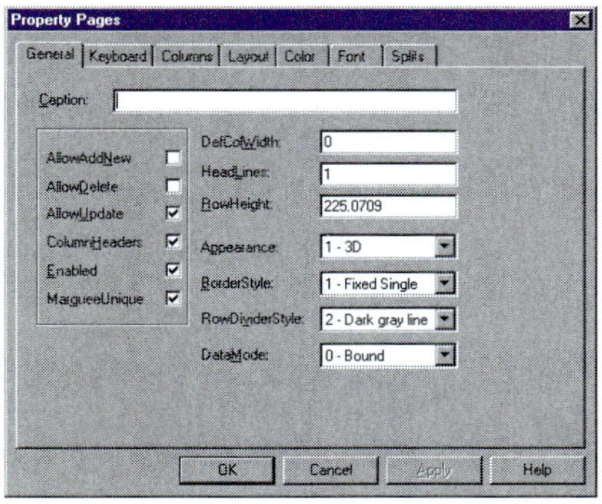

Modify the properties of the grid control using the custom Property Pages *dialog box.*

STEP 4: On the *General* tab select *AllowAddNew* and *AllowDelete*. Change the *Row Height* entry to *450* (approximately double the default entry).

STEP 5: Change to the *Columns* tab and make these changes:

Column4 (Subject_Code)
  Caption: *Subject*
Column5 (Shelf_Location)
  Caption: *Shelf*
Column6 (Fiction)
  Number Format: *Yes/No*

STEP 6: Click *Apply* to apply the changes without closing the *Property Pages* dialog box.

STEP 7: Change to the *Layout* tab and make the following changes. You may want to click *Apply* after each change.

Column0 (ISBN)
Locked: Checked
Width: *1200* (measurements in twips)
Column1 (Title)
WrapText: Checked
Width: *2000*
Column2 (Author)
WrapText: Checked
Width: *2000*
Column3 (Publisher)
WrapText: Checked
Width: *2000*
Column4 (Subject_Code)
Width: *700*
Column5 (Shelf_Location)
Width: *700*

STEP 8: Click OK to close the custom *Property Pages* dialog box.
STEP 9: Resize the form and data control as you wish.

Write the Exit Procedure

STEP 1: Code the mnuFileExit_Click procedure with an `End` statement.

You could run the project now and have a functioning database grid. However, we are going to add one more feature to the project and make the record number appear in the data control.

> **Tip**
> Quickly switch back and forth between the Code window and the Form window using keyboard shortcuts. F7 takes you to the Code window; Shift + F7 switches to the Form window.

Displaying the Record Number and Record Count

Often it is useful to display the record number and record count when viewing database records. You can use the **RecordCount** and **AbsolutePosition properties** of the data control's recordset to display both, for example: *Record 10 of 45.*

The RecordCount and AbsolutePosition Properties

The RecordCount property holds the number of records in a recordset; the AbsolutePosition holds the position of the current record in the recordset. However, AbsolutePosition is zero based; that is, the first record has an AbsolutePosition of zero. Therefore you must add one to the property to produce the record number.

Example

```
iCurrentRecord = datBooks.Recordset.AbsolutePosition + 1
```

If the recordset is at BOF or EOF, the AbsolutePosition property has a value of 0. *Note:* You cannot use the AbsolutePosition property as a record number because the position number changes as records are added and deleted.

To display the record number and count in the caption of the data control, you can create a sub procedure and use this code:

```
Private Sub SetRecordNumber()
    'Display the record number
    Dim iRecordCount     As Integer
    Dim iCurrentRecord   As Integer

    iRecordCount = datBooks.Recordset.RecordCount
    iCurrentRecord = datBooks.Recordset.AbsolutePosition + 1
    If datBooks.Recordset.EOF Then
        datBooks.Caption = "EOF"
    Else
     datBooks.Caption = "Record " & iCurrentRecord & " of " & iRecordCount
    End If
End Sub
```

Note: This technique for displaying the record number works only for a dynaset or snapshot type recordset, not for a table recordset. See *Recordsets* later in this chapter.

Opening the Database

When you run a project with a data control, the database file is opened automatically. The actual file open occurs *after* the Form_Load event finishes. If you want to do any initialization steps for the database file, you can explicitly open the file in the Form_Load event procedure. Use the data control's **Refresh method** to open the database.

The Refresh Method—General Form

```
datControlName.Refresh
```

The Refresh Method—Example

```
datBooks.Refresh
```

The `Refresh` method opens or reopens the database specified by the data control.

You can use the Form_Load event procedure to open the database and call the SetRecordNumber sub procedure illustrated earlier. When the database is first opened, the recordset's RecordCount property does not yet know the total number of records. Use a `MoveLast` method, which updates the RecordCount; then use a `MoveFirst` to return to the beginning of the recordset.

```
Private Sub Form_Load()
    'Open the database and display the record count

    With datBooks
        .Refresh                'Open the database
        .Recordset.MoveLast     'Get the record count
        .Recordset.MoveFirst
    End With
    SetRecordNumber
End Sub
```

The Reposition Event

The previous code displays the record number and count when the database is first opened. To display the record number as the user moves from record to record, use the data control's **Reposition event**. The Reposition event occurs each time a new record becomes current; it also occurs at BOF and EOF.

```
Private Sub datBooks_Reposition()
    'Display the record number

    SetRecordNumber
End Sub
```

Putting it Together

Now that you have seen the code for explicitly opening the database and displaying the record number, add the steps to your DB Grid project. Code the Form_Load and datBook_Reposition event procedures and the SetRecord-Number sub procedure.

The Code for the DB Grid Example

```
'Program Name:  R 'n R Book List Grid
'Programmer:    J.C. Bradley
'Date:          December 1997
'Purpose:       Display and update book information in the
'               R 'n R Book database using a grid control.
'Folder:        Ch1101

Option Explicit
________________________________________________________________

Private Sub datBooks_Reposition()
    'Display the record number

    SetRecordNumber
End Sub
________________________________________________________________
```

```
Private Sub Form_Load()
     'Open the database and display the record count

     With datBooks
          .Refresh                     'Open the database
          .Recordset.MoveLast          'Get the record count
          .Recordset.MoveFirst
     End With
     SetRecordNumber
End Sub
```

```
Private Sub mnuFileExit_Click()
     'Exit the project

     End
End Sub
```

```
Private Sub SetRecordNumber()
     'Display the record number
     Dim iRecordCount       As Integer
     Dim iCurrentRecord     As Integer

     iRecordCount = datBooks.Recordset.RecordCount
     iCurrentRecord = datBooks.Recordset.AbsolutePosition + 1
     If datBooks.Recordset.EOF Then
          datBooks.Caption = "EOF"
     Else
          datBooks.Caption = "Record " & iCurrentRecord & " of " & iRecordCount
     End If
End Sub
```

Validation and Error Trapping

When a computer program aborts and displays a cryptic system error message, who is to blame? the user? the programmer? the computer? Programmers sometimes tend to blame "stupid" users who just don't know what they are doing, but an amazing fact is that *really* good programmers seem to have "smarter" users who use programs correctly and make fewer errors. To become a good programmer, you must anticipate all possible actions of users (who don't have the benefit of your excellent logic abilities). Any action that it is possible for your program to take will be tried by some user. If your form has a button or command that shouldn't be pressed in some situations, be assured that one of your users will press it.

In Chapters 9 and 10 you learned to disable and enable command buttons to shield the user. In this section you will learn to use the database Validation event to check for some user errors, trap database errors using the `On Error` statement, and give your user a chance to recover after some errors, such as a missing or misplaced data file.

The programming examples in this section build on the hands-on project in Chapter 10. We will add data validation and error-trapping routines and incorporate other techniques to try to keep the user from making errors.

Locking Text Boxes

In prevous projects you disabled controls that you didn't want the user to select. In the case of text boxes, you can also lock them, which prevents any changes without making the control appear disabled. Set a text box's **Locked property** to True to lock it and to False to unlock it.

In the R 'n R Book List example, we don't want the user to change the ISBN, since that is the key field. However, we don't want to use a label for the ISBN, since we need to be able to type in an ISBN during an Add operation. Therefore, we will keep txtISBN locked most of the time and unlock it when an Add is in progress.

In the procedure to begin an Add (cmdAdd_Click), include this statement:

```
txtISBN.Locked = False
```

Because the only two actions that the user can take after beginning an Add are Save and Cancel, you should include the following statement in both routines:

```
txtISBN.Locked = True
```

Validating Data in the Validate Event

When you want to make sure that a required field has an entry or that a field has valid data, the Validate event is a good location to check. If the field is not valid, you can display an error message and cancel the operation.

The data control's Validate event occurs just before a new record becomes current (with a Move) or when an Update, AddNew, Delete, or Close occurs. You can do some checking before allowing the operation to complete.

The Validate Event—General Form

```
Private Sub DataControl_Validate(Action As Integer, Save As Integer)
```

The Validate Event—Example

```
Private Sub datBooks_Validate(Action As Integer, Save As Integer)
```

The values for the Action and Save arguments are passed to the sub procedure. You can check and/or modify their values inside the procedure. Both Action and Save are passed as integer values; you can use the actual numbers or the Visual Basic constants.

Action: The setting of the Action argument indicates the operation that occurred to cause the Validate event. You can change the value of Action. For example, change Action to 0 (vbDataActionCancel) to cancel the operation when the Sub terminates.

Constant	Integer Setting	Action That Caused Validate Event
vbDataActionCancel	0	Cancel when Sub exits
vbDataActionMoveFirst	1	MoveFirst
vbDataActionMovePrevious	2	MovePrevious
vbDataActionMoveNext	3	MoveNext
vbDataActionMoveLast	4	MoveLast
vbDataActionAddNew	5	AddNew
vbDataActionUpdate	6	Update
vbDataActionDelete	7	Delete
vbDataActionFind	8	Find
vbDataActionBookMark	9	Bookmark set
vbDataActionClose	10	Close
vbDataActionUnload	11	Form is being unloaded

Save: The value of the Save argument is set to True if any data have changed in a bound control on the form, meaning that the changed data should be saved in the file. You can set the value of Save to False if you don't want any changes to be saved.

Allowable Operations

There are some things you can do inside the Validate event procedure and some things you cannot. You *can* tell it to complete or cancel the operation and to save or not save any changes. But you *cannot* execute any other database methods during the Validate event. For example, you may determine that you need to do a Move or an AddNew. Rather than place the method in the Validate event (which causes an error), set a module-level Boolean variable to indicate the condition and check that variable after the current operation finishes. In the Validate procedure that follows, the variable mbValidationError is set to False at the top of the procedure and set to True if a validation error occurs. A little later in the chapter you will see that the cmdSave_Click procedure checks the value of mbValidationError.

Example Validate Event Procedure

The following example adds validation to the R 'n R database project from Chapter 10. In this example we want to make sure that the user enters 13 characters for the ISBN, since any other length is invalid. If an Add is in progress (the action is Update) and the length of txtISBN.Text is not exactly 13, an error condition occurs. We display a message box, reset the focus and select the text, set the Boolean variable mbValidationError to True, set the procedure's Action argument to cancel the operation, and set the Save argument to not save any changed data. *Note:* The variable mbValidationError must be dimensioned in the General Declarations Section.

```
Private Sub datBooks_Validate(Action As Integer, Save As Integer)
    'This sub is entered for every action in the database.
    'Validate the data for an Add operation
    Dim stMessage As String

    mbValidationError = False               'Set flag for no errors
    If Action = vbDataActionUpdate Then     'A new add is being saved
        With txtISBN
            If Len(.Text) <> 13 Then        'All ISBNs must be 13 characters
                stMessage = "Invalid ISBN"
                MsgBox stMessage, vbExclamation, "Data Entry Error"
                .SetFocus
                .SelStart = 0
                .SelLength = Len(.Text)
                mbValidationError = True
                Action = vbDataActionCancel
                Save = False
            End If
        End With
    End If
End Sub
```

Using the LostFocus Event

Another good time to check the contents of a control is in the control's **LostFocus event** procedure. This event occurs if the control has the focus and then loses it, usually when the user tabs to a new field or clicks on a button. In the previous example the check for a valid ISBN could be coded in the LostFocus event rather than in the Validate event.

```
Private Sub txtISBN_LostFocus()
    'Check the validity of the control during an Add
    'Note: the control is locked at all times except during an Add

    With txtISBN
        If Len(.Text) <> 13 Then        'All ISBNs must be 13 characters
            stMessage = "Invalid ISBN"
            MsgBox stMessage, vbExclamation, "Data Entry Error"
        End If
    End With
End Sub
```

You may notice that this example does not reset the focus in the text box after the error, as was done in the Validate event example. Before you code validation in the LostFocus event, you need to consider all possible actions that the user can take. The LostFocus event occurs when the user tabs out of the field *or* selects any other control. If the user clicks the Cancel button or chooses *File/Exit*, this procedure executes. If you reset the focus to the text box when the data are not valid, you may trap the user, requiring him or her to make a valid entry before canceling or exiting.

Trap Errors with On Error

Error trapping with `On Error` is very important when working with database files. You need to include the `On Error` in every procedure that accesses the database, such as the Add, Delete, Update, and all Moves. In each case trap for any errors you think are likely. For many routines you can just code an `On Error Resume Next`, which ignores the error and continues execution.

```
Private Sub cmdFirst_Click()
    'Move to first record

    On Error Resume Next
    datBooks.Recordset.MoveFirst
End Sub
```

Handling Error Conditions that Cancel an Operation

If an error occurs that will cancel an operation, such as a Delete or Add operation, the user should be notified. You can display a message and continue with program execution.

```
Private Sub cmdDelete_Click()
    'Delete the current record

    On Error GoTo HandleDeleteError
    With datBooks.Recordset
        .Delete                         'Delete the current record
        .MoveNext                       'Move to the following record
        If .EOF Then                    'If last record deleted
            .MovePrevious
            If .BOF Then                'If BOF and EOF true, no records remain
                MsgBox "The recordset is empty.", vbInformation, "No records"
                DisableButtons
            End If
        End If
    End With

cmdDelete_Click_Exit:
    Exit Sub
```

```
HandleDeleteError:
     Dim stMessage As String
     stMessage = "Cannot complete operation." & vbCrLf & vbCrLf _
               & Err.Description
     MsgBox stMessage, vbExclamation, "Database Error"
     On Error GoTo 0                        'Turn off error trapping
End Sub
```

Handling Errors after an Add Operation

When the user clicks *Save* after an Add operation, several errors are possible. A duplicate key will cause an error, as will a missing key field.

You must decide what action you want to take when the user has entered a complete new record and the ISBN duplicates one already in the file. Do you want to clear the data? Do you want to display a message and abort the operation? In this example we will allow the user to change the ISBN and continue with the Add if desired. To make this happen, you must save the contents of the controls on the screen, execute an AddNew method, and replace the contents of the controls. We will place this code in a separate sub procedure.

Note: You can find the complete list of error codes in the Help topic *Trappable Errors*.

```
Private Sub cmdSave_Click()
     'Save the current record

     On Error GoTo HandleSaveErrors
     datBooks.Recordset.Update
     If Not mbValidationError Then      'Passed the validation
         txtISBN.Locked = True          'Reset all
         EnableButtons
         cmdSave.Enabled = False
         cmdAdd.Caption = "&Add"
     End If

cmdSave_Click_Exit:
     Exit Sub

HandleSaveErrors:
     Dim stMessage As String
     Select Case Err.Number
         Case 3022                  'Duplicate key field
             stMessage = "Duplicate ISBN--Record not saved."
             MsgBox stMessage, vbExclamation, "Database Error"
             SetUpAddRecord         'Allow user to change ISBN and complete add
             On Error GoTo 0        'Turn off error trapping to allow completion
         Case 3058, 3315            'No entry in key field
             stMessage = "ISBN must be completed before save."
             MsgBox stMessage, vbExclamation, "Database Error"
             SetUpAddRecord         'Give another chance to complete record
             On Error GoTo 0        'Turn off error trapping to allow completion
```

```
        Case Else
            stMessage = "Record could not be saved." & vbCRLF _
                        & Err.Description
            MsgBox stMessage, vbExclamation, "Database Error"
            datBooks.Recordset.CancelUpdate
            Resume Next
    End Select
End Sub
```

```
Private Sub SetUpAddRecord()
    'Set up a new Add to allow the user another try
    Dim savISBN As String, savTitle As String, savAuthor As String
    Dim savPublisher As String, savSubject As String
    Dim savLocation As String, savFiction As Variant

    On Error Resume Next

    'Save the contents of the form controls
    savISBN = txtISBN.Text
    savTitle = txtTitle.Text
    savAuthor = txtAuthor.Text
    savPublisher = txtPublisher.Text
    savSubject = cboSubject.Text
    savLocation = cboLocation.Text
    savFiction = chkFiction.Value

    'Start a new Add
    datBooks.Recordset.AddNew

    'Place saved data back in form controls
    With txtISBN
        .Text = savISBN
        .SelStart = 0
        .SelLength = Len(.Text)
        .SetFocus
    End With
    txtTitle.Text = savTitle
    txtAuthor.Text = savAuthor
    txtPublisher.Text = savPublisher
    cboSubject.Text = savSubject
    cboLocation.Text = savLocation
    chkFiction.Value = savFiction
End Sub
```

Trapping File Open Errors

When your application begins, VB opens the database file that you specified in the data control's DatabaseName property. If the file or path cannot be found, a fatal error occurs.

Trapping for an open error is a little tricky because the database open does not occur in any of your event procedures. By default, the open executes after Form_Load finishes but before the Form_Paint event. The easiest way to trap for an error on the open is to explicitly open the database yourself in the Form_Load event. That way, you can include error trapping.

In this example we will open the database in the Form_Load event. If the database file isn't found, the `GetNewDatabaseName` function is called. In the `GetNewDatabaseName` function, we will display the *Open* common dialog box so the user can locate the file. If any other error occurs, the MsgBox displays the system error for the current error (Err.Description) and exits the project by calling the mnuFileExit_Click procedure.

```
Private Sub Form_Load()
     'Open the database

     On Error GoTo HandleFormLoadError
     datBooks.Refresh                       'Open the database

Form_Load_Exit:
     Exit Sub

HandleFormLoadError:
     Dim stNewDatabaseName     As String
     Select Case Err.Number
         Case 3004, 3024, 3044              'Database, file, or path not found
              stNewDatabaseName = GetNewDatabaseName
              If stNewDatabaseName = "" Then 'User canceled operation
                   mnuFileExit_Click
              Else
                   datBooks.DatabaseName = stNewDatabaseName
                   Resume                   'Reopen the database
              End If
         Case Else
              MsgBox Err.Description, vbOKOnly + vbExclamation, "Unexpected Error"
              mnuFileExit_Click             'Exit the project
     End Select
End Sub
```

In the `GetNewDatabaseName` function, notice the in-line error checking for the common dialog box. If the user clicks the Cancel button on the *Open* dialog box, error number 32755 occurs. The `On Error Resume Next` instructs Visual Basic to continue processing after the statement causing the error (the `dlgOpen.ShowOpen` statement). The next statement after ShowOpen should check the Err object to determine if the Cancel key was pressed.

```
Private Function GetNewDatabaseName() As String
    'Allow user to browse for the database
    Dim iResponse As Integer
    Dim stMsg     As String

    stMsg = "Database file not found." & vbCrLf & vbCrLf & _
          "Do you want to locate the file?"
    iResponse = MsgBox(stMsg, vbYesNo + vbQuestion, "File or Path not Found")
    If iResponse = vbNo Then
        GetNewDatabaseName = ""        'Set return filename to empty string
    Else                               'Allow browse for file name
        With dlgOpen
            .filename = datBooks.DatabaseName
            .Filter = "Database files (*.mdb)|*.mdb|All files (*.*)|*.*"
            On Error Resume Next                'Trap for the Cancel button
            .ShowOpen                           'Display Open dialog box
            If Err.Number = cdlCancel Then      'Cancel button pressed
                GetNewDatabaseName = ""         'Set return filename to empty string
            Else
                GetNewDatabaseName = .Filename  'Set return filename to selected file
            End If
        End With
    End If
End Function
```

Notice the actions taken after the user selects a new filename. The DatabaseName property of the data control is set to the Filename property of the common dialog control. However, that isn't enough to make the database open with the new filename—it must be opened with a `Refresh` method. Back in the Form_Load error handler, after getting the new filename, the `Resume` statement sends execution back to the statement that caused the original error.

Feedback 11.1

1. Write the statement(s) to display the record number in a label.
2. Write the statement(s) to instruct VB to ignore any error and just keep processing.
3. What statement(s) would appear in a data control's Validate event to prevent saving any changed data for all operations except an Update?
4. Write the statement(s) to check for an empty string in txtName (a data-bound control) in the txtName_LostFocus event procedure. If no data exists, display a message box.
5. Write an error-handling routine that executes a `Resume Next` for error numbers 3022, 3058, and 3109. For all other errors, display a message and exit the program.
6. Explain what will display for this statement:

```
MsgBox "Error " & Err.Number & ": " & Err.Description
```

Programming Example Showing Validation Techniques

This example starts with the hands-on programming example from Chapter 10 and adds numerous validation routines that combine many of the techniques discussed in the previous sections. Figure 11.7 shows the form for this project.

Figure 11.7

The form for the database validation example.

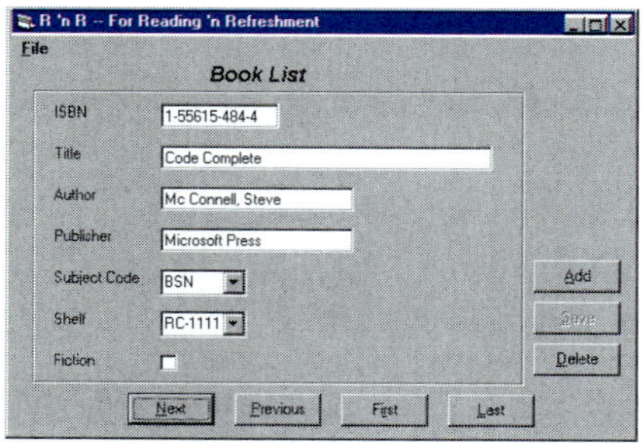


```
'Program Name:   R 'n R Book List Database
'Programmer:     J.C. Bradley
'Date:           September 1997
'Purpose:        Display and update book information in the
'                R 'n R Book database, using buttons for
'                navigation and combo boxes for field lookup
'Folder:         Ch1102

Option Explicit
Dim mbValidationError    As Boolean
```

```
Private Sub cmdAdd_Click()
    'Add a new record

    On Error GoTo HandleAddErrors
    If cmdAdd.Caption = "&Add" Then
        datBooks.Recordset.AddNew           'Clear out fields for new record
        txtISBN.Locked = False
        txtISBN.SetFocus
        DisableButtons                      'Disable navigation
        cmdSave.Enabled = True              'Enable the Save button
        cmdAdd.Caption = "&Cancel"          'Allow a Cancel option
    Else
        datBooks.Recordset.CancelUpdate     'Cancel the Add
        txtISBN.Locked = True
        EnableButtons                       'Enable navigation
        cmdSave.Enabled = False             'Disable the Save button
        cmdAdd.Caption = "&Add"             'Reset the Add button
    End If
```

```
cmdAdd_Click_Exit:
    Exit Sub

HandleAddErrors:
    Dim stMessage As String
    stMessage = "Cannot complete operation." & vbCrLf & vbCrLf _
            & Err.Description
    MsgBox stMessage, vbExclamation, "Database Error"
    On Error GoTo 0                    'Turn off error trapping
End Sub
```

```
Private Sub cmdDelete_Click()
    'Delete the current record

    On Error GoTo HandleDeleteError
    With datBooks.Recordset
        .Delete                  'Delete the current record
        .MoveNext                'Move to the following record
        If .EOF Then             'If last record deleted
            .MovePrevious
            If .BOF Then         'If BOF and EOF true, no records remain
                MsgBox "The recordset is empty.", vbInformation, "No records"
                DisableButtons
            End If
        End If
    End With

cmdDelete_Click_Exit:
    Exit Sub

HandleDeleteError:
    Dim stMessage As String
    stMessage = "Cannot complete operation." & vbCrLf & vbCrLf _
            & Err.Description
    MsgBox stMessage, vbExclamation, "Database Error"
    On Error GoTo 0                    'Turn off error trapping
End Sub
```

```
Private Sub cmdFirst_Click()
    'Move to first record

    On Error Resume Next
    datBooks.Recordset.MoveFirst
End Sub
```

```
Private Sub cmdLast_Click()
    'Move to last record

    On Error Resume Next
    datBooks.Recordset.MoveLast
End Sub
```

```
Private Sub cmdNext_Click()
    'Move to next record

    On Error Resume Next
    With datBooks.Recordset
        .MoveNext
        If .EOF Then
            .MoveFirst
        End If
    End With
End Sub
```

```
Private Sub cmdPrevious_Click()
    'Move to previous record

    On Error Resume Next
    With datBooks.Recordset
        .MovePrevious
        If .BOF Then
            .MoveLast
        End If
    End With
End Sub
```

```
Private Sub cmdSave_Click()
    'Save the current record

    On Error GoTo HandleSaveErrors
    datBooks.Recordset.Update
    If Not mbValidationError Then       'Passed the validation
        txtISBN.Locked = True           'Reset all
        EnableButtons
        cmdSave.Enabled = False
        cmdAdd.Caption = "&Add"
    End If

cmdSave_Click_Exit:
    Exit Sub

HandleSaveErrors:
    Dim stMessage As String
    Select Case Err.Number
    Case 3022                          'Duplicate key field
        stMessage = "Duplicate ISBN--Record not saved."
        MsgBox stMessage, vbExclamation, "Database Error"
        SetUpAddRecord               'Allow user to change ISBN and complete Add
        On Error GoTo 0              'Turn off error trapping to allow completion
```

```
    Case 3058, 3315              'No entry in key field
        stMessage = "ISBN must be completed before save."
        MsgBox stMessage, vbExclamation, "Database Error"
        SetUpAddRecord           'Give another chance to complete record
        On Error GoTo 0          'Turn off error trapping to allow completion
    Case Else
        stMessage = "Record could not be saved." & vbCrLf _
                    & Err.Description
        MsgBox stMessage, vbExclamation, "Database Error"
        datBooks.Recordset.CancelUpdate
        Resume Next
    End Select
End Sub
```

```
Private Sub datBooks_Validate(Action As Integer, Save As Integer)
    'This sub is entered for every action in the database.
    'Validate the data for an Add operation
    Dim stMessage As String

    mbValidationError = False                'Set flag for no errors
    If Action = vbDataActionUpdate Then      'A new Add is being saved
        With txtISBN
            If Len(.Text) <> 13 Then         'All ISBNs must be 13 characters
                stMessage = "Invalid ISBN"
                MsgBox stMessage, vbExclamation, "Data Entry Error"
                .SetFocus
                .SelStart = 0
                .SelLength = Len(.Text)
                mbValidationError = True
                Action = vbDataActionCancel
                Save = False
            End If
        End With
    End If
End Sub
```

```
Private Sub Form_Load()
    'Open the database

    On Error GoTo HandleFormLoadError
    datBooks.Refresh                         'Open the database

Form_Load_Exit:
    Exit Sub

HandleFormLoadError:
    Dim stNewDatabaseName   As String
```

```
    Select Case Err.Number
        Case 3004, 3024, 3044               'Database, file, or path not found
            stNewDatabaseName = GetNewDatabaseName
            If stNewDatabaseName = "" Then 'User canceled operation
                mnuFileExit_Click
            Else
                datBooks.DatabaseName = stNewDatabaseName
                Resume                      'Reopen the database
            End If
        Case Else
            MsgBox Err.Description, vbOKOnly + vbExclamation, "Unexpected Error"
            mnuFileExit_Click               'Exit the project
    End Select
End Sub
```

```
Private Sub mnuFileExit_Click()
    'Exit the project

    End
End Sub
```

```
Private Sub DisableButtons()
    'Disable navigation buttons

    cmdNext.Enabled = False
    cmdPrevious.Enabled = False
    cmdFirst.Enabled = False
    cmdLast.Enabled = False
    cmdDelete.Enabled = False
End Sub
```

```
Private Sub EnableButtons()
    'Enable navigation buttons

    cmdNext.Enabled = True
    cmdPrevious.Enabled = True
    cmdFirst.Enabled = True
    cmdLast.Enabled = True
    cmdDelete.Enabled = True
End Sub
```

```
Private Function GetNewDatabaseName() As String
     'Allow user to browse for the database
     Dim iResponse As Integer
     Dim stMsg     As String

     stMsg = "Database file not found." & vbCrLf & vbCrLf & _
             "Do you want to locate the file?"
     iResponse = MsgBox(stMsg, vbYesNo + vbQuestion, "File or Path not Found")
     If iResponse = vbNo Then
         GetNewDatabaseName = ""            'Set return filename to empty string
     Else                                   'Allow browse for file name
         With dlgOpen
             .filename = datBooks.DatabaseName
             .Filter = "Database files (*.mdb)|*.mdb|All files (*.*)|*.*"
             On Error Resume Next                'Trap for the Cancel button
             .ShowOpen                           'Display Open dialog box
             If Err.Number = cdlCancel Then      'Cancel button pressed
                 GetNewDatabaseName = ""         'Set return filename to empty string
             Else
                 GetNewDatabaseName = .filename  'Set return filename to selected file
             End If
         End With
     End If
End Function
```

```
Private Sub SetUpAddRecord()
     'Set up a new Add to allow the user another try
     Dim savISBN As String, savTitle As String, savAuthor As String
     Dim savPublisher As String, savSubject As String
     Dim savLocation As String, savFiction As Variant

     On Error Resume Next

     'Save the contents of the form controls
     savISBN = txtISBN.Text
     savTitle = txtTitle.Text
     savAuthor = txtAuthor.Text
     savPublisher = txtPublisher.Text
     savSubject = cboSubject.Text
     savLocation = cboLocation.Text
     savFiction = chkFiction.Value

     'Start a new Add
     datBooks.Recordset.AddNew
```

```
    'Place saved data back in form controls
    With txtISBN
        .Text = savISBN
        .SelStart = 0
        .SelLength = Len(.Text)
        .SetFocus
    End With
    txtTitle.Text = savTitle
    txtAuthor.Text = savAuthor
    txtPublisher.Text = savPublisher
    cboSubject.Text = savSubject
    cboLocation.Text = savLocation
    chkFiction.Value = savFiction
End Sub
```

Recordsets

Visual Basic supports three kinds of **recordsets**:

1. A **table recordset** represents a single table as it exists in a database file. Table recordsets are usually updateable, unless the file is locked or it is opened for ReadOnly.
2. A **dynaset** is a temporary set of data taken from one or more tables in the underlying file. A dynaset may be a query that was defined in an Access database, a single table, a subset of a table, or the result of joining multiple tables. Like a table, a dynaset is updateable if the file is not locked or opened for ReadOnly. The data in a dynaset are "live"—that is, any changes made to the data as your project is executing will appear in your recordset. *Note:* Some dynasets created from joining tables are nonupdateable; see "The SQL Select Statement—Examples" later in this chapter.
3. A **snapshot** recordset, like a dynaset, may be taken from one or more tables. The differences are that a snapshot is not updateable and also not live. You can think of a snapshot recordset like a photograph—a picture of reality at a given point in time.

The data control has a **RecordsetType property**, which you can set at design time or run time (Figure 11.8). The default type is dynaset. Table recordsets are faster than dynasets, but dynasets are more flexible, as you will see in the section "Creating a New Dynaset" later in this chapter. If you are planning to print a report, a snapshot is most efficient.

Figure 11.8

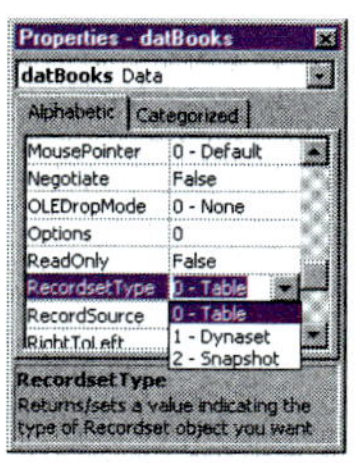

Set the RecordsetType property at design time or run time.

Searching for a Specific Record—Dynasets and Snapshots

You can search for a particular value in any field in a dynaset or snapshot. For example, you could request a certain name, account number, phone number, book title, author—any field stored in the database and bound to one of your controls. Use the **FindFirst**, **FindLast**, **FindNext**, and **FindPrevious methods** to locate any data.

The FindFirst, FindLast, FindNext, and FindPrevious Methods—General Form

```
datControl.Recordset.{FindFirst | FindLast | FindNext | FindPrevious} Criteria
```

The criteria specify the field name from the database and the contents for which you are searching. When we cover SQL statements later in this chapter, you will see that the criteria in a Find is like a Where clause in SQL, but without the word *Where*.

The Find methods may be used on a dynaset or a snapshot recordset, but not on a table recordset. (For tables, the `Seek` method is used. `Seek` is covered later in this chapter.)

The FindFirst, FindLast, FindNext, and FindPrevious Methods—Example

```
datBooks.Recordset.FindFirst "ISBN = '123-456-789-X'"
datMembers.Recordset.FindNext "FirstName = 'Dennis'"
datMembers.Recordset.FindFirst "FirstName = '" & txtName.Text & "'"
datMembers.Recordset.FindFirst "Amount > 100"
datMembers.Recordset.FindNext "Amount > " & txtAmount.Text
```

For a string search criterion, the string must be enclosed in single quotes, as in the first two examples. In the third example, the confusing mix of quotes produces the correct search string. If txtName.Text holds the name "Theresa", then the search string is `FirstName = 'Theresa'`.

When searching in a numeric field, do not enclose the numeric value in single quotes. The fourth example above includes a numeric constant, and the fifth example searches for the value entered in a text box. Assuming that the text box holds the number "123", the search string will be `Amount > 123`.

If you are searching a field which has any spaces in its name, the field name must be enclosed in square brackets:

```
datEmployees.Recordset.FindFirst "[Pay Rate] > 30000"
```

The `FindNext` and `FindPrevious` operations always begin with the current record and move in the direction indicated. `FindFirst` begins at the beginning of the file, and `FindLast` begins its search at the end of the file.

For the comparison operator, you may use =, >, <, <=, >=, <>, `Like`, `Between`, and `In`. To use the `Like` operator, use an asterisk as a wildcard character to match any character(s) in that position.

Examples

```
"PayRate <= 50000"
"LastName Like 'Br*'"          'Find all last names beginning with "Br"
"Amount Between 50 And 100"
"LastName Not Like 'A*'"       'All last names not beginning with "A"
"LastName In('Adams', 'Baker', 'Charles')   'All matching last names
```

The NoMatch Property

After you attempt to Find a record, always test the **NoMatch property** of the data control. When you begin a Find, NoMatch is set to False. If no record is found to meet your criteria, NoMatch is set to True. If a match is found, the record becomes current and is displayed in the data-bound controls. If no match is found, the current record number is unpredictable. A good way to take care of a no-match situation is to use a bookmark.

Bookmarks

You can set a bookmark on any record in a dynaset and use the bookmark later to return to that record. Set a variable equal to the recordset's **BookMark property** to save it for future reference. Any time you set the BookMark property to the variable name, the bookmarked record becomes the current record. *Note:* Use variant datatype for a variable to hold a bookmark.

```
'Make sure RecordsetType is set to Dynaset for this to work
 Dim vBookMark       As Variant

 vBookMark = datBooks.Recordset.BookMark       'Save record number _
                                                in bookmark variable
 datBooks.RecordSet.FindFirst "Title Like 'How*'"
 If datBooks.RecordSet.NoMatch = True Then
     MsgBox "No record was found.", vbInformation, "No Match"
     datBooks.Recordset.BookMark = vBookMark 'Return to bookmarked _
                                              record
 End If
```

Seeking with Table Indexes—Table Recordsets

The fastest way to search for a particular record is to use the **`Seek` method**, which can be used only with a Table recordset type. The `Seek` method uses indexes for the search, which is much faster than checking every record in the table as you do in a `Find`.

In order to do a `Seek`, the field (or fields) on which you search must be defined with an index. With the Learning Edition of Visual Basic and the data control, you can use only those indexes already defined in the database; with the Professional or Enterprise Edition, you can create your own indexes at run time using DAO (data access objects). *Note:* DAO is beyond the scope of this text.

The Seek Method—General Form

```
datControl.Recordset.Seek ComparisonOperator, FieldValue
```

The comparison operator must be enclosed in quotation marks and can be any one of these: "=", ">=",">","<=","<". The FieldValue is the actual value for which to search. String literals must be enclosed in quotation marks; numeric values must not be so enclosed.

The Seek Method—Examples

```
datBooks.Recordset.Seek  "=",  "0-671-66398-4"
datBills.Recordset.Seek  ">=", 1 'Find first record greater than or _
                         equal to 1 in the first position of the key
datCustomers.Recordset.Seek ">=", stSearchString
```

Before you can `Seek`, you *must* first set the recordset's **Index property** to the name of an index in your table. In an Access table, the index on the primary key is called *PrimaryKey.* If other indexes are also defined in the table, usually the index name is the same as the field name.

Notice in the following program example that you can also use the BookMark and NoMatch properties with the `Seek` method.

```
Private Sub cmdSearch_Click()
    'Search for a book, based on its ISBN (the primary key)
    'Make sure RecordsetType is set to Table for this to work
    Dim vBookMark       As Variant
    Dim stISBN          As String

    vBookMark = datBooks.Recordset.Bookmark
    stISBN = InputBox("Enter ISBN", "Find a Book")
    datBooks.Recordset.Index = "PrimaryKey"    'Set the index
    datBooks.Recordset.Seek ">=", stISBN       'Seek the record
    If datBooks.Recordset.NoMatch Then
        MsgBox "No match found", vbExclamation, "Find a book"
        datBooks.Recordset.Bookmark = vBookMark
    End If
End Sub
```

Reordering a Table Recordset

You saw in the preceding section that you can select an index field for a table recordset. Changing the current index effectively changes the order in which records are displayed. Although the physical order of the records does not change, as you navigate through a table the records appear in order by the index.

In the following example, the table may be displayed in ISBN order (the primary key), in Title order (a secondary index defined in the table), or in Entry order, which is the order in which the records were added to the table.

For this continuing Books table example for R 'n R, an *Organize* menu is added to the form (Figure 11.9). The user can choose to display the records in order by ISBN, by Title, or in Entry order.

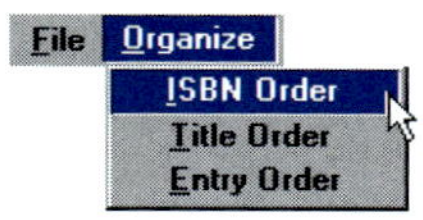

Figure 11.9

The Organize menu offers choices to display the Books table in three orders. Change the recordset's Index property to change the order.

```
Private Sub mnuOrgISBN_Click()
    'Set the index for ISBN Order

    On Error GoTo HandleErrors
    datBooks.Recordset.Index = "PrimaryKey"
    Exit Sub

HandleErrors:
    MsgBox "That index does not exist", vbExclamation, "Index Error"
    On Error GoTo 0
End Sub
```

```
Private Sub mnuOrgTitle_Click()
    'Set the index for Title Order

    On Error GoTo HandleErrors
    datBooks.Recordset.Index = "Title"
    Exit Sub

HandleErrors:
    MsgBox "That index does not exist", vbExclamation, "Index Error"
    On Error GoTo 0
End Sub
```

```
Private Sub mnuOrgEntry_Click()
    'Set the index for Data-entry Order

    On Error GoTo HandleErrors
    datBooks.Recordset.Index = ""
    Exit Sub
```

```
HandleErrors:
    MsgBox "That index does not exist", vbExclamation, "Index Error"
    On Error GoTo 0
End Sub
```

Feedback 11.2

1. What type(s) of recordset is always read-only? What type(s) may be updateable *or* read-only?
2. In what type(s) of recordset is the data "live;" that is, any changes will be automatically saved in the file?
3. In what type(s) of recordset can the `FindFirst`, `FindLast`, `FindNext`, and `FindPrevious` methods be used?
4. In what type(s) of recordset can the `Seek` method be used?
5. In what type(s) of recordset can you set the Index property to a different index?
6. Write the code statement using `FindFirst` to find the first record with a name beginning with "K" in a CustomerName field. Make up any needed control or variable names.
7. Write the code statement using `Seek` to find the first record with a name beginning with "K" in a CustomerName field. Make up any needed control or variable names; the table has an index defined for the CustomerName field.

Working with Database Fields

In the sections that follow, we will be referencing individual fields from a recordset by name, reading the contents of fields, loading field values into a list box, and selecting records using criteria.

Referring to Database Fields

At times you may want to refer to a single field in the current recordset. Use either of these formats to refer to a field:

```
datControl.Recordset!FieldName
```

or

```
datControl.Recordset("FieldName")
```

If the field name in the table is more than one word, you must enclose the name in quotes or square brackets:

```
datBiblio.Recordset![Year Published]
```

or

```
datBiblio.Recordset("Year Published")
```

or

```
datBiblio.Recordset!"Year Published"
```

Loading Database Fields into a List Box

In the earlier examples for `Find` and `Seek`, the user entered the search value into an input box. Two better approaches might be to offer a list of possible values or use a combo box that gives the user the opportunity to select *or* enter a new value. To fill a list with values from a recordset, use a `Do/Loop`. You can place the loop in the Form_Activate procedure or in the Form_Load procedure. Note that by default files are opened between the Load and Activate events. If you prefer to fill the list in the Form_Load procedure, use a `Refresh` method to open the file first. When you decide whether to fill the list in the Form_Load or Form_Activate procedure, remember that Form_Load occurs once, the first time you show a form. Form_Activate occurs each time you show the form. If the data might have changed since the form was last displayed, use the Form_Activate procedure.

```
Private Sub Form_Load()
     'Fill the Author list

     With datBooks
         .Refresh                    'Open database

         Do Until .Recordset.EOF 'Fill the list
             If .Recordset!Author <> "" Then
                 cboAuthor.AddItem .Recordset!Author
             End If
             .Recordset.MoveNext
         Loop
     End With
End Sub
```

Creating a New Dynaset

Recall that a dynaset is a temporary set of data from a database. It may be a complete table, a subset of only certain fields of a table, or only the records that match a given criterion. A dynaset may also be the result of joining the data from multiple tables. As an example of a joined dynaset, consider an application to produce invoices in which a customer number must be joined with name and address information and product codes must be joined with product description and pricing information.

Using SQL

Visual Basic uses Structured Query Language (SQL) to create new dynasets. **SQL** (pronounced either "sequel" or "S, Q, L") is an industry-standard language for accessing relational databases. Entire books and courses are devoted to using SQL. In this brief introduction, we will use SQL to select fields and records from a table and to join the fields from two tables. For more information, see Visual Basic's *Help* or one of the many books available, such as *The Practical SQL Handbook* by Bowman, Emerson, and Darnovsky.

Setting a New RecordSource

Creating a new dynaset is a two-step process. You must set the data control's RecordSource property to an SQL query and then reopen the recordset using the `Refresh` method.

In the following example the Author and Title fields are taken from the Books table, and the Subject is taken from the Subjects table. The Subject Code is used to match the records from the two tables.

```
Dim stSQL              As String

stSQL = "Select Author, Title, Subject From Books, Subjects " & _
            "Where Books.Subject_Code = Subjects.SubjectCode"
datBooks.Recordsource = stSQL        'Set new RecordSource
datBooks.Refresh                     'Open the recordset
```

Format of SQL Select Statements

SQL `Select` statements create a new recordset, based on the criteria you specify. `Select` statements can get quite complicated and can be used to join multiple tables or to group and sort the records. These examples will use some of the basic capabilities of SQL statements. (*Note:* Not all options of the `Select` statement are included here.)

The SQL Select Statement—General Form

```
Select [Distinct] FieldList From TableNames
 Where SearchConditions
 Group By FieldList
 Having GroupCriteria
 Order By FieldList
```

For the FieldList, you can list the field names or use an asterisk to indicate all fields from the named table(s). Multiple-word field names must be enclosed in square brackets.

The optional Distinct drops out duplicates so that no two records are alike.

The SQL Select Statement—Examples

```
Select * From Books

Select * From Books, Subjects
  Where Books.Subject_Code = Subjects.SubjectCode
  Order By Title
```

Note that the second example joins the Books and Subject tables so that the actual name of the subject, not just the Subject Code, can be displayed. This easy method for joining tables creates a recordset that is nonupdateable. To make a joined recordset updateable, you must use the Join clause of the SQL Select statement, which is not covered here.

Tip

For help writing SQL queries, see the Programming Hints at the end of this chapter.

Comparing Database Fields to Visual Basic Fields

The syntax for specifying a field name in an SQL Where clause depends on whether the field is in the table or is a Visual Basic variable or property. The following examples compare a table name to a variable and to a property:

```
'Compare to a string field
stSQL = "Select * From Books " & _
        "Where Subject = '" & stSubject & "'"
datBooks.Recordsource = stSQL
datBooks.Refresh

'Compare to a property
stSQL = "Select * From Books " & _
        "Where Title Like '" & txtSearchTitle.Text & "*'"
```

If you are joining multiple tables, specify field names preceded by the table name:

```
stSQL = "Select * From Books, Subjects " & _
        "Where Books.Title Like '" & txtSearchTitle.Text & "*'" & _
        "And Books.Subject_Code = Subjects.SubjectCode"
```

Check for an Empty Recordset

When you open a recordset, especially one in which the user is searching for particular values, it's quite possible for the recordset to be empty—that is, no records matched the criteria. If a recordset is empty, both BOF and EOF are True after the `Refresh` method.

```
stSQL = "Select * From Books " & _
        "Where Subject = '" & stSubject & "'"
datBooks.Recordsource = stSQL
datBooks.Refresh
If datBooks.Recordset.BOF and datBooks.Recordset.EOF Then
    MsgBox "No records match " & stSubject, vbExclamation, "No Match"
End If
```

Feedback 11.3

Use these two tables to answer the following questions. Assume that the form contains a data control called datInfo.

Table Names:

Fields:

Customers
Name
Address
ZIP
Phone

Cities
ZIPCode
City
State

1. Write the Visual Basic statements to open a recordset with just the Name and Phone fields from the Customers table.
2. Write the statements to open a recordset of all fields in the Cities table.
3. Write the statements to create a recordset combining all of the fields from the two tables. Include a Where clause to join the two tables on the ZIP code.
4. Write the statements to create a recordset combining the Name, Address, City, State, and ZIP.
5. Modify the code for the previous question to make sure there are no duplicate records.
6. Write the code to check for an empty recordset. Display a message box if the recordset is empty.

Your Hands-On Programming Example

In this project for R 'n R you will create a project that allows the user to select books by author or by subject. The main form displays the complete information about a book (including the complete Subject Name, not just the Code). A *Select* menu allows the user to choose *Select Records* or *All Records.* Be sure to include a check mark next to the currently selected option.

A second form holds dropdown combo boxes filled with the author names and subjects. The user can select either or both (or partial names), and the first form will reappear with only the requested books.

Hints: To have data-bound controls on two forms, both forms must have data controls. A data-bound control must be bound to a data control on the same form. In code you can refer to controls on other forms using the exclamation point:

```
frmBookData!datBooks.RecordSource = ...
```

Planning the Project

Sketch the main form (Figure 11.10) and the selection form (Figure 11.11). Your users check over the designs, and you are ready to proceed.

Figure 11.10

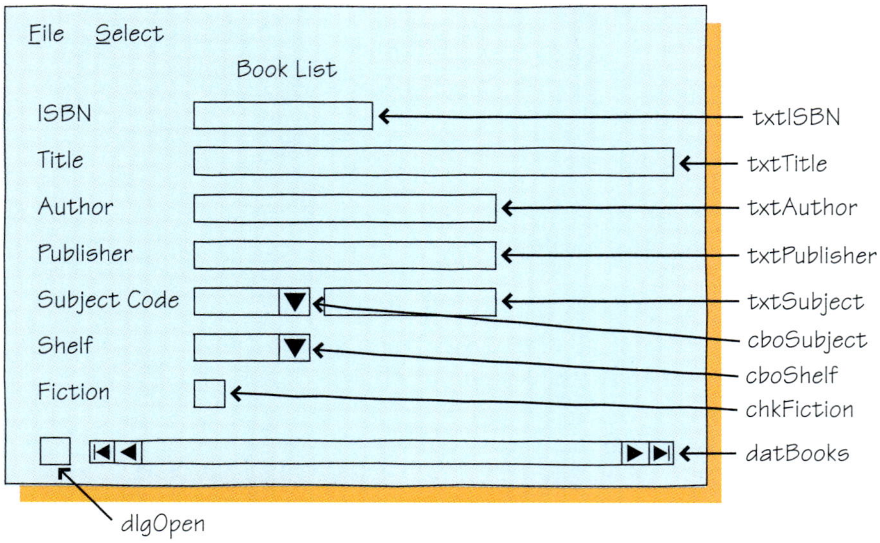

A planning sketch for the main form for the hands-on programming example.

Figure 11.11

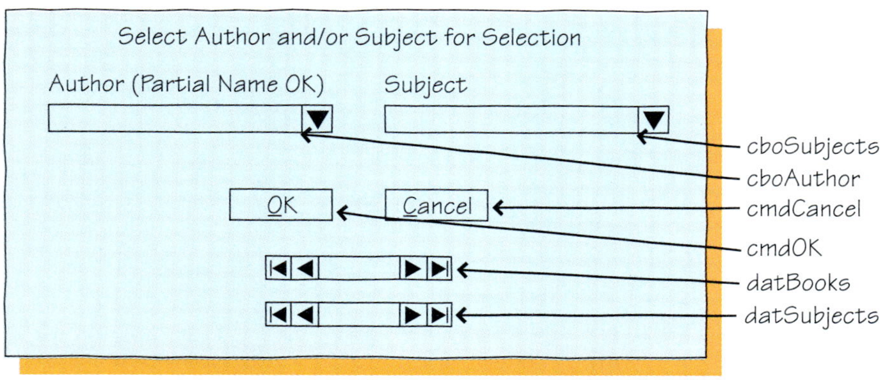

A planning sketch for the selection form for the hands-on programming example.

Plan the Objects and Properties: Main Form

Object	Property	Setting
frmBookData	Name	frmBookData
	Caption	R 'n R—for Reading 'n Refreshment
datBooks	Name	datBooks
	Connect	Access
	DatabaseName	RnRBooks.mdb
	RecordsetType	Dynaset
	RecordSource	Books
	Visible	True
Label1	Caption	ISBN
Label2	Caption	Title
Label3	Caption	Author
Label4	Caption	Publisher
Label5	Caption	Subject Code
Label6	Caption	Shelf
Label7	Caption	Fiction
txtISBN	Name	txtISBN
	Text	(blank)
	DataSource	datBooks
	DataField	ISBN
txtTitle	Name	txtTitle
	Text	(blank)
	DataSource	datBooks
	DataField	Title
txtAuthor	Name	txtAuthor
	Text	(blank)
	DataSource	datBooks
	DataField	Author
txtPublisher	Name	txtPublisher
	Text	(blank)
	DataSource	datBooks
	DataField	Publisher
cboSubject	Name	cboSubject
	Text	(blank)

(continued)

Object	Property	Setting
cboSubject (*cont'd*)	DataSource	datBooks
	DataField	Subject_Code
	List	ART BSS FNT RLG RMN HMR SCF BSN PHL EDC MST SLH
txtSubject	Name	txtSubject
	Text	(blank)
	DataSource	datBooks
	DataField	Subject (Not shown in list, must type it in.)
cboShelf	Name	cboShelf
	Text	(blank)
	DataSource	datBooks
	DataField	Shelf_Location
	List	RC-1111 RC-1112 RC-1113 RC-1114
chkFiction	Name	chkFiction
	Caption	(blank)
	DataSource	datBooks
	DataField	Fiction
dlgOpen	Name	dlgOpen
	DialogTitle	"Open Database File"
	CancelError	True
mnuFile	Name	mnuFile
	Caption	&File
mnuFileExit	Name	mnuFileExit
	Caption	E&xit

(*continued*)

Object	Property	Setting
mnuSelect	Name	mnuSelect
	Caption	&Select
mnuSelectRecords	Name	mnuSelectedRecords
	Caption	&Selected Records
mnuSelectAll	Name	mnuSelectAll
	Caption	Show &All Records
	Checked	True

Plan the Objects and Properties: Selection Form

Object	Property	Setting
frmSelect	Name	frmSelect
	Caption	Select Books
Label1	Caption	Select Author and/or Subject for Selection
Label2	Caption	Author (Partial Name OK)
Label3	Caption	Subject
datBooks	Name	datBooks
	Connect	Access
	DatabaseName	RnRbooks.mdb
	RecordsetType	Dynaset
	RecordSource	Books
	Visible	False
datSubjects	Name	datSubjects
	Connect	Access
	DatabaseName	RnRBooks.mdb
	RecordsetType	Dynaset
	RecordSource	Subjects
	Visible	False
cboAuthor	Name	cboAuthor

(continued)

Object	Property	Setting
cboAuthor *(cont'd)*	Style	0 - Dropdown Combo
	DataSource	datBooks
	DataField	Author
	Sorted	True
cboSubject	Name	cboSubject
	Style	0 - Dropdown Combo
	DataSource	datSubjects
	DataField	Subject
	Sorted	True
cmdCancel	Name	cmdCancel
	Caption	&Cancel
	Cancel	True
cmdOK	Name	cmdOK
	Caption	&OK
	Default	True

Plan the Event Procedures: Main Form

Object	Procedure	Actions
frmBookData	Form_Load	Call DisplayAllRecords.

mnuSelectRecords	Click	Display selection form as modal.
		If selection made Then
		  Check Selection menu command.
		  Uncheck All menu command.
		If empty recordset Then
		  Display error message.
		  Call DisplayAllRecords.

mnuSelectAll	Click	Call DisplayAllRecords.
mnuFileExit	Click	End.

(General)	DisplayAllRecords	Set RecordSource to SQL string.
		Refresh.
		Check All menu command.
		Uncheck Selected menu command.
		Error handler:
		  Case File not Found
		    Call GetNewDatabaseName.
		  Case Else
		    Display error message.
		  Call mnuFileExit_Click.

(continued)

Object	Procedure	Actions
	GetNewDatabaseName	Display MsgBox "Locate File?"

		If response is No Then
		 Set return filename to empty string.
		Else
		 Display Open dialog box.
		 If Cancel pressed
		  Set return filename to empty string.
		Else
		  Set return filename to selected file.

Plan the Event Procedures: Selection Form

Object	Procedure	Actions
frmSelect	Form_Activate	Clear cboAuthor.
		Set SQL string and open database.

		Do until EOF
		 If Author not empty Then
		  Add Author to cboAuthor.
		 End If
		 Move to next record.
		Loop

		Clear cboSubject.
		Open database.
		Do until EOF
		Add Subject to cboSubject.
		Loop
cmdCancel	Click	Set gbSelectionMade to False.
		Hide the select form.
cmdOK	Click	If Selection made from cboAuthor Then Set bSelectAuthor = True.
		If Selection made from cboSubject Then Set bSelectSubject = True.
		If both Author and Subject selected Then Set up SQL string. ElseIf only Author selected Then Set up SQL string. ElseIf only Subject selected Then Set up SQL string.
		If any selection was made Then Set Recordsource and open the database.
		Hide the form.
cmdCancel	Click	Set gbSelectionMade = False.
		Hide the form.

Write the Project

After completing the planning steps, it's time to create the forms, following the sketches in Figures 11.10 and 11.11. Figures 11.12 and 11.13 show the completed forms.

Figure 11.12

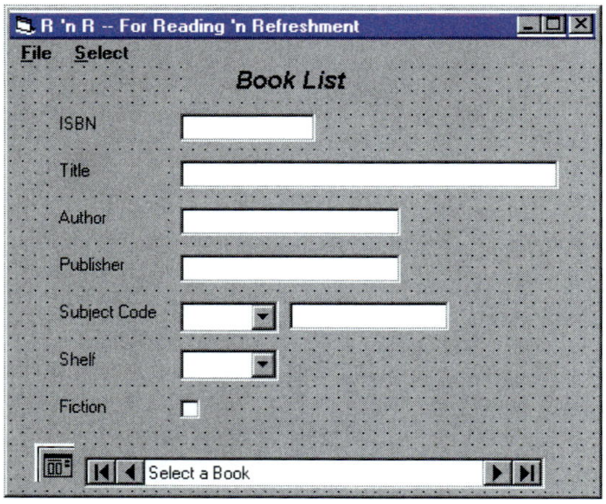

The main form for the hands-on programming example.

Figure 11.13

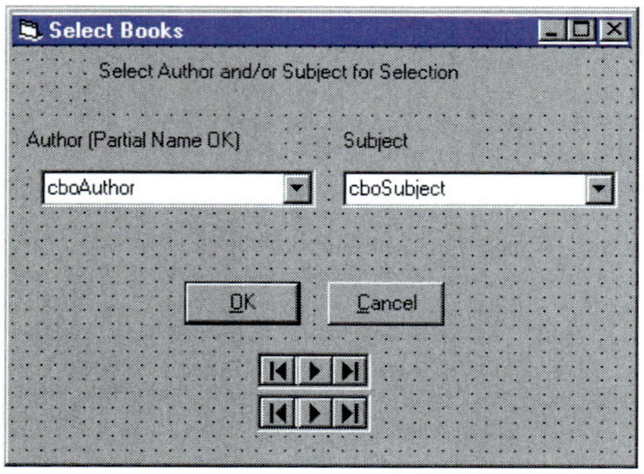

The selection form for the hands-on programming example.

- Set the properties of each of the objects, according to your plan.
- Write the code. Working from the pseudocode, write each event procedure.
- Thoroughly test the project. Make sure to set the data control to a nonexistant filename to test your file open routine. Test all varieties of selection, as well as canceling the selection form.

The Project Coding Solution

The Main Form

```
'Project:        R 'n R Book List Selection
'Programmer:     J.C. Bradley
'Date:           December 1997
'Purpose:        Display book information in the R 'n R Book database.
'                Combine fields from two tables on the main form.
'                Allow user to enter criteria and create new recordsets.
'Folder:         Ch1104

Option Explicit
```

```
Private Sub Form_Load()
     'Set the Recordsource for the data control

     DisplayAllRecords
End Sub
```

```
Private Sub mnuFileExit_Click()
     'Exit the project

     End
End Sub
```

```
Private Sub mnuSelectRecords_Click()
     'Display Selection form and setup Recordset
     Dim stSQL                As String

     frmSelect.Show vbModal                'Display the form as modal
     If gbSelectionMade = True Then        'Successful selection
          mnuSelectRecords.Checked = True
          mnuSelectAll.Checked = False
     End If
     If datBooks.Recordset.BOF And datBooks.Recordset.EOF Then
          MsgBox "No records match your criteria", vbExclamation, _
          "No Matching Records"
          DisplayAllRecords
     End If
End Sub
```

```
Private Sub mnuSelectAll_Click()
     'Display all records in table

     DisplayAllRecords
End Sub
```

```
Private Sub DisplayAllRecords()
     'Display all records in table
     Dim stSQL              As String
     Dim stMsg              As String
     Dim iResponse          As Integer

     On Error GoTo HandleErrors
     stSQL = "Select * From Books, Subjects " & _
             "Where Books.Subject_Code = Subjects.SubjectCode"
     datBooks.RecordSource = stSQL
     datBooks.Refresh
     mnuSelectAll.Checked = True
     mnuSelectRecords.Checked = False

DisplayAllRecordsExit:
     Exit Sub

HandleErrors:
     Select Case Err.Number
         Case 3004, 3024, 3044              'Database, file, or path not found
              gstNewDatabaseName = GetNewDatabaseName
              If gstNewDatabaseName = "" Then   'User canceled operation
                   mnuFileExit_Click
              Else
                  datBooks.DatabaseName = gstNewDatabaseName
                  Resume                     'Reopen the database
              End If
         Case Else
              MsgBox Err.Description, vbOKOnly + vbExclamation, "Unexpected Error"
              mnuFileExit_Click              'Exit the project
     End Select
End Sub
```

```
Private Function GetNewDatabaseName() As String
     'Allow user to browse for the database
     Dim iResponse          As Integer
     Dim stMsg              As String

     stMsg = "Database file not found." & vbCrLf & vbCrLf & _
           "Do you want to locate the file?"
     iResponse = MsgBox(stMsg, vbYesNo + vbQuestion, "File or Path not Found")
```

```
    If iResponse = vbNo Then
        GetNewDatabaseName = ""           'Set return filename to empty string
    Else                                  'Allow browse for file name
        With dlgOpen
            .filename = datBooks.DatabaseName
            .Filter = "Database files (*.mdb)|*.mdb|All files (*.*)|*.*"
            On Error Resume Next          'Trap for the Cancel button
            .ShowOpen                     'Display Open dialog box
            If Err.Number = cdlCancel Then   'Cancel button pressed
                GetNewDatabaseName = "" 'Set return filename to empty string
            Else
                GetNewDatabaseName = .filename 'Set return filename to selected file
            End If
        End With
    End If
End Function
```

The Selection Form

```
'Module:          Select.frm
'Programmer:      J.C. Bradley
'Date:            December 1997
'Purpose:         Form to allow selection of records in
'                 the R 'n R Books database using SQL queries.
'Folder:          Ch1104
Option Explicit
```

```
Private Sub cmdCancel_Click()
    'Exit the form

    gbSelectionMade = False                       'No selection made
    Me.Hide
End Sub
```

```
Private Sub cmdOK_Click()
    'Setup new Recordset based on selections

    Dim stSQL               As String
    Dim bSelectAuthor       As Boolean
    Dim bSelectSubject      As Boolean

    If cboAuthor.Text <> "" Then                  'New author selected
        bSelectAuthor = True
    End If
    If cboSubject.Text <> "" Then                 'New subject selected
        bSelectSubject = True
    End If
    gbSelectionMade = False                       'No selection made yet
```

```
    If bSelectAuthor And bSelectSubject Then     'Both selected
        stSQL = "Select * from Books, Subjects " & _
                "Where Books.Author Like '" & cboAuthor.Text & "*' " & _
                "And Subjects.Subject like '" & cboSubject.Text & "*' " & _
                "And Subjects.SubjectCode = Books.Subject_Code"
        gbSelectionMade = True                   'Successful selection
    ElseIf bSelectAuthor Then                    'Author only selected
        stSQL = "Select * from Books, Subjects " & _
                "Where Books.Author Like '" & cboAuthor.Text & "*' " & _
                "And Subjects.SubjectCode = Books.Subject_Code"
        gbSelectionMade = True                   'Successful selection
    ElseIf bSelectSubject Then                   'Subject only selected
        stSQL = "Select * from Books, Subjects " & _
                "Where Subjects.Subject Like '" & cboSubject.Text & "*' " & _
                "And Subjects.SubjectCode = Books.Subject_Code"
        gbSelectionMade = True                   'Successful selection
    End If
    If gbSelectionMade = True Then               'Successful selection
        frmBookData!datBooks.RecordSource = stSQL
        frmBookData!datBooks.Refresh             'Reopen main database
    End If
    Me.Hide                                      'Exit this form
End Sub
```

```
Private Sub Form_Activate()
    'Fill (or Refill) the lists

    Dim stSQL As String

    'Fill Author list
    cboAuthor.Clear                              'Clear out prior contents
    stSQL = "Select Distinct Author From Books "
    With datBooks
        .RecordSource = stSQL
        .Refresh                                 'Reopen table for authors
        Do Until .Recordset.EOF                  'Fill the list
            If .Recordset!Author <> "" Then
                cboAuthor.AddItem .Recordset!Author
            End If
            .Recordset.MoveNext
        Loop
    End With

    'Fill Subject list
    cboSubject.Clear                             'Clear out prior contents
    With datSubjects
        .Refresh                                 'Reopen table for subjects
        Do Until .Recordset.EOF                  'Fill the list
            cboSubject.AddItem .Recordset!Subject
            .Recordset.MoveNext
        Loop
    End With
End Sub
```

```
Private Sub Form_Load()
    'Get new database filename if changed

    If gstNewDatabaseName <> "" Then            'New file selected
        datBooks.DatabaseName = gstNewDatabaseName
        datSubjects.DatabaseName = gstNewDatabaseName
    End If
End Sub
```

The Standard Code Module

```
'Module:        Books.Bas
'Programmer:    J.C. Bradley
'Date:          December 1997
'Purpose:       Declare global variables for Book database.
'Folder:     Ch1104
Option Explicit

Public gbSelectionMade      As Boolean
Public gstNewDatabaseName   As String
```

Programming Hints

Trapping Database Errors

It's important to place an `On Error` statement in any procedure that does database access. You can write one error-handling sub procedure and include it in a standard code module to be used by all forms in your project. You might consider writing one fairly robust error-handling code module and adding it to all your database projects.

You must pass the error number to the error-handling procedure. Also consider passing a variable that indicates whether a `Resume`, `Resume Next`, `On Error Go To 0`, or program cancellation is needed.

You will still need considerable coding in your database to handle subs. You might consider setting up a template for the error handling and copying it into all routines that do database access. Then you can modify the action you take in each sub, depending on the situation.

Here is a suggested starting place for error handling:

```
Private Sub DatabaseAccess()
    On Error GoTo HandleErrors
    'Do database processing here

DatabaseAccessExit:
    Exit Sub
```

```
HandleErrors:
    Dim ErrorNumber    As Integer
    Dim ErrorOutcome   As Integer
    ErrorNumber = Err.Number
    HandleAllErrors ErrorNumber, ErrorOutcome   'Call Handler
    Select Case ErrorOutcome
        Case Outcome_Resume
            Resume
        Case OutcomeResumeNext
            Resume Next
        Case OutcomeGoTo0
            On Error GoTo 0
        Case OutcomeCancel
            mnuFileExit_Click
    End Select
End Sub
```

```
'Module:        Error handler standard code module
Public Const OUTCOME_RESUME = 0
Public Const OUTCOME_RESUMENEXT = 1
Public Const OUTCOME_GOTO0 = 2
Public Const OUTCOME_CANCEL = 3

Sub HandleAllErrors(ErrorNumber, ErrorOutcome)
    Select Case ErrorNumber
        Case 3004, 3024 'File not found
            ErrorOutcome = OUTCOME_CANCEL
        Case 3021       'No current record
            ErrorOutcome = OUTCOME_RESUMENEXT
    '...
End Sub
```

Advanced Database Processing

If you plan to do serious database application development, you will want to purchase the VB Professional Edition or Enterprise Edition. With these versions you can define and use Data Access Objects; create a new database; modify the structure of a database, including adding and deleting fields; create a new index; and use open database connectivity (ODBC) to connect to external databases.

Get Help Coding SQL Statements

You can get some help writing SQL queries. If you have Microsoft Access installed on your computer, you can open the database in Access and create a query that displays the data you want. Then click the SQL button in Query Design and view the SQL statement. You can copy and paste the statement into Visual Basic (where it will require a little modification). You can also give the Access Query a name, save the file, and then use the query name for the RecordSource property of the data control.

The VisData Add-In to VB can also help you write and test SQL statements. Open VisData, open your database, and write your SQL queries in the SQL window. When you have a query that works correctly, copy and paste it into your VB code.

Summary

1. The DB Grid control can be used to display and/or update database recordsets. The grid displays records in rows and columns, resembling a spreadsheet.
2. Use the data control's `Refresh` method to open or reopen the database.
3. The data control's RecordCount property holds the number of records in a recordset; the AbsolutePosition property holds the record number of the current record. AbsolutePosition is zero based.
4. The data control's Reposition event occurs each time a new record becomes current. Use the event procedure to perform any checking on the individual record.
5. The Locked property of a text box can be set to prevent any changes to the contents.
6. Use the data control's Validate event to check for errors. You can use the Action argument to cancel the operation and the Save argument to prevent changed data from being written into the file.
7. A good location to validate the contents of a text box is the control's LostFocus event.
8. Most procedures that perform database access need error trapping with an `On Error` statement.
9. When the user clicks Save after an Add operation, you must trap for a duplicate or missing key field.
10. The three types of recordsets are tables, dynasets, and snapshots. Tables and dynasets are live and can be updated; snapshots represent an unchangeable picture of the data at one point in time.
11. The `FindFirst`, `FindLast`, `FindNext`, and `FindPrevious` methods may be used to search for any value in any field of a dynaset or snapshot recordset. The NoMatch property is set to True if a match is not made.
12. Use the recordset's Bookmark property to store or set the current record number.
13. To search for a particular record in a table recordset, set the recordset's Index property to an existing index name and Seek for a matching value in the key field.
14. Display a table recordset in a different order by changing the Index property to an existing index name.
15. Visual Basic uses SQL to create new recordsets. Set the data control's RecordSource property to an SQL query and execute a `Refresh` method.
16. You can write a generalized error-handling procedure in a standard code module, add it to each project that performs database access, and call the procedure when needed.

Key Terms

Review Questions

1. When would it be a good idea use a grid control?
2. When does the Validate event occur? What are the Action and Save arguments passed by the Validate procedure?
3. Explain the differences among tables, dynasets, and snapshots.
4. For which type(s) of recordsets is a Find valid (`FindFirst`, `FindNext`, `FindLast`, or `FindPrevious`)? What types of data can be searched for with a Find?
5. For which type(s) of recordsets is a `Seek` valid? Which fields in a recordset can be searched with a `Seek`?
6. What is SQL and how is it used in Visual Basic?

Programming Exercises

11.1 *Grid*: Write a project that will display the Publishers table in a grid. Use the Biblio.mdb sample database that comes with Visual Basic. Make sure that the grid cells are large enough to display all the data, and display the record number and record count in the caption of the data control.

The Biblio.mdb database should be in the VB folder, the folder where Visual Basic is installed on your system.

Note: The Biblio.mdb database included with VB4 was 288 KB, small enough to easily fit on a diskette. The version included with VB5 is 3.5 MB—too large for a diskette. The older version is included on your Student Diskette. The two versions of the file have the same structure; the size difference is due to the large number of records added to the newer version.

11.2 *Validation*: Modify project 10.2 or 10.3, which maintain the Subjects table in the R 'n R database. Validation required: Do not allow the user to change the Subject Code (the primary key) except during an Add. If the database isn't found on the open, display an error message and the *Open File* dialog box so the user can select another file. Make sure that no error can cause a run-time error. Do not allow a duplicate key field or deletion of the last record to cancel the project.

If you are modifying Exercise 10.2, add a Cancel button to allow the user to back out of an Add operation.

11.3 *Validation and Find*: Modify project 10.5, which maintains the Publishers table in the Biblio.mdb sample database. Include validation: Do not allow any run-time errors; the primary key field (PubID) cannot be changed except during an Add. Do not allow a duplicate key field or deletion of the last record to cancel the project.

Include menu choices or command buttons to search for a name or a company name using a Find.

Note: See the note in Exercise 11.1 about the size of the file.

11.4 *Reorder by Index:* Write a project that will display a table in order by one of three fields. Use the Titles table in the Biblio.mdb sample database, which comes with Visual Basic. Allow the user to select Title Order, ISBN Order, or Publisher's ID Order.

Display the following fields from the Titles table:

Title	(indexed)
Year Published	
ISBN	(PrimaryKey)
PubID	(indexed)

Note: See the note in Exercise 11.1 about the size of the file.

11.5 *SQL Dynaset*: This project displays fields from the Titles table and the Publishers table in the Biblio.mdb database. The layout of the Publishers table (shown in project 10.4) has a primary key of PubID; the Titles table (described in project 11.4) includes a PubID field, which can be used to join the two tables.

The form should contain these fields:

Titles table: Title, ISBN, Year Published
Publishers table: PubID, Company Name, City
Note: See the note in Exercise 11.1 about the size of the file.

11.6 *SQL Dynaset; Selection from List:* Modify project 11.5 to allow the user to select a subset of the data by Publisher. Include a second form holding a list of publishers. (Do not allow a publisher to be listed more than once.) When the user selects a publisher name from the list, return to the first form to display all records from that publisher.

Include menu choices to select by publisher or display all records. The currently selected option should be checked.

Note: See the note in Exercise 11.1 about the size of the file.

CASE STUDIES

VB Mail Order

Grid

Display the Product table of VBMail.mdb in a grid. Include the record number and record count either in the caption of the data control or in a label. Make sure the grid cells are large enough to display all the data.

Allow the user to make Adds and Deletions to the table.

Validation: Table type recordset

Modify the VB Mail Order database project from Chapter 10. The new menu will add choices to seek for a customer by last name or by customer ID. An *Organize* menu will allow the user to display the information in order by LastName or CustomerID.

Do not allow the user to change the CustomerID field (the primary key) except during an Add operation. If the database isn't found on the open, display an error message and the *Open File* dialog box so the user can select another file. Make sure that no error can cause a run-time error.

Include a Cancel button to allow the user to back out of an Add operation.

Note: This exercise uses indexes. The recordset must be table type.

SQL Dynaset

In this project for VB Mail Order, you will create an application that allows the user to select products by catalog name or by description from VBMail.mdb. The main form displays the product number, description, price, weight, and catalog name.

A *Select* menu allows the user to choose *Select Records* or *All Records*. Be sure to include a check mark next to the currently selected option.

A second form holds dropdown combo boxes filled with the catalog names and product descriptions (display only one list entry for each description—no duplicates). The user can select either or both (or partial names), and the first form will reappear with only the requested products.

Tables

Product
ProductNumber (indexed) (compound primary key)
Catalog Number (indexed) (compound primary key)
Description
Price
Weight

Catalog
Number (primary key)
Name (indexed)
Phone

Hints: To have data-bound controls on two forms, both must have data controls. A data-bound control must be bound to a data control on the same form. In code you can refer to controls on other forms by using the exclamation point.

VB Auto Center

Grid

Display the Vehicle table of VBAuto.mdb in a grid. Include the record number and record count either in the caption of the data control or in a label. Make sure the grid cells are large enough to display all the data.

Allow the user to make Adds and Deletions to the table.

Validation; Table type recordset

Modify the VB Auto database project from Chapter 10. The new menu will add choices to seek for a vehicle by inventory ID or by manufacturer. An *Organize* menu will allow the user to display the information in order by Manufacturer or InventoryID. *Note:* You must use a table type recordset.

Do not allow the user to change the InventoryID field (the primary key) except during an Add. If the database isn't found on the open, display an error message and the *Open File* dialog box so the user can select another file. Make sure that no error can cause a run-time error.

Include a Cancel button to allow the user to back out of an Add operation.

SQL Dynaset

Note: This project is a modification of the Chapter 10 assignment; it may not be combined with the previous validation exercises, since the recordset will not be updateable.

In this project for VB Auto Center, you will create a project that allows the user to select products by CustomerName or by InventoryIDNumber. The main form displays the InventoryIDNumber, Manufacturer, ModelName, Year, VehicleIDNumber, CostValue, and the CustomerName. A *Select* menu allows the user to choose *Select Records* or *All Records*. Be sure to include a check mark next to the currently selected option.

A second form holds dropdown combo boxes filled with the customer names (display only one list entry for each description—no duplicates) and inventory ID numbers. The user can select either or both, and the first form will reappear with only the requested products.

Tables

Vehicle
InventoryID (indexed) (primary key)
Manufacturer
Model
Year
CostValue
VehicleID

Customer
Number (primary key)
Name (indexed)
InventoryIDNumber

Hints: To have data-bound controls on two forms, both must have data controls. A data-bound control must be bound to a data control on the same form. In code you can refer to controls on other forms by using the exclamation point.

CHAPTER

12

Drag-and-Drop

At the completion of this chapter, you will be able to . . .

1. Explain the difference between the source and target in a drag-and-drop operation.

2. Code a program that incorporates drag-and-drop.

One of the handy visual tools of Windows is the drag-and-drop operation. In this chapter you will learn how to incorporate drag-and-drop into your programs.

Drag-and-Drop Terminology

Before you are ready to code a drag-and-drop operation, you need to know some terminology. Also, you need to understand the properties that must be set and the difference between a DragOver event and a DragDrop event.

The Source and the Target

In a drag-and-drop operation, an object is moved from one location to another. The object being moved (dragged) is called the **source**; the location to which it is moved is called the **target**. Figure 12.1 shows a form with a source image and a target image. In the example imgPaper is the source and imgTrash is the target.

Figure 12.1

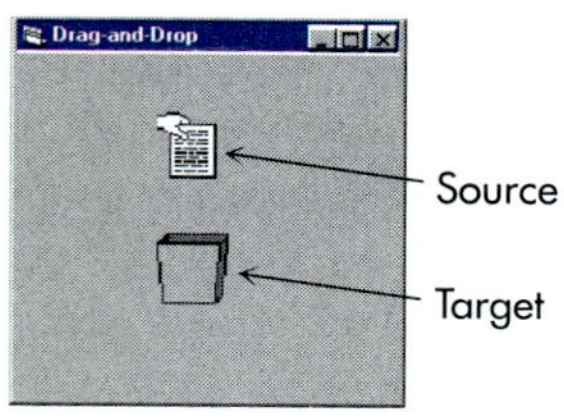

The Source object is dragged to the Target.

Source Object Properties

To make a source object movable, set its **DragMode property** to 1-Automatic. You will also want to set the **DragIcon property** to display an icon; otherwise, when you drag the object, you see only an outline.

DragOver and DragDrop Events

As an object is dragged across a form, events are occurring. The events are for the target objects, not the source. For example, as you drag an image across a form, the form's **DragOver event** occurs. If you drag the image across a control, such as a command button, the command button's DragOver event occurs. As long as you keep the mouse button down and keep moving, DragOver events occur for the form and every control over which you move. When you release the mouse button with the image over a control, the control's **DragDrop event** occurs; of course, if you release the mouse button over the form, the *form's* DragDrop event occurs.

Therefore, for any drag-and-drop operation, multiple DragOver events may occur. Only one DragDrop event occurs—when the operation is complete. All the events occur to the target objects, not to the source object.

Note: You can also code for events that occur for the source object, such as the Click event and the MouseDown, MouseUp, and MouseMove events. This brief introduction focuses on the events for the target objects.

A Step-by-Step Example

In this example you will develop a small application that allows the user to drag the airplane icon into the hangar (use your imagination for the hanger). Notice that Figure 12.2 contains two airplane icons—the source (imgPlane) and another inside the target (imgPlaneParked). The second image has its Visible property set to False, so it won't be seen until the plane is inside the hangar.

This example uses a picturebox control. For further information about pictureboxes, see Chapter 13.

Figure 12.2

The form for the airplane step-by-step example.

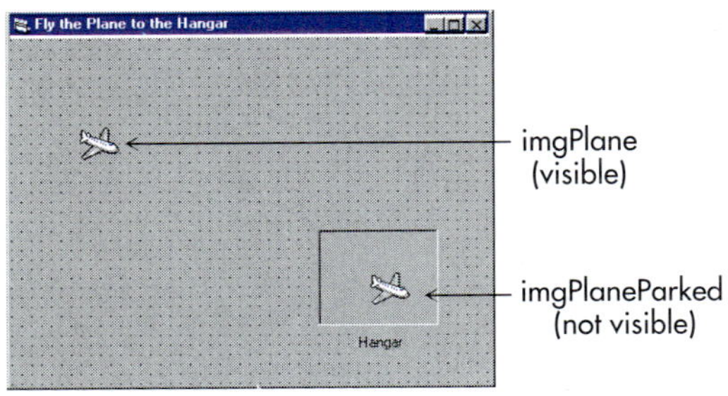

Create the User Interface

STEP 1: Begin a new project and place the picturebox and the two image controls (for the two airplanes) on the form. Make sure to create the second airplane image *inside* the picturebox, which is its container. (If you try to drag the image on top of the picturebox, it will disappear behind the control because of the way the graphic controls are layered on the form. You can either draw the image inside the picturebox or cut-and-paste it inside; dragging does not place the image inside the picturebox.)

STEP 2: Create the label under the picturebox (the one captioned Hangar).

Set the Properties

STEP 1: Set the properties for the form.

Property	Value
Name	frmPlane
Caption	Fly the Plane to the Hangar

STEP 2: Set the properties for the first airplane image.

Property	Value
Name	imgPlane
Stretch	True
Picture	Vb\Graphics\Icons\Industry\Plane.ico
DragIcon	Vb\Graphics\Icons\Industry\Plane.ico
DragMode	1 - Automatic

STEP 3: Set the properties for the second airplane image.

Property	Value
Name	imgPlaneParked
Stretch	True
Picture	Vb\Graphics\Icons\Industry\Plane.ico
Visible	False

STEP 4: Set the Name property of the picturebox to picHangar.
STEP 5: Set the Caption property of the label to Hangar.

Write the Code

STEP 1: Try a test run of the program before you write any code. Click the Run button and try dragging the plane image.

You should see an icon as you drag, but the original image still appears (Figure 12.3). The next step will be to make the source image invisible as you begin to drag the image over the form.

Figure 12.3

The icon moves as you drag it, but the original image is still visible.

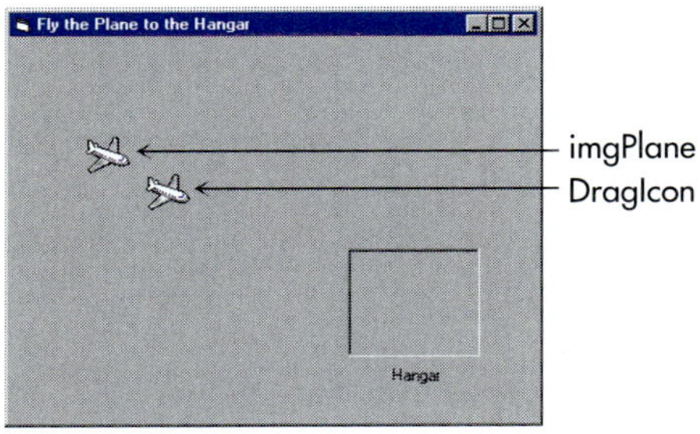

STEP 2: Click the Stop button to halt program operation.

Code the Drag Operation

STEP 3: In the Code window, click on *Form* for the object and sanserif-*DragOver* for the procedure.

STEP 4: Code the following remark and line of code in the Form_DragOver event.

```
'Make the plane invisible

imgPlane.Visible = False
```

STEP 5: Run the program again. When you begin dragging the plane image, the original should disappear, so that it looks like you are actually dragging the image (Figure 12.4). Try dropping it anywhere. (Disappears, doesn't it?) Now it's time to take care of the drop operation.

Figure 12.4

For a proper drag, the original image should disappear.

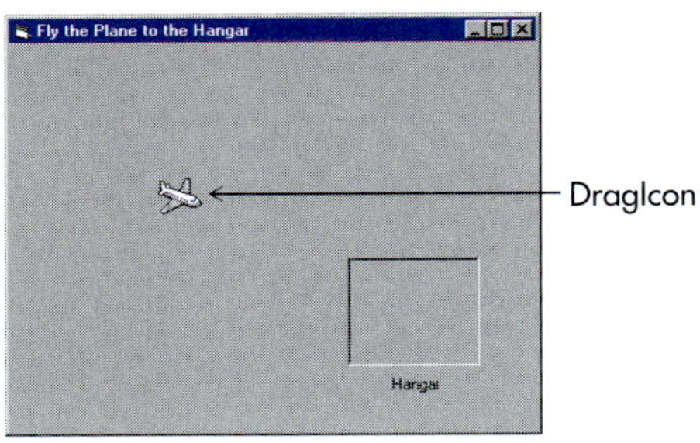

Click on the Stop button to halt program operation.

Code the Drop Operation

A DragDrop event may occur for the intended target (the picturebox), but perhaps the user misses (how?) or has a change of heart. If a DragDrop event occurs for the form or for any control other than the intended target, the drop is in error and the original image must become visible again.

STEP 6: Code the DragDrop event for the picturebox (picHangar).

```
Private Sub picHangar_DragDrop(Source As Control, X As Single, Y As Single)
    'Good Drop

    imgPlaneParked.Visible = True
End Sub
```

STEP 7: Code the DragDrop event for the form.

```
Private Sub Form_DragDrop(Source As Control, X As Single, Y As Single)
    'Bad Drop

    imgPlane.Visible = True
End Sub
```

STEP 8: Code a DragDrop event for the label control. If the user drops the plane on the label, it's another bad drop.

```
Private Sub Label1_DragDrop(Source As Control, X As Single, Y As Single)
    'Bad Drop

    imgPlane.Visible = True
End Sub
```

Run the Project

STEP 1: Start the project running. Try dragging and dropping the plane on the hangar (Figure 12.5). Then stop the project; restart and try dropping on the form. Stop, restart, and try dropping on the label. For each bad drop, the plane should reappear in its original location.

If you have problems, check the event procedure names. You must code the DragDrop event for the picturebox, the form, and the label.

Figure 12.5

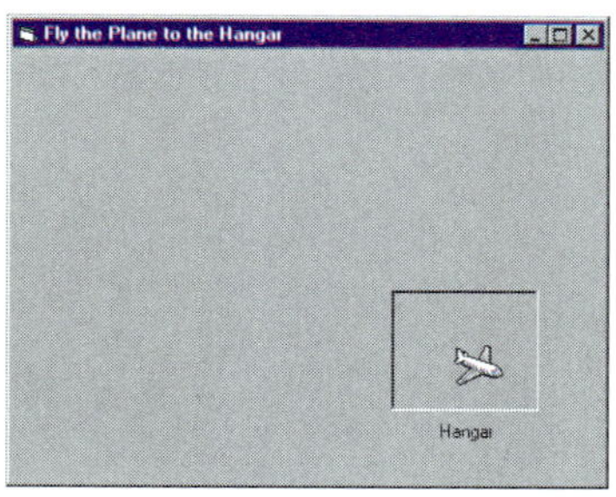

A good drag-and-drop with the airplane in the hangar.

Wouldn't it be helpful to have command buttons to exit the project and to reset the image to its original location?

Add Command Buttons

STEP 1: Add two command buttons to the form (Figure 12.6) and set their properties.

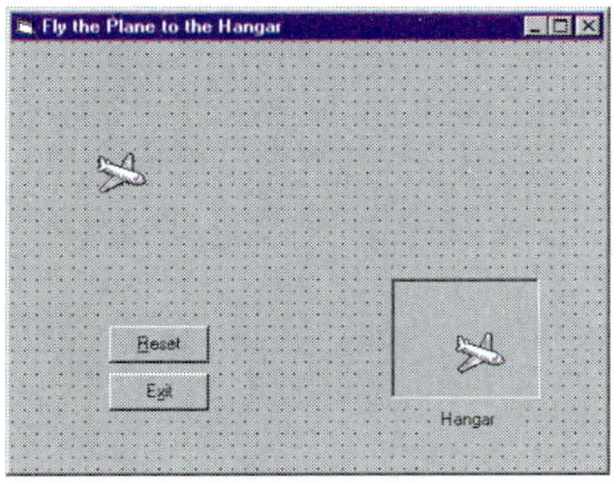

Figure 12.6

Add a Reset and an Exit command button to the form.

Object	Property	Value
cmdReset	Name	cmdReset
	Caption	&Reset
cmdExit	Name	cmdExit
	Caption	E&xit

STEP 2: Code the cmdReset_Click event.

```
Private Sub cmdReset_Click()
    'Reset to original condition

    imgPlaneParked.Visible = False
    imgPlane.Visible = True
End Sub
```

STEP 3: Code the cmdExit_Click event.

```
Private Sub cmdExit_Click()
     'Exit the project

     End
End Sub
```

You *could* test the project to see what happens when you drop the plane on a command button now, but the plane would disappear from the screen (from radar?). A better practice is to code the DragDrop event for the two command buttons first.

STEP 4: Copy and paste the statements from the Form_DragDrop event procedure into the cmdReset_DragDrop event procedure.

```
Private Sub cmdReset_DragDrop(Source As Control, X As Single, Y As Single)
    'Bad Drop

    imgPlane.Visible = True
End Sub
```

STEP 5: Paste another copy into the DragDrop event for the cmdExit button.

```
Private Sub cmdExit_DragDrop(Source As Control, X As Single, Y As Single)
    'Bad Drop

    imgPlane.Visible = True
End Sub
```

Run the Completed Project

STEP 1: Try each option. Drag the plane and drop it anywhere on the form. Drag it to its hangar and try the Reset button. Then test your Exit button.

Dragging and Dropping Multiple Objects

In the previous example only one object was enabled for drag-and-drop. Recall that the source object becomes invisible in the form's DragOver event procedure. What if the form has more than one possible source object (as in Figure 12.7)? Which object should become invisible? Fortunately, there's an easy answer. Notice the first line of the DragOver event procedure:

```
Private Sub cmdExit_DragOver(Source As Control, X As Single, Y As Single)
```

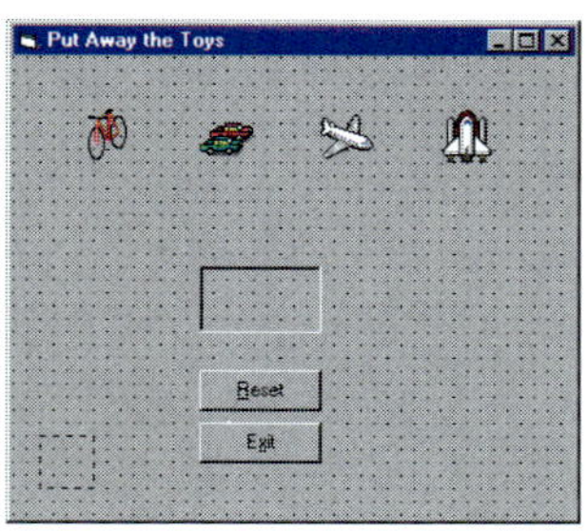

Figure 12.7

All four toy icons on this form can be dragged to the target (a toybox).

The Source argument holds the name of the control that caused the DragOver event to occur. You can use the name *Source* to reference the source control in code.

```
Source.Visible = False
```

Passing the Source Argument

There may be times when you want to call another procedure from a DragOver or a DragDrop event procedure. Recall from the previous example that if a source object is dropped on any control other than the target, it is considered a "bad drop." In a bad drop, the source control must be made visible again. Rather than place identical code in the DragDrop event for all other controls on the form, consider writing one BadDrop sub procedure and calling it wherever necessary. The Source argument that is passed to the DragDrop event procedure can be passed along to the BadDrop sub procedure.

```
Private Sub cmdExit_DragDrop(Source As Control, X As Single, Y As Single)
    'Bad drop

    BadDrop Source          'Call the BadDrop procedure and pass along Source
End Sub
```

```
Private Sub cmdReset_DragDrop(Source As Control, X As Single, Y As Single)
    'Bad drop

    BadDrop Source          'Call the BadDrop procedure and pass along Source
End Sub
```

```
Private Sub BadDrop(Source)
    'Make source control visible

    Source.Visible = True
End Sub
```

Note: In this example the BadDrop sub procedure has only one line of code, so it could be argued that it is efficient to place that line in each DragDrop event. In many situations, such as the chapter hands-on programming example, there are several things to do for a bad drop. In that case it is best to create a separate general sub procedure.

Changing the Icon of the Target Image

In the airplane step-by-step example, a successful drag-and-drop operation caused a second image to become visible. Another approach is to change the icon of the target image. Continuing with the toybox example (Figure 12.7), when a successful drop is made, the icon of the target changes. Notice in the following code how the Picture property of the target is changed to match the Picture property of the source.

```
Private Sub imgTarget_DragDrop(Source As Control, X As Single, Y As Single)
    'Got a hit

    imgTarget.Picture = Source.Picture
End Sub
```

Setting the DragIcon Property of Source Controls

In most cases you want the DragIcon of a source control to be the same as its Picture property. You can set both properties to the same filename in the Properties window, as you did in the earlier step-by-step example. But a better approach is to set only the Picture property at design time. Then in the Form_Load event set the control's DragIcon property to its Picture property. That way the file is loaded from disk only once.

```
imgPlane.DragIcon = imgPlane.Picture
```

If you have multiple images that can be dragged, consider making them a control array. In the toybox example, the four images are named imgToy(0), imgToy(1), imgToy(2), and imgToy(3). A loop in the Form_Load event procedure will set the DragIcon property for all images. (Note that the number of lines of code remains the same for 15 or 20 or 4 toy images.)

```
Private Sub Form_Load()
     'Setup DragIcon properties
     Dim iCounter

     For iCounter = 0 To 3
         imgToy(iCounter).DragIcon = imgToy(iCounter).Picture
      Next iCounter
End Sub
```

Blanking Out an Image

If you want to remove an icon from an image, you have two choices. You can either use the LoadPicture function with a blank filename or set the image's Picture property to another (blank) image. The second approach is the more efficient but requires you to place an extra image, with no Picture property, on the form.

Method 1

```
imgTarget.Picture = LoadPicture("")
```

Method 2

```
imgTarget.Picture = imgBlank.Picture
```

Feedback 12.1

1. Name two properties of the source object that should be changed for drag-and-drop operations.

2. To what object does the DragDrop event belong?
3. What object does the Source argument of the DragOver event contain?

The Toybox Program

Here are the entire program specifications for the toybox example shown in Figure 12.7. Try entering and running it.

Object	Property	Setting
frmToys	Name	frmToys
	Caption	Put Away the Toys
imgToy(0)	Name	imgToy(0)
	DragMode	1 - Automatic
	Picture	Vb\Graphics\Icons\Industry\Bicycle.ico
imgToy(1)	Name	imgToy(1)
	DragMode	1 - Automatic
	Picture	Vb\Graphics\Icons\Industry\Cars.ico
imgToy(2)	Name	imgToy(2)
	DragMode	1 - Automatic
	Picture	Vb\Graphics\Icons\Industry\Plane.ico
imgToy(3)	Name	imgToy(3)
	DragMode	1 - Automatic
	Picture	Vb\Graphics\Icons\Industry\Rocket.ico
imgTarget	Name	imgTarget
	BorderStyle	1 - Fixed Single
	Stretch	True
imgBlank	Name	imgBlank
cmdReset	Name	cmdReset
	Caption	&Reset
cmdExit	Name	cmdExit
	Caption	E&xit

The Procedures

Object	Procedure	Actions
frmToys	Load	Set DragIcon to Picture property for all four images.
	DragOver	Set source control invisible.
	DragDrop	Call BadDrop procedure.
imgTarget	DragDrop	Set Picture property to picture of source.
cmdExit	Click	Exit the project.
	DragDrop	Call BadDrop procedure.
cmdReset	Click	Set Visible = True for all four images. Set Picture property of target to blank.
	DragDrop	Call BadDrop procedure.
General	BadDrop	Set Visible = True for source image.

The Project Coding Solution

```
'Program:      Toybox Drag-and-Drop Example
'Programmer:   J.C. Bradley
'Date:         December 1997
'Purpose:      Drag-and-drop multiple objects.
'Folder:       Ch1202
Option Explicit
```

```
Private Sub cmdExit_Click()
    'Exit the project

    End
End Sub
```

```
Private Sub cmdExit_DragDrop(Source As Control, X As Single, Y As Single)
    'Bad drop

    BadDrop Source
End Sub
```

```
Private Sub cmdReset_Click()
    'Replace images
    Dim iCounter As Integer

    For iCounter = 0 To 3
        imgToy(iCounter).Visible = True
    Next iCounter
    imgTarget.Picture = imgBlank.Picture
End Sub
```

```
Private Sub cmdReset_DragDrop(Source As Control, X As Single, Y As Single)
    'Bad drop

    BadDrop Source
End Sub
```

```
Private Sub Form_DragDrop(Source As Control, X As Single, Y As Single)
    'Bad drop

    BadDrop Source
End Sub
```

```
Private Sub Form_DragOver(Source As Control, X As Single, _
        Y As Single, State As Integer)
    'Make the source control invisible

    Source.Visible = False
End Sub
```

```
Private Sub Form_Load()
    'Setup DragIcon properties
    Dim iCounter

    For iCounter = 0 To 3
        imgToy(iCounter).DragIcon = imgToy(iCounter).Picture
    Next iCounter
End Sub
```

```
Private Sub BadDrop(Source)
    'Make source control visible

    Source.Visible = True
End Sub
```

```
Private Sub imgTarget_DragDrop(Source As Control, X As Single, Y As Single)
    'Got a hit

    imgTarget.Picture = Source.Picture
End Sub
```

Your Hands-On Programming Example

This drag-and-drop example combines many of the techniques from the chapter. In addition, you must change target icons more than once. Figure 12.8 shows a sketch of the form; Figures 12.9, 12.10, and 12.11 show the form during run time.

Figure 12.8

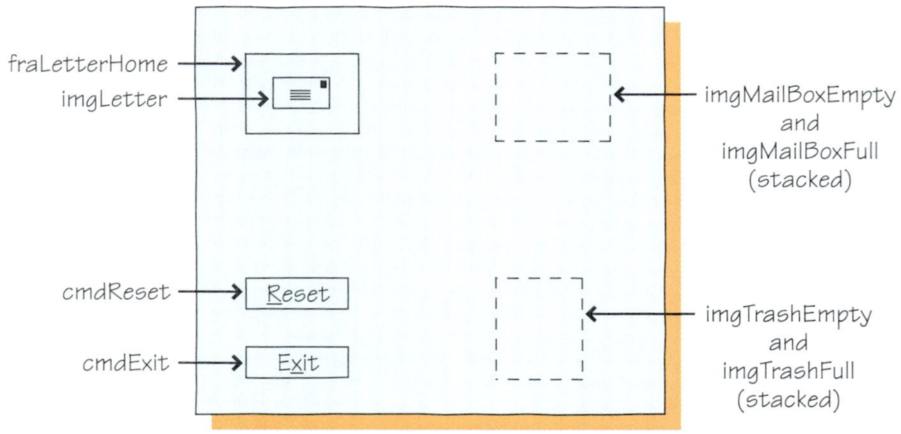

The planning sketch for the hands-on programming example.

Figure 12.9

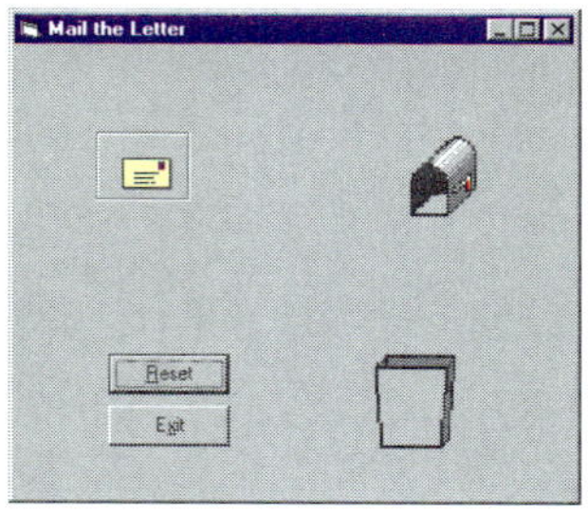

The form as it appears when the project begins execution.

Figure 12.10

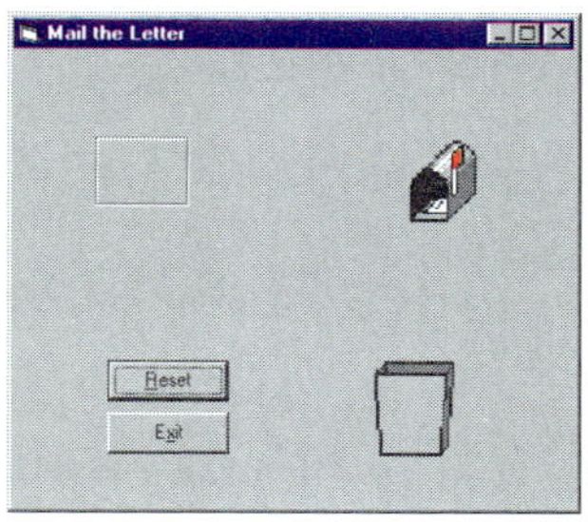

When the letter is placed in the mailbox, the flag goes up.

Figure 12.11

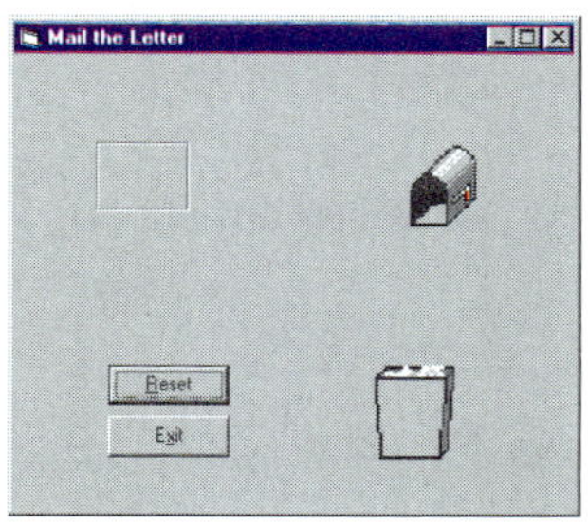

When the letter is placed in the trash can, the trash is visible.

When the letter is dropped on the mailbox, the icon changes to a mailbox with the flag up and a letter inside. The letter can be dragged from the mailbox and dropped in the trash can or back in its original frame. When the letter is dropped in the trash can, the icon changes to a trash can with visible trash inside. The letter can also be dragged out of the trash can and dropped either on the mailbox or on the letter's original frame.

Since you want to drag a letter from the mailbox or the trash can, the DragIcon property of each must be set to the same icon as the letter image. (You want to drag a picture of a letter, not a picture of a trash can.)

The two icons for the mailbox are stored in two image controls—one visible and one invisible. Manipulating the two images gets a little tricky, but remember what you learned about multiple controls: You can select multiple controls by dragging a selection box around them or Ctrl-click on them, or you can set similar properties on multiple selected controls in the Properties window (such as their Top, Left, and Width properties). You can also select one control and choose *Send to Back* or *Bring to Front* on the *Edit* menu.

The two image controls for the trash cans are developed in the same way as the mailboxes.

Planning the Project

Sketch the form, which is shown in Figure 12.8.

Plan the Objects and Properties

Object	Property	Setting
frmMail	Name	frmMail
	Caption	Mail the Letter
fraLetterHome	Name	fraLetterHome
	Caption	(blank)
imgLetter	Name	imgLetter
	DragMode	1 - Automatic
	Stretch	True
	Icon	Vb\Graphics\Icons\Mail\Mail02a.ico
imgMailBoxEmpty	Name	imgMailBoxEmpty
	Stretch	True
	Picture	Vb\Graphics\Icons\Mail\mail16a.ico
imgMailBoxFull	Name	imgMailBoxFull
	Stretch	True
	Picture	Vb\Graphics\Icons\Mail\mail16b.ico
	DragMode	1 - Automatic
	Visible	False

(continued)

Object	Property	Setting
imgTrashEmpty	Name	imgTrashEmpty
	Stretch	True
	Picture	Vb\Graphics\Icons\Computer\Trash04b.ico
imgTrashFull	Name	imgTrashFull
	Stretch	True
	Picture	Vb\Graphics\Icons\Computer\Trash04a.ico
	DragMode	1 - Automatic
	Visible	False
cmdReset	Name	cmdReset
	Caption	&Reset
cmdExit	Name	cmdExit
	Caption	E&xit

Plan the Event Procedures

Plan the actions for the event procedures.

Object	Procedure	Actions
frmMail	Load	Set DragIcon of imgLetter, imgMailboxFull, and imgTrashFull to imgLetter.Picture.
	DragOver	Case imgLetter Set Visible = False for imgLetter. Case imgTrashFull Set Visible = False for imgTrashFull. Set Visible = True for imgTrashEmpty. Case imgMailBoxFull Set Visible = False for imgMailBoxFull. Set Visible = True for imgMailBoxEmpty.
	DragDrop	Call BadDrop procedure.
imgMailBoxEmpty	DragDrop	Set Visible = False for imgMailBoxEmpty. Set Visible = True for imgMailBoxFull.
imgTrashEmpty	DragDrop	Set Visible = False for imgTrashEmpty. Set Visible = True for imgTrashFull.
fraLetterHome	DragDrop	Set Visible = True for imgLetter.
cmdExit	Click	Exit the project.
	DragDrop	Call BadDrop procedure.
cmdReset	Click	Set Visible = True for imgLetter, imgMailBoxEmpty, and imgTrashEmpty. Set Visible = False for imgMailBoxFull and imgTrashFull
	DragDrop	Call BadDrop procedure.

(continued)

Object	**Procedure**	**Actions**
General sub procedure	BadDrop	Case imgLetter Set Visible = True for imgLetter. Case imgTrashFull Set Visible = True for imgTrashFull. Set Visible = False for imgTrashEmpty. Case imgMailBoxFull Set Visible = True for imgMailBoxFull. Set Visible = False for imgTrashEmpty.

Write the Project

Follow the sketch in Figure 12.8 to create the form. Figures 12.9, 12.10, and 12.11 show the completed form at different stages of run time.

Set the properties of each object according to your plan.

The next step is to write the code. Working from the pseudocode, write each event procedure.

When you complete the code, thoroughly test the project by dragging the letter to each target and resetting from each position.

The Project Coding Solution

```
'Program:       Drag-and-Drop Hands-On Example
'Programmer:    J.C. Bradley
'Date:          December 1997
'Purpose:       Mail or trash a letter using drag-and-drop.
'Folder:        Ch1203
Option Explicit
```

```
Private Sub cmdExit_Click()
    'Exit the project

    End
End Sub
```

```
Private Sub cmdExit_DragDrop(Source As Control, X As Single, Y As Single)
    'Bad drop

    BadDrop Source
End Sub
```

```
Private Sub cmdReset_Click()
    'Initialize setup

    imgLetter.Visible = True
    imgMailBoxEmpty.Visible = True
    imgMailboxFull.Visible = False
    imgTrashEmpty.Visible = True
    imgTrashFull.Visible = False
End Sub
```

```
Private Sub cmdReset_DragDrop(Source As Control, X As Single, Y As Single)
    'Bad drop

    BadDrop Source
End Sub
```

```
Private Sub Form_DragDrop(Source As Control, X As Single, Y As Single)
    'Bad drop

    BadDrop Source
End Sub
```

```
Private Sub Form_DragOver(Source As Control, X As Single, _
        Y As Single, State As Integer)
    'Check source of DragOver and determine action

    Select Case Source
        Case imgLetter
            imgLetter.Visible = False
        Case imgTrashFull
            imgTrashFull.Visible = False
            imgTrashEmpty.Visible = True
        Case imgMailboxFull
            imgMailboxFull.Visible = False
            imgMailBoxEmpty.Visible = True
    End Select
End Sub
```

```
Private Sub Form_Load()
    'Set DragIcon to Letter

    imgLetter.DragIcon = imgLetter.Picture
    imgMailboxFull.DragIcon = imgLetter.Picture
    imgTrashFull.DragIcon = imgLetter.Picture
End Sub
```

```
Private Sub fraLetterHome_DragDrop(Source As Control, X As Single, _
        Y As Single)
    'Good drop

    imgLetter.Visible = True
End Sub
```

```
Private Sub imgMailBoxEmpty_DragDrop(Source As Control, X As Single, _
        Y As Single)
    'Good drop

    imgMailBoxEmpty.Visible = False
    imgMailboxFull.Visible = True
End Sub
```

```
Private Sub imgTrashEmpty_DragDrop(Source As Control, X As Single, _
        Y As Single)
    'Good drop

    imgTrashEmpty.Visible = False
    imgTrashFull.Visible = True
End Sub
```

```
Private Sub BadDrop(Source As Control)
    'Reset source after a bad drop

    Select Case Source
        Case imgLetter
            imgLetter.Visible = True
        Case imgTrashFull
            imgTrashFull.Visible = True
            imgTrashEmpty.Visible = False
        Case imgMailboxFull
            imgMailboxFull.Visible = True
            imgMailBoxEmpty.Visible = False
    End Select
End Sub
```

Programming Hints

Manual Drag-and-Drop

Sometimes you don't want to set the DragMode property of controls to True, because then normal mouse clicks and keystrokes are not recognized for that control. You can use the **Drag method** to drag-and-drop in code. For example, you can begin a Drag operation in the MouseDown event for a control (a text box in this example).

```
Private Sub txtEntry_MouseDown(Button As Integer, Shift As Integer, _
        X As Single, Y As Single)
    txtEntry.Drag
End Sub
```

This action begins a drag operation that behaves just like the automatic dragging in the chapter examples.

Summary

1. In a drag-and-drop operation, the control being dragged is the source and the destination is the target.
2. Set the source control's DragMode property and DragIcon property.
3. The DragOver event and DragDrop event belong to the target control. DragOver occurs as the source control is moving over the target; DragDrop occurs when the mouse button is released over the target.
4. The system passes the name of the source control to the DragOver and DragDrop event procedures.

Key Terms

`Drag` method *465*
DragDrop event *448*
DragIcon property *448*
DragMode property *448*
DragOver event *448*
source *448*
target *448*

Review Questions

1. Explain the differences between the source and target in a drag-and-drop operation.
2. What properties must be set for the source control in order to do drag-and-drop?
3. An image of a car is dragged across the form and dropped on an image of a garage. Describe the events that occur (and the objects to which they belong) as the operation takes place.
4. In a form's DragOver event, it is necessary to make the source control invisible. How can you determine which control is the source control?

Programming Exercises

12.1 Write a drag-and-drop program to play a game of darts. Use the icon files Vb\Graphics\Icons\Misc\Bullseye.ico and Vb\Graphics\Icons\Point10.ico. Place an invisible dart in the center of the target and make it visible when the target is hit. Also, keep track of the number of hits and display a running count.

The Reset button should reset the dart to its starting location.

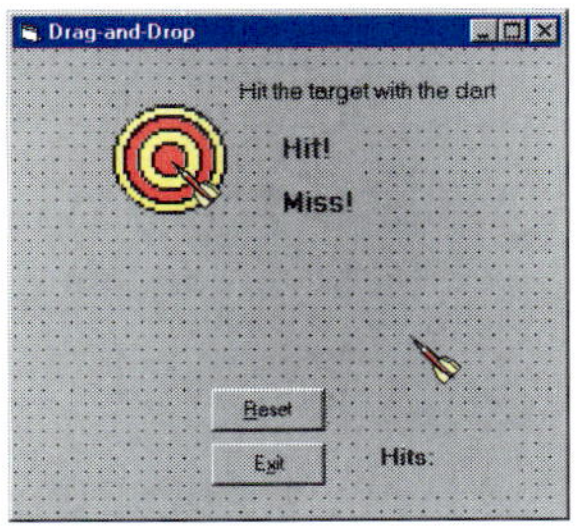

12.2 Create a project for a card suit guessing game. The user will drag the images to the boxes along the lower edge of the form. When the correct image is placed in a box, make the image remain there. When all four images are in the correct location, display a message box congratulating the user. The Reset button should replace the suit images at the top of the form and clear out the lower boxes. (*Hint:* For the boxes, use image controls with a border.) Consider using control arrays.

The four images are in the Vb\Graphics\Icons\Misc folder and are called Misc34.ico, Misc35.ico, Misc36.ico, and Misc37.ico.

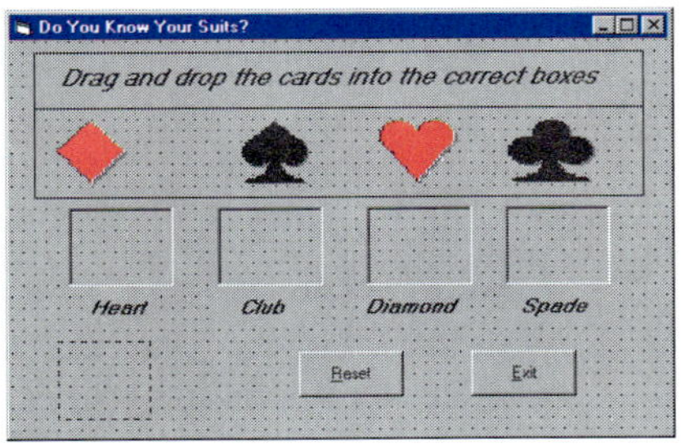

12.3 Create a project that keeps track of the food for the company picnic. The user will enter each person's name into the text box and then drag it to the correct list. Use drag-and-drop to move the names to the lists. (*Hint:* Use AddItem in the DragDrop event procedure.)

Do not allow a blank name to be added to a list; keep the three lists in alphabetic order; clear out the text box and set the focus after adding a name to one of the lists.

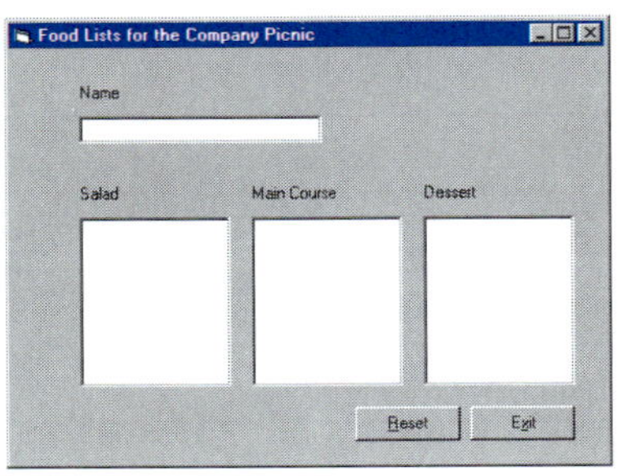

12.4 Modify project 12.3 to include a menu bar. Include a *Print* command with a submenu to select the item (Salads, Main Courses, or Desserts). Allow the user to print any of the lists, one at a time.

12.5 Create your own drag-and-drop application using graphic files available to you (or create your own using a draw or paint program). You can use files with the extensions .ico, .wmf, .bmp, .dib, .gif, .jpg, .emf, and .cur.

CASE STUDIES

VB Mail Order

Create a form that allows the user to select express delivery or freight through the use of drag-and-drop. Include a label that will display the words *Express Delivery—overnight* or *Freight—10 working days* after the user drops the appropriate icon in the mailbox.

For this project the empty mailbox (Mail16a.ico) is the empty target. The source will be Mail05b.ico for freight and Mail03.ico for express. When the selected type of delivery reaches the target, change the empty mailbox to have the flag up (Mail16b.ico).

VB Auto Center

Create a game project using drag-and-drop for the VB Auto Center. The form will contain the following images:

Vb\Graphics\Icons\Traffic\Trffc16.ico in the upper-left corner.

Vb\Graphics\Icons\Misc\Face01.ico in the upper-right corner (visible to begin).

Arranged horizontally across the center of the screen:

Vb\Graphics\Icons\Industry\Wrench.ico
Vb\Graphics\Icons\Industry\Gaspump.ico
Vb\Graphics\Icons\Elements\Water.ico

At the bottom of the screen:

Vb\Graphics\Icons\Misc\House.ico at the lower-left corner.

Vb\Graphics\Icons\Misc\Face03.ico at the lower-right corner (invisible to begin).

The car may be dragged to the icons only in the proper order before it goes home. The correct order: wrench for service, gas pump, and then water for the car wash. When the drops have been made in the proper order and the vehicle gets home, the top face becomes invisible and the lower face becomes visible.

CHAPTER

13

Graphics

At the completion of this chapter, you will be able to . . .

1. Understand the measurements in the graphics coordinate system.

2. Display and change colors using the `RGB` and `QBColor` functions.

3. Create graphics using graphics methods.

4. Understand the graphics-layering principles.

5. Load and change pictures at run time.

6. Create simple animation.

7. Use the timer control.

8. Use scroll bars to move and resize an image.

In past chapters you learned how to incorporate graphics using the shape, image, and line controls. In this chapter you will learn how to enhance the use of the controls and to use the graphics methods. New controls include the picturebox, the timer, and scroll bar controls.

The Graphics Environment

The measurement system you use in a project is known as the ***scale***. You can set the scale to twips, points, pixels, inches, or centimeters, or you can create your own scale.

The default scale is twips. A **twip** is a twentieth of a point. Since a **point** is a printer's measurement of 1/72nd of an inch, a twip is 1/1440th of an inch; in other words, an inch has 1,440 twips.

The term **pixel** is an abbreviation of *picture element,* a dot that makes up a picture. You are probably most familiar with pixels in the determination of the resolution of a monitor. A display of 1280 by 1024 is a reference to the number of pixels horizontally and vertically.

You can change the scale with the ScaleMode property. The examples in this chapter are based on twips.

The Coordinate System

Graphics are measured from a starting point of 0,0 for the *x* and *y* coordinates beginning in the upper-left corner. The *x* is the horizontal position, and *y* is the vertical measurement. The starting point depends on where the graphic is being placed. If the graphic is going directly on a form, the 0,0 coordinates are the upper-left corner of the form. You can also place graphics in containers, such as pictureboxes. In this case the picturebox has its own 0,0 **coordinate system** to be used as the starting point for measuring the location of items within the control (Figure 13.1).

Figure 13.1

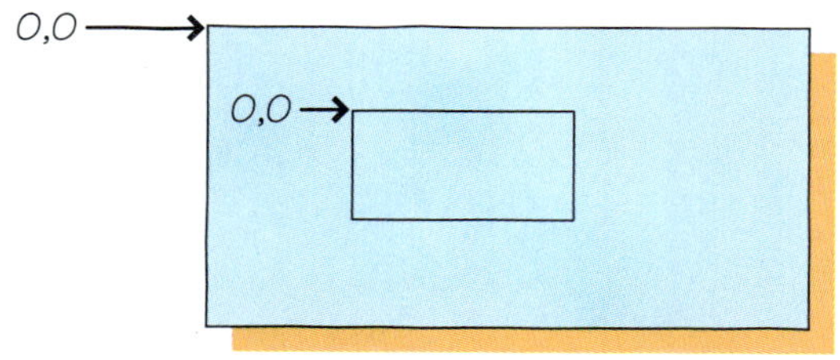

The coordinates for graphics begin with 0,0 in the upper-left corner of a form or container.

You can change the starting point of the coordinate system, the scale, or both. You control these with the ScaleLeft, ScaleTop, ScaleWidth, and ScaleHeight properties. For more information on changing these properties refer to the Help files in Visual Basic.

Picturebox Controls

The **picturebox control** is very similar to the image control, but a picturebox does not contain a Stretch property. However, it does have many other properties for graphics including those relating to the scale. Pictureboxes use more system resources than images use. For that reason, the recommended practice is to use an image control unless you need the added capabilities of a picturebox.

Figure 13.2 shows the toolbox tool for creating a picturebox, and Figure 13.3 shows a picturebox on a form. The three-character prefix for a picturebox name is "pic". Use the chart on the inside back cover of the text to compare the properties that apply to the image and to the picturebox.

Figure 13.2

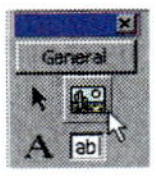

The picturebox tool from the toolbox.

Figure 13.3

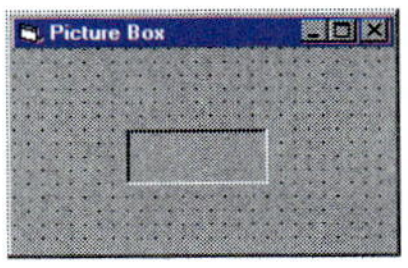

A picturebox control on a form.

Colors

You can specify colors for your graphics in a number of ways. The graphic controls have properties for ForeColor, BackColor, and FillColor. The VB graphics methods use the RGB color functions or the intrinsic color constants (such as vbRed and vbBlue).

The RGB Function

The **RGB function** specifies the quantities of red, green, and blue for the largest variety of colors. The value for each color ranges from 0 to 255, with 0 being the least intense. The color arguments are in the same order as their letters in the function name—red, green, and then blue. You can use the function to assign a color to a property or specify the color in a graphics method. Table 13.1 shows the RGB values for a few colors.

Table 13.1

The RGB values for some standard colors.

Color	Red Value	Green Value	Blue Value
Black	0	0	0
Blue	0	0	255
Green	0	255	0
Cyan	0	255	255
Red	255	0	0
Magenta	255	0	255
Yellow	255	255	0
White	255	255	255

The RGB Function—General Form

```
RGB(RedValue, GreenValue, BlueValue)
```

The RGB Function—Examples

```
lblWarning.BackColor = RGB(255, 0, 0)              'Red
txtName.Forecolor = RGB(255, 0, 255)               'Blue and red make magenta
Line (0, 0) - (1000, 1000), RGB(100, 100, 100)     'A gray line
```

The Visual Basic Intrinsic Color Constants

You can use the VB color constants introduced in Chapter 2 to specify colors for properties and for drawing graphics using the graphic methods. The color constants:

vbBlack
vbBlue
vbGreen
vbCyan
vbRed
vbMagenta
vbYellow
vbWhite

The QBColor Function

For compatibility with older versions of Basic, VB allows you to use color numbers that range from 0 to 15. To use these color numbers you must use the **QBColor function**, which converts the color numbers to their RGB equivalent.

Example

```
frmMyForm.BackColor = QBColor(1)          'Blue
```

Table 13.2 shows the sixteen color numbers that you can use with the `QBColor` function.

Table 13.2

The `QBColor` numbers, included in VB for compatibility with older versions of Basic.

Number	Color
0	Black
1	Blue
2	Green
3	Cyan
4	Red
5	Magenta
6	Yellow
7	White
8	Gray
9	Light Blue
10	Light Green
11	Light Cyan
12	Light Red
13	Light Magenta
14	Light Yellow
15	Bright White

The Graphics Methods

You can use the graphics methods to draw in a Form object, a Picturebox object, or the Printer object. The object you choose to use is considered the **container** for your graphics. If you omit the name of the object, it defaults to the form.

Using the graphics methods, such as `Cls`, `Pset`, `Line`, and `Circle` to draw graphics differs from using the graphics controls. Controls, such as shapes, lines, and images, appear on the form as it is loaded. If the form is resized or covered by another window and redisplayed, the graphics controls reappear. But the graphics you draw with code display when the code is executed. They do not redraw automatically. Therefore, if you want your graphics to redisplay each time the form is redisplayed, place the statements in the Paint event for the form or picturebox. You may also place graphics methods in a user event such as a command button's Click event.

The Cls Method

The **`Cls` method** clears the specified object. You could use `Cls` to clear an existing picture and change the background color of the form or picturebox. Remember that if the object is omitted on any of the graphics methods, the default is the form.

The CLS Method—General Form

```
[Object].Cls
```

The CLS Method—Examples

```
Cls              'Clear the background of the form
picLogo.Cls      'Clear a picture box
```

The PSet Method

The **`PSet` method** places a single point on the object in the location specified by the *x* and *y* coordinates. You may also specify the color for the point.

The PSet Method—General Form

```
[Object].PSet (x, y)[, Color]
```

The PSet Method—Examples

```
picLogo.PSet (100,100)
PSet (1000,1000), vbCyan
```

When the color is omitted, the ForeColor property setting of the object is used. The *x* and *y* coordinates may also be variables.

The **`Rnd` function** returns "random" numbers between 0 and the upper limit specified. Try the following code from the Ch1301 programming example, which demonstrates the use of the `Rnd` function. Figure 13.4 shows the screen generated by this code.

Figure 13.4

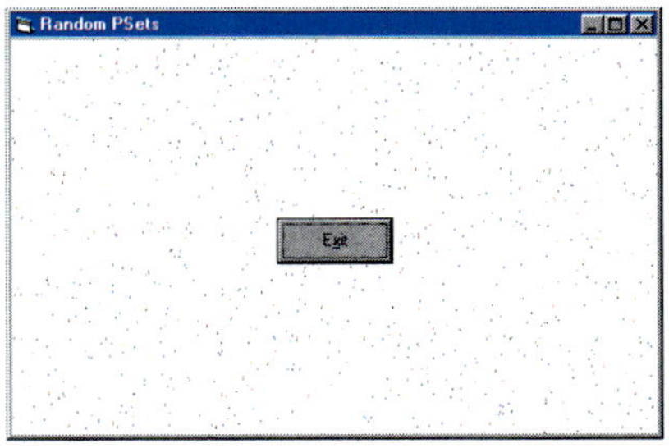

The screen for the random number PSet example, Ch1301.

```
'Program:       PSet
'Programmer:    A. Millspaugh
'Date:          December 1997
'Description:   Place colored dots randomly on the
'               form.
'Folder:        Ch1301
Option Explicit
```

```
Private Sub cmdExit_Click()
    'Terminate the Project

    End
End Sub
```

```
Private Sub Form_Paint()
    'Place random dots in random colors on form

    Dim iIndex As Integer
    Dim iColor As Integer
    Dim X, Y

    For iIndex = 1 To 1000
        X = Rnd * ScaleWidth
        Y = Rnd * ScaleHeight
        iColor = Rnd * 15
        PSet (X, Y), QBColor(iColor)
    Next iIndex
End Sub
```

The **DrawWidth property** determines the size of the point. Change the DrawWidth of the form in the Ch1301 PSet program to 5. Next try changing the form WindowState to Maximized and experiment with the ScaleHeight and ScaleWidth properties.

You can try this again, placing the dots within an object using Object.Width and Object.Height to control the upper limit.

If you wish to erase a point, place a new point on top of the old one using the BackColor property as the color.

The Line Method

Since a line is used to connect two points, the **Line method** needs two sets of coordinates specified for the line. If the first coordinate is not specified, the line is drawn from the last graphics point created on the screen.

The Line Method—General Form

```
[Object].Line [(x1, y1)]-(x2, y2)[, [Color][, B [ F ] ] ]
```

The Line Method—Examples

```
Printer.Line (5, 0)-(5,1000)
picLogo.Line - (500,100), QBColor(2)
picLogo.Line - (500,300), vbBlue
Line (iXStart, iYStart)-(iXEnd, iYEnd), iLineColor
```

Let's write a program to draw an *X* in a picturebox called picX. (See Figure 13.5.)

Figure 13.5

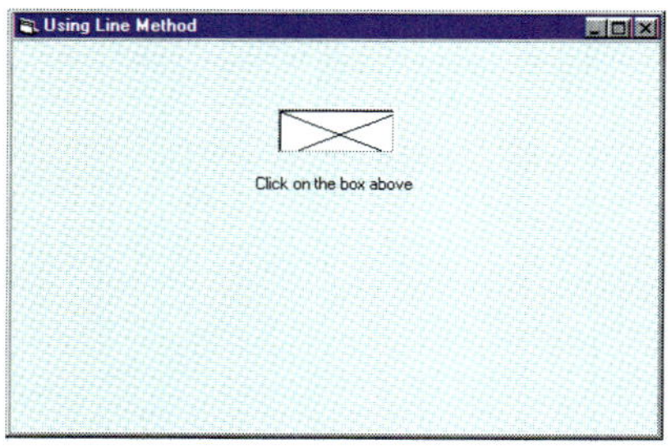

The screen for project Ch1302.

```
'Program:      Line
'Programmer:   A. Millspaugh
'Date:         December 1997
'Description:  Draw lines in a picture box.
'Folder:       Ch1302
Option Explicit
```

```
Private Sub picX_Click()
    'Create an X in the picture box

    picX.Line (0, 0)-(picX.Width, picX.Height)
    picX.Line (0, picX.Height)-(picX.Width, 0)
End Sub
```

Rectangles

You can also use the `Line` method to create boxes by adding the *B* parameter. The *B* stands for *box*. You can fill a box without specifying a color; the box will use the FillColor property. However, make sure to include the commas to indicate that the color argument is missing.

```
Line ( 0, 0)-(500, 500), ,B
```

The box may be filled with a solid color or a pattern, depending on the setting of the FillStyle property.

FillStyle	Name	Pattern
0	Solid	Uses the FillColor to fill the box.
1	Transparent (default)	No fill regardless of the FillColor setting.
2	Horizontal lines	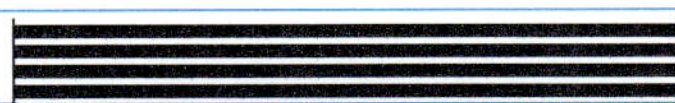
3	Vertical lines	
4	Upward diagonal lines	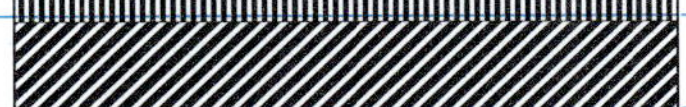
5	Downward diagonal lines	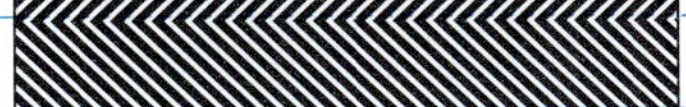
6	Crosshatch	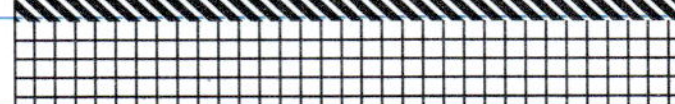
7	Diagonal crosshatch	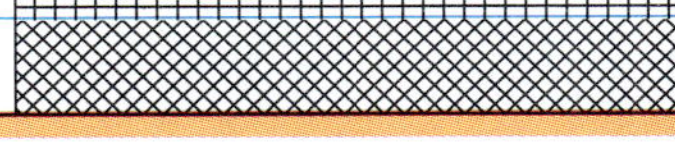

The *F* option listed in the general form of the `Line` method may be used to *fill* the box instead of using the FillStyle and the FillColor properties. You cannot use the *F* option without the *B*.

The Circle Method

You can draw rounded shapes using the **`Circle` method**. These shapes include circles, ovals, arcs, and pie-shaped wedges. To draw a circle, specify the coordinates of the center and the radius of the circle. You may also specify the color or let it default to the ForeColor.

```
picFace.Circle (160,100), 60
```

You can choose whether or not the circle is filled by setting the FillStyle property.

```
FillStyle = 0
Circle (1000,1000),500          'A filled circle
FillStyle = 1
Circle (2000,1000),500          'Outline of a circle
```

The full form of the `Circle` method includes an argument for start angle and end angle that will determine arcs and wedges. The aspect ratio argument is used to make ellipses (ovals).

The Circle Method—General Form

```
[Object].Circle (x, y), Radius [, Color [, StartAngle, EndAngle [, AspectRatio] ] ]
```

Arcs of a Circle

To draw parts of a circle, you can specify the beginning and ending points of the arc. The endpoints for the arc are determined by a measurement in radians, counterclockwise from 0 to 2 PI. The angle reference is illustrated below:

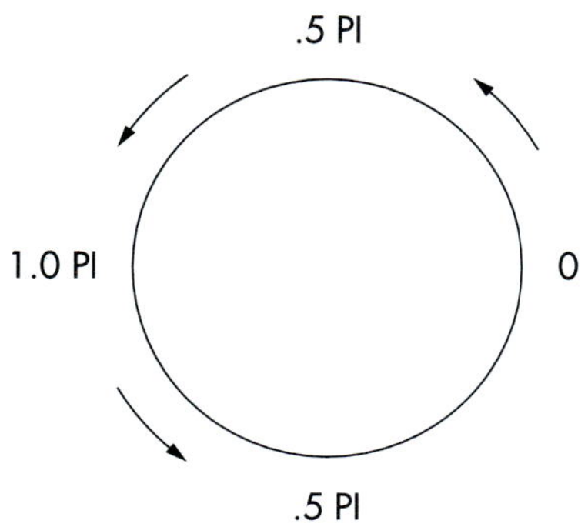

The statements

```
Const PI = 3.14159
Circle (500, 500), 500, , 0, PI
```

draw the top half of a circle, beginning at the right side (angle 0) and proceeding over the top to the left side (angle PI).

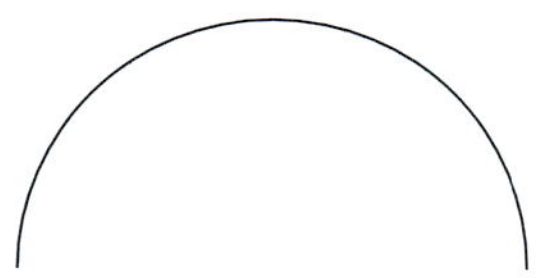

The following program uses circles and arcs to draw a happy face. Place the code in the form's Paint event. (See Figure 13.6.)

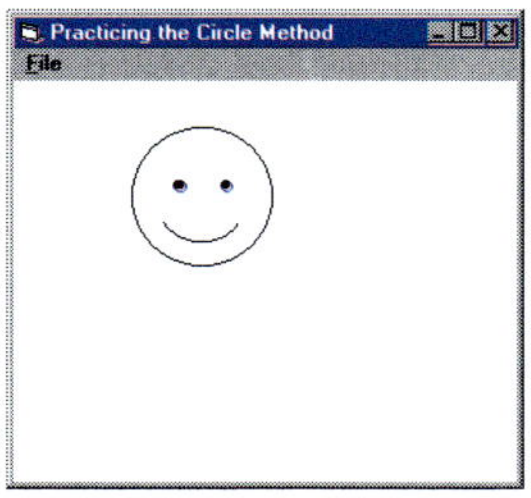

Figure 13.6

The screen for project Ch1303.

```
'Program:      Circle
'Programmer:   A. Millspaugh
'Date:         December 1997
'Description:  Draw a happy face.
'Folder:       Ch1303
Option Explicit
```

```
Private Sub Form_Paint()
    'Draw a happy face on the form
    Const PI = 3.14159

    FillStyle = 1
    Circle (1600, 1000), 600              'Outline of the face
    Circle (1600, 1000), 400, , PI * 1.2, PI * 1.8   'Smile
    FillStyle = 0
    Circle (1400, 900), 50, vbBlue        'Left eye
    Circle (1800, 900), 50, vbBlue        'Right eye
End Sub
```

```
Private Sub mnuFileExit_Click()
    'Terminate the project

    End
End Sub
```

Segments of a Pie

You can draw an arc with its endpoints connected to the center of the circle, creating a slice of pie. If you specify an endpoint as a negative number, a radius is drawn from the endpoint to the center point. *Note:* The minus sign preceding the endpoint specifies the radius; it does not indicate a negative angle.

```
Circle (50, 100), 30, , -PI / 2, -PI
```

will produce

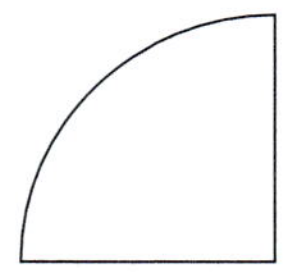

Ellipses

By setting the AspectRatio parameter of the `Circle` method, you can draw ellipses and elliptical arcs. The aspect ratio refers to the comparative length of a radius drawn on the horizontal to a radius drawn vertically. When this parameter is omitted, the aspect ratio is assumed to be one and the figure drawn is a circle. When the aspect ratio is less than one, the elliptical figure will be wider than it is tall. When the aspect ratio is greater than one, the ellipse will display taller than it is wide. (Notice the commas in the statements that indicate omitted parameters.)

```
Circle (1000,1000),1000, , , , .5       'Wide ellipse
Circle (3000,1000),1000, , , , 1.5      'Tall ellipse
```

Give the preceding lines of code a try.

The Step Keyword

Each graphics method discussed here can also use the **`Step` method**, which changes the coordinates from an absolute position to a relative position. Coordinates are normally measured from the starting point of the object (**absolute position**) on which they are drawn. By adding the `Step`, coordinates begin from the last point that was drawn, hence the starting point is a **relative position**.

A variation of the `PSet` method is the `PSet Step` statement that indicates that the x and y coordinates specified are relative to the last point drawn. The statement

```
PSet Step (100,100)
```

draws a point 100 twips to the right and 100 twips down from the last point specified in a graphics method. If there are no previous graphics methods, the offset is from the 0, 0 coordinate.

With the `Line` method you can give the second set of coordinates as an offset from the first.

```
Line -Step(1000, 1000)
```

Try the following lines of code:

```
PSet Step(100, 100)
Line -Step(1000, 1000)
Line -Step(2000, 0)
```

Feedback 13.1

1. Write the statement to draw a vertical line down the center of a form that has the following settings: ScaleWidth 6720, ScaleHeight 4230.
2. Write the statements to draw a "Pacman."

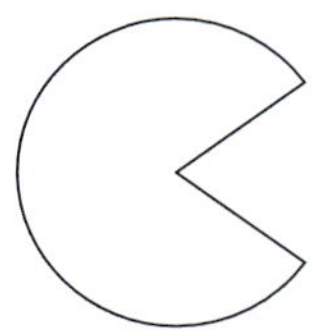

Layering

When displaying information on an object, different types of items are placed on different layers. The complete set of layers produces the output that we can see. (See Figure 13.7.)

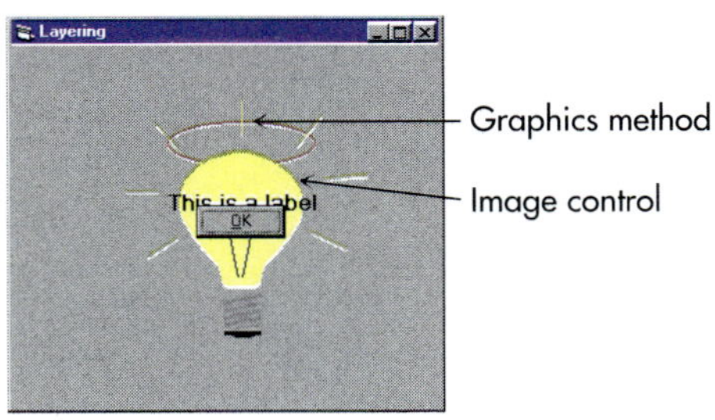

Figure 13.7

Most controls appear on the top layer, graphics controls appear on the middle layer, and graphics created with graphics methods appear on the bottom layer.

Layer	Contents
Front	Command buttons, check boxes, and other nongraphic controls.
Middle	Labels; graphics controls.
Back	Shapes created with graphics methods.

The items in the back layer are covered by items in the middle layer, which are then covered by controls in the front layer. Usually this arrangement is what you want, allowing your graphics to form a background for the controls. However, these default layers may act differently depending on the settings of the AutoRedraw and ClipControls properties, which contain Boolean values, and on whether the graphics methods are located in the Paint event or elsewhere.

If you set the **AutoRedraw property** to True, you will get **persistent graphics**, which save an image in memory so that it can be redisplayed. Although Windows takes care of windows and controls when objects are moved or resized, it is up to you to control the redraw for graphics. Although it sounds easy to just set AutoRedraw to True, there is a trade-off in performance because the process requires a large amount of memory. The default setting of AutoRedraw is False for forms and True for pictureboxes. It is to your advantage to place graphic images in pictureboxes rather than on forms because less memory is required.

One technique is to leave AutoRedraw set to False and call the Paint event procedure when needed.

The **clipping region** determines which portions of the screen will be painted. A form, frame, or picturebox has a **ClipControls property**. Setting ClipControls to False can also speed up the repainting process but may cause items to be mixed in the layering.

Use these guidelines for redrawing graphics:

1. When AutoRedraw is set to False, place graphics methods in the Paint event of the form or container.
2. Setting AutoRedraw to True will always provide normal layering but will slow the performance because too much memory is required. (Setting ClipControls to False may speed up the form display.)

You can also adjust the stacking order of items within a layer using the **`ZOrder` method**. This method can be used for forms or controls. Refer to Help for more information on the ZOrder method.

More Properties for Your Graphics Controls

You have used icons for the Picture property of an image control. Pictures in the form of bitmaps, icons, or metafiles may be added to a project during design time or at run time. You can create your own pictures in a Paint or Draw program and then copy and paste them using the Clipboard. Pictures may be placed in an image control, a picturebox control, or a form.

Controlling Pictures at Design Time

All three controls that can contain a picture have a Picture property. If you set the Picture property of a form, the graphic displays behind the controls. An advantage of using the image control rather than the picturebox control is that an image has a Stretch property that can be used to adjust the size of the picture when set to True.

Another way to insert a picture in a control is by using the Clipboard. First copy a picture from clip art or one that you created into the Clipboard. Then switch to Visual Basic and the *Paste* command on the *Edit* menu will be available to transfer the picture from the Clipboard onto the control.

To remove a picture, double-click the setting in the Picture property and press the Delete key.

Controlling Pictures at Run Time

You may also want to add or change a picture at run time. You can do so by having images or pictures that have their original Visible property set to False or by using the **LoadPicture function**.

If you store a picture in an invisible control, you can change the Visible setting to True; or you may decide to copy it to another control.

```
picLogo.Visible = True
imgLogo.Picture = picLogo.Picture
```

The `LoadPicture` function can be used in code to retrieve a file during run time. The problem with this method is that the path must be known. When you are running an application on multiple systems the path names may be different.

```
picLogo.Picture = LoadPicture("C:\VB\LOGO.BMP")
```

To remove a picture from the display, either hide it or use the `LoadPicture` function with empty quotes.

```
imgLogo.Visible = False
picLogo.Picture = LoadPicture("")
```

Moving a Picture

You can move picture controls by changing the values of the Left and Top properties. Another choice is the **Move method**. Since line controls do not have Top and Left properties, you must use the `Move` method to move them. The `Move` method produces a smoother appearing move than changing the Top and Left properties of controls.

The Move Method—General Form

```
[Object].Move Left [, Top[, Width[, Height]]]
```

Only the new setting for the Left property is required, but the Top, Width, and Height may also be changed. If no object is specified, the move applies to the current form.

The Move Method—Examples

```
Move 100                          'Changes the Left property of the current form
imgLogo.Move 100, 200
imgLogo.Move imgMove.Left + 50    'Moves relative to current position
```

Notice that a move can be relative to the current location by performing calculations in the `Move` method.

Simple Animation

Animation can be created by toggling between two pictures, moving a picture, or rotating through a series of pictures. You can also create graphics with the various graphics methods.

Many of the icons in the icon library have similar sizes but opposite states such as a closed file cabinet and an open file cabinet; a mail box with the flag up and with the flag down; a closed envelope and an open envelope; or a traffic light in red, yellow, or green. In Chapter 2 you used the two light bulbs: LightOn and LightOff.

The sample program demonstrates changing between two phone icons (a phone and a phone being held). The two icons are phone12.ico and phone13.ico in the Vb\Graphics\Icons\Comm folder. Two images, imgWithHand and imgNoHand, are set to invisible (Visible = False) and then assigned to imgPhone at run time. (See Figure 13.8.)

Figure 13.8

The screen for project Ch1304.

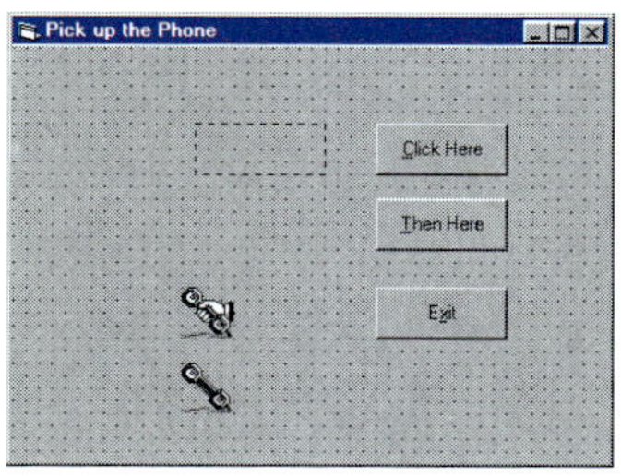


```
'Program:      Phones
'Programmer:   A. Millspaugh
'Date:         December 1997
'Description:  Change a picture of a phone to
'              show someone holding it.
'Folder:       Ch1304
Option Explicit
```

```
Private Sub cmdChange_Click()
    'Change the phones

    imgPhone.Picture = imgWithHand.Picture
End Sub
```

```
Private Sub cmdExit_Click()
    'Terminate the project

    End
End Sub
```

```
Private Sub cmdStart_Click()
    'Display the phone

    imgPhone.Picture = imgNoHand.Picture
End Sub
```

Several interesting procedures are supplied in a sample project called Blanker that comes with Visual Basic. The path for Blanker is usually Program Files\DevStudio\VB\Samples\PGuide\Blanker.

Try creating a picturebox, name it picAnimate, place one line control inside (called Line1), and use the following code for a command button:

```
Dim X, Y
For Y = 1 to 25
      picAnimate.Cls
      line1.X1 = Int(PicAnimate.Width * Rnd)
      line1.Y1 = Int(PicAnimate.Height * Rnd)
      line1.X2 = Int(PicAnimate.Width * Rnd)
      line1.Y2 = Int(PicAnimate.Height * Rnd)
      For X = 1 To 5000
      Next X              'Keep on screen awhile
Next Y
```

A nicer way to control the delay in the previous example is to use the timer control.

The Timer Control

You can build in a delay with a set interval using the **timer control** and its Timer event. You can place the control anywhere on the form; it is invisible at run time. The tool for the timer control is represented by the little stop-watch in the toolbox (Figure 13.9). The three-character prefix for naming a timer is "tmr".

Figure 13.9

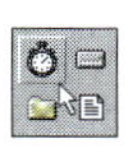

The tool for the timer control.

When you have a timer control on a form, it "fires" each time an interval elapses. You can place any desired code in the Timer event procedure; the code will execute each time the event occurs. You choose the interval for the timer by setting its **Interval property**, which can have a value of 0 to 65,535. This value specifies the number of milliseconds between the calls to the Timer event. One second is equivalent to 1,000 milliseconds. Therefore, for a three-second delay, set the timer's Interval property to 3,000. You can set the value at run time or at design time.

You can keep the Timer event from occurring by setting its **Enabled property** to False. The default value is True.

Your Hands-On Programming Example

In this project you will use a timer control to create simple animation. Place an airplane icon in an image control, move it across the screen, and also make it appear larger as it goes.

First, sketch a plan of the form (Figure 13.10).

Figure 13.10

A planning sketch for the hands-on programming example.

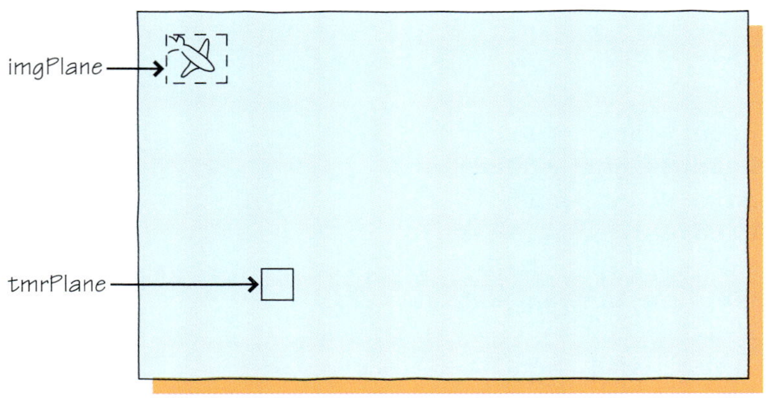

Plan the Objects and Properties

Object	Property	Setting
frmPlane	Name	frmPlane
	Caption	Fly the Plane
tmrPlane	Name	tmrPlane
	Interval	50
imgPlane	Name	imgPlane
	Icon	Vb\Graphics\Icons\Industry\Plane.ico

Plan the Event Proecedures

Plan the actions for the event procedure.

Procedure	Actions
tmrPlane_Timer	Move the plane. Adjust the size.

Write the Project

- Follow the sketch in Figure 13.10 to create the form. Figure 13.11 shows the completed form.

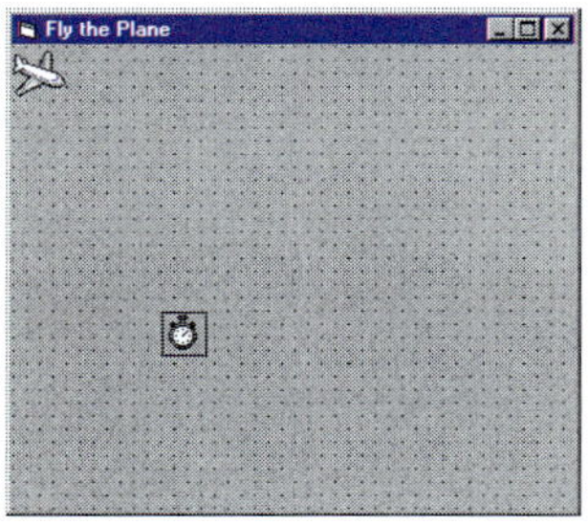

Figure 13.11

The form for the hands-on programming example.

- Set the properties of each object according to your plan.
- Write the code. Working from the pseudocode, write each event procedure.
- Thoroughly test the project.

The Programming Coding Solution

```
'Program:      Plane
'Programmer:   A. Millspaugh
'Date:         December 1997
'Description:  Move a plane with the timer.
'Folder:       Ch1305
Option Explicit
```

```
Private Sub TmrPlane_Timer()
    'Fly the Plane

    imgPlane.Move imgPlane.Left + 10, _
                  imgPlane.Top + 10, _
                  imgPlane.Width + 2, _
                  imgPlane.Height + 2
End Sub
```

More Graphics Techniques

Custom Coordinate Systems

You can specify a custom scale for your graphics by changing the coordinate system. Perhaps you would like the upper-left corner to start at 0,0 and the lower-right corner to be 100,100. Then all of your coordinates for graphics will be between 0 and 100. This change can be accomplished with the `Scale` method.

The Scale Method—General Form

```
[Object].Scale (x1 , y1) - (x2, y2)
```

The Scale Method—Example

```
picLogo.Scale (0, 0) - (100, 100)
```

The handy result of this statement is that you could then use ratios. The midpoint would be (50, 50).

The `Scale` method performs the same function as individually altering the settings in ScaleLeft, ScaleTop, ScaleWidth, and ScaleHeight.

PaintPicture Method

Another graphics method that you have available is the `PaintPicture` method, which can be used to place a graphic file on a form, the printer object, or in a picturebox.

This method is faster than moving picture controls around and can be used to copy graphics, such as when tiling a picture on the screen. By making the destination width a negative number, the graphic file can be flipped horizontally.

The PaintPicture Method—General Form

```
[Object].PaintPicture Picture, x1, y1[, DestinationWidth,_
DestinationHeight]
```

The PaintPicture Method—Example

```
PaintPicture picLogo.Picture, 100, 100
```

The following program creates a tiled image on the form (Figure 13.12).

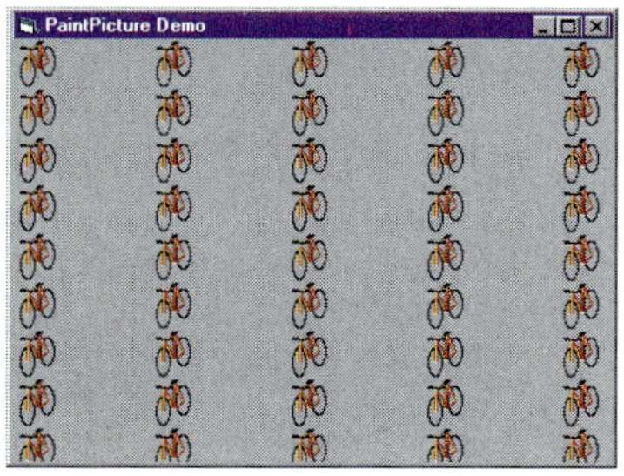

Figure 13.12

The form for example Ch1306.

```
'Program:     Tile
'Programmer:  A. Millspaugh
'Date:        December 1997
'Description: Create a tiled background on a form.
'Folder:      Ch1306
Option Explicit
________________________________________________

Private Sub Form_Paint()
    'Tile the background of the form
    Dim iIndex1 As Integer
    Dim iIndex2 As Integer

    For iIndex1 = 0 To 10
        For iIndex2 = 0 To 10
            frmTile.PaintPicture picTile.picture, _
                iIndex2 * picTile.Width, _
                iIndex1 * picTile.Height
        Next iIndex2
    Next iIndex1
End Sub
```

The Scroll Bar Controls

You can add **horizontal scroll bars** and **vertical scroll bars** to your form (Figure 13.13). These **scroll bar controls** are similar to the scroll bars in Windows that can be used to scroll through a document or window. Often scroll bars are used to control sound level, color, size, and other values that can be changed in small amounts or large increments.

Figure 13.13

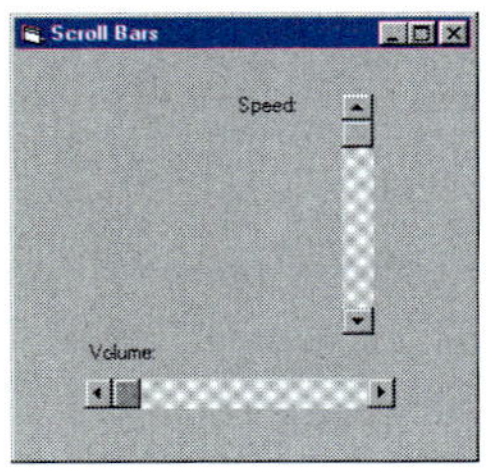

Horizontal scroll bars and vertical scroll bars can be used to select a value over a given range.

Properties for scroll bars are somewhat different than the controls we have worked with previously. Because the scroll bars represent a range of values, they have the following properties: **Min** for the minimum value, **Max** for the maximum value, **SmallChange** for the distance to move when the user clicks on the scroll arrows, and **LargeChange** for the distance to move when the user clicks on the gray area of the scroll bar (Figure 13.14).

Figure 13.14

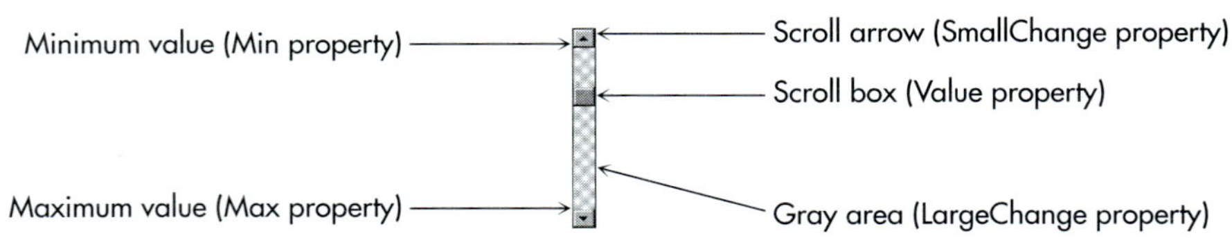

Clicking on the scroll arrow changes the Value property by SmallChange amount; clicking on the gray area of the scroll bar changes the Value property by LargeChange amount.

The Value property indicates the current position of the scroll box and its corresponding value within the scroll bar. When the user clicks the up arrow of a vertical scroll bar, the Value property decreases by the amount of SmallChange (if the Min value has not been reached). Clicking the down arrow causes the Value property to increase by the amount of SmallChange.

When naming scroll bars, use a prefix of "hsb" for horizontal scroll bars and "vsb" for vertical scroll bars. Figure 13.15 shows the horizontal scroll bar tool and vertical scroll bar tool from the toolbox.

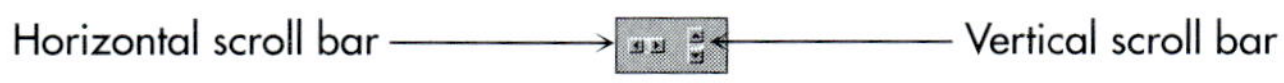

Figure 13.15

The toolbox tools for horizontal scroll bars and vertical scroll bars.

Scroll Bar Events

The events that occur for scroll bars differ from the ones used for other controls. Although a user might click on the scroll bar, there is no Click event; rather there are two events: a Change event and a Scroll event.

When the user clicks on a scroll arrow or the gray area of the scroll bar, a **Change event** occurs. If the user drags the scroll box instead, a **Scroll event** occurs. In fact, multiple scroll events occur, as long as the user continues to drag the scroll box. As soon as the user releases the mouse button, the Scroll events cease and a Change event occurs. When you write code for a scroll bar, usually you will want to code both a Change event procedure and a Scroll event procedure.

A Fun Programming Example

You can try the scroll bars and the shape controls with this little exercise. Open a new project and create a rectangle on the form using a shape control. Make a note of the shape's Location properties—Left, Top, Width, and Height. Then create an image inside the rectangle with its Picture property set to an icon of a car.

A horizontal scroll bar will make the image move sideways in the rectangle, and the vertical scroll bar will make it move up and down. Make sure that you set the Max and Min properties of the scroll bar to reflect the screen location of the rectangle. The SmallChange and LargeChange also need to be set.

Design and Create the Form

Figure 13.16 shows the form for this scroll bar example.

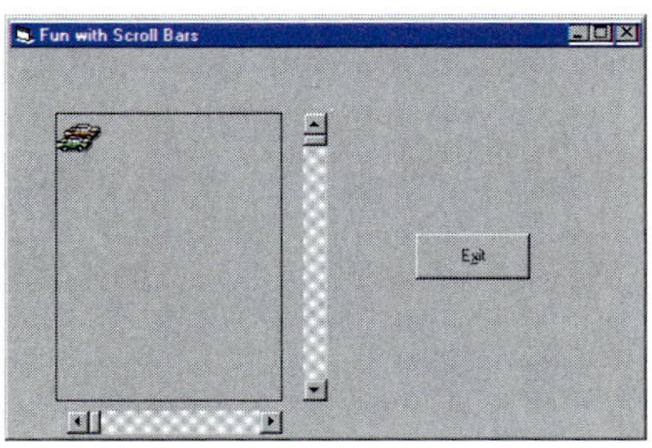

Figure 13.16

The form for the scroll bar programming example.

Set the Properties

Control	Property	Setting
Form1	Caption	Fun with Scroll Bars
	Name	frmScroll
shpRectangle	Name	shpRectangle
	Shape	0 - Rectangle
	Height	3135
	Left	480
	Top	720
	Width	2415
imgCar	Name	imgCar
	Picture	Vb\Graphics\Icons\Industry\Cars.ico
	Height	480
	Width	480
hsbMoveCar	Name	hsbMoveCar
	Min	480
	Max	1935 (rectangle width - image width)
	LargeChange	50
	SmallChange	10
vsbMoveCar	Name	vsbMoveCar
	Min	720 (top of rectangle)
	Max	3135 (rectangle height)
	LargeChange	50
	SmallChange	10
cmdExit	Name	cmdExit
	Caption	E&xit

Write the Code

Procedure	Actions
cmdExit_Click	Terminate the project.
vsbMoveCar_Change	Assign the scroll bar Value to the Top property of the image.
vsbMoveCar_Scroll	Assign the scroll bar Value to the Top property of the image.
hsbMoveCar_Change	Assign the scroll bar Value to the Left property of the image.
hsbMoveCar_Scroll	Assign the scroll bar Value to the Left property of the image.

The Project Coding Solution

```
'Program:       Scroll
'Programmer:    A. Millspaugh
'Date:          December 1997
'Description:   Use scroll bars to move an image
'               horizontally and vertically within the
'               limits of a rectangle.
'Folder:        Ch1307
Option Explicit
```

```
Private Sub cmdExit_Click()
    'Terminate the project

    End
End Sub
```

```
Private Sub hsbMoveCar_Change()
    'Controls the side to side movement
    'Used for arrow clicks

    imgCar.Left = hsbMoveCar.Value
End Sub
```

```
Private Sub hsbMoveCar_Scroll()
    'Controls the side to side movement
    'Used for scroll box movement

    imgCar.Left = hsbMoveCar.Value
End Sub
```

```
Private Sub vsbMoveCar_Change()
    'Positions the up and down movement
    'Used when arrow is clicked

    imgCar.Top = vsbMoveCar.Value
End Sub
```

```
Private Sub vsbMoveCar_Scroll()
    'Positions the up and down movement
    'Used when the scroll box is moved

    imgCar.Top = vsbMoveCar.Value
End Sub
```

Summary

1. Graphics may be measured in twips, points, pixels, inches, or centimeters. The measurement is known as the scale.
2. The coordinate system normally begins with 0,0 at the upper-left corner of the container object.
3. Colors are available using the `RGB` function, the intrinsic color constants, and the `QBColor` function.
4. The graphics methods include `PSet`, `Line`, and `Circle`. You can use the `Line` method to create a rectangular shape. The `Circle` method may be used for ellipses, arcs, and wedges.
5. Graphics and controls are created in three layers that produce a single display. The AutoRedraw and ClipControls properties affect the order of the layering.
6. Pictures can be loaded, moved, and resized at run time.
7. Animation effects can be created by using similar pictures and by controlling the location and visibility of controls.
8. The timer control can enable a Timer event that occurs at specified intervals.
9. Scroll bar controls are available for both horizontal and vertical control. Properties include Min, Max, SmallChange, and LargeChange. Scroll and Change events are used to control the action.

Key Terms

absolute position *480*
AutoRedraw property *482*
Change event *491*
`Circle` method *477*
ClipControls property *482*
clipping region *482*
`Cls` method *474*
container *473*
coordinate system *470*
DrawWidth property *475*
Enabled property *486*
horizontal scroll bars *490*
Interval property *486*
LargeChange property *490*
`Line` method *476*
`LoadPicture` function *483*
Max property *490*
Min property *490*
`Move` method *483*
persistent graphics *482*
picturebox control *471*
pixel *470*
point *470*
`PSet` method *474*
`QBColor` function *472*
relative position *480*
`RGB` function *471*
`Rnd` function *474*
scale *470*
Scroll bar control *490*
Scroll event *491*
SmallChange property *490*
`Step` method *480*
timer control *485*
twip *470*
vertical scroll bars *490*
`ZOrder` method *482*

Review Questions

1. How big is a twip?
2. To which controls do the graphics methods apply?
3. What happens when no object is specified for a graphics method such as `PSet` or `Cls`?
4. Name three methods available for graphics.
5. How is a pie-shaped wedge created?
6. What is the advantage to setting the AutoRedraw to True? to False?
7. What function is used to load a picture at run time?
8. How is a picture removed at run time?
9. What steps are necessary to change an image that contains a turned-off light bulb to a turned-on light bulb?
10. What is the purpose of the timer control?

Programming Exercises

13.1 Create a project that contains a picturebox and two buttons labeled *Smile* and *Frown.* The Smile button will display a happy face in the picturebox; Frown will display a sad face. Use graphics methods to draw the two faces.

13.2 Use graphics methods to create the background of a form. Draw a picture of a house, including a front door, a window, and a chimney.

13.3 Use an image control with a .bmp file from Windows. Set the Stretch property to True. Use a scroll bar to change the size of the image.

13.4 Use graphics from a clip art collection to create a project that has a command button for each month of the year. Have an appropriate image display in a picturebox for each month.

13.5 Use the bicycle icon from Visual Basic and a timer control to move the bicycle around the screen. Add a Start button and a Stop button. The Stop button will position the bicycle back to its original position. (The bicycle icon is stored as Vb\Graphics\Icons\Industry\Bicycle.ico.)

CASE STUDIES

VB Mail Order

Create a logo for VB Mail Order using graphics methods. Place the logo in the startup form for the project from Chapter 6. Add appropriate images and graphics to enhance each form. The graphics may come from .bmp files, clip art, or your own creation from Paintbrush.

VB Auto Center

Have the startup screen initially fill with random dots in random colors. Draw an Auto Center advertisement using graphics methods that will appear on the screen. Have various appropriate images (icons) appear in different locations, remain momentarily, and then disappear.

CHAPTER

14

Advanced Topics in Visual Basic

At the completion of this chapter, you will be able to...

1. Use ActiveX controls to extend the functionality of your projects.
2. Create a link from a Visual Basic project to a Web site.
3. Include procedures from dynamic link libraries (DLLs) in your projects.
4. Realize the potential for programming using the Windows API.
5. Use an OLE container control for linking or embedding objects.
6. Recognize the relationship between Visual Basic and VBA.
7. Understand the concepts of an object and a class.
8. Create a report using Crystal Reports.

In addition to the large variety of controls, statements, and functions that are a part of the language, as a Visual Basic programmer you have the opportunity to reach many other sources for your application needs. Controls have been referred to as *objects.* Objects go far beyond the controls that are a part of Visual Basic. Think of **objects** as programming components. You can create your own objects or incorporate those available from word processors, spreadsheets, graphics programs, and the multitude of software available.

Programs that run under Windows have access to other applications' objects through ActiveX controls, the object linking and embedding (OLE) container control, and through dynamic link libraries (DLLs). This chapter introduces these topics as well as some components designed specifically for use with Visual Basic.

ActiveX

The term **ActiveX** was originally used to refer to controls that could be used with the Internet. Since then the term has been expanded to refer to executable files, controls (COM, or Component Object Model, objects), and DLLs that are used by multiple applications. These controls were called *OLE controls* for a period of time, but the term OLE currently refers only to the process of object linking and embedding. The terminology has been changing rapidly and likely will change somewhat in the next few years as the use of the Internet expands.

Using ActiveX Controls

You have used many controls built into Visual Basic, plus some others, such as the grid and the common dialog box, that had to be added to the Visual Basic environment. In general, Microsoft refers to any controls as *ActiveX controls.* These controls may be part of Visual Basic or created by other companies, or you may create your own. The controls that are part of Visual Basic are called *intrinsic controls*; those that must be added later are called *components.* Many ActiveX controls are available in the Professional and Enterprise Editions of Visual Basic, as well as from other software developers.

A large selection of ActiveX controls is available to solve many problems. You can purchase controls to display various types of gauges and indicators, display data in grids, send and receive faxes, display video, scan bar codes, display calendars and appointments, and perform many other functions. Many ActiveX controls are available as shareware, and a few are freeware. Many can be downloaded from various Web sites.

The files for ActiveX controls have extensions of .OCX or .VBX. (Any controls developed for Visual Basic 4.0 or later should be .OCX files.)

Tip

To include objects that are available from other applications, use the *References* dialog box, which you can select from the *Project* menu.

When you select the *Components* command from the *Project* menu, you see a list of the controls available on the system (Figure 14.1). As you select a component name from the list, a line at the bottom of the dialog box shows the name and location of the selected control file. In most cases the file extension will be .OCX.

Figure 14.1

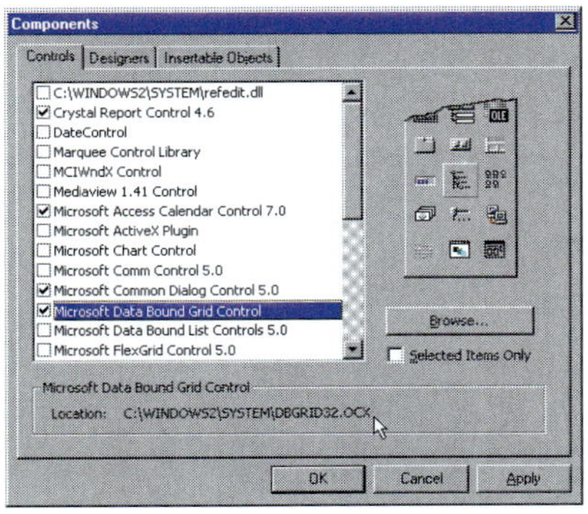

Available ActiveX controls appear in the Components dialog box.

The Tabbed Dialog Control

One of the handy extra controls that comes with Visual Basic is the Microsoft Tabbed Dialog Control 5.0. The tabbed dialog is a convenient way for placing a large amount of related material in one dialog box. You can find many examples of tabbed dialogs in Visual Basic, such as the *Components* dialog box that has three tabs: *Controls*, *Designers*, and *Insertable Objects*. Figure 14.2 shows a dialog box with a **Tabbed Dialog control**.

Figure 14.2

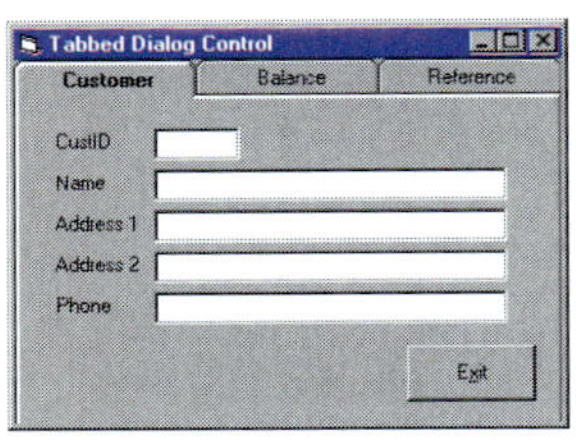

The tabs in this form were created with the Tabbed Dialog control.

To add a Tabbed Dialog control to your project, you must first add the control to your toolbox. Select *Microsoft Tabbed Dialog Control 5.0* from the *Components* dialog box (Figure 14.3). Figure 14.4 shows the Tabbed Dialog tool in the toolbox and a control on a form.

Figure 14.3

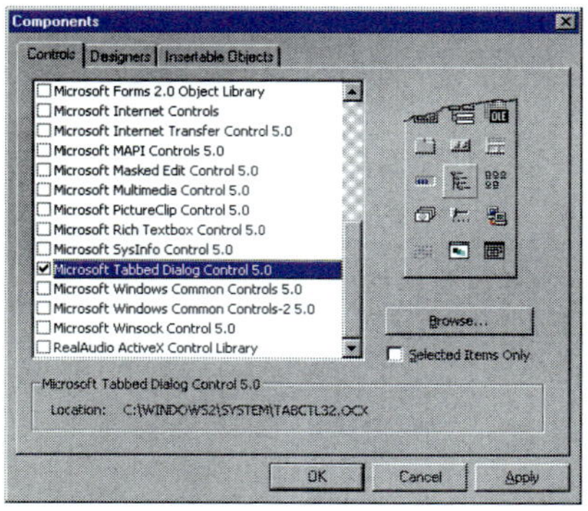

Select the Tabbed Dialog control from the Components *dialog box.*

Figure 14.4

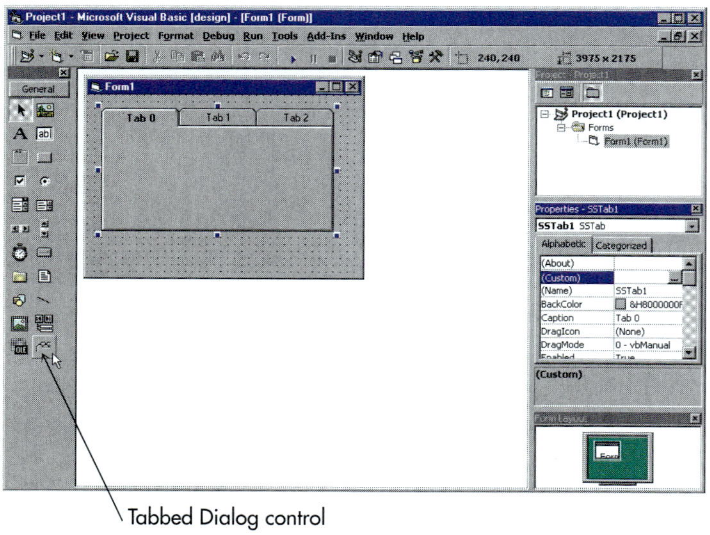

The tool for the Tabbed Dialog control as it appear in the toolbox and a control on a form.

The Tabbed Dialog control has many properties and methods that you can set or check at run time or at design time. The default name of the tab is SSTab1. Use the prefix "tab" when naming your control.

The easiest way to initially set up the control is to use the custom *Property Pages* dialog box (Figure 14.5). To display this dialog box, either click on the builder button for *Custom* in the control's Properties window (Figure 14.6) or right-click the control and select *Properties* from the shortcut menu (Figure 14.7). In this dialog box you can specify the number of tabs, tabs per row, and the tab caption of each tab. *Note:* The first tab is tab 0, the next is tab 1, and so forth.

Figure 14.5

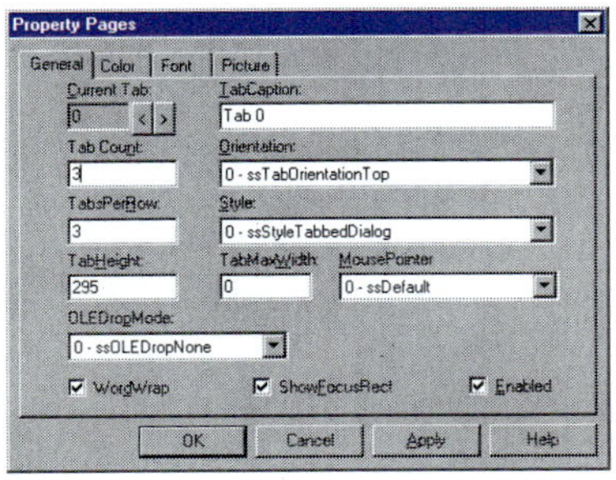

Set the properties for the Tabbed Dialog control in its custom Property Pages *dialog box.*

Figure 14.6

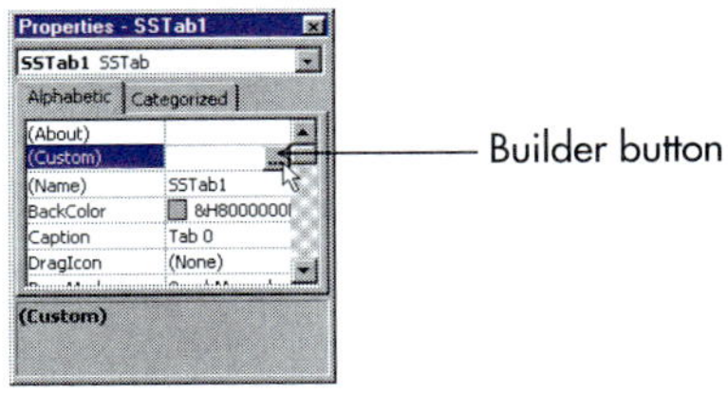

One way to display the Property Pages *dialog box is to click on the builder button for the* Custom *entry in the* Property *window.*

Figure 14.7

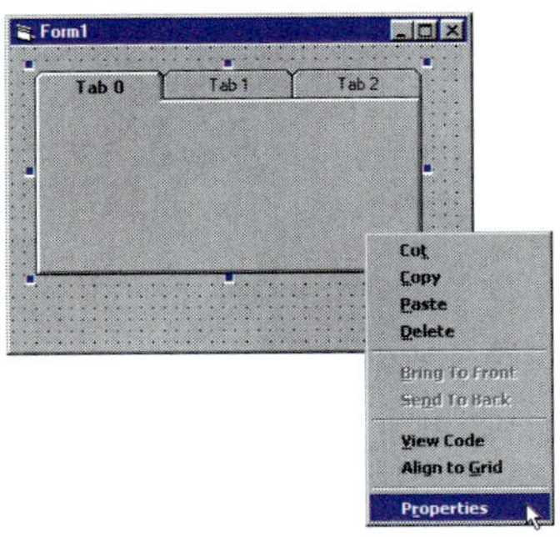

You can display the Property Pages *dialog box by right-clicking on the control to display the shortcut menu and selecting* Properties.

You can also set up the Tabbed Dialog control using the Properties window. To set the tab captions, click on each tab to select it and then change the caption in the Properties window.

Placing Controls on the Tab Sheets of a Tabbed Control

When you place controls such as text boxes and labels on top of a tabbed dialog control, usually you want the controls to appear only on the one tab page. Select the desired control's toolbox tool and manually draw the new control on top of the tabbed dialog control (do not double-click to place the control). If you double-click on a control in the toolbox, you are actually placing the control on the form and the control will appear on every tab. (This process is similar to the way you place controls inside frame controls; the Tabbed Dialog control is a container for the controls that "belong to" it.) If you *do* want a control to appear on all tabs, such as an Exit button, then place the control by double-clicking.

The Tabbed Dialog control for R 'n R has a *Coffee* tab with a list box and another tab containing a combo box. See Figures 14.8 and 14.9.

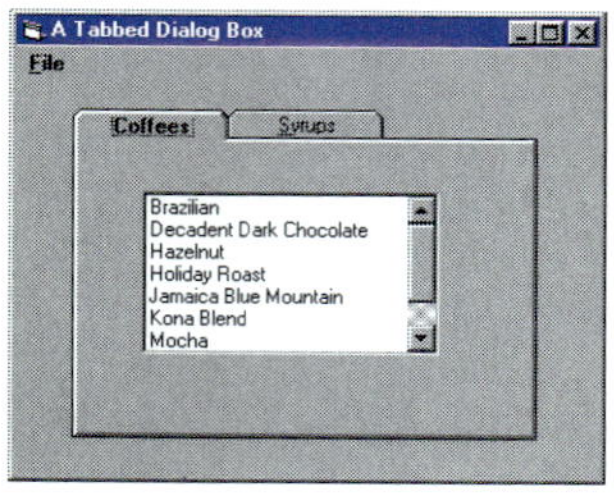

Figure 14.8

The form for R 'n R has a Tabbed Dialog control with two tabs.

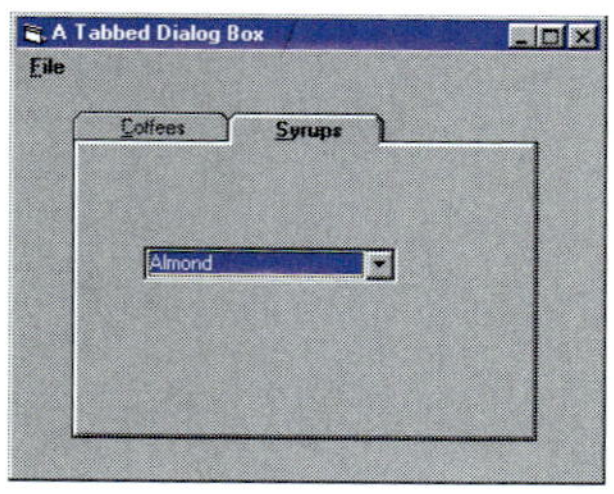

Figure 14.9

The second tab on the form for R 'n R holds a different list from the first tab.

Browsing the Web from a Visual Basic Project

New to VB 5!

Another ActiveX control available on the *Components* dialog box is the **Web browser control** (Figure 14.10). To add this control to your toolbox, place a check on the Microsoft Internet Controls in the *Components* selection of the *Project* menu. You can now link your Visual Basic application to the Internet.

Figure 14.10

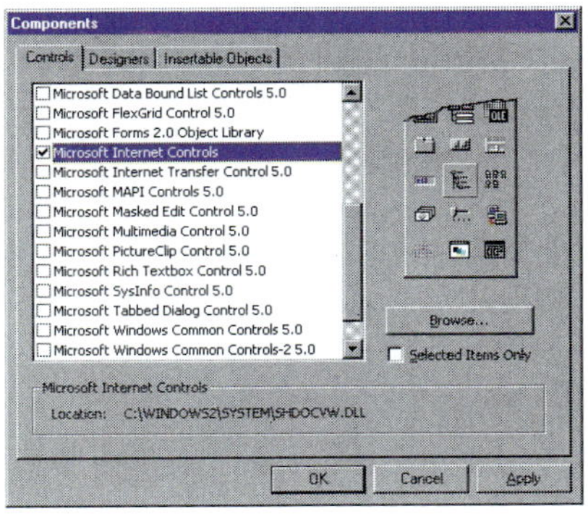

Add a Web browser control to a project by selecting Microsoft Internet Controls *in the* Components *dialog box.*

When you add this control to your project, a new window is created (Figure 14.11). Web pages will appear in this window on your form. The default name is WebBrowser1. When naming your control use the prefix "web".

Figure 14.11

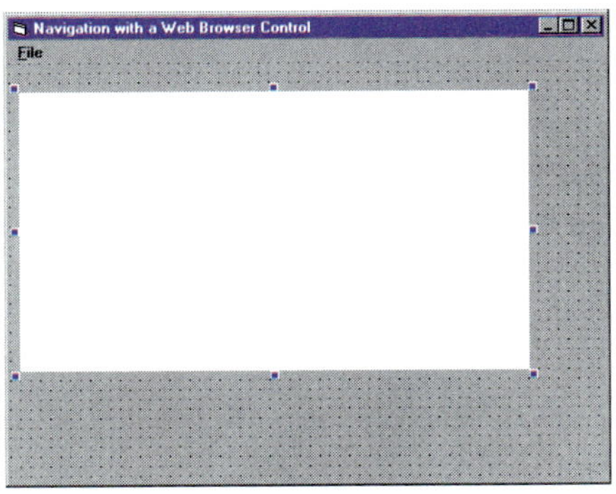

A Web browser control on a form. Web pages will appear in the window created by the control.

One of the methods of the control is `Navigate` that allows you to specify a specific Web site URL. Place the link as a string following the call to the method. The following code will bring up the Microsoft home page if there is a current connection to the Internet:

```
webBrowser.Navigate "Microsoft.com"
```

The computer system must be connected through an Internet provider for this control to work. If no browser is open, the project will attempt to open Internet Explorer. The program will work using Netscape Navigator; open the browser before executing your Visual Basic project.

Creating Your Own ActiveX Controls

In VB5 it is easy to create your own controls. In the *New Project* dialog box, you can choose to begin a new project for an ActiveX control, an ActiveX EXE, or an ActiveX DLL.

New to VB 5!

An ActiveX Control Project Using the Calendar Control

We will create a new ActiveX control that contains a Microsoft calendar control, a text box, and a command button. The user will enter a date in the text box and click the command button, and the corresponding date will appear on the calendar. Figure 14.12 shows the custom control; the following steps explain how to create it.

Figure 14.12

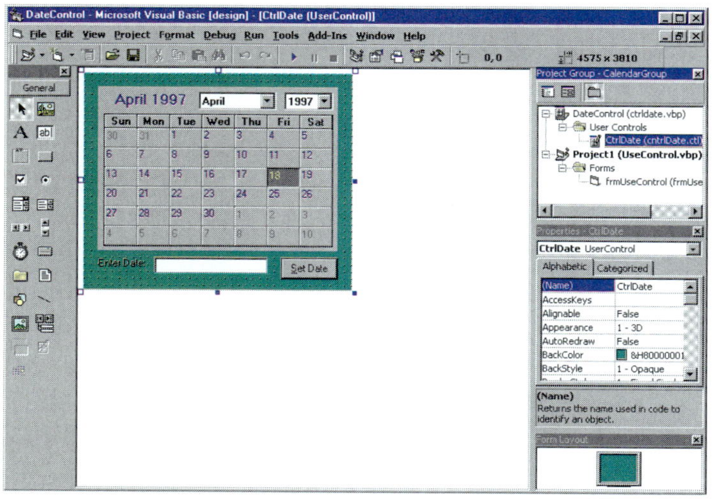

This form and controls make up a new custom control created with VB.

STEP 1: Open a new project selecting the ActiveX control option (Figure 14.13).

Figure 14.13

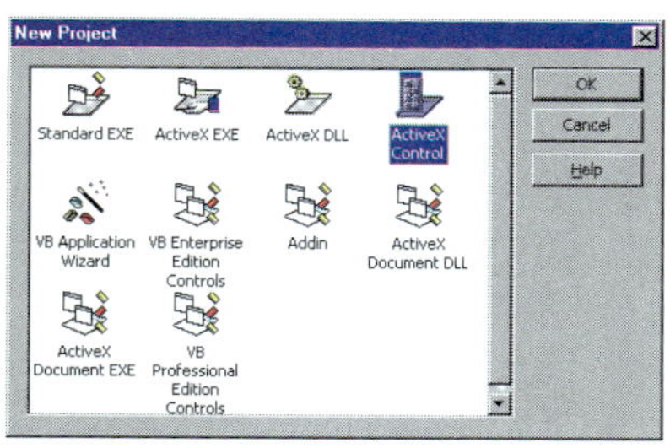

Select New Project from the File menu and select ActiveX Control to create a new control.

STEP 2: Use the *Components* dialog box to add *Microsoft Access Calendar Control 7.0* to your project and form (Figure 14.14).

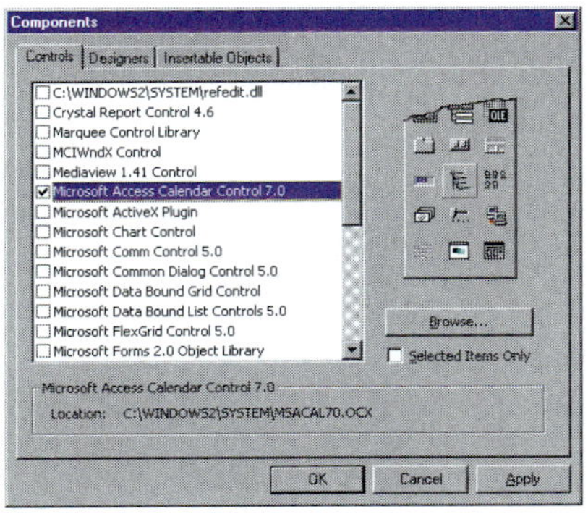

Figure 14.14

Select Microsoft Access Calendar Control 7.0 in the Components dialog box to add the control to your toolbox.

STEP 3: Design the interface and the code as you would for any other project (Figure 14.15).

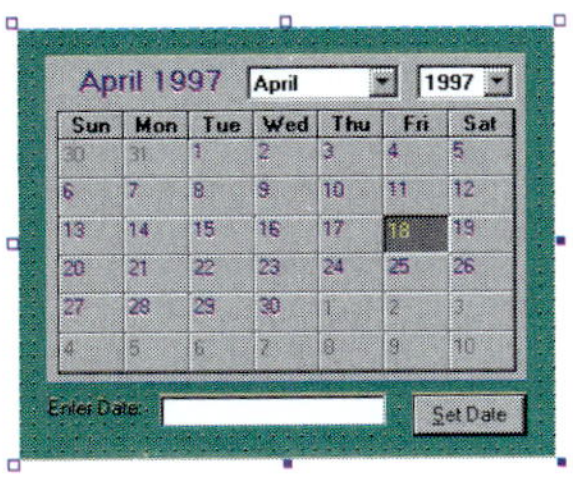

Figure 14.15

Set up the form and controls for the new custom control.

STEP 4: Select *Make .OCX* from the *File* menu to compile the code. Name your new control calDate.ocx; the control will automatically be placed in the *Components* dialog box.

STEP 5: Close the window for the control project before adding your new control to a regular VB project.

The Code for the ActiveX Control

The following program code converts the contents of the text box to a date data type. Date functions extract the year, month, and day from the date data type. Setting the properties of the calendar control (calDate) makes the date appear in the calendar.

```
'Project:        Calendar Activex
'Programmer:     A. Millspaugh
'Date:           August 1997
'Description:    Create an ActiveX control
'                that displays the date entered
'                in a text box.
'Folder:         Ch1403
```

```
Private Sub cmdDate_Click()
    'Use the date in the text box
    ' to set the calendar
    Dim dDate As Date

    If IsDate(txtDate.Text) Then
        dDate = txtDate.Text              'Convert the text box to a date data type
        calDate.Year = Year(dDate)        'Find the year and assign to calendar year
        calDate.Month = Month(dDate)      'Find the month and assign to calendar month
        calDate.Day = Day(dDate)          'Find the day and assign to calendar day
        calDate.Refresh                   'Display the Calendar again
    Else
        MsgBox "Not a valid date", vbOKOnly, "Date Check"
    End If
End Sub
```

Using Your New ActiveX Control

The steps for using the new control in a project are the same for using any other control. If your new control does not appear in the toolbox, open the *Components* dialog box; you will find its name there. Select the new control name, and the control will appear in your toolbox. Then add your new control to a form and test the control.

Dynamic Link Libraries

Libraries store commonly used procedures. As a project executes, it can call procedures from libraries. This is especially useful for procedures used by multiple projects; only one copy of the library is kept in memory and its procedures can be called by more than one project. Windows uses **dynamic link libraries (DLLs)** to store collections of procedures. The DLL file is then linked to your project when it runs. *Note:* Look at the list of library selections in the Visual Basic *References* dialog box from the *Project* menu. The line near the bottom of the dialog box shows the path including the .DLL extension (Figure 14.16). Use the Windows Explorer to look in the Windows and Windows\System folders; you will see many library files with the .DLL extension.

Figure 14.16

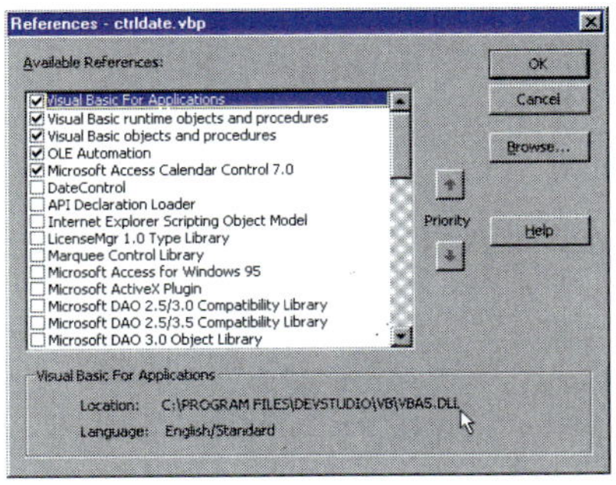

Select a DLL file from the References *dialog box. The DLL file names appear at the lower edge of the form.*

Windows applications routinely use DLLs. A project can call a function from the library and pass arguments if needed. The function is maintained separately from the programs that call it. Therefore, changes are made to the internal workings of a function in a dynamic link library without having to recode all the projects that call the function.

One extremely useful feature of Visual Basic is that a project can call and use library procedures used by the Windows system. Consequently, functions available in Windows but not available in Visual Basic can still be used. The DLLs that Windows applications use for such tasks as moving and resizing windows are referred to as the Windows application programming interface (**API**). Visual Basic uses many API DLLs to create the Visual Basic environment.

Most of the Windows DLL code is written in the C language and requires some use of C syntax. Don't worry if you don't know C. You don't have to write any C statements; you only have to pass arguments to the library procedures.

Two steps are required for using a DLL. Any time you call a procedure that is in a library, you must include a **`Declare` statement**. `Declare` statements tell Visual Basic the name of the procedure and the library where it can be found, along with the arguments the procedure needs. Once you have included the `Declare`, you can call the procedure as you would one of your own. You can call both sub procedures and function procedures from DLLs; the `Declare` statement specifies the type of procedure. (Recall that a function returns a value.)

The Declare Statement

`Declare` statements appear at the module level. You can include them in the General Declarations section of a form module or in a standard code module. Calls to the library procedures may appear in any module.

The Declare Statement—General Form

```
Declare Sub Name Lib LibName$ [Alias AliasName$] _
      ([ArgumentList]) [As Datatype]
Declare Function Name Lib LibName$ [Alias AliasName$] _
      ([ArgumentList]) [As Datatype]
```

The Name parameter refers to the name of the procedure. If the name of the procedure is the same as a reserved word in Visual Basic or one of your existing procedures, you will need to use an alias to give the procedure a new name within your project. The word *Lib* precedes the name of the DLL library file. The argument list specifies the arguments expected by the procedure.

In the first of the following examples, the function procedure is called *sndPlaySound* from the MMSystem library.

The Declare Statement—Examples

```
Declare Function sndPlaySound Lib "winmm" Alias "sndPlaySoundA" _
     (ByVal lpszSoundName As String, ByVal uFlags As Long) As Long

Declare Function GetWindowsDirectory Lib "kernel32" Alias GetWindowsDirectoryA" _
     (ByVal lpBuffer As String, ByVal nSize As Long) As Long
```

The arguments may have a datatype specified and can be passed ByVal or ByRef.

Passing Arguments ByVal and ByRef

Arguments may be passed to a called procedure by value or by reference. When passed **ByVal**, only a copy of the original value is passed; the called procedure cannot alter the original value. When items are passed **ByRef**, the memory address of the original value is passed to the procedure, allowing the procedure to change the original value. You will pass ByVal or ByRef based upon the requirements of the specific DLL. If no specification is made, the default is ByRef.

When you are calling Windows API procedures, always declare a string argument ByVal. Visual Basic and C do not store strings in the same way. A Visual Basic string holds the length of the string at the beginning; strings in C are variable in length and terminated by a NULL character. C does not actually have a string data type, but treats strings as an array of characters.

String arguments and array arguments are treated differently than other (nonarray) arguments. You should declare them as passing ByVal, but what is actually passed is the address of the first element of the array.

Calling a DLL Procedure

You can call a DLL procedure from within any procedure in the scope of the `Declare` statement. The call will look the same as calls to procedures that you have written. The passed arguments may be either variables or constants.

The following procedure uses the sndPlaySound function to play a sound wave file (.WAV extension). This shareware wave file sounds like the Laurel and Hardy "Look at the fine mess you've gotten us into now" routine. Although this example plays the sound when a command button is clicked, you might consider playing it in a validation routine when the user makes a mistake.

```
Private Sub cmdsound_Click()
    'Play a sound file
    Dim iTalk As Integer

    Const SYNC = 1
    iTalk = sndPlaySound(ByVal CStr("d:\sharwar\l&h.wav"), SYNC)
End Sub
```

The first parameter converts the path and filename string to a "C string" by using the CStr function. The second argument being passed is an integer constant. Compare these arguments with the Declare used for this DLL procedure. (*Note:* The path indicated must be valid for your system. This shareware file is included on your Student Diskette.)

```
Declare Function sndPlaySound Lib "winmm" Alias "sndPlaySoundA" _
  (ByVal lpszSoundName As String, ByVal uFlags As Long) As Long
```

The sndPlaySound function is very useful for including sounds in a multimedia type of program. You might consider scanning in your own pictures, recording a voice description, and playing back the sound file when the appropriate selection is made from a menu or command button.

Finding the Reference Information for DLLs

You are not expected to learn the names and arguments for DLL procedures. You will find small code samples in magazines, in articles that present tips, or in question-and-answer features. If you ask a "How do I do . . ." question online, the answer you receive may include a few lines of code that include a Declare and a call to the procedure.

Visual Basic comes with a reference database for the procedures in the Windows API. You can use the API Viewer VB Add-In to look up the names of library files, procedures, constants, and the format of the Declare for each call. In order to use the Add-In, it must be selected when you install VB on your system. Then select *Add-Ins/Add-In Manager* and select *VB API Viewer* from the dialog box to add the API Viewer to the *Add-Ins* menu. Open the viewer and open its text file. The text file should be located in the folder Program Files\DevStudio\VB\Winapi. After you locate the desired Declare and Const statements, you can copy and paste them into your project.

Accessing System Information with a DLL

Your project may need to know the specific hardware or software on the computer system running the program. Windows maintains this information, and you can access it with a DLL. The following program will determine the current version of Windows and the video configuration.

Figure 14.17 shows the form for this program example.

Figure 14.17

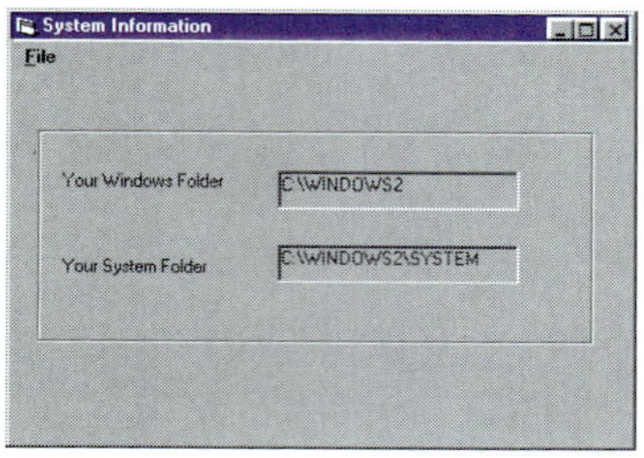

The form for the system information example program using a Windows API DLL.

```
'Project:      Ch1404.bas - Standard code module
'Programmer:   A. Millspaugh
'Date:         December 1997
'Description:  Declares the DLL procedures to find the
'              Windows and system folders.
'Folder:       Ch1404

     'Declare the DLL procedures
     Declare Function GetWindowsDirectory _
       Lib "kernel32" Alias "GetWindowsDirectoryA" _
       (ByVal lpBuffer As String, ByVal nSize As Long) _
       As Long
     Declare Function GetSystemDirectory Lib _
       "kernel32" Alias "GetSystemDirectoryA" _
       (ByVal lpBuffer As String, ByVal nSize As Long) _
       As Long
```

```
'Project:      Ch1404 frmSysInfo
'Programmer:   A. Millspaugh
'Date:         December 1997
'Description:  Uses DLL procedures to find the Windows
'              and system folders.
'Folder:       Ch1404
Option Explicit
```

```
Private Sub Form_Load()
     'Call the DLL procedures and assign return
     '   values to labels
     Dim stWinPath As String
     Dim vTemp
```

```
    'Create a string of 145 null characters
    stWinPath = String(145, Chr(0))
    'Fill the string with the path name
    vTemp = GetWindowsDirectory(stWinPath, 145)
    'Take the left characters up to the null
    lblWindowsDir.Caption = Left(stWinPath, InStr(stWinPath, Chr(0)) - 1)

    stWinPath = String(145, Chr(0))
    vTemp = GetSystemDirectory(stWinPath, 145)
    lblSystemDir.Caption = Left(stWinPath, InStr(stWinPath, Chr(0)) - 1)
End Sub
```

```
Private Sub mnuFileExit_Click()
    'Terminate the project

    End
End Sub
```

Placing Tabs for Columns in a List Box

Visual Basic list boxes and combo boxes do not have tab settings. At times you may want to fill a list with two or more columns. This example uses a Windows DLL to set tab stops in a list box. The project opens the Publishers table from the Visual Basic Biblio.mdb database and fills a list box with the data in three columns (Figure 14.18).

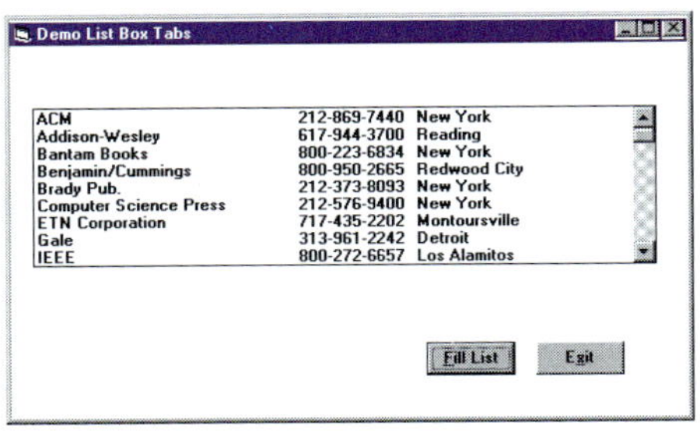

Figure 14.18

The columns in the list box created by using a Windows DLL to set tab stops.

```
'Project:       Demo Tabs
'Programmer:    J.C. Bradley
'Date:          August 1997
'Description:   Use a DLL to place tab stops in a list box.
'Folder:        Ch1405
Option Explicit
```

```
Private Declare Function SendMessage Lib "user32" Alias "SendMessageA" _
    (ByVal hwnd As Long, ByVal wMsg As Long, ByVal wParam As Long, _
    lParam As Any) As Long
Const LB_SETTABSTOPS = &H192
```

```
Private Sub cmdExit_Click()
    'Exit the project

    End
End Sub
```

```
Private Sub cmdFill_Click()
    'Fill the list box

    SetTabs lstData                         'Call procedure, passing name of list box
    Do Until datBiblio.Recordset.EOF
        '                                   'Chr$(9) is a Tab character
        lstData.AddItem datBiblio.Recordset!Name & Chr$(9) & _
                datBiblio.Recordset!Telephone & Chr$(9) & _
                datBiblio.Recordset!City
        datBiblio.Recordset.MoveNext
    Loop
End Sub
```

```
Private Sub SetTabs(Lst As ListBox)
    'Set the tab stops in a listbox

    ReDim iTabs(0 To 1) As Integer          'Two tab stops needed
    Dim lRtn            As Long             'DLL function returns a Long variable
    iTabs(0) = 110                          'Twips measurement for 1st tab stop
    iTabs(1) = 160                          'Twips measurement for 2nd tab stop
    lRtn = SendMessage(Lst.hwnd, LB_SETTABSTOPS, 2, iTabs(0))     'Set the stops
End Sub
```

Object Linking and Embedding

OLE enables you to link or embed objects from other applications into your project, either at run time or at design time. You can access objects from other types of applications without writing the code. Think how much time it would take to program a spreadsheet application. Why should you spend that time when excellent spreadsheets are available? OLE is the means by which each programmer can avoid "reinventing the wheel." The types of objects available to use in a project depend on the applications that are installed on your computer system or network.

Object Linking

Linking causes your program to access an object that is actually maintained by the application that creates it. A reference to the linked object is kept in your code, but the actual object is kept in the other application. This means that any application that has linking ability can access the linked object and change it. When your application runs, you can access the current state of the object.

An example of a linked object could be a spreadsheet showing the current status and costs for a project. The spreadsheet object could be included in a Visual Basic project, in a word processing document, as well as displayed from the spreadsheet application. The data in the linked spreadsheet can also be updated from each of the applications. Because each application is using the same object, any changes made to the spreadsheet would be available to all applications linked to it.

Object Embedding

Embedding places the object into your project. Hence, the object is maintainable only from within your project and cannot be accessed by other projects. Another result of embedding is that the Visual Basic project file becomes significantly larger because of the embedded code.

Consider a project that includes a spreadsheet object created in Excel. You can choose to create a new spreadsheet file or to include an existing spreadsheet. The steps to accomplish the two tasks are similar. First, create a new control on a form using the OLE tool from the toolbox (Figure 14.19); the *Insert Object* dialog box (Figure 14.20) appears automatically. Notice the option button for *Create New* or *Create from File.* Try clicking on the buttons and viewing the changes to the dialog box (Figure 14.21). If you want to create a new item within your project, you must make a selection from the *Object Type* list box.

Figure 14.19

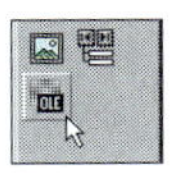

Use the OLE tool from the toolbox to link or embed an OLE object in a project.

Figure 14.20

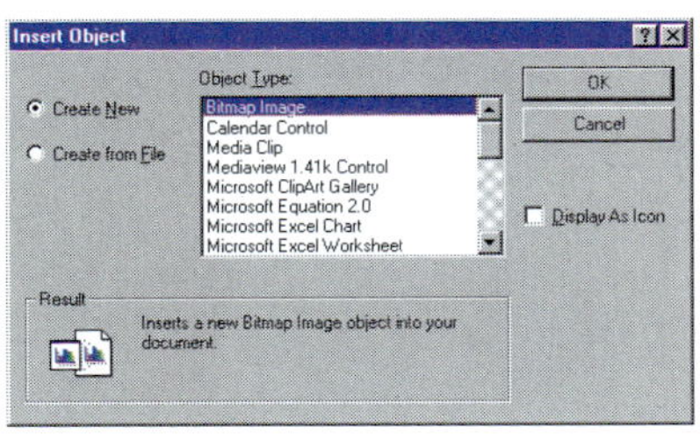

The Insert Object dialog box with its initial settings for creating a new object.

Figure 14.21

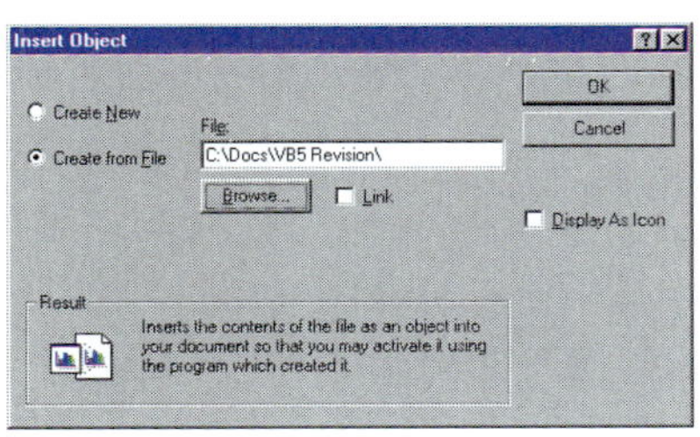

The Insert Object dialog box as it appears for Create from File.

The following example places an existing spreadsheet for R 'n R on a form as an embedded object. Figure 14.22 shows the form for this example. The steps are as follows:

Figure 14.22

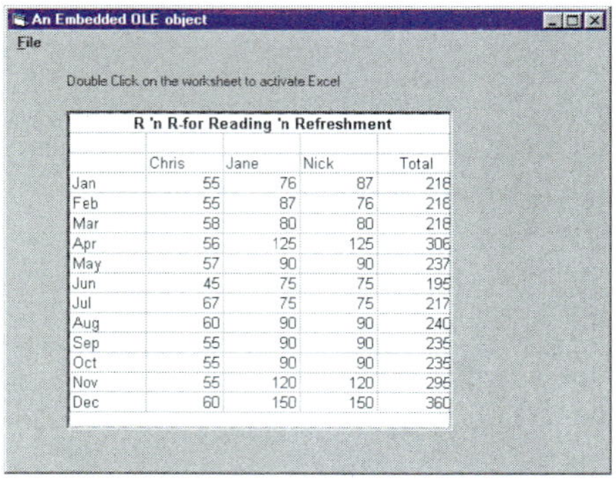

The form for the OLE example project showing an embedded Excel spreadsheet object.

STEP 1: Create a control on your form using the OLE tool from the toolbox; the *Insert Object* dialog box will display (refer to Figure 14.20).
STEP 2: Select the option button for *Create from File.*
STEP 3: Type the filename RNR.XLS in the File text box (or use the Browse button to locate the file in the Ch1406 folder).
STEP 4: Make sure that the Link check box is not selected so that the object will be embedded.

The project Ch1406 displays the interface shown in Figure 14.22 when the program is running.

Creating OLE Objects at Run Time

You can embed and link objects while a project is executing by using the properties and methods of the OLE control. You can create a link to an existing object by setting the control's SourceDoc property and using the `CreateLink` method. If you are linking to a datafile and want a specific range of the file, you can set the control's SourceItem property.

To embed an object, set the SourceDoc property and use the `CreateEmbed` method.

You can also allow the user to select the type of object to be linked or embedded as the project is running. Use the `InsertObjDlg` or the `PasteSpecialDlg` method. These methods display the *Object* dialog box or the *Paste Special* dialog box, respectively.

Visual Basic for Applications

Each Microsoft Office application, such as Excel, Word, PowerPoint, and Access, includes **Visual Basic for Applications (VBA)** for writing procedures. Most of the Visual Basic features that you have learned carry over to programming in VBA. Take a look at the Code window (Figure 14.23), the Visual Basic toolbar (Figure 14.24), and the Controls Toolbox toolbar (Figure 14.25) in Excel 97. You will find many items that look familiar.

Figure 14.23

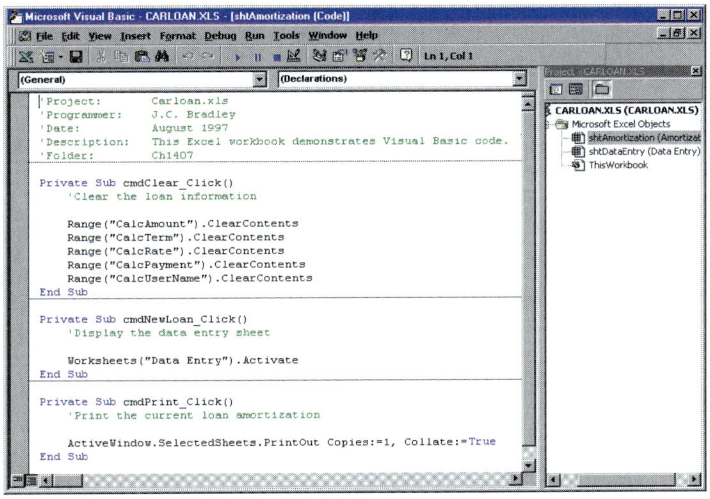

The Visual Basic Code window in Excel 97.

Figure 14.24

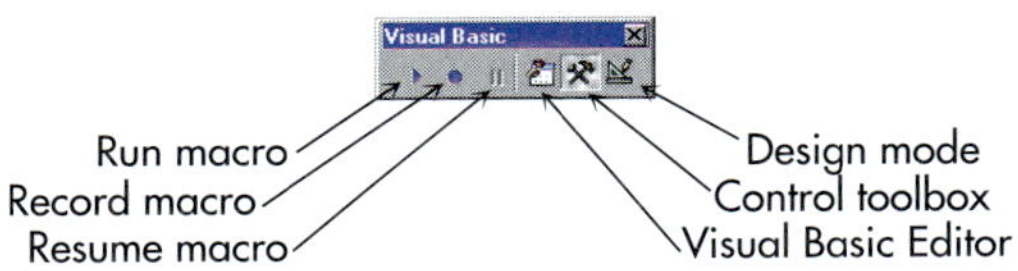

The Excel 97 Visual Basic toolbar.

Figure 14.25

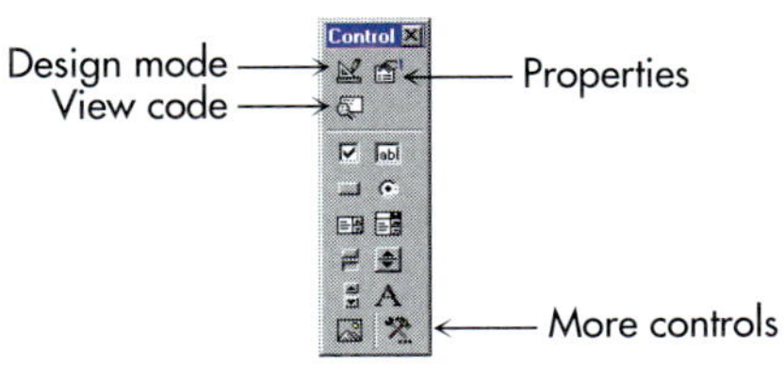

The Excel 97 Control Toolbox toolbar.

Recording an Excel Macro

If you have Excel 97 installed on your computer, you may be interested in trying the activities in this section. Start by recording an Excel macro: Select *Tools/Macros/Record New Macro*, and a dialog box will ask for the name of your macro. Give it the name *Demo;* a little Stop button appears in a toolbar. Then try typing something into your worksheet, such as your name and the date. Then click the Stop button.

Display the Visual Basic toolbar (*View/Toolbars*) and click on the Visual Basic Editor button (Figure 14.26). Then double-click on Module1 in the Project Explorer window. Your procedure (recorded macro) should appear in the Code window (Figure 14.27).

Figure 14.26

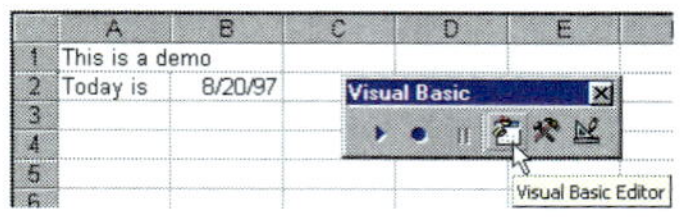

Click on the Visual Basic Editor button to display the Code window.

Figure 14.27

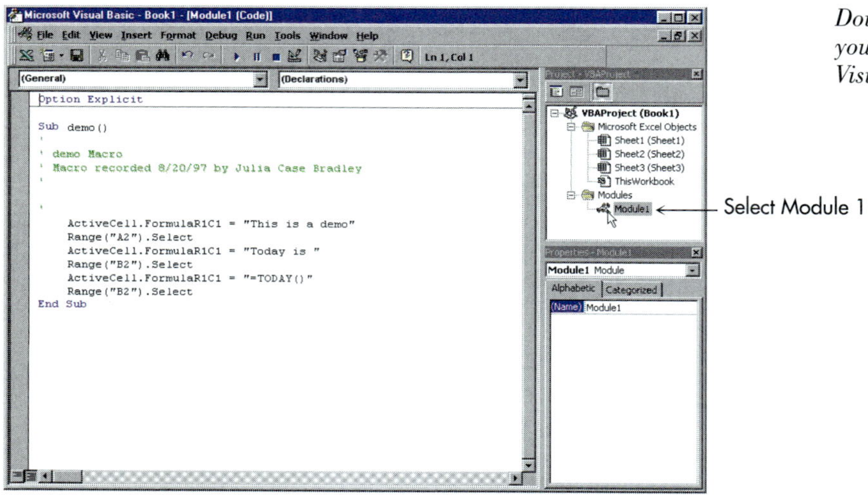

Double-click on Module1 and your new macro appears in the Visual Basic Code window.

Investigate the environment—the windows, the menus, and the toolbars. This environment is the same Visual Basic environment you are accustomed to. Now look at the code. The Visual Basic notation for remarks includes the name *Demo* that you called your macro. Notice the procedure begins with `Sub` and ends with `End Sub`. The statements inside the procedure reflect the steps you took while the macro was recording.

The structure of VBA is the same as the structure for Visual Basic. However, a spreadsheet has different objects, properties, events, and methods than Visual Basic has.

You can add objects with which you are familiar. Return to the Worksheet window by clicking on its Taskbar button. Then display the Control Toolbox toolbar (*View/Toolbars*). Create a command button. The tools are the same but you must click the tool and then draw it; the double-click method does not work in VBA.

After you create a new button, change to the design mode of Excel by clicking on the Design mode button on the Visual Basic toolbar. You can toggle between design mode and regular mode with the Design mode button. When you are in design mode, you can display the Properties window, change properties of controls, and write code.

A Sample Excel Visual Basic Application

Your student disk has a file called Carloan.xls for calculating loan payments and printing loan amortizations. It contains two sheets: a worksheet that resembles a dialog box for data entry (Figure 14.28*a*) and a second worksheet for the loan amortization (Figure 14.28*b*). The data entry worksheet has three command buttons: Calculate Payment, Display Amortization, and Clear. The loan amortization worksheet has buttons for Print, Clear, and New Loan. You can load the workbook file, run the application, and examine the Visual Basic procedures.

Note: Because there are no validation routines, you must enter all fields. The form is designed to print out the first three years of the loan.

Figure 14.28

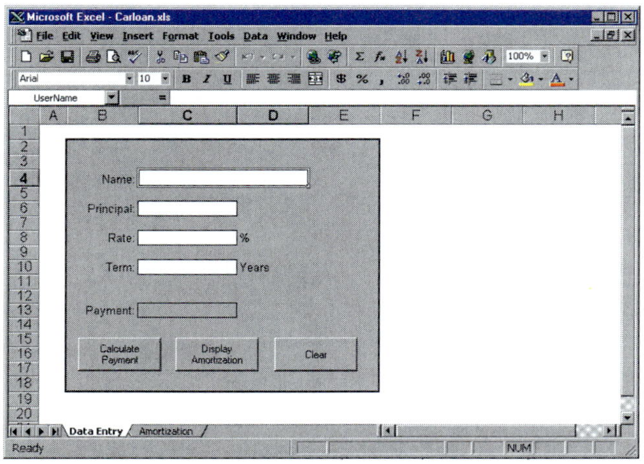

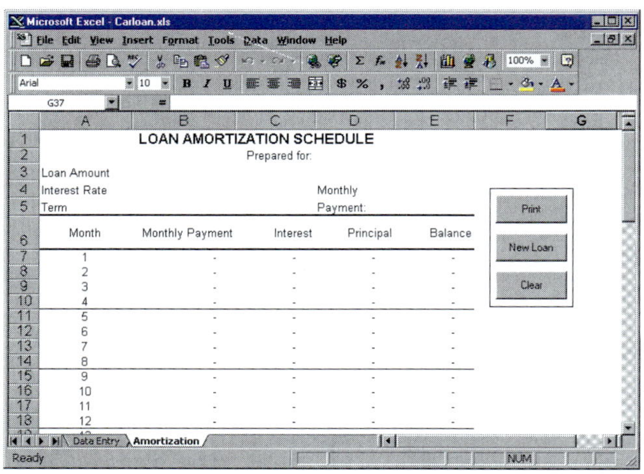

This Excel spreadsheet demonstrates using Visual Basic for Applications in Excel. This demo workbook has two worksheets: (a) The Data Entry sheet and (b) the Amortization sheet.

The Code for the Data Entry Worksheet

```
'Project:        Carloan.xls - Data Entry Sheet
'Programmer:     J.C. Bradley
'Date:           August 1997
'Description:    This Excel workbook file demonstrates using
'                Visual Basic in Excel 97.
'Folder:         Ch1407
Option Explicit
```

```
Private Sub cmdCalculateLoan_Click()
     'Calculate the payment

     Range("CalculatedPayment").Value = "=-PMT(YearlyRate/1200,_
         TermInYears*12, Principal)"
End Sub
```

```
Private Sub cmdClear_Click()
     'Clear the sheet

     Range("UserName").ClearContents
     Range("Principal").ClearContents
     Range("YearlyRate").ClearContents
     Range("TermInYears").ClearContents
     Range("CalculatedPayment").ClearContents
     Range("UserName").Select
End Sub
```

```
Private Sub cmdDisplay_Click()
     'Display Amortization worksheet

     cmdCalculateLoan_Click
     With Worksheets("Amortization")
          .Range("CalcAmount") = Range("Principal")
          .Range("CalcRate").Value = Range("YearlyRate") / 100
          .Range("CalcTerm").Value = Range("TermInYears")
          .Range("Payment").Value = Range("CalculatedPayment")
          .Range("CalcUserName").Value = Range("UserName")
          .Activate
     End With
End Sub
```

```
Private Sub Worksheet_Activate()
     'Set up the worksheet

     Range("UserName").Select
End Sub
```

The Code for the Loan Amortization Worksheet

```
'Project:      Carloan.xls - Loan Amortization Sheet
'Programmer:   J.C. Bradley
'Date:         August 1997
'Description:  This Excel workbook demonstrates Visual Basic code.
'Folder:       Ch1407
Option Explicit
```

```
Private Sub cmdClear_Click()
    'Clear the loan information

    Range("CalcAmount").ClearContents
    Range("CalcTerm").ClearContents
    Range("CalcRate").ClearContents
    Range("CalcPayment").ClearContents
    Range("CalcUserName").ClearContents
End Sub
```

```
Private Sub cmdNewLoan_Click()
    'Display the data entry sheet

    Worksheets("Data Entry").Activate
End Sub
```

```
Private Sub cmdPrint_Click()
    'Print the current loan amortization

    ActiveWindow.SelectedSheets.PrintOut Copies:=1, Collate:=True
End Sub
```

Help with Visual Basic in Excel

Another area that can help you learn more about VBA is Excel's *Help* menu. Under *Help/Contents* and *Index/Contents* select the topic *Microsoft Excel Visual Basic Reference* and expand the topics list. The Visual Basic section of *Help* gives a new index of topics that relate specifically to VB.

In addition to the Help screens, you can also try some demo programs that come with Excel.

Creating Your Own Objects

Beyond the many built-in choices you have for objects to include in your projects, Visual Basic allows you to create your own new object types by creating a **class module**. Just like other object types, your class may have both properties and methods. Remember: Properties are characteristics, and methods are actions that can be performed by a class of object.

Defining a class does not place an object in your form; it merely defines how an object of that type would act. To create a new object you specify the class type. For example, *command button* is a class but *cmdExit* is an actual occurrence or **instance** of the class; the instance is the object. Just as you may have multiple command buttons in a project, you may have many objects of a new class type.

Defining a Class

To create a new class, use the *Add Class Module* from the *Project* menu. You will see a code window similar to the code window for a standard code module. Any public variables that you declare will become the properties of the new class. The subs and functions are the methods.

```
Public cPrice         As Currency
Public iQuantity      As Integer
Public stDescription  As String
```

```
Public Function cInventoryValue() As Currency
    'Calculate the value of the inventory

    cInventoryValue = iQuantity * cPrice
End Function
```

This new class has the following properties: cPrice, iQuantity, and stDescription. The class has only one method: cInventoryValue.

Creating a New Object Using a New Class

Creating a class module only defines a new class; it does not create any objects. This process is similar to defining a new data type; you must then dimension variables of the new type. To create an object using your new class, you must create an instance of the class using the `New` keyword and specifying the class. This step is referred to as ***instantiating*** an object.

Dimensioning Objects Using the New Keyword—General Form

```
Dim Public|Private VariableName As New ClassName
```

Dimensioning Objects Using the New Keyword—Examples

```
Dim Emp As New Employee
Private MyInventory As New Inventory
Public NewForm As New frmMain
```

The **New keyword** is used to create a new instance of an object class. The object class can be a class that you create or standard Visual Basic objects such as forms.

Reusable Objects

An advantage of object-oriented code is the ability to reuse objects. When you create a new class by writing a class module, you can then use that class in multiple projects. Every object defined has its own set of properties, just like each control in your project has its own set of properties that act independently. For example, you may use two image objects: imgOne and imgTwo. Each has its own Visible property, which may have a different setting than the other.

You might want to create your own class to provide database access. You could include methods for adding and deleting data members. If you work frequently with sales, you might create an invoice class. The invoice class would likely have properties such as description, quantity, and cost. The methods would probably include finding the current value of the inventory.

Sample Project—Defining and Using a New Class

In this project we will create a new class called Inventory. Then, in a form module, we will dimension and use a new instance of the Inventory class.

Sample Code for Creating the Inventory Class

```
'Module         Class Module
'Programmer:    A. Millspaugh
'Date:          December 1997
'Description:   Declare properties and methods
'               for the inventory class.
'Folder:        Ch1408

Public cPrice        As Currency
Public iQuantity     As Integer
Public stDescription As String
_______________________________________________

Public Function cInventoryValue() As Currency
    'Calculate the value of the inventory

    cInventoryValue = iQuantity * cPrice
End Function
_______________________________________________
```

This example contains three properties defined as Public—cPrice, iQuantity, and stDescription. The method is cInventoryValue. Since the properties and methods are declared as public, they can be accessed from other modules. Private members of the class can be accessed only by procedures within the class module.

Defining and Using an Object of the Inventory Class

The code in this new form module creates an instance of the Inventory class defined in the preceding code. The properties and method are used in the mnuFileCalc_Click event.

```
'Project:       Calculate Inventory
'Programmer:    A. Millspaugh
'Date:          December 1997
'Description:   Calculate inventory amount using the Inventory class.
'               Instantiate the Inventory class as a new object.
'Folder:        Ch1408

Option Explicit
Private MyInventory As New Inventory
________________________________________________________________

Private Sub mnuFileCalc_Click()
    'Calculate the inventory value

    MyInventory.cPrice = txtPrice.Text
    MyInventory.iQuantity = txtQuantity.Text
    MyInventory.stDescription = txtDescription.Text
    lblInventoryValue.Caption = MyInventory.cInventoryValue()
End Sub
________________________________________________________________

Private Sub mnuFileExit_Click()
    'Terminate the project

    End
End Sub
________________________________________________________________
```

Crystal Reports

When you need to create a printed report based on a database, you can use the **Crystal Reports** add-in, available with the Professional and Enterprise Editions of VB. With Crystal Reports you design a report using the **Report Designer**. The report design is saved as a separate file on disk. Then you place a Crystal Reports ActiveX control on your form. You specify the name of the report file as one of the properties of the control. When your project runs, you can set the Action property of the Crystal Reports control, which sends the report to the printer or a Print Preview window on the screen.

To design your Crystal Report, you can run the Report Designer either as a stand-alone application or from within Visual Basic. To run Crystal Reports outside VB, run Crw32.exe in the Report folder beneath the VB folder. From within Visual Basic you will use the *Add-Ins* menu. The following step-by-step tutorial uses Crystal Reports from the VB *Add-Ins* menu.

Designing the Report

You will begin the report design from within VB. It isn't important whether or not you have a project open while you design the report.

STEP 1: Open the *Add-Ins* menu and select *Report Designer*. A new window opens for Crystal Reports Pro (Figure 14.29).

Note: If you see a registration form, click Done.

Figure 14.29

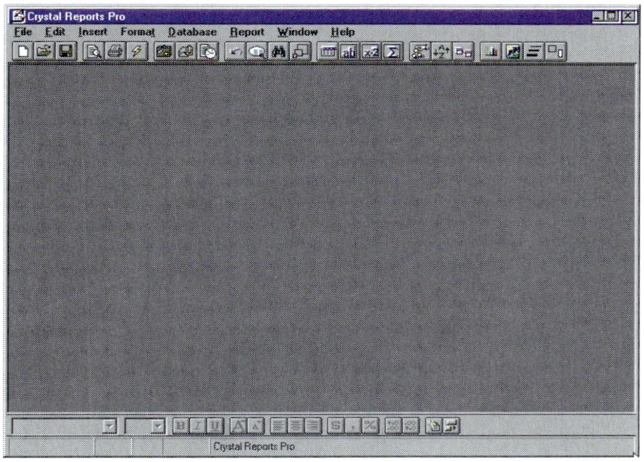

Create and modify reports using the Crystal Reports Pro window.

STEP 2: Select *File/New*, and the *Create New Report* dialog box appears (Figure 14.30). Click on the large button labeled Standard.

Figure 14.30

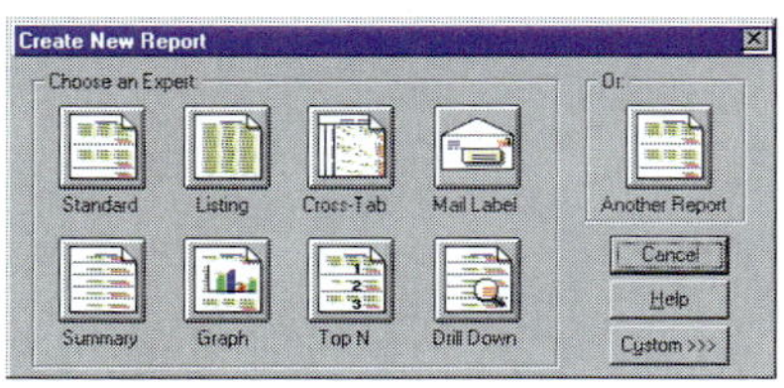

Choose your report type in the Create New Report dialog box.

The Create Report Expert wizard appears (Figure 14.31). You will use this wizard to select the database file and design the report. Notice that the wizard contains a tabbed dialog with numbered tabs for *Tables*, *Fields*, *Sort*, *Total*, *Select*, and *Style*.

Figure 14.31

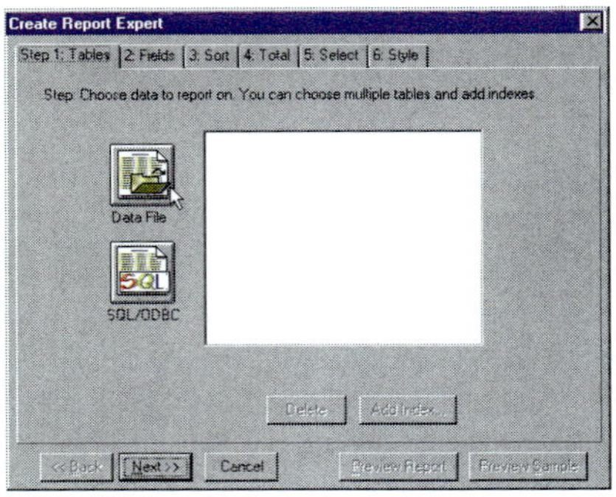

The Create Report Expert wizard can step you through creating a new report.

STEP 3: On the *Tables* tab click on the large Data File button. Specify the name and path of the RnrBooks.mdb database you will be using. After clicking on the Add button, click Done. A *Links* tab will appear.

STEP 4: Click on the Next command button.

STEP 5: On the *Fields* tab select the desired fields from the *Database Fields* list on the left and click the Add button to add the fields to the Report Fields list on the right (Figure 14.32). Select Author, Title, and Publisher, adding each to the report. Your completed list should look like Figure 14.32.

Figure 14.32

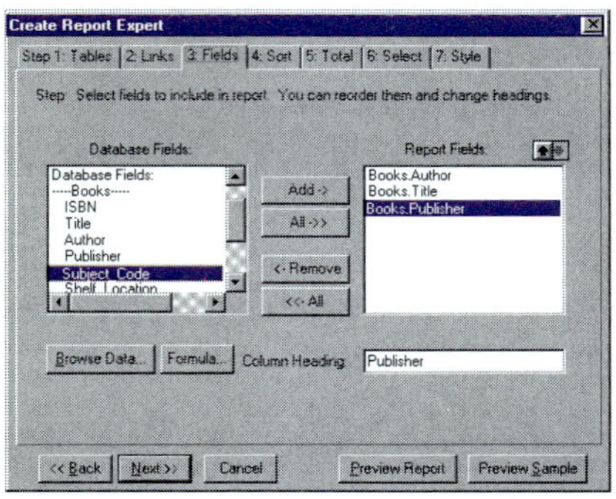

Select from the available fields to choose the fields to display on your report. The fields listed in Report Fields will appear on the report.

STEP 6: Click on the *Style* tab and type in your title. (Make up any title you wish. It's a good idea to include your name in the title if you are using a shared lab.)

You may want to investigate the other tabs now. As soon as you perform the next step, the wizard will disappear. After that point you must make any further changes in design view.

STEP 7: Click on the Preview Sample button to view the report.

You can click on the *Design* tab to see the design created by the wizard and/or modify it.

STEP 8: Choose *File/Save As*. Change to the folder that holds (or will hold) the Visual Basic project to display the report and name your report file *Rnr*. Crystal Reports will automatically add an extension of .RPT.

STEP 9: Select *File/Exit* to exit Crystal Reports and return to VB.

The report is saved as a file with an .RPT extension. It may now be printed or displayed from within a project.

Adding the Report to a Project

You can add a saved report to any VB project. You may have an application that displays and/or maintains a database, and you want to add report printing capability. You might also have a list of several reports from which the user can select.

To add the report, you add a Crystal Report control to your form. Just as with a Common Dialog control, the Crystal Report control appears on the form at design time, but not during run time. The control contains a variety of properties to control printing to the screen or to the printer and to connect to a specific .RPT file. Use "rpt" for the naming prefix of report controls.

In your VB code, you will set the Action property of the Crystal Report control to 1 to output the specified report. By default, the report goes to the printer, but you can specify the destination by first setting the control's Destination property. For the destination, you can use either the numeric literals or intrinsic constants:

Destination	Literal	Constant
Screen	0	crptToWindow
Printer	1	crptToPrinter

The following code sends a report to the screen for print preview:

```
rptRNR.Destination = crptToWindow
rptRNR.Action = 1
```

The following code sends a report to the printer:

```
rptRNR.Destination = crptToPrinter
rptRNR.Action = 1
```

Tip

You can display the *Components* dialog box by right-clicking on the toolbox.

Add Your Report to a Project

Follow these steps to add the previously created Rnr.RPT to a Visual Basic project:

STEP 1: Open a project (a new project or an existing project).

STEP 2: Open the *Components* dialog box and add *Crystal Report 4.6* to your toolbox. Add this control to your project (Figure 14.33).

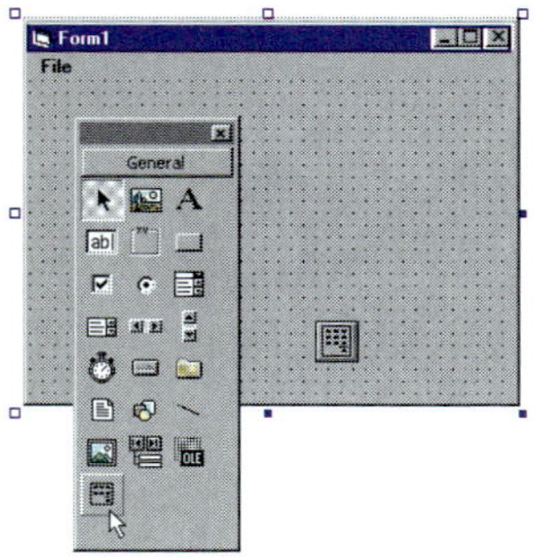

Figure 14.33

The Crystal Reports tool in the toolbox and a Crystal Reports control on the form.

STEP 3: Change the Name property of the new control to rptRnR.
STEP 4: Display the custom *Property Pages* dialog box from either the shortcut menu or the *(Custom)* entry in the Properties window.
STEP 5: On the *General* tab specify the path and filename of the .RPT file you created earlier. (You can click on the Build button to browse for the file.) Close the dialog box.
STEP 6: Create a menu bar with a *File* menu and commands for *Preview Report*, *Print Report*, and *Exit*. Code the mnuFileExit event procedure with an `End` statement.
STEP 7: Write the code to send the report to the screen and the printer. Referring to the code examples that appear before this section, set the Destination and Action properties for each option.
STEP 8: Test the project.

The Coding Solution

```
'Project:      Crystal Reports
'Programmer:   A. Millspaugh
'Date:         July 1997
'Description:  Use the Crystal Report control
'              to display or print a database report
'              created with Crystal Reports.
'Folder:       Ch1409

Private Sub mnuFileExit_Click()
    'Terminate the project

    End
End Sub
```

```
Private Sub mnuFilePreview_Click()
    'Send the report to the screen

    rptRnR.Destination = crptToWindow
    rptRnR.Action = 1
End Sub
```

```
Private Sub mnuFilePrint_Click()
    'Send the report to the printer

    rptRnR.Destination = crptToPrinter
    rptRnR.Action = 1
End Sub
```

Summary

1. ActiveX refers to controls and procedures that can be used by different applications. You can access objects other than the ones in the toolbox by selecting options from the *Components* or *Resources* dialog boxes from the commands on the *Project* menu.
2. The Visual Basic editor enables you to create new controls and to make the .OCX files that are registered in the *Components* dialog box.
3. Dynamic link libraries are procedures in library files, outside of Visual Basic, that can be linked and called when a project is running.
4. DLLs used by Windows are referred to as the Windows application programming interface (API).
5. DLL procedures may pass arguments by value (pass a copy of the value) or by reference (pass the address of the value).
6. Objects created by other applications can be linked to a Visual Basic project using the OLE container control. The object can appear on a Visual Basic form and be manipulated by the user of the Visual Basic project. Linked objects are actually maintained by the application that created them.
7. OLE embedded objects are similar to linked objects except that the files relating to the objects are stored with the Visual Basic project, which greatly increases the size of the project.
8. Visual Basic for Applications is the standard language used for generating procedures (macros) in other Microsoft application packages, such as Word, Excel, and Access.
9. A Visual Basic programmer can create new classes and use them to create new objects.
10. The Crystal Reports Report Designer add-in provides an easy method for designing reports for a database that can be printed from a VB project.

Key Terms

ActiveX *498*
API *507*
ByRef *508*
ByVal *508*
class module *519*
Crystal Reports *522*
`Declare` statement *507*
dynamic link libraries (DLL) *506*
embedding *513*
instance *520*
instantiating *520*
linking *512*
`New` keyword *521*
object *498*
OLE *512*
Report Designer *522*
Tabbed Dialog control *499*
Visual Basic for Applications (VBA) *514*
Web browser control *502*

Review Questions

1. What is an ActiveX control? Give an example.
2. What is a DLL?
3. What does *API* mean?
4. What are the purposes of a `Declare` statement?
5. Differentiate between ByVal and ByRef. When is each used?
6. Explain the difference between linking and embedding an object into a Visual Basic project.
7. What determines the list of objects that can be used with OLE in a particular system?
8. What does the term *object* mean?
9. What are the sources of objects?
10. How can a new type of object be created?

Programming Exercises

14.1 Add an OLE control to a form and select *Create New File.* Look over the list of OLE objects available on your system. Try linking and embedding an object and compare the file size of your projects.

14.2 Examine the .WAV files in your Windows directories. Write a project that prompts the user to guess a number. Have the project generate a random number from 1 to 100. Allow the user to enter a number. Display a message that indicates whether the response is too high or too low. If the user gives the correct answer, use the Tada.wav file to generate a sound.

14.3 If you have access to a multimedia system with a microphone, record a short message to a .WAV file. Write a project that plays back the sound file—a description of an item being displayed, for example.

14.4 Create a new class that calculates the commission to pay on a vehicle sale. The properties will include cost price and selling price. Create a method that calculates the commission as 40 percent of the profit. The profit is the selling price—the cost price. Test the class in a form that includes the vehicle information for the sale, the cost price, the selling price, and the commission.

CASE STUDIES

VB Mail Order

Create an ActiveX control to perform the actions VB Mail from Chapter 1. The class should display the name and telephone number for the contact person of the selected department.

Include command buttons for the Customer Relations, Marketing, Order Processing, and Shipping departments. When the user clicks on the button for a department, display the name and telephone number for the contact person in two labels. Also include identifying labels with Captions *Department Contact* and *Telephone Number.*

Test your control in a form that includes buttons to print the form and to exit.

Test Data

Department	Department Contact	Telephone Number
Customer Relations	Tricia Mills	500-1111
Marketing	Michelle Rigner	500-2222
Order Processing	Kenna DeVoss	500-3333
Shipping	Eric Andrews	500-4444

VB Auto Center

Create a new ActiveX control that includes a list box and a label. Selecting the department name from the list box should display the appropriate special in a label.

Create a form module that incorporates the new control.

Test Data

List Box	Special to Display in Label
Auto Sales	Family wagon, immaculate condition $12,995
Service Center	Lube, oil, filter $25.99
Detail Shop	Complete detail $79.95 for most cars
Employment Opportunities	Sales position: Contact Mr. Mann 551-2134 x475

APPENDIX

A

Answers to Feedback Questions

Feedback 2.1

Property	Setting
Name	imgBig
Stretch	True
Appearance	1 - 3D
BorderStyle	1 - Fixed Single
Visible	True

Feedback 2.2

1. `txtCompany.Text = ""`
   `txtCompany.SetFocus`
2. `lblCustomer.Caption = ""`
   `txtOrder.SetFocus`
3. (a) Check box is checked.
   (b) Option button is not selected.
   (c) Image is not visible.
   (d) The appearance is set to three dimensional; border style is fixed.
   (e) Assigns the value in txtCity.Text to lblCity.Caption.

Feedback 3.1

1. Does not indicate the data type with a prefix.
2. Cannot contain special characters such as #.
3. No blank spaces are allowed within an identifier.
4. The periods separate items such as object and property and should not be used in a variable identifier.
5. Cannot contain special characters such as `$`.
6. *Sub* is a reserved word in Visual Basic.
7. Valid name. Is it meaningful? That would depend upon the situation.
8. *Caption* is a property name and, as such, is a reserved word.
9. If the *c* is being used as a prefix for currency, the *O* should be capitalized to conform to the naming conventions.
10. A prefix should be used to specify the data type.
11. Valid.
12. Valid.

Feedback 3.2

Note: Answers may vary; make sure the prefix indicates the data type.

1. (a) sHoursWorked
   (b) stEmployeeName
   (c) stDepartmentNumber
2. (a) iQuantity
   (b) stDescription
   (c) stPartNumber
   (d) cCost
   (e) cSellingPrice

Feedback 3.3

Note: Answers may vary, make sure the prefix indicates the data type.

1. Dim mcTotal As Currency, declared at module level.
2. Const mcSALES_TAX_RATE As Currency = .07, declared at module level.
3. Dim miParticipantCount As Integer, declared at module level.

Feedback 3.4

1. 18
2. 1
3. 6
4. 5
5. 22
6. 4 to the power of 5; then multiply by 2 (2048).
7. 22
8. 38

Feedback 3.5

1. `lblAveragePay.Caption = Format$(mcAveragePay, "Currency")`
   $123.46
2. `lblPercentCorrect.Caption = Format$(sCorrect, "Percent")`
   76.00%
3. `lblTotal.Caption = Format$(mcTotalCollected, "Standard")`

Feedback 3.6

1. 1.35
2. 01.35
3. 1.3
4. $1
5. $1.3

Feedback 4.1

1. True
2. True
3. True
4. False
5. False
6. True
7. True
8. False
9. True
10. True

Feedback 4.2

1. The frogs option button on; the toads off.
2. It's the toads and the polliwogs.
3. It's false.
4.
```
If txtApples.Text > txtOranges.Text Then
     lblMost.Caption = "Apples"
Else
     lblMost.Caption = "Oranges"
End If
```
5.
```
If cBalance > 0 Then
    optFunds.Value = True
    cBalance = 0
    iCounter = iCounter + 1

Else
    optFunds.Value = False
End If
```

Feedback 5.1

1. Function procedure; a value is returned.
2.
```
Private Function iCalculateAverage (iValue1 As Integer, _
  iValue2 As Integer, iValue3 As Integer) As Integer
```

3. `iCalculateAverage = (iValue1 + iValue2 + iValue3) / 3`
4. The answer is assigned to a field with the name of the function.

Feedback 6.1

1. `Const miFAT_CALORIES As Integer = 9   'module level`
2. `Public gstNameHighest As String       'standard code module`
3. `Const gstCOMPANY_NAME As String = "Babs Bowling Service"`
   `'standard code module`
4. `Public gcTotalAmount As Currency      'standard code module`
5. `Public giPersonCount As Integer       'standard code module`
6. `Dim cTotal As Currency        'local to procedure`
7. (a) Module-level integer variable.
   (b) Standard code module currency variable.
   (c) Local currency variable.
   (d) Local currency constant.
   (e) Standard code module string constant.
   (f) Local string variable.
   (g) Module-level string variable.
   (h) Standard code module string variable.

Feedback 7.1

1. Tracks the physical number of elements in the list.
2. Stores the position of the currently selected item; has a value of −1 if nothing is selected.
3. String value of an item in the list.
4. Adds an item during run time.
5. Removes all items from the list.
6. Removes the selected or specified item from the list.
7. Displays the list in alphabetic order.

Feedback 7.2

```
bItemFound = False   'Set initial value of found flag to False
iItemIndex = 0                    'Initialize counter for index
'Loop until the item is found or the end of list is reached
Do Until bItemFound Or iItemIndex = lstItems.ListCount
    'Test if the text box entry matches item in list
    If txtNewItem.Text = lstItems.List(iItemIndex) Then
        bItemFound = True          'Set the found flag to True
    End If
    iItemIndex = iItemIndex + 1   'Increment counter for index
Loop
```

Feedback 7.3

1. **(a)** There should not be a comma after the ending value.
   (b) The `Next` statement must contain the control variable that follows the `For`, iIndex in this case.
   (c) The item following the word `For` must be a variable and must be the same as the one on the `Next` statement.
   (d) Valid.
   (e) Valid.
   (f) Will never execute; should have a negative Step argument.
2. **(a)** Will execute four times with an ending value in iCounter of 14.
   (b) Will execute 10 times with an ending value in iCounter of 0.
   (c) Will execute seven times with an ending value of 6.5.
   (d) Will not execute.
   (e) Will execute three times; iCounter will have an ending value of 4.

Feedback 7.4

```
1. Half a loaf is better than none
2. Half,             My Eye
3. Hawks0            Doves0
4.  1                 2                 3                 4                 5                 6
5.  1                 2                 3                 4                 5                 6
6.               3             5
7.                3                           5
```

Feedback 8.1

```
1. Select Case iTemp
           Case Is > 80
               lblComment.Caption = "It's Hot"
           Case Is > 32
               lblComment.Caption = "It's Freezing"
           Case Else
               lblComment.Caption = "It's Freezing"
   End Select
```

2.
```
'General Declarations
Dim mcCoffeePrice As Currency

Private Sub optCoffee_Click(Index As Integer)
    'Find the price
    Select Case iIndex
       Case 0
           mcCoffeePrice = 2
       Case 1
           mcCoffeePrice = 2.25
       Case 2
           mcCoffeePrice = 1.75
       Case 3
           mcCoffeePrice = 2.5
    End Select
End Sub
```
3. Use a Case Else:
```
Case Else
     MsgBox "You must select an option from the Coffee Selections"
```

Feedback 8.2

1. Valid.
2. Valid.
3. Valid.
4. Invalid, beyond the range.
5. Valid.
6. Invalid, negative number.
7. Yields a decimal number, but Basic will use the integer portion.
8. Valid.

Feedback 8.3

1.
```
Type StudentInfo
        stLastName        As String
        stFirstName       As String
        stStudentNumber   As String
        cUnits            As Currency
        cGPA              As Currency

End Type
```
2. `Dim Students(100) As StudentInfo`
3.
```
Type Project
        stName            As String
        stForm(10)        As String
        stSubdirectory    As String
End Type
```
4. `Dim MyProject As Project`
5. `Dim OurProjects(100) As Project`

Feedback 8.4

1. `Dim cTemperature(1 to 3, 1 to 5) As Currency`
2. ```
   For iColumn = 1 To 5
         cTemperature(1, iColumn) = 0
   Next iColumn
   ```
3. ```
   For iColumn = 1 To 5
          cTemperature(2, iColumn) = 75
   Next iColumn
   ```
4. ```
   For iColumn = 1 To 5
           cTemperature(3, iColumn) = cTemperature(1, _
               iColumn) + cTemperature(2, iColumn)
   Next Column
   ```
5. ```
   For Each vTemp in cTemperature
         Printer.Print vTemp
   Next vTemp
   ```

Feedback 9.1

1. (a) `Open "Vendor.Dat" For Output As #1`
   (b) ```
   For iIndex = 0 to lstVendor.ListCount - 1
         Write #1, lstVendor.List(iIndex)
   Next iIndex
   ```
   (c) `Close #1`
   (d) `Open "Vendor.Dat" For Input As #1`
   (e) ```
   Do Until EOF(1)
         Input #1, stVendor
         lstVendor.AddItem stVendor
   Loop
   ```
2. `EOF()`

Feedback 9.2

1. Turns off error trapping.
2. Branches execution to the line labeled `WhatToDo` when an error occurs.
3. Sets the error code to 53 and triggers the error condition so that the system will handle it.
4. Continues execution with the statement that caused the error.
5. Continues execution with the statement following the one that caused the error.

Feedback 9.3

1.
```
Type Inventory
        stDescription   As String * 30
        stPartNumber    As String * 5
        cPrice          As Currency
        iQuantity       As Integer
End Type
```
2. `Dim mInventoryRecord As Inventory`
3.
```
Open "C:\Inventory.Dat" For Random As #1 Len =
    Len(mInventoryRecord)
```
4. `iNumberRecords = LOF(1) / Len(mInventoryRecord)`
5. `Put #1, iRecordNumber, mInventoryRecord`
6. 6, the position number of the next record.
7. `Get #1, iRecordNumber, mInventoryRecord`

Feedback 10.1

datClasses.DatabaseName	CLASSES.MDB
datClasses.RecordSource	Teachers
txtTeacher.DataSource	datClasses
txtTeacher.DataField	Name
txtTeacher.Text	Not important—will display name from table

Feedback 11.1

1.
```
iRecordNumber = datControl.Recordset.AbsolutePosition + 1
If datControl.Recordset.EOF then
    lblRecordNumber.Caption = "EOF"
Else
    lblRecordNumber.Caption = iRecordNumber
End If
```
2. `On Error Resume Next`
3.
```
If Action <> vbDataActionUpdate then
    Save = False
End If
```
4.
```
If txtName.Text = "" Then
    MsgBox "Name required", vbExclamation, "Data Missing"
End If
```

5. ```
   HandleErrors:
        Select Case Err.Number
            Case 3022, 3058, 3109
                Resume Next
            Case Else
                MsgBox "Fatal error: " & Err.Description, vbCritical, _
                    "Error Condition"
                mnuFileExit_Click
        End Select
   ```
6. A message box will apear with the error number and the error description.

Feedback 11.2

1. Snapshots are always read-only. Tables and dynasets are usually updateable but may be set to read-only.
2. Tables and dynasets hold live data.
3. The `Find` methods can be used with dynasets and snapshots.
4. The `Seek` method can be used only for tables.
5. The Index property can be set only for tables.
6. `datCustomer.Recordset.FindFirst "CustomerName Like 'K*'"`
7. ```
   datCustomer.Recordset.Index = "CustomerName"
   datCustomer.Recordset.Seek ">=", "K"
   ```

Feedback 11.3

1. ```
   stSQL = "Select Name, Phone From Customers "
   datInfo.RecordSource = stSQL
   datInfo.Refresh
   ```
2. ```
   stSQL = "Select * From Cities"
   datInfo.RecordSource = stSQL
   datInfo.Refresh
   ```
3. ```
   stSQL = "Select * From Customers, Cities " & _
           "Where Customers.Zip = Cities.ZipCode"
   datInfo.RecordSource = stSQL
   datInfo.Refresh
   ```
4. ```
   stSQL = "Select Name, Address, City, State, ZIP " & _
            "From Customers, Cities " & _
            "Where Customers.Zip = Cities.ZipCode"
   datInfo.RecordSource = stSQL
   datInfo.Refresh
   ```
5. ```
   stSQL = "Select Distinct Name, Address, City, State, ZIP " & _
            "From Customers, Cities " & _
            "Where Customers.Zip = Cities.ZipCode"
   datInfo.RecordSource = stSQL
   datInfo.Refresh
   ```
6. ```
   If datInfo.RecordSet.BOF And datInfo.RecordSet.EOF Then
       MsgBox "No Records to Display"
   End If
   ```

Feedback 12.1

1. The DragMode property and the DragIcon property.
2. The target.
3. The name *Source* can be used to refer to the source control (the control being dragged over the target).

Feedback 13.1

1. `Line (3360, 0) - (3360, 4230)`
2. ```
   Const PI = 3.14159
   Circle (1600, 1000), 600, , -PI * 0.2, -PI * 1.8
   ```
   ```

APPENDIX

B

Functions for Working with Dates and Financial Calculations

Visual Basic includes a wealth of functions that you can use in your projects. The preceding chapters cover only a few of the available functions. Some of the string functions are covered in Chapter 7. Other functions that are covered include `MsgBox`, `Val`, `Ucase/Lcase`, and `Format`.

This appendix introduces some additional functions for handling dates and for performing financial calculations.

Date Functions

Visual Basic has several functions specifically for dealing with dates. The date functions can retrieve the system date, break down a date into component parts, test whether the contents of a field are compatible with the date data type, and convert other data types to a date.

Accessing the System Date

You can retrieve the system date from your computer with the `Date` function, which returns the current date, or the `Now` function which returns both the date and the time. These can be very handy in "time stamping" data or for inclusion in a report heading.

The Date and Now Functions—General Form

```
Now

Date
```

The Date and Now Functions—Examples

```
LblDate.Caption = Date          'Assign the system date to a label

Printer.Print Now
```

Date Variables

The date data type may hold values of many forms that represent a date. Examples could be May 22, 1998 or 5/22/98 or 5-22-1998. When a value is assigned to a date variable, it must be enclosed in # signs.

```
Dim dMyDate as Date
dMyDate = #3-1-97#
```

You can use the `Format$` function to format dates and times. To find the formats available search help for *Named Date/Time Formats.*

Converting Values to a Date Format

In order to store values in a date data type, you may need to convert the value of the data to a date type. You can accomplish this task with the `CDate` (convert to date) function.

The CDate Function—General Form

```
CDate(Variable or Property)
```

The CDate Function—Example

```
dMyDate = CDate(txtDate.Text)
```

When you want to compare two date fields from different sources, you can use the `CDate` function to assure that you are comparing compatible formats. This condition may occur when comparing a date from a database or file with the contents of a text box or date variable.

The DatePart Function

Another handy date function is the `DatePart` function, which can tell you if a date is a weekday, what day of the week, what month, and so on. The part of the date that you extract is determined by a part type (interval) according to the following chart:

Part Type/Interval	Part of Date
yyyy	Year
q	Quarter
m	Month
y	Day of year
d	Day
w	Weekday
ww	Week
h	Hour
n	Minute
s	Second

The DatePart Function—General Form

```
DatePart("PartType", Date)
```

The DatePart Function—Example

```
MsgBox "The Month is " & DatePart("m", dMyDate)
```

Notice in the example that the *m* for the part type is enclosed in quotes.

Finding the Difference Between Dates

You can use the `DateDiff` function to calculate with dates. The `DateDiff` function uses the same intervals as the DatePart function shown above. The `DateDiff` function uses two dates as arguments.

The DateDiff Function—General Form

```
DateDiff("Interval", Date1,Date2)
```

DateDiff Function—Example

```
MsgBox "It has been " & DateDiff("m", dMyDate, Now) & "months"
```

You could use this function to calculate the number of days prior to an event or how many days a payment is overdue.

Summary of Date Functions

Function	Purpose
`CDate`	Converts text data to date data type.
`Date`	Retrieves system date.
`DateDiff`	Finds the difference between two dates.
`DatePart`	Allows part of date to be accessed.
`IsDate`	Tests whether data can be converted to date data type.
`Now`	Retrieves system date and time.

Financial Functions

Visual Basic provides functions for many types of financial and accounting calculations, such as payment amount, depreciation, future value, and present value. When you use these functions, you eliminate the need to know and code the actual formulas yourself. Each financial function returns a value that you can assign to a variable, or to a property of a control.

Category	Purpose	Function
Depreciation	Double-declining balance.	DDB
	Straight line.	SLN
	Sum-of-the-years digits.	SYD
Payments	Payment.	Pmt
	Interest payment.	IPmt
	Principal payment.	PPmt
Return	Internal rate of return.	IRR
	Rate of return when payments and receipts are at different rates.	MIRR
Rate	Interest rate.	Rate
Future value	Future value of an annuity.	FV
Present value	Present value.	PV
	Present value when values are not constant.	NPV
Number of periods	Number of payments.	NPer

You must supply each function with the necessary values, called the *arguments*. You specify the name of the function, followed by parentheses that enclose the arguments.

The Visual Basic editor helps you type the arguments of functions. When you type the parentheses, the arguments will be specified in order. The one to be entered next is in bold. The order of the arguments is important because the function uses the values in the actual formula based on their position in the argument list. For example, the following `Pmt` function has three arguments: the interest rate, number of periods, and amount of loan. If you supply the values in a different order, the `Pmt` function will calculate with the wrong numbers.

The PMT Function

You can use the `Pmt` function to find the amount of each payment on a loan, if the interest rate, the number of periods, and the amount borrowed are known.

The Pmt Function—General Form

```
Pmt(interest rate per period, number of periods, amount of loan)
```

The interest rate must be specified as a decimal and adjusted to the interest rate per period. For example, if the loan is made with an annual rate of 10 percent and monthly payments, the interest rate must be converted to the monthly rate. Convert the annual rate to the monthly rate by dividing by the number of months in a year (.10/12).

The number of periods for the loan is the total number of payments. If you want to know the monthly payment for a five-year loan, you must convert the number of years to the number of months. Multiply the number of years by 12 months per year (12 * 5).

The Pmt Function—Example

```
cMonthlyRate = Val(txtRate.Text) * 12
cMonths = Val(txtYears.Text)/12
cAmount = Val(txtAmount.text)
lblMonthlyPayment.Caption = Pmt(cMonthlyRate, cMonths, cAmount)
```

Notice in the example that the fields used in the payment function are from text boxes that the user can enter, and the answer is displayed in a label. It would also be wise to use the `Format` function with these data.

The Rate Function

You can use the `Rate` function to determine the interest rate per period when the number of periods, the payment per period, and the original amount of the loan are known.

The Rate Function—General Form

```
Rate(number of periods, payment per period, loan amount)
```

The Rate Function—Example

```
cMonths = Val(txtYears.Text) * 12

cPayment = Val(txtPayment.Text)

cAmount = Val(txtAmount.Text)

msPeriodicRate = Rate(cMonths, cPayment, cAmount)
msAnnualRate = msPeriodicRate * 12
```

Functions to Calculate Depreciation

If you need to calculate the depreciation of an asset in a business, Visual Basic provides three functions: the double-declining-balance method, the straight-line method, and the sum-of-the-years-digits method.

The DDB function calculates the depreciation for a specific period within the life of the asset, using the double-declining-balance method formula. Once again, you do not need to know what the formula is but only in what order to enter the arguments. Incidentally, the *salvage value* is the value of the item when it is worn out.

The DDB (Double-Declining Balance) Function—General Form

```
DDB(original cost, salvage value, life of the asset, period)
```

The DDB Function—Example

```
cCost = Val(txtCost.Text)
cSalvage = Val(txtSalvage.Text)
cYears = Val(txtYears.Text)
cPeriod = Val(txtPeriod.Text)
lblDepreciation.Caption = DDB(cCost, cSalvage, cYears, cPeriod)
```

The other financial functions work in a similar manner. You can use the *Help* menu to find the argument list, an explanation, and an example.

Numeric Functions

Visual Basic includes functions for many mathematical operations.

Function	Returns
Abs(*x*)	The absolute value of x. $\lvert x \rvert = x$ if $x >= 0$ $\lvert x \rvert = -x$ if $x < 0$
Atn(*x*)	The angle in radians whose tangent is x.
Cint(*x*)	The integer closest to x (rounded).
Cos(*x*)	The cosine of x where x is in radians.
Exp(*x*)	The value of e raised to the power of x.
Fix(*x*)	The integer portion of x (truncated).
Int(*x*)	The largest integer $<= x$.
Log(*x*)	The natural logarithm of x, where $x > 0$.
Rnd	A random number in the range 0–1 (exclusive).
Sgn(*x*)	The sign of x. -1 if $x < 0$ 0 if $x = 0$ 1 if $x > 0$
Sin(*x*)	The sine of x where x is in radians.
Sqr(*x*)	The square root of x where x must be $>= 0$.
Tan(*x*)	The tangent of x where x is in radians.

Functions for Working With Strings

Visual Basic provides many string functions for working with text. Although several of the functions are covered in this text, many more are available.

Function	Returns
`Asc`(*StringExpression*)	The number corresponding to the ASCII code for the first character of String.
`Chr`(*NumericCode*)	A string character that corresponds to the ASCII code in the range 0–255. Reverse of the `Asc` function.
`Instr`([*StartingPosition*,] *StringExpression*, *SubString*)	A numeric value that is the position within the string where the substring begins; returns 0 if the substring is not found.
`LCase`(*StringExpression*)	The string converted to lowercase.
`Left`(*StringExpression*, *NumberOfCharacters*)	The left-most characters of the string for the indicated number of characters.
`Len`(*StringExpression*)	A numeric count of the number of characters in the string.
`Mid`(*StringExpression*, *StartingPosition* [, *NumberOfCharacters*])	A substring taken from the string, beginning at StartingPosition for the specified length.
`Right`(*StringExpression*, *NumberOfCharacters*)	The right-most characters of the string for the indicated number of characters.
`Space`(*NumerOfCharacters*)	A string of blank spaces for the specified number of characters.
`Str`(*NumericExpression*)	The string value of the numeric expression; used to convert numeric values to strings. Reverse of the `Val` function.
`String`(*NumerOfCharacters*, *StringExpression*)	A string of the named character(s) for a length of the specified number of characters.
`UCase`(*StringExpression*)	The string converted to uppercase.
`Val`(*StringExpression*)	The numeric value of the string expression; used to convert strings to numeric values. Reverse of the `Str` function.

APPENDIX

C

Tips and Shortcuts for Mastering the VB Environment

Set Up the Screen for Editing Convenience

As you work with the VB environment, you will find many ways to save time. Here are some tips and shortcuts that you can use to become more proficient using the environment to design, code, and run your projects.

Close Extra Windows

Arrange your screen for best advantage. While you are entering and editing code in the Code window, you don't need the toolbox, the Project Explorer window, the Properties window, or the Form Layout window. Click each window's close button; you can quickly and easily open each window again when you need it.

Display Windows Quickly

An easy way to display windows is to use the VB standard toolbar.

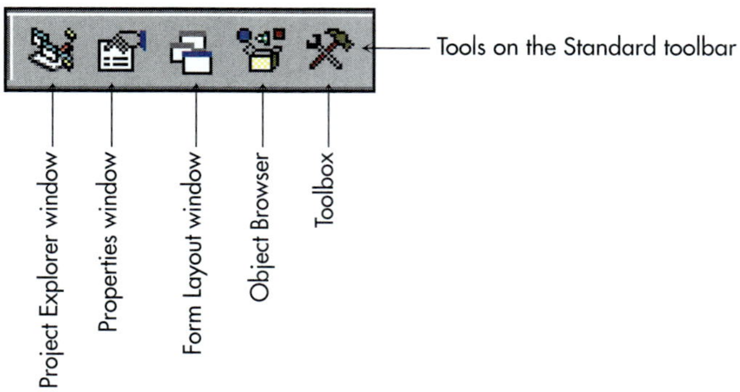

Display Windows Using Keyboard Shortcuts

Project Explorer window	Ctrl + R
Properties window	F4

Jump between the Form Window and Code Window

Form window	Shift + F7
Code window	F7
Jump back and forth	Ctrl + Tab

Dock and Float Windows for Your Convenience

All the toolbars and windows in the VB environment can be docked or floating. Windows toolbars can always be docked or floating; you can set the VB windows to be dockable or not on the *Docking* tab of the *Options* dialog box.

Moving Toolbars

You can drag a toolbar by pointing to a gray area of the toolbar (not on a button), press the mouse button, and drag to a new location. If you drop the toolbar somewhere in the middle of the screen, it will display as an independent window; the toolbar is *floating*. A docked toolbar is attached along one of the edges of the screen. You can dock a toolbar at the top; under the menu bar (the default); or along the bottom, the left, or the right edges of the screen.

Docking the VB Windows

Docking the VB Project Explorer, Properties, and Form Layout windows can be a challenge. Each can be docked independently along any edge of the screen. The windows can also be docked together, which is the default and the way the windows appear in most figures in this text. To dock the three windows along the right edge of the screen, first dock the Project Explorer window. Then drag the Properties window to the lower edge of the Project Explorer window and drop. Sometimes you need more than one try to dock a window correctly. You can watch the window's outline change shape to indicate its floating or docking position. Then drag the Form Layout window to the bottom of the Properties window and drop it. Again, you may need more than one try to dock the window in the right location.

After you dock the three windows, you can resize them by dragging on their borders.

Display the Edit Toolbar

You can save yourself time by displaying and using the Edit toolbar while you are editing code. Choose *View/Toolbars* to select the Edit toolbar. Or you can right-click on any toolbar to pop up a list of the available toolbars and turn any toolbar on or off.

Here is the recommended screen setup to use while entering and editing code in the Code window:

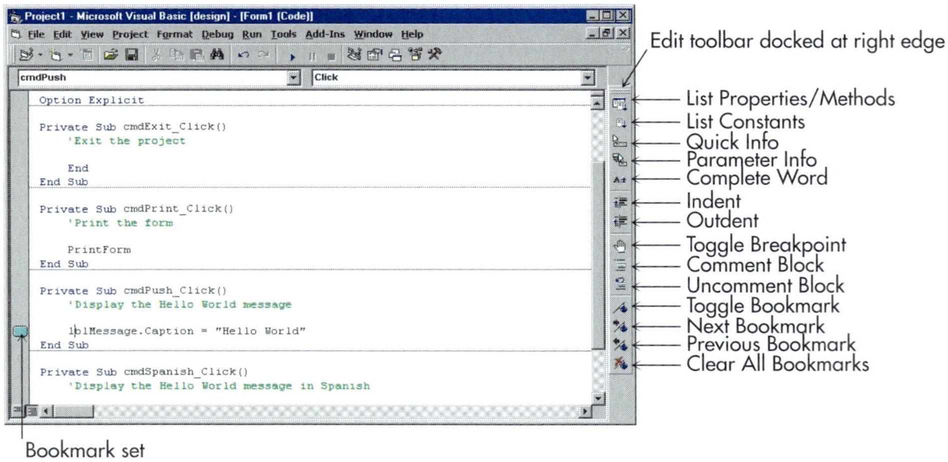

Block Comment: Use this command when you want to convert some code to comments, especially while you are testing and debugging projects. You can remove some lines from execution, to test the effect, without actually removing them. Select the lines and click the Block Comment button; each line will have an apostrophe appended at the left end.

Undo Block Comment: This command undoes the Block Comment command. Select some comment lines and click the Undo Block Comment button; the apostrophes at the beginning of the lines will be deleted.

Toggle Bookmark: This button sets and clears individual bookmarks. Bookmarks are useful when you are jumping around in the Code window. Set a bookmark on any line by clicking in the line and clicking the Toggle Bookmark button; you will see a mark in the margin area to the left of the marked line. You may want to set bookmarks in several procedures where you are editing or testing code.

Next Bookmark and *Previous Bookmark:* Use these buttons to quickly jump to the previous or next bookmark in the code.

Clear All Bookmarks: You can clear individual bookmarks with the Toggle Bookmark button or clear all bookmarks using this button.

Indent and *Outdent:* You can use these buttons to indent or outdent single lines or blocks of code. The buttons work the same way as the Tab and Shift + Tab keys.

The buttons for List Properties/Methods, List Constants, Quick Info, and Parameter Info can be helpful. By default, these options are turned on, and the lists automatically appear as you are typing code. You might prefer to keep the automatic features turned off and click the buttons when you actually want the lists to appear.

Try clicking the Complete Word button as you are typing the name of an object or a variable. If you have typed enough for the editor to identify the word, it will automatically fill in the rest.

Set Up Options for Your Convenience

The VB environment is customizable, and you may find that you prefer changing some of the options. Choose *Tools/Options* to display the *Options* dialog box. *Note:* If you are working in a shared lab, check with the instructor or lab technician before changing any options.

Editor Tab: For optimum editing, you will want to make sure that *Drag-and-Drop Text Editing*, *Default to Full Module View*, and *Procedure Separator* are selected.

General Tab: In the *Form Grid Settings* frame you can set up the way you want the grid to appear as you work on forms. You can turn the grid off or on, or modify the spacing of the grid dots.

Use Shortcuts When Editing Code

While you are editing code, save yourself time by using keyboard shortcuts.

Task	Shortcut
Delete the current line (insertion point anywhere in line).	Ctrl + Y
Delete from insertion point left to beginning of word.	Ctrl + Backspace
Delete from insertion point right to end of word.	Ctrl + Delete
Complete the word.	Ctrl + Spacebar
Jump to a procedure (insertion point on procedure name). Use this shortcut while working on the general sub procedures and functions that you write. For example, when writing a call to a function, you want to check the coding in the function. Point to the procedure name in the `Call` and press Shift + F2. After you finish looking at the function, press Ctrl + Shift + F2 to return to the original position (the `Call`).	Shift + F2
Jump back to original position after a jump.	Ctrl + Shift + F2
Jump to the top of the current module.	Ctrl + Home
Jump to the bottom of the current module.	Ctrl + End
Indent a block of code.	Highlight lines and use Edit toolbar button or Tab key.
Outdent (Un-indent) a block of code.	Highlight lines and use Edit toolbar button or Shift + Tab.

Split the Edit Window

You can view more than one procedure at a time by splitting the Code window. Point to the Split bar at the top of the vertical scroll bar and drag the bar down to the desired location. To remove the split, you can either drag the split bar back to the top or double-click the split bar.

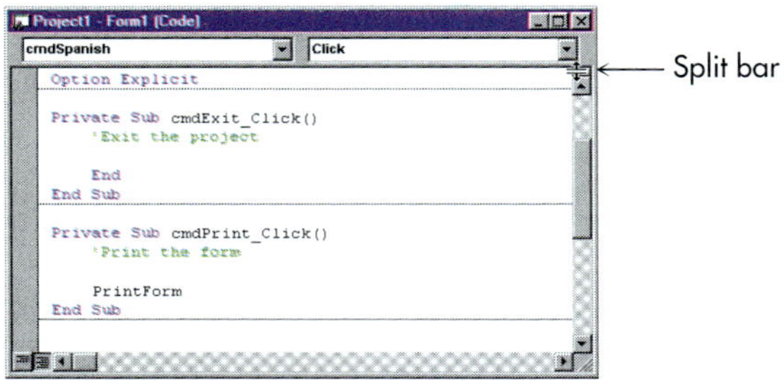

Use Drag-and-Drop Editing

You can use drag-and-drop to move or copy text to another location in the Code window, to the Code window for another project, to the Immediate window, or to the Watch window.

To move code, select the text, point to the selection, and drag it to a new location. You can copy text (rather than move it) by holding down the Ctrl key as you drag.

Use Shortcuts in the Form Window

You can save time while creating the user interface in the Form window by using shortcuts.

Create Multiple Controls of the Same Type

When you want to create several controls of the same class, you must select the toolbox tool each time you draw a new control. That is, unless you use this method: When you select the toolbox tool for the first control, hold down the Ctrl key as you click. After you create your first new control, the tool will stay selected so that you can create as many more controls of that class as you wish.

When you are finished, press Esc to deselect the tool or click on another toolbox tool.

Display the Form Editor Toolbar

You can display the Form Editor toolbar to save yourself time when working with multiple controls. Turn toolbars on and off from the *View/Toolbars* menu command or by right-clicking any toolbar.

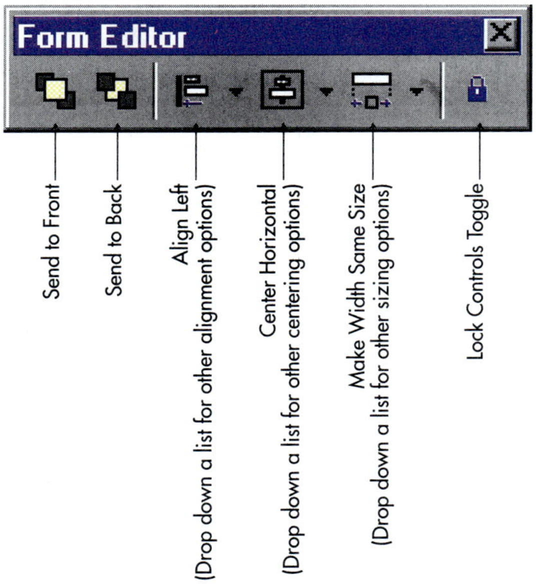

Nudge Controls into Place

Sometimes it is difficult to place controls exactly where you want them. Of course, you can use the alignment options on the *Format* menu or the Form Editor toolbar. You can also nudge controls in any direction by holding down the Ctrl key and pressing one of the arrow keys. *Nudging* moves a control one grid dot in the desired direction. If the grid is turned off, the control(s) moves by one pixel.

For example: Ctrl + Right Arrow moves a selected control one grid dot to the right.

Use Shortcuts to Execute a Project

You can use keyboard shortcuts to start and stop project execution.

Task	Shortcut
Run the current project (from Design time).	F5
Continue execution (from Break time).	F5
Restart execution from the beginning (from Break time).	Shift + F5
Stop execution.	Ctrl + Break
Begin execution, single-stepping through code.	F8

Use the Object Browser

The VB Object Browser can be a valuable source of information. You can use the Object Browser to examine objects, properties, methods, and events for VB objects; objects from other applications; and ActiveX controls. You can view a list of the objects, properties, procedures, and variable declarations in your project and jump to a section of your code.

Finding Lists of Constants

You can find listings of the VB constants using the Object Browser. The constants are grouped by function. Select *<All Libraries>* in the *Project/Library* box and then scroll the Classes list and click on the desired group; the constants will appear in the Members list. Or you can type something in the Search Text box and click the Search button.

This example shows the VB color constants:

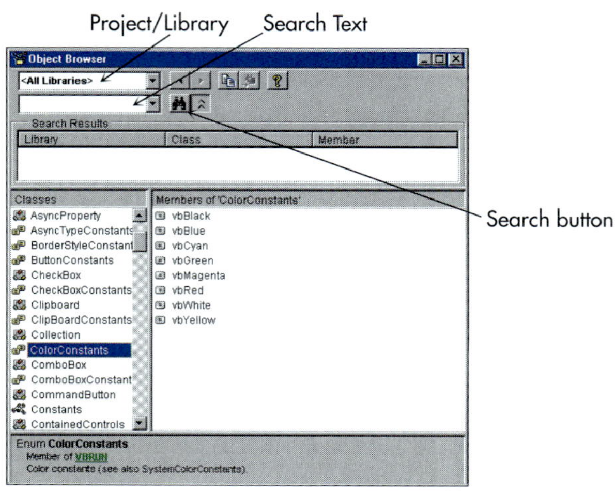

Learning About Objects

The Object Browser can show you all properties, methods, and events for an object. You can choose any of the VB objects; objects from other applications, such as Excel or Project; or an ActiveX control. Before you can display information about an object, it must be selected in the References list (*References* dialog box from the *Project* menu). *Note:* You can display the *References* dialog box directly from the Object Browser if you right-click to display the shortcut menu.

This example shows the listing for a vertical scroll bar control in the VB library.

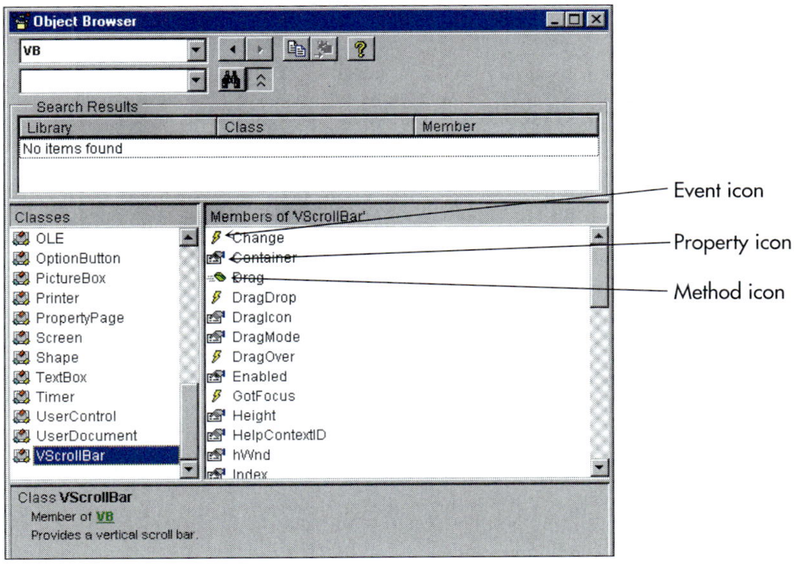

Jumping in Your Code

As soon as you develop a project with several modules, jumping to different sections of your code becomes more difficult. You can use the Object Browser for reference to recall the name you have given to any procedure, variable, or constant or to quickly jump to any position in your code.

Select your project name in the *Project/Library* box and the Classes list will show the modules in your project. The Members list displays all objects, properties, and coded procedures (the methods). To jump to any procedure listing, double-click on the desired name.

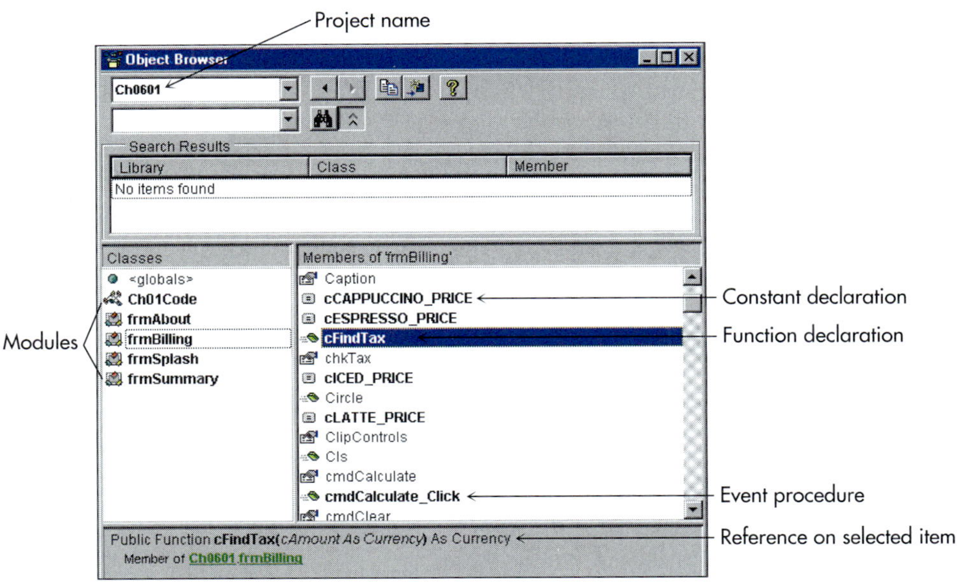

Glossary

About box A dialog box that contains information about a program.

absolute position Measurement from the starting point of a graphic object.

access key Key to press to activate a control rather than using the mouse. Also called keyboard shortcut.

ActiveX A custom control, program, or DLL that can be added to a project.

API Application program interface; a collection of DLLs used for Windows programming.

argument A value being passed to or from a procedure.

array A series of items, such as a control array or a variable array.

ASCII code The code used to represent characters on a microcomputer (American Standard Code for Information Interchange).

assignment statement Assigns a value to a variable or property of an object.

.BAS file File used to store standard code modules.

BOF Beginning of file, used for the Recordset object of the data control.

Boolean A data type that evaluates to True or False.

break time Temporary break in execution of a program used for debugging.

breakpoint Indicated point in project code where execution should break; used for debugging.

buffer Temporary storage area used for reading and writing data files. On a write, data are placed in the buffer until it is filled and then written to disk.

ByRef Declares that an argument passed to a procedure should be passed as the address of the data so that both calling and called procedures have access to the same memory location. Default type of argument used in DLLs.

ByVal Declares that an argument passed to a procedure should be passed as a copy of the data. The calling and called procedures do not have access to each other's variables.

cell Intersection of a row and a column; used for the grid control.

check box A control used to indicate a value that may be True or False. In any group of check boxes, any number may be selected.

checked Selected. A menu command preceded by a check mark or a check box containing an `X`.

class A prototype or blueprint for an object indicating the properties and methods.

class module Code used to define a new class of object.

clipping region Graphics area that defines the area to be redrawn.

code Programming statements in the Basic language.

Code window The Visual Basic window in which code is displayed and written.

color constant Predefined constants for specifying colors, such as vbRed and vbBlue.

column A vertical section of a grid control.

combo box control A control that is a combination of a list box and a text box.

command button A control used to activate a procedure.

common dialog boxes A set of Windows dialog boxes available to Visual Basic programmers for `Open`, `Save`, `Fonts`, `Print`, and `Color`.

compile error A syntax error (usually spelling or punctuation) found by the compiler before execution begins; causes Visual Basic to enter break time.

compound condition Multiple conditions combined with the use of the logical operators, `And` or `Or`.

concatenation Joining string (text) fields. The ampersand (&) is used to concatenate text.

condition An expression that will evaluate True or False. May be a comparison of two values (variables, properties, constants) using relational operators.

constant A value that cannot be changed during program execution.

context-sensitive Help Use of the F1 function key to directly access the Help topic related to the code containing the cursor.

control An object used on a graphical interface, such as an option button, text box, command button, or label.

control array A group of controls sharing the same name and event procedures.

coordinate system A measurement system used for creating graphics.

Crystal Reports A VB add-in that can be used to design and print reports for database files.

current record The position of the pointer in a database table or data file.

custom controls Additional controls that may be added to the toolbox for inclusion in a project. Also called *ActiveX* controls.

data element Unit within a user-defined data type or a data record. Also called a *field*.

data file Disk file that holds values for data records.

data tip A small label that displays the current value of a variable, property, or expression. Available only at break time by placing the pointer over the desired value.

data type Specifies the type of value to be stored in a variable or constant. May be used to indicate the return type for a function. Examples of data types are integer, currency, and string.

debug window A window that appears when a project is executed. It contains information about the status of the project and can be used to display or change program values.

debugging Finding and eliminating computer program errors.

declaration Nonexecutable code that sets up variables and constants, declares data types, and allocates memory. Can be used to set up arrays and specify the data type returned by a function. Example declaration statements are `Dim`, `Const`, `Static`, `Public`, and `Private`.

design time The status of the Visual Basic environment while a project is being developed, as opposed to run time or break time.

direct reference Accessing an element of an array by a subscript when the value of the subscript is known.

DLL Dynamic link library; a file with an extension of .DLL, used to hold procedures.

dropdown combo box A combo box control with a down-pointing arrow that allows the user to pull down the list. Allows efficient use of space on a form.

dropdown list A list box with a down-pointing arrow allowing the user to pull down the list. Allows efficient use of space on a form.

dynaset Temporary set of data taken from one or more tables in the underlying database file.

element Single item within a table, array, list, or grid.

embed An OLE action causing an object from a different application to be contained within a VB application. An embedded object cannot be modified from other applications.

empty string A string with a length of zero characters.

enabled A command button or menu command that is available to the user; indicated by a black Caption rather than a gray Caption.

EOF End of file; a condition that evaluates True when reading sequential files or accessing a database using a Recordset object of the data control.

Err object A special predefined Visual Basic object that stores the error number and its description when a run-time error occurs.

error trapping Coding to control the action when an error occurs.

event An action that may be taken by the user, such as a click, drag, key press, or scroll. Events can also be triggered by an internal action, such as repainting the form or validating a database action.

event-driven programming Applications designed to respond to actions taken by the user.

event procedure A procedure written to respond to an action taken by the user.

field A group of related characters used to represent one characteristic or attribute of an entity in a data file or database.

file mode Specification for the manner that data can be accessed from a disk file, including Input, Output, Append, Random, and Binary.

file number Buffer number used to read and write records in a data file.

file pointer Used to keep track of the current position when reading or writing a data file.

flag A variable, usually of Boolean type, used to indicate status, such as True or False, On or Off, Found or NotFound. Also called a *switch*.

focus The currently selected control, indicated by an I-beam, selected text, highlighted Caption, or a dotted border. The control with the focus is ready to receive user input.

form An object that acts as a container for the controls in a graphical interface.

form file A file with an .FRM extension; contains the code and control information for a single form.

form module The code related to a single form.

Form window The window in which the form is displayed at design time; can be displayed by pressing the Show Form button in the Project window.

format A specification for the way information will be displayed, including dollar signs, percent signs, and number of decimal positions.

format string A string of characters used to specify a custom-designed format.

frame A control used as a container to group other controls.

function A procedure that returns a value when it is called.

general declarations section The portion of a code module used to declare variables that will be available throughout that module.

global The scope of a variable, constant, or procedure that makes it available in all modules of a project.

graphical user interface (GUI) Program application containing icons, buttons, and menu bars.

grid control A control that has rows and columns and displays data in cells.

handle A small square on a selected control at design time; used to resize a control.

identifier A programmer-supplied name for a variable, constant, procedure, or control.

image A control that can contain a picture; has a stretch property to adjust the size of the contained graphic.

index A variable or a property that stores the position number of the elements in a series; used for list box controls, control arrays, variable arrays, and database records.

instant watch A debugging feature that allows you to quickly see the current value of a variable or expression.

intrinsic constants Constants supplied with a language or application such as vbBlue.

intrinsic controls Basic controls provided in the toolbox.

iteration A single pass through the body of a loop.

key field The field (or fields) on which a data file is organized; used to search for a record.

label A control that displays text as a Caption; cannot be altered by the user.

line-continuation character A space and underscore; used in program code to indicate that a Basic statement continues on the next line.

link An OLE relationship that places an object in your project but allows other applications to access and modify the object. A linked OLE object is not stored inside your project and is maintained by the creating application.

list box control A control that holds a list of values; the user cannot add new values at run time.

literal A string expression enclosed in quotation marks.

local The scope of a variable or constant that limits its visibility to the current procedure.

logic error An error in a project that does not halt execution but causes erroneous results in the output.

logical operator The operators `And`, `Or`, and `Not`; used to construct compound conditions and to reverse the truth of a condition.

lookup An operation that searches a table or an array to find a value when the subscript is not directly known.

loop A control structure providing for the repetition of statements.

loop index A counter variable used in a `For/Next` loop.

menu A list of choices; the available commands displayed in a menu bar.

message box A dialog box displaying a message to the user. The `MsgBox` function returns a value indicating the user's response.

method Predefined actions (procedures) provided with objects.

modal A form that requires the user to respond before transferring to any other form in the project.

modeless A form that does not prevent the user from accessing any other form before responding.

module A collection of procedures; may be a form module, a standard code module, or a class module. Each file in a project is a separate module.

navigation Stepping through the records of a database file: next record, previous record, first record, or last record.

nested A statement completely contained within another statement, such as a loop within a loop or a decision within a decision.

object An occurrence of a class type that has properties and methods. A specific instance of a control type or form.

object-oriented programming (OOP) An approach to programming that uses objects and their properties. Each type of object behaves in a certain way. Applications are built by combining objects and coding the actions to be taken when events occur. Visual Basic has many (but not all) of the characteristics of an object-oriented language.

OLE Object linking and embedding; a process used to share objects among applications.

option button A control used to indicate a value that may be True or False (selected or not selected). In any group of option buttons, only one button may be selected.

order of precedence Hierarchy of mathematical operations; the order in which operations are performed.

persistent graphics Graphics that are saved in memory and can be redisplayed.

picturebox A control used as a container; may hold graphics, pictures, text, or other controls.

pixel Picture element; a single dot on the screen; a unit of measurement for displaying graphics.

point A printer's measure used to define the size of a font; 1/72 of an inch.

posttest A loop that has its test condition after the body of the loop; the statements within the loop will always be executed at least once.

pretest A loop that has its test condition at the top; the statements inside the loop may never be executed.

print zone Preset column width used with the Printer object.

private Specifies local scope in a declaration. A procedure declared as private can be called only from another procedure in that module. A private variable is available only in the module in which it is declared.

procedure A unit of code; may be a sub procedure or a function procedure.

Professional Edition A version of Visual Basic that includes more controls than the Standard Edition and allows more robust database programming.

project file A file with a .VBP extension; used to store the information displayed in the Project window.

Project window A window that displays a list of the forms and standard code modules used for a project.

Properties window A window that shows the properties for each object in a form.

property Characteristic or attribute of an object; value may be set at design time or run time depending on the specific property.

public Specifies scope as global. A procedure declared as public can be called from other modules; a public variable is available in other modules in the project.

random file A data file that may be read or written in any order; has fixed-length records.

record A group of related fields; relates to data files and database tables.

recordset The current group of records associated with a data control; may be a table recordset, a dynaset, or a snapshot.

relational operator Comparison operators, including <, >, and =.

relative position In graphics, the position in relation to the last point drawn.

remark A Basic statement used for documentation; not interpreted by the compiler; also called a *comment*.

row A horizontal section of a grid control.

run time While a project is executing.

run-time error An error that occurs as a program executes; causes execution to break.

scope The extent of visibility of a variable or constant. The scope may be global, module level, or local.

search argument The value to be matched in a lookup operation.

separator bar A horizontal line used to separate groups of menu commands.

simple combo box A control that combines a text box and a list box, with no dropdown capability.

single step A debugging feature that executes the project code one line at a time and displays each line.

snapshot A temporary set of data from a database file that is not updateable or "live."

source The object being dragged in a drag-and-drop operation.

SQL Structured Query Language; an industry-standard database language available in Visual Basic.

standard code module A file with a .BAS extension used to declare global variables and constants; can contain procedures that will be called from multiple forms.

startup form The first form to appear when a project begins execution; a project must have a startup form.

statement A line of Visual Basic code.

static A setting for local variables that retains the value for multiple calls to the procedure.

string literal A constant enclosed in quotation marks.

sub procedure A procedure that takes actions but does not return a value.

subscript The position of an element within an array.

subscripted variable An element of an array.

switch See *flag*.

tabbed dialog A control that adds tabs that resemble folder tabs. Used to increase the usable portion of a window and to organize functions.

table A two-dimensional array.

table recordset A recordset defined using a single table in a database file.

text box A control for data entry; its value can be entered and changed by the user. Also called an *edit box*.

third-party control A custom control produced by a company other than Microsoft.

timer control A control that can be made to fire an event at a specified interval; can be used to perform actions repeatedly.

toolbar The group of buttons beneath the menu bar; used as shortcuts for menu commands.

toolbox A window that holds buttons used to create controls on a form.

twip A unit of measure for the display screen; 1/20 of a point or 1/1440 of an inch.

user-defined data type Grouping of data elements to create a new data type that can be used in declaration statements.

user interface The display and commands seen by a user; how the user interacts with an application. In Windows, the graphical display of an application containing controls and menus.

validation Verification of the values entered by the user. Validation may include checking for a range of values, checking for specific values, or verifying the data type.

variable A memory location referred to by a name. The value of a variable can change during execution of an application.

Visual Basic environment The Visual Basic elements used for program development at design time; includes the menu bar, toolbar, toolbox, Form window, Property window, Project window, and Menu editor.

Visual Basic for Applications (VBA) A version of Visual Basic that is included in many Microsoft application programs, such as Excel and PowerPoint.

watch A debugging tool that allows the programmer to view the value of a variable or expression as the project executes.

Web browser A control that has methods to navigate the Internet.

ZOrder method Changes the stacking order of graphical elements.

Index

A

B

C

G

OBJECTS/PROPERTIES

Object	Control?	Naming prefix	Align	Alignment	Appearance	AutoRedraw	AutoSize	BackColor	Bold	BorderColor	BorderStyle	BorderWidth	Caption	CellSelected	Clip	ClipControls	ColAlignment/Col/Cols	Color	Columns	Connect	ColWidth	ControlBox	CurrentX/CurrentY	DataBase/DatabaseName	DataField/DataSource	Default/Cancel	DragIcon/DragMode	DrawStyle/DrawWidth	Enabled	FillColor/FillStyle	FixedCols/FixedRows	Flags	Font
CheckBox	x	chk		x	x			x					x												x		x		x				x
ComboBox	x	cbo			x			x																	x		x		x				x
CommandButton	x	cmd			x			x					x													x	x		x				x
CommonDialog	x	dlg																x														x	
Data	x	dat	x		x			x					x							x				x			x		x				x
Err																																	
Font									x																								
Form		frm			x	x		x			x		x			x						x	x					x	x	x			x
Frame	x	fra			x			x			x		x			x											x		x				x
Grid	x	grd			x			x			x				x		x				x						x		x	x	x		
HScrollBar	x	hsb																									x		x				
Image	x	img			x						x														x		x		x				
Label	x	lbl		x	x		x	x			x		x												x		x		x				x
Line	x	lin								x	x	x																					
ListBox	x	lst			x			x											x						x		x		x				x
OLE	x	ole			x			x			x														x		x		x				
OptionButton	x	opt		x	x			x					x														x		x				x
PictureBox	x	pic	x		x	x	x	x			x					x							x		x		x	x	x	x			x
Printer																							x					x		x			x
Shape	x	shp						x		x	x	x																		x			
TextBox	x	txt		x	x			x		x															x		x		x				x
Timer	x	tmr																											x				
VScrollBar	x	vsb																									x		x				

OBJECTS/PROPERTIES (continued)

Object	ForeColor	Height	Icon	Image	ItemData	LargeChange	Left	LinkItem	LinkMode/LinkTopic	List/ListCount/ListIndex	MaxButton/MinButton	MultiLine	Name	Number	Picture	Row/Rows	ScaleHeight/Left/Mode/Top	ScrollBars	SelCount	Selected	SelEnd(Start)Row/Col	Shape	SmallChange	SourceItem	Stretch	TabIndex	TabStop	Text	Top	Value	Visible	Width	WindowState
CheckBox	x	x					x						x		x						x					x	x		x	x	x	x	
ComboBox	x	x			x		x			x			x													x	x	x	x		x	x	
CommandButton		x					x						x		x											x	x		x	x	x	x	
CommonDialog													x																				
Data	x	x					x						x																x		x	x	
Err														x																			
Font													x																				
Form	x	x	x	x			x		x		x		x		x		x												x		x	x	x
Frame	x	x					x						x													x			x		x	x	
Grid	x	x					x						x		x	x		x			x					x	x	x	x		x	x	
HScrollBar		x				x	x						x										x			x	x		x	x	x	x	
Image		x					x						x		x										x				x		x	x	
Label	x	x					x	x	x				x													x			x		x	x	
Line													x																		x		
ListBox	x	x			x		x			x			x						x	x						x	x	x	x		x	x	
OLE		x					x						x		x									x		x	x		x		x	x	
OptionButton	x	x					x						x		x											x	x		x	x	x	x	
PictureBox	x	x		x			x	x	x				x		x		x									x	x		x		x	x	
Printer	x	x															x															x	
Shape		x					x						x									x							x		x	x	
TextBox	x	x					x	x	x			x	x					x			x					x	x	x	x		x	x	
Timer													x																				
VScrollBar		x				x	x						x										x			x	x		x	x	x	x	